Anatomy & Physiology for Emergency Care

Frederic H. Martini, Ph.D.
Edwin F. Bartholomew, M.S.
Bryan E. Bledsoe, D.O., F.A.C.E.P., F.A.A.E.M., F.A.E.P., EMT-P
Emergency Care Contributions

with

William C. Ober, M.D.
Art Coordinator and Illustrator

Claire W. Garrison, R.N.
Illustrator

Kathleen Welch, M.D.
Clinical Consultant

Ralph T. Hutchings
Biomedical Photographer

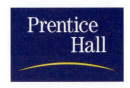

Prentice Hall

Upper Saddle River, New Jersey 07458

Library of Congress Cataloging-in-Publication Data

Martini, Frederic.
  Anatomy & physiology for emergency care/Frederic H. Martini,
Edwin F. Bartholomew; with William C. Ober ... [et al.].
    p. ; cm.
  "Enhanced edition of Essentials of anatomy & physiology"--Pref.
  Includes index.
  ISBN 0-13-042298-3
  1. Human physiology. 2. Human anatomy. 3. Emergency medical
services. I. Title: Anatomy and physiology for emergency care. II.
Bartholomew, Edwin F. III. Ober, William C. IV. Martini, Frederic.
Essentials of anatomy & physiology. V. Title.
  [DNLM: 1. Anatomy. 2. Emergency Medical Services. 3. Physiology.
QS 4 M3855a 2002]
  QP36 .M42 2002
  612--dc21

                                               2001053144

Dedication

To Kitty, P.K., Ivy, and Kate: We couldn't have done this without you. Thank you for your encouragement, patience, and understanding.

Notice on Care Procedures: It is the intent of the authors and publisher that this book be used as part of a formal EMS program taught by a licensed physician. The procedures described in this book are based upon consultation with EMS and medical authorities. The authors and publisher have taken care to make certain that these procedures reflect currently accepted clinical practice; however, they cannot be considered absolute recommendations.

The material in this book contains the most current information available at the time of publication. However, federal, state, and local guidelines concerning clinical practices, including, without limitation, those governing infection control and universal precautions, change rapidly. The reader should note, therefore, that the new regulations may require changes in some procedures.

It is the responsibility of the reader to familiarize himself or herself with the policies and procedures set by federal, state, and local agencies as well as the institution or agency where the reader is employed. The authors and publisher of this book disclaim any liability, loss, or risk resulting directly or indirectly from the suggested procedures and theory, from any undetected errors, or from the reader's misunderstanding of the text. It is the reader's responsibility to stay informed of any new changes or recommendations made by federal, state, or local agency as well as by his or her employing institution or agency.

Prentice Hall Engineering, Science, and Math
Editor in Chief for Science: Paul F. Corey
Senior Acquisitions Editor: Halee Dinsey
Senior Development Editor: Karen Karlin
Production Editor: Shari Toron
Assistant Vice President of Production and Manufacturing:
  David W. Riccardi
Executive Managing Editor: Kathleen Schiaparelli
Editor in Chief of Development: Carol Trueheart
Creative Director: Paul Belfanti
Executive Marketing Manager for Biology: Jennifer Welchans
Interior Design: Judith M. Coniglio
Cover Illustration: Abraham Echevarria
Manufacturing Manager: Trudy Pisciotti
Illustrators: William C. Ober, M.D., Claire W. Garrison, R.N.
Associate Creative Director: Amy Rosen
Art Director: Heather Scott
Assistant to Art Director: John Christiana
Art Manager: Gus Vibal
Editorial Assistant: Damian Hill

Pearson Education LTD.
Pearson Education Australia PTY, Limited
Pearson Education Singapore, Pte. Ltd
Pearson Education North Asia Ltd
Pearson Education Canada, Ltd.
Pearson Educación de Mexico, S.A. de C.V.
Pearson Education – Japan
Pearson Education Malaysia, Pte. Ltd

Brady/Prentice Hall Health
Publisher: Julie Levin Alexander
Executive Editor: Greg Vis
Managing Development Editor: Lois Berlowitz
Development Editor: John Joerschke
Director of Production and Manufacturing: Bruce Johnson
Managing Production Editor: Patrick Walsh
Production Liaison: Danielle Newhouse
Production Editor: Lori Dalberg, Carlisle Publishers Services
Manufacturing Manager: Ilene Sanford
Managing Photography Editor: Michal Heron
Design Director: Cheryl Asherman
Design Coordinator: Maria Guglielmo
Interior Design (Emergency Care Applications): Wanda España
Electronic Art Creation (Emergency Care Applications):
  Rolin Graphics, Inc.
Marketing Manager: Tiffany Price
Cover Designer: Rob Richman, LaFortezza Design
Product Information Manager: Rachele Triano
Printer/Binder: Von Hoffmann Press
Cover Printer: Phoenix Color
Composition: Carlisle Publishers Services

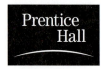

10 9 8 7 6

ISBN 0-13-042298-3

Contents in Brief

Contents

Chapter 1
An Introduction to Anatomy
and Physiology 2

Chapter 2
The Chemical Level
of Organization 28

Chapter 3
Cell Structure and Function 52

Chapter 4
The Tissue Level of Organization 80

EMERGENCY CARE APPLICATIONS A3-1

EMERGENCY CARE APPLICATIONS A4-1

Chapter 5
The Integumentary System 106

INTRODUCTION 108

EMERGENCY CARE APPLICATIONS A5-1

Chapter 6
The Skeletal System   120

EMERGENCY CARE APPLICATIONS A6-1

Chapter 7
The Muscular System 166

Chapter 8
Neural Tissue and the Central
Nervous System   214

Chapter 9
The Peripheral Nervous System and
Integrated Neural Functions 250

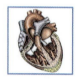

Chapter 10
Sensory Function 270

EMERGENCY CARE APPLICATIONS A10-1

Chapter 11
The Endocrine System 304

EMERGENCY CARE APPLICATIONS A11-1

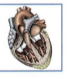

Chapter 12
Blood 332

x   Contents

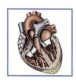

Chapter 13
The Heart 354

Chapter 14
Blood Vessels and Circulation 374

EMERGENCY CARE APPLICATIONS A14-1

Chapter 15
The Lymphatic System and
Immunity 410

EMERGENCY CARE APPLICATIONS A15-1

Chapter 16
The Respiratory System 436

EMERGENCY CARE APPLICATIONS A16-1

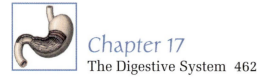

Chapter 17
The Digestive System 462

INTRODUCTION 464

Chapter 18
Nutrition and Metabolism 494

Chapter 19
The Urinary System 516

Chapter 20
The Reproductive System 546

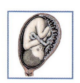

Chapter 21
Development and Inheritance 576

Preface to the Student

HOW TO SIMPLIFY YOUR LIFE: Getting the Most Out of This Book

This textbook was designed to help you master the terminology, basic concepts, and principles important to an understanding of the human body. It has three primary goals:

1. Building a foundation of essential knowledge (What structure is that? How does it work? What happens when it doesn't work?). Such a foundation will support further courses dealing with specific topics in human anatomy and physiology.

2. Providing a framework for interpreting and applying related information obtained outside the classroom. This framework should make it possible for you to utilize what you learn in this course in analyzing everyday problems and situations.

3. Providing an introduction to common emergency medical problems through discussion of relevant pathophysiology in conjunction with the presentation of normal anatomy and physiology. This will allow you to better understand the physiological basis of disease and will be continually reinforced as you undertake clinical courses that prepare you for actual patient care.

In addition, the need for well-trained professionals in the allied health field is greater than ever. To succeed in an allied health career, you must master the same skills that you need to succeed in this course. You must do more than develop a large technical vocabulary and retain a large volume of detailed information. You must **learn how to learn**—how to organize new information, connect it to what you already know, and then apply it as needed.

Can a text simplify this process? No textbook can give you more time. A text can, however, help you make better use of your time. By presenting the material in a clear, logical way that stresses concept organization, this text provides you with a strong foundation of essential knowledge and a framework for integrating and applying that knowledge. For example, certain themes and patterns appear again and again in the study of anatomy and physiology. The conceptual material will be much easier to deal with if you learn to recognize those patterns and organize the information accordingly. With this realization in mind, we've taken extra care to highlight the important patterns, create a sensible framework, and organize new information around that framework.

The User's Guide that follows this page describes the many learning aids that are built into this text. If you use them, they will help you improve your study skills and will make you more efficient at learning and integrating new information. These features were developed through feedback from students and instructors on campuses across the United States, Canada, Australia, New Zealand, and Europe. Many students, in person or by phone or e-mail, have told us that this system really works for them when other presentation styles have not. **Take the time to examine this User's Guide carefully**, and ask your instructor if you have questions about any of this book's learning aids. If you invest the time *now*, you can learn to use the book properly from the outset. Doing so will ensure that you will get the most from the time you invest in this course. In addition, becoming a more efficient learner will set you forth on a lifetime of learning that will make you a more valuable future professional, constantly improving and growing long after you've taken your last exam.

Good luck and best wishes,

Frederic H. Martini
Haiku, Hawaii

Edwin F. Bartholomew
Lahaina, Hawaii

Bryan E. Bledsoe
Midlothian, Texas

Emphasizing Concepts

Chapter Outline and Objectives

Each chapter opens with an outline that gives you an overview of the concepts. Integrated objectives help you structure your reading and keep your attention focused on the key points.

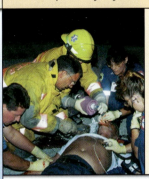

16 The Respiratory System

436

Your initial task in any medical emergency is to evaluate the status of the patient's airway. However, you can learn little about the status of the airway if the patient is not breathing. The respiratory system is a major body system that is closely interfaced with the circulatory system. A change in the respiratory system is often one of the earliest indicators of deterioration in a patient's condition. Such change should prompt immediate and detailed reevaluation.

Chapter Outline and Objectives

437

Vocabulary Development

alveolus, a hollow cavity; *alveolus, alveolar duct*
ateles, imperfect; *atelectasis*
*bronchus, windpipe, airway; *bronchitis*
cricoid, ring-shaped; *cricoid cartilage*
ektasis, expansion; *atelectasis*
-ia, condition; *pneumonia*
kentesis, puncture; *thoracentesis*
oris, mouth; *oropharynx*
*pneuma, air; *pneumothorax*
pneumon, lung; *pneumonia*
stoma, mouth; *tracheostomy*
thorac-, chest; *thoracentesis*
thyroid, shield-shaped; *thyroid cartilage*

---

168 The Muscular System

It is hard to imagine what life would be like without muscle tissue. We would be unable to sit, stand, walk, speak, or grasp objects. Blood would not circulate, because there would be no heartbeat to propel it through the vessels. The lungs could not rhythmically empty and fill, nor could food move through the digestive tract. Muscle tissue, one of the four primary tissue types, consists chiefly of elongated muscle cells that are highly specialized for contraction. The three types of muscle tissue—*skeletal muscle, cardiac muscle,* and *smooth muscle*—were introduced in Chapter 4. ∞ *p. 97* These muscle tissues share four basic properties:

1. **Excitability:** the ability to respond to stimulation. For example, skeletal muscles normally respond to stimulation by the nervous system, and some smooth muscles respond to circulating hormones.
2. **Contractility:** the ability to shorten actively and exert a pull, or tension, that can be harnessed by connective tissues.
3. **Extensibility:** the ability to continue to contract over a range of resting lengths. For example, a smooth muscle cell can be stretched to several times its original length and still contract on stimulation.
4. **Elasticity:** the ability of a muscle to rebound toward its original length after a contraction.

This chapter begins with the organization of skeletal muscle tissue. Although most of the muscle tissue in the body is skeletal muscle, this section will also consider cardiac and smooth muscle tissue. We will then proceed to a consideration of the functional organization of the muscular system.

FUNCTIONS OF SKELETAL MUSCLE

Skeletal muscle tissue, connective tissues, and neural tissue combine to form **skeletal muscles,** contractile organs that are directly or indirectly attached to bones. The muscular system includes approximately 700 skeletal muscles. These muscles perform the following functions:

1. **Produce movement.** Muscle contractions pull on tendons and move the bones of the skeleton.
2. **Maintain posture and body position.** Without constant muscular tension, you could not sit upright without collapsing or stand without toppling over.
3. **Support soft tissues.** The abdominal wall and the floor of the pelvic cavity consist of layers of muscle that support the weight of visceral organs and shield internal tissues from injury.
4. **Guard entrances and exits.** Skeletal muscles guard openings to the digestive and urinary tracts and provide voluntary control over swallowing, defecation, and urination.

5. **Maintain body temperature.** Muscle contractions require energy, and whenever energy is used in the body, some of it is converted to heat. The heat lost by working muscles keeps the body temperature in the normal range.

THE ANATOMY OF SKELETAL MUSCLES

When naming structural features of muscles and their components, anatomists often used the Greek words *sarkos* (flesh) and *mys* (muscle). These word roots will be encountered in the following discussions of the anatomy of skeletal muscle.

Gross Anatomy

Figure 7-1• illustrates the appearance and organization of a typical skeletal muscle. A skeletal muscle contains connective tissues, blood vessels, nerves, and skeletal muscle tissue.

Connective Tissue Organization

Three layers of connective tissue are part of each muscle: an outer epimysium, a central perimysium, and an inner endomysium (Figure 7-1•). The entire muscle is surrounded by the **epimysium** (ep-i-MIS-ē-um; *epi-,* on + *mys,* muscle), a layer of collagen fibers that separates the muscle from surrounding tissues and organs.

At each end of the muscle, the epimysial fibers come together to form **tendons,** bands of collagen fibers that attach skeletal muscles to bones. ∞ *p. 92* The tendon fibers are interwoven into the periosteum of the bone, providing a firm attachment. Any contraction of the muscle will exert a pull on its tendon and in turn on the attached bone.

The connective tissue fibers of the **perimysium** (per-i-MIS-ē-um; *peri-,* around) divide the skeletal muscle into a series of compartments, each containing a bundle of muscle fibers called a **fascicle** (FA-sik-ul; *fasciculus,* a bundle). In addition to collagen and elastic fibers, the perimysium contains blood vessels and nerves that supply the fascicles.

Within a fascicle, the **endomysium** (en-dō-MIS-ē-um; *endo-,* inside) surrounds each skeletal muscle fiber and ties adjacent muscle fibers together. Stem cells scattered among the fibers help repair damaged muscle tissue.

Nerves and Blood Vessels

Skeletal muscles are often called *voluntary muscles* because their contractions can occur under voluntary control. Many of these skeletal muscles may also be controlled involuntarily. For example, skeletal muscles involved with breathing, such as the *diaphragm,* usually work under involuntary control. Each skeletal

---

Vocabulary Aids:

Vocabulary Development

This section lists the important word roots that form the basis of the vocabulary in the chapter.

Key Terms

The most important new terms are highlighted in **bold type** and often include the pronunciation. All key terms are also listed at the end of the chapter for easy review.

Concept Links

The chain-link icon provides a quick visual signal that new material being presented is related to or builds on earlier discussions.

Visualizing Structure & Function

Outstanding Anatomy Art and Photos

To understand physiology, you must be able to visualize structures in the human body. Macro-to-micro drawings, coupled with histology or electron micrographs, make the details of anatomy easy to understand.

Figure Reference Locators

Red dots serve as place markers, making it easy to return to your spot in the narrative after you've studied an illustration.

Conceptual Diagrams Show Physiology

Physiological processes are easier to understand with flowcharts and diagrams that link structure and function.

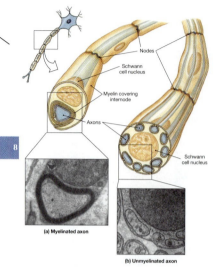

220 Neural Tissue and the Central Nervous System

8

Nodes

Schwann cell nucleus

Myelin covering internode

Axons

Schwann cell nucleus

(a) Myelinated axon

(b) Unmyelinated axon

•FIGURE 8-5   Schwann Cells and Peripheral Axons
(a) A single Schwann cell forms the myelin sheath around a portion of a single axon. This arrangement differs from the way myelin forms in the CNS; compare with Figure 8-4 (TEM × 14,048). (b) A single Schwann cell can encircle several unmyelinated axons. Unlike the situation in the CNS (Figure 8-4), every axon in the PNS is completely enclosed by glial cells.

NEUROPHYSIOLOGY

The sensory, integrative, and motor functions of the nervous system are dynamic and ever-changing. All of the important communications between neurons and other cells occur at membrane surfaces, through changes in the membrane potential. These membrane changes are electrical events that proceed at great speed.

The Membrane Potential

The cell membrane of an undisturbed cell has an excess of positive charges on the outside and an excess of negative charges on the inside. Such an uneven distribution of charges is known as a *potential difference*, and the size of the potential difference is measured in *volts*. Because the charges are separated by a cell membrane, the potential difference across the cell membrane of a living cell is called a **membrane potential**, or *transmembrane potential*. The **resting potential**, or membrane potential of an undisturbed cell, is very small. For example, the resting potential of a neuron averages about 0.070 volts, versus around 1.5 volts for a flashlight battery. Because they are so small, membrane potentials are usually reported in *millivolts* (mV, thousandths of volts) rather than volts. The resting potential of a neuron is −70 mV, with the minus sign indicating that the inside of the cell membrane contains an excess of negative charges as compared with the outside.

Factors Responsible for the Membrane Potential

As noted in earlier chapters, the intracellular and extracellular fluids differ markedly in ionic composition. For example, the extracellular fluid contains relatively high concentrations of sodium ions (Na^+) and chloride ions (Cl^-), whereas the intracellular fluid contains high concentrations of potassium ions (K^+) and negatively charged proteins (Pr^-).

The intracellular and extracellular fluids are separated by the cell membrane. The proteins cannot cross the membrane, and the ions can enter or leave the cell only by passing through membrane channels. ∞ *p. 59* There are many different types of channels in the membrane; some are always open (leak channels), and others open or close under specific circumstances (gated channels).

conduction. A Schwann cell may surround portions of several different unmyelinated axons (Figure 8-5b•).

✓ What would damage to the afferent division of the nervous system affect?

✓ Examination of a tissue sample shows unipolar neurons. Are these more likely to be sensory neurons or motor neurons?

✓ Which type of glial cell would you expect to be present in large numbers in brain tissue from a person suffering from an infection of the central nervous system?

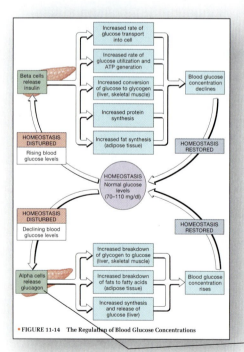

Beta cells release insulin

Increased rate of glucose transport into cell

Increased rate of glucose utilization and ATP generation

Increased conversion of glucose to glycogen (liver, skeletal muscle)

Increased protein synthesis

Increased fat synthesis (adipose tissue)

Blood glucose concentration declines

HOMEOSTASIS DISTURBED
Rising blood glucose levels

HOMEOSTASIS RESTORED

HOMEOSTASIS
Normal glucose levels (70–110 mg/dl)

HOMEOSTASIS DISTURBED
Declining blood glucose levels

HOMEOSTASIS RESTORED

Alpha cells release glucagon

Increased breakdown of glycogen to glucose (liver, skeletal muscle)

Increased breakdown of fats to fatty acids (adipose tissue)

Increased synthesis and release of glucose (liver)

Blood glucose concentration rises

•FIGURE 11-14   The Regulation of Blood Glucose Concentrations

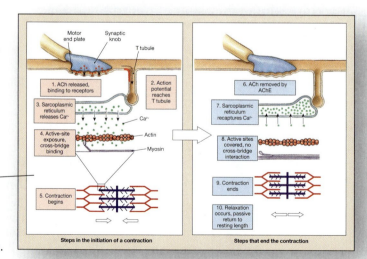

Motor end plate
Synaptic knob
T tubule

1. ACh released, binding to receptors

2. Action potential reaches T tubule

3. Sarcoplasmic reticulum releases Ca^{2+}

Ca^{2+}

4. Active-site exposure, cross-bridge binding

Actin

Myosin

5. Contraction begins

Steps in the initiation of a contraction

6. ACh removed by AChE

7. Sarcoplasmic reticulum recaptures Ca^{2+}

8. Active sites covered, no cross-bridge interaction

9. Contraction ends

10. Relaxation occurs, passive return to resting length

Steps that end the contraction

Integrating Concepts

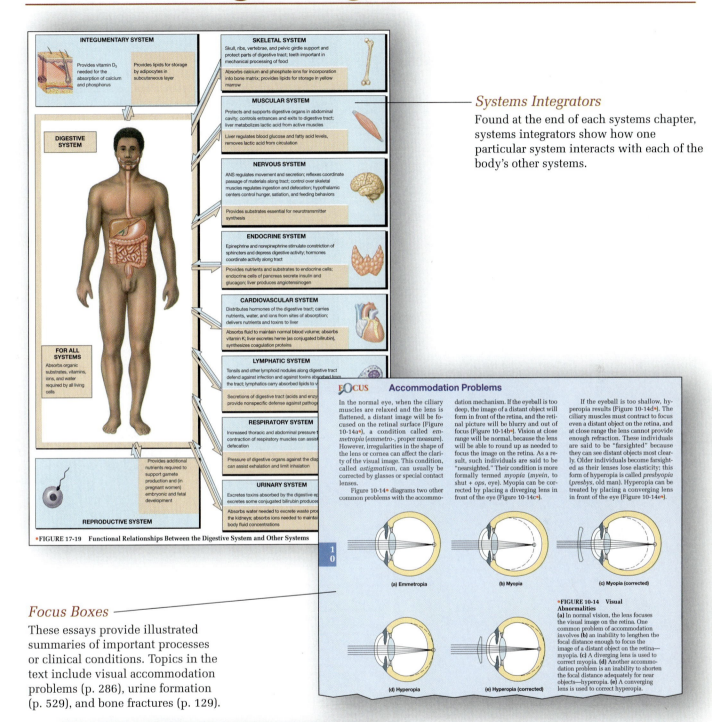

•FIGURE 17-19 Functional Relationships Between the Digestive System and Other Systems

Systems Integrators

Found at the end of each systems chapter, systems integrators show how one particular system interacts with each of the body's other systems.

Focus Boxes

These essays provide illustrated summaries of important processes or clinical conditions. Topics in the text include visual accommodation problems (p. 286), urine formation (p. 529), and bone fractures (p. 129).

Concept Check Questions

These questions, located at the ends of major sections in the narrative, will help you assess your understanding of the basic concepts addressed in the previous pages. Answers are provided at the end of each chapter.

Relating Clinical Examples

CLINICAL NOTE   **VITAL SIGNS**

Vital signs are outward indicators of what is going on inside the body. They include blood pressure (BP), heart rate, respiratory rate, and temperature. These measurements provide a great deal of information about a patient's condition and should be measured frequently.

The *pulse rate* is a measure of the number of times the heart beats per minute. The pulse is best measured where an artery lies close to the body's surface and crosses over a bone. Common locations for pulse determination are illustrated in Figure 14-6a. To measure the pulse rate, locate a suitable site and palpate the pulse. Then, count the number of pulse waves that occur in one minute. Alternatively, you can count the number of pulse waves in 30 seconds and multiply by two. In order to ensure accuracy, it is not recommended that intervals less than 30 seconds be measured.

The *respiratory rate* is a measure of the number of times a person breathes in one minute. To measure the respiratory rate, have the patient assume a comfortable position. While the patient is at rest, count the number of respirations that occur in one minute. People will alter their respiratory pattern if they feel it is being watched, so it is best to distract the patient. Skilled personnel will often take a patient's wrist and measure the pulse. Then, while still holding the wrist, they will count the respiratory rate while the patient thinks that the pulse is being measured.

The *blood pressure* is a function of the amount of blood being pumped by the heart (cardiac output) and the peripheral vascular resistance. To determine the blood pressure, a *blood pressure cuff (sphygmomanometer)* is placed on the arm 3–4 centimeters above the elbow (Figure 14-6b). A stethoscope is placed over the brachial artery. The blood pressure cuff is inflated to approximately 30 mm Hg above the point where it occludes the brachial artery and stops the flow of blood. Then, the pressure in the cuff is slowly released. When the pressure in the cuff falls below systolic pressure, blood flow resumes in the artery and produces *Korotkoff sounds*. As the pressure falls, the vessel remains open longer and the sounds in the artery change. When the cuff pressure falls below the diastolic pressure, blood flow becomes continuous and the Korotkoff sounds disappear completely.

The *temperature* is not often measured in EMS. However, electronic thermometers have made this a simple procedure. The temperature is measured in the mouth (under the tongue), rectally, or through the ear (tympanic membrane). Normal body temperature is 37° C (98.6° F).

1 4

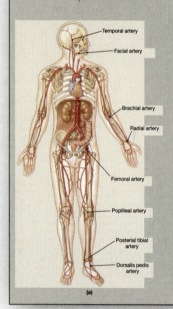

Temporal artery

Facial artery

Brachial artery

Radial artery

Femoral artery

Popliteal artery

Posterial tibial artery

Dorsalis pedis artery

(a)

•FIGURE 14-6 Checking the Pulse and Blood P[ressure] (a) Pressure points used to check the presence an[d rate] of the pulse. (b) The use of a sphygmomanometer [to measure] arterial blood pressure.

(b)

Clinical Note

Clinical or health-related topics of particular importance are presented in boxes set off from the main text. These essays cover major diseases, such as lung cancer and AIDS, in addition to other subjects of special interest, such as clinical procedures.

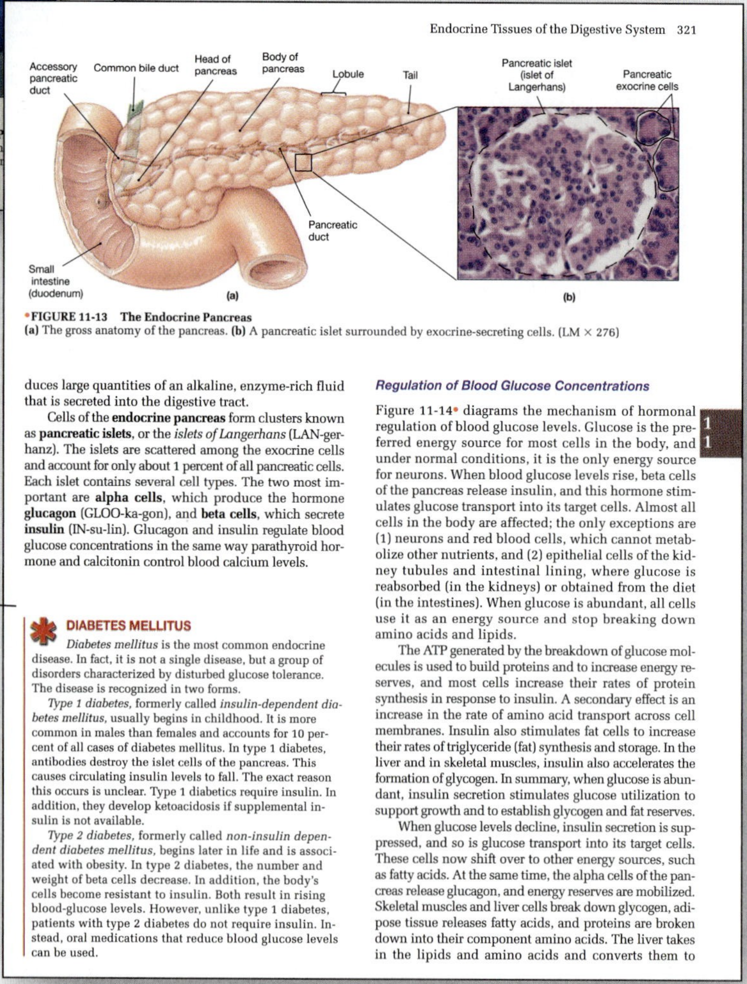

Accessory pancreatic duct   Common bile duct   Head of pancreas   Body of pancreas   Lobule   Tail   Pancreatic islet (islet of Langerhans)   Pancreatic exocrine cells

Pancreatic duct

Small intestine (duodenum)

(a)   **(b)**

•FIGURE 11-13 The Endocrine Pancreas
(a) The gross anatomy of the pancreas. (b) A pancreatic islet surrounded by exocrine-secreting cells. (LM × 276)

duces large quantities of an alkaline, enzyme-rich fluid that is secreted into the digestive tract.

Cells of the **endocrine pancreas** form clusters known as **pancreatic islets**, or the *islets of Langerhans* (LAN-gerhanz). The islets are scattered among the exocrine cells and account for only about 1 percent of all pancreatic cells. Each islet contains several cell types. The two most important are **alpha cells**, which produce the hormone **glucagon** (GLOO-ka-gon), and **beta cells**, which secrete **insulin** (IN-su-lin). Glucagon and insulin regulate blood glucose concentrations in the same way parathyroid hormone and calcitonin control blood calcium levels.

DIABETES MELLITUS

Diabetes mellitus is the most common endocrine disease. In fact, it is not a single disease, but a group of disorders characterized by disturbed glucose tolerance. The disease is recognized in two forms.

Type 1 diabetes, formerly called *insulin-dependent diabetes mellitus*, usually begins in childhood. It is more common in males than females and accounts for 10 percent of all cases of diabetes mellitus. In type 1 diabetes, antibodies destroy the islet cells of the pancreas. This causes circulating insulin levels to fall. The exact reason this occurs is unclear. Type 1 diabetics require insulin. In addition, they develop ketoacidosis if supplemental insulin is not available.

Type 2 diabetes, formerly called *non-insulin dependent diabetes mellitus*, begins later in life and is associated with obesity. In type 2 diabetes, the number and weight of beta cells decrease. In addition, the body's cells become resistant to insulin. Both result in rising blood-glucose levels. However, unlike type 1 diabetes, patients with type 2 diabetes do not require insulin. Instead, oral medications that reduce blood glucose levels can be used.

Regulation of Blood Glucose Concentrations

Figure 11-14• diagrams the mechanism of hormonal regulation of blood glucose levels. Glucose is the preferred energy source for most cells in the body, and under normal conditions, it is the only energy source for neurons. When blood glucose levels rise, beta cells of the pancreas release insulin, and this hormone stimulates glucose transport into its target cells. Almost all cells in the body are affected; the only exceptions are (1) neurons and red blood cells, which cannot metabolize other nutrients, and (2) epithelial cells of the kidney tubules and intestinal lining, where glucose is reabsorbed (in the kidneys) or obtained from the diet (in the intestines). When glucose is abundant, all cells use it as an energy source and stop breaking down amino acids and lipids.

1 1

The ATP generated by the breakdown of glucose molecules is used to build proteins and to increase energy reserves, and most cells increase their rates of protein synthesis in response to insulin. A secondary effect is an increase in the rate of amino acid transport across cell membranes. Insulin also stimulates fat cells to increase their rates of triglyceride (fat) synthesis and storage. In the liver and in skeletal muscles, insulin also accelerates the formation of glycogen. In summary, when glucose is abundant, insulin secretion stimulates glucose utilization to support growth and to establish glycogen and fat reserves.

When glucose levels decline, insulin secretion is suppressed, and so is glucose transport into its target cells. These cells now shift over to other energy sources, such as fatty acids. At the same time, the alpha cells of the pancreas release glucagon, and energy reserves are mobilized. Skeletal muscles and liver cells break down glycogen, adipose tissue releases fatty acids, and proteins are broken down into their component amino acids. The liver takes in the lipids and amino acids and converts them to

---

Clinical Discussions

Important clinical topics presented in context are set off by an icon, title, and vertical red bar. These topics have been selected not only for their medical importance, but also to show how an understanding of abnormal conditions can shed light on normal functions, and vice versa.

Reviewing the Concepts

Key Terms
Important terms introduced in the chapter are listed here with a page reference for quick review in context with the relevant material.

Summary Outline
This outline provides a detailed summary of all the sections in the chapter—including page references and all corresponding figure and table numbers.

Chapter Review

KEY TERMS

amphiarthrosis, p. 149
appendicular skeleton, p. 130
articulation, p. 149
axial skeleton, p. 130
bursa, p. 150
compact bone, p. 123
diaphysis, p. 123
diarthrosis, p. 149

epiphysis, p. 123
fracture, p. 127
ligament, p. 150
marrow, p. 123
meniscus, p. 150
ossification, p. 125
osteoblast, p. 124
osteoclast, p. 124

osteocyte, p. 123
osteon, p. 123
periosteum, p. 123
spongy bone, p. 123
synarthrosis, p. 149
synovial fluid, p. 150

SUMMARY OUTLINE

INTRODUCTION p. 122
1. The skeletal system includes the bones of the skeleton and the cartilages, ligaments, and other connective tissues that stabilize or interconnect bones. Its functions include structural support, storage, blood cell production, protection, and leverage.

THE STRUCTURE OF BONE p. 122
1. Bone, or osseous tissue, is a supporting connective tissue with a solid *matrix*.

Macroscopic Features of Bone p. 122
2. General categories of bones are **long bones**, **short bones**, **flat bones**, and **irregular bones**. *(Figure 6-1)*
3. The features of a long bone include a **diaphysis**, **epiphyses**, and a central *marrow cavity*. *(Figure 6-2)*
4. The two types of bone tissue are **compact**, or *dense*, **bone** and **spongy**, or *cancellous*, **bone**.
5. A bone is covered by a **periosteum** and lined with an **endosteum**.

Microscopic Features of Bone p. 123
6. Both types of bone contain **osteocytes** in **lacunae**. Layers of calcified matrix are **lamellae**, interconnected by **canaliculi**. *(Figure 6-3)*
7. The basic functional unit of compact bone is the **osteon**, containing osteocytes arranged around a **central canal**.
8. Spongy bone contains **trabeculae**, often in an open network.
9. Compact bone is located where stresses come from a limited range of directions; spongy bone is located where stresses are few or come from many different directions.
10. Cells other than osteocytes are also present in bone. **Osteoclasts** dissolve the bony matrix through the process of *osteolysis*. **Osteoblasts** synthesize the matrix in the process of *osteogenesis*.

BONE DEVELOPMENT AND GROWTH p. 125
1. **Ossification** is the process of converting other tissues to bone.

Intramembranous Ossification p. 125
2. **Intramembranous ossification** begins when stem cells in connective tissue differentiate into osteoblasts and can produce spongy or compact bone.

Endochondral Ossification p. 125
3. **Endochondral ossification** begins by the formation of a cartilage model of a bone that is gradually replaced by bone. *(Figure 6-4)*

Bone Growth and Body Proportions p.
4. There are differences between bones and viduals regarding the timing of epiphyseal clos

Requirements for Normal Bone Growth
5. Normal osteogenesis requires a reliable so als, vitamins, and hormones.

REMODELING AND HOMEOSTATIC ME p. 127
1. The organic and mineral components of tinuously recycled and renewed through the **remodeling**.

Remodeling and Support p. 127
2. The shapes and thicknesses of bones refle applied to them. Mineral turnover allows bo new stresses.

Homeostasis and Mineral Storage p. 12
3. Calcium is the most abundant mineral body, with roughly 99 percent of it located in The skeleton acts as a calcium reserve.

Injury and Repair p. 127
4. A **fracture** is a crack or break in a bone. R ture involves the formation of a **fracture he ternal callus**, and an **internal callus**. *(Figure Classification of Fractures)*

Aging and the Skeletal System p. 128
5. The effects of aging on the skeleton ca **teopenia** and **osteoporosis**.

Review Questions
Questions are organized in a three-tiered system to help you build your knowledge:

Level 1 questions allow you to test your recall of the chapter's basic information and terminology.

Level 2 questions help you check your grasp of concepts and your ability to integrate ideas presented in different parts of the chapter.

Level 3 questions let you develop your powers of reasoning and analysis by applying chapter material to plausible real-world and clinical situations.

Answers to Concept Check Questions
For easy reference, the concept check questions are answered at the end of each chapter.

---

3 REVIEW QUESTIONS

LEVEL 1   Reviewing Facts and Terms

Match each item in column A with the most closely related item in column B. Use letters for answers in the spaces provided.

Column A	Column B
___ 1. filtration	a. water out of cell
___ 2. osmosis	b. passive carrier-mediated transport
___ 3. hypotonic solution	c. endocytosis, exocytosis
___ 4. hypertonic solution	d. movement of water
___ 5. isotonic solution	e. hydrostatic pressure
___ 6. facilitated diffusion	f. normal saline
___ 7. carrier proteins	g. ion pump
___ 8. vesicular transport	h. water into cell
___ 9. cytosol	i. manufacture proteins
___10. cytoskeleton	j. digestive enzymes
___11. microvilli	k. internal protein framework
___12. ribosomes	l. control center for cellular operations
___13. mitochondria	m. intracellular fluid
___14. lysosomes	n. DNA strands
___15. nucleus	o. cristae
___16. chromosomes	p. synthesize components of ribosomes
___17. nucleoli	q. increase cell surface area

18. The study of the structure and function of cells is called:
(a) histology
(b) cytology
(c) physiology
(d) biology

19. The proteins in the cell membranes may function as:
(a) receptors and channels

22. Structures that perform specific functions within the cell are:
(a) organs
(b) organisms
(c) organelles
(d) chromosomes

23. The construction of a functional protein using the infor

LEVEL 2   Reviewing Concepts

29. Diffusion is important in body fluids because this process tends to:
(a) increase local concentration gradients
(b) eliminate local concentration gradients
(c) move substances against their concentration gradients
(d) create concentration gradients

30. When placed in a _____ solution, a cell will lose water through osmosis. The process results in the _____ of red blood cells.
(a) hypotonic, crenation
(b) hypertonic, crenation
(c) isotonic, hemolysis
(d) hypotonic, hemolysis

LEVEL 3   Critical Thinking and Clinical Applications

38. Experimental evidence shows that the transport of a certain molecule exhibits the following characteristics: (1) The molecule moves along its concentration gradient; (2) at concentrations above a given level, there is no increase in the rate of transport; and (3) cellular energy is not required for transport to occur. Which type of transport process is at work?

39. Two solutions, A and B, are separated by a selectively permeable barrier. Over a period of time, the level of fluid on side A increases. Which solution initially had the higher concentration of solute?

ANSWERS TO CONCEPT CHECK QUESTIONS

Page 64
1. Active transport processes require the expenditure of cellular energy in the form of the high-energy bonds of ATP molecules. Passive transport processes (*diffusion, osmosis, filtration,* and *facilitated diffusion*) move ions and molecules across the cell membrane without any energy expenditure by the cell. 2. Energy must be expended to transport H⁺ ions against their concentration gradient—that is, from a region where they are less concentrated (the cells lining the stomach) to a region where they are more concentrated (the interior of the stomach). An active transport process must be involved. 3. This is an example of phagocytosis.

Page 66
1. The fingerlike projections on the surface of the intestinal cells are *microvilli*. They increase the cells' surface area so they can absorb nutrients more efficiently. 2. Cells that lack centrioles are unable to divide.

Page 69
1. The SER functions in the synthesis of lipids such as steroids. Ovaries and testes would be expected to have a great deal of SER because these organs produce large amounts of steroid hormones. 2. The function of mitochondria is to produce energy for the cell in the form of ATP molecules. A large number of mitochondria in a cell would indicate a high demand for energy.

Page 73
1. The nucleus of a cell contains DNA that codes for the production of all of the cell's proteins. Some of these proteins are structural proteins that are responsible for the shape and other physical characteristics of the cell. Other proteins are enzymes that govern cellular metabolism, direct the production of cell proteins, and control all of the cell's activities. 2. If a cell lacked the enzyme RNA polymerase it would not be able to transcribe RNA from DNA. 3. The deletion of a base from a coding sequence of DNA during transcription would alter the entire mRNA base sequence after the deletion point. This would result in different codons on the messenger RNA that was transcribed from the affected region, and this, in turn, would result in the incorporation of a different series of amino acids into the protein. Almost certainly the protein product would not be functional.

Page 75
1. Cells that are preparing to undergo mitosis manufacture additional organelles and duplicate sets of their DNA. 2. The four stages of mitosis are prophase, metaphase, anaphase, and telophase. 3. If spindle fibers failed to form during mitosis, the cell would not be able to separate the chromosomes into two sets. If cytokinesis occurred, the result would be one cell with two sets of chromosomes and one cell with none.

Emergency Care Applications

6 Emergency Care Applications

OVERVIEW

The skeletal system forms the underlying framework of the body. It consists of 206 or more bones and the associated ligaments and cartilage. Numerous emergencies can arise affecting the skeletal system. Most are due to trauma, although several disease processes also can lead to skeletal-system emergencies. The skeletal system's numerous important functions include support of the soft tissues, production of blood cells, storage of minerals and lipids, and movement of the body as a whole (in conjunction with the muscular system). Because of their integrated relationship, the skeletal system and the muscular system often are referred to jointly as the *musculoskeletal system*. Physicians who specialize in the treatment of bone-related problems are called *orthopedic surgeons*. *Rheumatologists* are physicians who specialize in the medical treatment of joint problems, especially those of autoimmune origin. The following is a discussion of common bone and related injuries encountered in the emergency setting.

SKELETAL INJURIES

There are four general types of skeletal and joint injuries: sprains, subluxations, dislocations, and fractures.

Sprains

The sprain is an injury that stretches or tears one or more ligaments within a joint. This tearing of ligaments weakens the joint. Stresses to a joint can extend the joint beyond its normal range of motion, causing ligamentous injury (Figure A6-1•). The injury results in acute pain at the site, followed shortly by inflammation and swelling. Sprains are classified, or graded, according to their severity, using the following criteria:
- *Grade I.* Minor and incomplete tear. The ligament is painful and tender, but there is no laxity. Swelling and ecchymosis are usually minimal. The joint is stable.

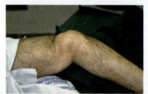

• FIGURE A6-1 Grade-2 Ankle Sprain Following Common Inversion Injury
The anterior tabofibular ligament appears completely torn, while the posterior tabofibular ligament is only partially torn. The vast majority of ankle sprains involve the lateral ligaments.

- *Grade II.* Significant but incomplete tear. There is laxity, but also an end-point beyond which no further opening of the joint occurs. Swelling and ecchymosis may be moderate to severe, and pain may range from moderate to severe. The joint is unstable but intact.
- *Grade III.* Complete tear and total failure of the ligament or ligaments involved. No end-point is felt when stress is applied to the ligament during examination of the joint. Pain and muscle spasm can often mask a grade III sprain, so the diagnosis is

easily missed. Due to severe pain and spasm, the injury may be mistaken for a fracture. A repeat examination several days later can help confirm the diagnosis. The joint is unstable.

Subluxation

A *subluxation*, also called a partial dislocation, is a partial displacement of a bone end from its position within a joint capsule. It occurs as the joint separates under stress, stretching the ligaments. A subluxation differs from a sprain in that it more significantly reduces the joint's integrity.

Dislocation

A *dislocation* is a complete displacement of bone ends from their normal position within a joint. The joint often fixes in an abnormal position with noticeable deformity (Figure A6-2•). This injury occurs when the bones of the joint move beyond their normal range of motion, usually with great force. It carries with it the danger of entrapping, compressing, or tearing nearby blood vessels and nerves. A dislocation should be suspected whenever a joint is deformed or does not move in a normal fashion.

Fracture

A *fracture* is an injury that interrupts the structural integrity of a bone. Most fractures are the result of significant trauma to a healthy bone. The bony cortex may be disrupted by many different forces including: a direct blow, angular (bending) forces, axial loading, twisting (torque) stress, or any combination of these.

Fractures also can occur in a bone that is diseased or otherwise abnormal. These pathological processes weaken the bone making it susceptible to fracture by forces that would, under normal circumstances, not typically disrupt the cortex. These fractures are called *pathological* fractures and can result from relatively minor trauma. Examples of pathological fractures include fractures through lytic metastatic (cancerous) lesions, fractures through benign bone cysts, and vertebral compression fractures in patients with advanced osteoporosis. Vertebral compression fractures are the most common type of pathological fracture.

Growth-Plate Injuries

Fractures can involve the epiphyseal growth plate in children. The cartilaginous epiphyseal plate, also called the physis, is readily injured because it is weaker than ossified bone or ligaments (Figure A6-3•). Damage to the epiphyseal plate during a child's growth may destroy all or part of the bone's ability to produce new bone, resulting in stunted or deformed growth thereafter. The potential for a growth disturbance from a growth-plate injury is re-

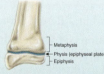

• FIGURE A6-2 Anterior Dislocation of the Knee
This rare injury poses a significant threat to blood vessels and nerves that transverse the knee. Immediate reduction is indicated.

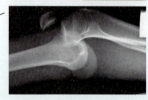

• FIGURE A6-3 Growth Plate in a Child's Long Bone
The growth plate is also called the physis or epiphyseal plate. The portion of bone proximal to the physis is the metaphysis; the segment distal to the physis is the epiphysis.

Metaphysis
Physis (epiphyseal plate)
Epiphysis

lated to the number of years the child has yet to grow. Thus, the older the child, the less time remains for a deformity to develop. The *Salter-Harris system* is often used to classify growth-plate injuries. The potential for growth disturbance increases as the classification number increases. The prognosis is best for type I fractures and

Emergency Care Applications   A6-2

A6-1

Emergency Care Applications

New *Emergency Care Applications* appear at the end of every chapter. These applications provide the focus to better prepare you for patient care.

Art and Photos

A careful selection of art and photos helps you to clearly understand the details of anatomy and physiology.

Preface to the Instructor

THE WORLD IS CHANGING...

The times in which we now live are full of change. The Information Age has brought an explosion in what we know, *how we know* what we know, and *how we share* what we know. The field of anatomy and physiology is an excellent case in point. New techniques and better communication have expanded our understanding of the intricate workings of the human body. New therapies and protocols have been developed to combat disease, reduce suffering, and promote good health. New methods of accessing and sharing information have linked health professionals around the world. Technology has facilitated the acquisition and distribution of information, and medical professionals have learned to use new technologies to increase their effectiveness as well as to improve the quality of medical care.

Demographic changes have also had a profound impact on the field of anatomy and physiology. With the average age of the population increasing, the demand for health services has increased strongly and will continue to do so for decades to come. As a result, there have never been greater opportunities for employment in applied-health related fields, from gerontology and nursing to sports training, from dietetics to occupational health and safety. Many students are interested in the field of emergency medical services.

These technological and demographic changes have created a strong demand for a well-trained, flexible work force. To be effective in almost any job today, you must know how to access and absorb new information, to use (or learn to use) available technology, and to solve problems. These requirements are especially apparent in the applied health fields. What we teach our students today will not include everything they will need to know 10 years from now. For those of us who prepare students for careers in the health sciences, it has become more important than ever to provide students not only with a specific set of skills and knowledge, but also with the skills needed for lifelong learning.

As the world has changed, so has the field of emergency medical services (EMS). The practice of emergency medicine is a bona fide medical specialty. Competent prehospital emergency care is now expected by the public. As the profession evolves, we are beginning to take a long and hard look at many of our practices and procedures using sound scientific principles. Quality research in EMS is being conducted in a great number of our medical schools and other institutions of higher learning. Also, technology has changed the face of emergency practice. Many procedures, once limited to the emergency department, are now possible in the ambulance. These include 12-lead ECGs, pulse oximetry, capnography, and many others. Likewise, the hospital practice of emergency medicine has changed. Bedside ultrasonography by the emergency physician has become the standard of care. Sophisticated diagnostic imaging, including CT, MRI, nuclear medicine, and other techniques are now available 24 hours a day, often within the confines of the emergency department. Although emergency medicine is becoming high tech, it is important to remember that it also should be "high touch." A comforting touch, a concerned ear, and a quiet voice can oftentimes provide more care than all of our technology combined. Always remember, treat the patient, not the monitor.

Anatomy & Physiology for Emergency Care is an enhanced edition of *Essentials of Anatomy & Physiology*, second edition (Martini/Bartholomew). It has been developed to meet the needs and interests of EMS students, who are eager to begin learning clinical information. "Emergency Care Applications," written specifically for EMS students, appear at the end of each chapter, enhancing the basic science material. Many illustrations within these applications sections detail actual emergency scenes. They contribute to a clinical focus and complement the high-quality anatomy and physiology art. In addition, clinical inserts and discussions throughout the text highlight important topics of interest to the EMS community.

SIMPLIFY

There have also been many changes in terms of the resources available to assist in the teaching of difficult concepts in anatomy and physiology. The use of animations and simulations, for instance, enables us to communicate abstract processes more effectively than ever before to students. Professionally developed lecture resources with a consistent style and terminology help us integrate new tools into our teaching in an efficient manner. On-line study tools can supplement office hours with 24-hour, on-demand remediation—ideal for today's students, many of whom are juggling work, family, and school responsibilities.

The focus of this text and learning system has been to simplify the processes of teaching and learning anatomy and physiology. Much as we would like to, we cannot create materials that will give any of us more time. But a carefully designed text and supplements package can help both instructors and students make better use of the time you do have. This is why we have developed a teaching/learning package to be as consistent and fully integrated as is possible.

Anatomy & Physiology for Emergency Care has been carefully designed to place information in a meaningful context and to help students develop their problem-solving skills. The *Preface to the Student* and *User's Guide* outline the specific pedagogical framework that is one of the hallmarks of this text. Encouraging your students to acquaint themselves with and to use this system of pedagogy will help them simplify their study process.

In this text, our aim has been to present information simply and clearly, with a suitable emphasis on the concrete, applied aspects of each topic. Those pursuing careers in the medical or allied health sciences will acquire the background needed to organize and integrate additional information. For those seeking careers outside the biomedical fields, the perception that anatomical and physiological processes are understandable, relevant, and logical should remain intact and valuable long after the origin and insertion of the latissimus dorsi muscle have been forgotten.

A consistent art style, close integration of text and art, and consistent terminology throughout are some of the additional ways in which we strive to simplify the teaching and learning process. Throughout this project, we have been fortunate to work with William Ober, M.D., a physician who is also an award-winning medical illustrator. Dr. Ober and his associate, Claire Garrison, R.N., played a key role in coordinating the art program for this textbook. Having a single illustration team responsible for the visual presentation of information throughout the book helps ensure that structures and processes are depicted in a consistent manner from figure to figure and chapter to chapter. This is the only essentials book with an art program created and managed by a medical illustrator.

INTEGRATED SUPPLEMENTS

The ancillary package for *Anatomy & Physiology for Emergency Care* has been designed to meet the needs of instructors and students. Consult your Brady sales representative regarding individual supplements.

For the Instructor

- **EMS Instructor's Resource Supplement**   Each chapter contains learning strategies for the application sections.

- **Multimedia Presentation Manager v.3.0**   This multimedia tool includes our image bank with all the art from the text as well as additional photographs, animations, and video clips. The easy-to-use navigation software enables you to build multimedia lectures or to integrate these resources into your own resources. This tool is fully compatible with Power Point and other graphics software.

- **300 Full-Color Transparency Acetates**   These acetates include key illustrations from the textbook.

- **Instructor's Resource Guide**   This useful guide provides lively, unique analogies and teaching tips as well as suggestions from other instructors across the United States.

- **Test Item File and Prentice Hall Custom Test Software**   Access a complete testing package with more than 3,000 questions. The testing package par-

allels the three-level learning system used in the textbook and also includes 200 pieces of unlabeled text art to allow you to create labeling exercises for exams.

- **Prentice Hall Laserdisc for Anatomy and Physiology** and **Bar Code Manual**   This laserdisc uses videodisc technology to feature high-quality animations based on art from the text.

- **Blackboard WebCT**   This courseware offers you all the advantages of a powerful course-management system while minimizing your need to develop primary content. The site is fully customizable, allowing you to teach just what you want to teach for the essentials level, and features numerous easy-to-use administrative tools.

For the Student

- **Companion Website for Essentials of Anatomy and Physiology**   An exciting new edition of Prentice Hall's Companion Website has been developed specifically for students using the second edition of *Essentials of Anatomy and Physiology*. In addition to multiple-choice, essay, and short-answer questions, this site's self-grading quizzes offer exercises in labeling and concept mapping for each chapter. Numerous interesting, related Websites are referenced and annotated in the Destinations sections, and our NetSearch offers students a convenient gateway to hundreds of other sites of interest.

- **Anatomy and Physiology Video Tutor**   This highly praised, 75-minute videotape focuses on the concepts that both instructors and students consistently identify as the most challenging. Physiological processes are demonstrated through the use of top-quality three-dimensional animations and video footage. On-camera narration and the accompanying frame-referenced study booklet allow for repeated concept review.

- **FAP-Interactive CD-ROM**   This interactive CD-ROM is ideal for students wanting a comprehensive electronic reference that can supplement the information provided in *Essentials of Anatomy and Physiology*. Many students are eager to see what they've learned in context. This CD-ROM offers two options to fulfill that need. First, it includes 20 **interactive tutorials** that use text graphics, animations, and audio to help students visualize difficult concepts. Embedded exercises require students to demonstrate their understanding. Second, it includes **cases** that let students practice their analytical and diagnostic skills in real-world situations. Audio and Internet links are accessed through embedded hot-links.

- **Applications Manual**   This unique supplement provides you with access to interesting and relevant clinical and diagnostic information. It includes introductory sections about the scientific method and the applications of chemistry and cell biology to clinical work, sections about each body system that parallel the textbook organization and provide more detailed clinical information, a full-color Surface Anatomy and Cadaver Atlas, and Critical-Thinking Questions for each body system. The *Applications Manual* is fully cross-referenced to the textbook to promote the integration of this material into the course.

- *Study Guide*   Designed to help you master the topics and concepts covered in the textbook, the study guide includes many labeling exercises, review questions, concept maps, and exercises that promote an understanding of body systems.

ACKNOWLEDGMENTS

Every textbook represents a group effort. Foremost on the list are the faculty and reviewers whose advice, comments, and collective wisdom helped shape both the first and second editions of *Essentials of Anatomy & Physiology*. Their interest in the subject, their concern for the accuracy and method of presentation, and their experience with students of widely varying abilities and backgrounds made the review process an educational experience. To these individuals, who carefully recorded their comments, opinions, and sources, we express our sincere thanks and best wishes.

In addition, we express thanks to the following individuals who reviewed the Emergency Care Applications and clincial inserts for *Anatomy & Physiology for Emergency Care.*

Howard A. Werman, M.D.
Associate Professor of Clinical Emergency Medicine
The Ohio State University College of Medicine and
   Public Health
Columbus, Ohio
Medical Director, MedFlight

Brenda M. Beasley, RN, BS, EMT-P
Department Chair, Allied Health/EMS Director of
   Education
Calhoun College
Decatur, Alabama

Robert A. De Lorenzo, M.D., F.A.C.E.P.
Lieut. Colonel, US Army
Brooke Army Medical Center
Ft. Sam Houston, Texas

Arthur Hsieh, NREMT-P, MA
EMS in Service Training, Chief
San Francisco Fire Department
San Franciso, California

Virtually without exception, reviewers stressed the importance of accurate, integrated, and visually attractive illustrations in helping students understand essential material. The art program was directed by Bill Ober, M.D. and Claire Garrison, R.N. Many of these illustrations include color photographs or micrographs collected from a variety of sources. Much of the work in tracking down these materials was performed by Stuart Kenter, whose efforts are greatly appreciated. Many of the light micrographs prepared by the senior author used commercially available slides obtained with the assistance of Carolina Biological Supply and Wards Scientific. The cadaver images and organ photos were provided in large part by Ralph Hutchings, whose artistic abilities and fine eye for detail are both envied and appreciated.

Any errors or oversights in this text are strictly those of the authors, not of the reviewers, artists, or editors. Any and all comments and suggestions will be deeply appreciated and carefully considered in the preparation of future editions.

Frederic H. Martini
Haiku, Hawaii

Edwin F. Bartholomew
Lahaina, Hawaii

Bryan E. Bledsoe
Midlothian, Texas

1

An Introduction to Anatomy and Physiology

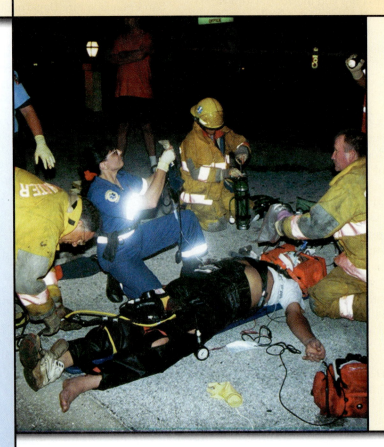

"Our patient has a single gunshot to the right hemithorax. The entrance wound is in the fourth intercostal space at the right midclavicular line, and the exit wound is in the sixth intercostal space at the right posterior axillary line." This radio report accurately describes the entrance and exit wounds of an EMS patient who has been shot in the chest. The description allows hospital personnel to form an accurate mental picture of the patient's injuries. As a member of the emergency care team, it is important to have a thorough understanding of human anatomy and physiology. Before you learn abnormal pathophysiology, you must first understand normal anatomy and physiology. This chapter introduces you to the fundamental aspects of human anatomy and physiology, including body organization, homeostasis, and topographical anatomy.

Chapter Outline and Objectives

Vocabulary Development

*ante-, before; *anterior*
bios, life; *biology*
cardium, heart; *pericardium*
*cephal-, head; *cephalic*
*cranio-, skull; *cranial*
dorsum, back; *dorsal*
homeo-, unchanging; *homeostasis*
-logy, study of; *biology*
medianus, situated in the middle; *median*
paries, wall; *parietal*
pathos, disease; *pathology*
peri-, around; *perimeter*
*post-, after; *posterior*
pronus, inclined forward; *prone*
*super-, above; *superior*
supinus, lying on the back; *supine*
-stasis, standing; *homeostasis*
venter, belly or abdomen; *ventral*

The world around us contains an enormous diversity of living organisms that vary widely in appearance and lifestyle. Despite their obvious differences, however, all living things perform the same basic functions:

- **Responsiveness**. Organisms respond to changes in their immediate environment; this property is also called *irritability*. You move your hand away from a hot stove, your dog barks at approaching strangers, fish are scared by loud noises, and tiny amoebas glide toward potential prey. Organisms also make longer-term changes as they adjust to their environments. For example, an animal may grow a heavier coat of fur as winter approaches, or it may migrate to a warmer climate. The capacity to make such adjustments is termed *adaptability*.

- **Growth**. Over a lifetime, organisms grow larger, increasing in size through an increase in the size or number of *cells*, the simplest units of life. Familiar organisms, such as dogs, cats, and people, are composed of billions of cells. In such multicellular organisms, the individual cells become specialized to perform particular functions. This specialization is called *differentiation*.

- **Reproduction**. Organisms reproduce, creating subsequent generations of similar organisms.

- **Movement**. Organisms are capable of producing movement, which may be internal (transporting food, blood, or other materials inside the body) or external (moving through the environment).

- **Metabolism**. Organisms rely on complex chemical reactions to provide the energy for responsiveness, growth, reproduction, and movement. They must also synthesize complex chemicals, such as proteins. *Metabolism* refers to all of the chemical operations under way in the body. Normal metabolic operations require the absorption of materials from the environment. To generate energy efficiently, most cells require various nutrients, as well as oxygen, a gas. *Respiration* refers to the absorption, transport, and use of oxygen by cells. Metabolic operations often generate unneeded or potentially harmful waste products that must be eliminated through the process of *excretion*.

For very small organisms, absorption, respiration, and excretion involve the movement of materials across exposed surfaces. But creatures larger than a few millimeters thick seldom absorb nutrients directly from their environment. For example, humans cannot absorb steaks, apples, or ice cream without processing them first. That processing, called *digestion*, occurs in specialized areas where complex foods are broken down into simpler components that can be absorbed easily.

Respiration and excretion are also more complicated for large organisms. Humans have specialized structures responsible for gas exchange (lungs) and excretion (kidneys). Although digestion, respiration, and excretion occur in different parts of the body, the cells of the body cannot travel to one place for nutrients, another for oxygen, and a third to get rid of waste products. Instead, individual cells remain where they are but communicate with other areas of the body through an internal transport system, or *circulation*. For example, your blood absorbs the waste products released by each of your cells and carries those wastes to the kidneys for excretion.

Biology, the study of life, includes a number of subspecialties. This text considers two biological subjects: anatomy and physiology. Over the course of 21 chapters, you will become familiar with the basic anatomy and physiology of the human body.

THE SCIENCES OF ANATOMY AND PHYSIOLOGY

The word *anatomy* has Greek origins, as do many other anatomical terms and phrases. A literal translation would be "a cutting open." **Anatomy** is the study of internal and external structure and the physical relationships between body parts. **Physiology**, another word derived from Greek, is the study of how living organisms perform their vital functions. The two subjects are interrelated. Anatomical information provides clues about probable functions, and physiological mechanisms can be explained only in terms of the underlying anatomy.

The link between structure and function is always present but not always understood. For example, the anatomy of the heart was clearly described in the fifteenth century, but almost 200 years passed before anyone realized that it pumped blood. Yet we knew details of cell physiology decades before improved microscopes enabled us to find the associated anatomical structures. This text will familiarize you with basic anatomy and give you an appreciation of the physiological processes that make human life possible. This knowledge should enable you to understand many kinds of disease processes and make informed decisions about your personal health.

Anatomical Perspectives

Anatomy can be categorized as microscopic anatomy or macroscopic (gross) anatomy on the basis of the degree of structural detail under consideration. Other anatomical specialties focus on specific processes or medical applications.

Microscopic Anatomy

Microscopic anatomy considers structures that cannot be seen without magnification. The boundaries of microscopic anatomy are established by the limits of the equipment used. A light microscope reveals basic details about cell structure, whereas an electron microscope can visualize individual molecules only a few nanometers (nm) across. As we proceed through the text, we will be considering details at all levels, from macroscopic to microscopic. (If you are unfamiliar with the terms used to describe measurements and weights over this size range, consult the tables in Appendix III.)

Microscopic anatomy can be subdivided into specialties that consider features within a characteristic range of sizes. **Cytology** (sī-TOL-o-jē) analyzes the internal structure of individual **cells**. The trillions of living cells in our bodies are composed of chemical substances in various combinations, and our lives depend on the chemical processes occurring in those cells. For this reason we will consider basic chemistry (Chapter 2) before examining cell structure (Chapter 3).

Histology (his-TOL-o-jē) takes a broader perspective and examines **tissues**, groups of specialized cells and cell products that work together to perform a particular function. The trillions of cells in the human body can be assigned to four major tissue types, and these tissues are the focus of Chapter 4. Tissues combine to form **organs**, such as the heart, kidney, liver, and brain. Many organs can be examined without a microscope, and at this level we cross the boundary into gross anatomy.

Gross Anatomy

Gross anatomy considers features visible with the unaided eye. There are many ways to approach gross anatomy. **Surface anatomy** refers to the study of general form and superficial markings. **Regional anatomy** considers all of the superficial and internal features in a specific region of the body, such as the head, neck, or trunk. **Systemic anatomy** considers the structure of major *organ systems*, which are groups of organs that function together to produce coordinated effects. For example, the heart, blood, and blood vessels form the *cardiovascular system*, which circulates oxygen and nutrients throughout the body.

Physiology

Physiology examines the function of anatomical structures; it considers the physical and chemical processes responsible for the characteristics of life, or vital functions. Because these vital functions are complex and much more difficult to examine than are most anatomical structures, the science of physiology includes even more specialties than does the science of anatomy.

Human physiology is the study of the functions of the human body. The cornerstone of human physiology is **cell physiology**, the study of the functions of living cells. Cell physiology includes events at the chemical and molecular levels—both chemical processes within cells and chemical interactions between cells. **Special physiology** is the study of the physiology of specific organs. Examples are renal physiology (kidney function) and cardiac physiology (heart function). **System physiology** considers all aspects of the function of specific organ systems. Respiratory physiology and reproductive physiology are examples. **Pathological physiology**, or **pathology**, studies the effects of diseases on organ or system functions. (The Greek word *pathos* means disease.) Modern medicine depends on an understanding of both normal and pathological physiology; the practitioner must know not only what is wrong but how to correct it.

Special topics in physiology address specific functions of the human body as a whole. These specialties focus on physiological interactions between multiple-organ systems. For example, exercise physiology studies the physiological adjustments to exercise. Many other such applied topics are discussed in boxes throughout the book.

✓ How are vital functions such as growth, responsiveness, reproduction, and movement dependent on metabolism?

✓ Would a histologist more likely be considered a specialist in microscopic anatomy or in gross anatomy? Why?

LEVELS OF ORGANIZATION

When considering events from the microscopic to macroscopic scales, we are examining several levels of organization. Figure 1-1• presents the relationships among the various levels of organization using the cardiovascular system as an example.

- **Chemical, or Molecular, Level**. Atoms, the smallest stable units of matter, combine to form *molecules* with complex shapes. Even at this simplest level, the specialized shape of a molecule determines its function. This is the chemical, or molecular, level of organization.

1

•FIGURE 1-1   **Levels of Organization**

Interacting atoms form molecules that combine to form cells, such as heart muscle cells. Groups of similar cells combine to form tissues with specific functions, such as heart muscle tissue. Organs, such as the heart, are composed of different tissues. The heart is one component of the cardiovascular system, which also includes the blood and blood vessels. All of the organ systems combine and interact to create an organism, a living human being.

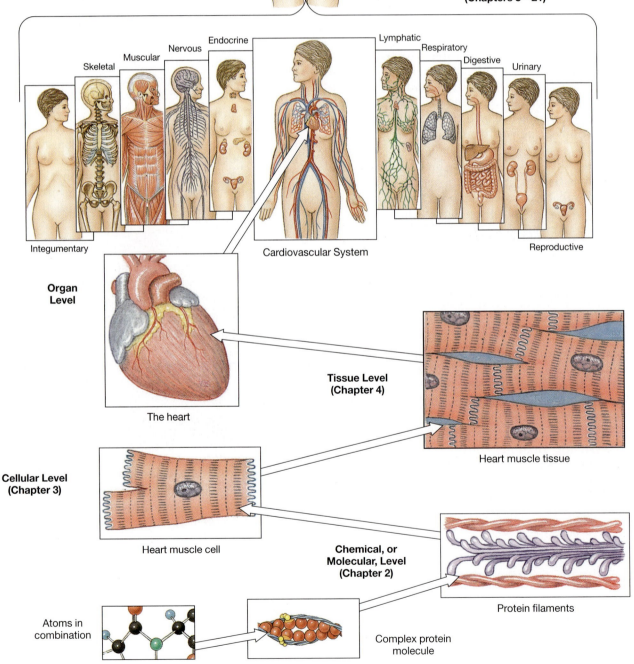

Organism Level

Organ System Level (Chapters 5 – 21)

Skeletal   Muscular   Nervous   Endocrine   Lymphatic   Respiratory   Digestive   Urinary

Integumentary   Cardiovascular System   Reproductive

Organ Level

The heart

Tissue Level (Chapter 4)

Heart muscle tissue

Cellular Level (Chapter 3)

Heart muscle cell

Chemical, or Molecular, Level (Chapter 2)

Protein filaments

Atoms in combination

Complex protein molecule

- **Cellular Level**. Different molecules interact to form *organelles*, such as the protein filaments found in muscle cells. Each type of organelle has a specific function. For example, interactions among protein filaments give muscle cells the ability to contract, or shorten. Organelles perform the vital functions that keep cells alive. Cells, the smallest living units in the body, represent the cellular level of organization.

- **Tissue Level**. A tissue is composed of similar cells working together to perform a specific function. Heart muscle cells form *cardiac muscle tissue*, an example of the tissue level of organization.

- **Organ Level**. An organ consists of two or more different tissues that work together to perform specific functions. Layers of muscle and other tissues form the wall of the heart, a hollow, three-dimensional organ. This is an example of the organ level of organization.

- **Organ System Level**. Each time it contracts, the heart pushes blood into a network of blood vessels. Together, the heart, blood, and blood vessels form the *cardiovascular system*, an example of the organ system level of organization.

- **Organism Level**. All of the organ systems of the body work together to maintain life and health. This brings us to the highest level of organization, that of the organism—in this case, a human being.

Each level of organization depends on the others, and damage at the cellular, tissue, or organ level can affect the entire system. For example, a chemical change in heart muscle cells can cause abnormal contractions or even stop the heartbeat. Physical damage to the muscle tissue, as in a chest wound, can make the heart ineffective even when most of the heart muscle cells are intact and uninjured. An inherited abnormality in heart structure can make it an ineffective pump, although the muscle cells and muscle tissue are perfectly normal. Because all parts of a system are interdependent, damage to one component will ultimately affect the system as a whole. For example, the heart cannot pump blood effectively after a massive blood loss if there is not enough blood to fill the circulatory system. If the heart cannot pump and blood cannot flow, oxygen and nutrients cannot be distributed. In a very short time, the cardiac muscle tissue begins to break down as individual muscle cells die from oxygen and nutrient starvation. Finally, because all of the body systems are interdependent, disruption of one system will affect all others. If the heart stops pumping blood, the damage will not be restricted to the cardiovascular system; unless something is done quickly, the person will die from the resulting damage to cells, tissues, and organs throughout the body.

AN INTRODUCTION TO ORGAN SYSTEMS

Figure 1-2• introduces the 11 organ systems in the human body and indicates their major functions. Figure 1-3• provides an overview of these individual organ systems and their major components.

Organ System		Major Functions
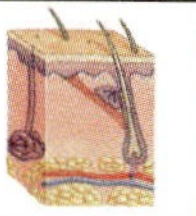	Integumentary system	Protection from environmental hazards, temperature control
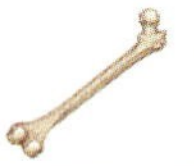	Skeletal system	Support, protection of soft tissues, mineral storage, blood formation
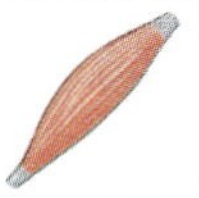	Muscular system	Locomotion, support, heat production
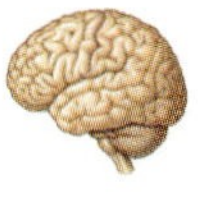	Nervous system	Directing immediate responses to stimuli, usually by coordinating the activities of other organ systems
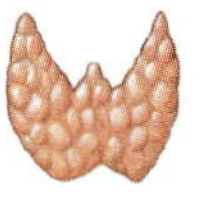	Endocrine system	Directing long-term changes in the activities of other organ systems
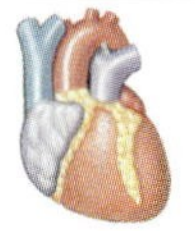	Cardiovascular system	Internal transport of cells and dissolved materials, including nutrients, wastes, and gases
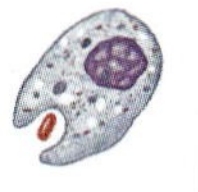	Lymphatic system	Defense against infection and disease
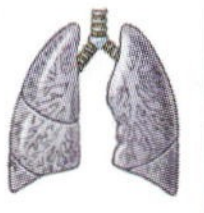	Respiratory system	Delivery of air to sites where gas exchange can occur between the air and circulating blood
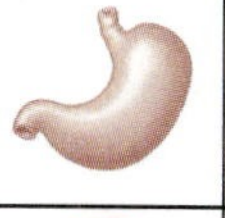	Digestive system	Processing of food and absorption of nutrients, minerals, vitamins, and water
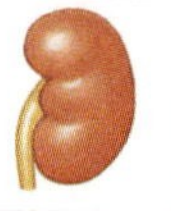	Urinary system	Elimination of excess water, salts, and waste products
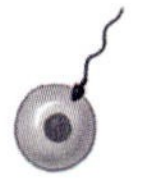	Reproductive system	Production of sex cells and hormones

•**FIGURE 1-2   An Introduction to Organ Systems**

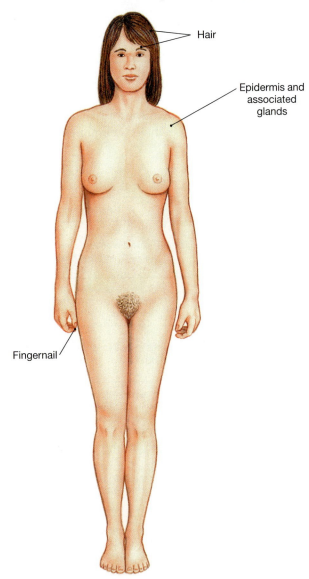

Hair

Epidermis and associated glands

Fingernail

(a) The Integumentary System

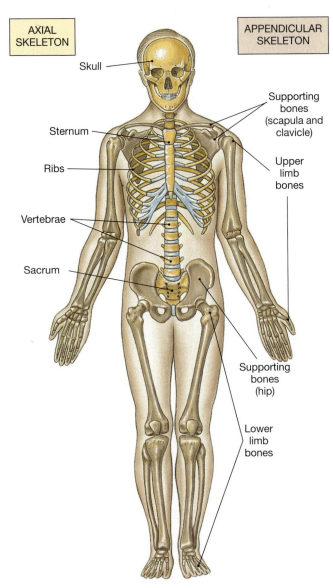

AXIAL SKELETON

APPENDICULAR SKELETON

Skull

Supporting bones (scapula and clavicle)

Sternum

Upper limb bones

Ribs

Vertebrae

Sacrum

Supporting bones (hip)

Lower limb bones

(b) The Skeletal System

Organ	Primary Functions
CUTANEOUS MEMBRANE	
Epidermis	Covers surface; protects underlying tissues
Dermis	Nourishes epidermis; provides strength; contains glands
HAIR FOLLICLES	Produce hair
Hairs	Provide sensation; provide some protection for head
Sebaceous glands	Secrete oil that lubricates hair
SWEAT GLANDS	Produce perspiration for evaporative cooling
NAILS	Protect and stiffen tips of fingers and toes
SENSORY RECEPTORS	Provide sensations of touch, pressure, temperature, pain

Organ	Primary Functions
BONES (206), CARTILAGES, AND LIGAMENTS	Support, protect soft tissues; store minerals
Axial skeleton (skull, vertebrae, sacrum, ribs, sternum)	Protects brain, spinal cord, sense organs, and soft tissues of chest cavity; supports the body weight over the legs
Appendicular skeleton (limbs and supporting bones)	Provides internal support and positioning of arms and legs; supports and moves axial skeleton
BONE MARROW	Primary site of blood cell production

• **FIGURE 1-3   The Organ Systems of the Human Body**

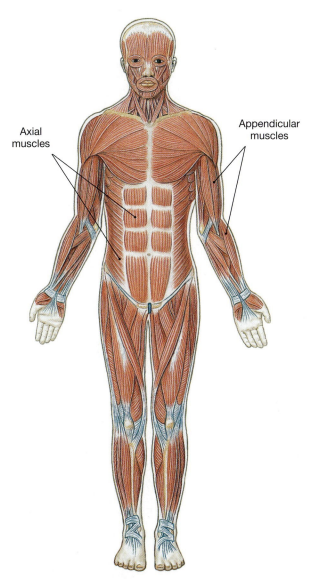

Axial muscles

Appendicular muscles

(c) The Muscular System

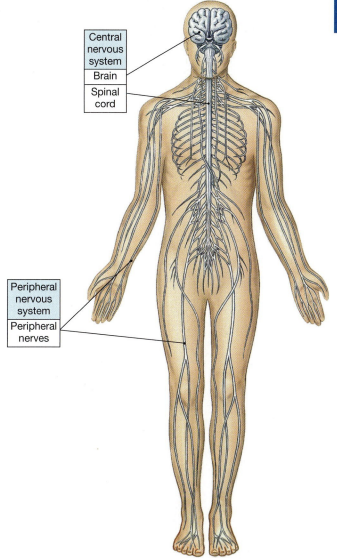

Central nervous system

Brain

Spinal cord

Peripheral nervous system

Peripheral nerves

(d) The Nervous System

Organ	Primary Functions
SKELETAL MUSCLES (700)	Provide skeletal movement; control entrances and exits of digestive tract; produce heat; support skeletal position; protect soft tissues
Axial muscles	Support and position axial skeleton
Appendicular muscles	Support, move, and brace limbs

Organ	Primary Functions
CENTRAL NERVOUS SYSTEM (CNS)	Acts as control center for nervous system; processes information; provides short-term control over activities of other systems
Brain	Performs complex integrative functions; controls voluntary activities
Spinal Cord	Relays information to and from the brain; performs less complex integrative functions; directs many simple involuntary activities
PERIPHERAL NERVOUS SYSTEM (PNS)	Links CNS with other systems and with sense organs

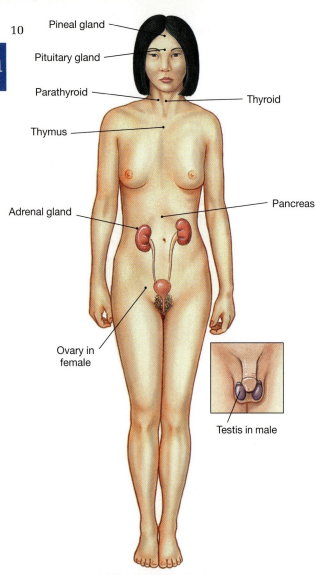

Pineal gland

Pituitary gland

Parathyroid

Thyroid

Thymus

Adrenal gland

Pancreas

Ovary in female

Testis in male

(e) The Endocrine System

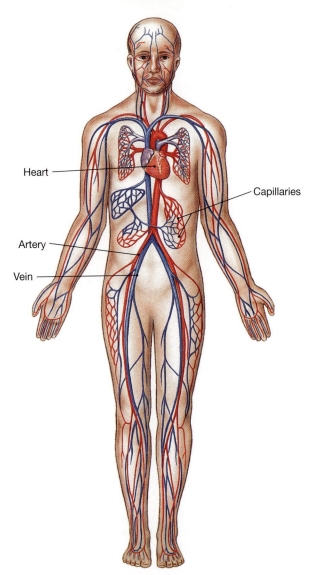

Heart

Capillaries

Artery

Vein

(f) The Cardiovascular System

Organ	Primary Functions
PINEAL GLAND	May control timing of sexual maturation and set day/night rhythms
PITUITARY GLAND	Controls other glands; regulates growth and fluid balance
THYROID GLAND	Controls tissue metabolic rate; regulates calcium levels
PARATHYROID GLAND	Regulates calcium levels (with thyroid)
THYMUS	Controls white blood cell maturation
ADRENAL GLANDS	Adjust water balance, tissue metabolism, cardiovascular and respiratory activities
KIDNEYS	Control red blood cell production; elevate blood pressure
PANCREAS	Regulates blood glucose levels
GONADS	*(see Figures 1-3k and 1-3l)*
Testes	Support male sexual characteristics and reproductive functions
Ovaries	Support female sexual characteristics and reproductive functions

Organ	Primary Functions
HEART	Propels blood; maintains blood pressure
BLOOD VESSELS	Distribute blood around the body
Arteries	Carry blood from heart to capillaries
Capillaries	Site of exchange between blood and interstitial fluids
Veins	Return blood from capillaries to heart
BLOOD	Transports oxygen and carbon dioxide; delivers nutrients and hormones; removes waste products; assists in defense against disease

• **FIGURE 1-3   continued**

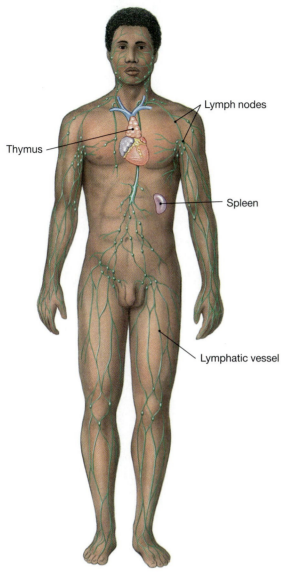

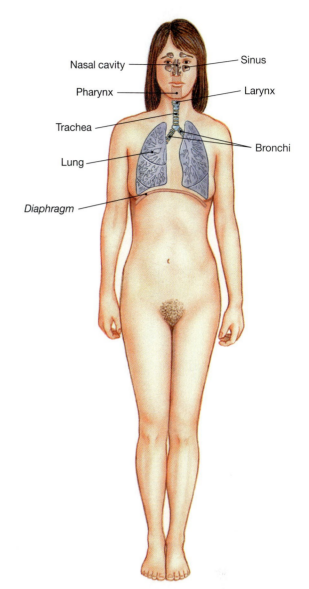

(g) The Lymphatic System

(h) The Respiratory System

Organ	Primary Functions
LYMPHATIC VESSELS	Carry lymph (water and proteins) from peripheral tissues to the veins of the cardiovascular system
LYMPH NODES	Monitor the composition of lymph; stimulate immune response
SPLEEN	Monitors circulating blood; stimulates immune response
THYMUS	Controls development and maintenance of one class of white blood cells (T cells)

Organ	Primary Functions
NASAL CAVITIES AND SINUSES	Filter, warm, humidify air; detect smells
PHARYNX	Chamber shared with digestive tract; conducts air to larynx
LARYNX	Protects opening to trachea and contains vocal cords
TRACHEA	Filters air, traps particles in mucus; cartilages keep airway open
BRONCHI	Same functions as trachea
LUNGS	Include airways and alveoli; volume changes responsible for air movement
Alveoli	Sites of gas exchange between air and blood

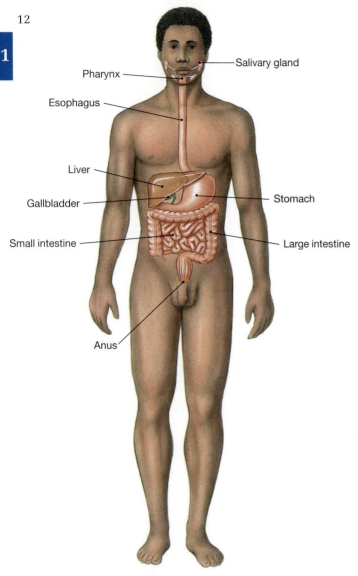

Salivary gland

Pharynx

Esophagus

Liver

Gallbladder

Stomach

Small intestine

Large intestine

Anus

(i) The Digestive System

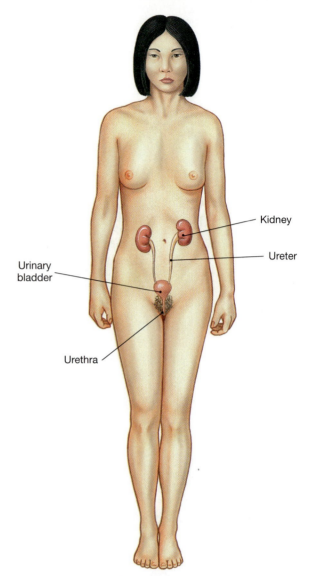

Kidney

Ureter

Urinary
bladder

Urethra

(j) The Urinary System

Organ	Primary Functions
SALIVARY GLANDS	Provide buffers and lubrication; produce enzymes that begin digestion
PHARYNX	Passageway connected to esophagus and trachea
ESOPHAGUS	Delivers food to stomach
STOMACH	Secretes acids and enzymes
SMALL INTESTINE	Secretes digestive enzymes and buffers, absorbs nutrients
LIVER	Secretes bile; regulates blood composition of nutrients
GALLBLADDER	Stores bile for release into small intestine
PANCREAS	Secretes digestive enzymes and buffers; contains endocrine cells (see Figure 1-3e)
LARGE INTESTINE	Removes water from fecal material; stores wastes

Organ	Primary Functions
KIDNEYS	Form and concentrate urine; regulate chemical composition of the blood
URETERS	Conduct urine from kidneys to urinary bladder
URINARY BLADDER	Stores urine for eventual elimination
URETHRA	Conducts urine to exterior

• **FIGURE 1-3** continued

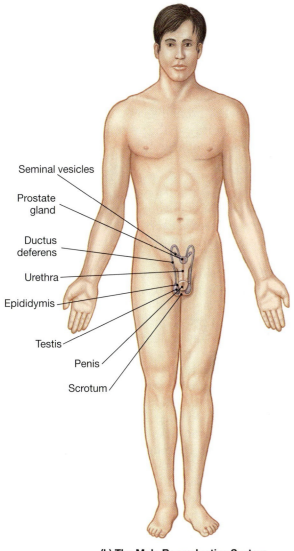

(k) The Male Reproductive System

Seminal vesicles
Prostate gland
Ductus deferens
Urethra
Epididymis
Testis
Penis
Scrotum

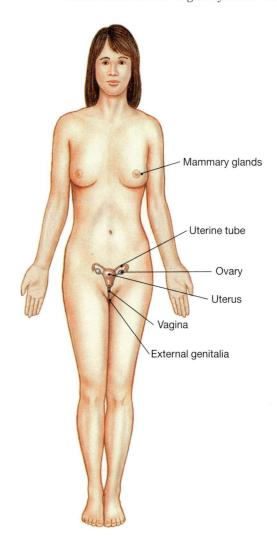

(l) The Female Reproductive System

Mammary glands
Uterine tube
Ovary
Uterus
Vagina
External genitalia

Organ	Primary Functions
TESTES	Produce sperm and hormones *(see Figure 1-3e)*
ACCESSORY ORGANS	
Epididymis	Site of sperm maturation
Ductus deferens (sperm duct)	Conducts sperm between epididymis and prostate
Seminal vesicles	Secrete fluid that makes up much of the volume of semen
Prostate gland	Secretes buffers and fluid
Urethra	Conducts semen to exterior
EXTERNAL GENITALIA	
Penis	Erectile organ used to deposit sperm in the vagina of a female; produces pleasurable sensations during sexual act
Scrotum	Surrounds and positions the testes

Organ	Primary Functions
OVARIES	Produce oocytes and hormones *(see Figure 1-3e)*
UTERINE TUBES	Deliver oocyte or embryo to uterus; normal site of fertilization
UTERUS	Site of embryonic development and diffusion between maternal and embryonic bloodstreams
VAGINA	Site of sperm deposition; birth canal at delivery; provides passage of fluids during menstruation
EXTERNAL GENITALIA	
Clitoris	Erectile organ that produces pleasurable sensations during sexual act
Labia	Contain glands that lubricate entrance to vagina
MAMMARY GLANDS	Produce milk that nourishes newborn infant

1 HOMEOSTASIS AND SYSTEM INTEGRATION

Organ systems are interdependent, interconnected, and packaged together in a relatively small space. The cells, tissues, organs, and systems of the body live together in a shared environment, like the inhabitants of a large city. City dwellers breathe the city air and drink the water provided by the local water company; cells in the human body absorb oxygen from the body fluids that surround them. All living cells are in contact with blood or some other body fluid, and any change in the composition of these fluids will affect them in some way. For example, changes in the temperature or salt content of the blood could cause anything from a minor adjustment (heart muscle tissue contracts more often, and the heart rate goes up) to a total disaster (the heart stops beating altogether).

Homeostatic Regulation

A variety of physiological mechanisms act to prevent potentially dangerous changes in the environment inside the body. **Homeostasis** (*homeo*, unchanging + *stasis*, standing) refers to the existence of a stable internal environment. To survive, every living organism must maintain homeostasis. The term **homeostatic regulation** refers to the adjustments in physiological systems that preserve homeostasis.

Homeostatic regulation usually involves (1) a **receptor** sensitive to a particular environmental change, or *stimulus*; (2) a **control center**, or *integration center*, which receives and processes the information from the receptor; and (3) an **effector**, which responds to the commands of the control center and whose activity opposes or enhances the stimulus. You are probably already familiar with several examples of homeostatic regulation, although not in those terms. As an example, consider the operation of the thermostat in a house or apartment (Figure 1-4•).

The thermostat is a control center that monitors room temperature. The gauge on the thermostat establishes the *set point*, the "ideal" room temperature. In our example, the set point is 22° C (around 72° F). The function of the thermostat is to keep room temperature within acceptable limits, usually within a degree or so of the set point. The thermostat receives information from a receptor, a thermometer exposed to air in the room, and it controls two effectors: a heater and an air conditioner. The principle is simple: The heater turns on if the room becomes too cold, and the air conditioner turns on if the room becomes too warm.

When the temperature at the thermometer increases outside of the normal range, the thermostat turns on the air conditioner. The air conditioner then cools the room. When temperature at the thermometer approaches the set point, the thermostat turns off the air conditioner (Figure 1-4a•).

A comparable pattern of events occurs if the temperature drops below normal levels: Temperature falls, and the thermostat turns on the heater; the temperature then rises, and the thermostat turns off the heater.

Negative Feedback

Regardless of whether the temperature at the receptor rises or falls, *a variation outside normal limits triggers an automatic response that corrects the situation.* This method of homeostatic regulation is called **negative feedback** because the effector that is activated by the control center opposes the stimulus.

Most homeostatic mechanisms in the body involve negative feedback. For example, consider the control of body temperature, a process called *thermoregulation*. Thermoregulation involves altering the relationship between heat loss, which occurs primarily at the body surface, and heat production, which occurs in all active tissues. In the human body, skeletal muscles are the most important generators of body heat.

The cells of the thermoregulatory control center are located in the brain. Temperature receptors are located in the skin, and the cells in the control center are sensitive to local body temperature. The thermoregulatory center has a set point near 37° C (98.6° F) (Figure 1-4b•). If temperature at the thermoregulatory center rises above 37.2° C, activity in the control center targets two different effectors: (1) smooth muscles in the walls of blood vessels supplying the skin and (2) sweat glands. The blood vessels dilate, increasing blood flow at the body surface, and the sweat glands accelerate their secretion. The skin then acts like a radiator, losing heat to the environment, and the evaporation of sweat speeds the process. When body temperature returns to normal, the control center becomes inactive, and superficial blood flow and sweat gland activity decrease to normal resting levels.

If temperature at the control center falls below 36.7° C, the control center targets the same two effectors, but this time blood flow to the skin declines, and sweat gland activity decreases. This combination reduces the rate of heat loss to the environment. Because heat production continues, body temperature gradually rises; once an acceptable temperature has been reached, the thermoregulatory center turns itself "off," and both blood flow and sweat gland activity in the skin increase to normal resting levels.

Homeostatic mechanisms using negative feedback usually ignore minor variations, and they maintain a normal range rather than a fixed value. In the example above, body temperature oscillates around the ideal set-point temperature. Thus any measured value, such as body temperature, can vary from moment to moment or day to day for any single individual. The variability between individuals is even greater, for each person has

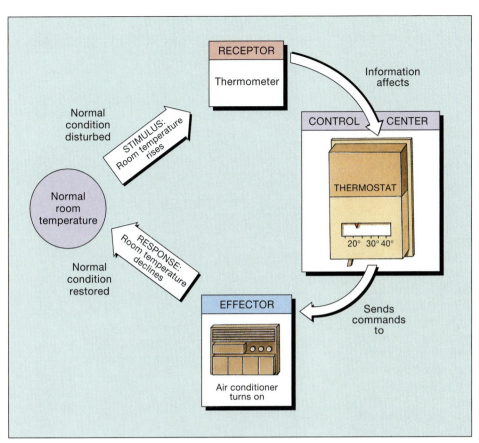

• FIGURE 1-4   Negative Feedback
In negative feedback, a stimulus
produces a response that opposes
the original stimulus. **(a)** A thermostat controls heating and cooling
systems to keep temperatures within acceptable limits. When the room
temperature rises or falls, the thermostat (a control center) triggers an
effector response that restores normal temperature. **(b)** Body temperature is regulated by a control center
in the brain that functions as a thermostat with a set point of 37° C. If
body temperature climbs above
37.2° C, heat loss is increased
through enhanced blood flow to the
skin and increased sweating.

RECEPTOR

Thermometer

Information
affects

CONTROL   CENTER

THERMOSTAT

20° 30° 40°

Normal
condition
disturbed

STIMULUS:
Room temperature
rises

Normal
room
temperature

RESPONSE:
Room temperature
declines

Normal
condition
restored

EFFECTOR

Air conditioner
turns on

Sends
commands
to

(a)

RECEPTORS

Temperature
sensors in skin
and cells of
thermoregulatory
center

Information
affects

CONTROL   CENTER

Thermoregulatory
center
of brain

Normal
temperature
disturbed

STIMULUS:
Rising body
temperature

HOMEOSTASIS
Normal
body
temperature

RESPONSE:
Increased heat
loss through
radiation and
evaporation

Normal
temperature
restored

EFFECTORS

Blood
vessels in
skin dilate

Sweat glands
in skin
increase
secretion

Sends
commands
to

(b)

1

slightly different homeostatic set points. It is therefore impractical to define "normal" homeostatic conditions very precisely. By convention, physiological values are reported either as averages, the average value obtained by sampling a large number of individuals, or as a range that includes 95 percent or more of the sample population. For instance, 5 percent of normal adults have a body temperature outside the "normal" range (below 36.7° C or above 37.2° C). But these temperatures are perfectly normal for them, and the variations have no clinical significance.

Positive Feedback

In **positive feedback**, *the initial stimulus produces a response that reinforces the stimulus*. For example, suppose the thermostat was wired so that when the temperature rose, it would turn on the heater rather than the air conditioner. In that case, the initial stimulus (rising room temperature) would cause a response (heater turns on) that would strengthen the stimulus. The room temperature would continue to rise until some external factor switched off the thermostat, unplugged the heater, or intervened in some other way before the house caught fire and burned down.

Negative feedback provides long-term regulatory control that results in relatively stable internal conditions. Positive feedback (Figure 1-5•) is important in driving a potentially dangerous or stressful process to completion. For example, the immediate danger from a severe cut is the loss of blood, which can lower blood pressure and reduce the efficiency of the heart. Damage to the blood vessel wall releases chemicals that begin the process of blood clotting. As clotting gets under way, each step releases chemicals that accelerate the process. This kind of cycle, a *positive feedback loop*, can be broken only by some external force or process—in this case, the formation of a blood clot that patches the vessel wall and stops the bleeding. The process of blood clotting will be examined more closely in Chapter 12. Labor and delivery, another example of positive feedback in action, will be discussed in Chapter 21.

Homeostasis and Disease

Physiological mechanisms do a remarkably good job of stabilizing internal conditions, regardless of our on-going activities. But when homeostatic regulation fails, organ systems begin to malfunction and the individual experiences the symptoms of illness, or **disease**.

✓ Why is homeostatic regulation important to humans?

✓ How is positive feedback helpful in producing necessary changes in individuals?

✓ What happens to the body when homeostasis breaks down?

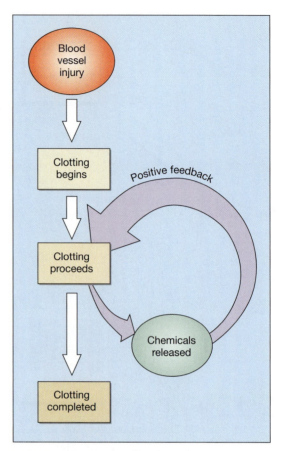

• FIGURE 1-5   Positive Feedback
In positive feedback, a stimulus produces a response that reinforces the original stimulus. Positive feedback is important in accelerating processes that must proceed to completion rapidly. In this example, positive feedback accelerates blood clotting until bleeding stops.

THE LANGUAGE OF ANATOMY

Early anatomists faced serious communication problems. For example, stating that a bump is "on the back" does not give very precise information about its location. Therefore, anatomists created maps of the human body, using prominent anatomical structures as landmarks, specialized directional terms, and reporting distances in centimeters or inches. In effect, anatomy uses a special language that must be learned almost at the start.

A familiarity with Latin and Greek word roots and their combinations makes anatomical terms more understandable. As new terms are introduced in the text, notes on their pronunciation and the relevant word roots will be provided. The Vocabulary Development lists at the start of each chapter are helpful aids in understanding the language of anatomy.

Latin and Greek terms are not the only foreign words imported into the anatomical vocabulary over the centuries, and the vocabulary continues to expand. Many anatomical structures and clinical conditions were initially named after either the discoverer or, in the case of diseases, the most famous victim. Although most such commemorative names, or *eponyms*, have been replaced by more precise terms, many are still in use.

Surface Anatomy

With the exception of the skin, none of the organ systems can be seen from the body surface. Therefore, you must create your own mental maps and extract information from the terms given in Figures 1-6• and 1-7•. Learning these terms now will help you make sense of many discussions in this book.

Anatomical Landmarks

Standard anatomical illustrations show the human form in the **anatomical position**, with the hands at the sides and the palms facing forward (Figure 1-6•). A person lying down in the anatomical position is said to be **supine** (sū-PĪN) when lying face up and **prone** when lying face down.

Important anatomical landmarks are also presented in Figure 1-6•. The anatomical terms are given in boldface, the common names in plain type, and the anatomical adjectives in parentheses. Become familiar with all three forms of a term. For example, the term *brachium* refers to the arm, and later chapters will

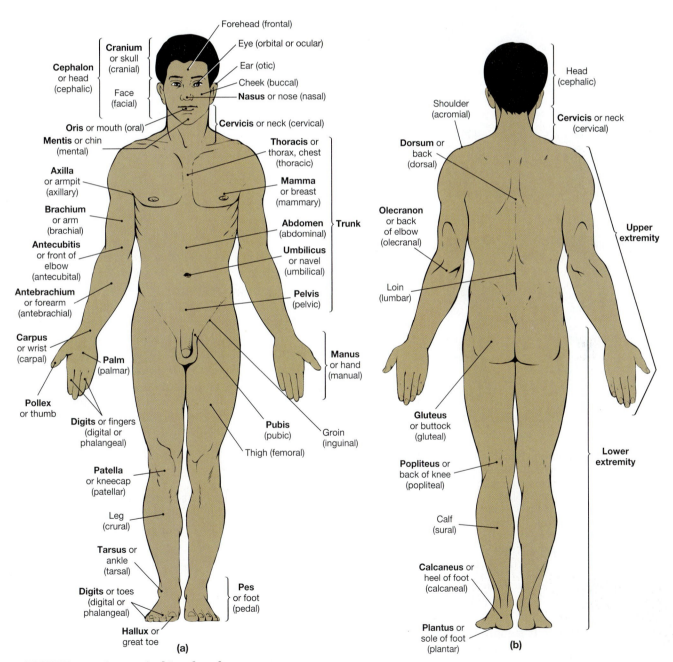

•FIGURE 1-6   Anatomical Landmarks
Anatomical terms are in boldface type, common names are in plain type, and anatomical adjectives are in parentheses.

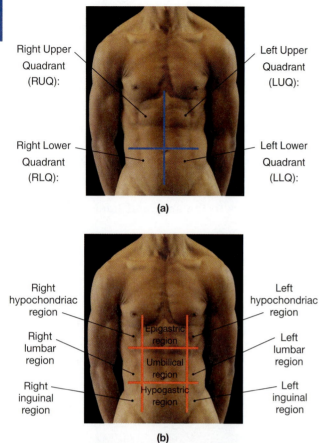

Right Upper Quadrant (RUQ):

Left Upper Quadrant (LUQ):

Right Lower Quadrant (RLQ):

Left Lower Quadrant (LLQ):

(a)

Right hypochondriac region

Left hypochondriac region

Right lumbar region

Epigastric region

Left lumbar region

Umbilical region

Right inguinal region

Hypogastric region

Left inguinal region

(b)

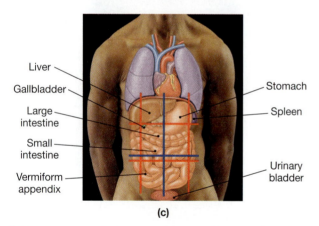

Liver

Gallbladder

Large intestine

Small intestine

Vermiform appendix

Stomach

Spleen

Urinary bladder

(c)

• **FIGURE 1-7   Abdominopelvic Quadrants and Regions**
(a) Abdominopelvic quadrants divide the area into four sections. These terms, or their abbreviations, are most often used in clinical discussions. **(b)** More precise regional descriptions are provided by reference to the appropriate abdominopelvic region. **(c)** Quadrants or regions are useful because there is a known relationship between superficial anatomical landmarks and underlying organs.

discuss the brachial artery, brachial nerve, and so forth. You might remember this term more easily if you know that the Latin word *brachium* is also the source of Old English and French words meaning "to embrace." Understanding the terms and their origins can help you remember the location of a particular structure, as well as its name.

TABLE 1-1	Regions of the Human Body (see Figure 1-6)
Structure	*Area*
Cephalon (head)	Cephalic region
Cervicis (neck)	Cervical region
Thoracis (chest)	Thoracic region
Abdomen	Abdominal region
Pelvis	Pelvic region
Loin (lower back)	Lumbar region
Buttock	Gluteal region
Pubis (anterior pelvis)	Pubic region
Groin	Inguinal region
Axilla (armpit)	Axillary region
Brachium (arm)	Brachial region
Antebrachium (forearm)	Antebrachial region
Manus (hand)	Manual region
Thigh	Femoral region
Leg (anterior)	Crural region
Calf	Sural region
Pes (foot)	Pedal region

Anatomical Regions

Major regions of the body are listed in Table 1-1 and shown in Figure 1-6•. Anatomists and clinicians often need to use regional terms as well as specific landmarks to describe a general area of interest or injury. Two methods are used to specify locations on the abdominal surface. Clinicians refer to the **abdominopelvic quadrants**: four segments divided by imaginary lines that intersect at the *umbilicus* (navel). This simple method, shown in Figure 1-7a•, is useful for describing aches, pains, and injuries. The location can help a doctor decide the possible cause. For example, tenderness in the right lower quadrant (RLQ) is a symptom of appendicitis, whereas tenderness in the right upper quadrant (RUQ) may indicate gallbladder or liver problems.

Anatomists like to use more precise regional distinctions to describe the location and orientation of internal organs. They recognize nine **abdominopelvic regions** (Figure 1-7b•). Figure 1-7c• shows the relationship between quadrants, regions, and internal organs.

Anatomical Directions

Figure 1-8• and Table 1-2 show the principal directional terms and examples of their use. There are many different directional terms, and some can be used interchangeably. For example, *anterior* refers to the front

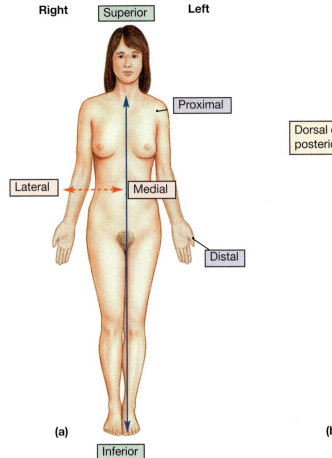

(a)

Right   Superior   Left

Proximal

Lateral   ←---→   Medial

Distal

Inferior

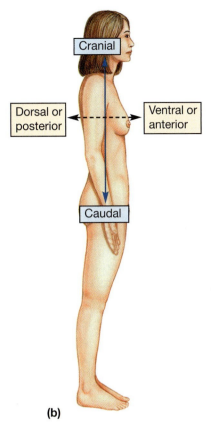

(b)

Cranial

Dorsal or posterior   ←--→   Ventral or anterior

Caudal

● **FIGURE 1-8   Directional References**
Important directional terms used in this text are indicated by arrows; definitions and descriptions are included in Table 1-2.

TABLE 1-2	Directional Terms (see Figure 1-8)	
Term	*Region or Reference*	*Example*
Anterior	The front; before	The navel is on the *anterior (ventral)* surface of the trunk.
Ventral	The belly side (equivalent to anterior when referring to human body)	
Posterior	The back; behind	The shoulder blade is located *posterior (dorsal)* to the rib cage.
Dorsal	The back (equivalent to posterior when referring to human body)	The *dorsal* body cavity encloses the brain and spinal cord.
Cranial or cephalic	The head	The *cranial*, or *cephalic*, border of the pelvis is superior to the thigh.
Superior	Above; at a higher level (in human body, toward the head)	The nose is *superior* to the chin.
Caudal	The tail (coccyx in humans)	The hips are *caudal* to the waist.
Inferior	Below; at a lower level	The knees are *inferior* to the hips.
Medial	Toward the body's longitudinal axis	The *medial* surfaces of the thighs may be in contact; moving medially from the arm across the chest surface brings you to the sternum.
Lateral	Away from the body's longitudinal axis	The thigh articulates with the *lateral* surface of the pelvis; moving laterally from the nose brings you to the eyes.
Proximal	Toward an attached base	The thigh is *proximal* to the foot; moving proximally from the wrist brings you to the elbow.
Distal	Away from an attached base	The fingers are *distal* to the wrist; moving distally from the elbow brings you to the wrist.
Superficial	At, near, or relatively close to the body surface	The skin is *superficial* to underlying structures.
Deep	Farther from the body surface	The bone of the thigh is *deep* to the surrounding skeletal muscles.

of the body, when viewed in the anatomical position; in human beings, this term is equivalent to *ventral*, which actually refers to the belly. Likewise, *posterior* and *dorsal* are terms that refer to the back of the human body. Although your instructor may have additional recommendations, these are the terms that appear frequently in later chapters. Remember that *left* and *right* always refer to the left and right sides of the subject, not of the observer.

Sectional Anatomy

A presentation in sectional view is sometimes the only way to illustrate the relationships between the parts of a three-dimensional object. An understanding of sectional views has become increasingly important since the development of procedures that enable us to see inside the living body without resorting to surgery (see Figure 1-12• for representative views).

Planes and Sections

Any slice through a three-dimensional object can be described with reference to three **sectional planes**, indicated in Figure 1-9• and Table 1-3:

1. *Transverse Plane.* The **transverse plane** lies at right angles to the long (head-foot) axis of the body, dividing it into **superior** and **inferior** sections. A cut in this plane is called a **transverse section**, a **horizontal section**, or a *cross section*.

2. *Frontal Plane.* The **frontal plane**, or **coronal plane**, parallels the long axis of the body. The frontal plane extends from side to side, dividing the body into **anterior** and **posterior** sections.

3. *Sagittal Plane.* The **sagittal plane** also parallels the long axis of the body, but it extends from front to back. A sagittal plane divides the body into *left* and *right* sections. A cut that passes along the midline and divides the body into left and right halves is a **midsagittal section**.

   Frontal and sagittal sections are often called *longitudinal sections*.

Body Cavities

Viewed in sections, the human body is not a solid object, like a rock, in which all of the parts are fused together. Many vital organs are suspended in internal

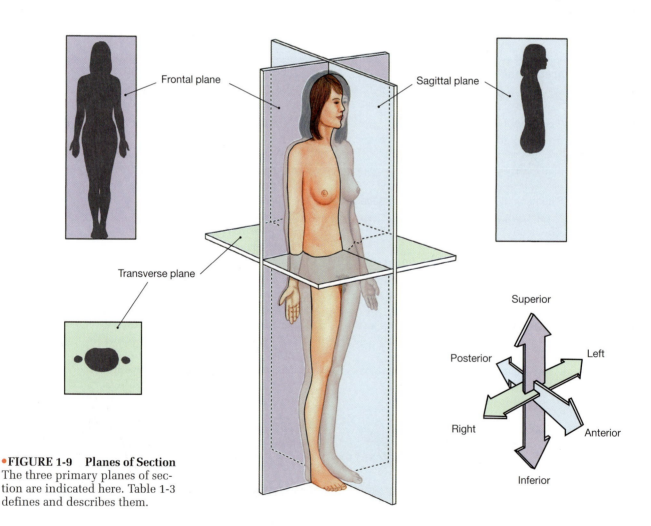

Frontal plane

Sagittal plane

Transverse plane

Superior

Posterior

Left

Right

Anterior

Inferior

•**FIGURE 1-9   Planes of Section**
The three primary planes of section are indicated here. Table 1-3 defines and describes them.

		Directional	
Orientation of Plane	Adjective	Reference	Description
Parallel to long axis	Sagittal	Sagittally	A *sagittal section* separates right and left portions. You examine a sagittal section, but you section sagittally.
	Midsagittal		In a *midsagittal section*, the plane passes through the midline, dividing the body in half and separating right and left sides.
	Frontal or coronal	Frontally or coronally	A *frontal*, or *coronal*, *section* separates anterior and posterior portions of the body; *coronal* usually refers to sections passing through the skull.
Perpendicular to long axis	Transverse or horizontal	Transversely or horizontally	A *transverse*, or *horizontal*, *section* separates superior and inferior portions of the body.

TABLE 1-3   **Terms That Indicate Planes of Section (see Figure 1-9)**

chambers called *body cavities*. These cavities have two essential functions:

1. They protect delicate organs, such as the brain and spinal cord, from accidental shocks and cushion them from the thumps and bumps that occur during walking, jumping, and running.
2. They permit significant changes in the size and shape of visceral organs. For example, because they are situated within body cavities, the lungs, heart, stomach, intestines, urinary bladder, and many other organs can expand and contract without distorting surrounding tissues and disrupting the activities of nearby organs.

Two body cavities form during embryonic development. A **dorsal body cavity** surrounds the brain and spinal cord, and a much larger **ventral body cavity** surrounds developing organs of the respiratory, cardiovascular, digestive, urinary, and reproductive systems.

Dorsal Body Cavities. The dorsal body cavity is a fluid-filled space whose limits are established by the **cranium**, the bones of the skull that surround the brain, and the spinal vertebrae (Figure 1-10a•). The dorsal body cavity is subdivided into the **cranial cavity**, which encloses the brain, and the **spinal cavity**, which surrounds the spinal cord.

Ventral Body Cavities. As development proceeds, internal organs grow and change their relative positions. These changes lead to the subdivision of the ventral body cavity. The **diaphragm** (DĪ-a-fram), a flat muscular sheet, divides the ventral body cavity into a superior **thoracic cavity**, enclosed by the chest wall, and an inferior **abdominopelvic cavity**, enclosed by the abdomen and pelvic girdle. The abdominopelvic cavity has two

subdivisions. The **abdominal cavity** extends from the inferior surface of the diaphragm to an imaginary line drawn from the inferior surface of the lowest spinal vertebra to the anterior and superior margin of the pelvic girdle. The portion of the ventral body cavity inferior to this imaginary line is the **pelvic cavity**.

The thoracic and abdominopelvic cavities contain spaces lined by a shiny, slippery, and delicate *serous membrane*. The parietal portion of a serous membrane forms the outer wall of the body cavity. The visceral portion covers the surfaces of internal organs, or **viscera** (VIS-e-ra), where they project into the body cavity. Many visceral organs undergo periodic changes in size and shape; the lungs inflate and deflate with each breath, and the volume of the heart changes during each heartbeat. A covering of serous membrane prevents friction between adjacent viscera and between the visceral organs and the body wall. The spaces between opposing membranes are very small, but they are separated by a thin layer of fluid.

To understand the relationship between a visceral organ and the serous membrane, consider the example in Figure 1-10b•. The heart projects into a space known as the **pericardial cavity**. The relationship resembles that of a fist pushing into a balloon. The wrist corresponds to the base of the heart, and the balloon corresponds to the serous membrane lining the pericardial cavity. The serous membrane is called the **pericardium** (*peri-*, around + *cardium*, heart). The layer covering the heart is the **visceral pericardium**, and the opposing surface is the **parietal pericardium**.

The thoracic cavity contains two **pleural cavities**, each surrounding a lung (Figure 1-10c•). The spatial relationships between the lungs and the pleural cavities resemble that between the heart and pericardium. The serous membrane lining the pleural cavities is called the **pleura** (PLOO-ra). The region between the two pleural cavities is known as the **mediastinum**

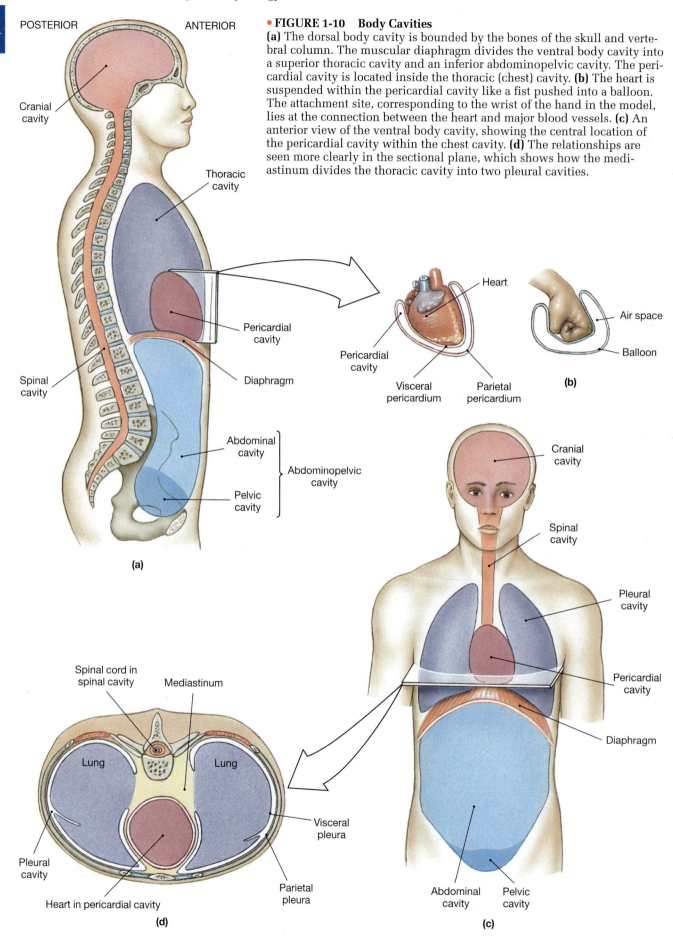

POSTERIOR   ANTERIOR

Cranial
cavity

Thoracic
cavity

Spinal
cavity

Pericardial
cavity

Diaphragm

Abdominal
cavity

Abdominopelvic
cavity

Pelvic
cavity

(a)

Heart

Pericardial
cavity

Air space

Balloon

Pericardial
cavity

Visceral
pericardium

Parietal
pericardium

(b)

Cranial
cavity

Spinal
cavity

Pleural
cavity

Pericardial
cavity

Diaphragm

Abdominal
cavity

Pelvic
cavity

(c)

Spinal cord in
spinal cavity

Mediastinum

Lung

Lung

Pleural
cavity

Heart in pericardial cavity

Visceral
pleura

Parietal
pleura

(d)

● **FIGURE 1-10   Body Cavities**
(a) The dorsal body cavity is bounded by the bones of the skull and verte-bral column. The muscular diaphragm divides the ventral body cavity into a superior thoracic cavity and an inferior abdominopelvic cavity. The peri-cardial cavity is located inside the thoracic (chest) cavity. **(b)** The heart is suspended within the pericardial cavity like a fist pushed into a balloon. The attachment site, corresponding to the wrist of the hand in the model, lies at the connection between the heart and major blood vessels. **(c)** An anterior view of the ventral body cavity, showing the central location of the pericardial cavity within the chest cavity. **(d)** The relationships are seen more clearly in the sectional plane, which shows how the medi-astinum divides the thoracic cavity into two pleural cavities.

(mē-dē-as-TĪ-num or mē-dē-AS-ti-num) (Figure 1-10d•). The mediastinum contains the thymus, trachea, esophagus, the large arteries and veins attached to the heart, and the pericardial cavity.

Most of the visceral organs in the abdominopelvic cavity project into the **peritoneal** (per-i-tō-NĒ-al) **cavity**. The serous membrane lining this cavity is the **peritoneum** (per-i-tō-NĒ-um). Organs such as the stomach, small intestine, and portions of the large intestine are suspended within the peritoneal cavity by double sheets of peritoneum, called **mesenteries** (MES-en-ter-ēz). Mesenteries provide support and stability while permitting limited movement.

This chapter provided an overview of the locations and functions of the major components of each organ system. It also introduced the anatomical vocabulary needed to follow more detailed anatomical descriptions in later chapters. Modern methods of visualizing anatomical structures in living individuals are summarized on pp. 23–24. Many of the figures in later chapters contain images produced by the procedures outlined in that section.

✓ What type of section would separate the two eyes?

✓ If a surgeon makes an incision just inferior to the diaphragm, what body cavity will be opened?

FOCUS   ## Sectional Anatomy and Clinical Technology

The term **radiological procedures** includes not only those scanning techniques that involve radioisotopes but also methods that employ radiation sources outside the body. Physicians who specialize in the performance and analysis of these procedures are called **radiologists**. Radiological procedures can provide detailed information about internal systems. Figures 1-11• and 1-12• compare the views provided by several different techniques. These figures include examples of X-rays, CT scans, MRI scans, and ultrasound images. Other examples of clinical technology will be found in later chapters.

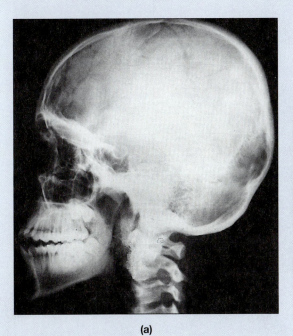

(a)

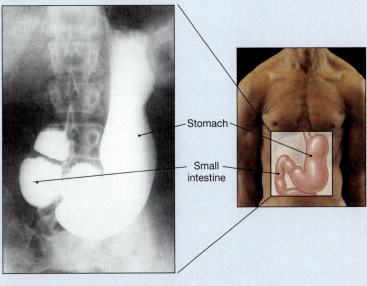

Stomach

Small intestine

(b)

• **FIGURE 1-11   X-rays**
(a) An X-ray of the skull, taken from the left side. **X-rays** are a form of high-energy radiation that can penetrate living tissues. In the most familiar procedure, a beam of X-rays travels through the body and strikes a photographic plate. All of the projected X-rays do not arrive at the film; some are absorbed or deflected as they pass through the body. The resistance to X-ray penetration is called **radiodensity**. In the human body, the order of increasing radiodensity is as follows: air, fat, liver, blood, muscle, bone. The result is an image with radiodense tissues, such as bone, appearing in white, and less dense tissues in shades of gray to black. The picture is a two-dimensional image of a three-dimensional object; in this image it is difficult to decide whether a particular feature is on the left side (toward the viewer) or on the right side (away from the viewer). **(b)** A barium-contrast X-ray of the upper digestive tract. Barium is very dense, and the contours of the gastric and intestinal lining can be seen outlined against the white of the barium solution.

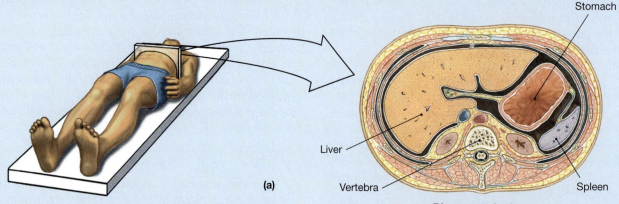

Stomach

Liver

Vertebra

Spleen

Diagrammatic view

(a)

• FIGURE 1-12   Scanning Techniques
(a) Diagrammatic views showing the relative position and orientation of the scans shown in parts (b) and (c).

(b) A color-enhanced CT scan of the abdomen. **CT** (*com*-puted *t*omography), formerly called **CAT** (*c*omputed *a*xial *t*omography), uses computers to reconstruct sectional views. A single X-ray source rotates around the body and the X-ray beam strikes a sensor monitored by the computer. The source completes one revolution around the body every few seconds; it then moves a short distance and repeats the process. The result is usually displayed as a sectional view in black and white, but it can be colorized for visual effect. CT scans show three-dimensional relationships and soft tissue structure more clearly than standard X-rays.

(c) A color-enhanced **MRI** scan of the same region. *M*agnetic *r*esonance *i*maging surrounds part or all of the body with a magnetic field about 3000 times as strong as that of the earth. Pulses of radio waves then cause tissues to release energy used to create an image. Details of soft tissue structure are usually much more clearly detailed than in CT scans. Note the differences in detail between this image, the CT scan, and the ultrasound image.

(d) An ultrasound scan of the abdomen. In **ultrasound** procedures, a small transmitter contacting the skin broadcasts a brief, narrow burst of high-frequency sound and then picks up the echoes. The sound waves are reflected by internal structures, and a picture, or **echogram**, can be assembled from the pattern of echoes. These images lack the clarity of other procedures, but no adverse affects have been reported, and fetal development can be monitored without a significant risk of birth defects. Special methods of transmission and processing permit analysis of the beating heart, without the complications that can accompany dye injections.

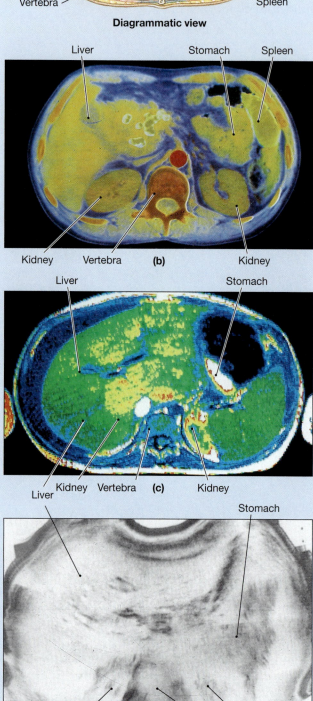

Liver   Stomach   Spleen

Kidney   Vertebra   (b)   Kidney

Liver   Stomach

Liver   Kidney   Vertebra   (c)   Kidney

Stomach

Kidney   Vertebra   Kidney

(d)

Chapter Review

KEY TERMS

anatomical position, *p. 17*	homeostasis, *p. 14*	positive feedback, *p. 16*
anatomy, *p. 4*	negative feedback, *p. 14*	sagittal plane, *p. 20*
diaphragm, *p. 21*	peritoneum, *p. 23*	transverse plane, *p. 20*
frontal plane, *p. 20*	physiology, *p. 4*	viscera, *p. 21*

SUMMARY OUTLINE

INTRODUCTION *p. 4*

1. **Biology** is the study of life; one of its goals is to discover the unity and patterns that underlie the diversity of living organisms.

2. All living things, from single *cells* to large multicellular organisms, perform the same basic functions: they respond to changes in their environment; they grow and reproduce to create future generations; they are capable of producing movement; and they absorb materials from the environment. Organisms absorb and consume oxygen during respiration, and they discharge waste products during excretion. Digestion occurs in specialized areas of the body to break down complex foods. The circulation forms an internal transportation system between areas of the body.

THE SCIENCES OF ANATOMY AND PHYSIOLOGY *p. 4*

Anatomical Perspectives *p. 4*

1. **Anatomy** is the study of internal and external structure and the physical relationships between body parts. **Physiology** is the study of how living organisms perform vital functions. All specific functions are performed by specific structures.

2. The boundaries of **microscopic anatomy** are established by the equipment used. **Cytology** analyzes the internal structure of individual **cells**. **Histology** examines **tissues** (groups of cells that have specific functional roles). Tissues combine to form **organs**, anatomical units with multiple functions.

3. **Gross (macroscopic) anatomy** considers features visible without a microscope. It includes **surface anatomy** (general form and superficial markings); **regional anatomy** (superficial and internal features in a specific area of the body); and **systemic anatomy** (structure of major organ systems).

Physiology *p. 5*

4. **Human physiology** is the study of the functions of the human body. It is based on **cell physiology**, the study of the functions of living cells. **Special physiology** studies the physiology of specific organs. **System physiology** considers all aspects of the function of specific organ systems. **Pathological physiology (pathology)** studies the effects of diseases on organ or system functions.

LEVELS OF ORGANIZATION *p. 5*

1. Anatomical structures and physiological mechanisms are arranged in a series of interacting levels of organization. *(Figure 1-1)*

AN INTRODUCTION TO ORGAN SYSTEMS *p. 7*

1. The major organs of the human body are arranged into 11 organ systems. The organ systems of the human body are the *integumentary, skeletal, muscular, nervous, endocrine, cardiovascular, lymphatic, respiratory, digestive, urinary,* and *reproductive systems*. *(Figures 1-2, 1-3)*

HOMEOSTASIS AND SYSTEM INTEGRATION *p. 14*

1. **Homeostasis** is the tendency for physiological systems to stabilize internal conditions; through **homeostatic regulation** these systems adjust to preserve homeostasis.

Homeostatic Regulation *p. 14*

2. Homeostatic regulation usually involves a **receptor** sensitive to a particular stimulus and an **effector** whose activity affects the same stimulus.

3. **Negative feedback** is a corrective mechanism involving an action that directly opposes a variation from normal limits. *(Figure 1-4)*

4. In **positive feedback** the initial stimulus produces a response that reinforces the stimulus. *(Figure 1-5)*

Homeostasis and Disease *p. 16*

5. Symptoms of **disease** appear when failure of homeostatic regulation causes organ systems to malfunction.

THE LANGUAGE OF ANATOMY *p. 16*

Surface Anatomy *p. 17*

1. Standard anatomical illustrations show the body in the **anatomical position**. If the figure is shown lying down, it can be either **supine** (face up) or **prone** (face down). *(Figure 1-6; Table 1-1)*

2. **Abdominopelvic quadrants** and **abdominopelvic regions** represent two different approaches to describing anatomical regions of the body. *(Figure 1-7)*

3. The use of special directional terms provides clarity when describing anatomical structures. *(Figure 1-8; Table 1-2)*

Sectional Anatomy *p. 20*

4. The three **sectional planes** (**frontal** or **coronal plane, sagittal plane,** and **transverse plane**) describe relationships between the parts of the three-dimensional human body. *(Figure 1-9; Table 1-3)*

5. **Body cavities** protect delicate organs and permit changes in the size and shape of visceral organs. The **dorsal body cavity** contains the **cranial cavity** (enclosing the brain) and **spinal cavity** (surrounding the spinal cord). The **ventral body cavity** surrounds developing respiratory,

cardiovascular, digestive, urinary, and reproductive organs. *(Figure 1-10a)*

6. During development the **diaphragm** divides the ventral body cavity into the superior **thoracic** and inferior **peritoneal cavities**. By birth, the thoracic cavity contains two **pleural cavities** (each containing a lung) and a **pericardial cavity** (which

surrounds the heart). The **abdominopelvic cavity** consists of the **abdominal cavity** and the **pelvic cavity**. *(Figure 1-10b,c,d)*

7. Important **radiological procedures** (which can provide detailed information about internal systems) include **X-rays, CT scans, MRI,** and **ultrasound**. Each technique has its advantages and disadvantages. *(Figures 1-11, 1-12)*

REVIEW QUESTIONS

LEVEL 1   Reviewing Facts and Terms

Match each item in column A with the most closely related item in column B. Use letters for answers in the spaces provided.

Column A

___ 1. cytology
___ 2. physiology
___ 3. histology
___ 4. metabolism
___ 5. homeostasis
___ 6. muscle
___ 7. heart
___ 8. endocrine
___ 9. temperature regulation
___10. blood clot formation
___11. supine
___12. prone
___13. ventral body cavity
___14. dorsal body cavity
___15. pericardium

Column B

a. study of tissues
b. constant internal environment
c. face up
d. study of functions
e. positive feedback
f. system
g. study of cells
h. negative feedback
i. brain and spinal cord
j. all chemical activity in body
k. thoracic and abdominopelvic
l. tissue
m. serous membrane
n. organ
o. face down

16. The process by which an organism increases the size and/or number of cells is called:
    (a) reproduction
    (b) adaptation
    (c) growth
    (d) metabolism

17. The terms that apply to the front of the body when in anatomical position are:
    (a) posterior, dorsal
    (b) back, front
    (c) medial, lateral
    (d) anterior, ventral

18. A cut through the body that passes perpendicular to the long axis of the body and divides the body into a superior and inferior section is known as a:
    (a) sagittal section
    (b) transverse section
    (c) coronal section
    (d) frontal section

19. The cranial and spinal cavities are found in the:
    (a) ventral body cavity
    (b) thoracic cavity
    (c) dorsal body cavity
    (d) abdominopelvic cavity

20. The diaphragm, a flat muscular sheet, divides the ventral body cavity into a superior _____ cavity and an inferior _____ cavity.
    (a) pleural, pericardial
    (b) abdominal, pelvic
    (c) thoracic, abdominopelvic
    (d) cranial, thoracic

21. The mediastinum is the region between the:
    (a) lungs and heart
    (b) two pleural cavities
    (c) thorax and abdomen
    (d) heart and pericardium

LEVEL 2   Reviewing Concepts

22. What basic functions are performed by all living things?

23. Beginning with the molecular level, list in correct sequence the levels of organization from the simplest level to the most complex level.

24. What is homeostatic regulation, and what is its physiological importance?

25. How does negative feedback differ from positive feedback?

26. Describe the position of the body when it is in the anatomical position.

27. As a surgeon, you perform an invasive procedure that necessitates cutting through the peritoneum. Are you more likely to be operating on the heart or on the stomach?

28. In which body cavity would each of the following organs or systems be found?

    (a) brain and spinal cord

    (b) cardiovascular, digestive, and urinary systems

    (c) heart, lungs

    (d) stomach, intestines

LEVEL 3   Critical Thinking and Clinical Applications

29. A hormone called *calcitonin* from the thyroid gland is released in response to increased levels of calcium ions in the blood. If this hormone exerts negative feedback, what effect will its release have on blood calcium levels?

30. An anatomist wishes to make detailed comparisons of medial surfaces of the left and right sides of the brain. This work requires sections that will show the entire medial surface. Which kind of sections should be ordered from the lab for this investigation?

ANSWERS TO CONCEPT CHECK QUESTIONS

Page 5
1. *Metabolism* refers to all of the chemical operations under way in the body. Organisms rely on complex chemical reactions to provide the energy for responsiveness, growth, reproduction, and movement.   **2.** A *histologist* investigates the structure and properties of tissues. *Histology* is considered a form of microscopic anatomy because it requires the use of a microscope to reveal the cells that make up tissues.

Page 16
1. Physiological systems can function normally only under carefully controlled conditions. Homeostatic regulation prevents potentially disruptive changes in the body's internal environment.   **2.** Positive feedback is useful in processes that must move quickly to completion once they have begun, such as blood clotting. It is harmful in situations in which a stable condition must be maintained, because it increases any departure from the desired condition. For example, positive feedback in the regulation of body temperature would cause a slight fever to spiral out of control, with fatal results. For this reason, most physiological systems exhibit negative feedback, which tends to oppose any departure from the norm.   **3.** When homeostasis fails, organ systems function less efficiently or begin to malfunction. The result is the state that we call *disease*. If the situation is not corrected, death can result.

Page 23
1. The two eyes would be separated by a *midsagittal section*.   **2.** The body cavity inferior to the diaphragm is the *abdominopelvic* (or *peritoneal*) *cavity*.

OVERVIEW

Emergency personnel must have a good understanding of human anatomy and anatomical terms. In prehospital care, unlike other allied health care providers, EMTs and paramedics often work independently. Because of this, they must be able to accurately and rapidly describe wounds and injuries to hospital personnel.

DESCRIPTIVE AND TOPOGRAPHIC ANATOMY TERMINOLOGY

Surface anatomy, also called *topographic anatomy,* is the study of the surface of the body including visible and palpable landmarks. The fundamental aim of surface anatomy is to visualize structures that lie beneath the skin and are hidden by it. Surface anatomy is really *descriptive anatomy,* and emergency personnel must be able to accurately describe an injury or other problem in anatomical terms to a remote physician or hospital. Many anatomical terms are based on Latin or Greek words. Thus, an understanding of Latin and Greek word roots and their combinations helps to make anatomical terms more understandable.

Anatomical Position

By convention or agreement, the *anatomical position* has been adopted worldwide for giving anatomical descriptions. All descriptions of the body are based on the assumption that the person is in this position. The standard anatomical position is standing with the head, eyes, and toes directed forward. The arms are at the sides with the palms of the hands facing forward (Figure A1-1●). In the male, the penis is considered in the anatomical position when erect. A person lying down in the anatomical position is said to be *supine* when lying face up and *prone* when lying face down. A patient lying on his or her left or right side is in the *lateral recumbent position.* A person lying on his or her back with the upper part of the body elevated at a 45-degree or greater angle is said to be in a *Fowler's position.* A person in the same position but with the head elevated at an angle less than 45 degrees is said to be in a *Semi-Fowler's* position. In the *lithotomy position,* the patient is lying face upward with the legs flexed and the thighs abducted. A person lying on his or her back with the lower part of the body elevated approximately 12 inches is said to be in the *Trendelenburg position.*

General Descriptions

The body can be divided into regions for description. These include: the *head;* the *torso,* or *trunk;* the *lower extremities;* and the *upper extremities.* The extremities, in turn, can be di-

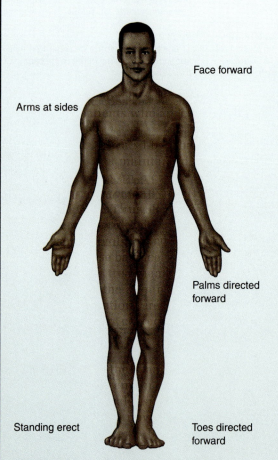

Face forward

Arms at sides

Palms directed forward

Standing erect

Toes directed forward

● **FIGURE A1-1   Normal Anatomical Position (anterior view)**

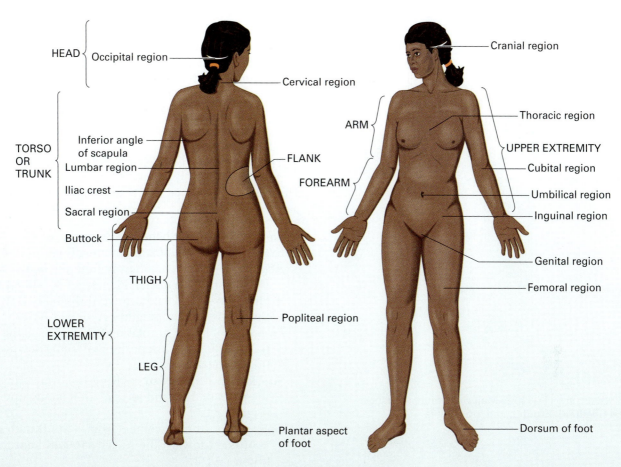

● **FIGURE A1-2   Regions of the Body and Important Topographical Landmarks**

vided into upper and lower parts. In the upper extremity, the elbow separates the upper and lower parts. The upper part of the upper extremity, from the shoulder to the elbow, is referred to as the *arm*. The lower part, extending from the elbow to the wrist, is considered the *forearm*. In the lower extremity, the knee is the dividing point. The portion of the lower extremity from the hip to the knee is called the *thigh*. The lower part of the lower extremity, from the knee to the foot, is called the *leg* (Figure A1-2●).

Anatomical Planes

Many descriptions are made using imaginary planes passing through the body in the anatomical position. Using these planes, directional terms can be developed that are useful in describing an injury or in conveying other information accurately and logically.

An imaginary plane that divides the body into right and left halves is called the *sagittal plane*. The sagittal plane is in the same plane as the sagittal suture of the skull. The sagittal plane that divides the body into equal left and right halves is called the *midsagittal* or *median*

plane. The plane oriented at a right angle to the median plane is the *coronal plane*. This divides the body into anterior (front) and posterior (back) portions. It is in the same plane as the coronal suture of the skull. Finally, the *horizontal,* or *transverse,* plane passes through the body at right angles to both the median and the coronal planes. It divides the body into superior (upper) and inferior (lower) portions (Figure A1-3●).

Directional Terms

The following topographical anatomical terms relate to direction:

Anterior—toward the front of the body
Ventral—toward the front of the body
Posterior—toward the back of the body
Dorsal—toward the back of the body
Lateral—away from the midline of the body
Medial—toward the midline of the body
Cranial—toward the head
Cephalic—toward the head

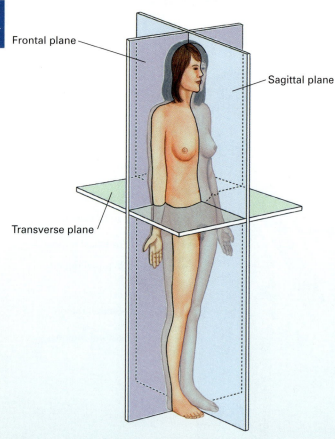

Frontal plane

Sagittal plane

Transverse plane

• **FIGURE A1-3 The Three Major Anatomical Planes:**
Sagittal (median), Frontal, and Transverse

Caudal—toward the tail
Superior—toward the top of the body
Inferior—toward the bottom of the body
Superficial—toward the exterior of the body
Deep—toward the interior of the body
Internal—inside the body
External—outside the body
Proximal—nearer the trunk of the body compared to another point
Distal—farther from the trunk of the body compared to another point

Terms Related to Body Movement

The following terms pertain to movement of the body or parts of the body:

Flexion—the act of bending (Figure A1-4•)
Extension—the act of straightening (Figure A1-4)
Abduction—a movement away from the body (away from the median plane) (Figures A1-5• and A1-6•)
Adduction—a movement toward the body (toward the median plane) (Figures A1-5 and A1-6)
Pronation—the act of rotating the arm, bringing the palm of the hand to a position of facing downward (Figure A1-7•)
Supination—the act of rotating the arm, bringing the palm of the hand to a position facing upward (Figure A1-7)
Opposition—the movement where the thumb pad is brought toward the finger pad and held there (Figure A1-8•)

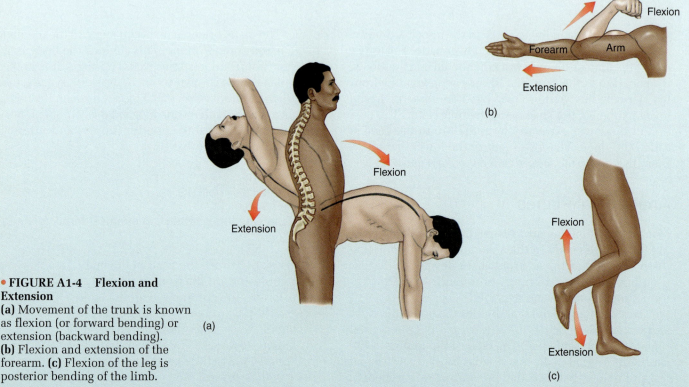

Flexion

Forearm   Arm

Extension

(b)

Flexion

Extension

Flexion

Extension

• **FIGURE A1-4   Flexion and**
Extension
(a) Movement of the trunk is known
as flexion (or forward bending) or
extension (backward bending).
(b) Flexion and extension of the
forearm. **(c)** Flexion of the leg is
posterior bending of the limb.

(a)

(c)

A1-3   An Introduction to Anatomy and Physiology

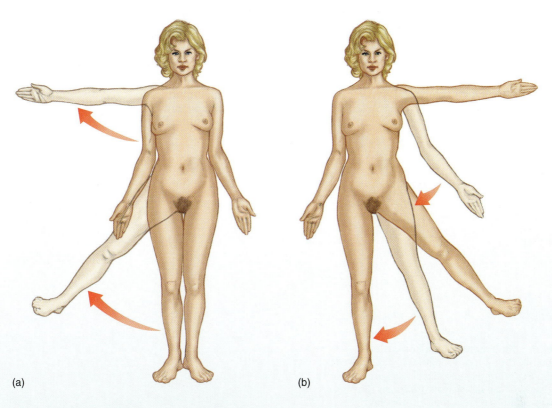

(a)

(b)

● **FIGURE A1-5   Abduction and Adduction**
(a) *Abduction* of the right limbs. **(b)** *Adduction* of the left limbs.

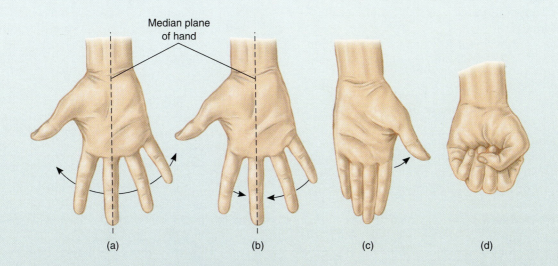

Median plane
of hand

(a)   (b)   (c)   (d)

● **FIGURE A1-6   Movements of the Fingers and the Thumb**
(a) Abduction of the fingers. **(b)** Adduction of the fingers. **(c)** Extension of the thumb and fingers.
(d) Flexion of the fingers and thumb. Note the median plane of the hand passes through the midline of the middle finger. The median plane of the foot passes through the second toe.

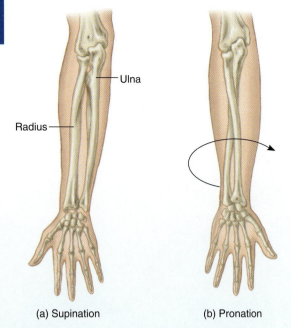

(a) Supination   (b) Pronation

• FIGURE A1-7   Movements of the Forearm
(a) Supination. **(b)** Pronation. Pronation is a medial rotation of the radius from its anatomical position so that the dorsum (back) of the hand faces anteriorly. Supination returns the hand to its anatomical position.

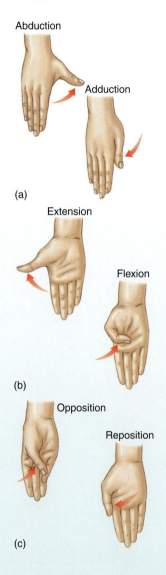

• FIGURE A1-8
Movements of the Thumb
(a) Abduction and adduction of the thumb.
(b) Flexion and extension of the thumb.
(c) Opposition and reposition of the thumb.

Reposition—the movement of the thumb from a position of opposition back to its anatomical position (Figure A1-8)

Protraction—a movement forward (as occurs when the jaw moves forward or the shoulders are drawn forward)

Retraction—a movement backward (as occurs with moving the jaw backward or drawing the shoulders backward)

Circumduction—to draw around, or to form a circle (a combination of successive movements of flexion, abduction, extension, and adduction) (Figure A1-9•)

Dorsiflexion of the foot—flexion of the foot at the ankle (Figure A1-10•)

Plantarflexion of the foot—extension of the foot at the ankle (as if standing on the tiptoes) (Figure A1-10)

Eversion of the foot—movement of the plantar surface away from the median plane of the body (Figure A1-10)

Inversion of the foot—movement of the plantar surface of the foot toward the median plane (Figure A1-10)

Rotation—the turning or revolving of a part of the body or a bone around its long axis (such as the rotation of the humerus at the shoulder joint)

Lateral rotation—rotation away from the median plane (Figure A1-11•)

Medial rotation—rotation toward the median plane (Figure A1-11)

TOPOGRAPHICAL ANATOMY OF THE CHEST

The exterior of the chest can be described with standard anatomical lines (Figures A1-12•, A1-13•, and A1-14•). A vertical line drawn from the midaxilla downward separates the anterior chest from the posterior chest. This is called the *midaxillary line.* A vertical line drawn from the center of the manubrium (the top of the sternum) to the xiphoid process (the bottom of the sternum) is called the *midsternal line.* It separates the right anterior chest from the left anterior chest. A vertical line drawn along the spine is the *mid-*

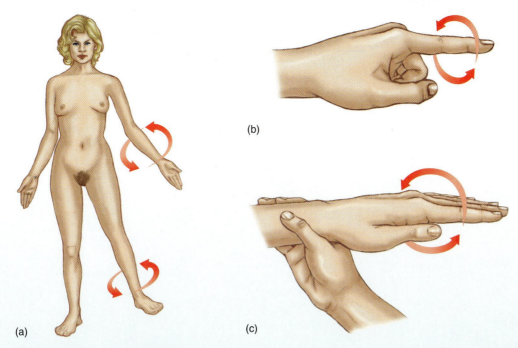

(b)

(c)

(a)

● **FIGURE A1-9   Circumduction**
(a) Circumduction of the left upper and left lower extremities at the shoulder and hip joints, respectively. **(b)** Circumduction of the index finger. **(c)** Circumduction of the hand at the wrist joint.

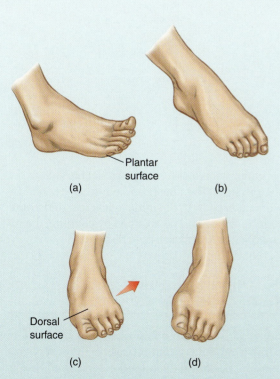

Plantar surface

(a)

(b)

Dorsal surface

(c)

(d)

● **FIGURE A1-10   Movements of the Foot**
(a) Dorsiflexion. **(b)** Plantarflexion. **(c)** Eversion. **(d)** Inversion.

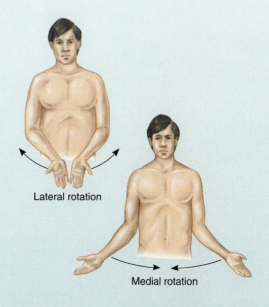

Lateral rotation

Medial rotation

● **FIGURE A1-11   Shoulder Joint Movements**
Note that the forearms are flexed at 90 degrees during rotation at this joint.

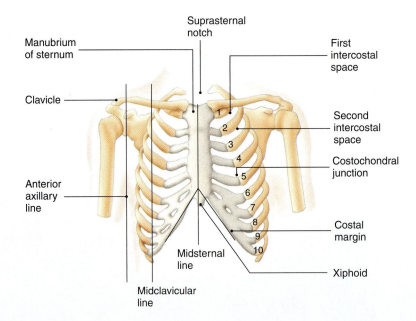

● **FIGURE A1-12**
Topographical Anatomy of the Anterior Chest

- Manubrium of sternum
- Clavicle
- Anterior axillary line
- Suprasternal notch
- First intercostal space
- Second intercostal space
- Costochondral junction
- Costal margin
- Xiphoid
- Midsternal line
- Midclavicular line

● **FIGURE A1-13**
Topographical Anatomy of the Posterior Chest

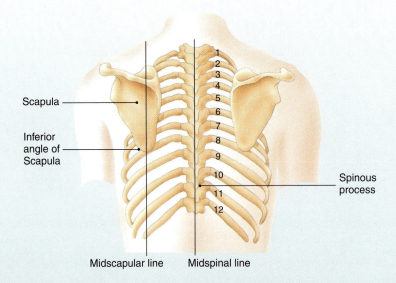

- Scapula
- Inferior angle of Scapula
- Spinous process
- Midscapular line
- Midspinal line

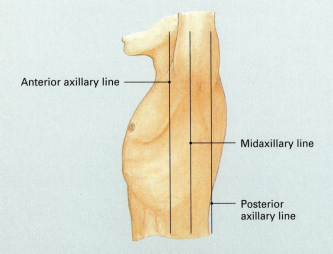

- Anterior axillary line
- Midaxillary line
- Posterior axillary line

● **FIGURE A1-14   Topographical Anatomy of the Lateral Chest**

spinal line, which separates the left posterior chest from the right posterior chest. The chest can be further divided by drawing vertical lines from the midclavicle and midscapula. Further localization can be obtained by counting the intercostal spaces (the spaces between the ribs).

TOPOGRAPHICAL ANATOMY OF THE ABDOMEN

The abdomen is divided into four quadrants by drawing a vertical line from the xiphoid process to the symphysis pubis. This line is then halved, and a horizontal line is drawn to separate the upper abdomen from the lower. The back is also part of the abdomen. It should be considered when referring to the abdomen. The point where

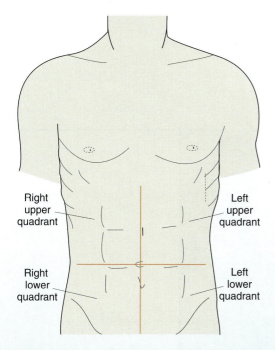

● **FIGURE A1-15   Topographical Anatomy of the Anterior Abdomen**

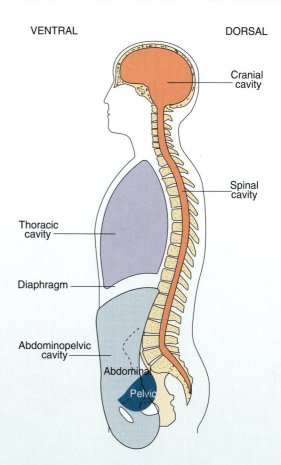

● **FIGURE A1-16   The Body Cavities**

the twelfth ribs attach to the twelfth vertebra is called the *costovertebral angle (CVA).* It is an important point in physical examination as it overlies the kidneys. The lateral aspect of the abdomen is often called the *flank.*

Organs contained within the abdominal quadrants include the following (Figure A1-15●):

- *Left upper quadrant:* spleen, tail of the pancreas, stomach, left kidney, and part of the colon.
- *Right upper quadrant:* liver, gall bladder, head of the pancreas, part of the duodenum, right kidney, and part of the colon.
- *Right lower quadrant:* appendix, ascending colon, small intestine, and the right ovary and fallopian tube.
- *Left lower quadrant:* small intestine, descending colon, and left ovary and fallopian tube.

BODY CAVITIES

The body contains several compartments, referred to as cavities. (Figure A1-16●). The superior-most cavity is the *cranium,* or *cranial vault,* which contains the brain. The *thoracic cavity* is the compartment that contains the heart, lungs, and mediastinum. It is bordered superiorly by the root of the neck and inferiorly by the diaphragm. The *abdominal cavity* is bordered by the diaphragm superiorly and by the pelvic inlet inferiorly. It contains the liver, gall bladder, stomach, pancreas, spleen, intestines,

kidneys, and adrenal glands. The *pelvic cavity* is bordered superiorly by the pelvic inlet and inferiorly by the pelvic floor. It contains the bladder, rectum, ovaries, fallopian tubes, and uterus. Because there is no anatomical division between the abdomen and the pelvis, they are often referred to jointly as the *abdominopelvic cavity.* The *spinal cavity* extends from the base of the skull down through the spinal canal to the sacrum. It contains the spinal cord and associated structures.

SUMMARY

It is essential that emergency medical personnel have a thorough understanding of topographical and descriptive anatomy. Patient reports and run reports must accurately reflect patient injuries or physical examination findings. Using accepted descriptive anatomical terms allows other health care workers to immediately mentally visualize your patient's condition. Some topographical anatomical terms are less frequently used. These should be periodically reviewed so that they can be properly used when the need arises.

2 The Chemical Level of Organization

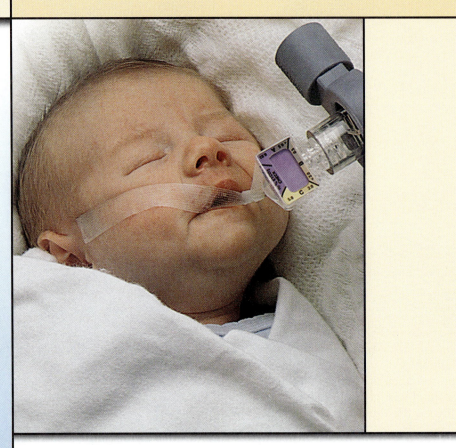

The human body is a mass of complex biochemical processes that constantly strive for homeostasis. Medical practitioners often must evaluate and measure the quantity of fundamental body chemicals, such as oxygen and carbon dioxide. For example, continuous measurement of end-tidal (exhaled) carbon dioxide as part of a mechanical ventilation system helps to assure that the endotracheal tube is placed properly and that biochemical processes that generate carbon dioxide are functioning properly.

Chapter Outline and Objectives

Vocabulary Development

anabole, a building up; *anabolism*
endo-, inside; *endergonic*
exo-, outside; *exergonic*
glyco-, sugar; *glycogen*
*hemo-, blood; *hemoglobin*
hydro-, water + lysis, breakdown; *hydrolysis*
katabole, a throwing down; *catabolism*
katalysis, dissolution; *catalysis*
lipos, fat; *lipids*
metabole, change; *metabolism*
sakcharon, sugar
+ **mono-**, single; *monosaccharide*
+ **di-**, two; *disaccharide*
+ **poly-**, many; *polysaccharide*

2 Our study of the human body begins at the most basic level of organization, that of individual atoms and molecules. The characteristics of all living and nonliving things—people, elephants, oranges, oceans, rocks, and air—result from the types of atoms involved and the ways in which those atoms combine and interact. The branch of science that deals with such interactions is **chemistry**. A familiarity with basic chemistry will help us understand how the properties of atoms can affect the anatomy and physiology of the cells, tissues, organs, and organ systems that make up the human body.

ATOMS AND MOLECULES

Matter is anything that occupies space and has *mass*, a property that, on earth, determines its weight. Matter occurs in one of three familiar states: solid (such as a rock), liquid (such as water), or gas (such as the atmosphere). All matter is composed of substances called **elements,** which cannot be broken down by heating or other ordinary physical means. The smallest piece of an element, and the simplest unit of matter, is an **atom**. Although physicists can split atoms apart, chemical reactions cannot change the basic identity of an atom. Atoms are so small that atomic measurements are most conveniently reported in billionths of a meter. The very largest atoms approach half of 1 billionth of a meter (0.5 nanometers) in diameter. One million atoms placed end to end would be no longer than a period on this page.

Atoms contain three major types of subatomic particles: protons, neutrons, and electrons. Protons and neutrons are similar in size and mass, but **protons** have a positive electrical charge (p^+), and **neutrons** are neutral—that is, uncharged (n^0). **Electrons** are much lighter, only

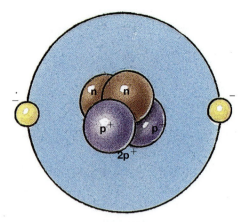

Helium (He)

● **FIGURE 2-1   Atomic Structure**
An atom of helium contains two of each subatomic particles; two protons, two neutrons, and two electrons.

1/1836th as massive as protons, and have a negative electrical charge (e^-). Figure 2-1● is a diagrammatic view of a simple atom of the element *helium*. This atom contains two protons, two neutrons, and two electrons.

The Structure of an Atom

All atoms contain protons and electrons, normally in equal numbers. The number of protons in an atom is known as its **atomic number**. A chemical element is a substance that consists entirely of atoms with the same atomic number.

Table 2-1 lists the important elements in the human body. Each element is universally known by its own abbreviation, or chemical symbol. Most of the symbols are

TABLE 2-1	The Principal Elements in the Human Body
Element (% of body weight)	*Significance*
Hydrogen (H) (9.7)	A component of water and most other compounds in the body
Oxygen (O) (65)	A component of water and other compounds; oxygen gas essential for respiration
Carbon (C) (18.6)	Found in all organic molecules
Nitrogen (N) (3.2)	Found in proteins, nucleic acids, and other organic compounds
Calcium (Ca) (1.8)	Found in bones and teeth; important for membrane function, nerve impulses, muscle contraction, and blood clotting
Phosphorus (P) (1)	Found in bones and teeth, nucleic acids, and high-energy compounds
Potassium (K) (0.4)	Important for proper membrane function, nerve impulses, and muscle contraction
Sodium (Na) (0.2)	Important for membrane function, nerve impulses, and muscle contraction
Chlorine (Cl) (0.2)	Important for membrane function and water absorption
Magnesium (Mg) (0.06)	Required for activation of several enzymes
Sulfur (S) (0.04)	Found in many proteins
Iron (Fe) (0.007)	Essential for oxygen transport and energy capture
Iodine (I) (0.0002)	A component of hormones of the thyroid gland

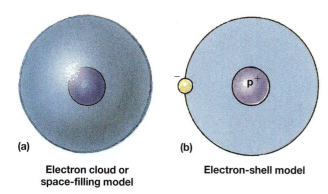

(a) Electron cloud or space-filling model

(b) Electron-shell model

• **FIGURE 2-2   Hydrogen Atoms**
(a) The electron cloud of a hydrogen atom is formed by the orbiting of an electron around the nucleus. **(b)** A two-dimensional model depicting the electron in an electron shell makes it easier to visualize the atom's components. A typical hydrogen nucleus contains a single proton and no neutrons.

easily connected with the names of the elements, but a few, such as Na for sodium, are abbreviations of their original Latin names, in this case *natrium*.

Hydrogen, the simplest element, has an atomic number of 1 because its atom contains one proton. The proton is located in the center of the atom and forms the **nucleus**. A single electron whirls around the nucleus at high speed, forming an **electron cloud** (Figure 2-2a•). To simplify matters, this cloud is usually represented as a spherical **electron shell** (Figure 2-2b•).

Isotopes

Neutrons are not always present in an atom, but when they are, they are found in the nucleus together with the protons. Unlike protons, neutrons can vary in number, even among atoms of the same element. Atoms of an element whose nuclei contain different numbers of neutrons are called **isotopes**. The presence or absence of neutrons generally has no effect on the chemical properties of an atom of a particular element. As a result, isotopes can be distinguished from one another only by their **mass number**—the total number of protons and neutrons. The nuclei of some isotopes may be unstable. Unstable isotopes are radioactive; that is, they spontaneously emit subatomic particles. These *radioisotopes* are sometimes used in diagnostic procedures.

Atomic Weight

Atomic mass numbers are useful because they tell us the number of protons and neutrons in the nuclei of different atoms. However, they do not tell us the *actual* mass of an atom, because they do not take into account the masses of electrons and the slight difference between the masses of a proton and neutron. They also don't tell us the mass of a "typical" atom, since any element consists of a mixture of isotopes. It is therefore useful to know the *average mass* of an atom, and this

value is an element's **atomic weight**. Atomic weight takes into account the mass of the subatomic particles and the relative proportions of any isotopes. For example, even though the atomic number of hydrogen is 1, the atomic weight of hydrogen is 1.0079. In this case, the atomic number and atomic weight differ primarily because a few hydrogen atoms have a mass number of 2 (one proton plus one neutron) and an even smaller number have a mass number of 3 (one proton plus two neutrons). The atomic weights of all 112 elements are included in Appendix II.

Electrons and Electron Shells

Atoms are electrically neutral because every positively charged proton is balanced by a negatively charged electron. These electrons occupy an orderly series of electron shells, and only the electrons in the outer shell can interact with other atoms. *The number and arrangement of electrons in an atom's outer electron shell determine the chemical properties of that element.*

The stability of the outer electron shell depends on the number of electrons it contains. An atom with a stable outer shell will not interact with other atoms. The first electron shell is filled when it contains two electrons. A hydrogen atom has one electron in this electron shell (Figure 2-2b•), and hydrogen atoms can react with many other atoms. A helium atom has two electrons in this electron shell (Figure 2-1•). Helium is called an inert gas because the outer electron shell is full and therefore stable. Helium atoms will neither react with one another nor combine with atoms of other elements.

The second electron shell can contain up to eight electrons. Carbon, with an atomic number of 6, has six electrons. In a carbon atom the first shell is filled (two electrons), and the second shell contains four electrons (Figure 2-3a•). In a neon atom (atomic number 10), the second shell is filled; neon is another inert gas (Figure 2-3b•).

Chemical Bonds and Chemical Compounds

An atom with a full outer electron shell is very stable and not reactive. Atoms with unfilled outer electron shells can achieve stability by sharing, gaining, or losing electrons through chemical reactions. Many of these chemical reactions produce **molecules**, chemical structures each containing more than one atom. Molecules called **compounds** contain atoms of more than one element. A compound is a new chemical substance with properties that can be quite different from those of its component elements. For example, a mixture of hydrogen and oxygen gases is highly flammable, but chemically combining hydrogen and oxygen atoms produces a compound, water, that can put out fires.

2

● **FIGURE 2-3   Atoms and Electron Shells**
(a) The first electron shell can hold only two electrons. In a carbon atom, with six protons and six
electrons, the third through sixth electrons occupy
the second electron shell. **(b)** The second shell can
hold up to eight electrons. A neon atom has 10
protons and 10 electrons; thus both the first and
second electron shells are filled. Notice that the
nuclei of helium, carbon, and neon contain neutrons as well as protons.

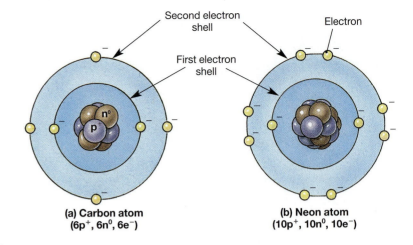

(a) **Carbon atom**
($6p^+$, $6n^0$, $6e^-$)

(b) **Neon atom**
($10p^+$, $10n^0$, $10e^-$)

Ionic Bonds

Atoms are electrically neutral because the number of
protons (each with a +1 charge) is equal to the number
of electrons (each with a −1 charge). If an atom loses an
electron, it will exhibit a charge of +1 because there
will be one proton without a corresponding electron;
losing a second electron would leave the atom with a
charge of +2. Similarly, adding one or two extra electrons to the atom will give it a respective charge of −1
or −2. Atoms or molecules that have a (+) or (−) charge
are called **ions**. Ions with a positive charge are **cations**
(KAT-ī-ons); those with a negative charge are **anions**
(AN-ī-ons). Table 2-2 lists several important ions in
body fluids.

In an **ionic** (ī-ON-ik) **bond**, anions and cations are
held together by the attraction between positive and negative charges. An example of a substance held together
by ionic bonds is ordinary table salt (Figure 2-4b●).

The steps in the formation of an ionic bond are illustrated in Figure 2-4a●. In this process, a sodium atom
donates an electron to a chlorine atom. This loss of an
electron creates a *sodium ion* with a +1 charge and a
chloride ion with a −1 charge. The two ions do not
move apart after the electron transfer, because the positively charged sodium ion is attracted to the negatively charged chloride ion. The combination of oppositely
charged ions forms the ionic compound *sodium chloride*, the chemical name for table salt.

Covalent Bonds

Another way atoms can complete their outer electron
shells is by sharing electrons with other atoms. The result
is a molecule held together by **covalent** (kō-VĀ-lent) **bonds**.

For example, individual hydrogen atoms, as diagrammed in Figure 2-2●, are not found in nature. Instead,
we find hydrogen molecules (Figure 2-5a●). Molecular hydrogen is a gas present in the atmosphere in very small
quantities. The two hydrogen atoms share their electrons,
with each electron whirling around both nuclei. The sharing of one pair of electrons creates a **single covalent bond**.

Oxygen, with an atomic number of 8, has two electrons in its first energy level and six in the second. Oxygen atoms (Figure 2-5b●) reach stability by pooling their
resources and sharing two pairs of electrons, forming a
double covalent bond. Molecular oxygen is an atmospheric gas that is very important to living organisms;
our cells would die without a constant supply of oxygen.

The chemical reactions in our bodies that consume
oxygen also produce a waste product, carbon dioxide.
The oxygen atoms in a carbon dioxide molecule form
double covalent bonds with the carbon atom, as shown
in Figure 2-5c●.

Covalent bonds are very strong because the electrons
tie the atoms together. In most covalent bonds the atoms
remain electrically neutral because the electrons are shared
equally. Such equal sharing between carbon atoms creates
the stable framework of the large molecules that make up
most of the structural components of the human body.

Elements differ in how strongly they hold shared
electrons. An unequal sharing creates a **polar covalent bond**. For example, in a molecule of water, an
oxygen atom forms covalent bonds with two hydrogen
atoms. The oxygen atom has a much stronger attraction for the shared electrons than do the hydrogen
atoms, so their electrons spend most of their time with
the oxygen atom. Because of the two extra electrons,
the oxygen atom develops a slight negative charge. At
the same time, the hydrogen atoms develop a slight
positive charge, because their electrons are away part
of the time.

TABLE 2-2	The Most Common Ions in Body Fluids
Cations	*Anions*
Na$^+$ (sodium)	**Cl$^-$** (chloride)
K$^+$ (potassium)	**HCO$_3^-$** (bicarbonate)
Ca^{2+} (calcium)	**HPO$_4^{2-}$** (biphosphate)
Mg^{2+} (magnesium)	**SO$_4^{2-}$** (sulfate)

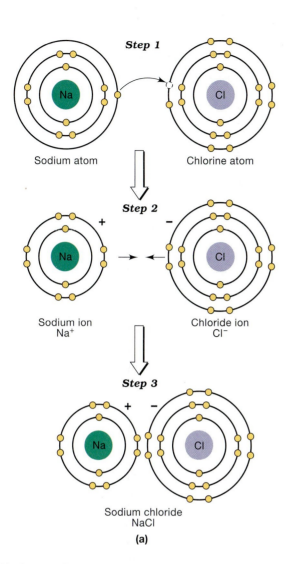

Step 1

Sodium atom   Chlorine atom

Step 2

Sodium ion
Na⁺

Chloride ion
Cl⁻

Step 3

Sodium chloride
NaCl

(a)

• FIGURE 2-4   Ionic Bonding
(a) Step 1: A sodium atom loses an electron, which is accepted by a chlorine atom. **Step 2**: Because the sodium (Na⁺) and chloride (Cl⁻) ions have opposite charges, they are attracted to one another. **Step 3**: The association of sodium and chloride ions forms the ionic compound sodium chloride. **(b)** Large numbers of sodium and chloride ions form a crystal of sodium chloride.

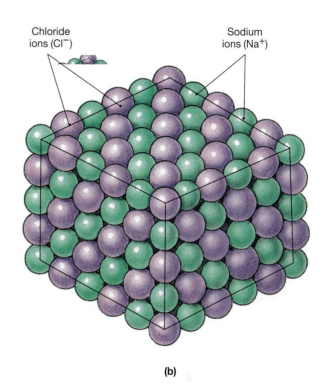

Chloride
ions (Cl⁻)

Sodium
ions (Na⁺)

(b)

Hydrogen Bonds

In addition to ionic and covalent bonds, weaker attractive forces act between atoms within different parts of a large molecule as well as between adjacent molecules. Hydrogen bonds are the most important of these attractive forces.

Hydrogen atoms often form polar covalent bonds with the atoms of elements such as oxygen, nitrogen, or both. In the process, the hydrogen atom develops a slight positive charge and its partner develops a weak negative charge. A **hydrogen bond** is the attraction between such a hydrogen atom and a negatively

	ELECTRON-SHELL MODEL AND STRUCTURAL FORMULA	SPACE-FILLING MODEL
(a) Hydrogen (H₂)	**H–H**	
(b) Oxygen (O₂)	**O=O**	
(c) Carbon dioxide (CO₂)	**O=C=O**	

• FIGURE 2-5   Covalent Bonds
(a) In a molecule of hydrogen, two hydrogen atoms share their electrons such that each has a filled outer electron shell. This sharing creates a single covalent bond. **(b)** A molecule of oxygen consists of two oxygen atoms that share two pairs of electrons. The result is a double covalent bond. **(c)** In a molecule of carbon dioxide, a central carbon atom forms double covalent bonds with a pair of oxygen atoms.

• **FIGURE 2-6 Hydrogen Bonds**
(a) The unequal sharing of electrons in a water molecule causes each of its two hydrogen atoms to have a slight positive charge and its oxygen atom to have a slight negative charge. Attraction between a hydrogen atom of one water molecule and the oxygen atom of another is a hydrogen bond (indicated by dashed lines). (b) Hydrogen bonding between water molecules at a free surface restricts evaporation and creates surface tension.

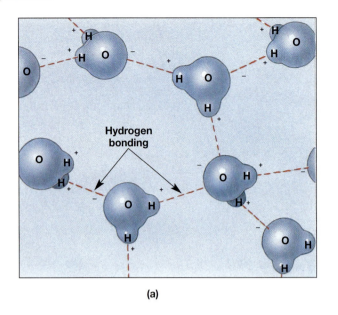

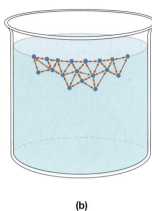

(a)

(b)

charged atom in another molecule or at another site within the same molecule. Hydrogen bonds do not create molecules, but they can alter molecular shapes or pull molecules together. For example, the hydrogen bonding between water molecules slows its rate of evaporation and creates its high surface tension (Figure 2-6●).

✓ Oxygen and neon are both gases at room temperature. Oxygen combines readily with other elements, but neon does not. Why?

✓ How is it possible for two samples of hydrogen to contain the same number of atoms but have different weights?

✓ Which kind of bond holds atoms in a water molecule together? Which kind of bond attracts water molecules to each other?

CHEMICAL NOTATION

Complex chemical compounds and reactions are most easily described with a simple form of "chemical shorthand" known as **chemical notation**. The rules of chemical notation are summarized in Table 2-3.

CHEMICAL REACTIONS

Living cells remain alive by controlling internal chemical reactions. In every **chemical reaction**, bonds between atoms are broken, and atoms are rearranged into new combinations. In effect, each cell is a chemical factory, carrying out the complex chemical reactions needed to sustain life. **Metabolism** (meh-TAB-ō-lizm;

metabole, change) refers to all of the chemical reactions in the body. These reactions release, store, and use energy to maintain homeostasis and perform essential functions.

Basic Energy Concepts

Most people are familiar with the concepts of work, energy, and heat. **Work** is movement or a change in physical structure. **Energy** is the capacity to perform work; movement or physical change will not occur unless energy is provided. There are two major types of energy: *kinetic energy* and *potential energy*.

Kinetic energy is the energy of motion. When a car hits a tree, it is kinetic energy that does the damage. **Potential energy** is stored energy. It may result from the position of an object (as when a book sits on a high shelf) or its physical structure (as when a spring is compressed or stretched). Kinetic energy had to be used to lift the book and stretch or compress the spring. The potential energy is converted back into kinetic energy when the book falls or the spring returns to its resting length; the energy released can be used to perform work.

A conversion between potential energy and kinetic energy is not 100 percent efficient. Each time an energy exchange occurs, some of the energy produces **heat**, an increase in random molecular motion. The temperature of an object is directly related to its heat content.

Living cells perform work in many forms. For example, the contraction of a skeletal muscle is a process that requires energy and generates large amounts of heat. The energy comes from the breaking of covalent bonds, utilizing the potential energy contained in the food we eat.

TABLE 2-3	Rules of Chemical Notation

1.   The abbreviation of an element indicates one atom of that element:

H = an atom of hydrogen; O = an atom of oxygen

2.   A number preceding the abbreviation of an element indicates more than one atom:

2 H = two individual atoms of hydrogen

2 O = two individual atoms of oxygen

3.   A subscript following the abbreviation of an element indicates a molecule with that number of atoms:

H_2 = a hydrogen molecule composed of two hydrogen atoms

O_2 = an oxygen molecule composed of two oxygen atoms

4.   In a description of a chemical reaction, the interacting participants are called *reactants*, and the reaction generates one or more *products*. An arrow indicates the direction of the reaction, from reactants (usually on the left) to products (usually on the right). In the reaction below, two atoms of hydrogen combine with one atom of oxygen to produce a single molecule of water.

$$2\,H + O \rightarrow H_2O$$

5.   A superscript plus or minus sign following the abbreviation for an element indicates an ion. A single plus sign indicates an ion with a charge of +1 (loss of one electron). A single minus sign indicates an ion with a charge of –1 (gain of one electron). If more than one electron has been lost or gained, the charge on the ion is indicated by a number preceding the plus or minus.

Na^+ = one sodium ion (has lost 1 electron)

Cl^- = one chloride ion (has gained 1 electron)

Ca^{2+} = one calcium ion (has lost 2 electrons)

6.   Chemical reactions neither create nor destroy atoms—they merely rearrange them into new combinations. Therefore, the numbers of atoms of each element must always be the same on both sides of the equation. When this is the case, the equation is *balanced*.

Unbalanced: $H_2 + O_2 \rightarrow H_2O$

Balanced: $2\,H_2 + O_2 \rightarrow 2\,H_2O$

Classes of Reactions

Three classes of chemical reactions are important to the study of physiology: *decomposition reactions, synthesis reactions,* and *exchange reactions.*

Decomposition

A **decomposition reaction** breaks a molecule into smaller fragments. Such reactions occur during digestion when food molecules are broken into smaller pieces. You could diagram a typical decomposition reaction as:

$$AB \rightarrow A + B$$

Catabolism (kah-TAB-o-lizm; *katabole*, a throwing down) refers to the breakdown of complex molecules within cells. A chemical bond contains potential energy that is released when that bond is broken. Our cells can capture some of that energy and use it to power essential functions such as growth, repair, movement, and reproduction.

Synthesis

Synthesis (SIN-the-sis) is the opposite of decomposition. A synthesis reaction assembles larger molecules from smaller components. These relatively simple reactions could be diagrammed as:

$$A + B \rightarrow AB$$

A and B could be individual atoms that combine to form a molecule, or they could be individual molecules combining to form larger, more complex structures. Synthesis always involves the formation of new chemical bonds, whether the reactants are atoms or molecules.

Anabolism (a-NAB-o-lizm; *anabole*, a building up) is the synthesis of new compounds in the body. Because it takes energy to create a chemical bond, anabolism usually represents an uphill struggle. Living cells are constantly balancing their chemical activities, with catabolism providing the energy needed to support synthesis as well as other vital functions.

2

Exchange Reactions

In an **exchange reaction**, parts of the reacting molecules are shuffled around, as in:

$$AB + CD \rightarrow AD + CB$$

You will notice that there are two products and two reactants. Although the reactants and products contain the same components (A, B, C, and D), they are present in different combinations. In an exchange reaction, the reactant molecules AB and CD break apart (a decomposition) before they interact with one another to form AD and CB (a synthesis). An example of such a reaction is the exchange of the components of sodium hydroxide (NaOH) and hydrochloric acid (HCl) to make table salt and water:

$$NaOH + HCl \rightarrow NaCl + H_2O$$

If breaking the old bonds releases more energy than it takes to create the new ones, the exchange reaction will release energy, usually in the form of heat. Such reactions are said to be **exergonic** (*exo-*, outside). If the energy required for synthesis exceeds the amount released by the associated decomposition reaction, additional energy (usually heat) must be provided. Such reactions are called **endergonic** (*endo-*, inside) because they absorb heat.

Reversible Reactions

Many important biological reactions are freely reversible. Such reactions can be diagrammed as:

$$A + B \leftrightarrow AB$$

This reaction reminds you that there are really two reactions occurring simultaneously, one a synthesis (A + B → AB) and the other a decomposition (AB→ A + B). At **equilibrium** (ē-kwi-LIB-rē-um) the two rates are in balance. As fast as a molecule of AB forms, another degrades into A + B. As a result, the number of A, B, and AB molecules present at any given moment does not change. Altering the concentrations of one or more of these molecules will temporarily upset the equilibrium. For example, adding additional molecules of A and B will accelerate the synthesis reaction (A + B → AB). As the concentration of AB rises, however, so does the rate of the decomposition reaction (AB → A + B), until a new equilibrium is established.

✓ In living cells, glucose, a six-carbon molecule, is converted into two three-carbon molecules by a reaction that yields energy. How would you classify this reaction?

✓ If the product of a reversible reaction is continuously removed, what do you think the effect will be on the equilibrium?

Acids and Bases

An **acid** is any substance that dissociates to *release* hydrogen ions. (Because a hydrogen ion consists solely of a naked proton, hydrogen ions are often referred to simply as protons, and acids as "proton donors.") Hydrochloric acid (HCl) is an excellent example:

$$HCl \rightarrow H^+ + Cl^-$$

The stomach produces this powerful acid to assist in the breakdown of food.

A **base** is a substance that removes hydrogen ions from a solution. Many common bases are compounds that dissociate in solution to liberate a hydroxide ion (OH^-). Hydroxide ions have a strong affinity for hydrogen ions and quickly react with them, tying them up as water molecules, thereby removing them from solution. For example, sodium hydroxide (NaOH) dissociates in solution as:

$$NaOH \rightarrow Na^+ + OH^-$$

Strong bases have a variety of industrial and household uses; drain openers and lye are two familiar examples. The human body contains weak bases that are important in counteracting acids produced by cellular metabolism.

pH

The concentration of hydrogen ions in blood or other body fluids is important because hydrogen ions are extremely reactive. In excessive numbers they can disrupt cell and tissue function by breaking chemical bonds and changing the shapes of complex molecules. The concentration of hydrogen ions must therefore be regulated within relatively narrow limits.

The concentration of hydrogen ions is usually reported in terms of the **pH** of the solution. The pH value is a number between 0 and 14. Pure water has a pH of 7. A solution with a pH of 7 is called *neutral*, because it contains equal numbers of hydrogen and hydroxide ions. A solution with a pH below 7 is called *acidic* (a-SI-dik), because there are more hydrogen ions than hydroxide ions. A pH above 7 is called *basic*, or *alkaline* (AL-kah-lin), because hydroxide ions outnumber hydrogen ions.

The pH values of some common liquids are indicated in Figure 2-7●. The pH of the blood normally ranges from 7.35 to 7.45. Variations in pH outside this range can damage cells and disrupt normal cellular functions. For example, a blood pH below 7 can produce coma, and a blood pH higher than 7.8 usually causes uncontrollable, sustained muscular contractions.

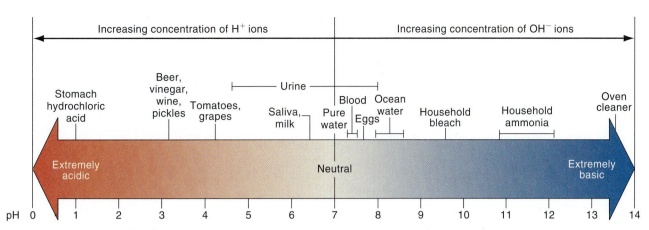

• **FIGURE 2-7   pH and Hydrogen Ion Concentration**
An increase or decrease of one unit corresponds to a tenfold change in H^+ concentration.

Buffers and pH

Buffers are compounds that stabilize pH by removing or replacing hydrogen ions. Antacids such as Alka-Seltzer®, Rolaids®, and Tums® are buffers that tie up excess hydrogen ions in the stomach. The normal pH of most body fluids ranges from 7.35 to 7.45. A variety of buffers, including sodium bicarbonate, are responsible for regulating pH. We will consider the role of buffers and pH control in Chapter 19.

✓ What is the difference between an acid and a base?

✓ Why would an extreme change in pH of body fluids be undesirable?

✓ How does an antacid decrease stomach discomfort?

The rest of this chapter focuses on nutrients and metabolites (me-TAB-o-līts). *Nutrients* are the essential elements and molecules absorbed from food. *Metabolites* include all of the molecules synthesized or broken down by chemical reactions inside our bodies. Like all chemical substances, nutrients and metabolites can be broadly categorized as *inorganic* or *organic*. Generally speaking, **inorganic compounds** are small molecules that do not contain carbon atoms. (The only exception is carbon dioxide.) **Organic compounds** are primarily composed of carbon atoms, and they can be much larger and more complex than inorganic compounds.

INORGANIC COMPOUNDS

The most important inorganic substances in the human body are carbon dioxide, oxygen, water, inorganic acids and bases, and salts.

Carbon Dioxide and Oxygen

Carbon dioxide (CO_2) is produced by cells through normal metabolic activity. It is transported in the blood and released into the air in the lungs. Oxygen (O_2), an atmospheric gas, is absorbed at the lungs, transported in the blood, and consumed by cells throughout the body. The chemical structures of these compounds were introduced earlier in the chapter.

Water and Its Properties

Water, H_2O, is the single most important constituent of the body, accounting for almost two-thirds of its total weight. A drastic change in body water content can have fatal consequences because virtually all physiological systems will be affected.

Three general properties of water are particularly important to our discussion of the human body:

- *Water is an excellent solvent.* Water dissolves a remarkable variety of inorganic and organic molecules, creating a *solution.* As they dissolve, the molecules break apart, releasing ions or molecules that become uniformly dispersed throughout the solution. The chemical reactions within living cells occur in solution, and the watery component, or plasma, of blood carries dissolved nutrients and waste products throughout the body. Most chemical reactions in the body take place in solution.

- *Water has a very high heat capacity.* It takes a lot of energy to make water boil, and a large amount of energy must be removed before water will freeze. As a result, the water in our cells remains a liquid over a wide range of environmental temperatures. Furthermore, it circulates within the body as the blood transports and

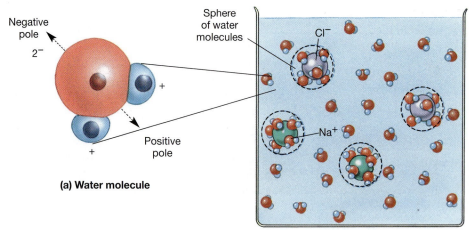

• FIGURE 2-8   Water Molecules and Solutions
(a) In a water molecule, oxygen forms polar covalent bonds with two hydrogen atoms. Because the hydrogen atoms are positioned toward one end of the molecule, the molecule has an uneven distribution of charges. This creates positive and negative poles. (b) Ionic compounds dissociate in water as the polar water molecules disrupt the ionic bonds. The ions remain in solution because the surrounding water molecules prevent the ionic bonds from re-forming.

redistributes heat. For example, heat absorbed as the blood flows through active muscles will be released when the blood reaches vessels in the relatively cool body surface.

- *Water is an essential reactant in the chemical reactions of living systems.* In such reactions, water is commonly involved in the synthesis and decomposition of various organic compounds. Water molecules are released during the synthesis of large organic molecules and absorbed during their decomposition.

Solutions

A **solution** consists of a fluid *solvent* and dissolved *solutes.* In biological solutions, the solvent is usually water and the solutes may be inorganic or organic. Inorganic compounds held together by ionic bonds undergo **ionization** (ī-on-i-ZĀ-shun), or *dissociation* (dis-sō-sē-Ā-shun), in solution. As shown in Figure 2-8•, ionic bonds are broken apart as individual ions form hydrogen bonds with water molecules. This process produces a mixture of cations and anions surrounded by so many water molecules that they are unable to re-form their original bonds.

Inorganic Acids and Bases

The discussion of acids and bases on p. 36 introduced an inorganic acid, hydrochloric acid (HCl), and an inorganic base, sodium hydroxide (NaOH). Several other inorganic acids are found in body fluids, including carbonic acid, sulfuric acid, and phosphoric acid. These acids, produced during normal metabolism, will be considered further in Chapters 16 and 19.

Salts

A **salt** is an inorganic compound consisting of a cation that is not a hydrogen ion and an anion that is not a

hydroxide ion. Salts are held together by ionic bonds, and in water they dissociate, releasing cations and anions. For example, table salt (NaCl) in solution dissociates into Na^+ and Cl^- ions; these are the most abundant ions in body fluids.

Salts are examples of **electrolytes** (ē-LEK-trō-līts), compounds whose ions will conduct an electrical current in solution. For example, sodium ions (Na^+), potassium ions (K^+), calcium ions (Ca^{2+}), and chloride ions (Cl^-) are released by the dissociation of electrolytes in blood and other body fluids. Alterations in the body fluid concentrations of these ions will disturb almost every vital function. For example, declining potassium levels will lead to a general muscular paralysis, and rising concentrations will cause weak and irregular heartbeats.

ORGANIC COMPOUNDS

Organic compounds contain the elements carbon and hydrogen, and usually oxygen as well. Organic molecules often contain long chains of carbon atoms linked by covalent bonds. These carbon atoms often form additional covalent bonds with hydrogen or oxygen atoms, and less often, with nitrogen, phosphorus, sulfur, iron, or other elements to produce the complex organic molecules characteristic of living organisms.

Although inorganic acids and bases were used as examples earlier in the chapter, there are also important organic acids and bases. For example, *lactic acid* is an organic acid generated by active muscle tissues.

This section focuses on four major classes of large organic molecules: *carbohydrates, lipids, proteins,* and *nucleic acids.* We will also consider the high-energy compounds that play a crucial role in many of the chemical reactions under way within our cells. In addition, the human body contains small quantities of many other organic compounds whose structures and functions will be considered in later chapters.

Carbohydrates

A **carbohydrate** (kar-bō-HĪ-drāt) is a molecule that contains carbon, hydrogen, and oxygen in a ratio near 1:2:1. Familiar carbohydrates include the sugars and starches that make up roughly half of the typical American diet. Our tissues can break down most carbohydrates, and although they sometimes have other functions, carbohydrates are most important as sources of energy. Despite their importance as an energy source, however, carbohydrates account for less than 3 percent of the total body weight. The three major types of carbohydrates are *monosaccharides, disaccharides,* and *polysaccharides.*

Monosaccharides

A **simple sugar**, or **monosaccharide** (mon-ō-SAK-ah-rīd; *mono-*, single + *sakcharon*, sugar), is a carbohydrate containing from three to seven carbon atoms. Included within this group is **glucose** (GLOO-kōs), $C_6H_{12}O_6$, the most important metabolic "fuel" in the body (Figure 2-9•).

Disaccharides and Polysaccharides

Carbohydrates other than simple sugars are complex molecules composed of monosaccharide building blocks. Through a **dehydration synthesis** reaction, the removal of water joins two simple sugars to form a **disaccharide** (dī-SAK-ah-rīd; *di-*, two) (Figure 2-10a•). Disaccharides such as **sucrose** (table sugar) have a sugary taste and are quite soluble. Many foods contain disaccharides, but they must be disassembled before they can be broken down to provide useful energy. The breakdown of a disaccharide into its component simple sugars is an example of **hydrolysis** (hī-DROL-i-sis; *hydro-*, water + *lysis*; breakdown) (Figure 2-10b•). Most junk foods, including candy and soft drinks, abound in simple sugars (often fructose) and disaccharides such as sucrose.

Larger carbohydrate molecules are called **polysaccharides** (pol-ē-SAK-ah-rīdz; *poly-*, many). *Starches* are glucose-based polysaccharides important in our diets. Most of the starches in our diet are synthesized by plants. The human digestive tract can break these molecules into simple sugars, and starches such as those found in potatoes and grains are important energy sources.

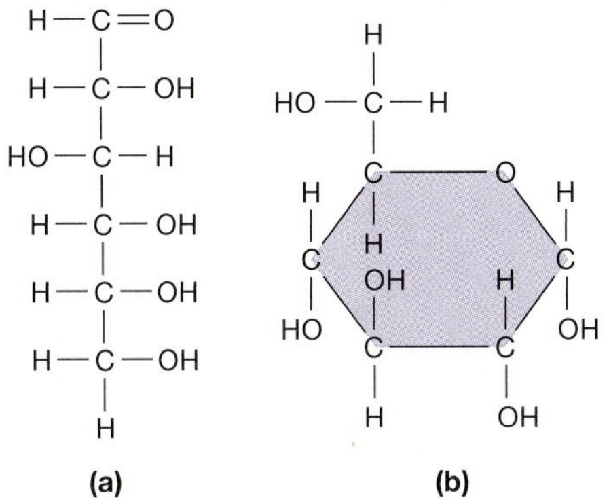

Glycogen (GLĪ-ko-jen), or *animal starch*, is a branched polysaccharide composed of interconnected glucose molecules (Figure 2-10c•). Like most other large polysaccharides, glycogen will not dissolve in water or other body fluids. Liver and muscle tissues manufacture and store significant amounts of glycogen. When these tissues have a high demand for energy, glycogen molecules are broken down into glucose; when demands are low, the tissues absorb or synthesize glucose and rebuild glycogen reserves.

Table 2-4 summarizes information concerning the carbohydrates.

Some people cannot tolerate sugar for medical reasons; others avoid it because they do not want to gain weight (excess sugars are stored as fat). Many of these people use artificial sweeteners in their foods and beverages. These compounds have a very sweet taste but either cannot be broken down in the body or are used in such small amounts that their breakdown does not contribute to the overall energy balance of the body.

Lipids

Lipids (*lipos*, fat) also contain carbon, hydrogen, and oxygen, but because they have relatively less oxygen than carbohydrates, the ratios do not approximate 1:2:1. In addition, lipids may contain small quantities of other elements, such as phosphorus, nitrogen, or sulfur. Familiar lipids include fats, oils, and waxes. Most lipids are insoluble in water, but special transport mechanisms carry them in the circulating blood.

Lipids form essential structural components of all cells. Lipid deposits also serve as energy sources and reserves. On average, lipids provide roughly twice as much energy as carbohydrates, gram for gram, when broken down in the body. For this reason there has been great interest in developing fat substitutes, such as Olestra®, that have the taste and texture of lipids but without the calories.

All together, lipids normally account for roughly 12 percent of our total body weight. There are many kinds of lipids in the body. The major types are *fatty acids, fats, steroids,* and *phospholipids* (Table 2-5, p. 41).

Fatty Acids

Fatty acids are long carbon chains with attached hydrogen atoms that end in a carboxyl group (—COOH). Because this group loses a H^+ in solution, it is also called a carboxylic acid group. While this group associates with water molecules, the rest of the carbon chain is relatively insoluble.

•FIGURE 2-9   Glucose
(a) The straight-chain structural formula. **(b)** The ring form that is most common in nature.

Dehydration synthesis

(a) During dehydration synthesis two molecules are joined by the removal of a water molecule.

Glucose Fructose → Sucrose + H_2O

Hydrolysis

(b) Hydrolysis reverses the steps of dehydration synthesis; a complex molecule is broken down by the addition of a water molecule.

Sucrose + H_2O → Glucose + Fructose

● **FIGURE 2-10   The Formation and Breakdown of Complex Sugars and Glycogen**

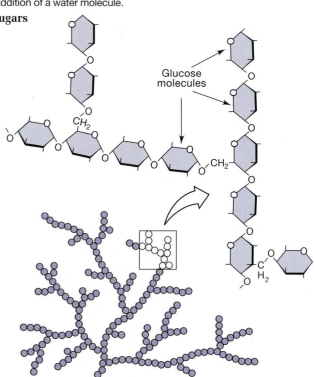

Glucose molecules

(c) Glycogen, a branching chain of glucose molecules, is stored in muscle cells and liver cells.

In a **saturated** fatty acid, each carbon atom has four single covalent bonds, enabling it to bond to a maximum number of hydrogen atoms. If any of the carbon-to-carbon bonds are double covalent bonds, then fewer hydrogen atoms are present and the fatty acid is **unsaturated**. The structure of saturated and unsaturated fatty acids is shown in the upper portion of Figure 2-11●. A **polyunsaturated** fatty acid contains multiple unsaturated bonds.

Both saturated and unsaturated fatty acids can be broken down for energy, but a diet containing large amounts of saturated fatty acids increases the risk of heart disease and other circulatory problems. Butter, fatty meat, and ice cream are popular dietary sources of saturated fatty acids. Vegetable oils such as olive oil or corn oil contain a mixture of unsaturated fatty acids.

Fats

Individual fatty acids cannot be strung together in a chain by dehydration synthesis, as simple sugars can. But they can be attached to another compound, **glycerol**

TABLE 2-4	Carbohydrates in the Body		
Structure	*Examples*	*Primary Functions*	*Remarks*
Monosaccharides (simple sugars)	Glucose, fructose	Energy source	Manufactured in the body and obtained from food; found in body fluids
Disaccharides	Sucrose, lactose, maltose	Energy source	Sucrose is table sugar, lactose is present in milk; all must be broken down to monosaccharides before absorption
Polysaccharides	Glycogen	Storage of glucose molecules	Glycogen is found in animal cells; other starches and cellulose in plant cells

TABLE 2-5	Representative Lipids and Their Functions in the Body		
Lipid Type	Examples	Primary Functions	Remarks
Fatty Acids	Lauric acid	Energy sources	Absorbed from food or synthesized in cells; transported in the blood for use in many tissues
Fats	Monoglycerides, diglycerides, triglycerides	Energy source, energy storage, insulation, and physical protection	Stored in fat deposits; must be broken down to fatty acids and glycerol before they can be used as an energy source
Steroids	Cholesterol	Structural component of cell membranes, hormones, digestive secretions in bile	All have the same carbon-ring framework
Phospholipids		Structural components of cell membranes	Composed of fatty acids and nonlipid molecules

(GLI-se-rol), to make a **fat**, through a similar reaction. In a **triglyceride** (trī-GLI-se-rīd), a glycerol molecule is attached to three fatty acids (see Figure 2-11●). Triglycerides, also known as *neutral fats*, are the most common fats in the body. In addition to serving as an energy reserve, fat deposits under the skin serve as insulation, and a mass of fat around a delicate organ, such as a kidney, provides a protective cushion. *Saturated fats,*

triglycerides containing saturated fatty acids, are usually solid at room temperature. *Unsaturated fats,* triglycerides containing unsaturated fatty acids, are usually liquid at room temperature.

Steroids

Steroids are large lipid molecules composed of four connected rings of carbon atoms, quite unlike the linear carbon chains of fatty acids. *Cholesterol* is probably the best-known steroid (Figure 2-12●). All of our cells are surrounded by *cell membranes* that contain cholesterol, and some chemical messengers, or *hormones,* are derived from cholesterol. Examples include the sex hormones testosterone and estrogen.

The cholesterol needed to maintain cell membranes and manufacture steroid hormones comes from two sources. One source is the diet; meat, cream, and egg yolks are especially rich in cholesterol. The second is the body itself, for the liver can synthesize large amounts of cholesterol. The ability of the body to synthesize this steroid can make it difficult to control blood cholesterol levels by dietary restriction alone. This difficulty can have serious repercussions because a strong

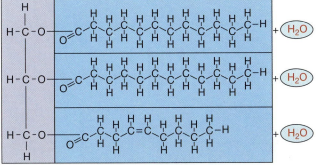

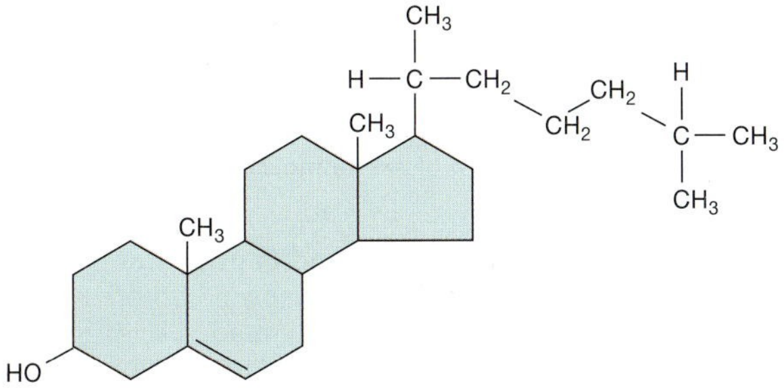

●**FIGURE 2-11   Triglyceride Formation**
The formation of a triglyceride involves the atttachment of three fatty acids to the carbons of a glycerol molecule. This example shows the attachment of one unsaturated and two saturated fatty acids to a glycerol molecule.

●**FIGURE 2-12**
A Cholesterol Molecule
Cholesterol, like all steroids, contains a complex four-ring structure.

2

link exists between high blood cholesterol concentrations and heart disease. Current nutritional advice suggests reducing cholesterol intake to under 300 mg per day; this amount represents a 40 percent reduction for the average American adult. The connection between blood cholesterol levels and heart disease will be examined more closely in Chapters 12 and 13.

Phospholipids

Phospholipids (FOS-fō-lip-ids) consist of a diglyceride attached to a molecule containing a phosphate group (PO_4^{3-}). The nonlipid portion is soluble in water, whereas the fatty acid portion is relatively insoluble. Phospholipids are the most abundant lipid components of cell membranes.

Proteins

Proteins are the most abundant and diverse organic components of the human body. There are roughly 100,000 different kinds of proteins, and they account for about 20 percent of the total body weight. All proteins contain carbon, hydrogen, oxygen, and nitrogen; smaller quantities of sulfur may also be present.

Protein Function

Proteins perform a variety of functions in seven major categories:

1. *Support.* **Structural proteins** create a three-dimensional supporting framework for the body, providing strength, organization, and support for cells, tissues, and organs.

2. *Movement.* **Contractile proteins** are responsible for muscular contraction; related proteins are responsible for the movement of individual cells.

3. *Transport.* Insoluble lipids, respiratory gases, special minerals, such as iron, and several hormones are carried in the blood attached to special **transport proteins**. Other specialized proteins transport materials from one part of a cell to another.

4. *Buffering.* Proteins provide a considerable buffering action, helping to restrict alterations in pH.

5. *Metabolic regulation.* **Enzymes** accelerate chemical reactions in living cells. The sensitivity of enzymes to environmental factors is extremely important in controlling the pace and direction of metabolic operations.

6. *Coordination, communication,* and *control.* Protein hormones can influence the metabolic activities of every cell in the body or affect the function of specific organs or organ systems.

7. *Defense.* The tough, waterproof proteins of the skin, hair, and nails protect the body from environmental hazards. In addition, proteins known as **antibodies** protect us from disease, and special clotting proteins restrict bleeding following an injury to the circulatory system.

Protein Structure

Proteins are chains of small organic molecules called **amino acids**. The human body contains significant quantities of 20 different amino acids. Each amino acid consists of a central carbon atom bonded to a hydrogen atom, an amino group (—NH₂), a carboxylic acid group (—COOH), and a variable R group (Figure 2-13a•). The R group may be a straight chain or a ring of atoms. A typical protein

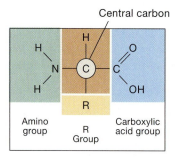

(a) Structure of an amino acid

•**FIGURE 2-13   Amino Acids and Peptide Bonds**
(a) Each amino acid consists of a central carbon atom to which four different groups are attached: a hydrogen atom, an amino group (—NH₂), a carboxylic acid group (—COOH), and a variable group generally designated R.
(b) Peptides form when a dehydration synthesis creates a peptide bond between the carboxyl group of one amino acid and the amino group of another. In this example, glycine and alanine are linked to form a dipeptide.

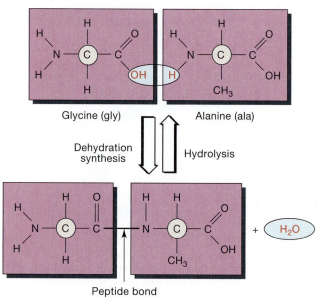

(b) Peptide bond formation

contains 1000 amino acids, but the largest protein complexes may have 100,000 or more. The individual amino acids are strung together like beads on a string, with the carboxylic acid group of one amino acid attached to the amino group of another. This connection is called a **peptide bond** (Figure 2-13b•). If a molecule consists of two amino acids, it is called a *dipeptide*. The chain can be lengthened by the addition of more amino acids. *Polypeptides* are long chains of amino acids. Proteins are polypeptide chains containing over 100 amino acids.

The shape of a short peptide chain primarily depends on interactions between amino acids at different sites along the peptide chain (Figure 2-14a•). Large proteins can have complex three-dimensional shapes. In a *globular protein*, such as *myoglobin*, the peptide chain folds back on itself, creating a rounded mass (Figure 2-14b•). Myoglobin is a protein found in muscle cells. Complex proteins may consist of several protein subunits. Examples are *hemoglobin*, a globular protein found inside red blood cells (Figure 2-13c•), and keratin (Figure 2-13d•), the tough, water-resistant protein found in skin, nails, and hair. Keratin is an example of a *fibrous protein*. In fibrous proteins the polypeptide strands are wound together as in a rope. Fibrous proteins are flexible but very strong.

The shape of a protein determines its functional properties, and the primary determinant of shape is the sequence of amino acids. Combining the 20 amino acids in various ways creates an almost limitless variety of proteins. Small differences can have large effects; changing one amino acid in a protein containing 10,000 or more amino acids may make it incapable of performing its normal function.

The shape of a protein—and thus its function—can be altered by small changes in the ionic composition, temperature, or pH of its surroundings. For example, very high body temperatures (over 43°C, or 110°F) cause death because at these temperatures proteins undergo **denaturation**, a change in their three-dimensional shape. Denatured proteins are nonfunctional, and the loss of structural proteins and enzymes causes irreparable damage to organs and organ systems. You see denaturation in progress each time you fry an egg, because the clear egg white contains abundant dissolved proteins. As the temperature rises, the protein structure changes and eventually the egg proteins form an insoluble white mass.

Enzymes and Chemical Reactions

Most chemical reactions do not occur spontaneously, because they require energy to activate the reactant molecules before a reaction can begin. **Activation energy** is the amount of energy required to start a reaction.

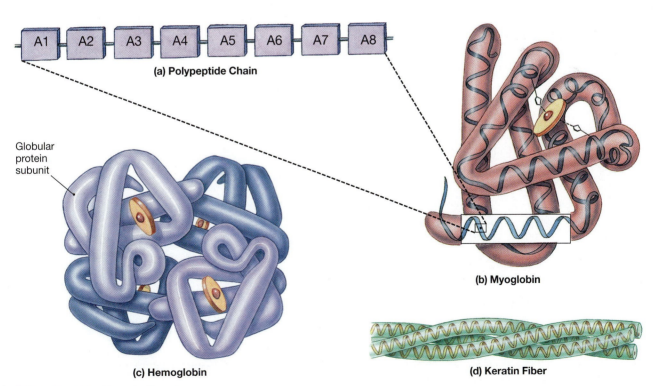

(a) Polypeptide Chain

Globular protein subunit

(b) Myoglobin

(c) Hemoglobin

(d) Keratin Fiber

•**FIGURE 2-14   Protein Structure**
(a) The shape of a polypeptide is determined by its sequence of amino acids. **(b)** Attraction between R groups plays a large role in forming globular proteins. Myoglobin is a globular protein involved in the storage of oxygen in muscle tissue. **(c)** A single hemoglobin molecule contains four globular subunits, each structurally similar to myoglobin. Hemoglobin transports oxygen in the blood. **(d)** In keratin, three fibrous subunits intertwine like the strands of a rope.

2

Figure 2-15a● diagrams the activation energy needed for a typical reaction. Although many reactions can be activated by changes in temperature or pH, such changes are deadly to cells. For example, to break down a complex sugar in the laboratory, you must boil it in an acid solution. Cells, however, avoid such harsh requirements by using special proteins called *enzymes* to speed up the reactions that support life. Enzymes belong to a class of substances called *catalysts* (KAT-ah-lists; *katalysis*, dissolution), compounds that accelerate chemical reactions without themselves being permanently changed. Living cells create specific enzymes to promote vital reactions.

Figure 2-15b● diagrams the effect of an enzyme on the activation energy of a typical reaction. Lowering the activation energy affects only the rate of a reaction, not the direction of the reaction or the products that will be formed. An enzyme cannot bring about a reaction that would otherwise be impossible.

Figure 2-16● shows a simple model of enzyme function. The reactants in an enzymatic reaction, called **substrates**, interact to form a specific **product**. Substrate molecules bind to the enzyme at a particular location called the **active site**. This binding depends on the complementary shapes of the two molecules, much as a key

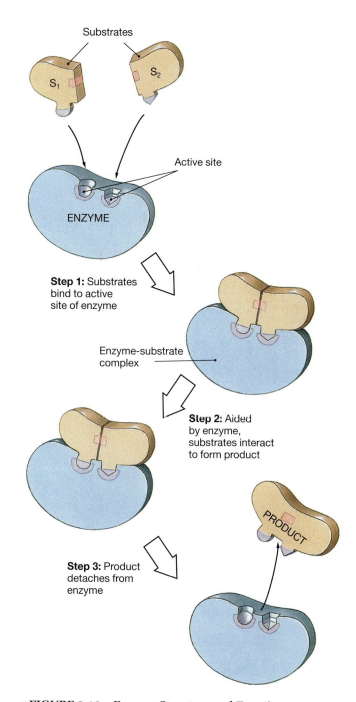

Step 1: Substrates bind to active site of enzyme

Step 2: Aided by enzyme, substrates interact to form product

Step 3: Product detaches from enzyme

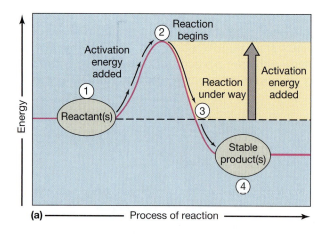

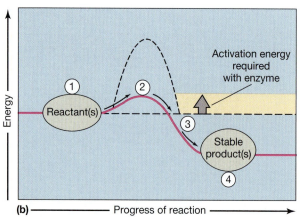

●**FIGURE 2-15   Activation Energy and Enzyme Function**
(a) Before a reaction can begin, considerable activation energy must be provided. In this diagram, the activation energy represents the energy required to proceed from point 1 to point 2. **(b)** The activation energy requirement of the reaction is much lower in the presence of an appropriate enzyme. This allows the reaction to take place much more rapidly, without the need for extreme conditions that would harm cells.

●**FIGURE 2-16   Enzyme Structure and Function**
Each enzyme contains a specific active site on its exposed surface. **Step 1:** A pair of substrate molecules (S_1 and S_2) binds to the active site. **Step 2:** The substrates interact, forming a new product. **Step 3:** The newly formed product detaches from the active site. Because the structure of the enzyme has not been affected, the entire cycle can be repeated.

fits into a lock. The shape of the active site is determined by the three-dimensional shape of the enzyme molecule. Once the reaction is completed and the products are released, the enzyme is free to catalyze another reaction.

Each enzyme works best at an optimal temperature and pH. As temperatures rise or pH shifts outside normal limits, proteins change shape and enzyme function deteriorates.

The complex reactions that support life proceed in a series of interlocking steps, each step controlled by a different enzyme. Such a reaction sequence is called a *metabolic pathway*. We will consider important metabolic pathways in later chapters.

Nucleic Acids

Nucleic (noo-KLĀ-ik) **acids** are large organic molecules composed of carbon, hydrogen, oxygen, nitrogen, and phosphorus. Nucleic acids store and process information at the molecular level inside living cells. There are two classes of nucleic acid molecules: **deoxyribonucleic** (dē-ok-se-rī-bō-noo-KLĀ-ik) **acid**, or **DNA**; and **ribonucleic** (rī-bō-noo-KLĀ-ik) **acid**, or **RNA**.

The DNA in our cells determines our inherited characteristics, such as eye color, hair color, blood

type, and so on. It affects all aspects of body structure and function because DNA molecules encode the information needed to build proteins. By directing the synthesis of structural proteins, DNA controls the shape and physical characteristics of our bodies. By controlling the manufacture of enzymes, DNA regulates not only protein synthesis but all aspects of cellular metabolism, including the creation and destruction of lipids, carbohydrates, and other vital molecules.

Several forms of RNA cooperate to manufacture specific proteins using the information provided by DNA. The functional relationships between DNA and RNA will be detailed in Chapter 3.

Structure of Nucleic Acids

A nucleic acid is made up of **nucleotides**. A single nucleotide has three basic components: a *sugar*, a *phosphate group* (PO_4^{3-}), and a *nitrogenous (nitrogen-containing) base* (Figure 2-17a•). The sugar is always a five-carbon sugar, either **ribose** (in RNA) or **deoxyribose** (in DNA). There are five nitrogenous bases: **adenine (A)**, **guanine (G)**, **cytosine (C)**, **thymine (T)**, and **uracil (U)**. Both RNA and DNA contain adenine, guanine, and cytosine. Uracil is found only in RNA, and thymine only in DNA.

•**FIGURE 2-17**
Nucleic Acids: RNA and DNA

Nucleic acids are long chains of nucleotides. Each molecule starts at the sugar-nitrogenous base of the first nucleotide and ends at the phosphate group of the last member of the chain. **(a)** An RNA molecule consists of a single nucleotide chain. Its shape is determined by the sequence of nucleotides and the interactions between them. **(b)** A DNA molecule consists of a pair of nucleotide chains linked by hydrogen bonding between complementary base pairs. **(c)** A three-dimensional model of a DNA molecule shows the double helix formed by the two DNA strands.

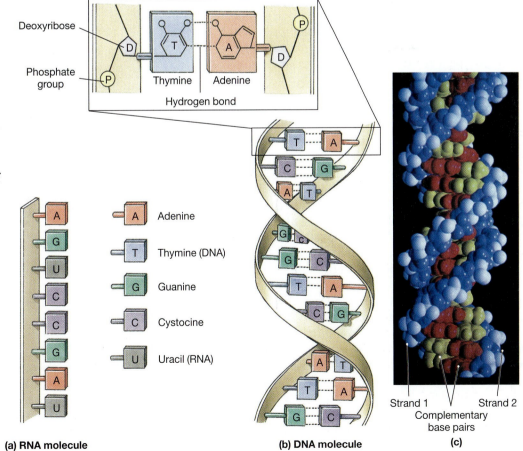

Deoxyribose

Phosphate group

Thymine   Adenine

Hydrogen bond

A Adenine

T Thymine (DNA)

G Guanine

C Cystocine

U Uracil (RNA)

(a) RNA molecule

(b) DNA molecule

Strand 1   Strand 2
Complementary base pairs

(c)

2

TABLE 2-6   **A Comparison of RNA and DNA**

Characteristic	RNA	DNA
Sugar	Ribose	Deoxyribose
Nitrogenous Bases	Adenine	Adenine
	Guanine	Guanine
	Cytosine	Cytosine
	Uracil	Thymine
Number of Nucleotides in a Typical Molecule	Varies from under 100 nucleotides to around 50,000	Always over 45 million nucleotides
Shape of Molecule	Single strand	Paired strands coiled in a double helix
Function	Performs protein synthesis as directed by DNA	Stores genetic information that controls protein synthesis by RNA

Important structural differences between RNA and DNA are listed in Table 2-6. A molecule of RNA consists of a single chain of nucleotides (Figure 2-17a•). A DNA molecule consists of a pair of nucleotide chains held together by weak bonds between the opposing nitrogen bases (Figure 2-17b•). Because of their shapes, adenine can bond only with thymine, and cytosine only with guanine. As a result, adenine-thymine and cytosine-guanine are known as **complementary base pairs**.

The two strands of DNA twist around one another in a **double helix** that resembles a spiral staircase, with the stair steps corresponding to the nitrogen base pairs. Figure 2-17c• presents this three-dimensional view of a DNA molecule.

High-Energy Compounds

Catabolism releases energy, and living cells can use that energy in constructive ways. Part of the energy released by catabolic reactions is captured in the creation of **high-energy bonds**. A high-energy bond is a covalent bond that stores an unusually large amount of energy (as would a tightly wound rubber band attached to the propeller of a model airplane). When that bond is later broken, perhaps in a distant portion of the cell, the energy will be released under controlled conditions (as when the propeller is turned by the unwinding rubber band). In our cells, a high-energy bond usually connects a phosphate group (PO_4^{3-}) to an organic molecule, resulting in a **high-energy compound**. One of the most important high-energy compounds in the body is **adenosine triphosphate**, or **ATP**.

Figure 2-18• details the structure of ATP. Within our cells the conversion of ADP to ATP represents the primary method of energy storage, and the reverse reac-

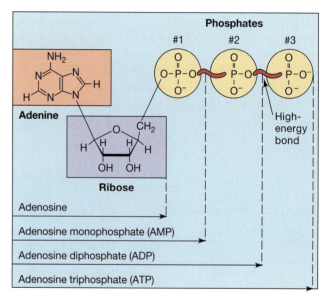

•**FIGURE 2-18   The Structure of ATP**
The ATP molecule is made up of an adenosine (adenine and sugar) molecule to which three phosphate groups have been joined. Both the second and third phosphates are bound to the molecule by high-energy bonds. Cells most often store energy by attaching a third phosphate group to ADP. Removing the phosphate group releases the energy for cellular work, including the synthesis of other molecules.

tion provides a mechanism for controlled energy release. The arrangement can be summarized as:

$$ATP \leftrightarrow ADP + phosphate\ group + energy$$

When energy sources are available, our cells make ATP from ADP and a phosphate group; when energy is required, the reverse reaction occurs.

CHEMICALS AND LIVING CELLS

Figure 2-19• and Table 2-7 review the major chemical components we have discussed in this chapter. But the human body is more than a collection of chemicals. Biochemical building blocks form cells. Each cell behaves like a miniature organism, responding to internal and external stimuli. A lipid membrane separates the cell from its environment, and internal membranes create compartments with specific functions. Proteins form an internal supporting framework and act as enzymes to accelerate and control the chemical reactions that maintain homeostasis. Nucleic acids direct the synthesis of all cellular proteins, including the enzymes that enable the cell to synthesize a wide variety of other substances. Carbohydrates provide energy for vital activities and form part of specialized compounds, in combination with proteins or lipids. The next chapter considers the combination of these compounds within a living, functional cell.

✓ A food contains organic molecules with the elements C, H, and O in a ratio of 1:2:1. What type of compound is this?

✓ Why does boiling a protein affect its structural and functional properties?

✓ How are DNA and RNA similar?

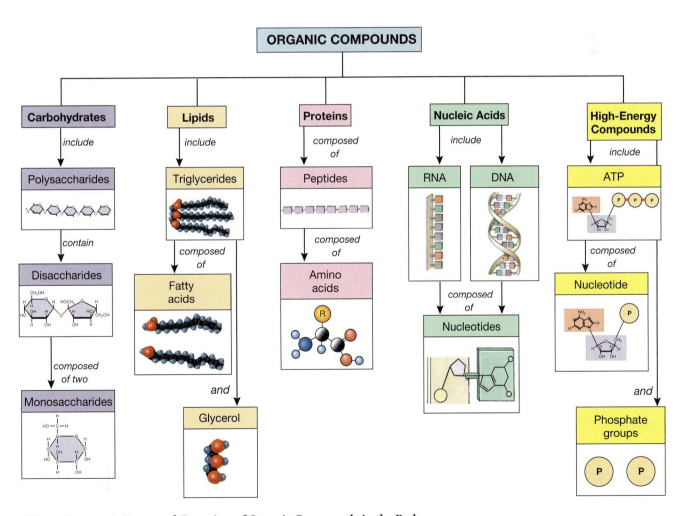

• **FIGURE 2-19   A Structural Overview of Organic Compounds in the Body**
Each of the classes of organic compounds is composed of simple structural subunits. Specific compounds within each class are listed above the basic subunits. Fatty acids are the main subunits of all lipids except steroids, such as cholesterol; only one type of lipid, the triglyceride, is represented here.

| TABLE 2-7 | The Structure and Function of Biologically Important Compounds | | |

Class	Building Blocks	Sources	Functions
INORGANIC **Water**	Hydrogen and oxygen atoms	Absorbed as liquid water or generated via metabolism	Solvent; transport medium for dissolved materials and heat; cooling through evaporation; medium for chemical reactions; reactant in hydrolysis
Acids, bases, salts	H^+, OH^-, various anions and cations	Obtained from the diet or generated via metabolism	Structural components; buffers; sources of ions
Dissolved gases	Oxygen, carbon, nitrogen, and other atoms	Atmosphere	O_2 required for normal cellular metabolism CO_2 generated by cells as a waste product
ORGANIC **Carbohydrates**	C, H, and O; CHO in a 1:2:1 ratio	Obtained in diet or manufactured in the body	Energy source; some structural role when attached to lipids or proteins; energy storage
Lipids	C, H, O, sometimes N or P; CHO not in 1:2:1 ratio	Obtained in diet or manufactured in the body	Energy source; energy storage; insulation; structural components; chemical messengers; physical protection
Proteins	C, H, O, N, often S	20 common amino acids; roughly half can be manufactured in the body, others must be obtained in the diet	Catalysts for metabolic reactions; structural components; movement; transport; buffers; defense; control and coordination of activities
Nucleic acids	C, H, O, N, and P; nucleotides composed of phosphates, sugars, and nitrogenous bases	Obtained in diet or manufactured	Storage and processing of genetic information
High-energy compounds	Nucleotides joined to phosphates by high-energy bonds	Synthesized by all cells	Storage or transfer of energy

Chapter Review
KEY TERMS

atom, p. 30	**electron**, p. 30	**metabolism**, p. 34
buffer, p. 37	**element**, p. 30	**molecule**, p. 31
carbohydrate, p. 39	**enzyme**, p. 42	**neutron**, p. 30
covalent bond, p. 32	**ion**, p. 32	**nucleic acid**, p. 45
decomposition reaction, p. 35	**isotope**, p. 31	**protein**, p. 42
electrolytes, p. 38	**lipid**, p. 39	**proton**, p. 30

SUMMARY OUTLINE

INTRODUCTION *p. 30*

ATOMS AND MOLECULES *p. 30*

1. Atoms are the smallest units of matter; they consist of **protons**, **neutrons**, and **electrons**. *(Figure 2-1)*

The Structure of an Atom *p. 30*

2. An **element** consists entirely of atoms with the same number of protons (**atomic number**). Within an atom, an **electron cloud** surrounds the nucleus. *(Figure 2-2; Table 2-1)*

3. The atomic mass of an atom is equal to the total number of protons and neutrons in its nucleus. **Isotopes** are atoms of the same element whose nuclei contain different numbers of neutrons. The **atomic weight** of an element takes into account the abundance of its various isotopes.

4. Electrons occupy a series of **electron shells** around the nucleus. The number of electrons in the outermost electron shell determine an atom's chemical properties. *(Figure 2-3)*

Chemical Bonds and Chemical Compounds *p. 31*

5. An **ionic bond** results from the attraction between **ions**: atoms that have gained or lost electrons. **Cations** are positively charged, and **anions** are negatively charged. *(Figure 2-4; Table 2-2)*

6. Atoms can combine to form a **molecule**; combinations of atoms of different elements form a **compound**. Some atoms share electrons to form a molecule held together by **covalent bonds**.

7. Sharing one pair of electrons creates a single covalent bond; sharing two pairs forms a **double covalent bond**. An unequal sharing of electrons creates a **polar covalent bond**. *(Figure 2-5)*

8. A **hydrogen bond** is the attraction between a hydrogen atom with a slight positive charge and a negatively charged atom in another molecule or within the same molecule. Hydrogen bonds can affect the shapes and properties of molecules. *(Figure 2-6)*

CHEMICAL NOTATION *p. 34*

1. Chemical notation allows us to describe reactions between reactants that generate one or more products. *(Table 2-3)*

CHEMICAL REACTIONS *p. 34*

1. Metabolism refers to all the **chemical reaction**s in the body. Our cells capture, store, and use energy to maintain homeostasis and support essential functions.

Basic Energy Concepts *p. 34*

2. Work involves movement of an object or a change in its physical structure, and **energy** is the capacity to perform work. There are two major types of energy: kinetic and potential.

3. Kinetic energy is the energy of motion. **Potential energy** is stored energy that results from the position or structure of an object. Conversions from potential to kinetic energy are not 100 percent efficient; every energy exchange produces **heat**.

Classes of Reactions *p. 35*

4. A chemical reaction may be classified as a **decomposition**, **synthesis**, or **exchange reaction**. **Exergonic** reactions release heat; **endergonic** reactions absorb heat.

5. Cells gain energy to power their functions by breaking down organic molecules, a process called **catabolism**. Much of this energy supports **anabolism**, the synthesis of new organic molecules.

Reversible Reactions *p. 36*

6. Reversible reactions consist of simultaneous synthesis and decomposition reactions. At **equilibrium** the rates of these two opposing reactions are in balance.

Acids and Bases *p. 36*

7. An **acid** releases hydrogen ions, and a **base** removes hydrogen ions from a solution.

pH *p. 36*

8. The **pH** of a solution indicates the concentration of hydrogen ions it contains. Solutions can be classified as neutral (pH = 7), acidic (pH < 7), or basic (alkaline) (pH > 7) on the basis of pH. *(Figure 2-7)*

9. Buffers maintain pH within normal limits (7.35–7.45 in most body fluids) by releasing or absorbing hydrogen ions.

10. Nutrients and metabolites can be broadly classified as organic (carbon-based) or inorganic.

INORGANIC COMPOUNDS *p. 37*
Carbon Dioxide and Oxygen *p. 37*

1. Living cells in the body generate carbon dioxide and consume oxygen.

Water and Its Properties p. *37*

2. Water is the most important inorganic component of the body.

3. Water is an excellent solvent, has a high heat capacity, and participates in the metabolic reactions of the body.

4. Many inorganic compounds will undergo **ionization**, or *dissociation*, in water to form ions. *(Figure 2-8)*

Inorganic Acids and Bases *p. 38*

5. Inorganic acids found in the body include hydrochloric acid, carbonic acid, sulfuric acid, and phosphoric acid. Sodium hydroxide is an inorganic base that may form within the body.

Salts *p. 38*

6. A **salt** is an inorganic compound whose cation is not H^+, and whose anion is not OH^-. Salts are **electrolytes**, compounds that dissociate in water and conduct an electrical current.

ORGANIC COMPOUNDS *p. 38*

1. Organic compounds contain carbon and hydrogen, and usually oxygen as well. Large and complex organic molecules include carbohydrates, lipids, proteins, and nucleic acids.

Carbohydrates *p. 39*

2. Carbohydrates are most important as an energy source for metabolic processes. The three major types are **monosaccharides** (simple sugars), **disaccharides**, and **polysaccharides**. *(Figures 2-9, 2-10; Table 2-4)*

Lipids *p. 39*

3. Lipids are water-insoluble molecules that include fats, oils, and waxes. There are four important classes of lipids: **fatty acids**, **fats**, **steroids**, and **phospholipids**. *(Table 2-5)*

2

4. Triglycerides (neutral fats) consist of three fatty acid molecules attached to a molecule of **glycerol**. *(Figure 2-11)*

5. *Cholesterol* is a precursor of steroid hormones and is an important component of cell membranes. *(Figure 2-12)*

Proteins *p. 42*

6. Proteins perform a great variety of functions in the body. Important types of proteins include **structural proteins, contractile proteins, transport proteins, enzymes,** hormones, and **antibodies.**

7. Proteins are chains of **amino acids** linked by **peptide bonds**. The sequence of amino acids and the interactions of their R groups influence the final shape of the protein molecule. *(Figures 2-13, 2-14)*

8. The shape of a protein determines its functional characteristics. Each protein works best at an optimal combination of temperature and pH.

9. Activation energy is the amount of energy required to start a reaction. Proteins called **enzymes** control many chemical reactions within our bodies. Enzymes are organic *catalysts*—substances that accelerate chemical reactions without themselves being permanently changed. *(Figure 2-15)*

10. The reactants in an enzymatic reaction, called **substrates**, interact to form a **product** by binding to the enzyme at the **active site**. *(Figure 2-16)*

Nucleic Acids *p. 45*

11. Nucleic acids store and process information at the molecular level. There are two kinds of nucleic acids: **deoxyribonucleic acid (DNA)** and **ribonucleic acid (RNA)**. *(Figure 2-17; Table 2-6)*

12. Nucleic acids are chains of nucleotides. Each nucleotide contains a sugar, a **phosphate group**, and a **nitrogenous base**. The sugar is always **ribose** or **deoxyribose**. The nitrogenous bases found in DNA are **adenine, guanine, cytosine,** and **thymine**. In RNA, **uracil** replaces thymine.

High-Energy Compounds *p. 46*

13. Cells store energy in **high-energy compounds**. The most important high-energy compound is **ATP (adenosine triphosphate)**. When energy is available, cells make ATP by adding a phosphate group to ADP. When energy is needed, ATP is broken down to ADP and phosphate. *(Figure 2-18)*

CHEMICALS AND LIVING CELLS *p. 47*

14. Biochemical building blocks form cells. *(Figure 2-19; Table 2-7)*

REVIEW QUESTIONS

LEVEL 1   Reviewing Facts and Terms

Match each item in column A with the most closely related item in column B. Use letters for answers in the spaces provided.

Column A

___ 1.   atomic number

___ 2.   covalent bond

___ 3.   ionic bond

___ 4.   catabolism

___ 5.   anabolism

___ 6.   exchange reaction

___ 7.   reversible reaction

___ 8.   acid

___ 9.   enzyme

___10.   buffer

___11.   organic compounds

___12.   inorganic compounds

Column B

a.   synthesis

b.   catalyst

c.   sharing of electrons

d. $A + B \longleftrightarrow AB$

e.   stabilize pH

f.   number of protons

g.   decomposition

h.   carbohydrates, lipids, proteins

i.   loss or gain of electrons

j.   water, salts

k. H^+ donor

l. $AB + CD \rightarrow AD + CB$

13. In atoms, protons and neutrons are found:
   (a) only in the nucleus
   (b) outside the nucleus
   (c) inside and outside the nucleus
   (d) in the electron cloud

14. The number and arrangement of electrons in an atom's outer electron shell determines its:
   (a) atomic weight
   (b) atomic number
   (c) electrical properties
   (d) chemical properties

15. The bond between sodium and chlorine in the compound sodium chloride (NaCl) is:
   (a) an ionic bond
   (b) a single covalent bond
   (c) a nonpolar covalent
   (d) a double covalent bondbond

16. What is the role of enzymes in chemical reactions?

17. List six elements found in abundance in the body.

18. What four major classes of organic compounds are found in the body?

19. List seven major functions performed by proteins.

LEVEL 2 Reviewing Concepts

20. Oxygen has 8 protons, 8 neutrons, and 8 electrons. What is the molecular weight of O_2?
    (a) 8
    (b) 16
    (c) 24
    (d) 32

21. Of the following selections, the one that contains only inorganic compounds is:
    (a) water, electrolytes, oxygen, carbon dioxide
    (b) oxygen, carbon dioxide, water, sugars
    (c) water, electrolytes, salts, nucleic acids
    (d) carbohydrates, lipids, proteins, vitamins

22. Glucose and fructose are examples of:
    (a) monosaccharides (simple sugars)
    (b) isotopes
    (c) lipids
    (d) a, b, and c are all correct

23. Explain the differences among (1) nonpolar covalent bonds, (2) polar covalent bonds, and (3) ionic bonds.

24. Why does pure water have a neutral pH?

25. A biologist analyzes a sample that contains an organic molecule and finds the following constituents: carbon, hydrogen, oxygen, nitrogen, and phosphorus. On the basis of this information, is the molecule a carbohydrate, a lipid, a protein, or a nucleic acid?

LEVEL 3 Critical Thinking and Clinical Applications

26. The element sulfur has an atomic number of 16 and an atomic weight of 32. How many neutrons are in the nucleus of a sulfur atom? Assuming that sulfur forms covalent bonds with hydrogen, how many hydrogen atoms could bond to one sulfur atom?

27. An important buffer system in the human body involves carbon dioxide (CO_2) and bicarbonate ions (HCO_3^-) as shown:

$$CO_2 + H_2O \longleftrightarrow H_2CO_3 \longleftrightarrow H^+ + HCO_3^-$$

If a person becomes excited and exhales large amounts of CO_2, how will his body's pH be affected?

ANSWERS TO CONCEPT CHECK QUESTIONS

Page 34
1. Atoms combine with each other so as to gain a complete set of eight electrons in their outer energy levels. Oxygen atoms do not have a full outer energy level and so will readily react with many other elements to attain this stable arrangement. Neon already has a full outer energy level and thus has little tendency to combine with other elements. **2.** Hydrogen can exist as three different isotopes: hydrogen-1, with a mass of 1; deuterium, with a mass of 2; and tritium, with a mass of 3. The heavier sample must contain a higher proportion of one or both of the heavier isotopes. **3.** A water molecule is formed by polar covalent bonds. Water molecules are attracted to one another by hydrogen bonds.

Page 36
1. Since this reaction involves a large molecule being broken down into two smaller ones, it is a decomposition reaction. Because energy is released in the process, the reaction can also be classified as exergonic. **2.** Removing the product of a reversible reaction would keep its concentration low compared with the concentration of the reactants. Thus the formation of product molecules would continue, but the reverse reaction would slow down, resulting in a shift in the equilibrium toward the product.

Page 37
1. An acid is a solute that releases H^+ ions in a solution; a base is a solute that removes H^+ from a solution. **2.** The normal pH range of body fluids is 7.35 to 7.45. Fluctuations in pH outside this range can break chemical bonds, alter the shape of molecules, and affect the functioning of cells, thereby harming cells and tissues. **3.** Stomach discomfort is often the result of excess stomach acidity ("acid indigestion"). Antacids contain a weak base that neutralizes the excessive acid.

Page 47
1. A C:H:O ratio of 1:2:1 would indicate that the molecule is a carbohydrate. The body uses carbohydrates chiefly as an energy source. **2.** The heat of boiling will break bonds that maintain the protein's tertiary structure, quaternary structure, or both. The resulting change in shape will affect the ability of the protein molecule to perform its normal biological functions. These alterations are known as denaturation. **3.** DNA and RNA are nucleic acids. Both are composed of sequences of nucleotides. Each nucleotide consists of a five-carbon sugar, a phosphate group (PO_4^{3-}), and a nitrogenous base.

2 Emergency Care Applications

OVERVIEW

The most fundamental components of any living organism are the various chemical compounds that form the basis for all physiological processes. The study of chemicals in a living organism is *biochemistry*. Scientists who study the various chemical processes of the body are *biochemists*. The chemistry of a living organism is exceedingly complex, and many biochemical processes are not completely understood.

The practice of medicine often involves detecting and treating problems or aberrations in the body's various biochemical processes. Because of this, medical personnel must have a good understanding of the major biochemical processes of the human body. In emergency medicine, time is often of the essence, and emergency personnel do not have time to consider all of the various biochemical processes involved in the problem at hand. However, there are several important chemical considerations in treating patients who are critically ill or injured. Among the more important of these is the body's acid-base balance, or pH. The pH must be maintained within very strict tolerances. An increase in acidity or alkalinity can worsen virtually any medical condition. Thus, it is essential that emergency personnel understand the complex issues involved in maintaining the body's acid-base balance.

Emergency treatment of many conditions involves the administration of medications. Medications are simply chemicals that modify or correct a biochemical abnormality. They exist in various chemical states, and emergency personnel must be familiar with the characteristics of each. Monitoring the amounts in the body of essential chemicals, such as oxygen and carbon dioxide, is now standard in emergency medical care. Because of this, it is important to understand the chemistry and technology behind these monitoring devices.

UNDERSTANDING PH

Acid-base balance is a dynamic relationship that reflects the relative concentration of hydrogen ions (H^+) in the body. Hydrogen ions are acidic, and their concentration must be maintained within fairly strict limits. Any deviation in the hydrogen ion concentration adversely affects all of the biochemical events in the body. Because of this, determination of the body's hydrogen ion concentration is important in emergency care.

Water molecules have a slight tendency to undergo reversible ionization to yield a *hydrogen ion (H^+)* and a *hydroxide ion (OH^-)* to form the following equilibrium:

$$H_2O \rightleftharpoons H^+ + OH^-$$

The ionization of water is very weak. In fact, only 1 out of every 10 million molecules of water is ionized at any given moment. Although water has only a very slight tendency to ionize, the products of ionization (H^+ and OH^-) have profound biological effects. The number of hydrogen ions and hydroxide ions in an aqueous (water) solution at 25° C (77° F) always equals the fixed number 1.0×10^{-14} M. When the concentrations of both hydrogen ions and hydroxide ions are exactly equal, as in pure water, the solution is said to be *neutral*. When neutral, the number of hydrogen ions equals 1.0×10^{-7} M and the number of hydroxide ions equals 1.0×10^{-7} M. Because of this, we know that when the number of hydrogen ions present is very high, then the concentration of hydroxide ions must be very low. Likewise, when the concentration of hydroxide ions is high, then the concentration of hydrogen ions must be low. Again, regardless of the balance between hydrogen ions and hydroxide ions, the total number of ions must be 1.0×10^{-14} M.

The need for a much simpler system of describing hydrogen ion concentrations quickly became evident. In 1909 the Swedish chemist H.P.L.Sørenson proposed that the hydrogen ion concentration be expressed in terms of the logarithm (log) of the reciprocal of the number. This system allows simple numbers to represent extremely large numbers of hydrogen

WHAT IS A LOGARITHM?

A *logarithm,* in mathematics, is the *exponent,* or *power,* to which a stated number, called the *base,* must be raised to yield a specific number. For example, in the expression $10^2 = 100$, the logarithm of 100 to the base 10 is 2. This is properly written as $\log_{10} 100 = 2$. Logarithms were initially created to help simplify arithmetical operations involving very large numbers. *Common logarithms* use the number 10 as the base number. However, logarithms can be used with base numbers other than 10. This can be illustrated by considering a sequence of powers to the number 2: 2^1, 2^2, 2^3, 2^4, 2^5, and 2^6, corresponding to the sequence of numbers 2, 4, 8, 16, 32, and 64. The exponents 1, 2, 3, 4, 5, and 6 are the logarithms of these numbers to the base 2.

In medicine, logarithms are used to describe chemical concentrations. Unless specified otherwise, always assume that a logarithm is in base 10 ($\log_{10}$). If another logarithm is being used, it will be specified in the notation (e.g., $\log_5$). The most frequent use of logarithms in medicine is in the pH system that describes the hydrogen ion concentration of a solution. In pure water, the hydrogen ion concentration is equal to 0.0000001, or 10^{-7}, moles per liter. Because the pH scale describes the reciprocal of the hydrogen ion concentration, the numbers are positive even though the concentration of hydrogen ions is less than 1. This simplifies discussion and calculations. Thus, a pH of 3.0 reflects a hydrogen ion concentration of 0.001, or 10^{-3} moles per liter. Likewise, a pH of 10 reflects a hydrogen ion concentration of 0.0000000001, or 10^{-10} moles per liter. A change in pH of 1 unit reflects a tenfold change in hydrogen ion concentration. Likewise, a change of 2 pH units indicates a hundredfold change in hydrogen ion concentration. Thus, the use of logarithms simplifies descriptions and calculations of these extremely large or small numbers.

ions. The system was called the pH system, which is an abbreviation for *potential of hydrogen.* Because of the large numbers involved, the use of logarithms simplifies discussion of hydrogen ion concentrations. It is important to remember that the pH system represents the reciprocal of the hydrogen ion concentration. Thus, the greater the number of hydrogen ions, the lower the pH. Conversely, the fewer the number of hydrogen ions, the higher the pH. The pH scale can be defined as:

$$pH = \log 1/[H^+]$$

Because the logarithm of 1 is 0, then the equation can be simplified as:

$$pH = -\log [H^+]$$

In a precisely neutral solution at 25° C (77° F), where the hydrogen ion concentration equals 1.0×10^{-7} M, the pH would be calculated as:

$$pH = \log 1/1.0 \times 10^{-7} = \log (1.0 \times 10^{-7}) = \log 1.0 + \log 10^7$$

$$pH = 0 + 7$$

$$pH = 7$$

TABLE A2-1 The pH Scale

Acidic Concentrations $[H^+]$, Moles	pH	Alkaline Concentrations $[OH]$, Moles	POH
1.0	0	10^{-14}	14
0.1	1	10^{-13}	13
0.01	2	10^{-12}	12
0.001	3	10^{-11}	11
10^{-4}	4	10^{-10}	10
10^{-5}	5	10^{-9}	9
10^{-6}	6	10^{-8}	8
10^{-7}	7	10^{-7}	7
10^{-8}	8	10^{-6}	6
10^{-9}	9	10^{-5}	5
10^{-10}	10	10^{-4}	4
10^{-11}	11	0.001	3
10^{-12}	12	0.01	2
10^{-13}	13	0.1	1
10^{-14}	14	1.0	0

Remember, the value of 7.0 for the pH of a precisely neutral solution is not an arbitrary number but is derived from the absolute value of the hydrogen ion concentration at 25° C. The pH scale varies from 0 to 14. A pH of 14 indicates that only hydroxide ions are present, while a pH of 0 indicates that only hydrogen ions are present.

Any pH greater than 7.0 is considered *alkaline* while any pH less than 7.0 is considered *acidic.* It is also important to note that the pH scale is logarithmic, not arithmetic. For example, if two solutions differ in pH by 1 pH unit, then one solution has 10 times the hydrogen ion concentration of the other. Thus, small changes in pH reflect massive changes in the number of hydrogen ions present.

Occasionally, the *pOH* is used to denote the alkalinity of a solution. pOH is similar to pH, except it represents the number of hydroxide ions present, not hydrogen ions (Table A2-1). It is helpful to remember that pH and pOH are related to each other in a very simple way:

$$pH + pOH = 14$$

The pH of the body is closely regulated between 7.35 and 7.45. Thus, alkalosis is a pH greater than 7.45, while acidosis is a pH of less than 7.35. Small changes in pH are corrected by the body's compensatory mechanisms, but significant changes are poorly tolerated. In fact, a change in pH of 0.5 units can be fatal.

In medical practice, the pH values of blood and urine are measured most frequently. Blood pH is obtained through an arterial blood gas (ABG) sample. For this, a small amount of arterial blood is removed from the radial, brachial, or femoral artery. This is quickly introduced into a blood gas machine where the pH is carefully measured. In the blood gas machine, a special glass electrode selectively measures hydrogen ion concentration. The signal from this electrode is amplified and compared with the signal generated by a control solution having a known pH. Based on this comparison, the pH can be determined. Because of this, it is important that ABG machines be carefully maintained and calibrated with the control solutions checked on a daily basis. In addition to pH, an ABG analysis measures the partial pressure of oxygen and carbon dioxide in the blood. Also, some machines will measure the bicarbonate concentration and the amount of hemoglobin present. A more detailed discussion of acid-base balance and the body's compensatory buffering mechanisms is presented in Chapter 19.

PHYSICAL PROPERTIES OF EMERGENCY MEDICATIONS

Many medications are used in prehospital care. Unlike in the hospital setting, medications used in the field are often exposed to environmental factors. In most cases, this rarely constitutes a problem. However, some medications are affected by environmental factors. Because of this, prehospital personnel must be familiar with the physical properties of the medications they use. Also, knowledge of the physical properties of prehospital medications helps in understanding their mechanism of action.

The three states of matter are *solid, liquid,* or *gas.* Two major factors affect the physical state of matter. The first factor is the intensity of the intermolecular forces of all kinds: solids have the strongest forces while gases have the weakest. The other factor is *temperature.* As the temperature rises, a substance will go from a solid to a liquid and then to a gaseous state.

As the material passes through these three phases from solid to liquid to gas, it absorbs heat, and its *enthalpy,* or heat content, increases. Thus, the enthalpy of a liquid is greater than that of its solid, and the enthalpy of a gas is greater than that of its liquid, because heat is absorbed during melting and vaporization. The temperature at which a solid becomes a liquid is its *melting point.* The temperature at which a liquid becomes a gas is its *boiling point.* However, prior to reaching the boiling point, some liquids will begin to convert to the gaseous state through *evaporation.* Chemicals vary in their tendency to change physical states. The tendency to assume the gaseous state is *volatility.* Chemicals with high volatility rapidly evaporate and assume the gaseous state, while chemicals with low volatility tend to remain in the liquid state.

Most medications used in prehospital care are in a liquid state. This allows the medication to be administered into the body without having to be absorbed by the gastrointestinal tract. The boiling point and the freezing point of most emergency medicines will not be encountered in routine usage. However, some medications pose

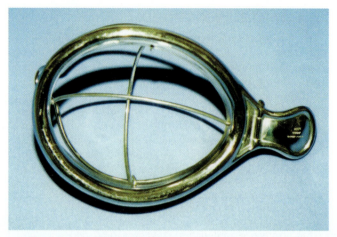

• **FIGURE A2-1   Ether Mask Used to Administer Ether as an Anesthetic Agent**
A cloth was placed in the frame and volatile ether was dripped onto the cloth for inhalation by the patient.

problems. For example, the medication mannitol is occasionally used in prehospital care to treat increased intracranial pressure, acute glaucoma, and blood transfusion reactions. Mannitol is a sugar and is used as an osmotic diuretic. It is supplied in liquid form in vials that contain a 20 percent solution. At temperatures less than 10° C (50° F), mannitol will begin to crystallize. Initially, these crystals cannot be seen by the naked eye. If the temperature of the drug drops below 5° C (40° F), the entire vial will crystallize as the drug changes to the solid state. The higher the concentration of mannitol, the greater its tendency to crystallize. Because of this, mannitol should always be administered through a filter to prevent any crystals, including microscopic crystals, from entering the patient's circulation. Remelting mannitol with boiling water or in a microwave oven can potentially damage the drug and should not be attempted. Mannitol, like all EMS medications, should be maintained at the appropriate temperature.

The volatility of certain drugs is important in emergency care. For example, the general anesthetic agents are highly volatile, which allows their rapid delivery to patients. For example, the initial prototype anesthetic, ether, is highly volatile. In early anesthetic practice, it was dripped slowly into an ether mask and the patient inhaled the drug, resulting in anesthesia (Figure A2-1•). However, because ether is extremely flammable and hazardous to surgical personnel, it is rarely used in modern medicine.

A commonly used anesthetic agent in modern medicine is *methoxyflurane (Pentrane).* In high doses, methoxyflurane is a general anesthetic, and in lower doses, it is an extremely effective analgesic agent. Although not approved for prehospital use in the United States, methoxyflurane is frequently used throughout Australian EMS as an analgesic agent. At room temper-

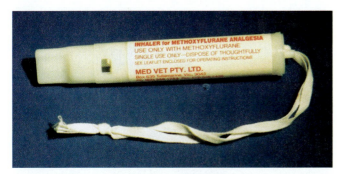

• FIGURE A2-2 Penthrane (methoxyflurane) Inhaler Used in Australia for Analgesia
Methoxyflurane, a volatile anesthetic and analgesic agent, is placed onto a wick in the device. The patient inhales through the mouthpiece. Supplemental oxygen can be provided.

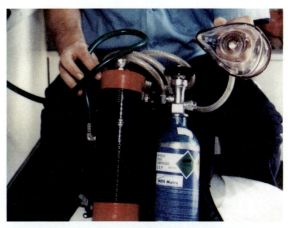

• FIGURE A2-3   Nitrous Oxide/Oxygen (Nitronox) System Used in United States Prehospital Care
Separate cylinders provide the gas to a blender, where it is mixed and delivered to the patient.

ature, methoxyflurane is a liquid; however, it is highly volatile and rapidly evaporates. For analgesia, 3 to 6 milliliters of a 0.5 percent solution of methoxyflurane are placed on the absorbent wick of a methoxyflurane (Penthrane) inhaler (Figure A2-2•). The inhaler is then handed to the patient, who breathes in and out through the mouthpiece. The onset of analgesia is rapid, and the effects of the drug quickly dissipate when removed. Because of this, it can be used in trauma, obstetrics, and other types of acute pain. A port on the methoxyflurane inhaler allows supplemental oxygen if required.

Nitrous oxide is another general anesthetic agent that has analgesic properties at lower concentrations. It is frequently used in the United States, Canada, and the United Kingdom for rapid analgesia. Because nitrous oxide can be an asphyxiant when used alone, it must always be administered with oxygen. Anesthesia is obtained when the level of nitrous oxide approaches 70 percent. Analgesia is obtained at a concentration of approximately 50 percent. In the United States, nitrous oxide and oxygen are administered from different cylinders. These gases are fed into a blender that mixes the correct 50 percent nitrous oxide/50 percent oxygen mixture (Figure A2-3•). If the level of oxygen falls below 50 percent, then the unit shuts down. Unfortunately, requiring separate oxygen and nitrous oxide cylinders makes the unit much heavier, bulkier, and harder to use in emergency care. In the Commonwealth countries, premixing nitrous oxide and oxygen into one cylinder is allowed (Entonox, Dolonox). This system is less bulky, less expensive, and easier to use in prehospital care.

One physical property of nitrous oxide affects its use in prehospital care. Nitrous oxide exists as a gas over liquid in pressurized steel containers at room temperature. However, at approximately -3.3° C (26° F), nitrous oxide returns to its liquid form. When this occurs, drug deliv-

ery ceases until the cylinder is warmed. Occasionally, inverting the cylinder two or three times may free enough gas to complete patient care. In the U.S. system (Nitronox), when nitrous oxide delivery ceases, the device allows the continued flow of pure oxygen. In the single-cylinder system, when the nitrous oxide liquefies, the mixture separates, and the gaseous oxygen occupies the top of the cylinder while the liquid nitrous oxide occupies the bottom of the cylinder. Administration of nitrous oxide through the single cylinder system in cold environments can cause decreased concentrations of the drug as it liquefies and leaves the mixture. Gentle rewarming of the cylinder at 20° C (68° F) and completely inverting the cylinder will restore the mixture.

BLOOD GASES

Oximetry

The measurement of oxygen levels in the body through *pulse oximetry* has become commonplace in emergency medicine. In fact, the oxygen saturation level, as determined through pulse oximetry, is often referred to as the "fifth vital sign." A pulse oximeter measures the hemoglobin oxygen saturation in peripheral tissues. It is noninvasive, rapidly applied, and easy to operate. Pulse oximetry readings are accurate and continually reflect any changes in peripheral oxygen delivery. In fact, oximetry often detects problems with oxygenation faster than standard physical assessment techniques.

Approximately 98 percent of oxygen is transported to the peripheral tissues bound to hemoglobin. Only 2 percent of oxygen is transported dissolved in the plasma. Normally, there is a fixed relationship between the partial pressure of oxygen and hemoglobin saturation.

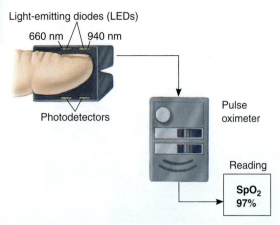

• FIGURE A2-4   Pulse Oximetry
Oxygen saturation can be determined by measuring the amounts of light absorbed by oxyhemoglobin and by reduced hemoglobin and then calculating the difference.

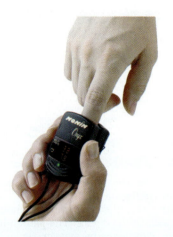

• FIGURE A2-5   Pulse Oximeter
Pulse-oximeter technology now allows accurate measurements of SpO_2 levels with devices smaller than a matchbox.

However, in certain disease processes, this relationship can be impaired. Pulse oximetry measures only the oxygen bound to hemoglobin.

Peripheral oxygen saturation is measured by placing a probe on a peripheral capillary bed such as the fingertip, toe, or earlobe. In infants, the sensor can be placed on the heel of the foot and secured with tape. The sensor contains two light-emitting diodes (LEDs) and two sensors (photodetectors). One LED emits light at 660 nm (red) and the other emits light at 940 nm (infrared). Photodetectors placed on the opposite side of a capillary bed (such as a fingertip) detect the amount of light transmitted through the capillary bed. The two wavelengths were chosen because one is absorbed by *oxyhemoglobin (hemoglobin with oxygen bound)* and the other is absorbed by *reduced hemoglobin (hemoglobin without oxygen bound).* The amount of light absorbed by these substances is constant with time and does not vary during the cardiac cycle. A small increase in arterial blood flow occurs with each heartbeat, resulting in increased light absorption. By comparing the ratio of pulsatile and baseline absorption of light at these two wavelengths, the ratio of oxyhemoglobin to reduced hemoglobin can be calculated (Figure A2-4•). This figure is the *oxygen-saturation percentage* or (SpO_2).

Pulse oximeters display the SpO_2 and the pulse rate as detected by the sensors. They show the SpO_2 either as a number or as a visual display that also shows the pulse's waveform. The relationship between the SpO_2 and the PaO_2 is very complex. However, the SpO_2 generally correlates with the PaO_2. The greater the PaO_2, the greater will be the oxygen saturation. Since hemoglobin carries 98 percent of oxygen in the blood while plasma carries only 2 percent, pulse oximetry accurately analyzes peripheral oxygen delivery (Figure A2-5•).

False readings with pulse oximetry are infrequent. When they do occur, the oximeter often generates an error signal or a blank screen. Causes of false readings include carbon monoxide poisoning, high-intensity lighting, and certain hemoglobin abnormalities. Nail polish, in certain cases, can interfere with oximetry function. This is particularly problematic with blue nail polish, which absorbs light at 960 nm, close to the wavelengths monitored by the oximeter. The absence of a pulse in an extremity also will cause a false reading. In hypovolemia and in severely anemic patients, the pulse oximetry reading can be misleading. While the SpO_2 reading may be normal, the total amount of hemoglobin available to carry oxygen may be so markedly decreased that the patient will remain hypoxic at the cellular level.

Capnography

Determining carbon dioxide (CO_2) levels has become a routine part of emergency care. CO_2 is the final product of the body's many biochemical processes and is eliminated by the respiratory system. The level of carbon dioxide in the blood can be determined with an arterial blood gas sample in the hospital setting, but this is unavailable in the prehospital environment. The two types of devices used to detect CO_2 levels in prehospital care are capnometers and end-tidal CO_2 ($ETCO_2$) detectors.

Continuous monitoring of exhaled CO_2 is possible with a capnometer. For this, the sensor is placed in-line with the endotracheal tube and bag-valve-mask unit. The sensor contains an infrared source and a photodetector. The presence of CO_2 affects the amount of infrared light that reaches the photodetector, allowing an accurate determination of exhaled CO_2 levels. Normally, the concentration of exhaled CO_2 is 5–6 percent (35–45 mm Hg). A fall in this level indicates a possible problem with perfusion or ventilation. In many critical care settings, and in the operating room,

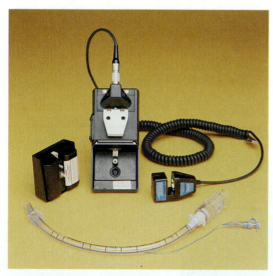

• **FIGURE A2-6   Electronic End-Tidal Carbon Dioxide Inhaler**

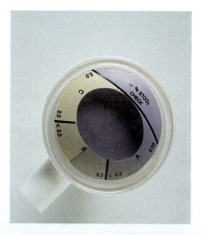

• **FIGURE A2-7   Colorimetric End-Tidal Carbon Dioxide Indicator Commonly Used in Prehospital Care**

monitoring of exhaled CO_2 has become the standard of care. Infrared $ETCO_2$ detectors are available for prehospital use (Figure A2-6•).

$ETCO_2$ detectors may also be used as an excellent indicator of proper endotracheal tube placement. If the endotracheal tube is placed properly into the trachea, then CO_2 should be present in the expired air. In EMS, a disposable colorimetric device is often used instead of an electronic infrared device. The colorimetric device is placed in-line with the endotracheal tube and ventilation device. If CO_2 is present, the detection paper turns from purple to yellow. The color changes have been further quantified to show that purple indicates a CO_2 concentration of less than 0.5 percent. Tan indicates a CO_2 concentration of 0.5 to 2.0 percent. Finally, yellow indicates a CO_2 concentration of greater than 2.0 percent. These devices monitor CO_2 levels breath-to-breath for up to 2 hours (Figure A2-7•). Recently, manufacturers of bag-valve-mask devices have added colorimetric CO_2 detectors to their devices as an added measure of safety. The

detection of CO_2 concentration in expired air is now a standard of care in prehospital medicine, especially to confirm proper endotracheal tube placement. It should be noted that the end-tidal CO_2 is unreliable for tube placement in cardiac arrest.

SUMMARY

It is essential that emergency personnel understand the fundamentals of the major chemical processes in the body. Abnormalities in any of the biochemical processes, such as a derangement in pH, can affect virtually every body system. Because of this, the pH should be maintained within normal limits. In addition, the physical properties of emergency drugs must be considered, given the environmental extremes encountered by field personnel. When indicated, adjustments must be made to assure that essential medications are maintained at the proper temperature and in the correct form. Monitoring oxygen saturation and carbon dioxide levels is now common in prehospital care. Emergency personnel must rapidly recognize any changes in these parameters and intervene accordingly.

3 Cell Structure and Function

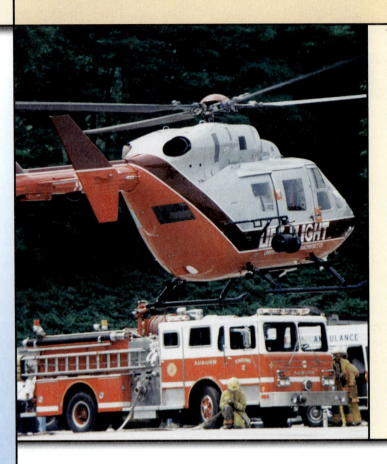

The cell is the fundamental unit of the body. Ultimately, all disease processes affect the cell. As an emergency care provider, it is important to have a thorough understanding of cellular structure and function. Many cells are highly specialized in their function. For example, the cells of the heart's electrical conductive system rapidly deliver the electrical impulse throughout the heart in a fraction of the time it would take for the impulse to move through normal heart muscle. Monitoring the heart's electrical conductive system is a fundamental part of advanced prehospital care. In addition, most of the fluids and medications used in emergency care directly affect the cells and their biochemical processes. Because of this, you must be familiar with the effects of emergency medications on cellular function.

Chapter Outline and Objectives

Vocabulary Development

aero-, air; *aerobic*
ana-, apart; *anaphase*
chondrion, granule; *mitochondrion*
chroma, color; *chromosome*
cyto-, cell; *cytoplasm*
endo-, inside; *endocytosis*
exo-, outside; *exocytosis*
hemo-, blood; *hemolysis*
hyper-, above; *hypertonic*
hypo-, below; *hypotonic*
inter-, between; *interphase*
interstitium, something standing
  between; *interstitial fluid*
iso-, equal; *isotonic*
kinesis, motion; *cytokinesis*
meta-, after; *metaphase*
micro-, small; *microtubules*
mitos, thread; *mitosis*
osmos, thrust; *osmosis*
phagein, to eat; *phagocyte*
pinein, to drink; *pinocytosis*
podon, foot; *pseudopod*
pro-, before; *prophase*
pseudo-, false; *pseudopod*
reticulum, network; *endoplasmic
  reticulum*
soma, body; *lysosome*
telos, end; *telophase*
tonos, tension; *isotonic*

3

As atoms are the building blocks of molecules, **cells** are the building blocks of the human body. Over the years, biologists have developed the **cell theory**, which includes the following four basic concepts:

1. Cells are the basic structural units of all plants and animals.
2. Cells are the smallest functioning units of life.
3. Cells are produced only by the division of preexisting cells.
4. Each cell maintains homeostasis.

An individual organism maintains homeostasis only through the combined and coordinated actions of many different types of cells. Figure 3-1● gives some examples of the range of cell sizes and shapes found in the human body.

Numbering in the trillions, the cells of the human body form and maintain anatomical structures and perform physiological functions as different as running and thinking. An understanding of how the human body functions thus requires a familiarity with the nature of cells.

STUDYING CELLS

The study of the structure and function of cells is called **cytology** (sī-TOL-ō-jē; cyto-, cell + -logy, the study of). What we have learned since the 1950s has given us new insights into the physiology of cells and their means of homeostatic control. Acquiring this knowledge depended upon developing better ways of viewing cells and applying new experimental techniques not only from biology but also from chemistry and physics.

The two most common methods used to study cell and tissue structure are light microscopy and electron microscopy. Before the 1950s most information was obtained through the use of light microscopy. Using a series of glass lenses, *light microscopy* can magnify cellular structures about 1000 times. Light microscopy typically involves looking at thin sections sliced from a larger piece of tissue. A photograph taken through a light microscope is called a *light micrograph (LM).* Many fine details of intracellular structure are too small to be seen with a light microscope. These details remained a mystery until investigators began using *electron microscopy,* a technique that replaced light with a focused beam of electrons. *Transmission electron micrographs (TEMs)* are photographs of very thin sections, and they can reveal fine details of cell membranes and intracellular structures. *Scanning electron micrographs (SEMs)* provide less magnification but reveal the three-dimensional nature of cell structures. An SEM provides a superficial view of a cell, a portion of a cell, or extracellular structures rather than a detailed sectional view.

You will see examples of light micrographs and both kinds of electron micrographs in figures through-

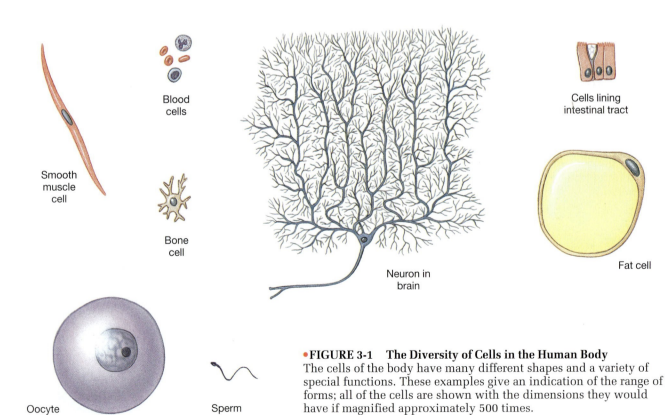

Smooth muscle cell

Blood cells

Bone cell

Neuron in brain

Cells lining intestinal tract

Fat cell

Oocyte

Sperm

●**FIGURE 3-1   The Diversity of Cells in the Human Body**
The cells of the body have many different shapes and a variety of special functions. These examples give an indication of the range of forms; all of the cells are shown with the dimensions they would have if magnified approximately 500 times.

out this text. The abbreviations LM, TEM, and SEM are followed by a number that indicates the total magnification of the image. For example, LM × 160 indicates that the structures in this light micrograph have been magnified 160 times.

An Overview of Cellular Anatomy

The "typical" cell is like the "average" person, so any description masks enormous individual variations. Our model cell will share features with most cells of the body without being identical to any. Figure 3-2• shows such a composite cell, and Table 3-1 provides an overview of the structures and functions of the parts of this cell.

A **cell membrane** separates the cell contents, or **cytoplasm**, from the watery medium that surrounds it, the **extracellular fluid**. The cytoplasm can be further subdivided into a fluid, the *cytosol*, intracellular structures collectively known as *organelles*, and *inclusions*, insoluble materials that may take the form of solid granules or lipid droplets.

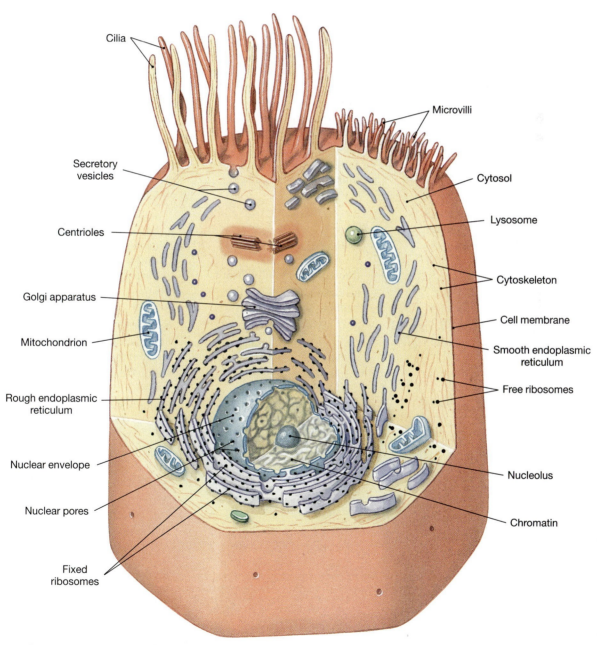

Cilia

Microvilli

Secretory
vesicles

Cytosol

Centrioles

Lysosome

Cytoskeleton

Golgi apparatus

Cell membrane

Mitochondrion

Smooth endoplasmic
reticulum

Free ribosomes

Rough endoplasmic
reticulum

Nuclear envelope

Nucleolus

Nuclear pores

Chromatin

Fixed
ribosomes

• **FIGURE 3-2   Anatomy of a Composite Cell**
See Table 3-1 for an overview of the functions associated with the various cell structures.

3 **TABLE 3-1** **Components of a Representative Cell**

Appearance	Structure	Composition	Function
	Cell membrane	Lipid bilayer, containing phospholipids, steroids, and proteins	Provides isolation, protection, sensitivity, and support; controls entrance/exit of materials
	Cytosol	Fluid component of cytoplasm	Distributes materials by diffusion
	NONMEMBRANOUS ORGANELLES		
	Cytoskeleton **Microtubule** **Microfilament**	Proteins organized in fine filaments or slender tubes	Provides strength; enables movement of cellular structures and materials
	Microvilli	Membrane extensions containing microfilaments	Increase surface area to facilitate absorption of extracellular materials
	Cilia	Membrane extensions containing microtubule doublets in a 9 + 2 array	Assist in movement of materials over surface
	Centrioles	Two centrioles, at right angles; each composed of 9 microtubule triplets	Enable movement of chromosomes during cell division
	Ribosomes	RNA + proteins; fixed ribosomes bound to endoplasmic reticulum, free ribosomes scattered in cytoplasm	Perform protein synthesis
	MEMBRANOUS ORGANELLES		
	Endoplasmic reticulum (ER)	Network of membranous channels extending throughout the cytoplasm	Synthesizes secretory products; provides intracellular storage and transport
	Rough ER	Has ribosomes attached to membranes	Synthesizes secretory proteins
	Smooth ER	Lacks attached ribosomes	Synthesizes lipids and carbohydrates
	Golgi apparatus	Stacks of flattened membranes containing chambers	Stores, alters, and packages secretory products; forms lysosomes
	Lysosomes	Vesicles containing powerful digestive enzymes	Remove damaged organelles or pathogens within cells
	Mitochondria	Double membrane, with inner folds (cristae) enclosing important metabolic enzymes	Produce 95% of the ATP required by the cell
	Nucleus	Nucleoplasm containing nucleotides, enzymes, and nucleoproteins; surrounded by double membrane (nuclear envelope)	Controls metabolism; stores and processes genetic information; controls protein synthesis
	Nucleolus	Dense region in nucleoplasm containing DNA and RNA	Synthesizes rRNA and assembles ribosomal subunits

THE CELL MEMBRANE

The outer boundary of the cell is formed by a cell membrane, or *plasma membrane*. Its four general functions are:

1. *Physical isolation*. The cell membrane is a physical barrier that separates the inside of the cell from the surrounding extracellular fluid.
2. *Regulation of exchange with the environment*. The cell membrane controls the entry of ions and nutrients, the elimination of wastes, and the release of secretory products.
3. *Sensitivity*. The cell membrane is the first part of the cell affected by changes in the extracellular fluid. It also contains a variety of receptors that allow the cell to recognize and respond to specific molecules in its environment. Any alteration in the cell membrane may affect all cellular activities.
4. *Structural support*. Specialized connections between cell membranes or between membranes and extracellular materials give tissues a stable structure.

Membrane Structure

The cell membrane is extremely thin and delicate. Its major components are lipids, proteins, and carbohydrates.

Membrane Lipids

Phospholipids are a major component of cell membranes. ∞ *p. 42* In a phospholipid, a phosphate group (PO_4^{3-}) serves as a link between a diglyceride (a glycerol backbone bonded to two fatty acid "tails") and a nonlipid "head." The phospholipids in a cell membrane lie in two distinct layers, with the heads on the outside and the tails on the inside. For this reason, the cell membrane is often called the **phospholipid bilayer** (see Figure 3-3•). Mixed in with the fatty acid tails are cholesterol molecules and small quantities of other lipids.

The lipid tails will not associate with water molecules, and this characteristic allows the cell membrane to act as a selective physical barrier. Ions and water-soluble compounds cannot cross the lipid portion of a cell membrane. Consequently, the cell membrane is very effective in isolating the cytoplasm from the surrounding extracellular fluid.

Membrane Proteins

Several types of proteins are associated with the cell membrane. They may be partially or totally embedded in the phospholipid bilayer or loosely bound to its inner or outer surface. Membrane proteins may function as *receptors, channels, carriers, enzymes, anchors,* or *identifiers*. Table 3-2 provides a functional description and example of each class of membrane protein.

Membrane structure is not rigid, and embedded proteins drift from place to place across the surface of the membrane like ice cubes in a punch bowl. In addition,

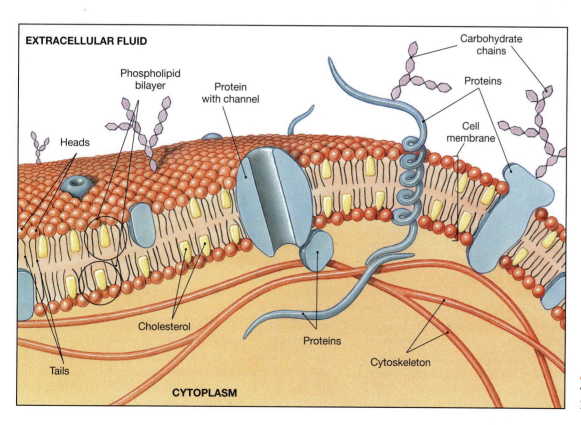

EXTRACELLULAR FLUID

Carbohydrate chains

Phospholipid bilayer

Protein with channel

Proteins

Heads

Cell membrane

Cholesterol

Proteins

Tails

Cytoskeleton

CYTOPLASM

• FIGURE 3-3
The Cell Membrane

TABLE 3-2	Types of Membrane Proteins	
Class	Function	Example
Receptor proteins	Sensitive to specific extracellular materials that bind to them and trigger a change in a cell's activity	Binding of the hormone insulin to membrane receptors increases the rate of glucose absorption by the cell.
Channel proteins	Central pore, or channel, permits water and solutes to bypass lipid portion of cell membrane.	Calcium ion movement through channels is involved in muscle contraction and the conduction of nerve impulses.
Carrier proteins	Bind and transport solutes across the cell membrane. This process may or may not require energy.	Carrier proteins bring glucose into the cytoplasm and also transport sodium, potassium, and calcium ions.
Enzymes	Catalyze reactions in the extracellular fluid or within the cell	Dipeptides are broken down into amino acids by enzymes on the membranes of cells lining the intestinal tract.
Anchor proteins	Attach the cell membrane to other structures and stabilize its position	Inside the cell, bound to the network of supporting filaments (the cytoskeleton); outside, attach the cell to extracellular protein fibers or to another cell
Identifier proteins	Identify a cell as self or nonself, normal or abnormal, to the immune system	One group of such recognition proteins is the major histocompatibility complex (MHC) discussed in Chapter 15.

the composition of the cell membrane can change over time, as membrane is added or removed through processes described later in this chapter.

Membrane Carbohydrates

Carbohydrates and lipids on the outer surface of the membrane (1) are important as cell lubricants and adhesives, (2) act as receptors for extracellular compounds, and (3) are part of a recognition system that keeps the immune system from attacking its own tissues.

Membrane Transport

Precisely which substances enter or leave the cytoplasm is determined by the **permeability** of the cell membrane. If nothing can cross the cell membrane, it is described as *impermeable*. If any substance at all can cross without difficulty, the membrane is *freely permeable*. Cell membranes are *selectively permeable*, permitting the free passage of some materials and restricting the passage of others. Passage selection is based on size, electrical charge, molecular shape, lipid solubility, or some combination of these factors.

Movement across the membrane may be passive or active. **Passive processes** move ions or molecules across the cell membrane without any energy expenditure by the cell. Passive processes include *diffusion, osmosis, filtration,* and *facilitated diffusion.* **Active processes,** discussed later in this chapter, require that the cell expend energy, usually in the form of ATP.

Diffusion

Ions and molecules are in constant motion, colliding and bouncing off one another and off any obstacles in their paths. **Diffusion** is the net movement of molecules from an area of relatively high concentration (or large number of collisions) to an area of relatively low concentration (or small number of collisions). The difference between the high and low concentrations represents a **concentration gradient**, and diffusion is often described as proceeding "down a concentration gradient" or "downhill." As a result of diffusion, solutes eventually become uniformly distributed, and concentration gradients are eliminated.

Diffusion occurs in air as well as in water. The smell of fresh flowers in a vase can sweeten the air in a large room, just as the molecules of a dissolved sugar cube can sweeten a cup of coffee. Each case begins with an extremely high concentration of molecules in a very localized area. Consider a cube of soluble solid material dropped into a beaker of water. As the material dissolves, its molecules establish a sharp concentration gradient with the surrounding clear water. Eventually, the dissolved molecules of the solid spread through the water until they are distributed evenly (Figure 3-4●).

Diffusion is important in body fluids because it tends to eliminate local concentration gradients. For example, each active cell in your body generates carbon dioxide, which diffuses out of the cell, and absorbs oxygen, which diffuses into the cell. As a result, the extracellular fluid around the cell develops a relatively high concentration

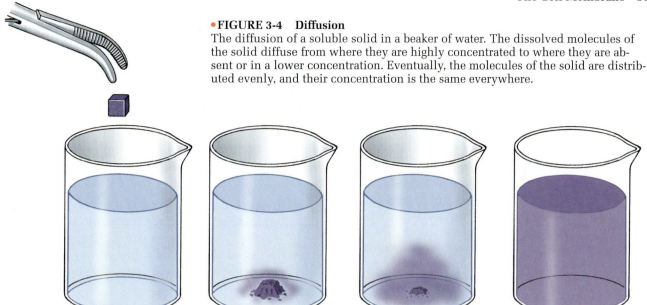

● **FIGURE 3-4   Diffusion**
The diffusion of a soluble solid in a beaker of water. The dissolved molecules of the solid diffuse from where they are highly concentrated to where they are absent or in a lower concentration. Eventually, the molecules of the solid are distributed evenly, and their concentration is the same everywhere.

of CO_2 and a relatively low concentration of O_2. Diffusion then distributes the carbon dioxide through the tissue and into the bloodstream. At the same time, oxygen diffuses out of the blood and into the tissue.

Diffusion Across Cell Membranes.   Water and dissolved solutes diffuse freely through the extracellular fluids of the body. The cell membrane, however, acts as a barrier that selectively restricts diffusion. Some substances can pass through easily, whereas others cannot penetrate the membrane at all. An ion or molecule can

independently diffuse across a cell membrane in one of two ways: (1) by moving across the lipid portion of the membrane or (2) by passing through a membrane channel. Therefore, the primary factors determining whether a substance can diffuse across a cell membrane are its lipid solubility and its size relative to the diameter of the membrane channels (Figure 3-5●).

Lipid solubility.   Alcohol, fatty acids, and steroids can enter cells easily because they can diffuse through the lipid portions of the membrane. Dissolved gases such as

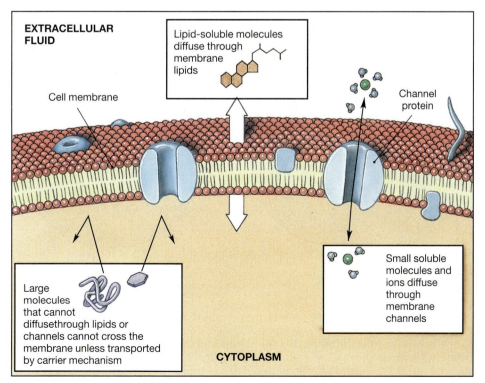

EXTRACELLULAR FLUID

Lipid-soluble molecules diffuse through membrane lipids

Cell membrane

Channel protein

Large molecules that cannot diffusethrough lipids or channels cannot cross the membrane unless transported by carrier mechanism

Small soluble molecules and ions diffuse through membrane channels

CYTOPLASM

● **FIGURE 3-5   Diffusion Across Cell Membranes**
The movement of a substance across the membrane depends on the lipid solubility and size of the substance.

oxygen and carbon dioxide also enter and leave our cells by diffusion through the lipid bilayer.

Size.   Water-soluble compounds must diffuse through channels in the membrane. These channels are very small, about 0.8 nm in diameter. Water molecules can enter or exit freely, but even a small organic molecule, such as glucose, is too big to fit through the channels.

Osmosis: A Special Type of Diffusion.   The diffusion of water across a membrane is called **osmosis** (oz-MŌ-sis; *osmos*, thrust). Both intracellular and extracellular fluids are solutions that contain a variety of dissolved materials, or **solutes**. Each solute tends to diffuse as if it were the only material in solution. For example, changes in the concentration of potassium ions will have no effect on the rate or direction of sodium ion diffusion. Some ions and molecules diffuse into the cytoplasm, others diffuse out, and a few, such as proteins, are unable to diffuse across a cell membrane. But if we ignore the individual identities and simply count the total number of solutes, we find that the *total* concentration of solutes on either side of the cell membrane stays the same.

This state of equilibrium persists because *the cell membrane is freely permeable to water.* Whenever a concentration gradient exists, water molecules will diffuse rapidly across the cell membrane until the gradient is eliminated. This movement, which eliminates differences in solute concentrations, occurs in response to a concentration gradient for water molecules.

Dissolved solute molecules occupy space that would otherwise be taken up by water molecules. Thus the higher the solute concentration, the lower the water concentration. As a result, *water molecules will tend to diffuse across a membrane toward the solution containing a higher solute concentration.*

Three characteristics of osmosis are of primary importance:

1. Osmosis is the diffusion of water molecules across a membrane.
2. Osmosis occurs across a selectively permeable membrane that is freely permeable to water but not to solutes.
3. In osmosis, water will flow across a membrane toward the solution that has the highest concentration of solutes.

Osmosis and Osmotic Pressure.   Figure 3-6• diagrams the process of osmosis. Step 1 shows two solutions (A and B) with differing solute concentrations separated by a selectively permeable membrane. As osmosis occurs, water molecules cross the membrane until the solute concentrations in the two solutions are identical (step 2a). Thus the volume of solution B increases at the expense of solution A. The greater the initial difference in solute concentrations, the stronger the osmotic flow. **Osmotic pressure** is the amount of pressure required to stop osmosis across a membrane.

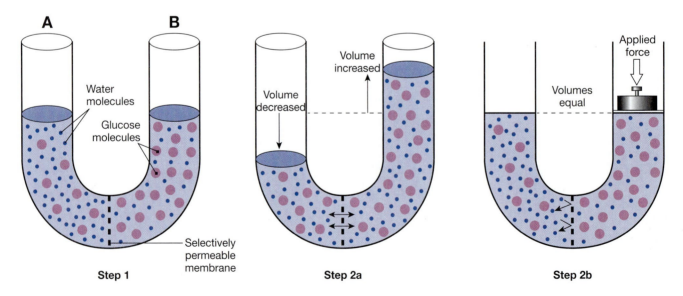

•**FIGURE 3-6   Osmosis**
Step 1: Two solutions containing different solute concentrations are separated by a selectively permeable membrane. Water molecules (small blue dots) begin to cross the membrane from solution A toward solution B, which has the higher concentration of solutes (larger pink circles). **Step 2a**: At equilibrium, the solute concentrations on the two sides of the membrane are equal. The volume of B has increased at the expense of that of A. **Step 2b**: Osmosis can be prevented by resisting the volume change. The osmotic pressure of B is equal to the amount of force required to stop the osmotic flow.

It is an indication of the force of water movement *into that solution* as a result of its solute concentration. As the solute concentration of a solution increases, so does its osmotic pressure. Osmotic pressure can be measured in several ways. For example, a strong enough opposing pressure can prevent the entry of water molecules. Pushing against a fluid generates *hydrostatic pressure*. In step 2b, hydrostatic pressure in solution B, created by the applied force, balances the osmotic pressure, and no net osmotic flow occurs.

Solutions of varying solute concentrations are described as *isotonic*, *hypotonic*, or *hypertonic* with regard to their effects on the shape or tension of the membrane of living cells. Although the effects of various osmotic solutions are difficult to see in most tissues, they are readily observed in red blood cells.

Figure 3-7a● shows the appearance of a red blood cell immersed in an isotonic solution. An **isotonic** (*iso-*, equal + *tonos*, tension) solution is one that will not cause a net movement of water into or out of the cell. In other words, an equilibrium exists, and as one water molecule moves out of the cell another moves in to replace it.

When a cell is placed in contact with a **hypotonic** (*hypo-*, below) solution, water will flow into the cytoplasm by osmosis. If the difference is substantial, the cell will swell up like a balloon, as shown in Figure 3-7b●. Ultimately the membrane may rupture, or *lyse*. In the case of red blood cells, this event, known as **hemolysis** (*hemo-*, blood + *lysis*, breakdown), leaves behind empty cell membranes known as red blood cell "ghosts."

When a cell is placed in contact with a **hypertonic** (*hyper-*, above) solution, water will flow out of the cell and into the surrounding medium by osmosis, and the cell will shrivel and dehydrate. In the case of red blood cells, this shrinking is called **crenation** (Figure 3-7c●).

It is often necessary to administer large volumes of fluid to people who have had a severe blood loss or who are dehydrated. A commonly administered fluid is a 0.9 percent (0.9 g/dl) solution of sodium chloride (NaCl), which approximates the normal osmotic concentration of the extracellular fluids. Called **normal saline**, this fluid is used because sodium and chloride are the most abundant ions in the body's extracellular fluid. Because there is little net movement of either type of ion across cell membranes, normal saline is essentially isotonic with respect to body cells.

Filtration

In **filtration**, water and small solute molecules are forced across a membrane because of a hydrostatic pressure gradient. Molecules of solute will be carried along with the water only if they are small enough to fit through the membrane pores. In the body, the heart pushes blood through the circulatory system and generates hydrostatic pressure, or *blood pressure*. Filtration occurs across the walls of small blood vessels, pushing water and dissolved nutrients into the tissues of the body. Filtration across specialized blood vessels in the kidneys is an essential step in the production of urine.

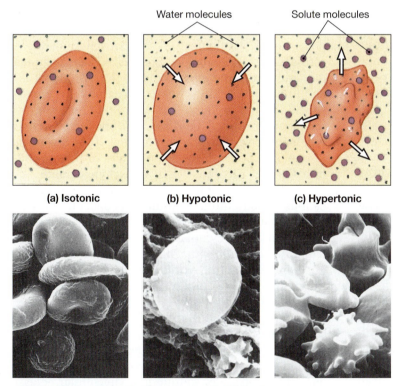

(a) Isotonic   **(b) Hypotonic**   **(c) Hypertonic**

●**FIGURE 3-7   Osmotic Flow Across Cell Membranes**
White arrows indicate the direction of osmotic water movement. **(a)** Because these red blood cells are immersed in an isotonic saline solution, no osmotic flow occurs and the cells have their normal appearance. **(b)** Immersion in a hypotonic saline solution results in the osmotic flow of water into the cells. The swelling may continue until the cell membrane ruptures. **(c)** Exposure to a hypertonic solution results in the movement of water out of the cells. The red blood cells shrivel and become crenated. (SEMs × 833)

Carrier-Mediated Transport

Carrier-mediated transport involves the activity of membrane proteins that bind specific ions or organic substrates and move them across the cell membrane. These proteins have several characteristics in common with enzymes. For example, they may be used over and over and are very selective about what they will bind and transport; the carrier protein that transports glucose will not carry other simple sugars.

Carrier-mediated transport can be passive (no ATP required) or active (ATP-dependent). In *passive transport*, solutes are typically

3

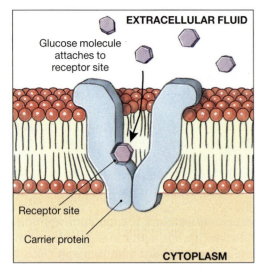

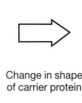

Change in shape
of carrier protein

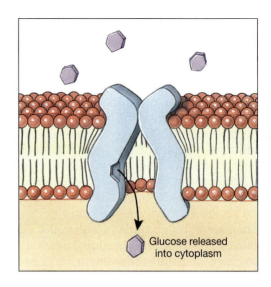

● **FIGURE 3-8   Facilitated Diffusion**
In this process, an extracellular molecule, such as glucose, binds to a receptor site on a carrier protein. The binding alters the shape of the protein, which then releases the molecule to diffuse into the cytoplasm.

carried from an area of high concentration to an area of low concentration. *Active transport* mechanisms may follow or oppose an existing concentration gradient.

Many carrier proteins transport one ion or molecule at a time, but some deal with two solutes simultaneously. In *cotransport*, the carrier transports the two substances in the same direction, either into or out of the cell. In *countertransport*, one substance moves into the cell while the other moves out.

Two major examples of carrier-mediated transport—*facilitated diffusion* and *active transport*—are discussed below.

Facilitated Diffusion.   Many essential nutrients, such as glucose or amino acids, are insoluble in lipids and too large to fit through membrane channels. However, these compounds can be passively transported across the membrane by carrier proteins in a process called **facilitated diffusion** (Figure 3-8●). The molecule to be transported first binds to a **receptor site** on the protein. It is then moved to the inside of the cell membrane and released into the cytoplasm.

As in the case of simple diffusion, no ATP is expended in facilitated diffusion, and the molecules move from an area of higher concentration to one of lower concentration. Facilitated diffusion differs from ordinary diffusion, however, because the rate of transport cannot increase indefinitely; only a limited number of carrier proteins are available in the membrane. Once all of them are operating, any further increase in the concentration of the solute will have no effect on the rate of movement into the cell.

Active Transport.   In **active transport**, the high-energy bond in ATP provides the energy needed to move ions or molecules across the membrane. The process is

complex, and specific enzymes must be present in addition to the carrier molecule. The advantage of active transport is that the cell can import or export specific materials *regardless of their intracellular or extracellular concentrations.*

All living cells contain carrier proteins called **ion pumps** that actively transport the cations sodium (Na^+), potassium (K^+), calcium (Ca^{2+}), and magnesium (Mg^{2+}) across their cell membranes. Specialized cells can transport additional ions such as iodide (I^-), chloride (Cl^-), and iron (Fe^{2+}). Many of these carrier proteins move a specific cation or anion in one direction only, either into or out of the cell. In a few cases, one carrier protein will move more than one ion at a time. If one ion moves in one direction and the other moves in the opposite direction, the carrier is called an **exchange pump**.

Sodium and potassium ions are the principal cations in body fluids. Sodium ion concentrations are high in the extracellular fluids, whereas sodium concentrations in the cytoplasm are relatively low. The distribution of potassium in the body is just the opposite—low in the extracellular fluids and high in the cytoplasm. As a result, sodium ions slowly diffuse into the cell, and potassium ions leak out.

Homeostasis within the cell depends on ejecting sodium ions and recapturing lost potassium ions. This exchange is accomplished through the activity of the **sodium-potassium exchange pump**. This ion pump exchanges intracellular sodium for extracellular potassium (Figure 3-9●).

Vesicular Transport

In **vesicular transport**, materials move into or out of the cell through the formation of vesicles, small membranous sacs. The two major categories of vesicular transport are *endocytosis* and *exocytosis*.

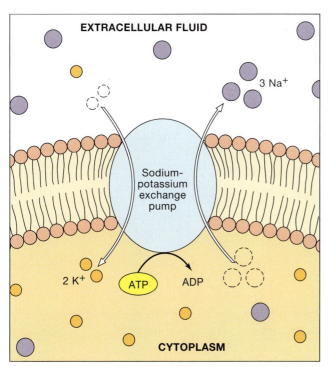

•FIGURE 3-9 The Sodium-Potassium Exchange Pump
The operation of the sodium-potassium exchange pump is an example of active transport because its operation requires the conversion of ATP to ADP.

Endocytosis. Endocytosis (EN-dō-sī-TŌ-sis; *endo-*, inside + *cyte*, cell) is the packaging of extracellular materials in a vesicle at the cell surface for importation *into* the cell. This process may involve relatively large volumes of extracellular material. There are two major types of endocytosis: *pinocytosis* and *phagocytosis*. Both are active processes that require ATP or other sources of energy.

- **Pinocytosis** (pi-nō-si-TŌ-sis; *pinein*, to drink), or "cell drinking," is the formation of small vesicles filled with extracellular fluid. In this process, common to all cells, a deep groove or pocket forms in the cell membrane and then pinches off.

- **Phagocytosis** (fa-gō-si-TŌ-sis; *phagein*, to eat), or "cell eating," produces vesicles containing solid objects (Figure 3-10•). Cytoplasmic extensions called **pseudopodia** (soo-dō-PŌ-dē-a; *pseudo-*, false + *podon*, foot) surround the object, and their membranes fuse to form a vesicle. The vesicle may then fuse with a *lysosome*, a membranous sac of digestive enzymes, whereupon its contents are broken down.

Most cells display pinocytosis, but phagocytosis, especially the entrapment of living or dead cells, is

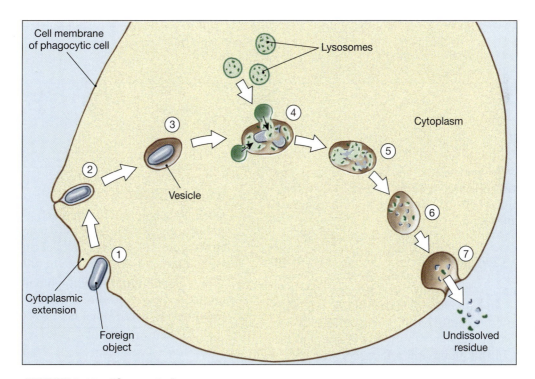

•FIGURE 3-10 Phagocytosis
(1) A phagocytic cell first comes in contact with the foreign object and sends cytoplasmic extensions around it. **(2)** The extensions approach one another and then **(3)** fuse to trap the material within a vesicle. **(4)** Lysosomes fuse with this vesicle, **(5–6)** activating digestive enzymes that gradually break down the structure of the phagocytized material. **(7)** Undissolved residue is then ejected from the cell by exocytosis.

TABLE 3-3 **A Summary of the Mechanisms Involved in Movement Across Cell Membranes**

Mechanism	Process	Factors Affecting Rate	Substances Involved
DIFFUSION	Molecular movement of solutes; direction determined by relative concentrations	Size of gradient, molecular size, charge, lipid solubility	Small inorganic ions, lipid-soluble materials (all cells)
Osmosis	Movement of water molecules toward solution containing relatively higher solute concentration; requires membrane	Concentration gradient, opposing osmotic or hydrostatic pressure	Water only (all cells)
FILTRATION	Movement of water, usually with solute, by hydrostatic pressure; requires filtration membrane	Amount of pressure, size of pores in filter	Water and small ions (blood vessels)
CARRIER-MEDIATED TRANSPORT			
Facilitated diffusion	Carrier molecules passively transport solutes down a concentration gradient	As above, plus availability of carrier protein	Glucose and amino acids (all cells)
Active transport	Carrier molecules actively transport solutes regardless of any concentration gradients	Availability of carrier proteins, substrate, and ATP	Na^+, K^+, Ca^{2+}, Mg^{2+} (all cells); other solutes by specialized cells
VESICULAR TRANSPORT			
Endocytosis	Creation of vesicles containing fluid or solid material	Stimulus and mechanics incompletely understood; requires ATP	Fluids, nutrients (all cells); debris, pathogens (specialized cells)
Exocytosis	Fusion of vesicles containing fluids and/or solids with the cell membrane	Stimulus and mechanics incompletely understood; requires ATP	Fluids, debris (all cells)

performed only by specialized cells of the immune system. Phagocytic cells will be considered in chapters dealing with blood cells (Chapter 12) and the immune response (Chapter 15).

Exocytosis. Exocytosis (EK-sō-sī-TŌ-sis; *exo-*, outside) is the functional reverse of endocytosis. In this process a vesicle created inside the cell fuses with the cell membrane and discharges its contents into the extracellular environment. The ejected material may be a secretory product, such as a hormone (a compound that circulates in the blood and affects cells in other parts of the body), mucus, or waste products remaining from the recycling of damaged organelles (Figure 3-10•).

Many of the transport mechanisms discussed above can be moving materials in and out of the cell at any given moment. These mechanisms are summarized in Table 3-3.

✓ What is the difference between active and passive transport processes?

✓ During digestion in the stomach, the concentration of hydrogen (H^+) ions rises to many times the concentration found in the cells of the stomach. What type of transport process could produce this result?

✓ When certain types of white blood cells encounter bacteria, they are able to engulf them and bring them into the cell. What is this process called?

THE CYTOPLASM

As explained earlier, *cytoplasm* is a general term for the material inside the cell between the cell membrane and the nucleus. The cytoplasm can be divided into the cytosol, organelles, and inclusions.

3

The Cytosol

The **cytosol** is the intracellular fluid, which contains dissolved nutrients, ions, soluble and insoluble proteins, and waste products. It differs in composition from the extracellular fluid that surrounds most of the cells in the body:

- The cytosol contains a high concentration of potassium ions, whereas extracellular fluid contains a high concentration of sodium ions.
- The cytosol contains a relatively high concentration of dissolved proteins, many of them enzymes that regulate metabolic operations. These proteins give the cytosol a consistency that varies between that of thin maple syrup and almost-set gelatin.
- The cytosol contains relatively small quantities of carbohydrates and large reserves of amino acids and lipids. The carbohydrates are broken down to provide energy, and the amino acids are used to manufacture proteins. The lipids stored in the cell are primarily used as an energy source when carbohydrates are unavailable.

The cytosol may also contain insoluble **inclusions**, such as stored nutrients. Examples include glycogen granules in muscle and liver cells and lipid droplets in fat cells.

Organelles

Organelles (or-gan-ELZ; "little organs") are structures that perform specific functions essential to normal cell structure, maintenance, and metabolism (see Table 3-1). Membrane-enclosed organelles include the *nucleus, mitochondria, endoplasmic reticulum, Golgi apparatus,* and *lysosomes.* The membrane isolates the organelle from the cytosol so the organelle can manufacture or store secretions, enzymes, or toxins that might otherwise damage the cell. The *cytoskeleton, microvilli, centrioles, cilia, flagella,* and *ribosomes* are organelles that are not surrounded by their own individual membranes.

The Cytoskeleton

The **cytoskeleton** is an internal protein framework of various threadlike filaments and hollow tubules that gives the cytoplasm strength and flexibility (Figure 3-11•). In most cells, the most important cytoskeletal elements are microfilaments and microtubules.

Microfilaments.   **Microfilaments** are the thinnest strands, usually composed of the protein **actin**. In most cells, they form a dense layer just inside the cell membrane. Microfilaments attach the cell membrane to the underlying cytoplasm by forming connections with proteins of the cell membrane. In addition, actin microfilaments can interact with thicker filaments made of

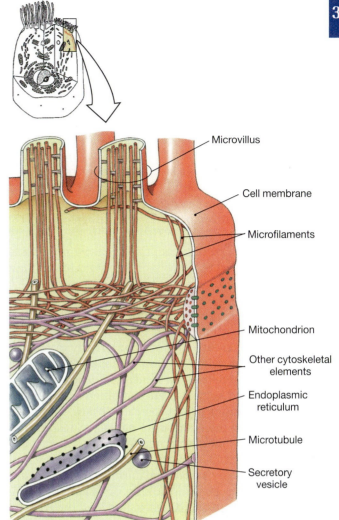

Microvillus

Cell membrane

Microfilaments

Mitochondrion

Other cytoskeletal elements

Endoplasmic reticulum

Microtubule

Secretory vesicle

•**FIGURE 3-11   The Cytoskeleton**
The cytoskeleton provides strength and structural support for the cell and its organelles. Interactions between cytoskeletal components are also important in moving organelles and changing the shape of the cell.

another protein, **myosin**, to produce active movement of a portion of a cell or to change the shape of the cell.

Microtubules.   **Microtubules**, found in all our cells, are hollow tubes built from the globular protein **tubulin**. Microtubules form the primary components of the cytoskeleton, giving the cell strength and rigidity and anchoring the position of major organelles.

During cell division, microtubules form the *spindle apparatus* that distributes the duplicated chromosomes to opposite ends of the dividing cell. This process will be considered in a later section.

Microvilli

Microvilli are small, finger-shaped projections of the cell membrane supported by microfilaments (see Figures 3-2• and 3-11•). Because they increase the surface area of the membrane, they are common features of cells actively engaged in absorbing materials from the extracellular fluid, such as the cells of the digestive tract and kidneys.

Centrioles, Cilia, and Flagella

In addition to functioning individually in the cytoskeleton, microtubules also interact to form more complex structures known as *centrioles*, *cilia*, and *flagella*.

Centrioles.   A **centriole** is a short cylindrical structure composed of microtubules (see Figure 3-2•, p. 55). All animal cells that are capable of dividing contain a pair of centrioles arranged perpendicular to each other. The centrioles create the spindle fibers that move DNA strands during cell division. Cells that do not divide, such as mature red blood cells and neurons of the brain, lack centrioles.

Cilia.   Cilia (singular *cilium*) are relatively long finger-shaped extensions of the cell membrane (see Figure 3-2•). They are supported internally by a cylindrical array of microtubules. Cilia undergo active movements that require ATP energy. Their movements are coordinated so that their combined efforts move fluids or secretions across the cell surface. For example, cilia lining the respiratory passageways beat in a synchronized manner to move sticky mucus and trapped dust particles toward the throat and away from delicate respiratory surfaces. If the cilia are damaged or immobilized by heavy smoking or some metabolic problem, the cleansing action is lost, and the irritants will no longer be removed. As a result, chronic respiratory infections develop.

Flagella.   Flagella (fla-JEL-ah; singular *flagellum*, whip) resemble cilia but are much longer. Flagella propel a cell through the surrounding fluid, rather than moving the fluid past a stationary cell. Flagella on *pathogenic* (disease-causing) *organisms* allow them to move through our tissues and body fluids. The sperm cell is the only human cell that has a flagellum. If the flagella are paralyzed or otherwise abnormal, the individual will be sterile, because immobile sperm cannot reach and fertilize an egg.

Ribosomes

Ribosomes are small organelles that manufacture proteins using information provided by the DNA of the nucleus. (This process will be discussed on p. 70). Each ribosome consists of ribosomal RNA and protein. Ribosomes are found in all cells, but their number varies depending on the type of cell and its activities. For example, liver cells, which manufacture blood proteins, have much greater numbers of ribosomes than do fat cells, which synthesize triglycerides.

There are two major types of ribosomes: free ribosomes and fixed ribosomes. **Free ribosomes** are scattered throughout the cytoplasm, and the proteins they manufacture enter the cytosol. **Fixed ribosomes** are attached to the endoplasmic reticulum, a membranous organelle discussed next. Proteins manufactured by fixed ribosomes enter the endoplasmic reticulum, where they are modified and packaged for export.

✓ Cells lining the small intestine have numerous fingerlike projections on their free surface. What are these structures, and what is their function?

✓ How would the absence of centrioles affect a cell?

The Endoplasmic Reticulum

The **endoplasmic reticulum** (en-dō-plaz-mik re-TIK-ū-lum; *reticulum*, a network), or **ER**, is a network of intracellular membranes that is connected to the membranous *nuclear envelope* surrounding the nucleus (see Figure 3-2•, p. 55). The ER has three major functions:

1. *Synthesis*. The membrane of the ER manufactures proteins, carbohydrates, and lipids.
2. *Storage*. The ER can hold or isolate synthesized molecules or materials absorbed from the cytosol that might otherwise affect other cellular operations.
3. *Transport*. Materials can travel from place to place within the cell without leaving the ER.

There are two distinct types of endoplasmic reticulum, **smooth endoplasmic reticulum (SER)** and **rough endoplasmic reticulum (RER)** (Figure 3-12•). The SER, which lacks ribosomes, is the site where lipids and carbohydrates are produced. The membranes of the RER are studded with ribosomes, indicating that they participate in protein synthesis. The amount of endoplasmic reticulum and the proportion of RER to SER vary depending on the type of cell and its ongoing activities. For example, pancreatic cells that manufacture digestive enzymes contain an extensive RER, and the SER is relatively small. The proportion is just the reverse in the cells that synthesize steroid hormones in the reproductive system.

The SER has a variety of functions, most of which involve the synthesis of lipids and carbohydrates. SER functions include (1) the synthesis of the phospholipids and cholesterol needed for maintenance and growth of the cell membrane, ER, nuclear membrane, and Golgi apparatus in all cells; (2) the synthesis of steroid hormones, such as *testosterone* and *estrogen* (sex hormones) in cells of the reproductive organs; and (3) the synthesis and storage of glycogen in skeletal muscle and liver cells.

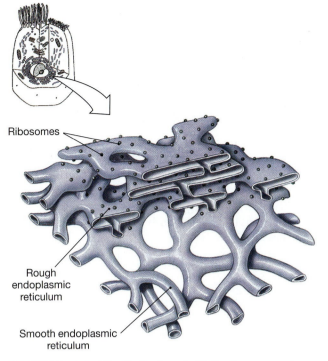

Ribosomes

Rough
endoplasmic
reticulum

Smooth endoplasmic
reticulum

• **FIGURE 3-12   The Endoplasmic Reticulum**
This diagrammatic sketch shows the three-dimensional relationships between the rough and smooth endoplasmic
reticula.

The lipids and carbohydrates produced by the SER
and the proteins produced by the ribosomes of the RER
may become incorporated into membranes or enter the
inner chambers of their respective endoplasmic reticulum. These molecules are then packaged into small

membrane sacs that pinch off from the tips of the ER.
The sacs, called *transport vesicles*, deliver them to the
Golgi apparatus, another membranous organelle, where
they are processed further.

The Golgi Apparatus

The **Golgi** (GOL-jē) **apparatus** consists of a set of five or
six flattened membrane discs. A single cell may contain several sets, each resembling a stack of dinner
plates (see Figure 3-2•, p. 55). The major functions of the
Golgi apparatus are: (1) the synthesis and packaging of
secretions, such as enzymes; (2) the renewal or modification of the cell membrane; and (3) the packaging of
special enzymes for use in the cytosol.

The various roles of the Golgi apparatus are diagrammed in Figure 3-13a•. The synthesis of proteins
and other substances occurs in the RER, and then transport vesicles move these products to the Golgi apparatus. Enzymes in the Golgi apparatus modify the newly
arrived molecules as other vesicles move them closer
to the cell surface through succeeding membranes. Ultimately, the modified materials are repackaged in vesicles that leave the Golgi apparatus. The Golgi apparatus
creates three classes of vesicles, each with a different
fate. One class of vesicles contains secretions that will
be discharged from the cell. These are called **secretory
vesicles**. The secretion occurs through exocytosis at the
cell surface (Figure 3-13b•). A second class of vesicles
does not contain secretions, but the vesicle membrane
will be incorporated into the cell membrane. Because
the Golgi apparatus continuously adds new membrane
to the cell surface in this way, the properties of the cell

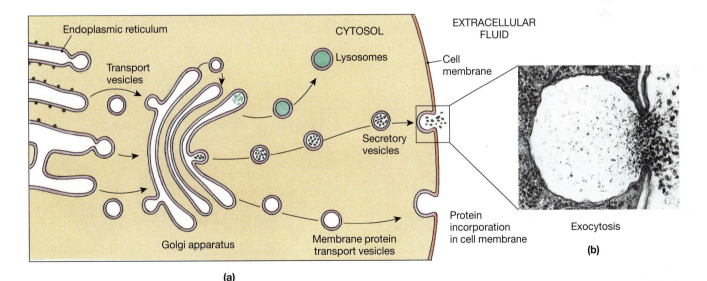

(a)

• **FIGURE 3-13   The Golgi Apparatus**
(a) Transport vesicles carry molecules manufactured in the endoplasmic reticulum to the Golgi apparatus, where these
molecules are modified and transported through succeeding membranes toward the cell surface. At the membrane closest
to the cell surface, three types of vesicles develop. Secretory vesicles carry secretions from the Golgi apparatus to the cell
surface, another group of vesicles adds additional membrane and protein to the cell membrane, and enzyme-filled lysosomes remain in the cytoplasm. **(b)** Exocytosis of secretions at the cell surface.

membrane can change. For example, receptors can be added or removed, making the cell more or less sensitive to a particular stimulus. A third class of vesicles will remain in the cytoplasm. These vesicles, called *lysosomes*, contain digestive enzymes.

Lysosomes

Lysosomes (LĪ-so-sōmz; *lyso-*, breakdown + *soma*, body) are vesicles filled with digestive enzymes. Lysosomes perform cleanup and recycling functions within the cell. Their enzymes are activated when they fuse with the membranes of damaged organelles, such as mitochondria or fragments of the endoplasmic reticulum. Then the enzymes break down the lysosomal contents. Nutrients reenter the cytosol through passive or active transport processes, and the remaining material is eliminated by exocytosis.

Lysosomes also function in the defense against disease. Through endocytosis, cells may engulf bacteria, fluids, and organic debris from their surroundings into vesicles formed at the cell surface. Lysosomes fuse with vesicles created in this way, and the digestive enzymes then break down the contents and release usable substances such as sugars or amino acids.

Lysosomes perform essential recycling functions by removing damaged or dead cells. Within such cells, lysosome membranes disintegrate, releasing active enzymes into the cytosol. These enzymes rapidly destroy the proteins and organelles of the cell, a process called **autolysis** (aw-TAH-li-sis; *auto-*, self). Because the breakdown of lysosomal membranes can destroy a cell, lysosomes have been called cellular "suicide packets." We do not know how to control lysosomal activities or why the enclosed enzymes do not digest the lysosomal membranes unless the cell is damaged.

Mitochondria

Mitochondria (mī-tō-KON-drē-ah; singular *mitochondrion*; *mitos*, thread + *chondrion*, granule) are small organelles containing enzymes that regulate the reactions that provide energy for the cell. Mitochondria have an unusual double membrane: an outer membrane surrounding the entire organelle and an inner membrane containing numerous folds, called *cristae*. The energy-producing enzymes reside on the cristae, which provide a large surface area for reactions to take place, and within the fluid they enclose, the *matrix* (Figure 3-14●). The number of mitochondria in a particular cell varies depending on its energy demands. For example, red blood cells have none, but mitochondria may account for 20 percent of the volume of an active liver cell.

Although most of the chemical reactions that release energy occur in the mitochondria, most of the cellular activities that require energy occur in the surrounding cytoplasm. Cells must therefore store energy in a form that can be moved from place to place. Energy is stored and transferred in the high-energy bond of ATP, as discussed in Chapter 2. ∞ *p. 46* Living cells break the high-energy phosphate bond under controlled conditions, reconverting ATP to ADP and releasing energy for their use.

Mitochondrial Energy Production.   Most cells generate ATP and other high-energy compounds through the breakdown of carbohydrates, especially glucose. Although most of the actual energy production occurs inside mitochondria, the first steps take place in the cytosol. In this reaction sequence, called *glycolysis*, six-carbon glucose molecules are broken down into three-carbon molecules of pyruvic acid. These molecules are then absorbed by the mitochondria. If glucose

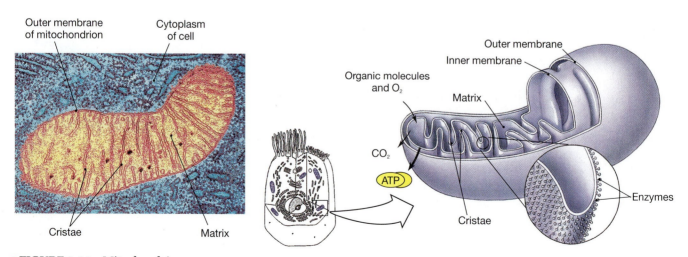

●**FIGURE 3-14   Mitochondria**
This TEM (× 43,200) shows a typical mitochondrion in section, and the sketch details its three-dimensional organization. Mitochondria absorb short carbon chains, ADP, P, and oxygen and generate carbon dioxide, water, and ATP.

or other carbohydrates are not available, mitochondria can absorb and utilize small carbon chains produced by the breakdown of proteins or lipids.

Because the key reactions involved in mitochondrial activity consume oxygen, the process of mitochondrial energy production is known as **aerobic** (*aero-*, air + *bios*, life) **metabolism**. Aerobic metabolism in mitochondria produces about 95 percent of the energy needed to keep a cell alive. Aerobic metabolism is discussed in more detail in Chapters 7 and 18.

Several inheritable disorders result from abnormal mitochondrial activity. The mitochondria involved have defective enzymes that reduce their ability to generate ATP. Cells throughout the body may be affected, but symptoms involving muscle cells, nerve cells, and the light receptor cells in the eye are most commonly seen because these cells have especially high energy demands.

✓ Cells in the ovaries and testes contain large amounts of smooth endoplasmic reticulum (SER). Why?

✓ Microscopic examination of a cell reveals that it contains many mitochondria. What does this observation imply about the cell's energy requirements?

THE NUCLEUS

The **nucleus** is the control center for cellular operations, for here is where the genetic information (DNA) is stored. Most cells contain a single nucleus, but there are exceptions. For example, skeletal muscle cells have many nuclei, and mature red blood cells have none. Figure 3-15• shows the structure of a typical nucleus. A **nuclear envelope** consisting of a double membrane surrounds the nucleus and its fluid contents, the **nucleoplasm**, from the cytosol. The nucleoplasm contains ions, enzymes, RNA and DNA nucleotides, proteins, small amounts of RNA, and DNA.

Chemical communication between the nucleus and the cytosol occurs through **nuclear pores**. These pores, which cover about 10 percent of the surface of the nucleus, are large enough to permit the movement of ions and small molecules but too small for the passage of proteins or DNA.

Chromosome Structure

The DNA in the cell nucleus interacts with special proteins to form complex structures known as **chromosomes** (*chroma*, color). Each nucleus contains 23 pairs of chromosomes; one member of each pair is derived from the mother and one from the father. The structure of a typical chromosome is shown in Figure 3-16•.

Each chromosome contains DNA strands bound to special proteins called *histones*. At intervals, the DNA strands wind around the histones, coiling up the DNA. The degree of coiling determines whether the chromosome is long and thin or short and fat. Chromosomes in a dividing cell are very tightly coiled, and they can be seen clearly as separate structures in light or electron micrographs. In cells that are not dividing, the DNA is loosely coiled, forming a tangle of fine filaments known as **chromatin**.

All vital cellular activities involve proteins, and proteins make up 15–30 percent of the weight of each cell. The nucleus controls cellular operations through its regulation of protein synthesis; the DNA strands of our chromosomes contain the information needed to synthesize at least 100,000 different proteins. (The

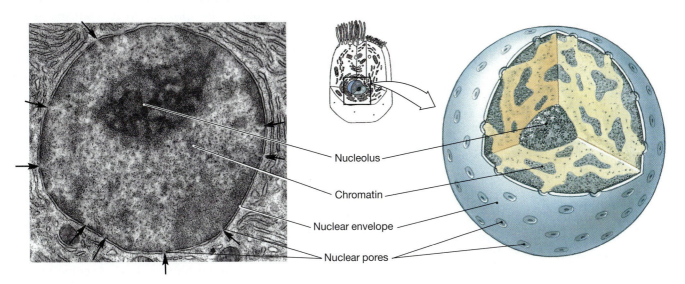

Nucleolus

Chromatin

Nuclear envelope

Nuclear pores

•FIGURE 3-15   The Nucleus
Electron micrograph and diagrammatic view showing important nuclear structures. The arrows indicate the locations of nuclear pores. (TEM × 4828)

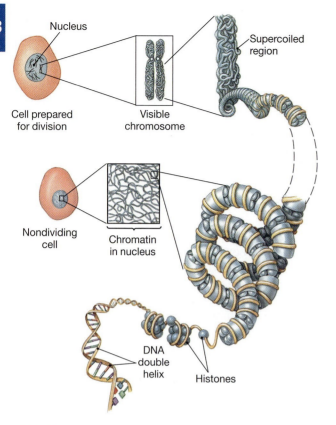

Nucleus

Supercoiled region

Cell prepared for division

Visible chromosome

Nondividing cell

Chromatin in nucleus

DNA double helix

Histones

•**FIGURE 3-16   Chromosome Structure**
DNA strands wound around histone proteins form coils that may be very tight or rather loose. In cells that are not dividing, the DNA is loosely coiled, forming a tangled network known as chromatin. When the coiling becomes tighter, as it does in preparation for cell division, the DNA becomes visible as distinct structures called chromosomes.

details of this process are discussed in the next section.) Most nuclei also contain one to four **nucleoli** (noo-KLĒ-ō-lī; singular *nucleolus*). Nucleoli are organelles that synthesize the components of ribosomes. For this reason, they are most prominent in cells that manufacture large amounts of proteins, such as muscle and liver cells.

The Genetic Code

The basic structure of nucleic acids was described in Chapter 2. ∞ *p. 45* A single DNA molecule consists of a pair of strands held together by hydrogen bonding between complementary nitrogenous bases. Information is stored in the sequence of nitrogenous bases (adenine, A; thymine, T; cytosine, C; and guanine, G) along the length of DNA strands. This information-storage system is known as the **genetic code**.

The genetic code is called a *triplet code* because a sequence of three nitrogenous bases can specify the identity of a single amino acid. Each **gene** consists of all the triplets needed to produce a specific protein. Be-

cause one triplet controls a single amino acid, the number of triplets (and the size of the gene) varies depending on the length of the protein that will be produced. Each gene also contains special segments responsible for regulating its own activity. In effect these triplets say, "Do (or do not) read this message," "Message starts here," and "Message ends here."

✳ DNA FINGERPRINTING

All of the nucleated cells in the body carry identical copies of the 46 chromosomes present in the fertilized egg at the time of conception. But the DNA nucleotide sequences do vary from individual to individual, and the chances of any two individuals, other than identical twins, having the same pattern is less than one in 9 billion. In other words, it is extremely unlikely that you will ever encounter someone else who has the same pattern of repeating nucleotide sequences present in your DNA.

An individual's identification can therefore be made on the basis of a pattern of DNA analysis, just as it can on the basis of a fingerprint. Skin scrapings, blood, semen, hair, or other tissues can be used as a sample source. Information from *DNA fingerprinting* has already been used to convict people who have committed violent crimes, such as rape or murder, and to free those who have been wrongly accused.

Protein Synthesis

Each molecule of DNA contains thousands of genes and therefore holds the information required to synthesize thousands of proteins. These genes are normally tightly coiled and bound to histones, which prevent their activation and, in doing so, prevent the synthesis of proteins. Before a specific gene can be activated, enzymes must temporarily break the weak bonds between its nitrogenous bases and detach it from the associated histones. Although the process that controls gene activation is only partially understood, more is known about protein synthesis. The process of **protein synthesis** is divided into *transcription*, the production of RNA from a single strand of DNA, and *translation*, the assembling of a protein by ribosomes, using the information carried by the RNA molecule. Transcription takes place within the nucleus, and translation occurs in the cytoplasm.

Transcription

Ribosomes, the organelles of protein synthesis, are found in the cytoplasm, whereas the genes remain in the nucleus. This separation between the manufacturing site and the DNA's protein blueprint is overcome by the movement of a molecular messenger, a single strand of RNA known as **messenger RNA (mRNA)**. The process of mRNA formation is called **transcription** because the

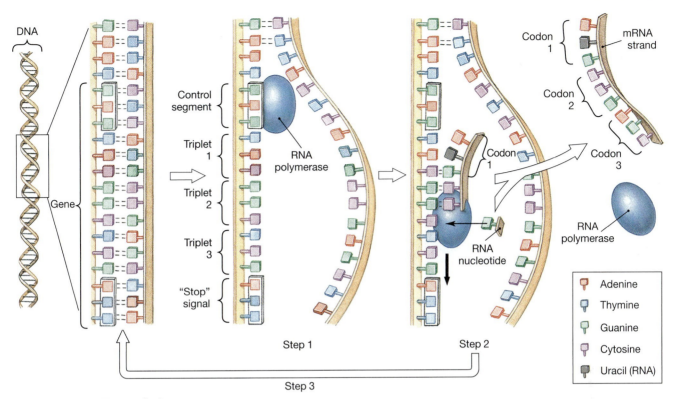

•FIGURE 3-17   Transcription

A small portion of a single DNA molecule, containing a single gene available for transcription. **Step 1:** The two DNA strands separate, and RNA polymerase binds to the control segment of the gene. **Step 2:** The RNA polymerase moves from one triplet to another along the length of the gene. At each site, complementary RNA nucleotides form hydrogen bonds with the DNA nucleotides of the gene. The RNA polymerase then strings the arriving nucleotides together into a strand of mRNA. **Step 3:** On reaching the stop signal at the end of the gene, the RNA polymerase and the mRNA strand detach, and the two DNA strands reattach.

newly formed mRNA is a copy of the information contained in the gene. Figure 3-17• details this process.

Each DNA strand contains thousands of individual genes. When a gene is activated, an enzyme, RNA polymerase, binds to the initial segments of the gene. This enzyme promotes the synthesis of an mRNA strand, using nucleotides complementary to those in the gene. The nucleotides involved are those characteristic of RNA, not DNA; RNA polymerase may attach adenine, guanine, cytosine, or uracil (U), but never thymine. Thus wherever an A occurs in the DNA strand, RNA polymerase will attach a U rather than a T. The mRNA strand thus contains a sequence of nitrogenous bases that are complementary to those of the gene. A sequence of three nitrogenous bases along the new mRNA strand represents a **codon** (KŌ-don) that is complementary to the corresponding triplet along the gene. At the DNA "stop" signal, the enzyme and the mRNA strand detach, and the complementary DNA strands reassociate.

The mRNA formed in this way may be altered before it leaves the nucleus. For example, some triplets may be removed, creating a shorter strand of mRNA. After modifications have been performed, the completed, functional mRNA strand passes through one of the nuclear pores and enters the cytoplasm.

Translation

Translation is the synthesis of a protein using the information provided by the sequence of codons along the mRNA strand. Every amino acid has at least one unique and specific codon; Table 3-4 includes several examples.

TABLE 3-4	Examples of the Genetic Code		
DNA Triplet	*mRNA Codon*	*tRNA Anticodon*	*Amino Acid or Instruction*
AAA	UUU	AAA	Phenylalanine
AAT	UUA	AAU	Leucine
ACA	UGU	ACA	Cysteine
CAA	GUU	CAA	Valine
GGG	CCC	GGG	Proline
CGA	GCU	CGA	Alanine
CGG	GCC	CGG	Alanine
CGC	GCG	CGC	Alanine
TAC	AUG	UAC	Start codon
ATT	UAA	[none]	Stop codon
ATC	UAG	[none]	Stop codon
ACT	UGA	[none]	Stop codon

3

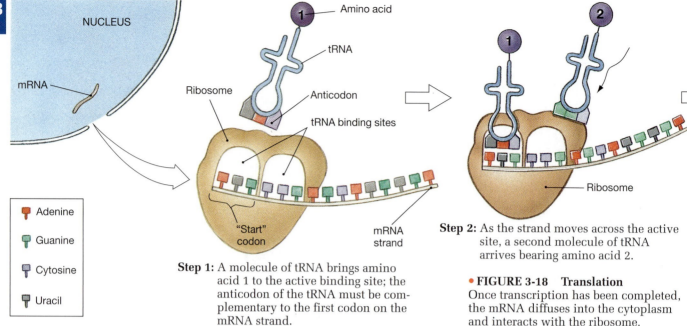

Step 1: A molecule of tRNA brings amino acid 1 to the active binding site; the anticodon of the tRNA must be complementary to the first codon on the mRNA strand.

Step 2: As the strand moves across the active site, a second molecule of tRNA arrives bearing amino acid 2.

• **FIGURE 3-18   Translation**
Once transcription has been completed, the mRNA diffuses into the cytoplasm and interacts with the ribosome.

During translation, the sequence of codons will determine the sequence of amino acids in the protein.

Translation is initiated when the newly synthesized mRNA binds with a ribosome (Figure 3-18•). Molecules of **transfer RNA (tRNA)** then deliver amino acids that will be used by the ribosome to assemble a protein. There are more than 20 different types of transfer RNA, at least one for each amino acid used in protein synthesis. Each tRNA molecule contains a complementary trio of nitrogenous bases, known as an **anticodon**, that will bind to a specific codon on the mRNA.

Step 1: Translation begins at the "start" codon of the mRNA strand, with the arrival and binding of the first tRNA. That tRNA carries a specific amino acid.

Step 2: A second tRNA then arrives, carrying a different amino acid, and binds to the second codon. Ribosomal enzymes now remove amino acid 1 from the first tRNA and attach it to amino acid 2 with a peptide bond. ∞ p. 43 The first tRNA then detaches from the ribosome and reenters the cytosol, where it can pick up another amino acid molecule and repeat the process. The ribosome now moves one codon farther along the length of the mRNA strand, and a third tRNA arrives, bearing amino acid 3.

Step 3: The ribosomal enzymes remove the dipeptide from the second tRNA and attach it to amino acid 3. The second tRNA is then released, and the ribosome moves one codon farther along the mRNA strand.

Step 4: Amino acids will continue to be added to the growing protein in this way until the ribosome reaches the "stop" codon. The ribosome then detaches, leaving an intact strand of mRNA and a completed polypeptide.

As you may recall from Chapter 2, a protein is a polypeptide containing 100 or more amino acids. ∞ p. 42 Translation proceeds swiftly, producing a typical protein (about 1000 amino acids) in around 20 seconds. The protein begins as a simple linear strand, but a more complex structure develops as it grows longer.

✱ RECOMBINANT DNA TECHNOLOGY

Many important medications are derived from animals. For example, insulin, an important hormone in glucose metabolism, was initially derived from swine or cattle. However, there are slight differences in the structure of human insulin and the structure of pork or beef insulin. The amino acid sequence in the animal insulin molecules differs slightly from human insulin. While animal insulin works well in humans, the body eventually begins to produce anti-insulin antibodies against the foreign part of the insulin molecule. Over time, humans on animal insulin require more and more insulin as their immune systems destroy increasing quantities of the animal insulin. This *insulin resistance* becomes a problem for long-term diabetics, as they require increasingly large doses of insulin.

However, scientists have developed a method of producing human insulin by a technique called *recombinant DNA technology*. With this technology, small fragments of human DNA that code for the production of insulin are inserted into specialized bacteria. These bacteria then begin producing insulin identical to human insulin. Diabetics can use this insulin without the risk of developing insulin resistance. Other medications produced by recombinant DNA technology include hepatitis B vaccines, "clot-busting" drugs (tPA) used in heart attacks, and others.

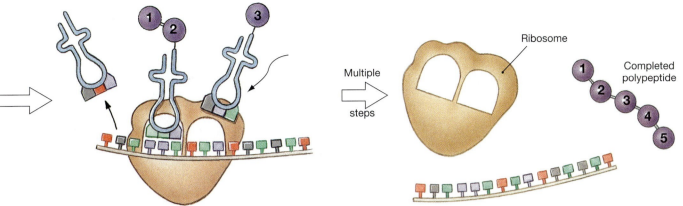

Step 3: Enzymes of the ribosome break the linkage between tRNA-1 and amino acid 1 and join amino acids 1 and 2 with a peptide bond. The ribosome shifts one codon to the right, tRNA-1 departs, and a third tRNA arrives.

Step 4: This process continues until the ribosome reaches the stop codon. The ribosome then breaks the connection between the last tRNA molecule and the polypeptide or protein. The ribosome disengages, leaving the mRNA strand intact.

✓ How does the nucleus control the cell's activities?

✓ What process would be affected by the lack of the enzyme RNA polymerase?

✓ During the process of transcription, a nucleotide was deleted from a mRNA sequence that coded for a protein. What effect would this deletion have on the amino acid sequence of the protein?

CELL DIVISION AND MITOSIS

Between fertilization and physical maturity, a human being goes from a single cell to roughly 75 trillion cells. This amazing increase in numbers occurs through a form of cellular reproduction called **cell division**. Even when development has been completed, cell division continues to be essential to survival as it replaces old and damaged cells.

Central to cell division is the accurate duplication of the cell's genetic material and its distribution to the two new daughter cells formed by division. This process is called **mitosis** (mī-TŌ-sis). Mitosis occurs during the division of the **somatic** (*soma*, body) **cells**, which include the vast majority of the cells in the body. Somatic cell division differs from the division of **reproductive cells**, the specialized cells in the testes and ovaries that give rise to sperm or ova (eggs), respectively. The production of sperm and ova involves a different form of cell division; this process, called **meiosis** (mī-Ō-sis), is described in Chapter 20.

Most cells spend only a small part of their life cycle engaged in cell division, or mitosis. For most of their lives, cells are in **interphase**, an interval of time between cell divisions when they perform normal functions.

Interphase

A somatic cell in interphase is not necessarily preparing for mitosis. Some mature cells, such as skeletal muscle cells and many nerve cells, never undergo mitosis or cell division. A cell that is going to divide must first manufacture enough organelles and cytosol to make two functional cells. These preparations may take hours, days, or weeks to complete, depending on the type of cell and the situation. For example, certain cells in the lining of the digestive tract divide every few days throughout life, whereas specialized cells in other tissues divide only under special circumstances, such as following an injury.

Once these preparations have been completed, the cell replicates the DNA in the nucleus, a process that takes 6–8 hours. The purpose of **DNA replication** is to copy the genetic information in the nucleus so that one set of chromosomes can be given to each of the two cells produced. This process starts when the complementary strands begin to separate and unwind (Figure 3-19●). Molecules of the enzyme *DNA polymerase* then bind to the exposed nitrogenous bases. As a result, complementary nucleotides in the nucleoplasm attach to the exposed nitrogenous bases of the DNA strand and form a pair of identical DNA molecules. Shortly after DNA replication has been completed, mitosis begins.

Mitosis

Mitosis is a process that separates and encloses the duplicated chromosomes of the original cell into two identical nuclei. Separation of the cytoplasm to form two separate and distinct cells involves a separate but related process known as **cytokinesis** (sī-tō-ki-NĒ-sis; *cyto-*, cell + *kinesis*, motion). Mitosis is divided into

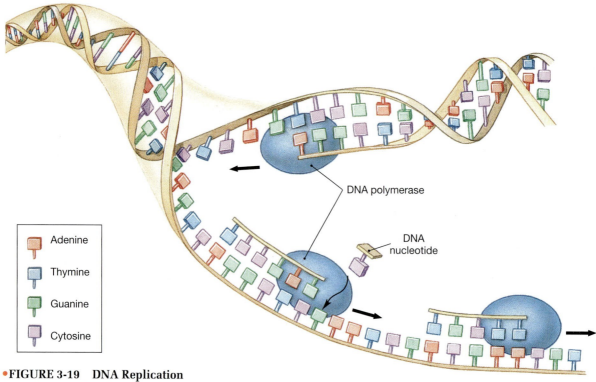

Legend:

■ Adenine

■ Thymine

■ Guanine

■ Cytosine

DNA polymerase

DNA nucleotide

•**FIGURE 3-19   DNA Replication**
In replication, the DNA strands unwind and DNA polymerase begins attaching complementary DNA nucleotides along each strand. Two identical copies of the original DNA molecule are produced.

four stages: *prophase*, *metaphase*, *anaphase*, and *telophase* (Figure 3-20•).

Stage 1: Prophase

Prophase (PRŌ-fāz; *pro-*, before) begins when the chromosomes coil so tightly that they become visible as individual structures. As a result of DNA replication, there are now two copies of each chromosome. Each copy, called a **chromatid** (KRŌ-ma-tid), is connected to its duplicate at a single point, the **centromere** (SEN-trō-mēr).

As the chromosomes appear, the two pairs of centrioles move toward opposite poles of the nucleus. An array of microtubules, called **spindle fibers**, extend between the centriole pairs. Prophase ends with the disappearance of the nuclear envelope.

Stage 2: Metaphase

Metaphase (MET-a-fāz; *meta-*, after) begins after the disintegration of the nuclear envelope. The spindle fibers now enter the nuclear region and the chromatids become attached to them. Once attachment has been completed, the chromatids move to a narrow central zone called the **metaphase plate**. Metaphase ends when all of the chromatids are aligned in the plane of the metaphase plate.

Stage 3: Anaphase

Anaphase (AN-uh-fāz; *ana-*, apart) begins when the centromere of each chromatid pair splits, and the chromatids separate. The two **daughter chromosomes** are now pulled toward opposite ends of the cell. Anaphase ends when the daughter chromosomes arrive near the centrioles at opposite ends of the cell.

Stage 4: Telophase

During **telophase** (TEL-o-fāz; *telos*, end), the cell prepares to return to the interphase state. The nuclear membranes form, the nuclei enlarge, and the chromosomes gradually uncoil. Once the chromosomes have unwound and the fine filaments of chromatin become visible, nucleoli reappear and the nuclei resemble those of interphase cells.

Cytokinesis

Telophase marks the end of mitosis proper, but the daughter cells have yet to complete their physical separation. This separation process, called **cytokinesis**, usually begins in late anaphase. As the daughter chromosomes near the ends of the spindle fibers, the cytoplasm constricts

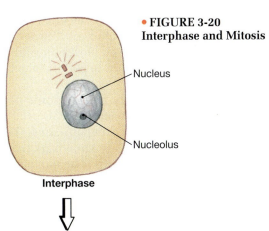

• FIGURE 3-20
Interphase and Mitosis

Nucleus

Nucleolus

Interphase

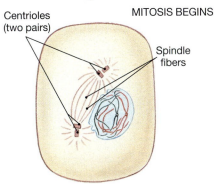

MITOSIS BEGINS

Centrioles
(two pairs)

Spindle
fibers

Early prophase

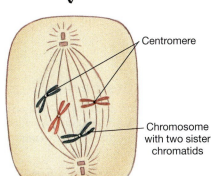

Centromere

Chromosome
with two sister
chromatids

Late prophase

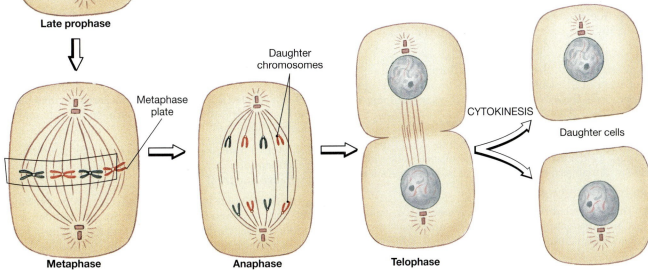

Metaphase
plate

Daughter
chromosomes

CYTOKINESIS

Daughter cells

Metaphase   **Anaphase**   **Telophase**

along the plane of the metaphase plate. This process continues throughout telophase and is usually completed sometime after the nuclear membrane has re-formed. The completion of cytokinesis marks the end of the process of cell division.

Cell Division and Cancer

Within normal tissues, the rate of cell division is balanced with the rate of cell loss. If this balance breaks down, abnormal cell growth and cell division will enlarge the tissue and form a **tumor**, or *neoplasm*. In a **benign tumor**, the abnormal cells remain consolidated and seldom threaten an individual's life. Surgery can usually remove the tumor if it begins to disturb the functions of the surrounding tissue.

Cells in a **malignant tumor**, however, no longer respond to normal control mechanisms. These cells spread not only into nearby tissue but also to other tissues and organs. This spread is called **metastasis** (me-TAS-ta-sis), a process quite difficult to control. Once in a new location, the metastatic cells produce secondary tumors.

The term **cancer** refers to an illness characterized by malignant cells. Such cancer cells lose their resemblance to normal cells and cause organs to dysfunction as their numbers increase. Cancer cells use energy less efficiently than normal cells, and they grow and multiply at the expense of normal tissues. The cancer cells steal nutrients from normal cells, and this accounts for the starved appearance of many patients in the late stages of cancer.

✓ What major event occurs during interphase of cells preparing to undergo mitosis?

✓ List the four stages of mitosis.

✓ What would happen if spindle fibers failed to form in a cell during mitosis?

---

3 CELL DIVERSITY AND DIFFERENTIATION

Fertilization produces a single cell with all of its genetic potential intact. A period of repeated cell divisions follows, ultimately producing trillions of cells. These cells are specialized to perform particular functions, and their specializations reflect the activation or deactivation of specific genes. The specialization process is called **differentiation**. For example, liver cells, fat cells, and neurons contain the same chromosomes and genes, but each cell type has a different set of genes available for transcription. The other genes in the nucleus have been deactivated, or "turned off." When a gene is deactivated, the cell loses the ability to create a particular protein and thus to perform any functions involving that protein.

Differentiation begins early in embryonic development, as the number of cells increases. It produces specialized cells with limited capabilities. These cells form organized collections known as *tissues*, each with discrete functional roles. The next chapter examines the structure and function of tissues and considers the role of tissue interactions in the maintenance of homeostasis.

Chapter Review

KEY TERMS

active transport, *p. 62*	**exocytosis**, *p. 64*	**phagocytosis**, *p. 63*
cells, *p. 54*	**gene**, *p. 70*	**protein synthesis**, *p. 70*
chromosomes, *p. 69*	**Golgi apparatus**, *p. 67*	**ribosome**, *p. 66*
cytoplasm, *p. 55*	**mitochondria**, *p. 68*	**transcription**, *p. 70*
cytosol, *p. 65*	**mitosis**, *p. 73*	**translation**, *p. 71*
diffusion, *p. 58*	**nucleus**, *p. 69*	**tumor**, *p. 75*
endocytosis, *p. 63*	**organelles**, *p. 65*	
endoplasmic reticulum, *p. 66*	**osmosis**, *p. 60*	

SUMMARY OUTLINE

INTRODUCTION *p. 54*

1. Contemporary **cell theory** incorporates several basic concepts: (1) **Cells** are the building blocks of all plants and animals; (2) cells are the smallest functioning units of life; (3) cells are produced by the division of preexisting cells; and (4) each cell maintains homeostasis. *(Figure 3-1)*

STUDYING CELLS *p. 54*

1. Electron microscopes are important tools used in **cytology**, the study of the structure and function of cells.

An Overview of Cellular Anatomy *p. 55*

2. A cell floats in the **extracellular fluid**. The cell's outer boundary, the **cell membrane**, separates the **cytoplasm**, or cell contents, from the extracellular fluid. *(Figure 3-2; Table 3-1)*

THE CELL MEMBRANE *p. 57*

1. The functions of the cell membrane include (1) physical isolation; (2) control of the exchange of materials with the cell's surroundings; (3) sensitivity; and (4) structural support.

Membrane Structure *p. 57*

2. The cell membrane, or *plasma membrane*, contains lipids, proteins, and carbohydrates. Its major components, lipid molecules, form a **phospholipid bilayer**. *(Figure 3-3)*

3. Membrane proteins may function as receptors, channels, carriers, enzymes, anchors, or identifiers. *(Table 3-2)*

Membrane Transport *p. 58*

4. Cell membranes are **selectively permeable**.

5. **Diffusion** is the net movement of material from an area where its concentration is relatively high to an area where its concentration is lower. Diffusion occurs until the **concentration gradient** is eliminated. *(Figures 3-4, 3-5)*

6. **Osmosis** is the diffusion of water across a membrane in response to differences in concentration. The force of movement is **osmotic pressure**. *(Figures 3-6, 3-7)*

7. In **filtration**, hydrostatic pressure forces water across a membrane; if membrane pores are large enough, molecules of solute will be carried along.

8. **Facilitated diffusion** is a type of **carrier-mediated transport** and requires the presence of carrier proteins in the membrane. *(Figure 3-8)*

9. **Active transport** mechanisms consume ATP but are independent of concentration gradients. Some **ion pumps** are **exchange pumps**. *(Figure 3-9)*

10. In **vesicular transport**, material moves into or out of a cell in membranous sacs. Movement into the cell occurs through **endocytosis**, an active process that includes **pinocytosis** ("cell-drinking") and **phagocytosis** ("cell-eating"). Movement out of the cell occurs through **exocytosis**. *(Figure 3-10; Table 3-3)*

THE CYTOPLASM *p. 64*

1. The cytoplasm surrounds the nucleus and contains a fluid **cytosol**, intracellular structures called *organelles*, and **inclusions**.

The Cytosol *p. 65*

2. The **cytosol** differs in composition from the extracellular fluid that surrounds most cells of the body.

Organelles *p. 65*

3. Membrane-enclosed **organelles** are surrounded by lipid membranes that isolate them from the cytosol. They include the endoplasmic reticulum, the nucleus, the Golgi apparatus, lysosomes, and mitochondria. *(Table 3-1)*

4. Organelles that are not membrane-enclosed are always in contact with the cytosol. They include the cytoskeleton, microvilli, centrioles, cilia, flagella, and ribosomes. *(Table 3-1)*

5. The **cytoskeleton** gives the cytoplasm strength and flexibility. Its two main components are **microfilaments** and **microtubules**. *(Figure 3-11)*

6. **Microvilli** are small projections of the cell membrane that increase the surface area exposed to the extracellular environment. *(Figure 3-11)*

7. **Centrioles** direct the movement of chromosomes during cell division.

8. **Cilia** beat rhythmically to move fluids or secretions across the cell surface.

9. **Flagella** move a cell through surrounding fluid rather than moving fluid past a stationary cell.

10. **Ribosomes** are intracellular factories that manufacture proteins. **Free ribosomes** float in the cytoplasm, and **fixed ribosomes** are attached to the endoplasmic reticulum.

11. The **endoplasmic reticulum (ER)** is a network of intracellular membranes. The two types are rough and smooth. **Rough endoplasmic reticulum (RER)** contains ribosomes and is involved in protein synthesis. **Smooth endoplasmic reticulum (SER)** does not contain ribosomes; it is involved in lipid and carbohydrate synthesis. *(Figure 3-12)*

12. The **Golgi apparatus** packages lysosomes and **secretory vesicles**. Secretions are discharged from the cell via exocytosis. *(Figure 3-13)*

13. **Lysosomes** are vesicles filled with digestive enzymes. Their functions include ridding the cell of bacteria and debris.

14. **Mitochondria** are double-membraned organelles responsible for 95 percent of the ATP production within a typical cell. High-energy bonds within adenosine triphosphate, or ATP, provide energy for cellular activities. The production of ATP in mitochondria involves **aerobic metabolism**. *(Figure 3-14)*

THE NUCLEUS *p. 69*

1. The **nucleus** is the control center for cellular operations. It is surrounded by a **nuclear envelope**, through which it communicates with the cytosol through **nuclear pores**. *(Figure 3-15)*

Chromosome Structure *p. 69*

2. The nucleus controls the cell by directing the synthesis of specific proteins using information stored in the DNA of **chromosomes**. *(Figure 3-16)*

The Genetic Code *p. 70*

3. The cell's information storage system, the **genetic code**, is called a *triplet code* because a sequence of three nitrogenous bases identifies a single amino acid. Each **gene** consists of all the triplets needed to produce a specific protein. *(Table 3-4)*

Protein Synthesis *p. 70*

4. **Protein synthesis** includes both *transcription*, which occurs in the nucleus, and *translation*, which occurs in the cytoplasm.

Transcription *p. 70*

5. During **transcription,** a strand of **messenger RNA (mRNA)** is formed and carries protein-making instructions from the nucleus to the cytoplasm. *(Figure 3-17)*

Translation *p. 71*

6. During **translation** a functional protein is constructed from the information contained in an mRNA strand. Each triplet of nitrogenous bases along the mRNA strand is a **codon**; the sequence of codons determines the sequence of amino acids in the protein. *(Figure 3-18)*

7. Molecules of **transfer RNA (tRNA)** bring amino acids to the ribosomes involved in translation. *(Figure 3-18)*

CELL DIVISION AND MITOSIS *p. 73*

1. **Mitosis** is the nuclear division of **somatic cells**. Meiosis is a form of nuclear division essential to the production of **reproductive cells** (sperm and ova).

Interphase *p. 73*

2. Most somatic cells are in **interphase** most of the time. Cells preparing for mitosis undergo **DNA replication** in this phase. *(Figure 3-19)*

Mitosis *p. 73*

3. Mitosis proceeds in four stages: **prophase**, **metaphase**, **anaphase**, and **telophase**. *(Figure 3-20)*

Cytokinesis *p. 74*

4. During **cytokinesis**, the cytoplasm divides, producing two identical daughter cells.

Cell Division and Cancer *p. 75*

5. Abnormal cell growth and division forms **benign tumors** or **malignant tumors** within a tissue. **Cancer** is a disease characterized by the presence of malignant tumors; over time, cancer cells tend to spread to new areas of the body.

CELL DIVERSITY AND DIFFERENTIATION *p. 76*

1. **Differentiation** is the specialization that produces cells with limited capabilities. These specialized cells form organized collections called *tissues*, each of which has specific functional roles.

3 REVIEW QUESTIONS

LEVEL 1 Reviewing Facts and Terms

Match each item in column A with the most closely related item in column B. Use letters for answers in the spaces provided.

Column A

___ 1. filtration
___ 2. osmosis
___ 3. hypotonic solution
___ 4. hypertonic solution
___ 5. isotonic solution
___ 6. facilitated diffusion
___ 7. carrier proteins
___ 8. vesicular transport
___ 9. cytosol
___10. cytoskeleton
___11. microvilli
___12. ribosomes
___13. mitochondria
___14. lysosomes
___15. nucleus
___16. chromosomes
___17. nucleoli

Column B

a. water out of cell
b. passive carrier-mediated transport
c. endocytosis, exocytosis
d. movement of water
e. hydrostatic pressure
f. normal saline
g. ion pump
h. water into cell
i. manufacture proteins
j. digestive enzymes
k. internal protein framework
l. control center for cellular operations
m. intracellular fluid
n. DNA strands
o. cristae
p. synthesize components of ribosomes
q. increase cell surface area

18. The study of the structure and function of cells is called:
    (a) histology
    (b) cytology
    (c) physiology
    (d) biology

19. The proteins in the cell membranes may function as:
    (a) receptors and channels
    (b) carriers and enzymes
    (c) anchors and identifiers
    (d) a, b, and c are correct

20. All of the following membrane transport mechanisms are passive processes except:
    (a) diffusion
    (b) facilitated diffusion
    (c) vesicular transport
    (d) filtration

21. _____ ion concentrations are high in the extracellular fluids, and _____ ion concentrations are high in the cytoplasm.
    (a) calcium, magnesium
    (b) chloride, sodium
    (c) potassium, sodium
    (d) sodium, potassium

22. Structures that perform specific functions within the cell are:
    (a) organs
    (b) organisms
    (c) organelles
    (d) chromosomes

23. The construction of a functional protein using the information provided by an mRNA strand is:
    (a) translation
    (b) transcription
    (c) replication
    (d) gene activation

24. The term *differentiation* refers to:
    (a) the loss of genes from cells
    (b) the acquisition of new functional capabilities by cells
    (c) the production of functionally specialized cells
    (d) the division of genes among different types of cells

25. What are the four general functions of the cell membrane?

26. By what four major transport mechanisms do substances get into and out of cells?

27. What are the three major functions of the endoplasmic reticulum?

28. List the four stages of mitosis in their correct sequence.

LEVEL 2 Reviewing Concepts

29. Diffusion is important in body fluids because this process tends to:
    (a) increase local concentration gradients
    (b) eliminate local concentration gradients
    (c) move substances against their concentration gradients
    (d) create concentration gradients

30. When placed in a _____ solution, a cell will lose water through osmosis. The process results in the _____ of red blood cells.
    (a) hypotonic, crenation
    (b) hypertonic, crenation
    (c) isotonic, hemolysis
    (d) hypotonic, hemolysis

31. Suppose that a DNA segment has the following nucleotide sequence: CTC ATA CGA TTC AAG TTA. Which of the following nucleotide sequences would be found in a complementary mRNA strand?
    (a) GAG UAU GAU AAC UUG AAU
    (b) GAG TAT GCT AAG TTC AAT
    (c) GAG UAU GCU AAG UUC AAU
    (d) GUG UAU GGA UUG AAC GGU

32. How many amino acids are coded in the DNA segment in the previous question?
    (a) 18
    (b) 9
    (c) 6
    (d) 3

33. What are the similarities between facilitated diffusion and active transport? What are the differences?

34. How does the cytosol differ in composition from the extracellular fluid?

35. Differentiate between transcription and translation.

36. List the stages of mitosis, and briefly describe the events that occur in each.

37. What is cytokinesis, and what role does it play in the cell cycle?

LEVEL 3   Critical Thinking and Clinical Applications

38. Experimental evidence shows that the transport of a certain molecule exhibits the following characteristics: (1) The molecule moves along its concentration gradient; (2) at concentrations above a given level, there is no increase in the rate of transport; and (3) cellular energy is not required for transport to occur. Which type of transport process is at work?

39. Two solutions, A and B, are separated by a selectively permeable barrier. Over a period of time, the level of fluid on side A increases. Which solution initially had the higher concentration of solute?

ANSWERS TO CONCEPT CHECK QUESTIONS

Page 64
1. Active transport processes require the expenditure of cellular energy in the form of the high-energy bonds of ATP molecules. Passive transport processes (*diffusion, osmosis, filtration,* and *facilitated diffusion*) move ions and molecules across the cell membrane without any energy expenditure by the cell.   **2.** Energy must be expended to transport H^+ ions against their concentration gradient—that is, from a region where they are less concentrated (the cells lining the stomach) to a region where they are more concentrated (the interior of the stomach). An active transport process must be involved.   **3.** This is an example of phagocytosis.

Page 66
1. The fingerlike projections on the surface of the intestinal cells are *microvilli.* They increase the cells' surface area so they can absorb nutrients more efficiently.   **2.** Cells that lack centrioles are unable to divide.

Page 69
1. The SER functions in the synthesis of lipids such as steroids. Ovaries and testes would be expected to have a great deal of SER because these organs produce large amounts of steroid hormones.   **2.** The function of mitochondria is to produce energy for the cell in the form of ATP molecules. A large number of mitochondria in a cell would indicate a high demand for energy.

Page 73
1. The nucleus of a cell contains DNA that codes for the production of all of the cell's proteins. Some of these proteins are structural proteins that are responsible for the shape and other physical characteristics of the cell. Other proteins are enzymes that govern cellular metabolism, direct the production of cell proteins, and control all of the cell's activities.   **2.** If a cell lacked the enzyme RNA polymerase it would not be able to transcribe RNA from DNA.   **3.** The deletion of a base from a coding sequence of DNA during transcription would alter the entire mRNA base sequence after the deletion point. This would result in different codons on the messenger RNA that was transcribed from the affected region, and this, in turn, would result in the incorporation of a different series of amino acids into the protein. Almost certainly the protein product would not be functional.

Page 75
1. Cells that are preparing to undergo mitosis manufacture additional organelles and duplicate sets of their DNA.   **2.** The four stages of mitosis are prophase, metaphase, anaphase, and telophase.   **3.** If spindle fibers failed to form during mitosis, the cell would not be able to separate the chromosomes into two sets. If cytokinesis occurred, the result would be one cell with two sets of chromosomes and one cell with none.

3 Emergency Care Applications

OVERVIEW

The fundamental unit of the body is the *cell.* The study of cell structure and function is called *cytology* or *cell biology.* Scientists who study cytology and cell biology are referred to as *cell biologists.* Cell biology and biochemistry are very closely related.

Emergency personnel must have a good understanding of human cellular function. Many of the fluids and medications used in emergency medicine directly affect the cells. A major component of emergency medical care is monitoring and replacing the various fluids and electrolytes of the body. A decrease in the absolute volume of body fluids is referred to as dehydration. An increase in fluid volume is called overhydration and can result in edema and heart failure. In addition to fluids, the concentration of essential electrolytes can be disturbed in injury and illness. Optimal body function depends on a normal concentration of body fluids and electrolytes. Because of this, the fluid and electrolyte balance of the body must be maintained within fairly narrow limits. In critical situations, such as shock, the rapid replacement of lost fluids can be life saving.

FLUID MOVEMENT

Water moves through the various membranes of the body by the process of *osmosis* (Figure A3-1•). The rate at which the fluid moves depends upon the differences in the concentration of solutes in the fluid (also called tonicity). The total number of particles in a solution is measured in terms of *osmoles.* In general, the osmole is too large a unit for expressing osmotic activity of solutes in the body fluids. Instead, the term *milliosmole (mOsm),* which equals 1/1000 osmole, is commonly used. Normal body tonicity is approximately 280–310 milliOsmoles/liter. The terms *osmolality* and *osmolarity* are often used to describe the number of solute particles in a solution. Osmolality is the number of osmoles per kilogram of water. *Osmolarity* is the number of osmoles per liter of solution. In dilute solutions, such as body fluids, these two terms can be used almost synonymously because the differences are small. In practice, *osmolarity* is used more frequently than *osmolality.*

Sodium, the most abundant ion in the extracellular fluid, is responsible for the osmotic balance of the extracellular fluid compartment. Water follows sodium in abundance in the extracellular fluid. Potassium is the

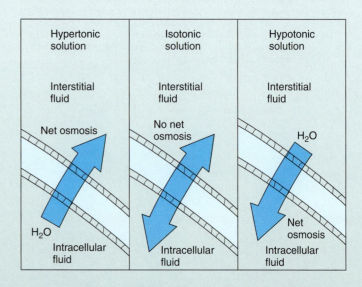

•FIGURE A3-1   Osmosis
Fluid movement between body fluid compartments depends upon the difference in solute concentrations. During osmosis, water moves from an area of low solute concentration to an area of high solute concentration (osmosis).

Hypertonic solution	Isotonic solution	Hypotonic solution
Interstitial fluid	Interstitial fluid	Interstitial fluid
Net osmosis	No net osmosis	H_2O
H_2O		Net osmosis
Intracellular fluid	Intracellular fluid	Intracellular fluid

most abundant ion in the intracellular fluid compartment. Generally, the osmolarity of intracellular fluid does not change very rapidly. However, when there is a change in the osmolarity of extracellular fluid, water will move from the intracellular to the extracellular compartment, or vice versa, until osmotic equilibrium is regained.

Within the extracellular compartment, movement of water between the plasma in the intravascular space and fluid in the interstitial space is primarily a function of forces at play in the capillary beds. In general, the movement of water and solutes across a cell membrane is governed by *osmotic pressure*. Osmotic pressure is the pressure exerted by the concentration of solutes on one side of a semipermeable membrane, such as a cell membrane or the thin wall of a capillary. Osmotic pressure can be thought of as a "pull" rather than a "push" because a hypertonic concentration of solutes tends to pull water from the other side of the membrane.

Generally, there is a "two-way street" as solutes move out of a space while water moves into the space to balance the concentration of solutes on both sides of the membrane. However, a somewhat different osmotic mechanism operates between the plasma inside a capillary and the fluid in the interstitial space outside of the capillary. Blood plasma generates *oncotic force,* which is sometimes called *colloid osmotic pressure.* Plasma proteins are colloids, large particles that do not readily move across the capillary membrane. The most abundant of these is the plasma protein *albumin.* Because of their size, colloids tend to remain within the capillary. At the same time, there is usually very little water in the interstitial space. The small amount of water that does get into the interstitial space is usually taken up by the lymphatic system. Therefore, because there is little water outside the capillary and because plasma proteins do not readily move outside of the capillary, the forces governing water's movement between the capillary and the interstitial space are almost all on one side, governed by the plasma on the inside of the capillary.

Another force inside the capillaries is *hydrostatic pressure,* which is the blood pressure, or force against the vessel walls, created by contractions of the heart. Hydrostatic pressure tends to force some water out of the plasma and across the capillary wall into the interstitial space, a process that is called *filtration.* Hydrostatic pressure (a force that favors filtration, pushing water out of the capillary) and *oncotic force* (a force opposing filtration, pulling water into the capillary) together are responsible for *net filtration,* which is described in *Starling's hypothesis:*

Net filtration = (forces favoring filtration) − (forces opposing filtration)

Net filtration in a capillary is normally zero. It works this way: as plasma enters the capillary at the arterial end, hydrostatic pressure forces water to cross the capillary membrane into the interstitial space. This loss of water increases the relative concentration of plasma proteins and hence the colloid osmotic pressure. By the time the plasma reaches the venous end of the capillary, the oncotic force exerted by the increased concentration of plasma proteins is great enough to pull the water from the interstitial space back into the capillary. The outcome is that water is retained in the intravascular space and does not remain in the interstitial space.

In prehospital emergency care, the exact concentration of fluid and electrolytes is not known. Because of this, intravenous (IV) replacement fluids whose fluid and electrolyte concentrations are similar to those of the body are used initially. Later, when the patient's fluid and electrolyte status is known, IV fluids that will correct any detected underlying fluid and electrolyte problems are administered.

IV FLUID THERAPY

IV fluid therapy is the introduction of fluids and other substances into the venous side of the circulatory system. An important part of emergency care, it is used to replace blood lost through hemorrhage, to replace electrolytes or fluids, and to introduce medications directly into the vascular system.

Numerous types of intravenous fluids are available, each designed to treat a particular type of fluid and electrolyte imbalance. The two primary reasons for starting an IV in the emergency setting are: (1) fluid volume replacement, and (2) intravenous access for drug administration. The following is a discussion of common intravenous fluids and their physiological actions after they enter the body.

IV Fluids

IV fluids are chemically prepared, sterile solutions tailored to the body's specific needs. They replace the body's lost fluids and/or aid in the delivery of IV medications. They also keep a vein patent when no fluid or drug therapy is required. IV fluids are supplied in four different forms: crystalloids, colloids, blood, and oxygen-carrying fluids.

Crystalloids

Crystalloids, the most commonly used IV fluid type in emergency medicine, contain water and electrolytes. They are classified based upon their tonicity and their relation to the tonicity of the body. Table A3-1 illustrates the electrolyte concentration and tonicity of common IV crystalloids. Note that the tonicity of the fluids is measured in terms of osmolarity (reflected as milliOsmoles per liter). Classes of crystalloids include:

- *Isotonic solutions.* Isotonic solutions have a tonicity equal to that of blood plasma. In a normally hydrated patient, they will not cause any significant fluid or electrolyte shift.

TABLE A3-1 Contents and Characteristics of Common Emergency Intravenous Fluids

Approximate Ionic Concentrations (mEq/l) and Calories per Liter

	Ionic Concentrations (mEq/l)							
	Sodium	Potassium	Calcium	Chloride	Lactate	Calories per liter	Osmolarity[a] (mOsm/l)	pH Range[b]
5% Dextrose Injection, USP	0	0	0	0	0	170	252	3.5–6.5
10% Dextrose Injection, USP	0	0	0	0	0	340	505	3.5–6.5
0.9% Sodium Chloride Injection, USP	154	0	0	154	0	0	308	4.5–7.0
Sodium Lactate Injection, USP (M/6 Sodium Lactate)	167	0	0	0	167	54	334	6.0–7.3
2.5% Dextrose & 0.45% Sodium Chloride Injection, USP	77	0	0	77	0	85	280	3.5–6.0
5% Dextrose & 0.2% Sodium Chloride Injection, USP	34	0	0	34	0	170	321	3.5–6.0
5% Dextrose & 0.33% Sodium Chloride Injection, USP	56	0	0	56	0	170	365	3.5–6.0
5% Dextrose & 0.45% Sodium Chloride Injection, USP	77	0	0	77	0	170	406	3.5–6.0
5% Dextrose & 0.9% Sodium Chloride Injection, USP	154	0	0	154	0	170	560	3.5–6.0
10% Dextrose & 0.9% Sodium Chloride Injection, USP	154	0	0	154	0	340	813	3.5–6.0
Ringer's Injection, USP	147.5	4	4.5	156	0	0	309	5.0–7.5
Lactated Ringer's Injection	130	4	3	109	28	9	273	6.0–7.5
5% Dextrose in Ringer's Injection	147.5	4	4.5	156	0	170	561	3.5–6.5
Lactated Ringer's with 5% Dextrose	130	4	3	109	28	180	525	4.0–6.5

*Normal physiological isotonicity range is approximately 280–310 mOsm/l. Administration of substantially hypotonic solutions may cause hemolysis, and administration of substantially hypertonic solutions may cause vein damage.
[b]pH ranges are USP for applicable solution, corporate specification for non-USP solutions.

- *Hypertonic solutions.* Hypertonic solutions have a higher solute concentration than do the body's cells. When administered to a normally hydrated patient, they cause a fluid shift from the intracellular compartment into the extracellular compartment. Later, solutes will diffuse in the opposite direction.
- *Hypotonic solutions.* Hypotonic solutions have a lower solute concentration than do the body's cells. When administered to a normally hydrated patient, they cause a fluid shift from the extracellular compartment into the intracellular compartment. Later, solutes will diffuse in the opposite direction.

The type of IV fluid used depends upon the patient's needs. In the prehospital setting, isotonic fluids are usually used, as the patient's underlying electrolyte and hydration status is unknown (Figure A3-2•). However, once the patient arrives in the emergency department, blood electrolyte studies are used to guide fluid selection and administration. The IV fluids most frequently used in prehospital care include:

- *Lactated Ringer's.* Lactated Ringer's solution is an isotonic electrolyte solution that contains sodium chloride, potassium chloride, calcium chloride, and sodium lactate in water.
- *Normal saline.* Normal saline is an isotonic electrolyte solution that contains sodium chloride in water.
- *5% dextrose in water (D_5W).* D_5W is a hypotonic glucose solution used to keep a vein patent and to dilute concentrated medications. While D_5W initially increases intravascular volume, glucose molecules rapidly diffuse across the vascular membrane and increase the amount of free water.

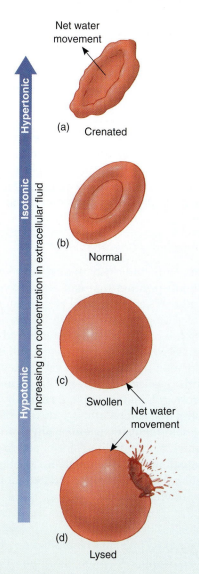

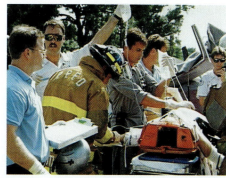

• FIGURE A3-3   Emergency Fluid Resuscitation
Administering IV fluids in the prehospital setting can often mean the difference between life and death for the victim of shock.

containing solutions will also contain electrolytes, usually sodium and chloride. Examples of these include:

- 2.5% dextrose and 0.45% sodium chloride ($D_{2.5}NS$)
- 5% dextrose and 0.20% sodium chloride (D_5NS)
- 5% dextrose and 0.33% sodium chloride (D_5NS)
- 5% dextrose and 0.45% sodium chloride (D_5NS)
- 5% dextrose and 0.9% sodium chloride (D_5NS)
- 10% dextrose and 0.9% sodium chloride ($D_{10}NS$)
- 5% dextrose in lactated Ringer's (D_5LR)

The high-concentration solutions, such as $D_{50}W$ and $D_{25}W$, are used for glucose replacement in documented hypoglycemia. $D_{10}W$ is used in patients such as chronic alcoholics who require calorie replacement in addition to water and electrolytes. D_5W and similar solutions are usually used for diluting intravenous medications and for conditions where an IV is started at a "to keep open" (TKO) or "keep vein open" (KVO) rate.

The solubility of dextrose is 1 gram per milliliter of water. Based on this property, dextrose-containing solutions are usually measured in *weight-in-volume percentages.* This system of measurement indicates the number of grams of dextrose in 100 mL of solution (water). A fully saturated solution contains 100 grams of dextrose per 100 mL of water and is considered a 100% solution ($D_{100}W$). $D_{50}W$, commonly used in prehospital care, contains 25 grams of glucose in 50 mL of water. Likewise, $D_{25}W$ contains 12.5 grams of glucose in 50 mL of water. $D_{25}W$ is preferred over $D_{50}W$ when administering intravenous dextrose to infants and children. $D_{25}W$ can be prepared by diluting 25 mL of $D_{50}W$ with 25 mL of sterile water for injection. This results in a solution that contains 12.5 grams of dextrose in 50 mL of water.

When considering glucose content, it is best to consider the amount of dextrose per mL of water. With a 50% dextrose solution, 1 mL of solution contains 0.5 grams of dextrose. Likewise, in a 25% dextrose solution, 1 mL of solution contains 0.25 grams of dextrose. A 100% dextrose solution would contain 1 gram/mL. A solution of 5% dextrose in water contains 0.05 grams of dextrose per mL.

• FIGURE A3-2   Effects of IV Fluids on Circulating Red Blood Cells (Erthrocytes)
Hypertonic fluids cause cell shrinkage (crenation), while hypotonic fluids cause intracellular swelling that eventually leads to cell rupture.

Both lactated Ringer's and normal saline are used for fluid replacement because of their immediate ability to expand the circulating fluid volume. However, due to the movement of electrolytes and water, two-thirds of either solution will be lost to the extravascular space within one hour (Figure A3-3•).

Dextrose-Containing Solutions

Several IV fluids contain dextrose (*d*-glucose) in varying concentrations. The most commonly used of these are 50% dextrose ($D_{50}W$) and 5% dextrose in water (D_5W). Other dextrose solutions include 25% dextrose ($D_{25}W$) and 10% dextrose and water ($D_{10}W$). Some dextrose-

Most intravenous fluids contain 5% dextrose in water or an electrolyte solution. When administered at a TKO or KVO rate, the amount of dextrose delivered to the patient is negligible. However, if IV solutions containing 5% dextrose are used for volume replacement, then the amount of dextrose administered can be potentially dangerous for the patient. A 1,000 mL bag of D_5W contains 50 grams of dextrose. This is equivalent to two prefilled syringes of $D_{50}W$. In multiple trauma, it is not uncommon to administer 2–3 liters of IV fluid in the prehospital setting. If D_5W were used, this would constitute a very high dextrose load. Infants and children are at increased risk of accidental overdose with dextrose. In documented hypoglycemia, the standard dose of dextrose is 0.5 grams per kilogram body weight. A child who weighs 10 kilograms, for example, would receive 5 grams of dextrose for documented hypoglycemia (10 mL of $D_{50}W$ or 20 mL of $D_{25}W$). The amount of IV fluid administered to children who are dehydrated or in shock is 20 mL/kg of an isotonic crystalloid solution such as normal saline or lactated Ringer's. If D_5W were used by accident, 20 mL of fluid would provide 1 gram of dextrose per kilogram body weight. This is twice the recommended dose for documented hypoglycemia. Avoid using dextrose-containing solutions for any situation where volume replacement must be provided.

Colloids

Colloid solutions contain large proteins that cannot pass through the capillary membrane. Consequently, they remain in the intravascular compartment for a period of time. In addition, colloids have osmotic properties that attract water into the intravascular compartment. Thus, a small quantity of colloid can significantly increase intravascular volume. Common colloids include:

- *Plasma protein fraction (Plasmanate).* Plasmanate is a protein-containing colloid solution. Its principle protein, albumin, is suspended in a saline solvent.
- *Salt-poor albumin.* Salt-poor albumin contains only human albumin. Each gram of albumin will retain approximately 18 mL of water in the intravascular space.
- *Dextran.* Dextran is not a protein but a large sugar molecule with osmotic properties similar to albumin's. It is supplied in two molecular weights: 40,000 and 70,000 Daltons. Dextran 40 has from two to two and a half times the colloidal osmotic pressure of albumin.
- *Hetastarch (Hespan).* Like Dextran, hetastarch is a sugar molecule with osmotic properties similar to those of proteins such as albumin.

Although colloids help to maintain intravascular volume, their use in the field is impractical. Their high cost, short shelf life, and specific storage requirements suit them better to the hospital setting.

Blood

The most desirable fluid for replacement is whole blood. Unlike colloids and crystalloids, the hemoglobin available in blood carries oxygen. Blood, however, is a precious commodity and must be conserved so that it can be of benefit to the most people. Its use in the field is usually limited to aeromedical operations or mass-casualty incidents. O-negative blood does not contain any antigenic proteins and is thus considered the "universal donor" type.

Oxygen-Containing Solutions

Intense research is underway to develop a synthetic, or artificial, blood product that can carry oxygen. These products, although experimental at present, show great promise for treating hypovolemia in the prehospital setting. Among the products being investigated are *perfluorocarbons (PFCs)*, which carry oxygen and other gases. The gases are retained on the carrying molecule by a surfactant, in this case lecithin. Several PFCs are being studied. Other research is directed at developing new types of hemoglobin that can be infused into the bloodstream. The hemoglobin molecule is either physically or chemically modified in order to limit side effects from infusion of pure hemoglobin. The hemoglobin is obtained from recombinant DNA synthesis, outdated human blood products, or bovine sources.

SUMMARY

The body requires a steady balance in fluid and electrolyte concentrations. Through homeostatic mechanisms, the body immediately reacts to any change in the fluid or electrolyte concentrationin order to return the concentration to normal. In emergencies, fluid and electrolyte administration can be lifesaving. In severe hemorrhage, crystalloid IV fluids can support necessary physiological functions until the underlying problem can be corrected or until blood or blood products can be administered. Likewise, access to the vascular system allows the rapid administration of essential emergency medications. Fluid and electrolyte therapy is a fundamental component of emergency care. All emergency personnel must be familiar with this therapy's underlying physiological processes as well as with the commonly used intravenous replacement fluids.

4 The Tissue Level of Organization

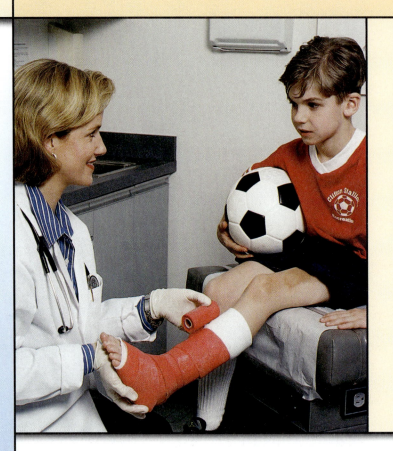

Much of modern medical practice involves aiding the body's own homeostatic mechanisms. The human body has a tremendous capacity to heal itself. For example, the child with a leg fracture will be able to bear full weight in 5–6 weeks. Within a year, the fracture site will no longer be visible on X-rays. Except for the liver, bone is unique among all body tissues in that it will form new bone, not scar tissue, when it heals after a fracture.

Chapter Outline and Objectives

Vocabulary Development

a-, without *avascular*
apo-, from; *apocrine*
*cardio-, heart; *cardiology*
cardium, heart; *pericardium*
chondros, cartilage; *perichondrium*
dendron, tree; *dendrites*
*derm-, skin; *dermotology*
desmos, ligament; *desmosome*
*endo-, inside; *endocrinology*
*gastr-, stomach; *gastroenterology*
glia, glue; *neuroglia*
*hemato-, blood; *hematology*
histos, tissue; *histology*
holos, entire; *holocrine*
hyalos, glass; *hyaline cartilage*
inter-, between; *interstitial*
krinein, to secrete; *exocrine*
lacus, pool; *lacunae*
meros, part; *merocrine*
*nephr-, kidney; *nephrology*
neuro, nerve; *neuron*
*ophthalm-, eye; *ophthamology*
*orth-, straight; *orthopedic*
os, bone; *osseous tissue*
*oto-, ear; *otolaryngology*
*patho-, disease; *pathology*
*pedia-, child; *pediatrics*
peri-, around; *perichondrium*
phagein, to eat; *macrophage*
pleura, rib; *pleural membrane*
pseudes, false; *pseudostratified*
*pulmo-, lung; *pulmonary*
sistere, to set; *interstitial*
soma, body; *desmosome*
squama, plate or scale; *squamous*
syn-, together; *synapse*
*thorac-, chest; *thoracic*
*uro-, urine; *urology*
vas, vessel; *vascular*

4

No single cell is able to perform the many functions of the human body. But through the process of differentiation, each cell specializes to perform a relatively restricted range of functions. Although there are trillions of individual cells in the human body, there are only about 200 different types of cells. These cell types combine to form **tissues**, collections of specialized cells and cell products that perform a limited range of functions. Tissues are categorized into four **primary tissue types**: *epithelial tissue, connective tissue, muscle tissue,* and *neural tissue* (Figure 4-1●).

The study of tissues, **histology** (*histos,* tissue), provides beautiful examples of the interplay of form and function. This chapter will examine the characteristics of each major tissue type and the relationship between their highly diverse cells and tissue function. Later chapters will consider the patterns of tissue interaction in various organs and systems in greater detail.

EPITHELIAL TISSUE

Epithelial tissue consists of epithelia (e-pi-THĒ-lē-a) and **glands**, secreting cells derived from epithelia. An **epithelium** is a layer of cells that forms a barrier with specific properties. Important characteristics of epithelia include the following:

- A free surface exposed to the environment or to some internal chamber or passageway.
- Attachment to underlying connective tissue by a *basement membrane.*
- The absence of blood vessels. Because of this **avascular** (ā-VAS-kū-lar; *a-*, without + *vas,* vessel) condition, epithelial cells must obtain nutrients from deeper tissues or from their exposed surfaces.

Epithelia cover both external and internal body surfaces. In addition to covering the skin, epithelia line internal passageways that communicate with the outside world, such as the digestive, respiratory, reproductive, and urinary tracts. These epithelia form selective barriers that separate the deep tissues of the body from the external environment.

Epithelia also line internal cavities and passageways, such as the chest cavity, fluid-filled chambers in the brain, eye, and inner ear, and the inner surfaces of blood vessels and the heart. These epithelia prevent friction, regulate the fluid composition of internal cavities, and restrict communication between the blood and tissue fluids.

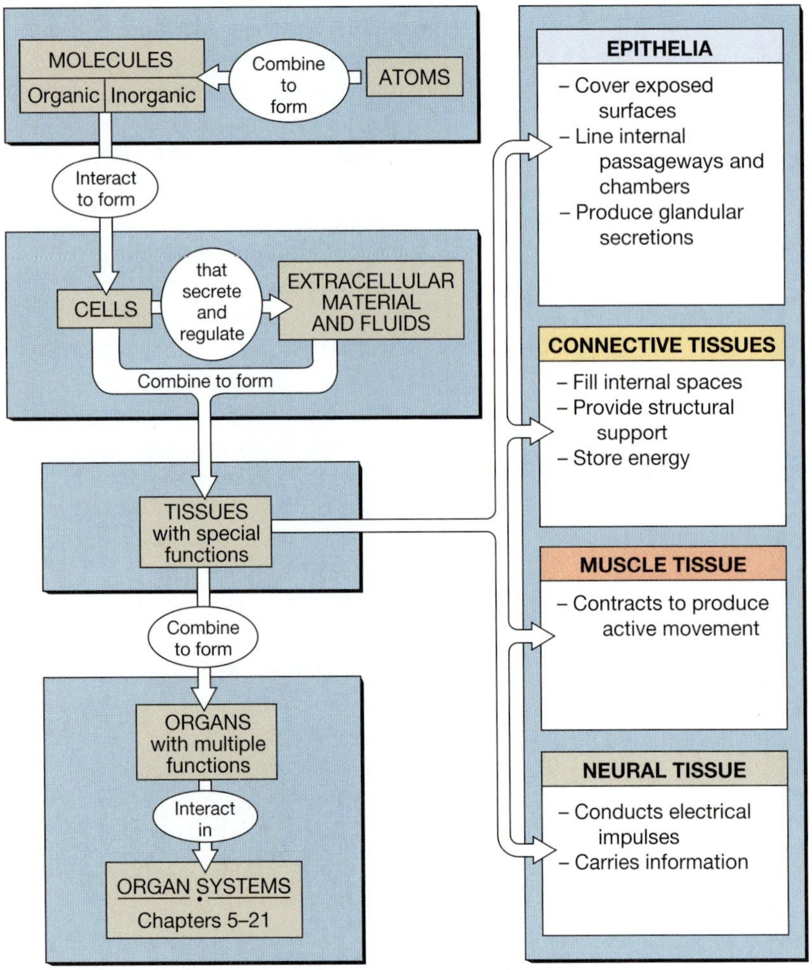

Functions of Epithelia

Epithelia perform four essential functions that can be summarized as follows:

1. *Providing physical protection.* Epithelia protect exposed and internal surfaces from abrasion, dehydration, and destruction by chemical or biological agents. For example, as long as it remains intact, the epithelium of your skin resists impacts and scrapes, restricts water loss, and prevents invasion of underlying structures by bacteria.

2. *Controlling permeability.* Any substance that enters or leaves the body must cross an epithelium. Some epithelia are relatively impermeable, whereas others are easily crossed by compounds as large as proteins.

3. *Providing sensations.* Specialized epithelial cells can detect changes in the environment and relay information about such changes to the nervous system. For example, touch receptors in the deepest layers of the epithelium of the skin respond by stimulating neighboring sensory nerves.

●**FIGURE 4-1   An Orientation to the Tissues of the Body**

4. *Producing specialized secretions.* Epithelial cells that produce secretions are called **gland cells**. In a **glandular epithelium**, most or all of the cells actively produce secretions. These secretions are classified according to their discharge location:

- **Exocrine** (*exo-*, outside + *krinein*, to secrete) secretions are discharged onto the surface of the skin or other epithelial surface. Enzymes entering the digestive tract, perspiration on the skin, and milk produced by mammary glands are examples.

- **Endocrine** (*endo-*, inside) secretions are released into the surrounding tissues and blood. These secretions, called *hormones*, regulate or coordinate the activities of other tissues, organs, and organ systems. (Hormones are discussed further in Chapter 11.) Endocrine secretions are produced in organs such as the pancreas, thyroid, and pituitary gland.

Intercellular Connections

To be effective in protecting other tissues, epithelial cells must remain attached to one another. If an epithelium is damaged or the connections are broken, it is no longer an effective barrier. For example, when the epithelium of the skin is damaged by a burn or abrasion, disease-causing bacteria can enter underlying tissues and cause an infection. Undamaged epithelia form effective barriers because the epithelial cells are held together by an intercellular cement (composed of a protein-polysaccharide mixture) and a variety of cell attachments, or junctions. Three such junctions are *gap junctions*, *tight junctions*, and *desmosomes*.

At a **gap junction**, two cells are held together by interlocked membrane proteins (Figure 4-2a•). Because these are channel proteins, the result is a narrow passageway that lets small solutes, such as ions, pass from cell to cell. Gap junctions interconnect cells in some epithelia, but they are most abundant in cardiac muscle and smooth muscle tissue, where they link adjacent muscle cells.

At a **tight junction**, the outermost lipid layers of adjacent cell membranes are tightly pressed together by interlocking proteins (Figure 4-2b•). Tight junctions prevent the passage of water and solutes between the cells. These junctions are common between epithelial cells exposed to harsh chemicals or powerful enzymes. For example, tight junctions between epithelial cells lining the digestive tract keep digestive enzymes, stomach acids, or waste products from damaging underlying tissues.

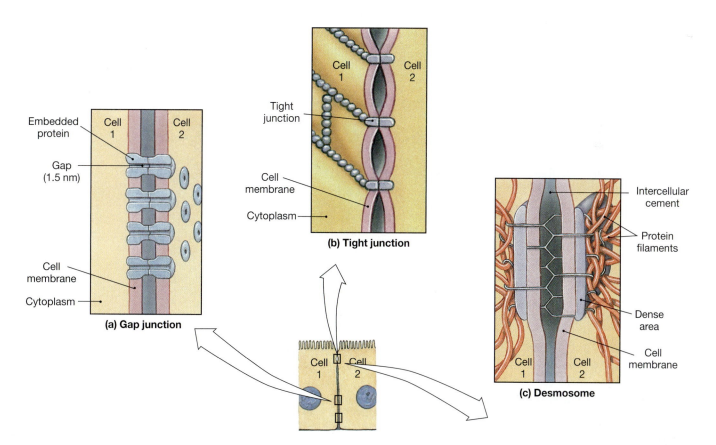

•**FIGURE 4-2   Cell Attachments**
(a) At a gap junction, the binding of membrane proteins containing channels creates a cytoplasmic connection between two cells. **(b)** A tight junction is formed when proteins bind together the outer layers of the two cell membranes. **(c)** A desmosome has a highly organized network of protein filaments.

4

At **desmosomes** (DEZ-mō-sōmz; *desmos*, ligament + *soma*, body), two cell membranes are locked together by intercellular cement and a network of fine protein filaments (Figure 4-2c•). Desmosomes are very strong, and the connection can resist stretching and twisting. In the skin, these links are so strong that dead cells are usually shed in thick sheets, rather than individually.

The Epithelial Surface

Many epithelia have microvilli on their exposed surfaces. ∞ *p. 65* They may vary in number from just a few to so many that they carpet the entire surface (Figure 4-3•). Microvilli are especially abundant on epithelial surfaces where absorption and secretion take place, such as along portions of the digestive and urinary tracts. These epithelial cells specialize in the active and passive transport of materials across their cell membranes. ∞ *p. 58* A cell with microvilli has at least 20 times the surface area of a cell without them; the greater the surface area of the cell membrane, the more transport proteins will be exposed to the extracellular environment. The diagram in Figure 4-3• also shows elongated microvilli, called *stereocilia*. Stereocilia are found only on very specialized cells in the male reproductive tract and in the inner ear. The stereocilia on inner ear cells are essential to our sensations of equilibrium and balance.

Some epithelia contain cilia on their exposed surfaces. ∞ *p. 66* A typical cell within a *ciliated epithelium* has roughly 250 cilia that beat in a coordinated fashion to move materials across the epithelial surface. For example, the ciliated epithelium that lines the respiratory tract moves mucus-trapped irritants away from the lungs and toward the throat.

The Basement Membrane

Epithelial cells not only must hold onto one another but also must remain firmly connected to the rest of the body. This function is performed by the **basement membrane**, which lies between the epithelium and underlying connective tissues (Figure 4-3a•). There are no cells within the basement membrane, which consists of a network of protein fibers. The epithelial cells adjacent to the basement membrane are firmly attached to its protein fibers. In addition to providing strength and resisting distortion, the basement membrane also provides a barrier that restricts the movement of proteins and other large molecules from the underlying connective tissue into the epithelium.

Epithelial Renewal and Repair

To maintain its structure, the epithelium must continually repair and renew itself by replacing exposed cells.

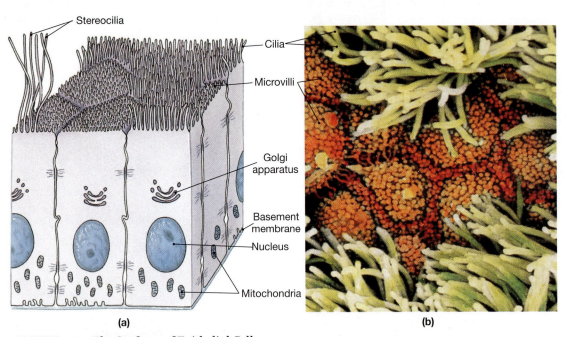

(a) (b)

•**FIGURE 4-3   The Surfaces of Epithelial Cells**
(a) The inner and outer surfaces of most epithelia are specialized for specific functions. The free surface often bears microvilli; less commonly, this surface has cilia or (very rarely) stereocilia. (Stereocilia and microvilli are seldom found on the same cell, but they are shown together here so you can easily compare their proportions.) Mitochondria are typically concentrated near the base of the cell, probably to provide energy for the cell's transport activities. **(b)** An SEM showing the surface of a ciliated epithelium that lines most of the respiratory tract. The small, bristly areas are microvilli on the exposed surfaces of mucus-producing cells that are scattered among the ciliated epithelial cells. (SEM × 13,469)

Epithelial cells may survive for just a day or two, because they are lost or destroyed by exposure to disruptive enzymes, toxic chemicals, pathogenic bacteria, or mechanical abrasion. The only way the epithelium can survive is by replacing itself over time through the continual division of unspecialized cells known as **stem cells**, or *germinative cells*. These are found in the deepest layers of the epithelium, near the basement membrane.

Classifying Epithelia

Epithelia are classified according to the number of cell layers and the shape of the exposed cells. This classification scheme recognizes two types of layering—*simple* and *stratified*—and three cell shapes—*squamous*, *cuboidal*, and *columnar*.

Cell Layers

A **simple epithelium** consists of a single layer of cells covering the basement membrane. Simple epithelia are relatively thin, and the nuclei of the individual cells form a rough line above the basement membrane. Since a single layer of cells cannot provide much mechanical protection, simple epithelia are found only in protected areas inside the body. They line internal compartments and passageways, including the body cavities and the interior of the heart and blood vessels.

Simple epithelia, shown in Figure 4-4•, are characteristic of regions where secretion or absorption occurs, such as the lining of the digestive and urinary tracts and the gas-exchange surfaces of the lungs. In such places, thinness is an advantage, for it reduces the diffusion time for materials crossing the epithelial barrier.

A **stratified epithelium** provides a greater degree of protection because it has several layers of cells above the basement membrane. Stratified epithelia are usually found in areas subject to mechanical or chemical stresses, such as the surface of the skin and the linings of the mouth and anus.

Cell Shape

In sectional view, the cells at the surface of the epithelium usually have one of three basic shapes.

1. *Squamous.* In a **squamous epithelium** (SKWĀ-mus; *squama*, a plate or scale), the cells are thin and flat and the nucleus occupies the thickest portion of each cell. Viewed from the surface, the cells look like fried eggs laid side by side.
2. *Cuboidal.* The cells of a **cuboidal epithelium** resemble little hexagonal boxes when seen in three dimensions, but in typical sectional view, they appear

square. The nuclei lie near the center of each cell, and they form a neat row.

3. *Columnar.* In a **columnar epithelium**, the cells are also hexagonal, but taller and more slender. The nuclei are crowded into a narrow band close to the basement membrane, and the height of the epithelium is several times the distance between two nuclei.

The two basic epithelial arrangements (simple and stratified) and the three possible cell shapes (squamous, cuboidal, and columnar) enable one to describe almost every epithelium in the body. We will focus here on only a few major types of epithelia; additional examples will be encountered in later chapters.

Simple Squamous Epithelia

A delicate **simple squamous epithelium** is found in protected regions where absorption takes place or where a slick, slippery surface reduces friction (Figure 4-4a•). Examples are portions of the kidney tubules, the exchange surfaces of the lungs, the lining of body cavities, and the lining of blood vessels and the heart.

Simple Cuboidal Epithelia

A **simple cuboidal epithelium** provides limited protection and occurs in regions where secretion or absorption takes place (Figure 4-4b•). These functions are enhanced by larger cells that have more room for the necessary organelles. Simple cuboidal epithelia secrete enzymes and buffers in the pancreas and salivary glands and line the ducts that discharge these secretions. Simple cuboidal epithelia also line portions of the kidney tubules involved in the production of urine.

Simple Columnar Epithelia

A **simple columnar epithelium** provides some protection and may also occur in areas of absorption or secretion (Figure 4-4c•). This type of epithelium lines the stomach, the intestinal tract, and many excretory ducts.

Pseudostratified Epithelia

Portions of the respiratory tract contain a columnar epithelium that includes a mixture of cell types. Because the nuclei are situated at varying distances from the surface, the epithelium has a layered appearance. Yet it is not a stratified epithelium, because all of the cells contact the basement membrane. Because it looks stratified but is not, it is known as a **pseudostratified columnar epithelium** (Figure 4-5a•, p. 87). The figure also shows the cilia that this tissue typically possesses. A ciliated pseudostratified columnar epithelium lines most of the nasal cavity, the trachea (windpipe) and bronchi, and portions of the male reproductive tract.

4

SIMPLE SQUAMOUS EPITHELIUM

LOCATIONS: Epithelia lining ventral body cavities; lining of heart and blood vessels; portions of kidney tubules (thin sections of loop of Henle), inner lining of cornea, exchange surfaces of lungs

FUNCTIONS: Reduces friction, controls vessel permeability, performs absorption and secretion

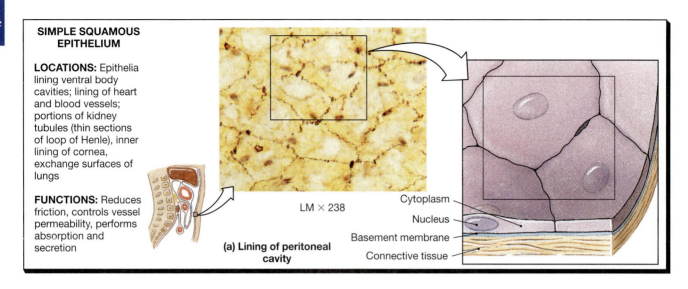

LM × 238

(a) Lining of peritoneal cavity

Cytoplasm
Nucleus
Basement membrane
Connective tissue

SIMPLE CUBOIDAL EPITHELIUM

LOCATIONS: Glands, ducts, portions of kidney tubules, thyroid gland

FUNCTIONS: Limited protection, secretion and/or absorption

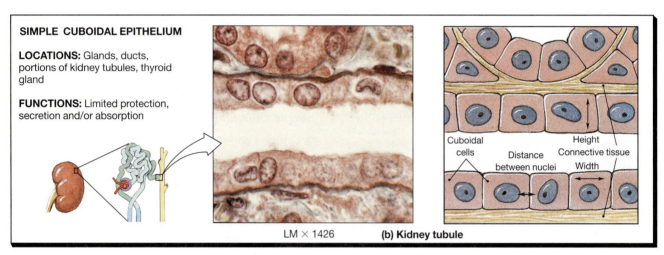

LM × 1426

(b) Kidney tubule

Cuboidal cells
Distance between nuclei
Height
Connective tissue
Width

SIMPLE COLUMNAR EPITHELIUM

LOCATIONS: Lining of stomach, intestine, gallbladder, uterine tubes, collecting ducts of kidneys

FUNCTIONS: Protection, secretion, absorption

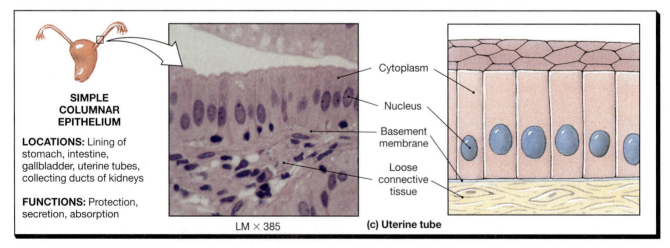

LM × 385

Cytoplasm
Nucleus
Basement membrane
Loose connective tissue

(c) Uterine tube

● **FIGURE 4-4   Simple Epithelia**
(a) A superficial view of the simple squamous epithelium that lines the peritoneal cavity. The three-dimensional drawing shows the epithelium in superficial and sectional views. **(b)** A section through the cuboidal epithelial cells of a kidney tubule. The diagrammatic view emphasizes structural details that permit the classification of an epithelium as cuboidal. **(c)** A micrograph showing the characteristics of simple columnar epithelium. In the diagrammatic sketch, note the relationships between the height and width of each cell; the relative size, shape, and location of nuclei; and the distance between adjacent nuclei. Compare with Figure 4-4b.

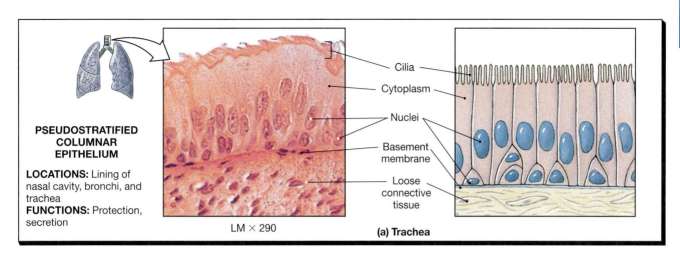

PSEUDOSTRATIFIED COLUMNAR EPITHELIUM

LOCATIONS: Lining of nasal cavity, bronchi, and trachea
FUNCTIONS: Protection, secretion

LM × 290

Cilia
Cytoplasm
Nuclei
Basement membrane
Loose connective tissue

(a) Trachea

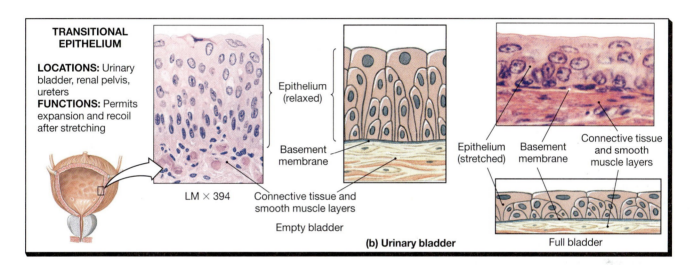

TRANSITIONAL EPITHELIUM

LOCATIONS: Urinary bladder, renal pelvis, ureters
FUNCTIONS: Permits expansion and recoil after stretching

LM × 394

Epithelium (relaxed)

Basement membrane

Connective tissue and smooth muscle layers

Empty bladder

Epithelium (stretched)   Basement membrane   Connective tissue and smooth muscle layers

Full bladder

(b) Urinary bladder

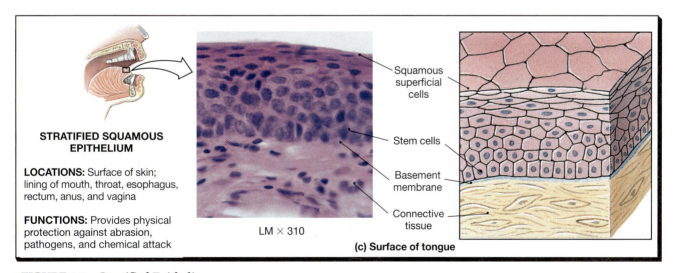

STRATIFIED SQUAMOUS EPITHELIUM

LOCATIONS: Surface of skin; lining of mouth, throat, esophagus, rectum, anus, and vagina

FUNCTIONS: Provides physical protection against abrasion, pathogens, and chemical attack

LM × 310

Squamous superficial cells
Stem cells
Basement membrane
Connective tissue

(c) Surface of tongue

● **FIGURE 4-5   Stratified Epithelia**
(a) The pseudostratified, ciliated, columnar epithelium of the respiratory tract. Note the uneven layering of the nuclei.
(b) At left, the lining of the empty urinary bladder, showing a transitional epithelium in the relaxed state. At right, the lining of the full bladder, showing the effects of stretching on the arrangement of cells in the epithelium. **(c)** A sectional view of the stratified squamous epithelium that covers the tongue.

4

Transitional Epithelia

A **transitional epithelium** lines the ureters and urinary bladder, where significant changes in volume occur (Figure 4-5b•). In an empty urinary bladder, the epithelium seems to have many layers, and the outermost cells appear rounded or cuboidal. The layered appearance results from overcrowding; the actual structure of the epithelium can be seen in the full bladder, when the pressure of the urine has stretched the lining to its natural thickness.

Stratified Squamous Epithelia

A **stratified squamous epithelium** is found where mechanical stresses are severe (Figure 4-5c•). The surface of the skin and the lining of the mouth, tongue, esophagus, and anus are good examples.

✳ CELLULAR ADAPTATION

Cells can change or adapt to their environment in order to protect themselves from injury. This process, called *cellular adaptation,* is a common and central aspect of many disease states. Cells can adapt by decreasing their size (*atrophy*), increasing their size (*hypertrophy*), increasing their numbers (*hyperplasia*), or by reversibly replacing one mature cell type with another, less mature type (*metaplasia*).

A good example of metaplasia is the response of bronchial (airway) tissues to prolonged exposure to cigarette smoke. In this process, normal columnar ciliated epithelial cells of the bronchial lining are replaced with stratified squamous epithelial cells. The newly formed replacement cells do not have cilia and do not secrete mucus. This results in a loss of two important pulmonary protective mechanisms. Bronchial metaplasia can often be reversed if the offending stimulus, usually cigarette smoke, is removed. When this occurs, normal columnar ciliated epithelial cells begin replacing cells changed through the metaplastic process.

In addition to metaplasia, continued, prolonged exposure to cigarette smoke can result in the cancerous transformation of bronchial epithelial cells (*dysplasia*). Bronchogenic (lung) cancers are a major health problem in industrialized countries. The mortality rate is high, causing 32 percent of all cancer deaths.

Glandular Epithelia

Many epithelia contain gland cells that produce exocrine or endocrine secretions. Exocrine secretions are produced by exocrine glands that discharge their products through a *duct*, or tube, onto some external or internal surface. Endocrine secretions (*hormones*) are produced by ductless glands and released into blood or tissue fluids. Exocrine glands are often described in terms of their *mode of secretion* or the *type of secretion*. Table 4-1 summarizes this information and provides specific examples.

Mode of Secretion

A glandular epithelial cell may use one of three methods to release its secretions: *merocrine secretion, apocrine secretion,* or *holocrine secretion.*

In **merocrine secretion** (MER-o-krin; *meros,* part + *krinein,* to secrete) the product is released through exocytosis. ∞ *p. 64* This method is the most common mode of secretion (Figure 4-6a•). **Apocrine secretion** (AP-ō-krin; *apo-,* off) involves the loss of both cytoplasm and the secretory product (Figure 4-6b•). The outermost portion of the cytoplasm becomes packed with secretory vesicles before it is shed. Whereas merocrine and apocrine secretions leave the cell intact and able to continue secreting, **holocrine secretion** (HOL-ō-krin; *holos,* entire) does not (Figure 4-6c•). Instead, the entire cell becomes packed with secretions and then bursts apart and dies.

Type of Secretion

There are many kinds of exocrine secretions, all performing a variety of functions. Examples are enzymes entering the digestive tract, perspiration on the skin, and the milk produced by mammary glands.

Exocrine glands may be categorized by the type or types of secretions produced. For example, *serous glands* secrete a watery solution containing enzymes,

---

TABLE 4-1	A Classification of Exocrine Glands	
Feature	*Description*	*Example*
MODE OF SECRETION		
Merocrine	Secretion occurs through exocytosis.	Mucus in digestive and respiratory tracts
Apocrine	Secretion occurs through loss of cytoplasm containing secretory product.	Milk in breasts; viscous underarm perspiration
Holocrine	Secretion occurs through loss of entire cell containing secretory product.	Skin oils and waxy coating of hair (produced by sebaceous glands of the skin)
TYPE OF SECRETION		
Serous	Watery solution containing enzymes	Parotid salivary gland
Mucous	Thick, slippery mucus	Sublingual salivary gland
Mixed	Produces more than one type of secretion	Submandibular salivary gland (serous and mucous)

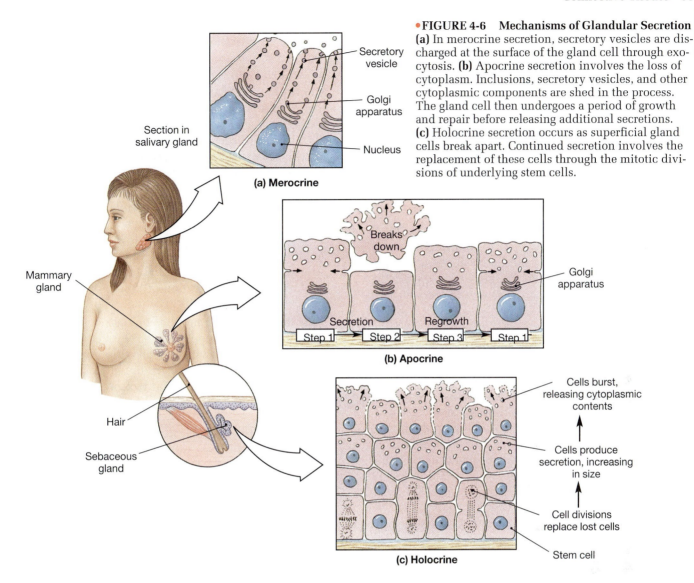

•FIGURE 4-6   Mechanisms of Glandular Secretion
(a) In merocrine secretion, secretory vesicles are discharged at the surface of the gland cell through exocytosis. **(b)** Apocrine secretion involves the loss of cytoplasm. Inclusions, secretory vesicles, and other cytoplasmic components are shed in the process. The gland cell then undergoes a period of growth and repair before releasing additional secretions. **(c)** Holocrine secretion occurs as superficial gland cells break apart. Continued secretion involves the replacement of these cells through the mitotic divisions of underlying stem cells.

Section in salivary gland

Secretory vesicle

Golgi apparatus

Nucleus

(a) Merocrine

Breaks down

Secretion

Regrowth

Golgi apparatus

Step 1   Step 2   Step 3   Step 1

(b) Apocrine

Mammary gland

Hair

Sebaceous gland

Cells burst, releasing cytoplasmic contents

Cells produce secretion, increasing in size

Cell divisions replace lost cells

Stem cell

(c) Holocrine

and *mucous glands* secrete a thick, slippery mucus. *Mixed glands* contain more than one type of gland cell and may produce two different exocrine secretions, or both exocrine and endocrine secretions.

✓ You look at a tissue under a microscope and see a simple squamous epithelium. Can it be a sample of the skin surface?

✓ Secretory cells associated with hair follicles fill with secretions and then rupture, releasing their contents. What kind of secretion is this?

✓ What physiological functions are enhanced by epithelial cells bearing microvilli and cilia?

CONNECTIVE TISSUES

Connective tissues are deep tissues that are never exposed to the environment outside the body. Their functions include:

- *Supporting and protecting.* The minerals and fibers produced by connective tissue cells establish a bony structural framework for the body, protect delicate organs, and surround and interconnect other tissue types.
- *Transporting materials.* Fluid connective tissue provides an efficient means of moving dissolved materials from one region of the body to another.
- *Storing energy reserves.* Fats are stored in connective tissue cells called *adipose cells* until needed.
- *Defending the body.* Specialized connective tissue cells respond to invasions by microorganisms through cell-to-cell interactions and the production of *antibodies.*

Connective tissues are the most diverse tissues of the body. Bone, blood, and fat are familiar connective tissues that have very different functions and properties. All connective tissues have three basic components: (1) specialized cells, (2) protein fibers, and (3) a

4

ground substance, a fluid that varies in consistency. The extracellular fibers and ground substance constitute the **matrix** that surrounds the cells. Whereas epithelial tissue consists almost entirely of cells, the extracellular matrix accounts for most of the volume of connective tissues.

Classifying Connective Tissues

Several classes of connective tissue are recognized on the basis of the physical properties of their ground substance (Figure 4-7•).

- **Connective tissue proper** refers to connective tissues with many types of cells and fibers surrounded by a syrupy ground substance. Examples are the tissue that underlies the skin, fatty tissue, and *tendons* and *ligaments*.
- **Fluid connective tissues** have a distinctive population of cells suspended in a watery ground substance that contains dissolved proteins. The two fluid connective tissues are *blood* and *lymph*.
- **Supporting connective tissues** are of two types, *cartilage* and *bone*. These tissues have a less diverse cell population than connective tissue proper and a matrix of dense ground substance and closely packed fibers. The fibrous matrix of bone is said to be *calcified* because it contains mineral deposits, primarily calcium salts, which give the bone strength and rigidity.

Connective Tissue Proper

Connective tissue proper contains fibers, a syrupy ground substance, and a varied cell population (Figure 4-8•). That population includes the following cell types:

- **Fibroblasts** (FĪ-brō-blasts) are the most abundant cells in connective tissue proper. They are responsible for the production and maintenance of the connective tissue fibers and the ground substance.
- **Macrophages** (MAK-rō-fā-jez; *phagein*, to eat) are scattered among the fibers. These cells engulf, or *phagocytize*, damaged cells or pathogens that enter the tissue and release chemicals that mobilize the immune system. ∞ *p. 63* When an infection occurs, additional macrophages are drawn to the affected area.
- **Fat cells** are known as *adipose cells*, or **adipocytes** (AD-i-pō-sīts). A typical adipocyte contains such a large droplet of lipid that the nucleus and other organelles are squeezed to one side of the cell. The number of fat cells varies from one connective tissue to another, from one region of the body to another, and from individual to individual.
- **Mast cells** are small, mobile connective tissue cells often found near blood vessels. The cytoplasm of a mast cell is packed with vesicles filled with chemicals that are released to begin the body's defensive activities after an injury or infection, as discussed later in the chapter.

In addition to mast cells and free macrophages, both phagocytic and antibody-producing white blood cells may move through the connective tissue. Their numbers increase markedly if the tissue is damaged, as does the production of **antibodies**, proteins that destroy invading microorganisms or foreign substances.

Connective Tissue Fibers

The three basic types of fibers—*collagen*, *elastic*, and *reticular*—are formed from protein subunits secreted by fibroblasts:

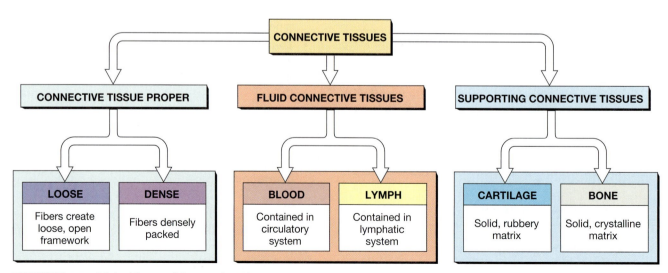

•FIGURE 4-7   **Major Types of Connective Tissue**

LOOSE CONNECTIVE TISSUE

LOCATIONS: Beneath dermis of skin, digestive tract, respiratory and urinary tracts; between muscles; around blood vessels, nerves, and around joints

FUNCTIONS: Cushions organs; provides support but permits independent movement; phagocytic cells provide defense against pathogens

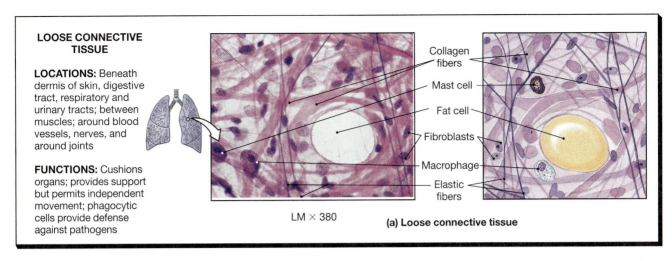

LM × 380

Collagen fibers

Mast cell

Fat cell

Fibroblasts

Macrophage

Elastic fibers

(a) Loose connective tissue

ADIPOSE TISSUE

LOCATIONS: Beneath skin, especially at sides, buttocks, breasts; behind eyeballs; around kidneys

FUNCTIONS: Provides padding and cushions shocks; insulates (reduces heat loss); stores energy reserves

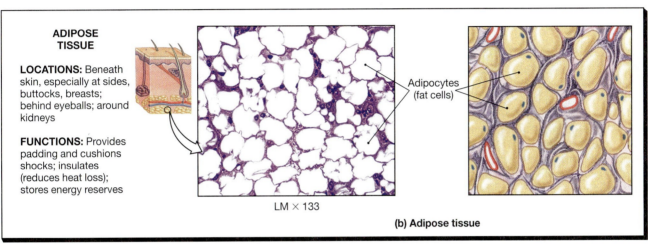

LM × 133

Adipocytes (fat cells)

(b) Adipose tissue

DENSE CONNECTIVE TISSUES

LOCATIONS: Between skeletal muscles and skeleton (tendons); between bones (ligaments); covering skeletal muscles; capsules of visceral organs

FUNCTIONS: Provide firm attachment; conduct pull of muscles; reduce friction between muscles; stabilize relative positions of bones; help prevent overexpansion of organs such as the urinary bladder

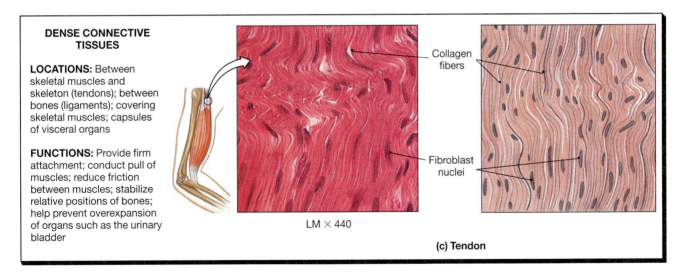

LM × 440

Collagen fibers

Fibroblast nuclei

(c) Tendon

●**FIGURE 4-8   Connective Tissue Proper: Loose and Dense Connective Tissues**
(a) All of the cells of connective tissue proper are found in loose connective tissue. **(b)** Adipose tissue is loose connective tissue dominated by adipocytes. In standard histological preparations, the tissue looks empty because the lipids in the fat cells dissolve during sectioning and staining. **(c)** The dense regular connective tissue in a tendon. Notice the densely packed, parallel bundles of collagen fibers. The fibroblast nuclei are flattened between the bundles.

4

- **Collagen fibers** are long, straight, and unbranched. The most common fibers in connective tissue proper, they are strong but flexible.
- **Elastic fibers** contain the protein *elastin*. They are branched and wavy, and after stretching will return to their original length.
- **Reticular fibers** (*reticulum*, a network), the least common of the three, are thinner than collagen fibers and commonly form a branching, interwoven framework in various organs.

Ground Substance

Ground substance fills all the spaces between cells and surrounds all the connective tissue fibers. In normal connective tissue proper, it is clear, colorless, and similar in consistency to maple syrup.

✳ **BLUNT CHEST TRAUMA**

The heart and great vessels are supported within the chest by strong connective tissues. These tissues allow limited movement of the heart and great vessels within the chest. The aortic arch is somewhat mobile, while the descending aorta is virtually immobile, particularly at the attachment of the fibrous *ligamentum arteriosum*. Vehicular trauma often involves a sudden and rapid deceleration, during which the heart continues to travel forward within the chest. This can place the aorta under great stress, often resulting in tearing and rupture, typically at the point where the *ligamentum arteriosum* attaches. Traumatic thoracic aortic rupture has a very high mortality rate with 80–90 percent of victims dying at the scene.

Connective tissue proper can be categorized as *loose connective tissues* and *dense connective tissues* on the basis of the relative proportions of cells, fibers, and ground substance. Loose connective tissues are the packing material of the body. These tissues fill spaces between organs, provide cushioning, and support epithelia. They also anchor blood vessels and nerves, store lipids, and provide a route for the diffusion of materials. Dense connective tissues are tough, strong, and durable. They resist tension and distortion and interconnect bones and muscles. Dense connective tissue also forms a thick layer, called a *capsule*, that surrounds visceral organs, such as the liver, kidneys, and spleen, and that also encloses joint cavities.

Loose Connective Tissue

Loose connective tissue, or *areolar tissue* (*areola*, little space), is the least specialized connective tissue in the adult body (Figure 4-8a•). It contains all of the cells and fibers found in any connective tissue proper, in addition to an extensive circulatory supply.

Loose connective tissue forms a layer that separates the skin from underlying muscles, providing both padding and a considerable amount of independent movement. For example, pinching the skin of the arm does not distort the underlying muscle. The ample blood supply in this tissue carries wandering cells to and from the tissue and provides for the metabolic needs of nearby epithelial tissue.

Adipose Tissue

Adipose tissue, or fat, is a loose connective tissue containing large numbers of fat cells, or adipocytes (Figure 4-8b•). The difference between loose connective tissue and adipose tissue is one of degree; a loose connective tissue is called adipose tissue when it becomes dominated by fat cells. Adipose tissue provides another source of padding and shock absorption for the body. It also acts as an insulating blanket that slows heat loss through the skin and functions in energy storage.

Adipose tissue is common under the skin of the sides, buttocks, and breasts. It fills the bony sockets behind the eyes, surrounds the kidneys, and dominates extensive areas of loose connective tissue in the pericardial and peritoneal (abdominal) cavities.

✳ **EMS AND OBESITY**

Emergency Medical Services (EMS) is thought of as an intense, exciting, and physically challenging profession. In actuality, EMS is a fairly sedentary job punctuated by short periods of intense activity. Because of this, EMS providers are at risk of gaining weight. In addition, they also run the risk of physical injury if they do not remain physically fit.

As an EMS provider, you should carefully monitor your weight and maintain a healthy lifestyle. This should include some form of regular physical exercise, rational eating, and adequate rest and relaxation. You cannot depend on the job alone to provide the exercise required to maintain optimal fitness. If your agency does not have an ongoing fitness program, encourage them to start one. The result is a healthier, safer, and more satisfying career.

Dense Connective Tissues

Dense connective tissues consist mostly of collagen fibers; they may also be called *fibrous tissues*. **Tendons** are cords of dense connective tissue that attach skeletal muscles to bones (Figure 4-8c•). Collagen fibers run along the length of the tendon and transfer the pull of the contracting muscle to the bone. **Ligaments** (LIG-a-ments) are bundles of fibers that connect one bone to another. Ligaments often contain elastic fibers as well as collagen fibers and thus can tolerate a modest amount of stretching.

Fluid Connective Tissues

Blood and **lymph** are connective tissues that contain distinctive collections of cells in a liquid matrix.

Under normal conditions, the proteins dissolved in this watery ground substance do not form large insoluble fibers.

A single cell type, the **red blood cell**, accounts for almost half the volume of blood. Red blood cells transport oxygen in the blood. The watery ground substance, called **plasma**, also contains small numbers of **white blood cells**, which are important components of the immune system, and **platelets**, cell fragments which function in blood clotting (Figure 4-9a•).

The extracellular fluid of the body is composed of plasma and **interstitial fluid** (in-ter-STISH-al; *inter*, between + *sistere*, to set), which surrounds the cells of other tissues. Plasma, confined to the vessels of the cardiovascular system, is kept in constant motion by contractions of the heart. A network of **arteries** carries blood away from the heart and toward fine, thin-walled vessels called **capillaries**. **Veins** collect and return blood to the heart, completing the circuit. In the tissues, filtration moves water and small solutes out of the capillaries and into the interstitial fluid.

Over time, interstitial fluid enters small passageways, or *lymphatics*, that return the fluid to the car-diovascular system. As the interstitial fluid flows along the lymphatic vessels, it contains large numbers of *lymphocytes*, cells responsible for the immune response. This combination of interstitial fluid and specialized cells forms lymph. Figure 4-9b• diagrams the movement of fluid from the plasma to the interstitial fluid and back again.

Supporting Connective Tissues

Cartilage and bone are called supporting connective tissues because they provide a strong framework that supports the rest of the body. In these connective tissues the matrix contains numerous fibers and, in some cases, deposits of insoluble calcium salts.

Cartilage

The matrix of **cartilage** consists of a firm gel containing embedded fibers. **Chondrocytes** (KON-drō-sīts), the only cells found within the matrix, live in small pockets known as *lacunae* (la-KOO-nē; *lacus*, pool). Because cartilage lacks blood vessels, chondrocytes must obtain

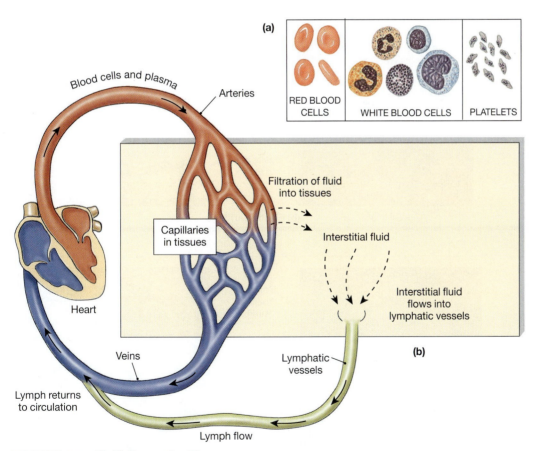

•**FIGURE 4-9   Fluid Connective Tissues**
(a) Specialized cells of the fluid connective tissues. **(b)** Blood travels through the circulatory system, pushed by the contractions of the heart. In capillaries, hydrostatic (blood) pressure forces fluid and dissolved solutes out of the circulatory system. This fluid mixes with the interstitial fluid already in the tissue. Interstitial fluid slowly enters lymphatic vessels; now called lymph, it travels along the lymphatics and reenters the circulatory system at one of the veins that returns blood to the heart.

4

nutrients and eliminate waste products by diffusion through the matrix. Structures of cartilage are covered and set apart from surrounding tissues by a **perichondrium** (per-i-KON-drē-um; *peri-*, around + *chondros*, cartilage), which contains blood vessels.

Types of Cartilage. The three major types of cartilage are *hyaline cartilage*, *elastic cartilage*, and *fibrocartilage*:

1. **Hyaline cartilage** (HĪ-a-lin; *hyalos*, glass) is the most common type of cartilage (Figure 4-10a●). Tough and

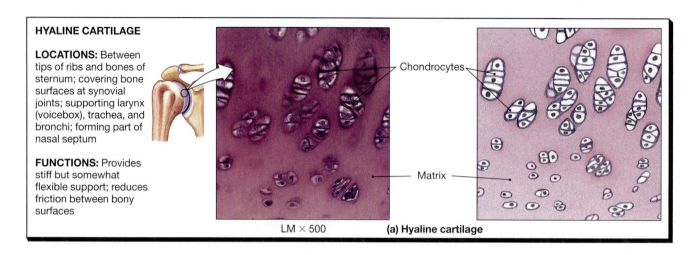

HYALINE CARTILAGE

LOCATIONS: Between tips of ribs and bones of sternum; covering bone surfaces at synovial joints; supporting larynx (voicebox), trachea, and bronchi; forming part of nasal septum

FUNCTIONS: Provides stiff but somewhat flexible support; reduces friction between bony surfaces

Chondrocytes

Matrix

LM × 500   **(a) Hyaline cartilage**

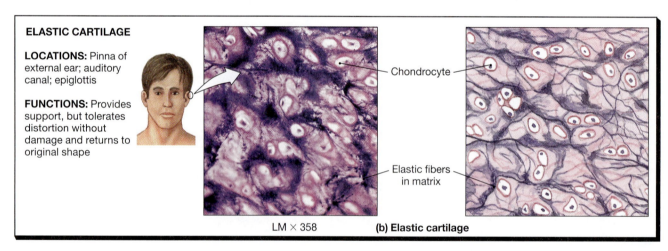

ELASTIC CARTILAGE

LOCATIONS: Pinna of external ear; auditory canal; epiglottis

FUNCTIONS: Provides support, but tolerates distortion without damage and returns to original shape

Chondrocyte

Elastic fibers in matrix

LM × 358   **(b) Elastic cartilage**

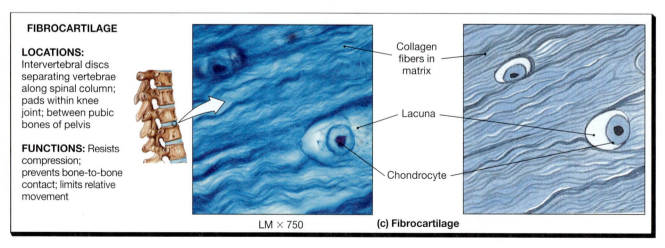

FIBROCARTILAGE

LOCATIONS: Intervertebral discs separating vertebrae along spinal column; pads within knee joint; between pubic bones of pelvis

FUNCTIONS: Resists compression; prevents bone-to-bone contact; limits relative movement

Collagen fibers in matrix

Lacuna

Chondrocyte

LM × 750   **(c) Fibrocartilage**

●**FIGURE 4-10   Types of Cartilage**
(a) Hyaline cartilage. Note the translucent matrix and the absence of prominent fibers. **(b)** Elastic cartilage. The closely packed elastic fibers are visible between the chondrocytes. **(c)** Fibrocartilage. The collagen fibers are extremely dense, and the chondrocytes are relatively far apart.

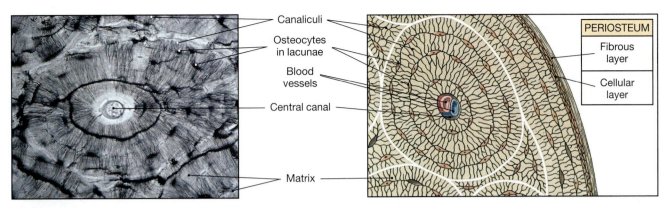

•FIGURE 4-11 Bone
The osteocytes in bone are usually organized in groups around a central space that contains blood vessels. For the micrograph, a sample of bone was ground thin enough to become transparent. Bone dust filled the lacunae and the central canal, making them appear dark.

somewhat flexible, this type of cartilage connects the ribs to the sternum (breastbone), supports the conducting passageways of the respiratory tract, and covers the surfaces of bones within joints.

2. **Elastic cartilage** (Figure 4-10b•) contains numerous elastic fibers that make it extremely resilient and flexible. Elastic cartilage supports the external flap (*pinna*) of the outer ear, the epiglottis, and the tip of the nose.

3. **Fibrocartilage** has little ground substance, and the matrix is dominated by collagen fibers (Figure 4-10c•). These fibers are densely interwoven, making this tissue extremely durable and tough. Fibrocartilaginous pads lie between the vertebrae of the spinal column, between the bones of the pelvis, and around or within a few joints and tendons. In these positions they resist compression, absorb shocks, and prevent damaging bone-to-bone contact. Cartilages in general heal poorly, and damaged fibrocartilages in joints such as the knee can interfere with normal movements.

✳ MENISCAL KNEE INJURIES

Sporting activities, particularly football, often result in knee injuries. A common knee injury is tearing or damaging one of the *menisci* (semilunar shaped) cartilages. These cartilages, which contain hyaline, cushion the bones in the joint and prevent bone contact. The medial and lateral menisci are located on the tibial plateau. During stress, these cartilages can be torn or otherwise damaged. As they are relatively avascular structures, they heal poorly and tend to be a source of ongoing problems for the patient.

Bone

Because the detailed histology of **bone**, or *osseous tissue* (OS-ē-us; *os*, bone), will be considered in Chapter 6, this discussion will focus on significant differences between cartilage and bone. The matrix of bone consists of hard calcium compounds and flexible collagen fibers. This combination gives bone truly remarkable

properties, making it both strong and resistant to shattering. In its overall properties, bone can compete with the best steel-reinforced concrete.

The general organization of bone is shown in Figure 4-11•. Lacunae within the matrix contain bone cells, or **osteocytes** (OS-tē-ō-sīts; *os*, bone + *cyte*, cell). The lacunae surround the blood vessels that branch through the bony matrix. Diffusion cannot occur through the bony matrix, but osteocytes obtain nutrients through cytoplasmic extensions that reach blood vessels and other osteocytes. The passageways through which these cytoplasmic processes run are called **canaliculi** (kan-a-LIK-ū-lē; little canals) because they form a branching network within the bony matrix.

Except within joint cavities, where opposing surfaces are coated with cartilage, each bone is surrounded by a fibrous **periosteum** (per-ē-OS-tē-um). Unlike cartilage, bone is constantly being changed, or remodeled, to such an extent that complete repairs can be made even after severe damage has occurred. Table 4-2 compares cartilage and bone.

✓ Lack of vitamin C in the diet interferes with the ability of fibroblasts to produce collagen. What effect might this interference have on connective tissue?

✓ Chemical analysis of a connective tissue reveals that the tissue contains primarily triglycerides. Which type of connective tissue is this?

✓ Why does cartilage heal so slowly?

MEMBRANES

Some anatomical terms have more than one meaning, depending on the context. One such term is *membrane*. For example, at the cellular level, membranes are lipid bilayers that restrict the passage of ions and other solutes. ∞ *p. 57* At the tissue level, membranes also form

TABLE 4-2	A Comparison of Cartilage and Bone	
Characteristic	Cartilage	Bone
STRUCTURAL FEATURES		
Cells	Chondrocytes in lacunae	Osteocytes in lacunae
Ground substance	Protein-polysaccharide gel	Insoluble salts (calcium phosphate and calcium carbonate)
Fibers	Collagen, elastic, reticular fibers (proportions vary)	Collagen fibers predominate
Vascularity	None	Extensive
Covering	Perichondrium	Periosteum
Strength	Limited: bends easily but hard to break	Strong: resists distortion until breaking point is reached
METABOLIC FEATURES		
Oxygen demands	Relatively low	Relatively high
Nutrient delivery	By diffusion through matrix	By diffusion through cytoplasm and fluid in canaliculi
Repair capabilities	Limited ability	Extensive ability

a barrier or an interface, such as the basement membranes that separate epithelia from connective tissues. At still another level, epithelia and connective tissues combine to form membranes that cover and protect other structures and tissues. The body has four such membranes: *mucous membranes*, *serous membranes*, the *cutaneous membrane*, and *synovial membranes* (Figure 4-12•).

Mucous Membranes

Mucous membranes line cavities that communicate with the exterior, including the digestive, respiratory, reproductive, and urinary tracts (Figure 4-12a•). The epithelial surfaces are kept moist at all times, typically by mucous secretions or by exposure to fluids such as urine or semen. The connective tissue portion of a mucous membrane is called the *lamina propria* (PRŌ-prē-uh).

Many mucous membranes are lined by simple epithelia that perform absorptive or secretory functions, such as the simple columnar epithelium of the digestive tract. However, other types of epithelia may be involved. For example, a stratified squamous epithelium covers the mucous membrane of the mouth, and the mucous membrane along most of the urinary tract contains a transitional epithelium.

Serous Membranes

Serous membranes line the sealed, internal cavities of the body. There are three serous membranes, each consisting of a simple epithelium supported by loose connective tissue (Figure 4-12b•). The **pleura** (PLOO-ra; *pleura*, rib) lines the pleural cavities and covers the lungs. The **peritoneum** (pe-ri-tō-NĒ-um; *peri*, around +

teinein, to stretch) lines the peritoneal (abdominal) cavity and covers the surfaces of enclosed organs such as the liver and stomach. The **pericardium** (pe-ri-KAR-dē-um) lines the pericardial cavity and covers the heart.

A serous membrane has *parietal* and *visceral* portions. ∞ *p. 21* The parietal portion lines the outer wall of the internal chamber, and the visceral portion covers organs within the body cavity. For example, the visceral pericardium covers the heart, and the parietal pericardium lines the inner surfaces of the pericardial sac that surrounds the pericardial cavity. *Serous fluid* covering the surfaces of the visceral and parietal membranes minimizes the friction between these opposing surfaces.

Cutaneous Membrane

The **cutaneous membrane** of the skin covers the surface of the body (Figure 4-12c•). It consists of a stratified squamous epithelium and the underlying connective tissues. In contrast to serous or mucous membranes, the cutaneous membrane is thick, relatively waterproof, and usually dry. The skin is discussed in detail in Chapter 5.

Synovial Membranes

Bones of the skeleton contact one another at joints, also called **articulations** (ar-tik-ū-LĀ-shuns). The type of connective tissue at a joint may restrict or enhance its movement. If the joint is mobile, the bony surfaces do not come into direct contact with one another. If they did, abrasion and impacts would damage the opposing surfaces, and smooth movement would be almost impossible. Instead, the ends of the bones are covered with hyaline cartilage and separated by a viscous *synovial*

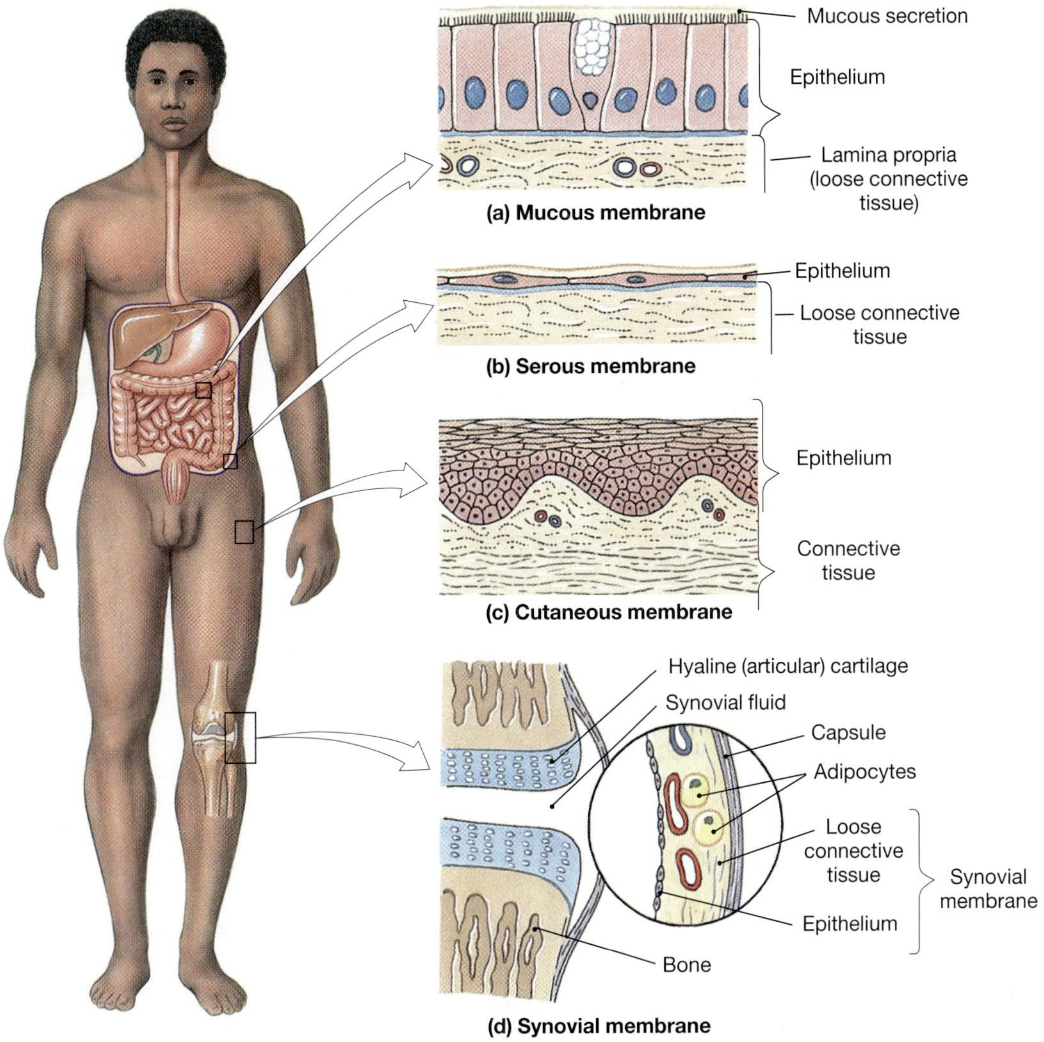

(a) Mucous membrane
- Mucous secretion
- Epithelium
- Lamina propria (loose connective tissue)

(b) Serous membrane
- Epithelium
- Loose connective tissue

(c) Cutaneous membrane
- Epithelium
- Connective tissue

(d) Synovial membrane
- Hyaline (articular) cartilage
- Synovial fluid
- Capsule
- Adipocytes
- Loose connective tissue
- Synovial membrane
- Epithelium
- Bone

•**FIGURE 4-12   Membranes**
(a) Mucous membranes are coated with the secretions of mucous glands. Mucous membranes with a simple columnar epithelium line most of the digestive and respiratory tracts and portions of the reproductive tract. **(b)** Serous membranes line the ventral body cavities (the peritoneal, pleural, and pericardial cavities). **(c)** The cutaneous membrane of the skin covers the outer surface of the body. **(d)** Synovial membranes line joint cavities and produce the fluid within the joint.

fluid produced by the **synovial** (sin-Ō-vē-al) **membrane**, which lines the joint cavity (Figure 4-12d•). The synovial fluid helps lubricate the joint and permits smooth movement. Unlike the other three membranes, the synovial membrane consists primarily of loose connective tissue, and the epithelial layer is incomplete.

✓ How does a cell membrane differ from a tissue-level membrane?

✓ Serous membranes produce fluids. What is their function?

✓ Why is the same epithelial organization found in the mucous membranes of the pharynx, esophagus, anus, and vagina?

MUSCLE TISSUE

Muscle tissue is specialized for contraction. A large skeletal muscle cell may be 100 micrometers (μm; 1 μm = 1/25,000 in.) in diameter and 25 cm (10 in.) long. Because skeletal muscle cells are relatively long and slender, they are usually called *muscle fibers*.

Muscle cell contraction involves interaction between filaments of *myosin* and *actin*, proteins found in the cytoskeletons of many cells. ∞ *p. 65* In muscle cells, however, the filaments are more numerous and arranged so that their interaction produces a contraction of the entire cell.

Figure 4-13• shows the three types of muscle tissue—*skeletal*, *cardiac*, and *smooth muscle tissues*.

4

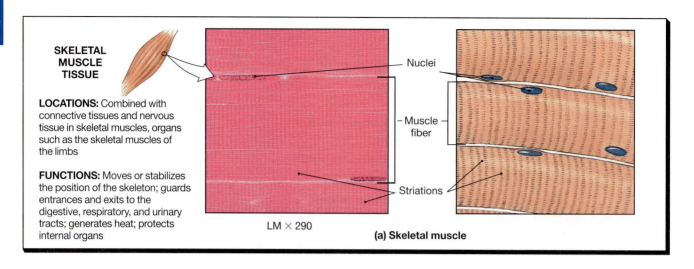

SKELETAL MUSCLE TISSUE

LOCATIONS: Combined with connective tissues and nervous tissue in skeletal muscles, organs such as the skeletal muscles of the limbs

FUNCTIONS: Moves or stabilizes the position of the skeleton; guards entrances and exits to the digestive, respiratory, and urinary tracts; generates heat; protects internal organs

Nuclei

Muscle fiber

Striations

LM × 290

(a) Skeletal muscle

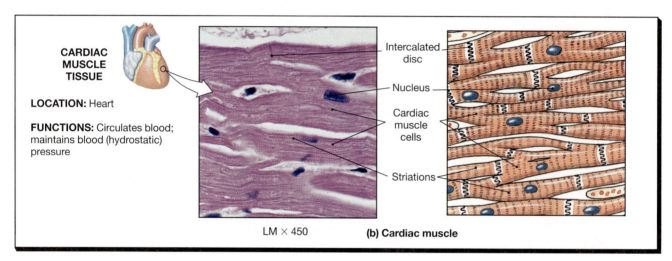

CARDIAC MUSCLE TISSUE

LOCATION: Heart

FUNCTIONS: Circulates blood; maintains blood (hydrostatic) pressure

Intercalated disc

Nucleus

Cardiac muscle cells

Striations

LM × 450

(b) Cardiac muscle

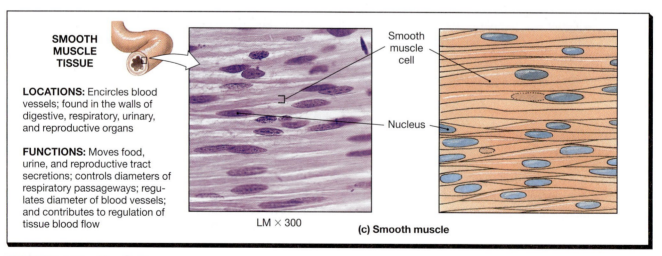

SMOOTH MUSCLE TISSUE

LOCATIONS: Encircles blood vessels; found in the walls of digestive, respiratory, urinary, and reproductive organs

FUNCTIONS: Moves food, urine, and reproductive tract secretions; controls diameters of respiratory passageways; regulates diameter of blood vessels; and contributes to regulation of tissue blood flow

Smooth muscle cell

Nucleus

LM × 300

(c) Smooth muscle

•**FIGURE 4-13   Muscle Tissue**
(a) Skeletal muscle fibers. Note the large fiber size, prominent banding pattern, multiple nuclei, and unbranched arrangement. **(b)** Cardiac muscle cells, which differ from skeletal muscle fibers in three major ways: size (cardiac muscle cells are smaller), organization (cardiac muscle cells branch), and number of nuclei (a typical cardiac muscle cell has one centrally placed nucleus). Both contain actin and myosin filaments in an organized array that produces striations. **(c)** Smooth muscle cells, which are small and spindle-shaped, with a central nucleus. They do not branch, and there are no striations.

The contraction mechanism is the same in all of them, but the organization of their actin and myosin filaments differs. Because each type will be examined in later chapters, notably Chapter 7, this discussion will focus on general characteristics rather than specific details.

Skeletal Muscle Tissue

Skeletal muscle tissue contains very large, multinucleated fibers (cells) tied together by loose connective tissue (Figure 4-13a•). The collagen and elastic fibers surrounding each cell and group of cells blend into those of a tendon that conducts the force of contraction, usually to a bone of the skeleton. Contractions of muscle tissue cause the bones to move.

Because the actin and myosin filaments are arranged in organized groups, skeletal muscle fibers appear to be marked by a series of bands known as *striations*. Skeletal muscle fibers will not usually contract unless stimulated by nerves. Since the nervous system provides voluntary control over its activities, skeletal muscle is described as *striated voluntary muscle*.

Cardiac Muscle Tissue

Cardiac muscle tissue is found only in the heart (Figure 4-13b•). Cardiac muscle cells are much smaller than skeletal muscle fibers, and each cardiac muscle cell usually has a single nucleus. Cardiac muscle cells are interconnected at **intercalated** (in-TER-ka-lā-ted) **discs**, specialized attachment sites containing gap junctions and desmosomes. The muscle cells branch, forming a network that efficiently conducts the force and stimulus for contraction from one area of the heart to another.

Unlike skeletal muscle, cardiac muscle does not rely on nerve activity to start a contraction. Instead, specialized cells, called *pacemaker cells*, establish a regular rate of contraction. Although the nervous system can alter the rate of pacemaker activity, it does not provide voluntary control over individual cardiac muscle cells. In short, cardiac muscle can be considered *striated involuntary muscle*.

Smooth Muscle Tissue

Smooth muscle tissue is found in the walls of blood vessels; around hollow organs such as the urinary bladder; and in layers around the respiratory, circulatory, digestive, and reproductive tracts (Figure 4-13c•).

A smooth muscle cell is small and slender, tapering to a point at each end; each smooth muscle cell has one nucleus. Unlike skeletal and cardiac muscle, the actin and myosin filaments in smooth muscle cells are scattered throughout the cytoplasm, and there are no striations.

Smooth muscle cells may contract on their own, or their contractions may be triggered by neural activity. The nervous system usually does not provide voluntary control over smooth muscle contractions, and smooth muscle is therefore categorized as *nonstriated involuntary muscle*.

NEURAL TISSUE

Neural tissue is specialized for the conduction of electrical impulses that convey information or instructions from one region of the body to another. Most of the neural tissue (98 percent) is concentrated in the brain and spinal cord, the control centers for the nervous system.

Neural tissue contains two basic types of cells: **neurons** (NOO-ronz; *neuro-*, nerve) and several different kinds of supporting cells, or **neuroglia** (noo-RŌG-lē-a; *glia*, glue). Neurons transmit the actual signals as electrical events affecting their cell membranes. The neuroglia provide physical support for neural tissue, maintain the chemical composition of the tissue fluids, and defend the tissue from infection.

A typical neuron has a cell body, or **soma** (SŌ-ma; *soma*, body), that contains the nucleus (Figure 4-14•). The stimulus that results in the production of an electrical impulse usually affects the cell membrane of one of the **dendrites** (DEN-drīts; *dendron*, tree). Stimulation alters the permeability of the cell membrane, eventually producing an electrical impulse that is conducted along the length of the axon. **Axons**, which may reach a meter in length, are often called *nerve fibers*. Each axon ends at *synaptic terminals*. Each terminal is part of a **synapse** (SIN-aps; *syn-*, together), a specialized site where the neuron communicates with another cell. Chapter 8, which considers the properties of neural tissue, provides more detail on the structure and function of synapses.

✓ What type of muscle tissue has small, spindle-shaped cells with single nuclei and no obvious banding pattern?

✓ Our voluntary control is restricted to which type of muscle tissue?

✓ Why are skeletal muscle cells and axons also called fibers?

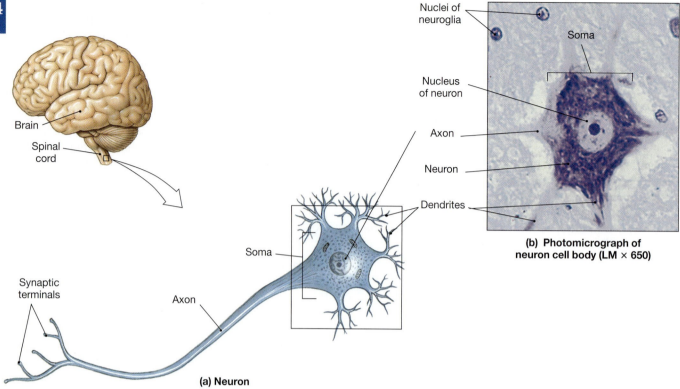

Brain

Spinal cord

Synaptic terminals

Soma

Axon

Nuclei of neuroglia

Soma

Nucleus of neuron

Axon

Neuron

Dendrites

Dendrites

(b) Photomicrograph of neuron cell body (LM × 650)

(a) Neuron

•**FIGURE 4-14   Neural Tissue**

TISSUE INJURIES AND REPAIRS

Tissues in the body are not independent of each other; they combine to form organs with diverse functions. Any injury to the body affects several tissue types simultaneously, and these tissues must respond in a coordinated manner to restore homeostasis.

The restoration of homeostasis following a tissue injury involves two related processes. First, the area is isolated from neighboring healthy tissue while damaged cells, tissue components, and any dangerous microorganisms are cleaned up. This phase, which coordinates the activities of several different tissues, is called **inflammation**, or the *inflammatory response*. Inflammation begins immediately after an injury and produces several familiar sensations, including swelling, warmth, redness, and pain. An inflammation can result from many stimuli, including impact, abrasion, chemical irritation, and infection by pathogens, such as bacteria or viruses.

Second, the damaged tissues are replaced or repaired to restore normal function. This repair process is called **regeneration**. Inflammation and regeneration are controlled at the tissue level. The two phases overlap; isolation of the area of damaged tissue establishes a framework that guides the cells responsible for recon-

struction, and repairs are under way well before cleanup operations have ended. Later chapters, especially Chapter 15, will examine inflammation and regeneration in more detail.

TISSUES AND AGING

Tissues change with age, and there is a decrease in the speed and effectiveness of tissue repairs. In general, repair and maintenance activities throughout the body slow down, and a combination of hormonal changes and alterations in lifestyle affect the structure and chemical composition of many tissues. Epithelia get thinner and connective tissues more fragile. Individuals bruise more easily and bones become brittle; joint pain and broken bones are common complaints among the elderly. Cardiac muscle fibers and neurons cannot be replaced, and cumulative losses from even relatively minor damage can contribute to major health problems, such as cardiovascular disease or deterioration in mental function.

In later chapters, we will consider the effects of aging on specific organs and systems. Some of these changes are genetically programmed. For example, as people age, their chondrocytes produce a slightly different form of the gelatinous compound making up the cartilage matrix. This difference in composition probably accounts for the increase in thickness and stiffness of cartilages that we observe in older people.

Other age-related changes in tissue structure have multiple causes. The age-related reduction in bone strength in women, a condition called *osteoporosis*, is often caused by a combination of inactivity, low dietary calcium levels, and a reduction in circulating estrogens (sex hormones). A program of exercise, calcium supplements, and hormonal replacement therapies can usually maintain normal bone structure for many years.

Aging and Cancer Incidence

4

Cancer rates increase with age, and roughly 25 percent of all Americans develop cancer at some point in their lives. It has been estimated that 70–80 percent of cancer cases result from chemical exposure, environmental factors, or some combination of the two, and 40 percent of these cancers are caused by cigarette smoke. Each year, over 500,000 Americans die of cancer, making this disease Public Health Enemy #2, second only to heart disease. Cancer development was discussed in Chapter 3. ∞ *p. 75*

Chapter Review

KEY TERMS

basement membrane, *p. 84*
blood, *p. 92*
bone, *p. 95*
cartilage, *p. 93*
connective tissue, *p. 89*
epithelium, *p. 82*
fibroblasts, *p. 90*

gap junction, *p. 83*
gland cells, *p. 83*
inflammation, *p. 100*
lymph, *p. 92*
macrophage, *p. 90*
mucous membrane, *p. 96*
muscle tissue, *p. 97*

neural tissue, *p. 99*
neuron, *p. 99*
serous membrane, *p. 96*
stem cells, *p. 85*
tissue, *p. 82*

SUMMARY OUTLINE

INTRODUCTION *p. 82*

1. **Tissues** are collections of specialized cells and cell products that are organized to perform a relatively limited number of functions. There are four **primary tissue types**: *epithelial tissue, connective tissues, muscle tissue,* and *neural tissue.* **Histology** is the study of tissues. *(Figure 4-1)*

EPITHELIAL TISSUE *p. 82*

1. An **epithelium** is an **avascular** layer of cells that forms a barrier that has certain properties.

Functions of Epithelia *p. 82*

2. Epithelia provide physical protection, control permeability, provide sensations, and produce specialized secretions. Gland cells are epithelial cells that produce secretions.

3. **Exocrine** secretions are released onto body surfaces; **endocrine** secretions, known as *hormones*, are released by gland cells into the surrounding tissues.

Intercellular Connections *p. 83*

4. The individual cells that make up tissues attach to one another or to extracellular protein fibers in three ways: *gap junctions, tight junctions,* and *desmosomes. (Figure 4-2)*

5. In a **gap junction**, two cells are held together by interlocked membrane proteins, forming a narrow passageway.

6. At a **tight junction**, the outer surfaces of the two cell membranes are bound tightly together; these are the strongest intercellular connections.

7. A **desmosome** has a very thin layer of intercellular cement between the cell membranes, reinforced by a network of protein fibers.

The Epithelial Surface *p. 84*

8. Epithelial cells may have cilia or microvilli. The coordinated beating of the cilia on a ciliated epithelium moves materials across the epithelial surface. *(Figure 4-3)*

The Basement Membrane *p. 84*

9. The inner surface of each epithelium is connected to a noncellular **basement membrane**.

Epithelial Renewal and Repair *p. 84*

10. Divisions by **stem cells**, or *germinative cells*, continually replace the short-lived epithelial cells.

Classifying Epithelia *p. 85*

11. Epithelia are classified on the basis of the number of cell layers and the shape of the exposed cells.

12. A **simple epithelium** has a single layer of cells covering the basement membrane; a **stratified epithelium** has several layers. In a **squamous epithelium** the cells are thin and flat. Cells in a **cuboidal epithelium** resemble little hexagonal boxes;

4

those in a **columnar epithelium** are taller and more slender. *(Figures 4-4, 4-5)*

Glandular Epithelia *p. 88*

13. A glandular epithelial cell may release its secretions through *merocrine*, *apocrine*, or *holocrine* mechanisms. *(Figure 4-6)*

14. In **merocrine secretion**, the most common method of secretion, the product is released through exocytosis. **Apocrine secretion** involves the loss of both secretory product and cytoplasm. Unlike the first two methods, **holocrine secretion** destroys the cell, which becomes packed with secretions and finally bursts.

15. Exocrine secretions may be *serous* (watery, usually containing enzymes), *mucous* (thick and slippery), or *mixed* (containing enzymes and lubricants). *(Table 4-1)*

CONNECTIVE TISSUES *p. 89*

1. **Connective tissues** are internal tissues with many important functions: establishing a structural framework; transporting fluids and dissolved materials; protecting delicate organs; supporting, surrounding, and interconnecting tissues; storing energy reserves; and defending the body from microorganisms.

2. All connective tissues have specialized cells, extracellular protein fibers, and a **ground substance**. The protein fibers and ground substance constitute the **matrix**.

Classifying Connective Tissues *p. 90*

3. **Connective tissue proper** refers to connective tissues that contain varied cell populations and fiber types surrounded by a syrupy ground substance. *(Figure 4-7)*

4. **Fluid connective tissues** have a distinctive population of cells suspended in a watery ground substance containing dissolved proteins. The two types are *blood* and *lymph*. *(Figure 4-7)*

5. **Supporting connective tissues** have a less diverse cell population than connective tissue proper and a dense matrix that contains closely packed fibers. The two types of supporting connective tissues are *cartilage* and *bone*. *(Figure 4-7)*

Connective Tissue Proper *p. 90*

6. Connective tissue proper contains fibers, a viscous ground substance, and a varied cell population.

7. There are three types of fiber in connective tissue: **collagen fibers**, **reticular fibers**, and **elastic fibers**.

8. Connective tissue proper is classified as **loose** or **dense connective tissues**. Loose connective tissues include loose connective tissue, or *areolar tissue*, and **adipose tissue**. *(Figure 4-8a,b)*

9. Most of the volume in dense connective tissue consists of fibers. Dense connective tissues form **tendons** and **ligaments**. *(Figure 4-8c)*

Fluid Connective Tissues *p. 92*

10. **Blood** and **lymph** are connective tissues that contain distinctive collections of cells in a fluid matrix. *(Figure 4-9)*

11. Blood contains **red blood cells**, **white blood cells**, and **platelets**. The watery ground substance of the blood is called **plasma**.

12. **Arteries** carry blood from the heart and toward **capillaries**, where water and small solutes move into the **interstitial fluid** of surrounding tissues. **Veins** return blood to the heart.

13. Lymph forms as interstitial fluid enters the **lymphatics**, which return lymph to the circulatory system.

Supporting Connective Tissues *p. 93*

14. Cartilage and bone are called supporting connective tissues because they support the rest of the body.

15. The matrix of **cartilage** consists of a firm gel and cells called **chondrocytes**. A fibrous **perichondrium** separates cartilage from surrounding tissues. The three types of cartilage are **hyaline cartilage**, **elastic cartilage**, and **fibrocartilage**. *(Figure 4-10)*

16. Chondrocytes rely on diffusion through the avascular matrix to obtain nutrients.

17. **Bone**, or *osseous tissue*, has a matrix consisting of collagen fibers and calcium salts, which give it unique properties. *(Figure 4-11; Table 4-2)*

18. **Osteocytes** depend on diffusion through **canaliculi** for nutrient intake.

19. Each bone is surrounded by a **periosteum**.

MEMBRANES *p. 95*

1. Membranes form a barrier or an interface. Epithelia and connective tissues combine to form membranes that cover and protect other structures and tissues. There are four types of membranes: *mucous*, *serous*, *cutaneous*, and *synovial*. *(Figure 4-12)*

Mucous Membranes *p. 96*

2. **Mucous membranes** line cavities that communicate with the exterior. Their surfaces are normally moistened by mucous secretions.

Serous Membranes *p. 96*

3. **Serous membranes** line internal cavities and are delicate, moist, and very permeable.

Cutaneous Membrane *p. 96*

4. The **cutaneous membrane** covers the body surface. Unlike serous and mucous membranes, it is relatively thick, waterproof, and usually dry.

Synovial Membranes *p. 96*

5. **Synovial membranes**, located at joints, or articulations, produce *synovial fluid* in joint cavities. Synovial fluid helps lubricate the joint and promotes smooth movement.

MUSCLE TISSUE p. 97

1. Muscle tissue, consisting of *muscle fibers*, is specialized for contraction. The three types of muscle tissue are *skeletal*, *cardiac*, and *smooth muscle tissues*. *(Figure 4-13)*

Skeletal Muscle Tissue *p. 99*

2. **Skeletal muscle tissue** contains very large fibers tied together by collagen and elastic fibers. Skeletal muscle fibers have a striped appearance because of the organization of contractile proteins. The stripes are called *striations*. Because we can control the contraction of skeletal muscle fibers through the nervous system, skeletal muscle can be considered *striated voluntary muscle*.

Cardiac Muscle Tissue *p. 99*

3. Cardiac muscle tissue is found only in the heart. The nervous system does not provide voluntary control over cardiac muscle cells. Thus, cardiac muscle is *striated involuntary muscle.*

Smooth Muscle Tissue *p. 99*

4. Smooth muscle tissue is found in the walls of blood vessels, around hollow organs, and in layers around various tracts. It is classified as *nonstriated involuntary muscle.*

NEURAL TISSUE *p. 99*

1. Neural tissue is specialized to conduct electrical impulses that convey information from one area of the body to another.

2. Cells in neural tissue are either neurons or neuroglia. **Neurons** transmit information as electrical impulses in their cell membranes. Several kinds of **neuroglia** serve both supporting and defense functions. *(Figure 4-14)*

3. A typical neuron has a **soma**, **dendrites**, and an **axon**, which ends at a **synapse**.

TISSUE INJURIES AND REPAIRS *p. 100*

1. Any injury affects several tissue types simultaneously, and they respond in a coordinated manner. Homeostasis is restored in two processes: *inflammation* and *regeneration.*

2. Inflammation, or the *inflammatory response*, isolates the injured area while damaged cells, tissue components, and any dangerous microorganisms are cleaned up.

3. Regeneration is the repair process that restores normal function.

TISSUES AND AGING *p. 100*

1. Tissues change with age. Repair and maintenance grow less efficient, and the structure and chemical composition of many tissues are altered.

Aging and Cancer Incidence *p. 101*

2. Cancer incidence increases with age, with roughly three-quarters of all cases caused by exposure to chemicals or environmental factors.

REVIEW QUESTIONS

LEVEL 1   Reviewing Facts and Terms

Match each item in column A with the most closely related item in column B. Use letters for answers in the spaces provided.

Column A

___ 1. histology
___ 2. microvilli
___ 3. gap junction
___ 4. tight junction
___ 5. germinative cells
___ 6. destroys gland cell
___ 7. hormones
___ 8. adipocytes
___ 9. bone-to-bone attachment
___10. muscle-to-bone attachment
___11. skeletal muscle
___12. cardiac muscle

Column B

a. repair and renewal
b. ligament
c. endocrine secretion
d. absorption and secretion
e. fat cells
f. holocrine secretion
g. study of tissues
h. tendon
i. intercellular connection
j. interlocking of membrane proteins
k. intercalated discs
l. striated, voluntary

13. The four basic tissue types found in the body are:
    (a) epithelia, connective, muscle, neural
    (b) simple, cuboidal, squamous, stratified
    (c) fibroblasts, adipocytes, melanocytes, mesenchymal
    (d) lymphocytes, macrophages, microphages, adipocytes

14. Long microvilli incapable of movement are called:
    (a) cilia
    (b) flagella
    (c) stereocilia
    (d) a, b, and c are correct

15. The most abundant connections between cells in the superficial layers of the skin are:
    (a) intermediate junctions
    (b) gap junctions
    (c) desmosomes
    (d) tight junctions

16. The three cell shapes making up epithelial tissue are:
    (a) simple, stratified, transitional
    (b) simple, stratified, pseudostratified
    (c) hexagonal, cuboidal, spherical
    (d) cuboidal, squamous, and columnar

17. The tissue that contains the fluid ground substance is
    (a) epithelial
    (b) neural
    (c) muscle
    (d) connective

18. The three major types of cartilage in the body are:
    (a) collagen, reticular, elastic
    (b) areolar, adipose, reticular
    (c) hyaline, elastic, fibrocartilage
    (d) keratin, reticular, elastic

4

19. The primary function of serous membranes in the body is:
    (a) to minimize friction between opposing surfaces
    (b) to line cavities that communicate with the exterior
    (c) to perform absorptive and secretory functions
    (d) to cover the surface of the body

20. Large muscle fibers that are multinucleated, striated, and voluntary are found in:
    (a) cardiac muscle tissue
    (b) skeletal muscle tissue
    (c) smooth muscle tissue
    (d) a, b, and c are correct

21. Intercalated discs and pacemaker cells are characteristic of:
    (a) smooth muscle tissue
    (b) cardiac muscle tissue
    (c) skeletal muscle tissue
    (d) a, b, and c are correct

22. Axons, dendrites, and a soma are characteristics of cells found in:
    (a) neural tissue
    (b) muscle tissue
    (c) connective tissue
    (d) epithelial tissue

23. What are the four essential functions of epithelial tissue?

24. What three types of layering make epithelial tissue recognizable?

25. What three basic components are found in connective tissues?

26. Which fluid connective tissues and supporting connective tissues are found in the human body?

27. Which four kinds of membranes composed of epithelial and connective tissues cover and protect other structures and tissues in the body?

28. What two cell populations make up neural tissue? What is the function of each?

LEVEL 2   Reviewing Concepts

29. In surfaces of the body where mechanical stresses are severe, the dominant epithelium is:
    (a) stratified squamous epithelium
    (b) simple cuboidal epithelium
    (c) simple columnar epithelium
    (d) stratified cuboidal epithelium

30. Why does holocrine secretion require continuous cell division?

31. What is the difference between an exocrine and an endocrine secretion?

32. A significant structural feature in the digestive system is the presence of tight junctions located near the exposed surfaces of cells lining the digestive tract. Why are these junctions so important?

33. Why are infections always a serious threat after a severe burn or abrasion?

34. What characteristics make the cutaneous membranes different from the serous and mucous membranes?

LEVEL 3   Critical Thinking and Clinical Applications

35. A biology student accidentally loses the labels of two prepared slides she is studying. One is a slide of animal intestine and the other of animal esophagus. You volunteer to help her sort them out. How would you decide which slide is which?

36. You are asked to develop a scheme that can be used to identify the three different types of muscle tissue in two steps. What would the two steps be?

ANSWERS TO CONCEPT CHECK QUESTIONS

Page 89

1. No. A simple squamous epithelium does not provide enough protection against infection, abrasion, and dehydration and is not found in the skin surface.   **2.** The process described is *holocrine secretion*.   **3.** The presence of microvilli on the free surface of epithelial cells greatly increases the surface area for absorption. Cilia function to move materials over the surface of epithelial cells.

Page 95

1. Collagen fibers add strength to connective tissue. We would therefore expect vitamin C deficiency to result in the production of connective tissue that is weaker and more prone to damage.   **2.** The tissue is adipose (fat) tissue.   **3.** Cartilage lacks a direct blood supply, which is necessary for proper healing to occur. Materials that are needed to repair damaged cartilage must diffuse from the blood to the chondroblasts. This diffusion process takes a long time and retards the healing process.

Page 97

1. Cell membranes are composed of lipid bilayers. Tissue membranes consist of a layer of epithelial tissue and a layer of connective tissue.   **2.** *Serous fluid* minimizes the friction between the serous membranes that cover the surfaces of organs and the surrounding body cavity.   **3.** All of these regions are subject to mechanical trauma and are abraded by food (pharynx and esophagus), feces (anus), or intercourse or childbirth (vagina).

Page 99

1. Since both cardiac and skeletal muscles are striated (banded), this must be *smooth muscle tissue*.   **2.** Only skeletal muscle tissue is voluntary.   **3.** Both skeletal muscle cells and neurons are called fibers because they are relatively long and slender.

4 Emergency Care Applications

Overview

A significant portion of the education of emergency medical personnel occurs in various hospital settings. Because of this, it is important for emergency care providers to understand the roles and responsibilities of other medical personnel as well as their own. The following discussion outlines the health care system and the roles and responsibilities of various health care providers.

The House of Medicine

Medicine is the science and art of diagnosing, treating, and preventing disease and injury. Disease has been one of humanity's greatest problems. Only during the last 100 years has medicine developed weapons to effectively fight disease. Physicians and other health care professionals use clues to identify, or diagnose, a specific disease or injury. This is usually accomplished by taking a medical history, performing a physical examination, and by assessing the results of laboratory tests and imaging exams. After making a diagnosis, physicians choose the best treatment for the patient. Some treatments cure a disease, others only relieve symptoms and do not cure the underlying disease.

Physicians

Physicians are practitioners who diagnose diseases and injuries, administer treatment, and provide advice on ways to stay healthy. The two kinds of physicians in the United States are the doctor of medicine (MD) and the doctor of osteopathy (DO). Both use medicines, surgery, and other standard methods of treating disease. DOs place special emphasis on problems involving the musculoskeletal system.

Patients may receive care from primary care physicians, specialists, or both. Primary care physicians include general practitioners, family practitioners, general internists, and general pediatricians. Obstetrician/gynecologists are sometimes considered primary care physicians as many women use them as their primary health care providers. Patients usually consult a primary care doctor when they first become ill or injured. Primary care physicians can treat most common disorders, providing comprehensive care for their patients.

Medical knowledge and technology have advanced so far that no one physician can master the entire field of medicine. Because of this, primary care physicians may refer patients with unusually complicated problems to specialists who have advanced training in a particular disease process or field of medicine. Specialists may even concentrate on one particular area and become subspecialists.

Medical Education

The education of a physician is long and demanding. In the United States, physicians usually complete four years of college before applying to medical school. The actual courses of study that students pursue in college vary, but students must complete a number of science and mathematics classes before applying. Of the 144 medical schools in the United States, 125 award the MD degree and 19 award the DO degree. Entrance to medical or osteopathic school is very competitive. Only students with excellent grades and high scores on the Medical College Admissions Test (MCAT) are accepted. In a recent year, close to 47,000 people applied for admission to medical school, but only 17,000 were accepted. Medical school consists of four years of intense study. Typically, the first two years emphasize basic science education including anatomy, physiology, pharmacology, pathology, microbiology, and much more. First- and second-year medical students are slowly introduced to the practice of medicine through classes in physical examination and through observation of practicing physicians. The last two years of medical school are devoted to learning the clinical sciences and are largely spent in a teaching hospital or clinic. Upon completion of medical school, the physician will be awarded the MD or DO degree. Medical graduates must successfully complete a medical licensure examination. In most states, MDs and DOs take the same exam.

However, the physician cannot be licensed until he or she has successfully completed a year of postgraduate training, formerly called an internship.

Upon graduation, physicians can choose to become primary care physicians or specialist physicians. They learn their chosen area of medicine by completing a residency in that field. Residencies may last from three to six years, depending on the field of study chosen. Residencies in the surgical fields are usually the longest. Some physicians still refer to the first year of residency training as an *internship* and refer to physicians in their first year of postgraduate training as *interns.* For the most part, however, physicians in postgraduate residencies are referred to as *residents.* They may also be classified by their year of postgraduate training (i.e., PGY-1, PGY-2). At the completion of residency, physicians take an examination in their chosen field and obtain board certification. Some physicians may choose to further specialize following residency training. In this case, they will enter a *fellowship* that may last from one to five years. Physicians in fellowship programs are referred to as *fellows.* Cardiothoracic surgeons, for example, must complete four years of college, four years of medical school, six years of surgical residency, and four years of cardiothoracic surgical fellowship. This totals 18 years of education after high school before they practice independently. Upon completion of their fellowship, they will take a board certification examination in their specialty.

In England, Australia, India, and many other foreign countries, students who have been accepted to medical school enter medical school immediately after high school. The medical school program in those countries is six years long. The first two years are similar to regular college courses, although the students begin to have some exposure to clinical medicine. The last four years are similar to U.S. medical schools. At the completion of medical school, students are awarded a bachelor of medicine, bachelor of surgery (MBBS) degree. Following this, they can enter general practice or enter into postgraduate training. The MBBS degree is not recognized in the United States. Thus, when physicians who have the MBBS enter the United States, they are labeled and licensed as MDs and use the MD degree after their name instead of MBBS.

Upon completion of residency and/or fellowship training, physicians enter the independent practice of medicine. Physicians who have completed their postgraduate training are referred to as *attending physicians.* In teaching hospitals, attending physicians supervise and are responsible for all patient care. Medical students report to residents, residents report to fellows, and fellows report to attendings. The level of training can sometimes be determined by the length of the lab coat worn by the physician. By tradition, medical students wear short lab coats (similar in look to a dinner jacket). Residents wear lab coats that extend to halfway down the thigh. Attending physicians wear full lab coats that extend nearly to the knee.

Medical Specialties

There are many different medical specialties. The American Board of Medical Specialties (ABMS), the principle accrediting board of MD training programs, recognizes 17 specialties. The American Osteopathic Association (AOA), the principle accrediting board of DO training programs, recognizes 18 major medical specialties and numerous subspecialties. A DO may be certified by an ABMS board if he or she completed an MD residency program or by an AOA board if he or she completed a DO residency. Some DOs are certified by both boards. The major medical specialties as recognized by the ABMS are:

- *Allergy and immunology.* Physicians who specialize in allergy and immunology study the diagnosis and treatment of allergic and immunological disorders. The physician must complete a three-year residency in either internal medicine or pediatrics and become board certified in that field. Then, he or she must complete a two-year fellowship in allergy and immunology before becoming board certified.

- *Anesthesiology.* Anesthesiologists are physicians who specialize in providing anesthesia for surgical patients. Many anesthesiologists also specialize in the management of acute and chronic pain. Anesthesiology residencies typically last four years. In addition, anesthesiologists can obtain subspecialty certification in critical care medicine and pain management.

- *Colon and rectal surgery.* Colon and rectal surgeons specialize in surgery of the large intestine and rectum. They must first complete a six-year general surgery residency and become board certified in general surgery. Then, they must complete a one-year fellowship in colon and rectal surgery.

- *Dermatology.* A dermatologist is a physician who specializes in diseases of the skin. Dermatologists must complete a four-year residency. In addition, they can obtain subspecialty certification in dermatopathology and dermatological immunology.

- *Emergency medicine.* Physicians who specialize in emergency medicine train to treat and stabilize emergency injuries and illnesses. Emergency physicians must complete a three- or four-year residency. They can obtain certificates of added qualification in medical toxicology, undersea and hyperbaric medicine, pediatric emergency medicine, and sports medicine through completion of a fellowship.

- *Family practice.* A family practitioner is a primary care physician trained in all aspects of medicine. He or she can manage the majority of problems encountered in general medical practice. Some family practitioners practice uncomplicated obstetrics. The family practice residency program is three years long. In addition, family practitioners can obtain certificates of added qualification in adolescent medicine, geriatric medicine, and sports medicine.

- *Internal medicine.* An internist is a physician who specializes in the diagnosis and treatment of diseases of the adult. Residency training for internal medicine is usually three years. There are ten subspecialties of internal medicine:
  - *Allergy and immunology.* Allergists must complete a two-year fellowship emphasizing treatment of allergic and immunological diseases.
  - *Cardiology.* Cardiologists must complete a three-year fellowship emphasizing the treatment of heart and related disorders. Cardiology is subdivided into *clinical cardiac electrophysiology* and *interventional cardiology.*
  - *Endocrinology, diabetes, and metabolism.* Endocrinologists must complete a two-year fellowship concentrating on diseases of the endocrine system, especially diabetes mellitus.
  - *Gastroenterology.* Gastroenterologists undergo a three-year fellowship concentrating on diseases of the gastrointestinal system and related organs. Significant emphasis is placed upon obtaining competence at fiber-optic endoscopy of the colon and stomach.
  - *Hematology.* Hematologists complete a two-year fellowship studying diseases of the blood and related disorders.
  - *Infectious disease.* Physicians interested in infectious disease must complete a two-year fellowship concentrating on disease spread by infectious agents such as bacteria or viruses.
  - *Medical oncology.* Medical oncologists must complete a two-year fellowship that concentrates on treatment, including chemotherapy, of malignant and similar diseases.
  - *Nephrology.* Nephrologists are physicians who study diseases of the kidneys and genitourinary system. The fellowship program lasts two years.
  - *Pulmonary disease.* Pulmonologists are physicians who complete a two-year fellowship concentrating on the treatment of diseases of the lungs and respiratory tract.
  - *Rheumatology.* Rheumatologists are physicians who treat diseases of the joints and diseases that are autoimmune in nature. The fellowship program is two years.

  In addition to these subspecialties, internists can seek certificates of added qualification in adolescent medicine, critical care medicine, geriatric medicine, and sports medicine.
- *Medical genetics.* Medical geneticists are physicians and scientists who specialize in treating inherited diseases and advising patients on disease possibilities. The residency program is four to five years long.
- *Neurological surgery.* Neurosurgeons specialize in the surgical treatment of injuries and illnesses in-

volving the brain, spinal cord, or peripheral nerves. Most neurosurgical residencies are five years long.
- *Nuclear medicine.* Nuclear medicine physicians use radioactive and stable substances in the diagnosis and treatment of disease. They must complete a two-year residency.
- *Obstetrics and gynecology.* Physicians who specialize in the treatment of diseases of women are called obstetricians and gynecologists. The residency program is usually four years. Subspecialty certification is available in gynecological oncology, maternal/fetal medicine, and reproductive endocrinology and fertility.
- *Ophthalmology.* Ophthalmologists are physicians who specialize in the medical and surgical treatment of eye disorders. They must complete a four-year residency program before sitting for the board certification exam.
- *Orthopedic surgery.* Surgeons who specialize in the treatment of bone and joint disorders are called orthopedic surgeons. They must complete an accredited orthopedic surgical residency, which usually lasts five to six years. A certificate of added qualification is available in hand surgery (Figure A4-1●).
- *Otolaryngology.* Physicians who specialize in the medical and surgical treatment of diseases and injuries of the ears, nose, and throat are otolaryngologists. The residency program is five years long.
- *Pathology.* Physicians who specialize in the laboratory study of disease are pathologists. Pathology residencies are at least four years long. Subspecialty certification is available for: blood banking/transfu-

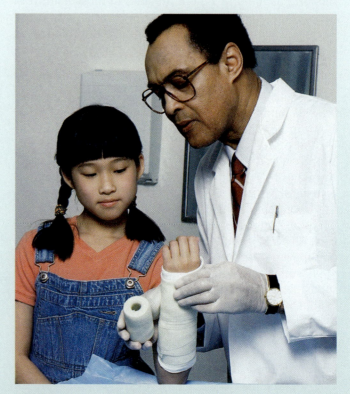

● **FIGURE A4-1   An Orthopedist**

sion medicine, chemical pathology, cytopathology, dermatopathology, forensic pathology, hematology, medical microbiology, molecular/genetic pathology, neuropathology, and pediatric pathology.

- *Pediatrics.* Pediatrics is the area of medicine devoted to the care of infants and children. The primary pediatric residency is three years. Subspecialty certification is available in: adolescent medicine, pediatric cardiology, pediatric critical care medicine, development/behavioral pediatrics, pediatric emergency medicine, pediatric endocrinology, pediatric gastroenterology, pediatric hematology/oncology, pediatric infectious diseases, neonatal/perinatal medicine, pediatric nephrology, neurodevelopmental disorders, pediatric pulmonology, and pediatric rheumatology.

- *Physical medicine and rehabilitation.* Physiatrists are physicians who have completed a four-year residency in physical medicine and rehabilitation. They concentrate on the assessment and rehabilitation of patients with physical disabilities. Subspecialty certification is available in spinal cord injury medicine, pain management, and pediatric rehabilitation medicine.

- *Plastic surgery.* Plastic surgeons are physicians who perform restorative or cosmetic surgery on the skin and associated structures. Residency training is five to six years. Subspecialty certification is available in hand surgery.

- *Preventative medicine.* Preventative medicine physicians typically will concentrate on aerospace medicine, occupational medicine, or general/preventive medicine. Residency programs are typically four years long. Subspecialty certification is available in undersea and hyperbaric medicine and medical toxicology.

- *Psychiatry and neurology.* Psychiatrists are physicians who specialize in the treatment of behavioral and mental disease. Neurologists treat medical conditions of the nervous system. Psychiatry residencies and neurology residencies are typically four years. Subspecialty certification for psychiatrists is available in addiction medicine, child and adolescent psychiatry, clinical neurophysiology, forensic psychiatry, geriatric psychiatry, and pain management. Neurologists can obtain subspecialty certification in clinical neurophysiology and pain management.

- *Radiology.* Radiology is the specialty of medicine that deals with diagnostic imaging through X-rays, ultrasound, magnetic resonance, and similar technologies. Residency programs are usually four years long. The subspecialties of radiology include: diagnostic radiology with special competence in nuclear radiology; certificates of added qualification in vascular and interventional radiology, neuroradiology, and pediatric radiology.

- *Surgery.* Physicians who provide surgical treatment of injuries and illness are called surgeons. Surgical residency programs are usually six years. The subspe-

cialties of surgery include: pediatric surgery, vascular surgery, surgical critical care, and surgery of the hand.

- *Thoracic Surgery.* Surgery of the thorax and its contents, including the heart, is the domain of a thoracic surgeon. Thoracic surgery residencies are typically six years long.

- *Urology.* Urology is the surgical treatment of diseases and illnesses of the genitourinary tract. Urologists must complete a six-year residency program.

Osteopathic Medicine

As previously discussed, MDs and DOs are the only complete physicians in the United States. Medicine as practiced by MDs is often referred to as allopathic medicine, while that practiced by DOs is called osteopathic medicine. Today, the difference between the two disciplines is minimal. DOs obtain additional undergraduate education in the musculoskeletal system and learn to perform osteopathic manipulation. In addition, DOs are trained to treat the "whole patient" instead of some disease entity.

The system of bones and muscles makes up about two-thirds of the body's mass. DOs know that the body's structure plays a critical role in its ability to function. They can use their eyes and hands to identify structural problems and to support the body's natural tendency toward health and self-healing.

Andrew Taylor Still, MD, developed osteopathic medicine in 1874. Dr. Still became dissatisfied with the effectiveness of nineteenth-century medicine after several of his children died of meningitis. He believed that many of the medications of his day were useless or even harmful. In response, he founded a philosophy of medicine based on ideas that dated back to Hippocrates. The philosophy focused on the unity of all body parts. He identified the musculoskeletal system as a key element of health. Recognizing the body's ability to heal itself, he stressed preventive medicine, eating well, and staying fit. He introduced the concept of osteopathic manipulative therapy where problems with the musculoskeletal system were corrected by applying various manual treatment techniques.

Osteopathic medicine was regarded as a cult until the middle of the twentieth century. Because DOs and MDs did not practice together, DOs established a parallel system of osteopathic hospitals where DOs could practice and schools where DOs could train. Following the Vietnam war, during which the U.S. military commissioned DOs as medical officers, the barriers between MDs and DOs were slowly broken down. Now, DOs have served as surgeon general of the army and as personal physicians for several presidents. Today, DOs and MDs practice together, and in many states, they take the same licensure examination. Unfortunately, because of the demands of medicine today, much of the uniqueness of osteopathic medicine has been lost. Many DOs complete MD residency programs and practice identically to MDs. Osteopathic medical schools now emphasize primary care, and because of this, approximately 64 percent of all DOs practice in primary care, many in rural areas.

Other Doctoral Health Care Providers

Although DOs and MDs are the only complete physicians in United States health care, there are several other doctoral level health care providers. These include dentists, podiatrists, optometrists, psychologists, chiropractors, and naturopaths.

Dentists

Dentists treat problems related to the teeth, gums, and related structures. They look beyond the mouth and treat people as individuals. Many systemic disease processes can be identified by examination of the mouth and teeth. Dentists detect and diagnose disease, provide for the aesthetic appearance of the teeth, provide surgical restoration of the teeth, and provide public information about prevention. Dentists perform surgery related to the mouth and can administer and prescribe medications as needed.

Dental school is four years long. Like medical and osteopathic school, students usually enter dental school after completion of a bachelor's degree, although some enter after two years of college. Dental school admission is highly selective. Students must have good college grades, perform well on the Dental Admissions Test (DAT), and show aptitude toward dentistry. Upon completion of dental school, students are awarded the doctor of dental surgery (DDS) or doctor of dental medicine (DMD) degree. Dentists who desire to practice general dentistry can enter practice after dental school. Those who desire to specialize will enter postgraduate training programs, usually lasting two years. The recognized specialties of dentistry include:

- *Dental public health.* The science and art of preventing and controlling dental diseases.
- *Endodontics.* The branch of dentistry that is concerned with the morphology, physiology, and pathology of the human dental pulp and periadicular tissues.
- *Oral and maxillofacial pathology.* The branch of dentistry that deals with the nature, identification, and management of oral and maxillofacial diseases.
- *Oral and maxillofacial surgery.* The specialty of dentistry that includes the diagnosis, surgical and adjunctive treatment of diseases, injuries, and defects involving the oral and maxillofacial region (also called oral surgeons).
- *Orthodontics and dentofacial orthopedics.* The area of dentistry that corrects the movement and location of teeth and related structures.
- *Pediatric dentistry.* The age-defined specialty of dentistry that is limited to infants and children.
- *Periodontics.* The branch of dentistry that treats the gums and other structures surrounding the teeth.

- *Prosthodontics.* The branch of dentistry that pertains to restoration or maintenance of oral functions, comfort, and appearance.
- *Oral and maxillofacial radiology.* Specialty of dentistry that involves imaging of the teeth and associated structures.

General dentists and most specialists are office based. Some of the surgical specialties of dentistry, such as oral and maxillofacial surgery, are hospital based. A physician will usually work with the oral surgeon to manage nondental related problems in hospitalized patients.

Podiatrists

Podiatrists are doctoral health care providers who concentrate on medical and surgical care of the feet. Most students entering podiatric medical school hold a bachelor's degree. Most podiatric medical schools require that students also write the Medical College Admissions Test (MCAT). Podiatric medical school is four years and similar to medical school, except that the emphasis is on the feet. Upon graduation from podiatric medical school, podiatrists are awarded the doctor of podiatric medicine (DPM) degree. Some will enter general practice and others will complete a one- to two-year residency, often in a teaching hospital. Podiatrists perform surgery on the feet and can prescribe medications for foot and related problems. Podiatrists can obtain specialty certification in podiatric orthopedics, podiatric surgery, or primary podiatric medicine.

Optometrists

Doctors of optometry (ODs) are health care providers who examine, diagnose, treat, and manage diseases and disorders of the visual system, the eye, and associated structures. Optometrists enter optometry school after two to four years of college. Optometry school is four years, and students earn the doctor of optometry (OD) degree upon graduation. Optometrists primarily perform refractive examinations of the eye. In some states, optometrists can prescribe a limited number of medications related to the eye. In other states they cannot prescribe. Optometrists are often confused with ophthalmologists. Ophthalmologists are MDs or DOs who have completed a four-year residency in the medical and surgical care of the eyes and related structures. Optometrists do not perform surgery.

Psychologists

Psychologists have completed a clinical psychology program and have been awarded the doctor of philosophy (Ph.D.) degree. They provide individual and family counseling for emotional and mental diseases. They also provide diagnostic testing and assessment. Psychologists cannot prescribe medications. The difference between psychiatrists and psychologists is often misunderstood. Psychiatrists are physicians (MD or DO) who have completed a four-year psychiatry residency. They treat emotional and mental illness with multiple modalities including medications. Often, psychiatrists and psychologists work together, with the psychologist providing much of the counseling while the psychiatrist manages medications and other problems.

Chiropractors

Chiropractic is a branch of the healing arts concerned with human health and disease processes. Central to chiropractic is the "vertebral subluxation," a condition in which a vertebra becomes slightly misaligned with an adjacent segment in such a way as to disturb nerve function. The objective of chiropractic is to locate, analyze, and correct vertebral subluxations, usually through spinal manipulation. One criticism of chiropractic is that the vertebral subluxation has never been scientifically proven to exist.

Some chiropractors limit their practice to spinal manipulation for back pain and related problems. Others believe that chiropractic manipulation can treat other conditions by removing impediments to nerve conduction. This is a major source of discord within the chiropractic profession. "Straight" chiropractors limit their practice to treatment of musculoskeletal problems and back pain. They refer patients to medical or osteopathic doctors for problems that are not of a musculoskeletal origin. "Mixer" chiropractors use spinal manipulation, also called chiropractic adjustments, to treat problems outside of the musculoskeletal system such as ear infections, ulcer disease, and gall bladder disease.

Chiropractic was founded in 1878 when Daniel David Palmer, a magnetic healer, applied force to a bump that he detected on the back of a janitor who had recently lost his hearing after working in a cramped, stooped position. As he applied the force, Palmer felt a "pop," and the bump disappeared. Several days later, the janitor's hearing returned and chiropractic was born.

Chiropractic colleges are usually three to four years long. Students usually enter chiropractic school after two years of college. Upon completion of the chiropractic curriculum, they are granted a doctor of chiropractic (DC) degree. They then take a state licensure exam and can begin independent practice. Chiropractors cannot perform surgery or prescribe medication. They can use X-rays for evaluation of the spine and can use various physical therapy modalities. In some states in the U.S., chiropractors can refer to themselves as chiropractic physicians.

Spinal manipulation has been found effective for the treatment of mechanical musculoskeletal back pain and similar conditions. Its effectiveness in treating other medical conditions has never been scientifically documented.

Naturopathic Physicians

A relatively new doctoral level health care provider is the naturopathic physician. Naturopathic schools have a four-year program that contains the same basic science courses as traditional medical schools. However, they also study clinical nutrition, acupuncture, homeopathic medicine, botanical medicine, psychology, and counseling. At the completion of their education, students receive a doctor of naturopathic medicine (ND) degree. Naturopathic physicians use holistic and nontoxic approaches to therapy with an emphasis on disease prevention and optimizing wellness. They cannot prescribe medications or practice surgery.

Midlevel Practitioners

With the advent of managed care, a need has arisen to use nonphysicians to assist in primary care roles. These health care providers, often called *midlevel practitioners,* work with licensed physicians. Physician assistants (PAs), nurse practitioners (NPs), and nurse anesthetists (CRNAs) are the most common midlevel practitioners.

PAs attend physician assistant programs that are usually located in medical schools. They enter after they have completed two years of college. PA school is usually two years long, and some PA programs now offer master's degrees. PAs practice under the direction of a licensed physician. However, the physician does not have to be physically present in the clinic. PAs can specialize in areas of medicine such as family practice, emergency medicine, and pediatrics.

Nurse practitioners are advanced nurses who have completed an approved nurse practitioner program. Nurse practitioners must have a bachelor's degree in nursing and experience as a registered nurse prior to entering NP school. NP school is usually two years long and trains the nurse for practice, usually in a clinic setting. NP programs can specialize in family practice, geriatrics, internal medicine, or pediatrics. NPs work under the direction of a licensed physician. However, the physician does not have to be physically present. NPs often staff rural and public health clinics and can consult with physicians by telephone if needed.

Certified registered nurse anesthetists (CRNAs) are nurses who have completed a two-year program in anesthesia. To enter the program, the nurse must have a bachelor's degree in nursing and several years of clinical nursing experience. Most CRNA programs award a master's degree upon completion. CRNAs work under the supervision of an MD or DO anesthesiologist (although this is being challenged). People often confuse anesthesiologists and anesthetists. Anesthesiologists are MD or DO physicians who have completed a residency program in anesthesiology. Anesthetists are nurses who have completed a nurse anesthesia program.

Nursing

Nurses provide the vast majority of actual patient care in this country. There are two major categories of nurses: registered nurses (RNs) and licensed practical nurses (LPNs). In some states, LPNs are referred to as licensed vocational nurses (LVNs) (Figure A4-2•).

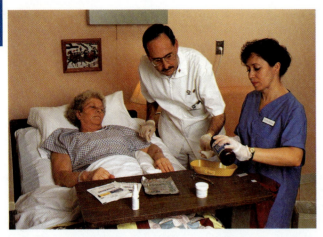

• **FIGURE A4-2** **The Nursing Assistant Helps the Nurse Care for the Patient**

LPNs undergo an intense one-year program that prepares them to provide bedside nursing care. The first part of the program is classroom-based and includes the basic sciences and nursing science. The latter parts of the class are conducted in the hospital, where the students learn and practice their skills. Upon completion of their training, they receive a certificate and are able to sit for the state licensure examination.

Registered nurses can complete one of three different program types. The shortest is a two-year associate's degree program. In this case, the student completes required prenursing classes, then studies nursing science in the classroom, and finally finishes by learning in the hospital setting. Upon completion of the program, students earn an associate degree in nursing (ADN). Although not common today, some programs still offer a diploma program. This is a three-year program that concentrates on prenursing, classroom, and clinical nursing instruction. Finally, many nursing programs offer a bachelor's degree. The first two years are prenursing courses, and the last two years are classroom and clinical nursing classes. Upon completion, the nurse receives a bachelor of science degree in nursing (BSN).

Graduate courses leading to a master's of science in nursing (MSN) and a Ph.D. in nursing are available. Many community colleges have begun to offer a paramedic-to-nurse bridge program for paramedics who want to become a nurse. Several programs provide nursing education by correspondence and over the Internet. These programs are popular with EMS personnel because of the difficult work schedules inherent in EMS.

Allied Health Personnel

For one person to be well versed in all aspects of health care is impossible. Because of this, numerous *allied health personnel* have evolved to assist physicians and

nurses in providing patient care. Examples of allied health personnel include:

- *Anesthesiologist assistant.* Assists anesthesiologist by preparing equipment and supplies and by monitoring patients.
- *Art therapist.* Provides art therapy as a rehabilitation tool.
- *Athletic Trainer.* Provides preventive and field care for various sporting teams and events.
- *Audiologist.* Provides hearing testing and fits hearing aids and similar devices.
- *Blood Bank Technologist.* Assures blood is gathered, stored, tested, and administered in a safe and proper manner.
- *Cardiovascular Technologist.* Performs cardiovascular diagnostic testing such as electrocardiograms, echocardiography, stress testing, and cardiac monitoring.
- *Clinical Laboratory Science/Medical Technology.* Staffs the medical laboratory and performs essential testing of body products.
- *Counseling-Related Occupations.* Provide counseling for mental health, substance abuse, rehabilitation, and similar patients.
- *Cytotechnologist.* Studies and prepares cells and tissues such as Pap smears.
- *Dental Assistant.* Chair-side assistant to a dentist in day-to-day practice.
- *Dental Hygienist.* Evaluates and cleans teeth in dental office and instructs the patient in preventive dental care.
- *Dental Laboratory Technician.* Works in dental lab making dentures, crowns, implants, and bridges.
- *Diagnostic Medical Sonographer.* Performs diagnostic ultrasound, usually in a hospital radiology department.
- *Dietetic Technician, Dietician.* Instructs patients in dietary health and supervises hospital nutrition programs.
- *Emergency Medical Technician, Paramedic.* Provides advanced emergency care to ill or injured patients.
- *Genetic Counselor.* Assists patients and families in regard to diagnosed or possible genetic or hereditary problems.
- *Health Information Management.* Organizes and controls all patient medical records in hospital or office setting.
- *Histologic Technician/Histotechnologist.* Prepares tissues for examination by pathologist.
- *Kinesiotherapist.* Assists patients in movement following injury or illness, often working with physical therapists.
- *Medical Assistant.* Medical office assistant who provides medical services for a practicing physician or midlevel provider.

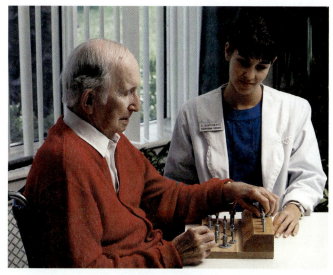

• FIGURE A4-3   Occupational Therapist

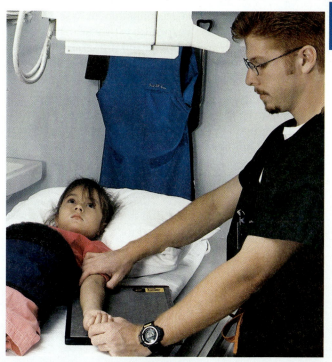

• FIGURE A4-4   X-ray Technician

- *Music Therapist.* Works with other rehabilitative specialists by providing music therapy to rehabilitation and mental health patients.
- *Nuclear Medical Technologist.* Prepares, administers, and monitors nuclear radioisotopes in a hospital nuclear medicine department.
- *Occupational Therapy.* Provides instruction and rehabilitation to patients following injury or illness so they can return to their chosen occupation (Figure A4-3•).
- *Ophthalmic Dispensing Optician.* Prepares and dispenses eyewear and contact lenses based upon prescription by an optometrist or ophthalmologist.
- *Ophthalmic Laboratory Technician/Technologist.* Technician who prepares prescription lenses in an ophthalmic laboratory.
- *Orthoptist.* Prepares braces and similar devices for patients who have had injuries or illnesses.
- *Orthotist and Prosthetic Technician.* Prepares artificial limbs and other body parts for patients who have undergone amputation or another body changing procedure.
- *Pathologist's Assistant.* Assists pathologist in the hospital laboratory and in the autopsy theater.
- *Perfusionist.* Operates cardiac bypass pump for patients undergoing open-heart surgery.
- *Physical Therapist/Physical Therapy Assistant.* A physical therapist is a person with a bachelor's or master's degree in physical therapy who prepares and supervises physical rehabilitation for a patient. A physical therapy assistant is a person with an associate's degree who assists a physical therapist in patient care including use of modalities.

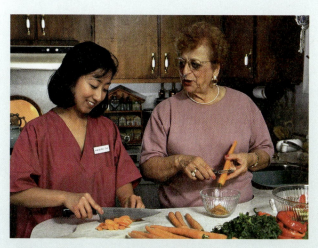

• FIGURE A4-5   Assisting a Patient at Home

- *Radiation Therapist/Radiographer.* Radiation therapist provides therapeutic radiation therapy to cancer patients. Radiographer or radiological technician performs medical imaging techniques such as X-rays, computed tomography (CT) scans, and magnetic resonance imaging (MRI) scans (Figure A4-4•).
- *Rehabilitation Counselor.* Oversees emotional and mental component of injury or illness rehabilitation (Figure A4-5•).

- *Respiratory Therapist.* Responsible for assessing and providing ordered respiratory procedures for patients. Is also responsible for the preparation and operation of ventilators and all respiratory devices found in a hospital.
- *Speech-Language Pathologist.* Assists patients, especially those who have had a stroke or head injury, in learning to speak and communicate.
- *Surgical Technologist.* Technologist who works in hospital setting assisting surgeons in performing surgical procedures.
- *Therapeutic Recreation Specialist.* Instructs and oversees patients' recreation needs, especially those patients who are hospitalized for a prolonged period.

SUMMARY

The house of medicine is indeed complex, and this discussion has not covered every aspect of health care provision. However, emergency medical personnel should be familiar with the various health care personnel they will encounter during the course of their hospital rotations, and later as they interact with hospital personnel as members of the emergency medical services system. Remember, emergency medical technicians and paramedics are essential parts of the health care system.

5

The Integumentary System

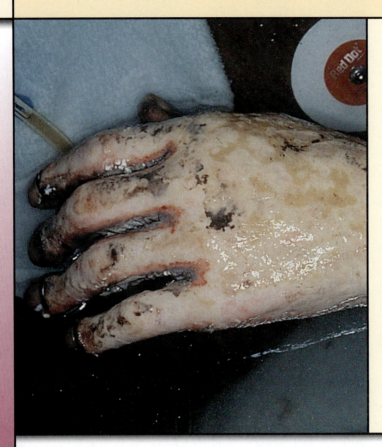

The integumentary system is the largest and most visible organ system of the body. It plays a major role in maintaining homeostasis and in protecting the organism from the environment. Any interruption in the skin poses a potential risk to the entire organism. Burns are some of the most painful and debilitating injuries encountered in emergency medical care. They can cause significant loss of body fluids and provide a direct route for the invasion of infectious organisms. In this chapter, we will examine the integumentary system and its many functions. In addition, we will discuss common illnesses and injuries that affect the skin.

Chapter Outline and Objectives

  1 *Describe the general functions of the integumentary system.*

  2 *Describe the main structural features of the epidermis, and explain their functional significance.*

  3 *Explain what accounts for individual and racial differences in skin, such as skin color.*

  4 *Describe how the integumentary system helps regulate body temperature.*

  5 *Discuss the effects of ultraviolet radiation on the skin and the role played by melanocytes.*

  6 *Discuss the functions of the skin's accessory structures.*

  7 *Describe the mechanisms that produce hair and that determine hair texture and color.*

  8 *Explain how the skin responds to injury and repairs itself.*

  9 *Summarize the effects of the aging process on the skin.*

Vocabulary Development

*angio-, vessel; *angioma*
cornu, horn; *stratum corneum*
cutis, skin; *cutaneous*
derma, skin; *dermis*
epi-, above or over; *epidermis*
facere, to make; *cornified*
germinare, to start growing;
    stratum germinativum
keros, horn; *keratin*
kyanos, blue; *cyanosis*
luna, moon; *lunula*
melas, black; *melanin*
onyx, nail; *eponychium*
papilla, a nipple-shaped mound;
    dermal papillae

5

The integumentary system, consisting of the skin, hair, nails, and various glands, is the most visible organ system of the body. Because of its visibility, we devote a lot of time to its upkeep. Washing the face and hands, brushing or trimming hair, clipping nails, taking showers, and applying deodorant are activities that modify the appearance or properties of the skin. And when something goes wrong with the skin, the effects are immediately apparent. Even a relatively minor skin condition, such as mild acne, will be noticed at once, whereas more serious problems in other systems are often ignored. The skin, however, may also provide visible signs of major systemic disorders through changes in its color, flexibility, or sensitivity.

This chapter focuses on the important structural and functional relationships in the skin. In the process, it demonstrates patterns that apply to tissue and organ interactions in other systems.

INTEGUMENTARY STRUCTURE AND FUNCTION

The **integumentary system**, or simply the **integument**, has two major components: the cutaneous membrane and the accessory structures. The **cutaneous membrane**, or *skin*, is an organ composed of the superficial epithelium, or **epidermis** (*epi-*, above), and the underlying connective tissues of the **dermis**. The **accessory structures** include hair, nails, and a variety of multicellular exocrine glands.

The general structure of the integument is shown in Figure 5-1•. Beneath the dermis, the loose connective tissue of the **subcutaneous layer**, or **hypodermis**, attaches the integument to deeper structures, such as muscles or bones. Although often not considered to be part of the integumentary system, this layer will be considered here because of its extensive interconnections with the dermis.

As we will see, the five major functions of the various parts of the integument are:

1. *Protection.* The skin covers and protects underlying tissues and organs from impacts, chemicals, and infections, and prevents the loss of body fluids.

2. *Temperature maintenance.* The skin maintains normal body temperature by regulating heat gain or loss to the environment.

3. *Storage of nutrients.* The deeper portions of the dermis typically contain a large reserve of lipids in the form of adipose tissue.

4. *Sensory reception.* Receptors in the integument detect touch, pressure, pain, and temperature stimuli and relay that information to the nervous system.

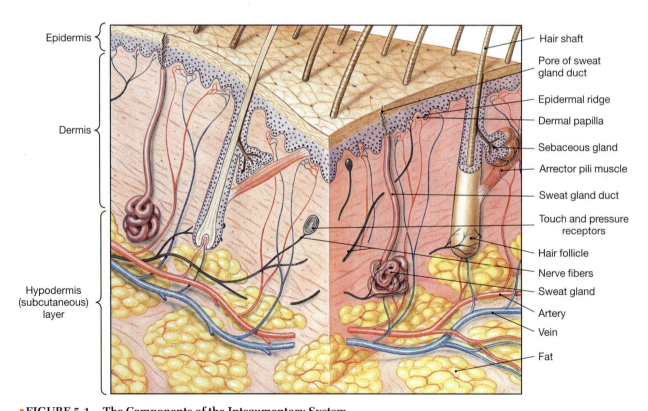

•**FIGURE 5-1   The Components of the Integumentary System**
The relationships among the major components of the integumentary system (with the exception of nails, shown in Figure 5-7).

5. *Excretion and secretion.* The integument excretes salts, water, and organic wastes, and produces milk, a specialized exocrine secretion.

Each of these functions will be explored more fully as we discuss the individual components of the system.

The Epidermis

The epidermis consists of a stratified squamous epithelium. ∞ *p. 88* Several different cell layers are present, but the precise boundaries between them are often difficult to see in a light micrograph. The majority of the body is covered by thin skin. In a sample of **thin skin**, the epidermis is a mere 0.08 mm thick. In **thick skin**, found on the palms of the hands and soles of the feet, the epidermis may be as much as six times thicker. The words *thin* and *thick* refer only to the relative thickness of the epidermis, not to the integument as a whole.

Layers of the Epidermis

Refer to Figure 5-2• as we describe the layers, or **strata** (singular *stratum*), in a section of thick skin. Beginning at the basement membrane and traveling toward the free surface, we find the *stratum germinativum*, the *stratum spinosum*, the *stratum granulosum*, the *stratum lucidum*, and the *stratum corneum*.

Stratum Germinativum. The deepest epidermal layer is called the **stratum germinativum** (STRA-tum jer-mi-na-TĒ-vum; *stratum*, layer + *germinare*, to start growing), or *stratum basale* (*basis*, base). This layer is firmly attached to the basement membrane, which separates the epidermis from the loose connective tissue of the adjacent dermis. The stratum germinativum forms **epidermal ridges**, which extend into the dermis, increasing the area of contact between the two regions. Epidermal ridges of the palms and soles improve our gripping ability and increase the skin's sensitivity. Dermal projections called *dermal papillae* (singular *papilla*, a nipple-shaped mound) extend between adjacent ridges (Figure 5-1•). Because there are no blood vessels in the epidermis, epidermal cells must obtain nutrients delivered by dermal blood vessels. The combination of ridges and papillae increases the surface area for diffusion between the dermis and epidermis.

The contours of the skin surface follow the ridge patterns. This pattern is most easily observed on the thick skin of the palms and soles, where the ridges form complex whorls. The superficial ridges on the palms and soles increase the surface area of the skin and increase friction, ensuring a secure grip. Ridge shapes are genetically determined; those of each person are unique and do not change over the course of a lifetime. Fingerprints are ridge patterns on the tips of the fingers that can be used to identify individuals; they have been used in criminal investigations for over a century.

Large stem cells dominate the stratum germinativum, making it the layer where new cells are generated and begin to grow. The divisions of these cells replace more superficial cells that are lost or shed at the epithelial surface. The stratum germinativum also contains *melanocytes*, cells whose cytoplasmic processes extend between epithelial cells in this layer, and receptors that provide information about objects touch-

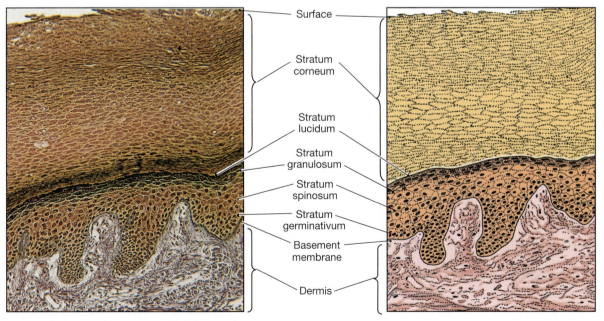

•**FIGURE 5-2 Layers of the Epidermis**
A profile of the epidermis in thick skin. (LM × 150)

5

ing the skin. Melanocytes synthesize *melanin*, a yellow-brown to black pigment that colors the epidermis.

Stratum Spinosum.

Each time a stem cell divides, one of the daughter cells enters the next layer, the **stratum spinosum** (spiny layer), where it may continue to divide. The stratum spinosum is several cells thick, and the cells are bound together by desmosomes. ∞ *p. 84* The name of this layer is based on the fact that the desmosomes and other cytoskeletal structures make the cells appear shrunken and spiny when prepared for viewing under a microscope.

Stratum Granulosum.

The **stratum granulosum** consists of cells displaced from the spinosum layer. By the time epithelial cells reach this layer, most have stopped dividing, and they begin manufacturing large quantities of proteins and enzymes.

Stratum Lucidum.

In the thick skin of the palms and soles, a glassy **stratum lucidum** (clear layer) covers the stratum granulosum. The cells in this layer are flattened and densely packed. The cytoplasm contains enzymes involved in the production of the fibrous protein **keratin** (KER-a-tin; *keros*, horn), introduced in Chapter 2. ∞ *p. 43*

Stratum Corneum.

The most superficial layer of the epidermis, the **stratum corneum** (KŌR-nē-um; *cornu*, horn), consists of flattened and dead epithelial cells that have accumulated large amounts of keratin.

Keratin is extremely strong, light, flexible, durable, and water-resistant. In the human body, keratin not only coats the surface of the skin but forms the basic structure of hair, calluses, and nails. In other animals, it is even more versatile, making up cow horns and hooves, bird feathers, reptile scales, porcupine quills, the armor of armadillos, and baleen plates in the mouths of whales.

It takes 2–4 weeks for a cell to move from the stratum germinativum to the stratum corneum. During this time, the cell is displaced from its oxygen and nutrient supply, becomes packed with keratin, and finally dies. The dead cells usually remain in the stratum corneum for an additional 2 weeks before they are shed or washed away. As superficial layers are lost, new layers arrive from the underlying strata. Thus the deeper layers of the epithelium and underlying tissues remain protected by superficial layers of dead, durable, and expendable cells.

Permeability of the Epidermis

An epithelium containing large amounts of keratin is said to be **keratinized** (ker-A-tin-īzed), or **cornified** (KŌR-ni-fīd; *cornu*, horn + *facere*, to make). A cornified epithelium is only around 1/100,000th as permeable to water and electrolytes as are other epithelia. Normally the stratum corneum is relatively dry; only around 10 percent of the cell weight is water. This dryness makes it unattractive to many bacteria, and thus a good protective barrier.

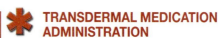

TRANSDERMAL MEDICATION ADMINISTRATION

Some drugs can be administered through the epidermis in a process called *transdermal medication administration.* Medications commonly administered by this route include nitroglycerin, female hormones, blood pressure medications, and narcotic pain relievers. Drug delivery systems have been developed that provide steady and prolonged delivery of the medication for as long as one week.

For transdermal administration, a predetermined amount of the drug is placed into an adhesive patch. These drugs must be lipid-soluble in order to penetrate the skin. Alternatively, the drug can be mixed with an inert solvent that is highly lipid-soluble. The resultant mixture is absorbed through the skin. The patch is applied to the skin, and the drug is slowly absorbed. Once the drug has penetrated the cell membranes in the *stratum corneum* and enters the underlying tissues, it is absorbed into the circulation. Transdermal administration provides significant patient convenience, as the drug is administered slowly and continuously over a long period, which helps minimize undesired side effects.

In the emergency setting, topical nitroglycerin preparations are among the drugs most frequently administered by the transdermal route. These can be rapidly applied to the patient's chest wall. Drug delivery begins promptly and continues at a steady rate. This minimizes many of the drug's unpleasant side effects (e.g., headache).

Skin Color

The color of the epidermis is caused by the interaction between (1) pigment composition and concentration and (2) the dermal blood supply.

Pigmentation. The epidermis contains variable quantities of two pigments, carotene and melanin. **Carotene** (KAR-ō-tēn) is an orange-yellow pigment that normally accumulates inside epidermal cells. Carotene pigments are found in a variety of orange-colored vegetables, such as carrots and squashes. **Melanin** is a brown, yellow-brown, or black pigment produced by melanocytes. **Melanocytes** manufacture and store melanin and inject that pigment into the epithelial cells of the stratum germinativum and stratum spinosum (Figure 5-3•). This transfer of pigmentation colors the entire epidermis. Melanocyte activity slowly increases in response to sunlight exposure, peaking around 10 days after the initial exposure.

Sunlight contains significant amounts of **ultraviolet (UV) radiation**. A small amount of UV radiation is beneficial, for it stimulates the synthesis of vitamin D_3 in the epidermis; this process is discussed in a later section. Too much ultraviolet radiation, however, produces immediate effects of mild or even serious burns. Melanin helps prevent skin damage by absorbing ultraviolet radiation before it reaches the deep layers of the epidermis and dermis. Within the epidermal cells,

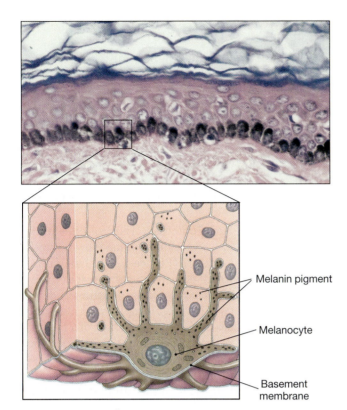

•FIGURE 5-3   Melanocytes
The location and orientation of melanocytes in the deepest layer of the epidermis (stratum germinativum) of a black person.

more pronounced. When the vessels are temporarily constricted, as when one is frightened, the skin becomes relatively pale. During a sustained reduction in circulatory supply, the blood in the skin loses oxygen and takes on a much deeper red tone. The skin then takes on a bluish coloration called **cyanosis** (sī-a-NŌ-sis; *kyanos*, blue). In individuals of any skin color, cyanosis is most apparent in areas of thin skin, such as the lips, ears, or beneath the nails. It can be a response to extreme cold or a result of circulatory or respiratory disorders, such as heart failure or severe asthma.

In general, pigment content can overshadow other factors; for example, circulatory changes have a less visible effect on skin color in dark-skinned individuals. But, although the skin pigments of such individuals may obscure localized inflammation or cyanosis, color changes can usually be seen through the nails, where the epidermis lacks dark pigments.

The Epidermis and Vitamin D₃

Although strong sunlight can damage epithelial cells and deeper tissues, limited exposure to sunlight is very beneficial. When exposed to ultraviolet radiation, epidermal cells in the stratum spinosum and stratum germinativum convert a steroid related to cholesterol into **vitamin D_3**. This product is absorbed, modified, and released by the liver and then converted by the kidneys into *calcitriol*, a hormone essential for the absorption of calcium and phosphorus by the small intestine. An inadequate supply of vitamin D_3 leads to impaired bone maintenance and growth.

✓ Excessive shedding of cells from the outer layer of skin in the scalp causes dandruff. What is the name of this layer of skin?

✓ As you pick up a piece of lumber, a splinter pierces the palm of your hand and lodges in the third layer of the epidermis. Identify this layer.

✓ Why does exposure to sunlight or tanning lamps cause the skin to become darker?

---

melanin concentrates around the nuclear envelope and absorbs the UV before it can damage the nuclear DNA.

Despite the presence of melanin, long-term damage can result from repeated exposure, even in darkly pigmented individuals. For example, alterations in the underlying connective tissues lead to premature wrinkling, and skin cancers can result from chromosomal damage in stem cells of the stratum germinativum or in melanocytes. One of the major consequences of the global depletion of the ozone layer in the upper atmosphere will be a sharp increase in the rate of skin cancers.

The ratio between melanocytes and stem (germinative) cells ranges between 1:4 and 1:20, depending on the region of the body surveyed. The observed differences in skin color between individuals and even races do not reflect different *numbers* of melanocytes, but merely different levels of melanin production. For example, in the inherited condition *albinism*, melanin pigment is not produced by the melanocytes, even though these cells are distributed normally. Individuals with this condition, known as *albinos*, have light-colored skin and hair.

Dermal Circulation.   Blood with abundant oxygen is bright red, and blood vessels in the dermis normally give the skin a reddish tint that is common in lightly pigmented individuals. When those vessels are dilated, as during inflammation, the red tones become much

The Dermis

The dermis lies beneath the epidermis. It has two major components: a superficial *papillary layer* and a deeper *reticular layer*.

Layers of the Dermis

The **papillary layer**, named after the dermal papillae, consists of loose connective tissue that supports and nourishes the epidermis. This region contains the capillaries and nerves supplying the surface of the skin.

The deeper **reticular layer** consists of an interwoven meshwork of dense, irregular connective tissue.

Bundles of collagen fibers leave the reticular layer to blend into those of the papillary layer above, so the boundary line between these layers is indistinct. Collagen fibers of the reticular layer also extend into the subcutaneous layer below. This layer provides support and attachment for the dermis while also allowing flexibility and independent movement.

Other Dermal Components

In addition to protein fibers, the dermis contains a mixed cell population that includes all of the cells of connective tissue proper. ∞ *p. 90* Accessory organs of epidermal origin, such as hair follicles and sweat glands, extend into the dermis (see Figure 5-1•, p. 108).

Other systems communicate with the skin through their connections to the dermis. For example, the reticular and papillary layers contain a network of blood vessels (cardiovascular system), lymphatics (lymphatic system), and nerve fibers (nervous system).

Blood vessels provide nutrients and oxygen and remove carbon dioxide and waste products. Both the blood vessels and the lymphatics help local tissues defend and repair themselves after an injury or infection. The nerve fibers control blood flow, adjust gland secretion rates, and monitor sensory receptors in the dermis and the deeper layers of the epidermis. These receptors, which provide sensations of touch, pain, pressure, and temperature, will be detailed in Chapter 10.

The Subcutaneous Layer

An extensive network of connective tissue fibers attaches the dermis to the subcutaneous layer. The boundary between these two layers is indistinct, and although the subcutaneous layer is not actually a part of the integument, it is important in stabilizing the position of the skin in relation to underlying tissues and organs.

The subcutaneous layer (hypodermis) consists of loose connective tissue with many fat cells. These adipose cells provide infants and small children with a layer of "body fat" over the entire body that reduces heat loss, provides an energy reserve, and absorbs shocks from inevitable tumbles.

As maturation proceeds, the distribution of subcutaneous fat changes. Men tend to accumulate such fat at the neck, upper arms, along the lower back, and over the buttocks, and women in the breasts, buttocks, hips, and thighs. Both women and men, however, may accumulate distressing amounts in the abdominal hypodermis, producing a prominent "pot belly."

The hypodermis is quite elastic. Below its superficial region with its large blood vessels, the hypodermis contains no vital organs and few capillaries. The lack of vital organs makes *subcutaneous injection* a useful method for administering drugs (thus the familiar term *hypodermic needle*).

Accessory Structures

Accessory structures include hair follicles, sebaceous glands, sweat glands, and nails.

Hair Follicles

Hairs project above the surface of the skin almost everywhere except over the sides and soles of the feet, the palms of the hands, the sides of the fingers and toes, the lips, and portions of the external genital organs. Hairs originate in complex organs called **hair follicles**.

The Structure of Hair Follicles. Hair follicles project deep into the dermis and often extend into the underlying subcutaneous layer (Figure 5-4•). The walls of each follicle contain all the cell layers found in the epidermis. Hair is formed at the deepest portion of the follicle, where stem cells divide. As keratinization occurs, the follicle produces the cylindrical **shaft** of a hair. The shaft of the hair that projects above the skin surface consists entirely of dead, keratinized cells.

Differences in the appearance of hair among individuals result from the size of the follicles, the activity of follicular cells, and the shapes of the hairs. For example, straight hairs are round in cross section, whereas curly ones are rather flattened.

Functions of Hair. The 5 million hairs on the human body have important functions. The roughly 100,000 hairs on the head protect the scalp from ultraviolet light, cushion light blows to the head, and provide insulating benefits for the skull. The hairs guarding the entrances to the nostrils and external ear canals help prevent the entry of foreign particles and insects, and eyelashes perform a similar function for the surface of the eye. A sensory nerve fiber is associated with the base of each hair follicle. As a result, the movement of the shaft of even a single hair can be felt consciously. This sensitivity provides an early-warning system that may help prevent injury. For example, you may be able to swat a mosquito before it reaches the skin surface.

Ribbons of smooth muscle, called **arrector pili** (a-REK-tōr PĪ-lī) muscles, extend from the papillary dermis to a connective tissue sheath that surrounds each hair follicle (Figure 5-4•). When stimulated, the arrector pili pull on the follicles and elevate the hairs. Contraction may be caused by emotional states, such as fear or rage. Contractions also occur as a response to cold, producing the characteristic "goose bumps" associated with shivering. In a furry mammal, this action increases the thickness of the insulating coat, rather like putting on an extra sweater. Although we do not receive any comparable insulating benefits, the reflex persists.

Hair Color. Hair color reflects differences in the type and amount of pigment produced by melanocytes at the

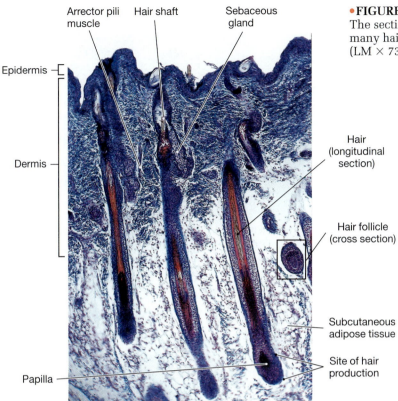

Arrector pili muscle   Hair shaft   Sebaceous gland

Epidermis

Dermis

Papilla

Hair (longitudinal section)

Hair follicle (cross section)

Subcutaneous adipose tissue

Site of hair production

•**FIGURE 5-4   Hair Follicles**
The sectional appearance of the skin of the scalp. Notice the many hair follicles and the way they extend into the dermis. (LM × 73)

5

✓ What condition is produced by the contraction of the arrector pili muscles?

✓ A person suffers a burn on the forearm that destroys the epidermis and the deep dermis. When the injury heals, would you expect to find hair growing again in the area of the injury?

✓ Describe the functions of the subcutaneous layer.

papilla. Although these characteristics are genetically determined, the condition of your hair may also be influenced by hormonal or environmental factors. As pigment production decreases with age, the color of hair lightens toward gray. White hair results from the presence of air bubbles within the hair shaft. Because the hair itself is dead and inert, changes in coloration are gradual. Unless bleach is used, it is not possible for hair to "turn white overnight," as some horror stories would have us believe.

✳ THE HAIR IN DISEASE

The hair is a tactile sensory organ that covers the entire body, with the exception of the palms, soles, and parts of the genitalia. Like other body organs, the hair can be affected by disease. Changes in hair growth or distribution can be an aid in the diagnostic process.

Loss of hair occurs with aging. Normally, about 50 hairs are lost each day. Losses of more than 100 hairs per day (*alopecia*) may indicate underlying disease. Severe malnutrition and chemotherapy can cause hair loss. Chemotherapy, often used to treat cancer, inhibits cell growth. This is especially apparent in cells that are rapidly dividing. Cells in the hair follicle divide more rapidly than other body cells. Thus, hair loss often results from chemotherapy.

Hair growth and distribution are primarily controlled by masculine hormones (*androgens*). Diseases that cause an increase in androgens often result in excessive hair growth (*hirsutism*). These include certain tumors, polycystic ovarian disease, and hyperplasia of the adrenal glands. Both hair loss and excessive hair growth should be investigated to determine the underlying cause.

Sebaceous Glands

The integument contains two types of exocrine glands: sebaceous glands and sweat glands. **Sebaceous** (sē-BĀ-shus) **glands** are holocrine glands that discharge a waxy, oily secretion into hair follicles (Figure 5-5•). Several sebaceous glands may communicate with a single follicle by means of short ducts. The gland cells manufacture large quantities of lipids as they mature, and their eventual death releases the lipids into the open passageway of the gland. The contraction of the arrector pili muscle that elevates the hair squeezes the sebaceous gland, forcing the waxy secretions onto the surface of the skin. This secretion, called **sebum** (SĒ-bum), lubricates the hair shaft to prevent its drying and breaking, and its low pH inhibits the growth of some types of bacteria.

Sebaceous glands are very sensitive to changes in the concentrations of sex hormones, and their secretory activities accelerate at puberty. For this reason, an individual with large sebaceous glands may be especially prone to develop **acne** during adolescence. In this condition, sebaceous ducts become blocked and secretions accumulate, causing inflammation and providing a fertile environment for bacterial infection.

Sweat Glands

The integument contains two different populations of sweat glands: *apocrine sweat glands* and *merocrine sweat glands*. The differences between apocrine secretion and merocrine secretion were discussed in Chapter 4 (see Table 4-1, p. 88), and both gland types are shown in Figure 5-6•.

Apocrine Sweat Glands.   In the armpits, around the nipples, and in the groin, **apocrine sweat glands** communicate with hair follicles. At puberty, these coiled

5

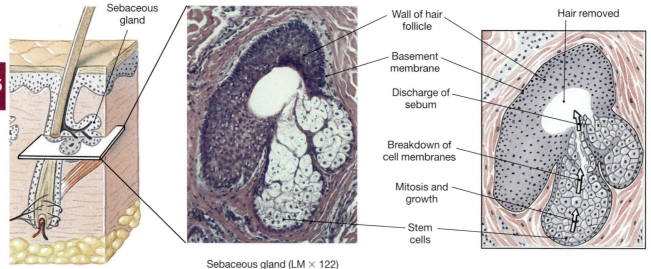

Sebaceous gland (LM × 122)

●**FIGURE 5-5   Sebaceous Glands and Hair Follicles**
The structure of a sebaceous gland and accompanying hair follicle.

tubular glands begin discharging a sticky, cloudy secretion that becomes odorous when broken down by bacteria. In other mammals, this odor is an important form of communication; in our culture, whatever function it has is masked by products such as deodorants. Other products, such as antiperspirants, contain astringent compounds that contract the skin and its sweat gland openings, thus decreasing the quantity of both apocrine and merocrine secretions.

Merocrine Sweat Glands.   Merocrine sweat glands, or *eccrine* (EK-rin) *sweat glands*, are far more numerous and widely distributed than apocrine glands. The adult integument contains around 3 million eccrine glands. Palms and soles have the highest numbers; it has been estimated that the palm of the hand has about 500 glands per square centimeter (3000 per square inch).

Merocrine sweat glands are coiled tubular glands that discharge their secretions directly onto the surface of the skin. The primary functions of their secretions, called *perspiration*, are to cool the surface of the skin and reduce body temperature. When a person sweats in the hot sun, all the merocrine glands are working together. The blood vessels beneath the epidermis are flushed with blood, and the skin assumes a reddish color. The skin surface is warm and wet, and as the moisture evaporates, the skin cools. If body temperature falls below normal, perspiration ceases, blood flow to the skin declines, and the cool, dry surfaces release little heat into the environment. The role of the skin in thermoregulation was considered in Chapter 1 (see p. 14); Chapter 18 will examine this process in greater detail.

The perspiration produced by merocrine glands is a clear secretion that is more than 99 percent water, but it does contain a mixture of electrolytes, metabolites, and waste products such as urea. The electrolytes give sweat its salty taste. When all of the merocrine sweat glands are working at maximum, the rate of perspiration may exceed a gallon (about 4 liters) per hour, and dangerous fluid and electrolyte losses can occur. For this reason, marathon runners and other endurance athletes must drink fluids at regular intervals.

Nails

Nails form at the fingers and toes, where they protect the exposed tips and help limit their distortion when you grasp an object, climb a tree, run, or apply pressure in other ways. The structure of a nail is shown in

●**FIGURE 5-6
Sweat Glands**

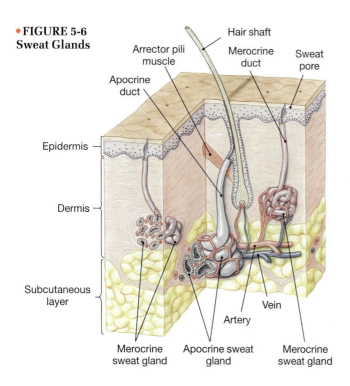

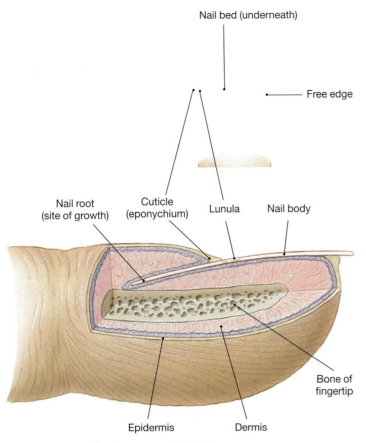

Nail bed (underneath)

Free edge

Nail root
(site of growth)

Cuticle
(eponychium)

Lunula

Nail body

Bone of
fingertip

Epidermis   Dermis

•FIGURE 5-7   The Structure of a Nail

(LOO-nū-la; *luna*, moon). The nail body is re-
cessed beneath the level of the surrounding epithelium.

INJURY AND REPAIR

The skin can regenerate effectively even after considerable damage has occurred. Skin regeneration
can take place because stem cells that persist in
both its epithelial and connective tissue components divide to replace lost epidermal and dermal
cells. This process can be slow, and when large
surface areas are involved, problems of infection
and fluid loss complicate the situation. The relative speed and effectiveness of skin repair vary depending on the type of wound. A slender, straight
cut, or *incision*, may heal relatively quickly compared with a deep scrape, or *abrasion*, which involves a much greater area. Burns are relatively
common injuries that result from exposure of the
skin to heat, radiation, electrical shock, or strong
chemical agents. The severity of the burn reflects
the depth of penetration and the total area affected. The most common descriptive terms refer to
the depth of penetration, and these are detailed in
Table 5-1. The larger the area affected, the greater
the impact on integumentary function.

Figure 5-7•. The visible **nail body** consists of a dense
mass of dead, keratinized cells. The body of the nail
covers the **nail bed**, but nail production occurs at the
nail root, an epithelial fold not visible from the surface. A portion of the stratum corneum of the fold extends over the exposed nail nearest the root, forming
the **cuticle**, or *eponychium* (ep-ō-NIK-ē-um; *epi-*, over
+ *onyx*, nail). Underlying blood vessels give the nail
its pink color, but near the root these vessels may be
obscured, leaving a pale crescent known as the **lunula**

AGING AND THE INTEGUMENTARY SYSTEM

Aging affects all the components of the integumentary
system. The major changes including the following:

- *Skin injuries and infections become more common.* Such problems are more likely because the
  epidermis thins as stem cell activity declines.

TABLE 5-1	A Classification of Burns	
Classification	Damage Report	Appearance and Sensation
First-degree burn	*Killed*: superficial cells of epidermis *Injured*: deeper layers of epidermis, papillary dermis	Inflamed; tender
Second-degree burn	*Killed*: superficial and deeper cells of epidermis; dermis may be affected *Injured*: damage may extend into reticular layer of the dermis, but many accessory structures unaffected	Blisters; very painful
Third-degree burn	*Killed*: all epidermal and dermal cells *Injured*: hypodermal and deeper tissues and organs	Charred; no sensation at all

- *The sensitivity of the immune system is reduced.* The number of macrophages and other cells of the immune system decreases to around 50 percent of levels seen at maturity. This loss further encourages skin damage and infection.
- *Muscles become weaker, and bone strength decreases.* Such changes are caused by a decline in vitamin D_3 production of around 75 percent.
- *Sensitivity to sun exposure increases.* Lesser amounts of melanin are produced because melanocyte activity declines. The skin of Caucasians becomes very pale.
- *The skin becomes dry and often scaly.* Glandular activity declines, reducing sebum production and perspiration (see below).
- *Hair thins and changes color.* Follicles stop functioning or produce thinner, finer hairs. With decreased melanocyte activity, these hairs are gray or white.
- *The integument weakens, and sagging and wrinkling occur.* The dermis becomes thinner, and the elastic fiber network decreases in size. The integument therefore becomes weaker and less resilient. These effects are most pronounced in areas exposed to the sun.
- *The ability to lose heat decreases.* The blood supply to the dermis is reduced at the same time that sweat glands become less active. This combination makes the elderly less able to lose body heat, and overexertion or overexposure to warm temperatures can cause dangerously high body temperatures.

- *Skin repairs proceed relatively slowly.* For example, it takes 3–4 weeks to complete the repairs to a blister site in a person age 18–25. The same repairs at age 65–75 take 6–8 weeks. Because repairs are slow, recurrent infections may occur.
- *Secondary sex characteristics in hair and body fat distribution begin to fade.* Because of lowered levels of sex hormones, people age 90–100 of both sexes and all races look very much alike.

✓ What will happen if the duct of an infected sebaceous gland becomes blocked?

✓ Deodorants are used to mask the effects of secretions from what type of skin gland?

✓ Older people do not tolerate the summer heat as well as they did when they were young, and they are more prone to heat-related illness. What accounts for this change?

INTEGRATION WITH OTHER SYSTEMS

Although the integumentary system can function independently, many of its activities are integrated with those of other systems. Figure 5-8• diagrams the major functional relationships. The role of the skin in temperature control, through interactions with the nervous and cardiovascular systems, was detailed in Chapter 1 (see Figure 1-4b•, p. 15).

Chapter Review

KEY TERMS

cutaneous membrane, *p. 108*	hair follicle, *p. 112*	nail, *p. 114*
dermis, *p. 108*	integument, *p. 108*	sebaceous glands, *p. 113*
epidermis, *p. 108*	keratin, *p. 110*	stratum germinativum, *p. 109*
hair *p. 112*	melanin, *p. 110*	subcutaneous layer, *p. 108*

SUMMARY OUTLINE

INTRODUCTION *p. 108*

INTEGUMENTARY STRUCTURE AND FUNCTION *p. 108*

1. The **integumentary system**, or **integument**, consists of the **cutaneous membrane**, which includes the **epidermis** and **dermis**, and the **accessory structures**. Underneath lies the **subcutaneous layer** (or **hypodermis**). *(Figure 5-1)*

The Epidermis *p. 109*

2. **Thin skin** covers most of the body; heavily abraded body surfaces may be covered by **thick skin**.

3. Cell divisions by the stem cells that make up the **stratum germinativum** replace more superficial cells.

4. As epidermal cells age, they pass through the **stratum spinosum**, the **stratum granulosum**, the **stratum lucidum** (in thick skin), and the **stratum corneum**. In the process, they

SKELETAL SYSTEM

Provides structural support

Synthesizes vitamin D₃, essential for calcium and phosphorus absorption (bone maintenance and growth)

THE INTEGUMENTARY SYSTEM

FOR ALL SYSTEMS

Provides mechanical protection against environmental hazards

MUSCULAR SYSTEM

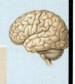

Contractions of skeletal muscles pull against skin of face, producing facial expressions important in communication

Synthesizes vitamin D₃, essential for normal calcium absorption (calcium ions play an essential role in muscle contraction)

NERVOUS SYSTEM

Controls blood flow and sweat gland activity for thermoregulation; stimulates contraction of arrector pili muscles to elevate hairs

Receptors in dermis and deep epidermis provide sensations of touch, pressure, vibration, temperature, and pain

ENDOCRINE SYSTEM

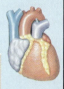

Sex hormones stimulate sebaceous gland activity; male and female sex hormones influence hair growth, distribution of subcutaneous fat, and apocrine sweat gland activity; adrenal hormones alter dermal blood flow and help mobilize lipids from adipocytes

Synthesizes vitamin D₃, precursor of calcitriol

CARDIOVASCULAR SYSTEM

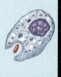

Provides O₂ and nutrients; delivers hormones and cells of immune system; carries away CO₂, waste products, and toxins; provides heat to maintain normal skin temperature

Stimulation by mast cells produces localized changes in blood flow and capillary permeability

LYMPHATIC SYSTEM

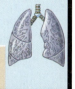

Assists in defending the integument by providing additional macrophages and mobilizing lymphocytes

Provides physical barriers that prevent pathogen entry; macrophages resist infection; mast cells trigger inflammation and initiate the immune response

RESPIRATORY SYSTEM

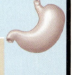

Provides oxygen and eliminates carbon dioxide

Hairs guard entrance to nasal cavity

DIGESTIVE SYSTEM

Provides nutrients for all cells and lipids for storage by adipocytes

Synthesizes vitamin D₃, needed for absorption of calcium and phosphorus

REPRODUCTIVE SYSTEM

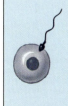

Covers external genitalia; provides sensations that stimulate sexual behaviors; mammary gland secretions provide nourishment for newborn infant

Sex hormones affect hair distribution, adipose tissue distribution in subcutaneous layer, and mammary gland development

URINARY SYSTEM

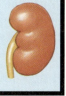

Excretes waste products, maintains normal body fluid pH and ion composition

Assists in elimination of water and solutes; keratinized epidermis limits fluid loss through skin

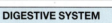

●FIGURE 5-8   Functional Relationships Between the Integumentary System and Other Systems

accumulate large amounts of **keratin**; the epithelium is thus said to be **keratinized**. Ultimately, the cells are shed or lost. *(Figure 5-2)*

5. **Epidermal ridges**, such as those on the palms and soles, improve our gripping ability and increase the skin's sensitivity.

6. The color of the epidermis depends on two factors: blood supply and pigment composition and concentration. **Melanocytes** protect the stem cells from **ultraviolet (UV) radiation**. *(Figure 5-3)*

7. Epidermal cells synthesize **vitamin D₃** when exposed to sunlight.

The Dermis *p. 111*

8. The dermis consists of the **papillary layer** and the deeper **reticular layer**.

9. The papillary layer of the dermis contains blood vessels, lymphatics, and sensory nerves. This layer supports and nourishes the overlying epidermis. The reticular layer consists of a meshwork of collagen and elastic fibers oriented to resist tension in the skin.

10. Components of other systems (cardiovascular, lymphatic, and nervous) that communicate with the skin are in the dermis.

The Subcutaneous Layer *p. 112*

11. The subcutaneous layer stabilizes the skin's position against underlying organs and tissues.

Accessory Structures *p. 112*

12. **Hairs** originate in complex organs called **hair follicles**. Each hair has a **shaft** composed of dead keratinized cells. *(Figure 5-4)*

13. The **arrector pili** muscles can elevate the hairs.

14. Our hairs grow and are shed according to a cyclic pattern. A single hair grows for 2–5 years and is subsequently shed.

15. **Sebaceous glands** discharge the waxy **sebum** into hair follicles. *(Figure 5-5)*

16. **Apocrine sweat glands** produce an odorous secretion; the more numerous **merocrine sweat glands** produce *perspiration*, a watery secretion. *(Figure 5-6)*

17. **Nails** are sheets of dense, keratinized cells. They provide support for the tips of the fingers and toes. Nail production occurs at the **nail root**. *(Figure 5-7)*

INJURY AND REPAIR *p. 115*

1. The skin can regenerate effectively even after considerable damage.

2. Burns are relatively common injuries characterized by damage to layers of the epidermis and perhaps the dermis. *(Table 5-1)*

AGING AND THE INTEGUMENTARY SYSTEM *p. 115*

1. Aging affects all the components of the integumentary system. *(Figure 5-8)*

INTEGRATION WITH OTHER SYSTEMS *p. 116*

1. Many of the integumentary system's functions are integrated with those of other systems.

REVIEW QUESTIONS

LEVEL 1   Reviewing Facts and Terms

Match each item in column A with the most closely related item in column B. Use letters for answers in the spaces provided.

Column A

___ 1. cutaneous membrane

___ 2. carotene

___ 3. melanocytes

___ 4. epidermal layer containing stem cells

___ 5. smooth muscle

___ 6. epidermal layer of flattened and dead cells

___ 7. bluish skin

___ 8. sebaceous glands

___ 9. merocrine (eccrine) glands

___10. vitamin D₃

Column B

a. arrector pili

b. cyanosis

c. perspiration

d. sebum

e. stratum corneum

f. skin

g. orange-yellow pigment

h. bone growth

i. pigment cells

j. stratum germinativum

11. The two major components of the integument are:
    (a) the cutaneous membrane and the accessory structures
    (b) the epidermis and the hypodermis
    (c) the hair and the nails
    (d) the dermis and the subcutaneous layer

12. The fibrous protein that forms the basic structural component of hair and nails is:
    (a) collagen
    (b) melanin
    (c) elastin
    (d) keratin

13. The two types of exocrine glands in the skin are:
    (a) merocrine and sweat glands
    (b) sebaceous and sweat glands
    (c) apocrine and sweat glands
    (d) eccrine and sweat glands

14. The following are all accessory structures of the integumentary system except:
    (a) nails
    (b) hair
    (c) dermal papillae
    (d) sweat glands

15. Sweat glands that communicate with hair follicles in the armpits and produce an odorous secretion are:
    (a) apocrine glands
    (b) merocrine glands
    (c) sebaceous glands
    (d) a, b, and c are correct

16. The reason older persons are more sensitive to sun exposure and more likely to experience sunburn is that with age:
    (a) melanocyte activity declines
    (b) vitamin D_3 production declines
    (c) glandular activity declines
    (d) skin thickness decreases

17. Which two skin pigments are found in the epidermis?

18. Which two major layers constitute the dermis, and what components are found in each layer?

19. Which two groups of sweat glands are contained in the integument?

LEVEL 2 Reviewing Concepts

20. During the transdermal administration of drugs, why are fat-soluble drugs more desirable than those that are water-soluble?

21. In our society, a tan body is associated with good health. However, medical research constantly warns about the dangers of excessive exposure to the sun. What are the benefits of a tan?

22. Why is a subcutaneous injection with a hypodermic needle a useful method for administering drugs?

23. Why does skin sag and wrinkle as a person ages?

LEVEL 3 Critical Thinking and Clinical Applications

24. A new mother notices that her 6-month-old child has a yellow-orange complexion. Fearful that the child may have jaundice (a condition caused by a toxic yellow-orange pigment in the blood), she takes him to her pediatrician. After examining the child, the pediatrician declares him perfectly healthy and advises the mother to watch the child's diet. Why?

25. Vanessa remarks that her 80-year-old grandmother keeps her thermostat set at 80° F and wears a sweater on balmy spring days. When she asks her grandmother why, her grandmother tells her that she is cold. Vanessa can't understand this and asks you for an explanation. What would you tell Vanessa?

ANSWERS TO CONCEPT CHECK QUESTIONS

Page 111
1. Cells are constantly shed from the *stratum corneum*.   **2.** The splinter is lodged in the *stratum granulosum*.   **3.** When exposed to the ultraviolet radiation in sunlight or tanning lamps, melanocytes in the epidermis and dermis synthesize the pigment melanin, darkening the skin.

Page 113
1. Contraction of the arrector pili muscles pulls the hair follicles erect, depressing the area at the base of the hair and making the surrounding skin appear higher. The result is known as "goose bumps" or "goose pimples."   **2.** Hair is a derivative of the epidermis, so if the epidermis is destroyed by the injury, no hair follicles would be available to produce new hair.   **3.** The subcutaneous layer stabilizes the position of the skin in relation to underlying tissues and organs; stores fat; and, because its lower region contains few capillaries and no vital organs, provides a useful site for the injection of drugs.

Page 116
1. If the duct of a sebaceous gland is blocked by infection, the result is a *furuncle* or *boil*.   **2.** Apocrine sweat glands produce a secretion containing several kinds of organic compounds. Some of these compounds have an odor, and others produce an odor when metabolized by skin bacteria. Deodorants are used to mask the odor of these secretions.   **3.** As a person ages, the blood supply to the dermis decreases and merocrine sweat glands become less active. These changes make it more difficult for the elderly to cool themselves in hot weather.

5 Emergency Care Applications

OVERVIEW

The integumentary system consists of the skin, hair, nails, and various glands. The largest and one of the most versatile organs of the body, it plays a major role in the maintenance of homeostasis. The study and treatment of diseases of the skin, hair, and nails is called *dermatology,* and physicians who specialize in the medical and surgical treatment of these disorders are called *dermatologists.* Dermatologists diagnose and treat skin, hair, and nail conditions and perform minor skin surgeries such as lesion removal. Physicians who perform major skin surgery are referred to as *plastic surgeons.* There are two general categories of plastic surgery: reconstructive and cosmetic (aesthetic). Reconstructive surgery corrects defects due to trauma, tumors, and disease, whereas cosmetic surgery is elective surgery that changes the physical appearance of a part of the body.

The integumentary system is essential to the body's continued maintenance of homeostasis. Its functions include:

- *Protection.* The skin is a barrier that prevents the entry of microorganisms and other harmful substances. It also prevents the loss of water from the body to the environment.
- *Temperature maintenance.* The integument plays a major role in temperature balance by regulating heat gain or heat loss to the environment.
- *Nutrient storage.* The subcutaneous tissues contain a large reserve of lipids for use in metabolism and hormone production.
- *Sensory reception.* The skin contains a vast network of sensory fibers and nerves that detect touch, pressure, pain, and temperature.
- *Excretion and secretion.* The skin secretes water, salt, and organic wastes as the body strives to maintain homeostasis. The skin is important in the synthesis of important chemicals and hormones including the production of Vitamin D.

The skin consists of the epidermis, the dermis, and the subcutaneous tissues. It is thickest on the lower back and thinnest on the genitalia. Various tensions on the skin cause it to be oriented into patterns called *cleavage lines* or *Langer's lines* (Figures A5-1● and A5-2●). Incisions and wounds perpendicular to cleavage lines tend to gape open, while incisions and wounds parallel to the cleavage lines tend to heal with a thin, less noticeable scar.

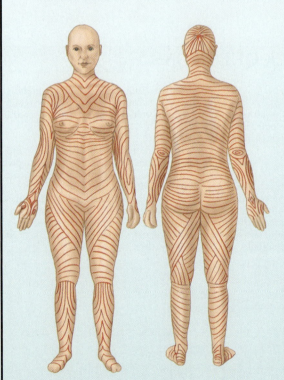

● **FIGURE A5-1   Cleavage Lines, or Langer's Lines**   These lines represent natural tension patterns in the skin. If possible, surgeons try to make their incisions parallel to the cleavage lines so that tension on the wound edges is kept to a minimum.

Skin Color

Skin color is an important indicator of body function and varies from person to person. Changes in skin color are often evidence of a systemic disease. Normal skin color in light-skinned people is pink, indicating adequate cardiorespiratory function and vascular in-

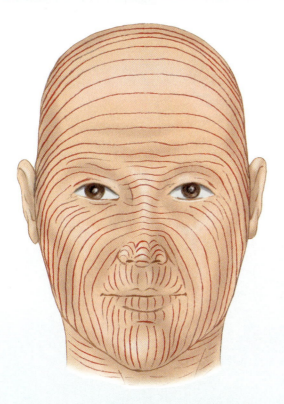

• **FIGURE A5-2**   **Cleavage Lines of the Face**

tegrity. In dark-skinned people, inspect the mucous membranes (such as the lips) to detect skin color changes. Paleness indicates decreased blood flow through the skin and results from anemia or conditions such as hypothermia or hypovolemia. A bluish discoloration of the skin is called *cyanosis* and is due to increased amounts of unoxygenated hemoglobin. The presence of cyanosis should alert care providers to an underlying problem adversely affecting oxygenation or perfusion. A yellowish discoloration of the skin, *jaundice* is due to the accumulation of bilirubin in the skin tissues. This is seen in liver diseases such as hepatitis and liver failure. A red coloration to the skin may be due to carbon monoxide poisoning. As carbon monoxide replaces oxygen on the hemoglobin molecules, the red color of the blood is enhanced, and this is evident in the skin.

Skin Lesions

A skin lesion is any disruption of normal skin tissue. The numerous types of skin lesions are usually classified as primary, arising in previously normal skin (Figure A5-3•); secondary, resulting from changes in primary lesions (Figure A5-4•); and vascular, involving a blood vessel (Figure 5-5•).

Primary Lesions

- Macule—circumscribed change in skin color without elevation or depression of the surface; less than 1 cm in diameter. Examples: freckles, flat moles, measles.

- Patch—circumscribed change in skin color without elevation or depression of the surface; greater than 1 cm diameter. Examples: birthmarks, Mongolian spots, café-au-lait spots.
- Papule—solid, elevated area that varies in size; usually less than 1 cm in diameter. Examples: warts, elevated moles, insect bites.
- Plaque—solid, elevated area that varies in size; usually greater than 1 cm in diameter. Examples: psoriasis, seborrheic keratosis.
- Wheal—circumscribed, flat-topped, firm elevation with well-defined, palpable margin. Examples: allergic reactions, hives, insect stings.
- Nodule—small lesion in the dermal or subcutaneous tissue. Examples: skin cysts, fatty tumors (lipoma).
- Tumor—elevated, solid lesion; may be clearly demarcated; often greater than 2 cm in diameter. Examples: skin cancers, lipomas.
- Vesicle—elevated, circumscribed, superficial lesion containing serous fluid; less than 1 cm in diameter. Examples: chicken pox (varicella), shingles (herpes zoster).
- Bulla—elevated, circumscribed, superficial lesion containing serous fluid; less than 2 cm in diameter. Examples: blisters, second-degree burns.
- Pustule—elevated, superficial lesion; similar to a vesicle, but filled with purulent fluid (pus). Examples: acne pimple, spider bite.
- Cyst—elevated, circumscribed, encapsulated lesion; in dermis or subcutaneous tissue, filled with liquid or semisolid material. Examples: cystic acne, sebaceous cyst.

Secondary Lesions

- Fissure—deep, linear crack or break from the epidermis that extends into the dermis; may be moist or dry. Examples: athlete's foot, cracks at corner of mouth.
- Erosion—loss of part of the epidermis, depressed, moist, glistening; often follows rupture of a vesicle or bulla. Examples: varicella (after rupture), second-degree burn (after rupture).
- Ulcer—loss of epidermis and dermis; concave; varies in size. Examples: decubitus ulcers (bed sores), stasis ulcers.
- Scar—area of replacement fibrosis of the dermis resulting from destruction of the dermis or subcutaneous layers. Examples: surgical scar, acne scars.
- Keloid—sharply elevated, irregularly shaped, progressively enlarging scar; caused by excessive collagen; more common in blacks and Orientals. Example: large scar from minor trauma, such as ear piercing.
- Excoriation—loss of the epidermis; linear, hollowed-out, crusted area. Examples: abrasions, scabies (mites).
- Scale—desiccated, thin plates of cornified epithelial cells; often due to abnormal keratinization. Example: psoriasis.

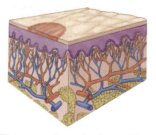

Macule – Flat spot, color varies from white to brown or from red to purple, diameter less than 1 cm

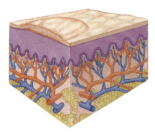

Plaque – Superficial papule, diameter more than 1 cm, rough texture

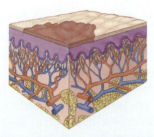

Patch – Irregular flat macule, diameter greater than 1 cm

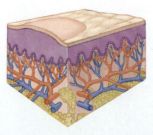

Wheal – Pink, irregular spot varying in size and shape

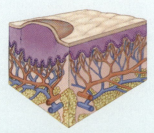

Papule – Elevated firm spot, color varies from brown to red or from pink to purplish red, diameter less than 1 cm

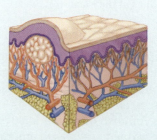

Nodule – Elevated firm spot, diameter 1–2 cm

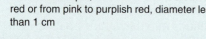 **FIGURE A5-3   Primary Skin Lesions**

- Crust—results from drying of serum, blood, sebum, or interstitial fluid over the epidermis. Examples: seborrheic dermatitis, impetigo.
- Lichenification—rough, thickened epidermis secondary to persistent rubbing, itching, or skin irritation; often involves flexor surface of extremity. Examples: chronic dermatitis, fungal infections.
- Atrophy—thinning of the skin surface and loss of skin markings; skin appears translucent and paperlike. Examples: aged skin, striae.

Vascular Lesions

- Purpura—reddish-purple patches due to blood in the dermis; greater than 0.5 cm in diameter. Example: idiopathic thrombocytopenia purpura (ITP).
- Petechiae—reddish-purple patches due to blood in the dermis; less than 0.5 cm in diameter (often pinpoint). Examples: Rocky Mountain spotted fever, acute meningiococcemia.
- Ecchymosis—reddish purple blotches due to leakage of blood from artery or vein; size varies. Example: bruising due to trauma.

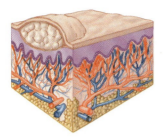

Tumor – Elevated solid, diameter more than 2 cm, may be same color as skin

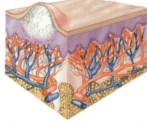

Pustule – Elevated area, diameter less than 1 cm, contains purulent fluid

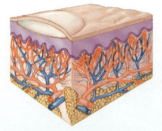

Vesicle – Elevated area, diameter less than 1 cm, contains serous fluid

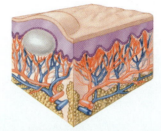

Cyst – Elevated, palpable area containing liquid or viscous matter

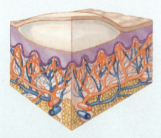

Bulla – Vesicle with diameter more than 1 cm

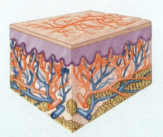

Telangiectasia – Red, threadlike line

• **FIGURE A5-3 Primary Skin Lesions** *(continued)*

- Spider angioma—dilation of superficial skin arteriole with central, reddish, pulsating punctum with dilating legs. Examples: pregnancy, alcoholic liver disease.
- Venous star—dilation of superficial skin vein; compressible punctum with dilating legs. Example: age-related (usually on the head and neck).
- Capillary hemangioma—irregular red spots due to capillary dilation; compressible. Examples: birthmarks in babies (often disappear by age 2 years).
- Telangiectasia—fine, irregular red lines due to dilated superficial blood vessels. Examples: vascular inflammation, rosacea.

MEDICAL CONDITIONS OF THE SKIN

Many diseases affect the skin. These can be localized to the skin or can involve other body organs and systems. Often, skin lesions are due to infections or problems elsewhere in the body.

Exanthems

Many of the viruses that infect humans cause characteristic skin rashes during the course of the infection. An *exanthem* is an acute, generalized skin eruption that can

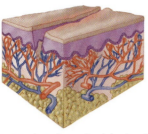

Fissure – Linear red crack ranging into dermis

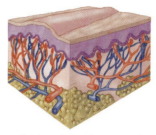

Scar – Fibrous, depth varies, color ranges from white to red

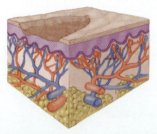

Erosion – Depression in epidermis, caused by tissue loss

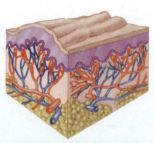

Keloid – Elevated scar, irregular shape, larger than original wound

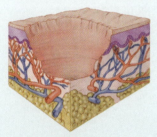

Ulcer – Red or purplish depression ranging into dermis, caused by tissue loss

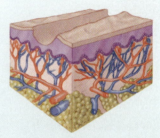

Excoriation – Linear, may be hollow or crusted, caused by loss of epidermis leaving dermis exposed

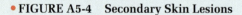

• **FIGURE A5-4   Secondary Skin Lesions**

be caused by drugs, viruses, or certain bacteria. Usually, the eruption causes macules or papules, although some will have vesicles. Most of the childhood viral infections are characterized by recognizable viral exanthems (Figure A5-6•). These include: *rubella (3-day, or German measles), rubeola (red measles), roseola,* and *varicella (chicken pox).* Certain bacterial infections also result in the development of an exanthem. The most common of these, *scarlet fever (scarletina),* is caused by group A beta-

hemolytic streptococcus infection, usually pharyngitis. The rash of scarlet fever feels like sandpaper, and the face is flushed with an obvious pallor around the mouth.

Many of the viral exanthems are asymptomatic. Some, however, can cause itching and pain. Varicella causes vesicles that can actually shed the virus. Exanthems do not require specific treatment. Instead, treatment is directed at the underlying cause or at the symptoms that are making the patient uncomfortable.

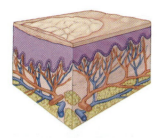

Scale – Elevated area of excessive exfoliation, varies in thickness, shape, and dryness, and ranges in color from white to silver or tan

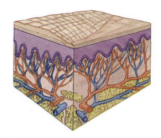

Lichenification – Thickening and hardening of epidermis with emphasized lines in skin, resembles lichen

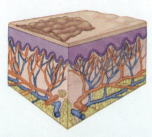

Crust – Reddish, brown, black, tan, or yellowish dried blood, serum, or pus

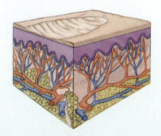

Atrophy – Skin surface thins and markings disappear, semitransparent parchment-like appearance

● **FIGURE A5-4   Secondary Skin Lesions** *(continued)*

Herpes Zoster

Herpes zoster (shingles) is a disease characterized by the eruption of groups of vesicles along the dermatome of a sensory nerve. The virus that causes varicella (chicken pox) and herpes zoster is the varicella-zoster virus (VZV). After the initial infection with VZV, the patient will develop varicella. This usually occurs during childhood. During the course of the varicella infection, the VZV enters the ganglia for the sensory nerve and remains there for life. Later in life, the virus becomes reactivated and spreads along the sensory nerve that it infected. Stress, disease, and immunosuppression appear to be causes of virus reactivation, although in most cases the cause is idiopathic (cannot be determined). Initially, zoster causes pain that is often severe, followed by redness of the affected area. The redness and rash are limited to the dermatome of the affected nerve, and the rash does not cross the midline of the body. Zoster infections can also affect the cranial nerves or involve the eye. Eventually, the vesicles will break out. Although antiviral drugs do not eradicate the virus, they are effective in decreasing the severity of the infection and the length of the outbreak, which may last for several weeks.

Staphylococcal Scalded Skin Syndrome

Staphylococcal scalded skin syndrome (SSSS) is most frequently seen in children less than 5 years of age. It is caused by infection with group II staphylococci, which produces a toxin that causes separation of the skin just below the granular layer of the epidermis. This results in sloughing of the skin in the affected areas. The toxin, an epidermolysin, is usually produced at a site other than the skin and is delivered to the skin via the circulatory system.

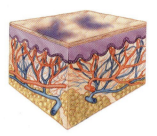

Purpura – Reddish-purple blotches,
diameter more than 0.5 cm

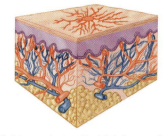

Spider angioma – Reddish legs radiate
from red spot

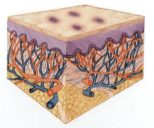

Petechiae – Reddish-purple spots,
diameter less than 0.5 cm

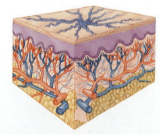

Venous star – Bluish legs radiate from
blue center

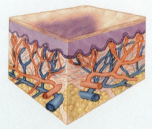

Ecchymoses – Reddish-purple blotch,
size varies

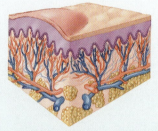

Capillary hemangioma – Irregular red spots

• **FIGURE A5-6   Examples of
Viral Exanthems Associated
with Childhood Illness:
Varicella, or Chicken Pox,
and Rubeola, or Red Measles.**

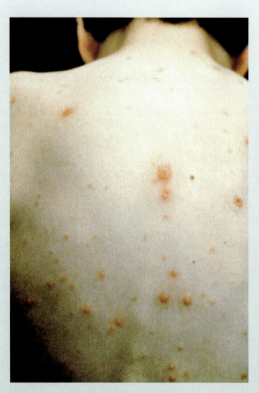

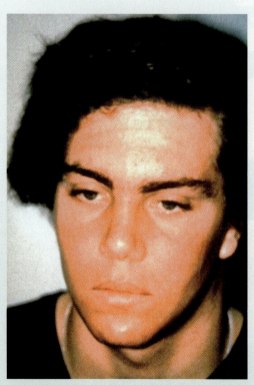

SSSS begins with fever, malaise, irritability, and runny nose, followed by generalized erythema (redness) with exquisite tenderness. The erythema spreads from the face and trunk to cover the entire body with the exception of the palms of the hands, soles of the feet, and mucous membranes. Within 48 hours, blisters and bullae may form and the pain becomes severe. As the blisters rupture, fluid is lost, resulting in dehydration. In severe cases, the skin of the entire body may slough. Treatment of SSSS includes antibiotics to eradicate the underlying infection and replacement fluids if needed. The skin should be treated the same as with a severe burn. Children with a large area of skin involvement are best treated in a burn center.

Toxic Epidermal Necrolysis

Toxic epidermal necrolysis (TEN) is a serious and sometimes fatal drug reaction that is similar to staphylococcal scalded skin syndrome. It primarily affects adults. Antibiotics of the sulfonamide class, nonsteroidal anti-inflammatory drugs, and anticonvulsants seem to be the cause of most cases of TEN. The skin eruption is preceded by fever, malaise, anorexia, and inflammation of the eyelids and mucous membranes. The skin becomes reddened and is very tender, first in the axillae and groin, then extending over the body surface. Blisters and bullae form, and the entire epidermis may be shed. TEN causes full-thickness necrosis (death) of the epidermis with subepidermal blister formations. Treatment is identical as for burns, and severe cases are best managed in a burn unit.

TRAUMATIC CONDITIONS OF THE SKIN

Traumatic disruption of the layers of the skin exposes the tissues underneath. This increases the likelihood of infection, loss of body fluids, and pain. Skin trauma can result from direct trauma (either sharp or blunt) or burns (either thermal or chemical).

Soft-Tissue Wounds

Trauma that results in the disruption of the layers of the skin is called a wound. There are several classifications of wounds. These include:

- Abrasion—is a simple scrape or scratch where the outer layer of skin is damaged but not all of the layers are penetrated (Figure A5-7●).
- Laceration—commonly called a cut, a laceration may be smooth or jagged (Figure A5-8●). Smooth wounds are usually caused by a sharp edge such as a razor blade or glass. Jagged wounds can be due to injury from duller objects such as jagged metal. They can also occur as a result of blunt trauma such as a blow or fall.

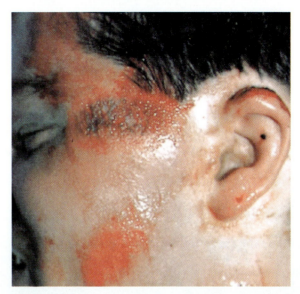

● **FIGURE A5-7   An Abrasion of the Left Side of the Face**

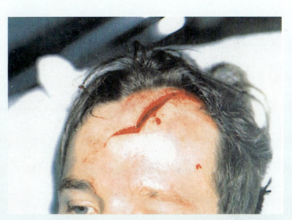

● **FIGURE A5-8   A Jagged Laceration of the Forehead**

- Puncture—occurs when a sharp, pointed object penetrates the skin or other tissues (Figure A5-9●). Common causes include such items as nails, ice picks, splinters, or knives. There are two types of puncture wounds, penetrating and perforating. *Penetrating puncture wounds* can be shallow or deep and can injure underlying tissues and blood vessels. Penetrating puncture wounds carry an increased incidence of infection as foreign material may be carried into the wound during injury and remain there due to sealing of the surface. *Perforating puncture wounds* have both an entrance wound and an exit wound. Often, the exit wound is more serious than the entrance wound. An example of a penetrating puncture wound is a gunshot wound.
- Avulsion—is an injury where a flap of skin and tissues are torn loose or pulled completely off (Figure A5-10●). Avulsions can cause serious tissue defects

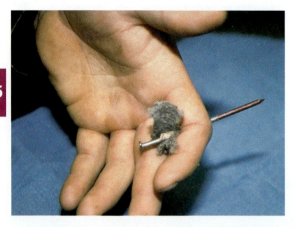

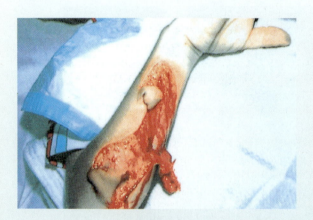

• FIGURE A5-9   Examples of Puncture Wounds

An impaled nail containing carpet fibers remains in place; gunshot wound to the thigh—the entry wound is on the left and the exit wound on the right.

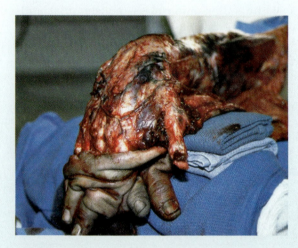

• FIGURE A5-10   Avulsion of the Skin of the Forearm

• FIGURE A5-11   Degloving Injury

and subsequent scarring. A special type of avulsion is the *degloving avulsion*. This is a potentially devastating wound where the skin, usually of the hand, is stripped off like a glove (Figure A5-11•).

- Amputation—occurs when an extremity, or part of an extremity is completely cut through or torn off (Figure A5-12•). Amputations often are caused by machinery and can be life-threatening. Today, using microsurgical techniques, amputated body parts can be replanted if the condition of the tissues is satisfactory.

- Crush injury—results when a body part, usually an extremity, becomes caught between heavy items such as parts of machinery. There is often massive damage to underlying blood vessels, nerves, and bone.

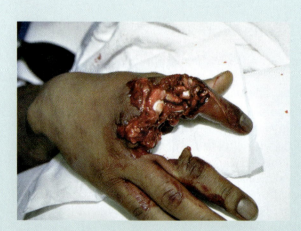

• FIGURE A5-12   Partial Amputation of the Right Hand

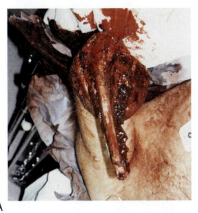
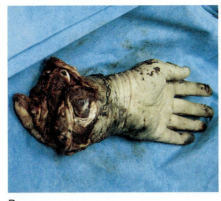
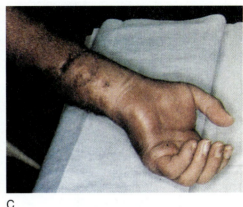

A B C

• **FIGURE A5-13 Amputation and Replantation**
(a) Complete amputation of the left forearm at the wrist caused by tractor power takeoff device (PTO)—contraction of the forearm muscles exposes the radius and ulna; **(b)** the amputated hand was found and retrieved by EMS personnel; **(c)** using microvascular surgical techniques, the hand was replanted.

Soft-tissue injuries are commonly encountered in emergency care. They are often grotesque and can distract from other patient care activities. Fortunately, they are rarely life threatening. In the prehospital setting, they are usually dressed to prevent further contamination, and definitive care, such as wound repair or surgery, is carried out at the hospital.

Limb Replantation

With the advent of microsurgical techniques, many body parts can be surgically reattached, or replanted, following amputation (Figure A5-13•). Amputated body parts should be located at the emergency scene and should accompany the patient to the hospital if at all possible. Even if an amputated part is too damaged for replantation, the tissues can be used to help repair the wound.

The separated body part should be cleaned of any gross debris, exposed areas covered with a lightly moistened gauze, and then placed into a sealed plastic bag. The bag should be immersed into saline with a few pieces of ice added. Packing the body part in ice, as was the old practice, caused tissue damage at a cellular level, adversely impacting limb survival. Many body parts have been successfully replanted including arms, hands, feet, legs, ears, the nose, and the penis. Patients with amputations where replantation is a possibility should be transported to medical centers with microsurgical replant capabilities.

The material placed directly on a wound is called a *dressing.* These are sterile and designed to control bleeding and protect the wound from contamination. A dressing is held in place by a *bandage.* Bandages can be made from gauze, elastic material, cloth, and many other materials. Sometimes, wounds require splinting. This is especially true in cases where there may be an associated fracture or where movement might cause the wound to open.

Injury and Repair

The skin is an amazingly resilient organ. It can regenerate effectively, even after considerable damage. This is due to stem cells in the epithelial and connective tissues. The rate of wound repair is related to several factors such as wound size, infection, fluid loss, vascular supply, and overall patient condition. Small lacerations may heal quickly while large avulsions and burns can take considerably more time.

Regeneration of a wound following injury involves several distinct stages (Figure A5-14•). If the wound extends through the epidermis and into the dermis or connective tissue, bleeding usually occurs. The blood at the site of the wound will collect and clot, eventually forming a *scab.* This serves to temporarily restore the integrity of the epidermis and limits the entry of additional organisms. Next, the cells of the stratum germinativum, the deepest layer of the epidermis, begin to undergo rapid division. As this occurs, they migrate along the sides of the wound, attempting to replace the lost epidermal cells. Scavenger, phagocytic cells remove debris from the wound. Additional phagocytic cells are transported to the injury site via the circulatory system.

If the wound is extensive or deep, repairs to the dermis must be under way before epithelial cells can be laid down. Fibroblast and mesenchymal cells begin to divide, producing mobile cells that penetrate the deeper areas of the wound. Damaged blood vessels begin to repair themselves through division of endothelial cells. These cells follow the fibroblasts into the deeper areas of the wound, providing a blood supply. Together, fibroblasts, the blood clot, and the developing capillary network are called *granulation tissue.* Ultimately, the clot dissolves and the number of capillaries declines

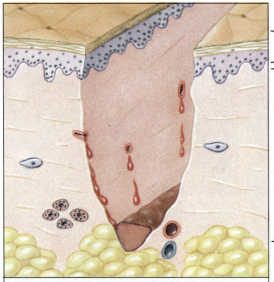

Epidermis

Dermis

Step 1: Bleeding occurs at the injury site immediately after the injury, and mast cells in the region trigger an inflammatory response.

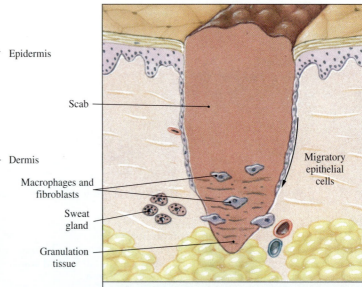

Scab

Migratory epithelial cells

Macrophages and fibroblasts

Sweat gland

Granulation tissue

Step 2: After several hours, a scab has formed and cells of the stratum germinativum are migrating along the edges of the wound. Phagocytic cells are removing debris, and more of these cells are arriving via the enhanced circulation. Clotting around the edges of the affected area partially isolates the region.

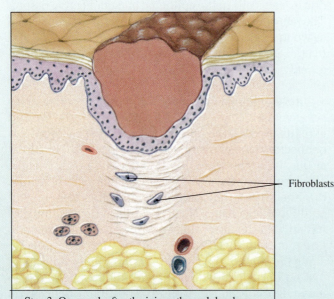

Fibroblasts

Step 3: One week after the injury, the scab has been undermined by epidermal cells migrating over the meshwork produced by fibroblast activity. Phagocytic activity around the site has almost ended, and the fibrin clot is disintegrating.

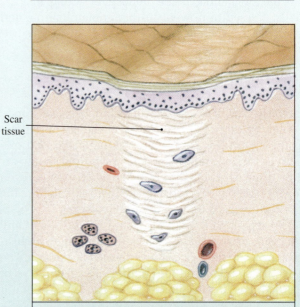

Scar tissue

Step 4: After several weeks, the scab has been shed, and the epidermis is complete. A shallow depression marks the injury site, but fibroblasts in the dermis continue to create scar tissue that will gradually elevate the overlying epidermis.

• FIGURE A5-14   The Process of Skin Repair

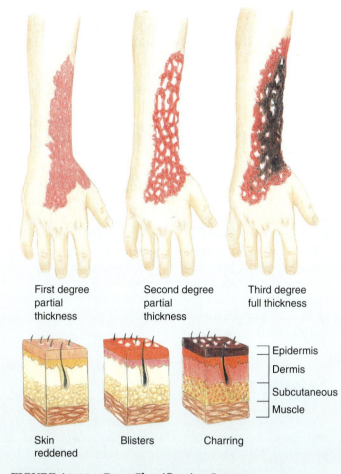

First degree partial thickness

Second degree partial thickness

Third degree full thickness

Epidermis
Dermis
Subcutaneous
Muscle

Skin reddened

Blisters

Charring

• FIGURE A5-15   Burn Classification System

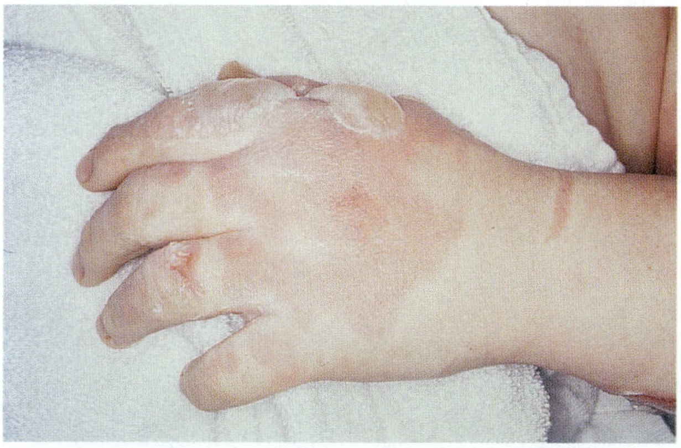

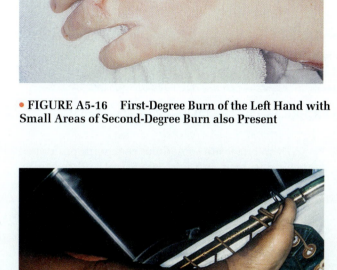

• FIGURE A5-16   First-Degree Burn of the Left Hand with Small Areas of Second-Degree Burn also Present

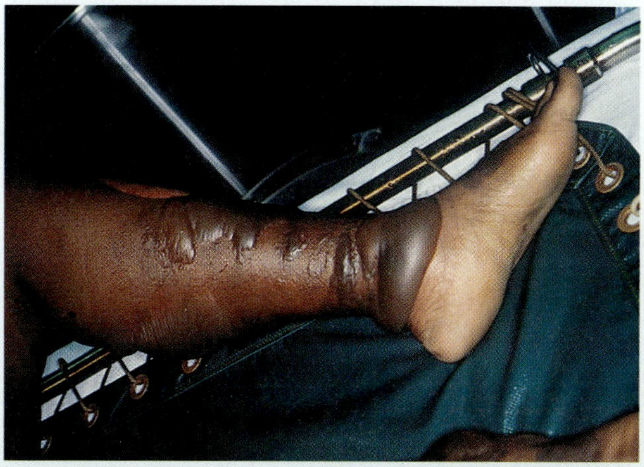

• FIGURE A5-17   Second-Degree Burn of the Left Leg

as the needs of the healing tissue decrease. Fibroblast activity leads to the formation of collagen fibers and *ground substance.*

The repaired wound is different from the original tissues. There is an increased number of collagen fibers and a decreased number of blood vessels resulting in *scar tissue.* This scar tissue varies based upon the type of wound and the age and health of the patient.

Burns

Skin injury caused by heat, chemicals, electricity, and radiation is called a *burn.* Although burns usually affect the skin, they can also affect underlying tissues such as the subcutaneous tissues, muscle, blood vessels, nerves, and even bone.

Burns are classified by depth and include the following (Figure A5-15•):

- *First-degree burns*—also called superficial burns, first-degree burns involve only the epidermis. They can be quite painful, as nerve fibers are uninjured. Example: sunburn (Figure A5-16•).
- *Second-degree burns*—also called partial thickness burns, the epidermis is burned through and the dermis is damaged (Figure A5-17•). There is usually intense pain and blistering. The blisters develop as plasma and interstitial fluids are released into the skin and elevate the top layer. Example: scald injury.
- *Third-degree burns*—also called full thickness burns, third-degree burns are characterized by damage to all layers of the skin (Figure A5-18•). The patient may not suffer as much pain as would be expected, as pain fibers in the skin may be destroyed by the injury. Third-degree burns are almost always accompanied by partial thickness burns and some degree of pain is usually present. Third-degree burns usually require skin grafting and are very disfiguring.

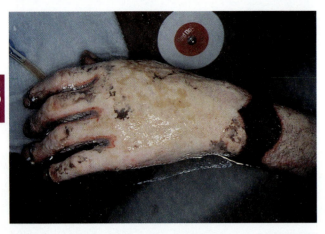

• **FIGURE A5-18**   **Third-Degree Burn of the Left Hand**

Deep burns are sometimes seen with prolonged exposure to heat and with electrical and lightning injuries. In some cases, muscle tissue and bone will be involved. Although these are technically considered full thickness burns, they are occasionally called fourth-degree burns to separate them from less severe injuries.

The severity of a burn is determined by consideration of the following factors:

• Body regions burned
• Depth of the burn
• Extent of the burn
• Agent or source of the burn
• Age of the patient
• Other associated illnesses and injuries

The agent or source of the burn can be significant. For example, electrical burns may cause only a small area of skin injury but cause massive injury to underlying tissues. Chemical burns are of special concern, as the chemical can remain on the skin and continue to burn for hours or even days.

The extent of a burn is important to determine. The amount of body surface area (BSA) involved can be quickly estimated by using the *rule of nines* (Figure A5-19•). In an adult, each of the following areas represents 9 percent of the BSA: head and neck, each upper extremity, chest, abdomen, upper back, lower back, the front of each lower extremity, and the back of each lower extremity. Together, these total 99 percent. The remaining 1 percent of BSA is assigned to the genital region. In children, the head is proportionally large compared to the body, and the body regions are adjusted accordingly. Another system of estimating the amount of BSA burned is the *palmar method*. The patient's palm equals about 1 percent of the patient's BSA. Considering this, the percentage of BSA burned can be quickly approximated. This system is particularly useful for smaller burns.

SUMMARY

The integumentary system is the largest organ of the body and plays a major role in maintaining homeostasis and in protecting the organism from the environment. Many disease and injury processes affect the skin, and emergency personnel must be able to detect and interpret skin changes secondary to injury or illness. Injuries to the skin are one of the most common emergency conditions encountered. Proper healing and a good cosmetic outcome are often dependent on care provided in the prehospital setting and in the emergency department.

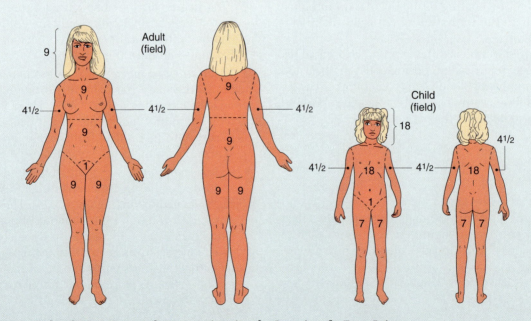

• **FIGURE A5-19**   **Rule-of-Nines System for Approximating the Severity of a Burn Injury**

6

The Skeletal System

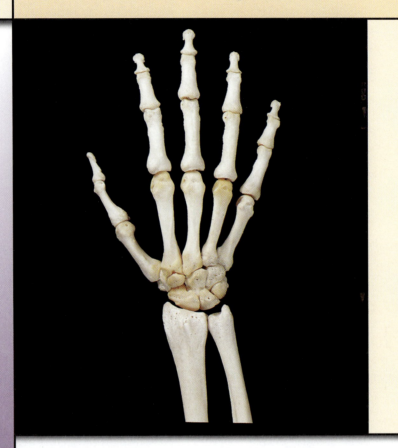

Skeletal injuries are a common reason people seek emergency medical care. Injuries to ligaments (sprains) and injuries to bones (fractures) occur with falls, sporting activities, motor-vehicle collisions, and numerous other activities. Evaluation of bone injuries is usually accomplished with X-rays. However, ligaments cannot be visualized with normal X-rays. Most ligamentous injuries can be detected with physical examination and range of motion testing. In severe injuries, or in cases where the ligamentous injury is uncertain, magnetic resonance imaging (MRI) can be used to detail the involved structures.

Chapter Outline and Objectives

Vocabulary Development

ab-, from; *abduction*
acetabulum, a vinegar cup; *acetabulum* of the hip joint
ad-, toward, to; *adduction*
amphi-, on both sides; *amphiarthrosis*
arthros, joint; *synarthrosis*
blast, precursor; *osteoblast*
circum-, around; *circumduction*
clast, break; *osteoclast*
clavius, clavicle; *clavicle*
concha, shell; middle *concha*
corona, crown; *coronoid fossa*
cranio-, skull; *cranium*
cribrum, sieve; *cribriform plate*
dens, tooth; *dens*
dia-, through; *diarthrosis*
duco, to lead; *adduction*
e-, out; *eversion*
gennan, to produce; *osteogenesis*
gomphosis, a bolting together; *gomphosis*
in-, into; *inversion*
infra-, beneath; *infraspinous fossa*
lacrimae, tears; *lacrimal* bones
lamella, thin plate; *lamellae* of bone
malleolus, little hammer; medial *malleolus*
meniscus, crescent; *menisci*
osteon, bone; *osteocytes*
penia, lacking; *osteopenia*
planta, sole; *plantar*
porosus, porous; *osteoporosis*
septum, wall; *nasal septum*
stylos, pillar; *styloid process*
supra-, above; *supraspinous fossa*
sutura, a sewing together; *suture*
teres, cylindrical; *ligamentum teres*
trabecula, wall; *trabeculae* in spongy bone
trochlea, pulley; *trochlea*
vertere, to turn; *inversion*

The skeleton has many functions, but the most obvious is supporting the weight of the body. This support is provided by bones, structures as strong as, or stronger than, reinforced concrete but considerably lighter. Unlike concrete, bones can be remodeled and reshaped to meet changing metabolic demands and patterns of activity. Bones work together with muscles to maintain body position and to produce controlled, precise movements. With the skeleton to pull against, contracting muscles can make us sit, stand, walk, or run.

The skeletal system includes the bones of the skeleton and the cartilages, ligaments, and other connective tissues that stabilize or connect them. This system performs the following functions:

1. *Support.* The skeletal system provides structural support for the entire body. Individual bones or groups of bones provide a framework for the attachment of soft tissues and organs.

2. *Leverage.* Bones of the skeleton function as *levers* that change the magnitude and direction of the forces generated by skeletal muscles. The resulting movements range from the delicate motion of a fingertip to powerful changes in the position of the entire body.

3. *Protection.* Delicate tissues and organs are often surrounded by skeletal elements. The ribs protect the heart and lungs, the skull encloses the brain, the vertebrae shield the spinal cord, and the pelvis cradles delicate digestive and reproductive organs.

4. *Storage.* The calcium salts of bone represent a valuable mineral reserve that maintains normal concentrations of calcium and phosphate ions in body fluids. In addition, fat cells in areas of *yellow marrow* store lipids as an energy reserve.

5. *Blood cell production.* Red blood cells and other blood elements are produced within the *red marrow,* which fills the internal cavities of many bones. The role of the bone marrow in blood cell formation will be discussed in later chapters dealing with the cardiovascular and lymphatic systems (Chapters 12–15).

THE STRUCTURE OF BONE

Bone, or **osseous tissue**, is one of the supporting connective tissues, and it contains specialized cells, extracellular fibers, and a ground substance. In supporting connective tissues, the fibers and ground substance interact to form a *matrix*. The distinctive solid, stony character of bone results from the deposition of calcium salts within the matrix. Calcium phosphate, $Ca_3(PO_4)_2$, accounts for almost two-thirds of the weight of bone. The remaining third is dominated by collagen fibers, with osteocytes and other cell types providing only around 2 percent of the mass of a bone.

Macroscopic Features of Bone

The bones of the human skeleton have four general shapes: long, short, flat, and irregular (Figure 6-1●). **Long bones** are longer than they are wide, whereas **short bones**

●FIGURE 6-1   Shapes of Bones

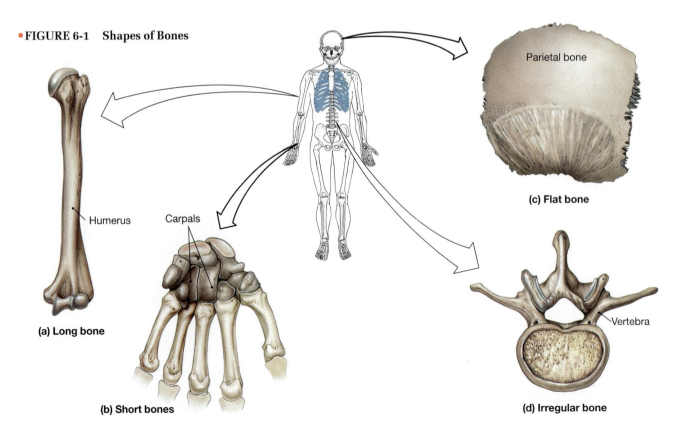

Parietal bone

(c) Flat bone

Humerus

Carpals

(a) Long bone

(b) Short bones

Vertebra

(d) Irregular bone

are of roughly equal dimensions. Examples of long bones are bones of the limbs, such as the bones of the arm (*humerus*) and thigh (*femur*). Short bones include the bones of the wrist (*carpal bones*) and ankles (*tarsal bones*). **Flat bones** are thin and relatively broad, such as the *parietal bones* of the skull, the ribs, and the shoulder blades (*scapulae*). **Irregular bones** have complex shapes that do not fit easily into any other category. An example is any of the *vertebrae* of the spinal column.

The typical features of a long bone such as the humerus are shown intact in Figure 6-1a• and in longitudinal section in Figure 6-2•. A long bone has a central shaft, or **diaphysis** (dī-A-fi-sis), and expanded ends, or **epiphyses** (ē-PIF-i-sēz). The diaphysis surrounds a central *marrow cavity*. The epiphyses of adjacent bones articulate with each other and are covered by *articular cartilages*. As will be discussed below, growth in the length of an immature long bone occurs at the junctions between the epiphyses and the diaphysis.

The two types of bone tissue are visible in Figure 6-2•: compact bone and spongy bone. **Compact bone**, or *dense bone*, is relatively solid, whereas **spongy bone**, or *cancellous* (KAN-sel-us) *bone*, resembles a network of bony rods or struts separated by spaces that are normally filled with bone **marrow**. Both compact and spongy bone are present in the humerus; compact bone forms the diaphysis, and spongy bone fills the epiphyses.

The outer surface of a bone is covered by a **periosteum**, which consists of a fibrous outer layer and a cellular inner layer (Figures 6-2•, 6-3•). The periosteum isolates the bone from surrounding tissues, provides a route for circulatory and nervous supply, and actively participates in bone growth and repair. The fibers of *tendons* and *ligaments* intermingle with those of the periosteum, attaching skeletal muscles to bones and one bone to another.

Inside the bone, a cellular **endosteum** lines the marrow cavity and other inner surfaces. The endosteum is active during bone growth and whenever repair or remodeling is under way.

Microscopic Features of Bone

The general histology of bone was introduced in Chapter 4 (see Figure 4-11•, p. 95). Both compact and spongy bone contain bone cells, or **osteocytes** (OS-tē-ō-sīts; *osteon*, bone), in small pockets called **lacunae** (la-KOO-nē). Lacunae are found between narrow sheets of calcified matrix that are known as **lamellae** (lah-MEL-lē; *lamella*, thin plate). Small channels, called **canaliculi** (ka-na-LIK-ū-lē), radiate through the matrix, interconnecting lacunae and linking them to nearby blood vessels. The canaliculi contain cytoplasmic extensions of the osteocytes. Nutrients from the blood and waste products from the osteocytes diffuse through the fluid that surrounds these cells and their extensions.

Compact and Spongy Bone

The basic functional unit of compact bone, the **osteon** (OS-tē-on), or *Haversian system*, is shown in Figure 6-3•. Within an osteon, the osteocytes are arranged in concentric layers around a **central canal**, or *Haversian canal*, that contains one or more blood vessels. The lamellae are cylindrical, oriented parallel to the long axis of the central canal. **Perforating canals**, or *canals of Volkmann*, provide passageways for linking the blood vessels of the central canals with those of the periosteum or the marrow cavity.

Spongy bone has a quite different lamellar arrangement and no osteons. Instead, the lamellae form rods or plates called **trabeculae** (tra-BEK-ū-lē; *trabecula*, wall). Frequent branchings of the thin trabeculae create an open network. Canaliculi radiating from the lacunae of spongy bone end at the exposed surfaces of the trabeculae, where nutrients and wastes diffuse between the marrow and osteocytes.

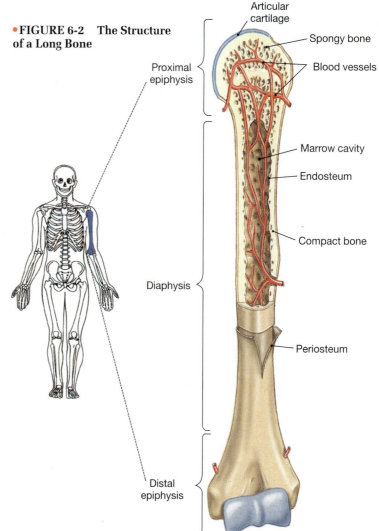

•**FIGURE 6-2   The Structure of a Long Bone**

- Articular cartilage
- Spongy bone
- Blood vessels
- Marrow cavity
- Endosteum
- Compact bone
- Periosteum

Proximal epiphysis

Diaphysis

Distal epiphysis

6

•**FIGURE 6-3   The Structure of a Typical Bone**
(a) A thin section through compact bone; in this procedure the intact matrix and central canals appear white, and the lacunae and canaliculi appear black. (LM × 272) © R.G. Kessell & R.H. Kardon "Tissues & Organs: A Text–Atlas of Scanning Electron Microscopy," W.H. Freeman & Co., 1979. All Rights Reserved.**(b)** A diagrammatic view of the structure of a typical bone, the humerus.

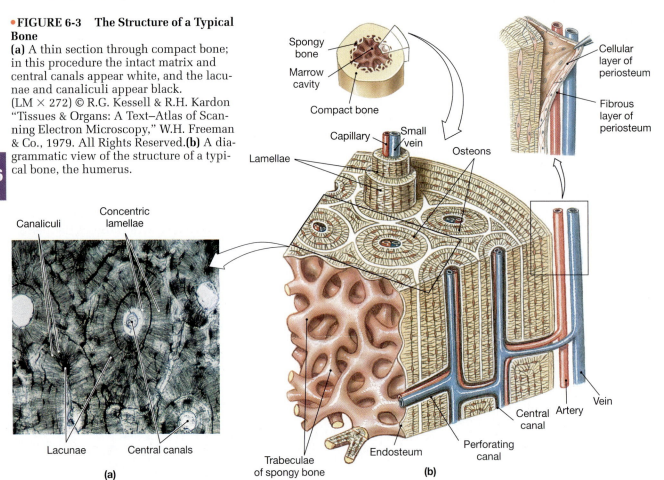

(a)

(b)

A layer of compact bone covers bone surfaces everywhere except inside *joint capsules*, where articular cartilages protect opposing surfaces. Compact bone is usually found where stresses come from a limited range of directions. The limb bones, for example, are built to withstand forces applied at either end. Because the osteons are parallel to the long axis of the shaft, a limb bone does not bend, even when a large force is applied to either end. However, a much smaller force applied to the side of the shaft can break the bone.

Bones do bend in disorders that reduce the amount of calcium salts in the skeleton. As the proportion of calcium to collagen decreases, the bones become very flexible, and they become less able to resist compression and tension. An example of such a condition is *rickets*, a childhood disorder that results from a deficiency of vitamin D_3. Affected individuals develop a bowlegged appearance as the leg bones bend under the weight of the body.

In contrast, spongy bone is found where bones are not heavily stressed or where stresses arrive from many directions. For example, spongy bone is present at the epiphyses of long bones, where stresses are transferred across joints. In addition, spongy bone is much lighter than compact bone. This reduces the weight of the skeleton and makes it easier for muscles to move the bones. Finally, the trabecular framework protects the cells of the bone marrow, and areas of spongy bone, such as the epiphyses of the femur, are important sites of blood cell formation.

Cells in Bone

Although osteocytes are the most abundant cells in bone, other cell types are also present. These cells, called *osteoclasts* and *osteoblasts*, are associated with the endosteum that lines the inner cavities of both compact and spongy bone and the cellular layer of the periosteum. Three primary cell types occur in bone:

1. Osteocytes, mature bone cells. Osteocytes maintain normal bone structure by recycling the calcium salts in the bony matrix around themselves and assisting in repairs.
2. **Osteoclasts** (OS-tē-ō-klasts; *clast*, break), giant cells with 50 or more nuclei. Acids secreted by osteoclasts dissolve the bony matrix through *osteolysis* and release the stored minerals. This process helps regulate calcium and phosphate concentrations in body fluids.
3. **Osteoblasts** (OS-tē-ō-blasts; *blast*, precursor), the cells responsible for the production of new bone, a process called *osteogenesis* (os-tē-ō-JEN-e-sis; *gennan*, to produce). At any given moment, osteoclasts

are removing matrix and osteoblasts are adding to it. When an osteoblast becomes completely surrounded by calcified matrix, it differentiates into an osteocyte.

✓ How would the strength of a bone be affected if the ratio of collagen to calcium increased?

✓ A sample of bone shows concentric layers surrounding a central canal. Is it from the shaft or the end of a long bone?

✓ If the activity of osteoclasts exceeds that of osteoblasts in a bone, how will the bone's mass be affected?

BONE DEVELOPMENT AND GROWTH

The growth of the skeleton determines the size and proportions of the body. Skeletal growth begins about 6 weeks after fertilization, when the embryo is about 12 mm long. (Before this time, all supporting elements are made of cartilage.) Bone growth continues through adolescence, and portions of the skeleton usually do not stop growing until age 18–25. This section considers the process of osteogenesis (bone formation) and growth. The next section examines the maintenance and turnover of mineral reserves in the adult skeleton.

During development, cartilage or fibrous connective tissue is replaced by bone. The process of replacing other tissues with bone is called **ossification**. There are two major forms of ossification. In *intramembranous ossification*, bone develops within sheets or membranes of connective tissue. In *endochondral ossification*, bone replaces existing cartilage.

Intramembranous Ossification

Intramembranous (in-tra-MEM-bra-nus) **ossification** begins when osteoblasts differentiate within fibrous connective tissue. Most often this differentiation occurs in the deep layers of the dermis. The osteoblasts cluster together and secrete the organic components of the matrix. This mixture then becomes mineralized through the crystallization of calcium salts. The place where ossification first occurs is called an **ossification center**. As ossification proceeds, some osteoblasts become trapped inside bony pockets and change into osteocytes.

Bone growth is an active process, and osteoblasts require oxygen and a reliable supply of nutrients. Blood vessels that branch in the embryonic connective tissue meet these demands and over time become trapped within the developing bone. Initially, the intramembranous bone resembles spongy bone, further remodeling around the trapped blood vessels can produce compact bone. Several flat bones of the skull, the lower jaw, and the collarbones (*clavicles*) form this way.

Endochondral Ossification

Most of the bones of the skeleton are formed through the **endochondral** (en-dō-KON-dral; *endo*, inside + *chondros*, cartilage) **ossification** of existing cartilage. The cartilages develop first; they are like miniature cartilage models of the future bone. By the time an embryo is 6 weeks old, the cartilage models of the future limb bones begin to be replaced by true bone. Steps in their growth and ossification are diagrammed in Figure 6-4●.

Bone formation begins near the middle of the shaft, at a *primary center of ossification*, and proceeds toward either end. Eventually, *secondary centers of ossification* develop in the epiphyses. At this stage, the bone of the shaft and the bone of each epiphysis are separated by areas of cartilage known as **epiphyseal plates**. On the shaft side of the epiphyseal plate, osteoblasts continuously invade the cartilage and convert it to bone. But on the epiphyseal side of the plate, *chondrocytes* produce new cartilage at the same rate. ∞ *p. 93* As a result, the shaft grows longer but the epiphyseal plate remains. This process could be compared to a jogger following someone on a bicycle. The jogger keeps advancing, but the bike stays a few feet ahead.

When sex hormone production increases at puberty, bone growth accelerates dramatically, and osteoblasts begin to produce bone faster than epiphyseal cartilage expands. In effect, the jogger speeds up, moving closer to the bicycle ahead. Over time, the epiphyseal plates narrow and finally ossify, or "close." This period of sudden growth ends as the individual reaches sexual and physical maturity. The location of the plate can still be detected in X-rays as a distinct *epiphyseal line* that remains after epiphyseal growth has ended.

While the bone elongates, it also grows larger in diameter. The diameter enlarges at its outer surface through a process called *appositional growth*. This enlargement occurs as cells of the periosteum develop into osteoblasts and produce additional bony matrix. As new bone is deposited on the outer surface of the shaft, the inner surface is eroded by osteoclasts, and the marrow cavity gradually enlarges.

Bone Growth and Body Proportions

The timing of epiphyseal closure varies from bone to bone and individual to individual. The toes may complete their ossification by age 11, whereas portions of the pelvis or the wrist may continue to enlarge until age 25. The epiphyseal plates in the arms and legs usually close by age 18 (women) or 20 (men). Differences in sex hormones account for variations in body size and proportions between men and women.

6

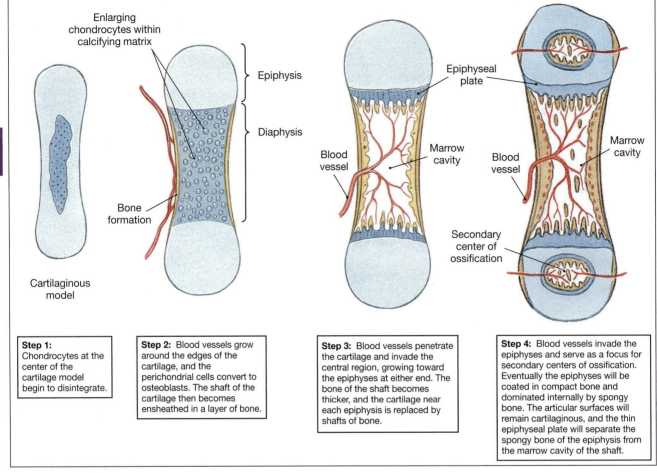

Enlarging chondrocytes within calcifying matrix

Epiphysis

Diaphysis

Bone formation

Cartilaginous model

Epiphyseal plate

Blood vessel

Marrow cavity

Blood vessel

Marrow cavity

Secondary center of ossification

Step 1: Chondrocytes at the center of the cartilage model begin to disintegrate.

Step 2: Blood vessels grow around the edges of the cartilage, and the perichondrial cells convert to osteoblasts. The shaft of the cartilage then becomes ensheathed in a layer of bone.

Step 3: Blood vessels penetrate the cartilage and invade the central region, growing toward the epiphyses at either end. The bone of the shaft becomes thicker, and the cartilage near each epiphysis is replaced by shafts of bone.

Step 4: Blood vessels invade the epiphyses and serve as a focus for secondary centers of ossification. Eventually the epiphyses will be coated in compact bone and dominated internally by spongy bone. The articular surfaces will remain cartilaginous, and the thin epiphyseal plate will separate the spongy bone of the epiphysis from the marrow cavity of the shaft.

• **FIGURE 6-4   Endochondral Ossification**

Requirements for Normal Bone Growth

Normal osteogenesis cannot occur without a reliable source of minerals, especially calcium salts. During pre-natal development these minerals are absorbed from the mother's bloodstream. The demands are so great that the maternal skeleton often loses bone mass during pregnancy. From infancy to adulthood, the diet must provide adequate amounts of calcium and phosphate, and the individual must be able to absorb and transport these minerals to sites of bone formation.

Vitamin D_3 plays an important role in normal calci-um metabolism by stimulating the absorption and trans-port of calcium and phosphate ions. This vitamin can be obtained from dietary supplements or manufactured by epidermal cells exposed to UV radiation. ∞ *p. 111* After vitamin D_3 has been processed in the liver, the kid-neys convert a derivative of this vitamin into *calcitriol*, a hormone that stimulates the absorption of calcium and phosphate ions across the intestinal lining. Rickets is marked by a softening and bending of bones that occurs in growing children, usually as a result of vitamin D_3 deficiency.

Vitamin A and *vitamin C* are also essential for nor-mal bone growth and remodeling. For example, a defi-ciency of vitamin C will cause *scurvy*. One of the primary symptoms of this condition is a reduction in osteoblast activity that leads to weak and brittle bones. In addition to vitamins, hormones such as growth hor-mone, thyroid hormones, sex hormones, and those in-volved with calcium metabolism are essential to normal skeletal growth and development.

✓ How could X-rays of the femur be used to deter-mine whether a person had reached full height?

✓ In the Middle Ages, choirboys were sometimes cas-trated (had their testes removed) to prevent their voices from changing. How would castration have affected their height?

✓ Why are pregnant women given calcium supple-ments and encouraged to drink milk even though their skeletons are fully formed?

REMODELING AND HOMEOSTATIC MECHANISMS

Of the five major functions of the skeleton discussed earlier in this chapter, support and storage depend on the dynamic nature of bone. In adults, osteocytes in lacunae maintain the surrounding matrix, continually removing and replacing the surrounding calcium salts. But osteoclasts and osteoblasts also remain active, even after the epiphyseal plates have closed. Normally their activities are balanced: As one osteon forms through the activity of osteoblasts, another is destroyed by osteoclasts. The turnover rate for bone is quite high, and in adults roughly 18 percent of the protein and mineral components are removed and replaced each year through the process of **remodeling**. Every part of every bone may not be affected, as there are regional and even local differences in the rate of turnover. For example, the spongy bone in the head of the femur may be replaced two or three times each year, whereas the compact bone along the shaft remains largely untouched.

Remodeling and Support

Regular mineral turnover gives each bone the ability to adapt to new stresses. Heavily stressed bones become thicker, stronger, and develop more pronounced surface ridges; bones not subjected to ordinary stresses become thin and brittle. Regular exercise is thus an important stimulus that maintains normal bone structure.

Degenerative changes in the skeleton occur after even brief periods of inactivity. For example, using a crutch while wearing a cast takes the weight off the injured leg. After a few weeks, the unstressed leg will lose up to about a third of its bone mass. The bones rebuild just as quickly when they again carry their normal weight.

Homeostasis and Mineral Storage

The bones of the skeleton are more than just racks to hang muscles on. They are important mineral reservoirs, and calcium is the most abundant mineral in the human body. A typical human body contains 1–2 kg (2.2–4.4 lb) of calcium, with 99 percent of it deposited in the skeleton.

Calcium ion concentrations must be closely controlled to prevent damage to essential physiological systems. Small variations from normal concentrations will have some effect on cellular operations, and larger changes can cause a clinical crisis. Neurons and muscle cells are particularly sensitive to changes in the concentration of calcium ions. If the calcium concentration in body fluids increases by 30 percent, neurons and muscle cells become relatively unresponsive. If calcium levels decrease by 35 percent, they become so excitable that convulsions may occur. A 50 percent reduction in calcium concentrations

usually causes death. Such gross disturbances in calcium metabolism are relatively rare, because calcium ion concentrations are so closely regulated that daily fluctuations of more than 10 percent are very unusual.

Parathyroid hormone (PTH) and *calcitriol* are hormones that work together to elevate calcium levels in body fluids. Their actions are opposed by *calcitonin*, which depresses calcium levels in body fluids. These hormones and their regulation are discussed further in Chapter 11.

By providing a calcium reserve, the skeleton helps maintain calcium homeostasis in body fluids. This function can directly affect the shape and strength of the bones in the skeleton. When large numbers of calcium ions are mobilized, bones become weaker; when calcium salts are deposited, bones become more massive.

Injury and Repair

Despite its mineral strength, bone cracks or even breaks if subjected to extreme loads, sudden impacts, or stresses from unusual directions. All such cracks and breaks in bones constitute a **fracture**. Fractures are classified according to their external appearance, the site of the fracture, and the nature of the break. Important fracture types are indicated in the Focus box on p. 129.

Bones will usually heal even after they have been severely damaged, as long as the circulatory supply and the cellular components of the endosteum and periosteum survive. Steps in the repair process, which may take from 4 months to well over a year following a fracture, are diagrammed in Figure 6-5•:

Step 1: In even a small fracture, many blood vessels are broken and extensive bleeding occurs. Pooling and clotting of the blood forms a swollen area called a **fracture hematoma** (*hemato-*, blood; + *tumere*, to swell), which closes off the injured blood vessels.

Step 2: Cells of the periosteum and endosteum migrate into the fracture zone. There they form localized thickenings—an **external callus** (*callum*, hard skin) and **internal callus**, respectively. At the center of the external callus, cells differentiate into chondrocytes and build blocks of cartilage.

Step 3: Osteoblasts replace the central cartilage of the external callus with spongy bone. When this process is complete, the external and internal calluses form a continuous brace of spongy bone at the fracture site.

Step 4: The remodeling of spongy bone at the fracture site may continue from a period of 4 months to well over a year. When the remodeling is complete, the fragments of dead bone and the spongy bone of the calluses will be gone, and only living compact bone will remain. The repair may be "good as new," with no sign that a fracture occurred, but the bone may be slightly thicker than normal at the fracture site.

6

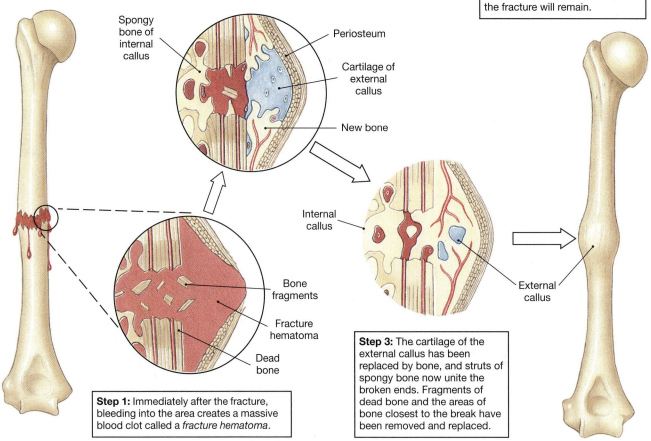

•FIGURE 6-5   Steps in the Repair of a Fracture

Step 2: An *internal callus* forms as a network of spongy bone unites the inner surfaces, and an *external callus* of cartilage and bone stabilizes the outer edges.

Step 4: A swelling initially marks the location of the fracture. Over time this region will be remodeled, and little evidence of the fracture will remain.

Spongy bone of internal callus

Periosteum

Cartilage of external callus

New bone

Internal callus

External callus

Bone fragments

Fracture hematoma

Dead bone

Step 1: Immediately after the fracture, bleeding into the area creates a massive blood clot called a *fracture hematoma*.

Step 3: The cartilage of the external callus has been replaced by bone, and struts of spongy bone now unite the broken ends. Fragments of dead bone and the areas of bone closest to the break have been removed and replaced.

AGING AND THE SKELETAL SYSTEM

The bones of the skeleton become thinner and relatively weaker as a normal part of the aging process. Inadequate ossification is called **osteopenia** (os-tē-ō-PĒ-nē-a; *penia*, lacking), and all people become slightly osteopenic as they age. The reduction in bone mass occurs because between the ages of 30 and 40, osteoblast activity begins to decline while osteoclast activity continues at normal levels. Once the reduction begins, women lose roughly 8 percent of their skeletal mass every decade, whereas men's skeletons deteriorate at about 3 percent per decade. All parts of the skeleton are not equally affected. Epiphyses, vertebrae, and the jaws lose more than their fair share, resulting in fragile limbs, a reduction in height, and the loss of teeth.

✳ COMPRESSION FRACTURES

Aging affects virtually every body system, and the skeletal system is no exception. Bone mass is normally lost with age in a process called *osteopenia*. However, some people will lose significantly more bone in a process called *osteoporosis.* In severe osteoporosis, over 50% of the bone mass can be lost. This is a particular problem in women following menopause where decreasing levels of female hormones (*estrogens*) results in loss of bone mass. This causes the bones to become weak and subject to fracture.

The weight-bearing parts of the spinal bones (*vertebral bodies*) are particularly vulnerable to osteoporosis. With advanced osteoporosis, relatively minor trauma, even as simple as rolling over in bed, can cause compression fractures. *Compression fractures* cause the vertebral body to collapse (much like crushing a soft drink can), resulting in pain, limited movement, and a loss in body height. Elderly patients with multiple compression fractures may actually lose several inches of body height.

✓ Why would you expect the arm bones of a weight lifter to be thicker and heavier than those of a jogger?

✓ Why is osteoporosis more common in older women than older men?

FOCUS   A Classification of Fractures

Fractures are classified according to their external appearance, the site of the fracture, and the nature of the crack or break in the bone. Important fracture types are indicated below, with representative X-rays. Many fractures fall into more than one category. For example, a Colles' fracture is a transverse fracture, but depending on the injury, it may also be a comminuted fracture that can be either open or closed. Closed, or simple, fractures are completely internal; they do not involve a break in the skin. Open, or compound, fractures project through the skin; they are more dangerous because of the possibility of infection or uncontrolled bleeding.

6

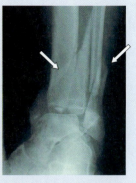

A **Pott's fracture** occurs at the ankle and affects both bones of the leg.

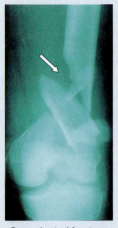

Comminuted fracture of distal femur

Comminuted fractures shatter the affected area into many, small bony fragments.

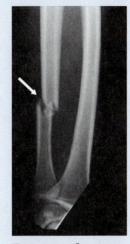

Transverse fractures break a shaft of a bone across its long axis.

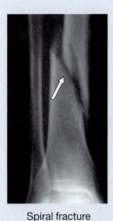

Spiral fracture of tibia

Spiral fractures, produced by twisting stresses, spread along the length of the bone.

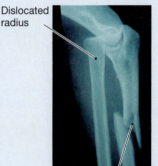

Dislocated radius

Displaced ulnar fracture

Displaced fractures produce new and abnormal arrangements of bony elements.

Nondisplaced fractures retain the normal alignment of the bone elements or fragments.

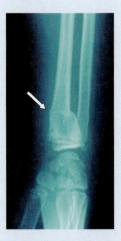

A **Colles' fracture** is a break in the distal portion of the radius, the slender bone of the forearm; it is often the result of reaching out to cushion a fall.

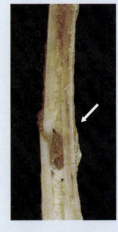

In a **greenstick fracture,** only one side of the shaft is broken, and the other is bent; this type usually occurs in children, whose long bones have yet to ossify fully.

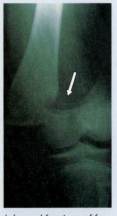

Epiphyseal fracture of femur

Epiphyseal fractures usually occur where the matrix is undergoing calcification and chondrocytes are dying. A clean transverse fracture along this line usually heals well. Fractures between the epiphysis and the epiphyseal plate can permanently halt further longitudinal growth unless carefully treated; often surgery is required.

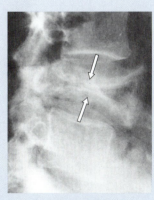

Compression fracture of vertebra

Compression fractures occur in vertebrae subjected to extreme stresses, as when landing on your seat after a fall.

AN OVERVIEW OF THE SKELETON

Skeletal Terminology

Each of the bones in the human skeleton not only has a distinctive shape but also has characteristic external features. For example, elevations or projections form where tendons and ligaments attach and where adjacent bones articulate. Depressions and openings indicate sites where blood vessels and nerves lie alongside or penetrate the bone. These external landmarks are called **bone markings**, or *surface features*. The most common terms used to describe bone markings are listed and illustrated in Table 6-1.

Skeletal Divisions

The skeletal system consists of 206 separate bones and a number of associated cartilages (Figure 6-6●, p. 132).

It consists of axial and appendicular divisions. The **axial skeleton** forms the longitudinal axis of the body. This division's 80 bones can be subdivided into (1) the 22 bones of the **skull**, plus associated bones (6 **auditory ossicles** and the **hyoid bone**); (2) the 26 bones of the **vertebral column**; and (3) the **thoracic cage** (*rib cage*), composed of 24 **ribs** and the **sternum**.

The **appendicular skeleton** includes the bones of the limbs and those of the **pectoral** and **pelvic girdles**, which attach the limbs to the trunk. All together there are 126 appendicular bones; 32 are associated with each upper limb, and 31 with each lower limb.

The sections that follow discuss the structure of a typical skeleton. When viewed in detail, however, no two skeletons are exactly alike, owing to differences in body size, weight, sex, race, medical history, and other factors. A detailed analysis of a skeleton can actually provide important information about an individual; for this reason, skeletal analysis plays an important role in anthropology, as well as in criminal investigations.

TABLE 6-1	An Introduction to Bone Markings	
General Description	*Anatomical Term*	*Definition*
Elevations and projections (general)	Ramus	An extension of a bone making an angle to the rest of the structure
Processes formed where tendons or ligaments attach	Trochanter	A large, rough projection
	Tuberosity	A smaller, rough projection
	Tubercle	A small, rounded projection
	Crest	A prominent ridge
	Line	A low ridge
Processes formed for articulation with adjacent bones	Head	The expanded articular end of an epiphysis, separated from the shaft by the neck
	Neck	A narrow connection between the epiphysis and diaphysis
	Condyle	A smooth, rounded articular process
	Trochlea	A smooth, grooved articular process shaped like a pulley
	Facet	A small, flat articular surface
	Spine	A pointed process
Depressions	Fossa	A shallow depression
	Sulcus	A narrow groove
Openings	Foramen	A rounded passageway for blood vessels and/or nerves
	Fissure	An elongate cleft
	Canal	A passageway through the substance of a bone
	Sinus	A chamber within a bone, normally filled with air

THE AXIAL DIVISION

The **axial skeleton** creates a framework that supports and protects organ systems in the dorsal and ventral body cavities. In addition, it provides an extensive surface area for the attachment of muscles that (1) adjust the positions of the head, neck, and trunk; (2) perform respiratory movements; and (3) stabilize or position elements of the appendicular skeleton.

The Skull

The bones of the skull protect the brain and support delicate sense organs involved with vision, hearing, balance, olfaction (smell), and gustation (taste). The skull is made up of 22 bones: 8 form the **cranium**, and 14 are associated with the face. Seven additional bones are associated with the skull: 6 *auditory ossicles*, tiny bones involved in sound detection, are encased by the *tem-*

poral bones of the cranium, and the *hyoid bone* has ligamentous connections to the inferior surface of the skull.

The cranium encloses the **cranial cavity**, a fluid-filled chamber that cushions and supports the brain. The outer surface of the cranium provides an extensive area for the attachment of muscles that move the eyes, jaws, and head.

The Bones of the Cranium

The Frontal Bone.   The **frontal bone** of the cranium forms the forehead and the superior surface of the **orbits**, the bony recesses that contain the eyes (Figures 6-7, p. 133, and 6-8•, p. 134). A **supraorbital foramen** is an opening that pierces the bony ridge above each orbit, forming a passageway for blood vessels and nerves passing to or from the forehead. (Sometimes the ridge has a deep groove, called a *supraorbital notch*, rather than a foramen, but the function is the same.) Above the orbit, the frontal bone contains air-filled internal chambers

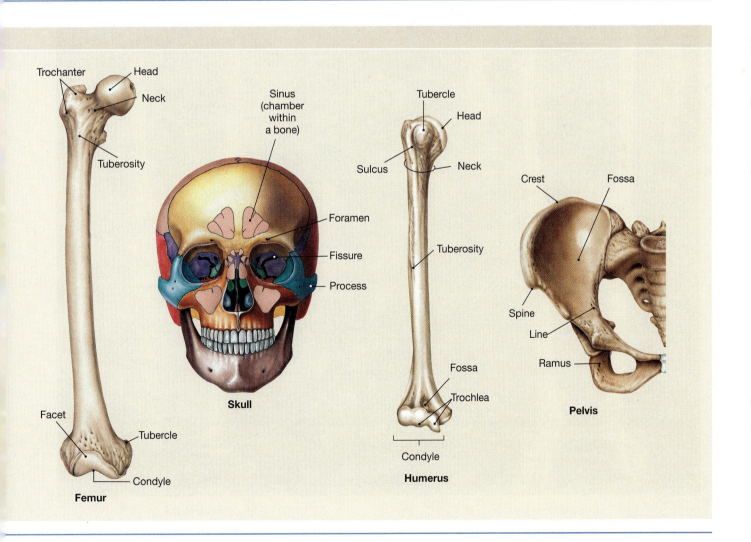

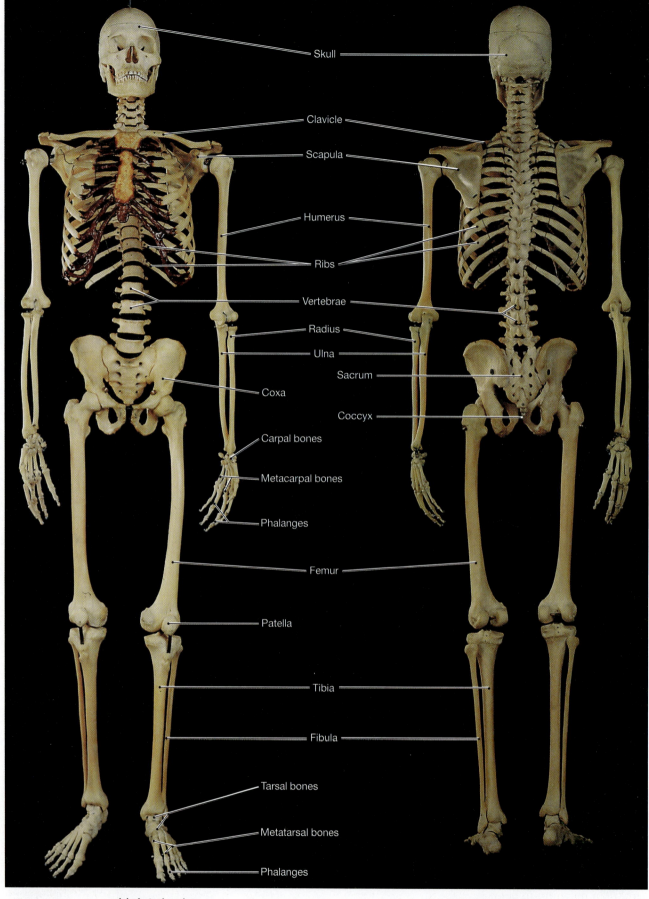

Skull

Clavicle

Scapula

Humerus

Ribs

Vertebrae

Radius

Ulna

Sacrum

Coxa

Coccyx

Carpal bones

Metacarpal bones

Phalanges

Femur

Patella

Tibia

Fibula

Tarsal bones

Metatarsal bones

Phalanges

(a) Anterior view

(b) Posterior view

•FIGURE 6-6   The Skeleton

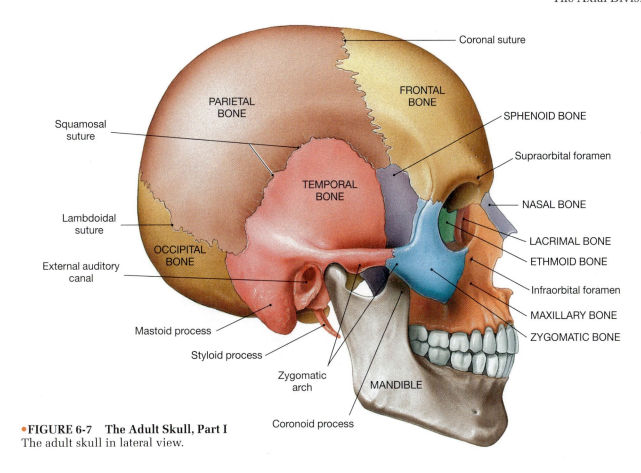

Coronal suture

FRONTAL BONE

PARIETAL BONE

SPHENOID BONE

Supraorbital foramen

NASAL BONE

LACRIMAL BONE

ETHMOID BONE

Infraorbital foramen

MAXILLARY BONE

ZYGOMATIC BONE

TEMPORAL BONE

Squamosal suture

Lambdoidal suture

OCCIPITAL BONE

External auditory canal

Mastoid process

Styloid process

Zygomatic arch

MANDIBLE

Coronoid process

•**FIGURE 6-7   The Adult Skull, Part I**
The adult skull in lateral view.

6

that communicate with the nasal cavity. These **frontal sinuses** make the bone lighter and produce mucus that cleans and moistens the nasal cavities (Figure 6-9b•, p. 135). The **infraorbital foramen** is an opening that marks the path of a major sensory nerve from the face.

The Parietal Bones.   On both sides of the skull, a **parietal** (pa-RĪ-e-tal) **bone** is posterior to the frontal bone (Figures 6-8, 6-9•). Together the parietal bones form the roof and the superior walls of the cranium. The parietal bones interlock along the **sagittal suture**, which extends along the midline of the cranium. Anteriorly, the two parietal bones articulate with the frontal bone along the **coronal suture**.

The Occipital Bone.   The **occipital bone** forms the posterior and inferior portions of the cranium. Along its superior margin, the occipital bone contacts the two parietal bones at the **lambdoidal** (lam-DOYD-al) **suture** (Figure 6-7•). Figure 6-8b• presents an inferior view of the skull, showing the orientation of the occipital bone and its relationships with other bones in the floor of the cranium. The occipital bone surrounds the **foramen magnum**, the opening that connects the cranial cavity with the spinal cavity. The spinal cord passes through the foramen magnum to connect with the inferior portion of the brain. On either side of the foramen mag-

num are the **occipital condyles**, the sites of articulation between the skull and the vertebral column.

The Temporal Bones.   Below the parietal bones and contributing to the sides and base of the cranium are the **temporal bones**. The temporal bones contact the parietal bones along the **squamosal suture** (Figure 6-7•).

The temporal bones display a number of distinctive anatomical landmarks. One of them, the **external auditory canal**, leads to the **tympanum,** or *eardrum.* The eardrum separates the external auditory canal from the *middle ear cavity,* which contains the *auditory ossicles,* or *ear bones.* The structure and function of the tympanum, middle ear cavity, and auditory ossicles will be considered in Chapter 10.

Anterior to the external auditory canal is a transverse depression, the **mandibular fossa**, which marks the point of articulation with the lower jaw (mandible) (Figure 6-8b•). The prominent bulge just posterior and inferior to the entrance to the external auditory canal is the **mastoid process**, which provides a site for the attachment of muscles that rotate or extend the head. Adjacent to the base of the mastoid process is the long, sharp **styloid** (STĪ-loyd; *stylos*, pillar) **process**. The styloid process anchors muscles and ligaments associated with the tongue and hyoid bone.

6

•FIGURE 6-8   The
Adult Skull, Part II

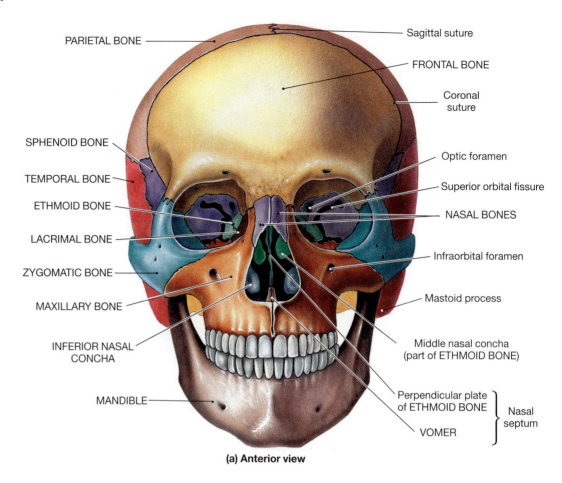

PARIETAL BONE

Sagittal suture

FRONTAL BONE

Coronal
suture

SPHENOID BONE

Optic foramen

TEMPORAL BONE

Superior orbital fissure

ETHMOID BONE

NASAL BONES

LACRIMAL BONE

Infraorbital foramen

ZYGOMATIC BONE

Mastoid process

MAXILLARY BONE

Middle nasal concha
(part of ETHMOID BONE)

INFERIOR NASAL
CONCHA

MANDIBLE

Perpendicular plate
of ETHMOID BONE

VOMER

Nasal
septum

(a) Anterior view

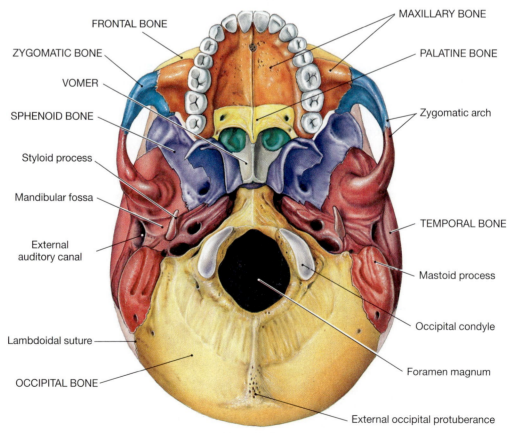

FRONTAL BONE

MAXILLARY BONE

ZYGOMATIC BONE

PALATINE BONE

VOMER

SPHENOID BONE

Zygomatic arch

Styloid process

Mandibular fossa

External
auditory canal

TEMPORAL BONE

Mastoid process

Occipital condyle

Lambdoidal suture

Foramen magnum

OCCIPITAL BONE

External occipital protuberance

(b) Inferior view

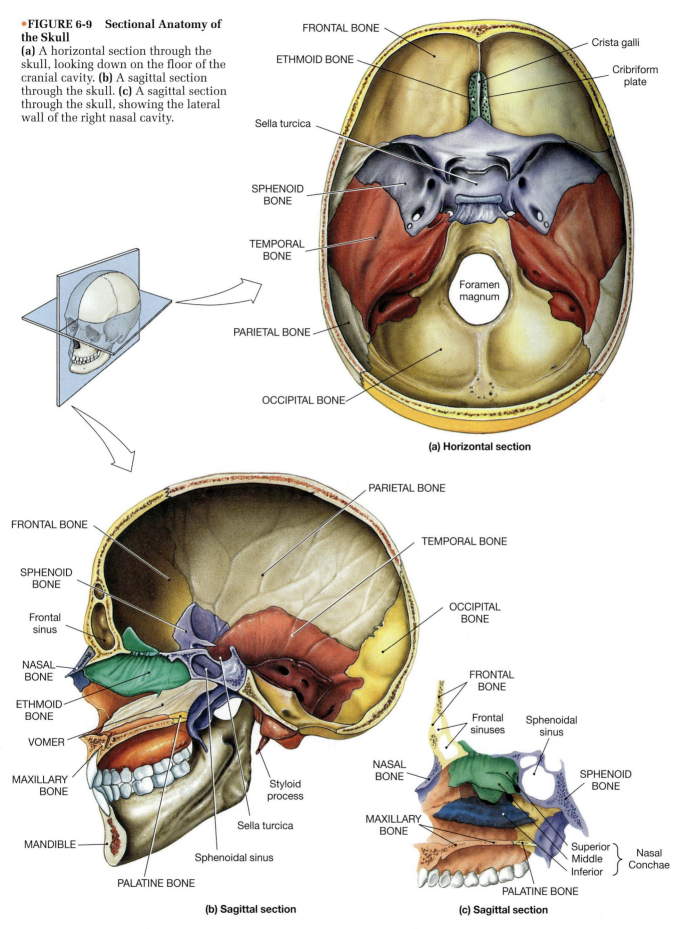

6

•FIGURE 6-9   **Sectional Anatomy of the Skull**
(a) A horizontal section through the skull, looking down on the floor of the cranial cavity. (b) A sagittal section through the skull. (c) A sagittal section through the skull, showing the lateral wall of the right nasal cavity.

FRONTAL BONE

ETHMOID BONE

Crista galli

Cribriform plate

Sella turcica

SPHENOID BONE

TEMPORAL BONE

Foramen magnum

PARIETAL BONE

OCCIPITAL BONE

(a) Horizontal section

PARIETAL BONE

FRONTAL BONE

TEMPORAL BONE

SPHENOID BONE

OCCIPITAL BONE

Frontal sinus

NASAL BONE

ETHMOID BONE

VOMER

MAXILLARY BONE

Styloid process

Sella turcica

MANDIBLE

Sphenoidal sinus

PALATINE BONE

(b) Sagittal section

FRONTAL BONE

Frontal sinuses

Sphenoidal sinus

NASAL BONE

SPHENOID BONE

MAXILLARY BONE

Superior
Middle
Inferior

Nasal Conchae

PALATINE BONE

(c) Sagittal section

6

The Sphenoid Bone.

The **sphenoid** (SFĒ-noyd) **bone** forms part of the floor of the cranium. It also acts like a bridge, uniting the cranial and facial bones, and it braces the sides of the skull. The general shape of the sphenoid has been compared to that of a giant bat with wings extended. The wings can be seen most clearly on the superior surface (Figure 6-9a•). From the front (Figure 6-8a•) or side (Figure 6-7•), it is covered by other bones. Like the frontal bone, the sphenoid bone also contains a pair of sinuses, called **sphenoidal sinuses** (Figure 6-9b•).

The lateral "wings" of the sphenoid extend to either side from a central depression called the **sella turcica** (TUR-si-ka) (Turk's saddle) (Figure 6-9a•). It encloses the pituitary gland, an endocrine organ that is connected to the inferior surface of the brain by a narrow stalk of neural tissue.

The Ethmoid Bone.

The **ethmoid bone** is anterior to the sphenoid bone. The ethmoid bone consists of two honeycombed masses of bone. It forms part of the cranial floor, contributes to the medial surfaces of the orbit of each eye, and forms the roof and sides of the nasal cavity (Figure 6-8a•). A prominent ridge, the **crista galli**, or "cock's comb," projects above the superior surface of the ethmoid (Figure 6-9a•). Holes in the **cribriform plate** (*cribrum*, sieve) on either side permit passage of sensory nerves traveling from olfactory (smell) receptors in the nasal cavity to the brain.

The lateral portions of the ethmoid bone contain the **ethmoidal sinuses** that drain into the nasal cavity. Projections called the **superior** and **middle nasal conchae** (KONG-kē; *concha*, shell) extend into the nasal cavity toward the *nasal septum* (*septum*, wall) that divides the nasal cavity into left and right portions (Figures 6-8a, 6-9b,c•). The nasal conchae slow the movement of air through the nasal cavity, allowing time for the air to become warm, moist, and clean before it reaches the delicate portions of the respiratory tract. The **perpendicular plate** of the ethmoid extends inferiorly from the crista galli, passing between the conchae to contribute to the nasal septum (Figure 6-8a•).

✓ The mastoid and styloid processes are found on which of the skull bones?

✓ What bone contains the depression called the sella turcica? What is located in the depression?

✓ Which bone of the cranium articulates directly with the vertebral column?

The Bones of the Face

The facial bones protect and support the entrances to the digestive and respiratory tracts. They also provide areas for the attachment of muscles that control our facial expressions and help us manipulate food. Of the 14 facial bones, only the lower jaw, or *mandible*, is movable.

The Maxillary Bones.

The **maxillary** (MAK-si-ler-ē) **bones**, or *maxillae*, articulate with all other facial bones except the mandible. The maxillary bones form (1) the floor and medial portion of the rim of the orbit (Figure 6-8a•); (2) the walls of the nasal cavity; and (3) the anterior roof of the mouth, or *hard palate* (Figure 6-9b•). The maxillary bones contain large **maxillary sinuses**, which lighten the portion of the maxillary bones above the embedded teeth. Infections of the gums or teeth can sometimes spread into the maxillary sinuses, increasing pain and making treatment more complicated.

The Palatine Bones.

The paired **palatine bones** form the posterior surface of the *bony palate*, or *hard palate*—the "roof of the mouth" (Figures 6-8b, 6-9b•). The superior surfaces of the horizontal portion of each palatine bone contribute to the floor of the nasal cavity. The superior tip of the vertical portion of each palatine bone forms a small portion of the inferior wall of the orbit.

The Vomer.

The inferior margin of the **vomer** articulates with the paired palatine bones. The vomer supports a prominent partition that forms part of the *nasal septum*, along with the ethmoid bone (Figures 6-8a, 6-9b•).

The Zygomatic Bones.

On each side of the skull, a **zygomatic** (zī-go-MA-tik) **bone** articulates with the frontal bone and the maxilla to complete the lateral wall of the orbit (Figures 6-7, 6-8a•). Along its lateral margin, each zygomatic bone gives rise to a slender bony extension that curves laterally and posteriorly to meet a process from the temporal bone. Together these processes form the **zygomatic arch**, or *cheekbone*.

The Nasal Bones.

Forming the bridge of the nose midway between the orbits, the **nasal bones** articulate with the superior frontal bone and the maxillary bones (Figures 6-7, 6-8a•).

The Lacrimal Bones.

The **lacrimal** (*lacrimae*, tears) **bones** are located within the orbit on its medial surface. They articulate with the frontal, ethmoid, and maxillary bones (Figures 6-7, 6-8a•).

The Inferior Nasal Conchae.

The paired **inferior nasal conchae** project from the lateral walls of the nasal cavity (Figure 6-8a•). Their shape helps slow airflow and deflects arriving air toward the olfactory (smell) receptors located near the upper portions of the nasal cavity.

The Nasal Complex.

The **nasal complex** includes the bones that form the superior and lateral walls of the nasal cavities and the sinuses that drain into them. The ethmoid bone and vomer form the bony portion of the **nasal septum** that separates the left and right portions of the nasal cavity (Figure 6-8a•). The frontal, sphenoid, ethmoid, palatine, and maxillary bones contain air-filled chambers collectively known as the **paranasal sinuses**. The paranasal sinuses are significant because (1) they reduce the weight of the skull, and (2) they are lined by an extensive area of mucous epithelium that connects to the nasal cavities. The mucous secretions are released into the nasal cavities, and the ciliated epithelium passes the mucus back toward the throat, where it is eventually swallowed. Incoming air is humidified and warmed as it flows across this carpet of mucus, and foreign particles, such as dust and bacteria, become trapped in the sticky mucus and swallowed. This mechanism helps protect more delicate portions of the respiratory tract.

The Mandible.   The broad **mandible** is the bone of the lower jaw. It forms a broad, horizontal curve with vertical processes at either end. The more posterior **condylar process** ends at the *mandibular condyle*, a smoothly curved surface that articulates with the mandibular fossa of the temporal bone on that side. This articulation is quite mobile, and the disadvantage of such mobility is that the jaw can easily be dislocated. The anterior **coronoid** (kō-RŌ-noyd) **process** is the attachment point for the *temporalis muscle*, a powerful muscle that closes the jaws.

The Hyoid Bone

The small, U-shaped hyoid bone hangs below the skull, suspended by ligaments from the styloid processes of the temporal bones. The hyoid (1) serves as a base for muscles associated with the tongue and *larynx* (voicebox) and (2) supports and stabilizes the position of the larynx.

✓ During baseball practice, a ball hits Casey in the eye, fracturing the bones directly above and below the orbit. Which bones were broken?

✓ What are the functions of the paranasal sinuses?

✓ Why would a fracture of the coronoid process of the mandible make it difficult to close the mouth?

✓ What symptoms would you expect to see in a person suffering from a fractured hyoid bone?

The Skulls of Infants and Children

Many centers of ossification are involved in the formation of the skull. As the fetus develops, the individual centers begin to fuse. This fusion produces a smaller number of composite bones. For example, the sphenoid begins as 14 separate ossification centers but ends as just one. At birth, the fusion has yet to be completed, and there are two frontal bones, four occipital bones, and several sphenoid and temporal elements.

The skull organizes around the developing brain, and as the time of birth approaches, the brain enlarges rapidly. Although the bones of the skull are also growing, they fail to keep pace, and at birth the cranial bones are connected by areas of fibrous connective tissue known as **fontanels** (fon-tah-NELZ). The fontanels, or "soft spots," are quite flexible and permit distortion of the skull without damage. Such distortion normally occurs during delivery and eases the passage of the infant along the birth canal. Figure 6-10• shows the prominent fontanels and the appearance of the skull at birth.

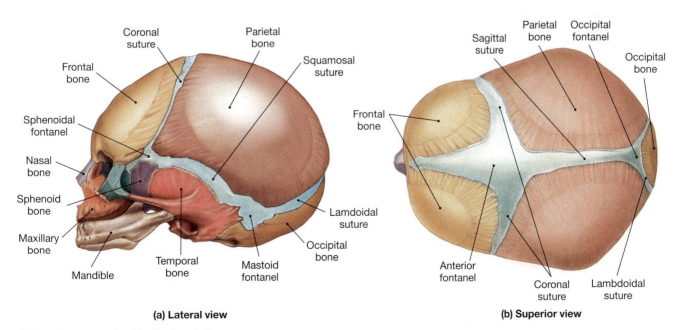

(a) Lateral view

(b) Superior view

•**FIGURE 6-10   The Skull of an Infant**
Infant skulls contain more individual bones than adult skulls. Many of these bones eventually fuse to create the adult skull. The flat bones of the skull are separated by areas of fibrous connective tissue called fontanels, which allow for cranial expansion and distortion during birth. By about age 4, these areas disappear, and skull growth is completed. **(a)** A lateral view. **(b)** A superior view.

The Neck and Trunk

The rest of the axial skeleton is subdivided on the basis of vertebral structure, as shown in Figure 6-11•. The **cervical region** of the vertebral column consists of the seven **cervical vertebrae** of the neck (abbreviated as C_1 to C_7). The cervical region begins at the articulation of C_1 with the occipital condyles of the skull and extends inferiorly to the articulation of C_7 with the first thoracic vertebra. The **thoracic region** consists of the 12 **thoracic vertebrae** (T_1 to T_{12}), each of which articulates with one or more pairs of ribs. The **lumbar region** contains the five **lumbar vertebrae** (L_1 to L_5). The first lumbar vertebra articulates with T_{12}, and the fifth lumbar vertebra articulates with the **sacrum** (SĀ-krum). The sacrum is a single bone formed by the fusion of the five embryonic vertebrae of the **sacral region**. The **coccygeal region** is made up of the small **coccyx** (KOK-siks), which also consists of fused vertebrae. The total length of the adult vertebral column averages 71 cm (28 in.).

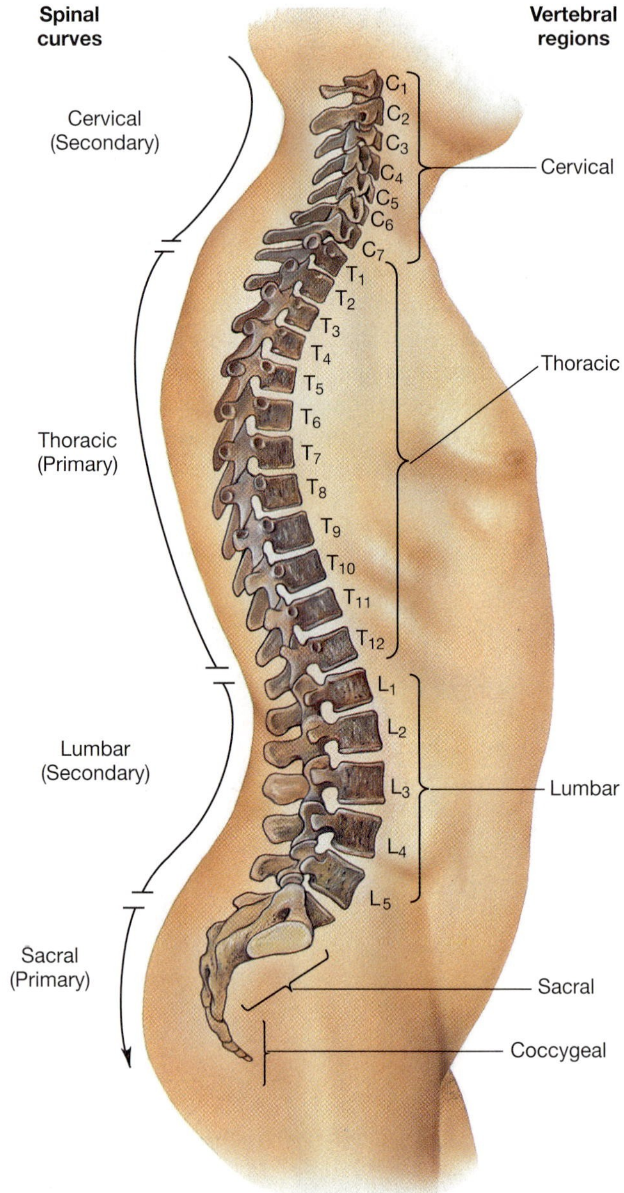

Spinal Curvature

The vertebrae do not form a straight and rigid structure. A side view of the spinal column reveals four **spinal curves** (Figure 6-11•). The *thoracic* and *sacral curves* are called **primary curves** because they appear late in fetal development, as the thoracic and abdominal organs enlarge. The *cervical* and *lumbar curves*, known as **secondary curves**, do not appear until months after birth. The cervical curve develops as the infant learns to balance the head upright, and the lumbar curve develops with the ability to stand. When standing, the weight of the body must be transmitted through the spinal column to the pelvic girdle and ultimately to the legs. Yet most of the body weight lies in front of the spinal column. The secondary curves bring that weight in line with the body axis. All four spinal curves are fully developed by the time a child is 10 years old.

Several abnormal distortions of spinal curvature may appear during childhood and adolescence. Examples are *kyphosis* (kī-FŌ-sis; exaggerated thoracic curvature), *lordosis* (lor-DŌ-sis; exaggerated lumbar curvature), and *scoliosis* (skō-lē-Ō-sis; an abnormal lateral curvature).

Vertebral Anatomy

Figure 6-12• shows representative vertebrae from different regions of the vertebral column. A comparison of these vertebrae reveals a large number of similar features. The more massive, weight-bearing portion of a vertebra is called the **body**. Extending posteriorly from the sides of the vertebral body are the **pedicles** (PE-di-kls). **Transverse processes** projecting laterally or dorsolaterally from the pedicles serve as sites for muscle attachment. The pedicle on each side supports a **lamina**, which unites with the lamina of the opposite side to form the **spinous process**, or *spinal process*. The spinous processes form the bumps that can be felt along the midline of your back. Like the transverse processes, *articular processes* arise at the junction between the pedicles and laminae. The articular processes of successive vertebrae contact one another at the **articular facets**.

The pedicles and laminae create the **vertebral arch**, which forms the lateral and posterior walls of the **vertebral foramen** (plural, *foramina*). The vertebral foramen encloses a portion of the **vertebral canal**, which

Spinal curves

Cervical (Secondary)

Thoracic (Primary)

Lumbar (Secondary)

Sacral (Primary)

Vertebral regions

C_1
C_2
C_3
C_4
C_5
C_6
C_7 — Cervical

T_1
T_2
T_3
T_4
T_5
T_6
T_7 — Thoracic
T_8
T_9
T_{10}
T_{11}
T_{12}

L_1
L_2
L_3 — Lumbar
L_4
L_5

— Sacral

— Coccygeal

•**FIGURE 6-11   The Vertebral Column**
The major divisions of the vertebral column, showing the four spinal curves.

•FIGURE 6-12   Typical Vertebrae of the
Cervical, Thoracic, and Lumbar Regions
Each vertebra is shown in superior view.

contains the spinal cord. **Intervertebral foramina** between successive vertebrae permit the passage of nerves running to or from the enclosed spinal cord.

Adjacent vertebrae are connected by longitudinal ligaments. The bony faces of the vertebral bodies usually do not contact one another, because an **intervertebral disc** of fibrocartilage lies between them. Intervertebral discs are not found in the sacrum and coccyx, where the vertebrae have fused, or between the first and second cervical vertebrae.

An intervertebral disc consists of an extensive region of fibrocartilage that surrounds a soft, gelatinous mass. Intervertebral discs act as shock absorbers, compressing and distorting when stressed. This change prevents bone-to-bone contact that might damage the vertebrae or jolt the spinal cord and brain. These discs make a significant contribution to an individual's height; they account for roughly one-quarter of the length of the spinal column above the sacrum. Part of the loss in height that accompanies aging results from the decreasing size and resiliency of intervertebral discs.

Although all vertebrae have many similar characteristics, some regional differences reflect differences in function. The structural differences among the vertebrae are discussed next.

The Cervical Vertebrae

The seven cervical vertebrae extend from the head to the thorax. A typical cervical vertebra is illustrated in Figure 6-12a•. Notice that the body of the vertebra is relatively small compared with the size of the vertebral foramen. At this level the spinal cord still contains most of the axons that connect the brain to the rest of the body. From the first thoracic vertebra to the sacrum, the diameter of the spinal cord decreases, and so does the size of the vertebral foramen. At the same time, the vertebral bodies gradually enlarge, because they must bear more weight.

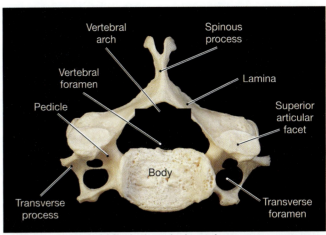

(a) Typical cervical vertebra

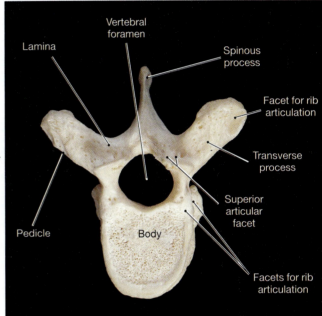

(b) Typical thoracic vertebra

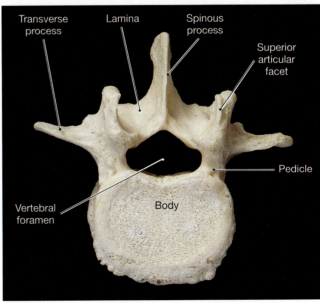

(c) Typical lumbar vertebra

6

Distinctive features of a typical cervical vertebra include: (1) an oval, concave vertebral body; (2) a relatively large vertebral foramen; (3) a stumpy spinous process, usually with a notched tip; and (4) round **transverse foramina** within the transverse processes. These foramina protect important blood vessels supplying the brain.

The first two vertebrae have unique characteristics that allow for specialized movements. The **atlas** (C_1) holds up the head, articulating with the occipital condyles of the skull. It is named after Atlas, the figure in Greek mythology who held up the world. The articulation between the occipital condyles and the atlas permits nodding (as when indicating "yes") but prevents twisting. The atlas in turn forms a pivot joint with the **axis** (C_2) through a projection on the axis called the **odontoid process**, or *dens* (*denz*; tooth). This articulation, which permits rotation (as when shaking the head to indicate "no"), is shown in Figure 6-13•.

The Thoracic Vertebrae

There are 12 thoracic vertebrae (Figure 6-12b•). Distinctive features of a thoracic vertebra include: (1) a characteristic heart-shaped body that is more massive than that of a cervical vertebra; (2) a large, slender spinous process that points inferiorly; and (3) articular surfaces on the body and, in most cases, on the transverse processes for articulation with one or more pairs of ribs.

The Lumbar Vertebrae

The distinctive features of lumbar vertebrae (Figure 6-12c•) include: (1) a vertebral body that is thicker and more oval than that of a thoracic vertebra; (2) a relatively massive, stumpy spinous process that projects posteriorly, providing surface area for the attachment of the lower back muscles; and (3) bladelike transverse processes that lack articulations for ribs.

The lumbar vertebrae are the most massive and least mobile, for they support most of the body weight. As you increase the weight on the vertebrae, the intervertebral discs become increasingly important as shock absorbers. The lumbar discs, which are subjected to the most pressure, are the thickest of all. The lumbar articulations restrict the stresses on the discs by limiting vertebral motion.

Shortly after physical maturity is reached, the gelatinous mass within each disc begins to degenerate, and the "cushion" becomes less effective. Over the same period, the outer fibrocartilage loses its elasticity. If the stresses are sufficient, the inner mass may break through the surrounding fibrocartilage and protrude beyond the intervertebral space. This condition, called a *herniated disc*, further reduces disc function. The term *slipped disc* is often used to describe this problem, although the disc does not actually slip.

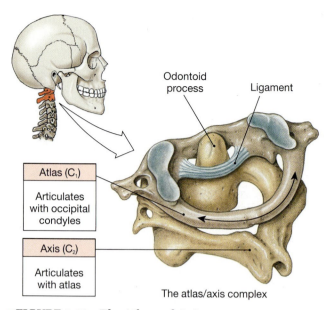

•**FIGURE 6-13   The Atlas and Axis**
The articulation between the atlas (C_1) and the axis (C_2).

The Sacrum and Coccyx

The sacrum consists of the fused elements of five sacral vertebrae. This structure protects the reproductive, digestive, and excretory organs and attaches the axial skeleton to the appendicular skeleton by articulation with the pelvic girdle. The broad surface area of the sacrum provides an extensive area for the attachment of muscles, especially those responsible for leg movement. Figure 6-14• shows the posterior and anterior surfaces of the sacrum.

Because the sacrum resembles a triangle, the narrow, caudal portion is called the **apex**, and the broad superior surface is the **base**. The **articular processes** form articulations with the last lumbar vertebra. The **sacral canal** begins between those processes and extends the length of the sacrum. Nerves and membranes that line the vertebral canal in the spinal cord continue into the sacral canal. A prominent bulge at the anterior tip of the base, the **sacral promontory**, is an important landmark during pelvic examinations and during labor and delivery.

Before birth, five vertebrae fuse to form the sacrum, and their spinal processes form a series of elevations along the *median sacral crest*. The inferior end of the sacral canal is covered by connective tissues. On either side of the sacrum, the **sacral foramina** penetrate the sacrum. The intervertebral foramina, now enclosed by the fused sacral bones, open into the sacral foramina. Along its lateral border, a thickened, flattened area marks the *sacroiliac joint*, the site of articulation with the *coxae* (hip bones).

The coccyx provides an attachment site for a muscle that closes the anal opening. The 3–5 (most often 4)

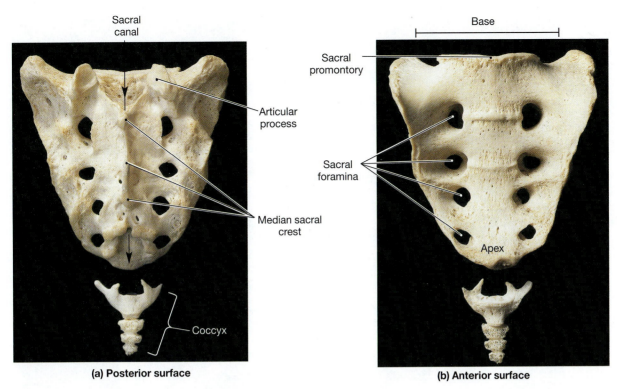

(a) Posterior surface

(b) Anterior surface

•**FIGURE 6-14   The Sacrum and Coccyx**

coccygeal vertebrae do not complete their fusion until late in adulthood. In elderly people, the coccyx may also fuse with the sacrum.

The Thorax

The skeleton of the chest, or thorax, consists of the thoracic vertebrae, the ribs, and the sternum. The ribs and the sternum form the thoracic cage, or rib cage, and establish the contours of the thoracic cavity. The thoracic cage protects the heart, lungs, and other internal organs and serves as a base for muscles involved with respiration.

The Ribs and Sternum.   Ribs, or *costal bones*, are elongate, flattened bones that originate on or between the thoracic vertebrae and end in the wall of the thoracic cavity. There are 12 pairs of ribs (Figure 6-15•). The first seven pairs are called **true ribs**. These ribs reach the anterior body wall and are connected to the sternum by separate cartilaginous extensions, the **costal cartilages**. Ribs 8–12 are called the **false ribs**, because they do not attach directly to the sternum. The costal cartilages of ribs 8–10 fuse together. This fused cartilage merges with the costal cartilage of rib 7 before it reaches the sternum. The last two pairs of ribs are called **floating ribs**, because they have no connection with the sternum.

The adult sternum has three parts. The broad, triangular **manubrium** (ma-NŪ-brē-um) articulates with the

clavicles of the appendicular skeleton and with the cartilages of the first pair of ribs. The *jugular notch* is the shallow indentation on the superior surface of the manubrium. The elongate **body** ends at the slender **xiphoid** (ZĪ-foyd) **process**. Ossification of the sternum begins at six to ten different centers, and fusion is not completed until at least age 25. The xiphoid process is usually the last of the sternal components to ossify and fuse. Impact or strong pressure can drive it into the liver, causing severe damage. Cardiopulmonary resuscitation (CPR) training strongly emphasizes the proper positioning of the hand to reduce the chances of breaking the xiphoid process or ribs.

With their complex musculature, dual articulations at the vertebrae, and flexible connection to the sternum, the ribs are quite mobile. Because they are curved, their movements affect both the width and the depth of the thoracic cage, increasing or decreasing its volume.

✓ Joe suffered a hairline fracture at the base of the odontoid process. Which bone is fractured, and where would you find it?

✓ Improper administration of CPR (cardiopulmonary resuscitation) could result in a fracture of which bone?

✓ In adults, five large vertebrae fuse to form what single structure?

6

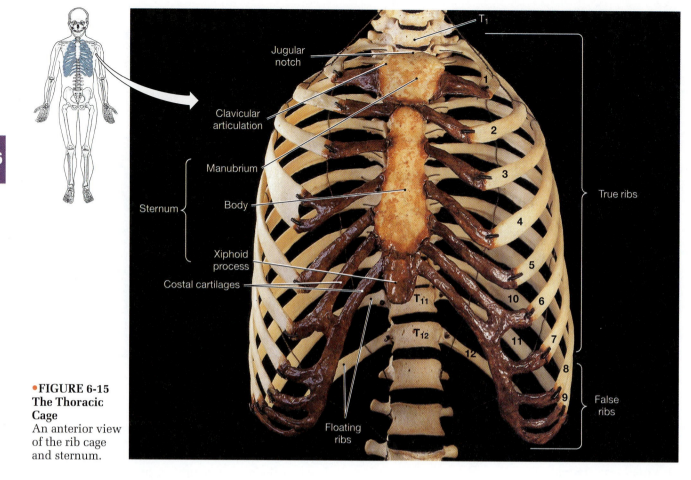

Jugular
notch

Clavicular
articulation

Manubrium

Sternum

Body

Xiphoid
process

Costal cartilages

T₁

1

2

3

4

5

10   6

T₁₁

T₁₂

11   7

12

8

9

True ribs

False
ribs

Floating
ribs

●**FIGURE 6-15**
**The Thoracic
Cage**
An anterior view
of the rib cage
and sternum.

THE APPENDICULAR DIVISION

The appendicular skeleton includes the bones of the upper and lower limbs and the pectoral and pelvic girdles that connect the limbs to the trunk.

The Pectoral Girdle

Each upper limb articulates with the trunk at the pectoral girdle, or *shoulder girdle*. The pectoral girdle consists of a broad, flat **scapula** (*shoulder blade*) and the slender, curving **clavicle** (*collarbone*). The clavicle articulates with the manubrium of the sternum; this is the *only* direct connection between the pectoral girdle and the axial skeleton. Skeletal muscles support and position the scapula, which has no bony or ligamentous bonds to the thoracic cage.

Movements of the clavicle and scapula position the shoulder joint and provide a base for arm movement. Once the shoulder joint is in position, muscles that originate on the pectoral girdle help to move the arm. The surfaces of the scapula and clavicle are therefore extremely important as sites for muscle attachment.

The Clavicle

The S-shaped clavicle bone, shown in Figure 6-16●, articulates with the manubrium component of the sternum and the *acromion* of the scapula. The smooth superior surface of the clavicle lies just beneath the skin. The rough inferior surface of the *acromial end* is marked by prominent lines and tubercles that indicate the attachment sites for muscles and ligaments.

The clavicle is the only firm attachment between the axial skeleton and the shoulder girdle and upper limb. It is small and light, and its curved shape makes it relatively fragile. As a result, clavicular fractures are very common injuries.

The clavicle limits the range of motion of the shoulder. People with inherited developmental abnormalities that reduce or eliminate the clavicles have completely mobile scapulae and can swing their shoulders medially almost far enough to meet in front of the sternum.

The Scapula

Figure 6-17● details the anatomy of the right scapula. Its anterior face forms a broad triangle bounded by the **superior**, **medial**, and **lateral borders**. Muscles that po-

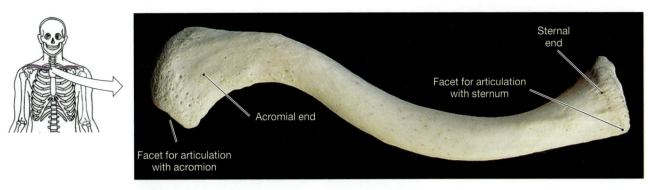

Sternal
end

Facet for articulation
with sternum

Acromial end

Facet for articulation
with acromion

6

•**FIGURE 6-16   The Clavicle**
A superior view of the right clavicle.

sition the scapula attach along these edges. The inter-section of the lateral and superior borders thickens into the shallow, cup-shaped **glenoid cavity**, or *glenoid fossa* (FOS-sah). ∞ *p. 130* At the glenoid cavity, the scapula articulates with the proximal end of the humerus to form the *shoulder joint*. The bone surrounding the gle-

noid cavity attaches to the body of the scapula at the *scapular neck*.

Figure 6-17b• shows a lateral view of the scapula and the two large processes that extend over the glenoid fossa. The smaller, anterior projection is the **coracoid** (kō-RA-koyd) **process**. The **acromion** (a-KRŌ-mē-on) is

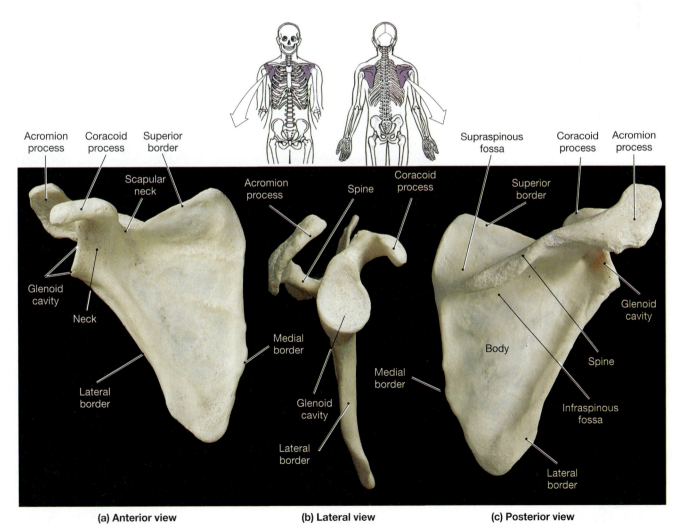

Acromion
process

Coracoid
process

Superior
border

Scapular
neck

Acromion
process

Spine

Coracoid
process

Supraspinous
fossa

Coracoid
process

Acromion
process

Superior
border

Glenoid
cavity

Neck

Medial
border

Glenoid
cavity

Medial
border

Body

Glenoid
cavity

Spine

Lateral
border

Lateral
border

Infraspinous
fossa

Lateral
border

(a) Anterior view

(b) Lateral view

(c) Posterior view

•**FIGURE 6-17   The Scapula**
Major landmarks on the right scapula.

the larger, posterior projection. If you run your fingers along the superior surface of the shoulder joint, you will feel this process. The acromion articulates with the distal end of the clavicle.

The **scapular spine** divides the posterior surface of the scapula into two regions (Figure 6-17c•). The area superior to the spine is the **supraspinous fossa** (*supra-*, above); the *supraspinatus muscle* attaches here. The region below the spine is the **infraspinous fossa** (*infra-*, beneath), home of the *infraspinatus muscle*. Both muscles are attached to the humerus, the proximal bone of the upper limb.

The Upper Limb

The upper limb consists of the arm and forearm. The arm contains a single bone, the **humerus**, which extends from the scapula to the elbow. At its proximal end, the round **head** of the humerus articulates with the scapula. At its distal end, it articulates with the bones of the forearm, the *radius* and *ulna*.

The Humerus

Figure 6-18• illustrates the anatomy of the humerus. The prominent **greater tubercle**, near the rounded head, establishes the contour of the shoulder. The **lesser tubercle** lies more anteriorly, separated from the greater tubercle by a deep groove. Muscles are attached to both tubercles, and a large tendon runs along the groove. The *anatomical neck* lies between the tubercles and below the surface of the head. Distal to the tubercles, the narrow *surgical neck* is the region of growing bone. It earned its name by being a common fracture site.

The proximal shaft of the humerus is round in section. The elevated **deltoid tuberosity** that runs along the lateral border of the shaft is named after the *deltoid muscle* that attaches to it.

Distally, the posterior surface of the shaft flattens and the humerus expands to either side, forming a broad triangle. **Medial** and **lateral epicondyles** project to either side, providing additional surface area for muscle attachment, and the smooth, articular **condyle** dominates the inferior surface of the humerus.

A low ridge crosses the condyle, dividing it into two distinct regions. The **trochlea** is the large medial portion shaped like a spool or pulley (*trochlea* is Latin for pulley). The trochlea extends from the base of the **coronoid** (KŌR-ō-noyd; *corona*, crown) **fossa** on the anterior surface to the **olecranon fossa** on the poste-

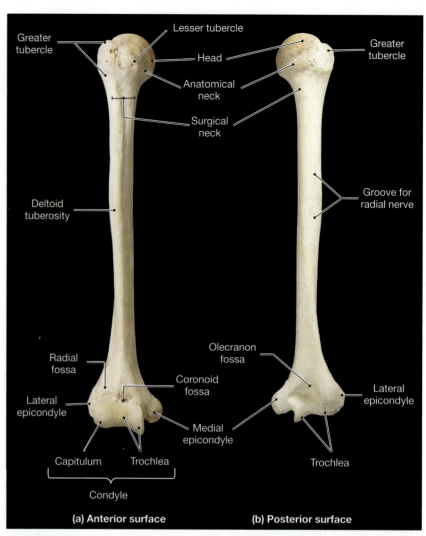

•**FIGURE 6-18   The Humerus**
Major landmarks on the right humerus.

rior surface. These depressions accept projections from the surface of the ulna as the elbow reaches its limits of motion. The **capitulum** forms the lateral region of the condyle. A shallow **radial fossa** proximal to the capitulum accommodates a small projection on the radius.

The Radius and Ulna

The **radius** and **ulna** are the bones of the forearm. In the anatomical position, the radius lies along the lateral (thumb) side of the forearm. The ulna forms the medial support of the forearm. The structure of these bones is shown in Figure 6-19a•.

The elbow is formed by the superior projection of the ulna, the **olecranon** (ō-LEK-ra-non) **process**. On its anterior surface, the **trochlear notch** articulates with the trochlea of the humerus to form the elbow joint. The olecranon process forms the superior lip of the notch, and the **coronoid process** provides a prominent inferior margin. When the elbow joint is fully extended, the arm and

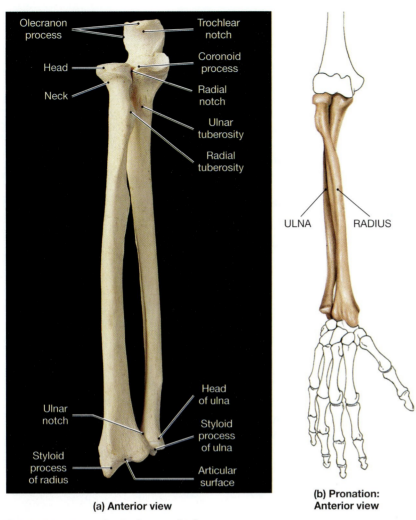

(a) Anterior view

(b) Pronation: Anterior view

•**FIGURE 6-19   The Radius and Ulna**
(a) An anterior view. **(b)** Notice the changes that occur during pronation.

tends from the tuberosity to the head of the radius. The disc-shaped head articulates with the capitulum of the humerus at the elbow joint and with the ulna at the radial notch. This proximal articulation with the ulna allows the radius to roll across the ulna, rotating the palm in a movement known as *pronation* (Figure 6-19b•). The reverse movement, which returns the forearm to the anatomical position, is called *supination*.

The Wrist and Hand

There are 27 bones in the hand, supporting the wrist, palm, and fingers (Figure 6-20•). The eight bones of the wrist, or *carpus*, form two rows. There are four proximal **carpal bones**: (1) the *scaphoid bone*, (2) the *lunate bone*, (3) the *triangular bone* (or *triquetral bone*), and (4) the *pisiform* (PI-si-form) *bone*. There are also four distal carpal bones: (1) the *trapezium*, (2) the *trapezoid bone*, (3) the *capitate bone*, and (4) the *hamate bone*. A fibrous capsule, reinforced by broad ligaments, surrounds the wrist complex and stabilizes the positions of the individual carpal bones.

Five **metacarpal** (met-a-KAR-pal) **bones** articulate with the distal carpal bones and form the palm of the hand. The metacarpal bones in turn articulate with the finger bones, or **phalanges** (fa-LAN-jēz). Each hand has 14 phalangeal bones. Four of the fingers contain three phalanges each (proximal, middle, and distal), but the thumb, or **pollex**, has only two (proximal and distal) phalanges.

✓ Why would a broken clavicle affect the mobility of the scapula?

✓ The rounded projections on either side of the elbow are parts of which bone?

forearm form a straight line, and the olecranon process swings into the olecranon fossa on the posterior face of the humerus. A muscle that attaches to the ulna at the **ulnar tuberosity** swings the forearm toward the arm, a movement called *flexion*. When the elbow is fully bent, the coronoid process projects into the coronoid fossa on the anterior surface of the humerus.

Lateral to the coronoid process, a smooth **radial notch** accommodates the head of the radius. A fibrous sheet connects the lateral margin of the ulna to the radius along its length. The ulnar shaft ends at a disc-shaped head whose posterior margin supports a short **styloid process**. The distal end of the ulna is separated from the wrist joint by a pad of cartilage, and only the expansive distal portion of the radius participates in the wrist joint. The styloid process of the radius assists in the stabilization of the joint by preventing lateral movement of the bones of the wrist (*carpal bones*).

Near the elbow, a prominent **radial tuberosity** marks the attachment site of another powerful muscle, the *biceps brachii*, that flexes the forearm. A narrow *neck* ex-

The Pelvic Girdle

The pelvic girdle articulates with the thigh bones. Because of the stresses involved in weight bearing and locomotion, the bones of the pelvic girdle and lower limbs are more massive than those of the pectoral complex. The pelvic girdle is also much more firmly attached to the axial skeleton. Dorsally, the two halves of the pelvic girdle contact the lateral surfaces of the sacrum. Ventrally, the pelvic elements are interconnected by a fibrocartilage pad.

6

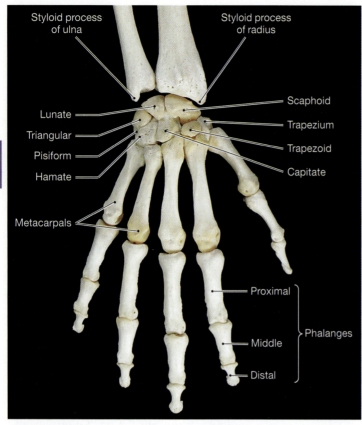

Styloid process of ulna

Styloid process of radius

Lunate

Triangular

Pisiform

Hamate

Metacarpals

Scaphoid

Trapezium

Trapezoid

Capitate

Proximal

Middle

Distal

Phalanges

•FIGURE 6-20   **Bones of the Wrist and Hand**
A posterior view.

The pelvic girdle consists of two large hip bones, or **coxae** (Figure 6-21a•). Each coxa forms through the fusion of three bones, an **ilium** (IL-ē-um), an **ischium** (IS-kē-um), and a **pubis** (PŪ-bis). Dorsally the hipbones articulate with the sacrum at the **sacroiliac joint**. Ventrally the coxae are connected at the *pubic symphysis*. At the hip joint on either side, the head of the femur (thighbone) articulates with the curved surface of the **acetabulum** (a-se-TAB-ū-lum; *acetabulum*, a vinegar cup) (Figure 6-21b•).

The Coxa

The ilium is the most superior and largest coxal bone. Above the acetabulum, the ilium forms a broad, curved surface that provides an extensive area for the attachment of muscles, tendons, and ligaments. The superior margin of the ilium, the **iliac crest**, marks the sites of attachments of both ligaments and muscles. Near the superior and posterior margin of the acetabulum, the ilium fuses with the ischium. The roughened inferior surface of the ischium supports the body's weight when sitting.

The fusion of a narrow branch of the ischium with a branch of the pubis completes the encirclement of the **obturator** (OB-tū-rā-tor) **foramen**. This space is closed by a sheet of collagen fibers whose inner and outer surfaces provide a firm base for the attachment of muscles and visceral structures.

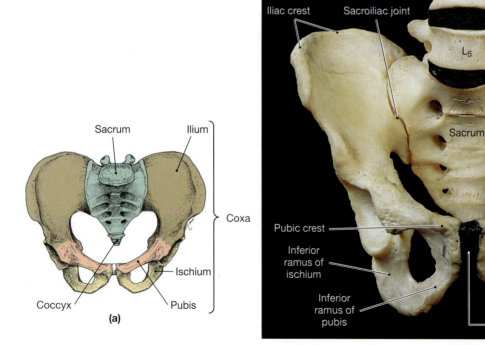

Sacrum

Ilium

Coxa

Ischium

Coccyx

Pubis

(a)

Iliac crest

Sacroiliac joint

L₅

Sacrum

Pubic crest

Inferior ramus of ischium

Inferior ramus of pubis

Acetabulum

Obturator foramen

Pubic symphysis

(b) Anterior view

•FIGURE 6-21   **The Pelvis**
(a) The components of the pelvis. **(b)** An anterior view of the pelvis of an adult male.

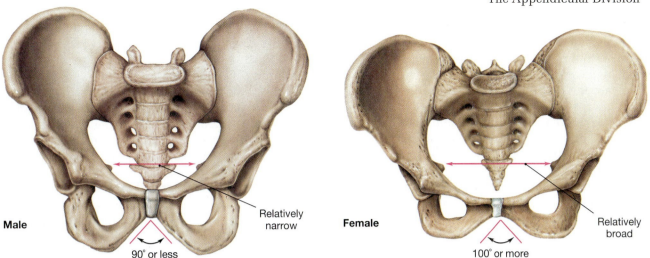

Male

Relatively narrow

90° or less

Female

Relatively broad

100° or more

•**FIGURE 6-22   Gender Differences in the Anatomy of the Pelvis**

6

The anterior and medial surface of the pubis contains a roughened area that marks the **pubic symphysis**, an articulation with the pubis of the opposite side. The pubic symphysis limits movement between the two pubic bones.

The Pelvis

The **pelvis** consists of the coxae, the sacrum, and the coccyx (see Figure 6-21a•). It is thus a composite structure that includes portions of both the appendicular and axial skeletons. An extensive network of ligaments connects the lateral borders of the sacrum with the iliac crests, the inferior surfaces of the ischia, and the superior border of the pubic bones. Other ligaments tie the ilia to the posterior lumbar vertebrae. These interconnections increase the structural stability of the pelvis.

The shape of the pelvis of a female is somewhat different from that of a male (Figure 6-22•). Some of the differences are the result of variations in body size and muscle mass. Others are adaptations for childbearing and are necessary to support the weight of the developing fetus and to ease passage of the newborn through the pelvis during delivery.

The Lower Limb

The skeleton of the lower limb includes (1) the *femur*, the bone of the thigh; (2) the *tibia* and *fibula*, the bones of the leg; and (3) the bones of the ankle and foot.

The Femur

The **femur**, or *thighbone*, is the longest, heaviest, and strongest bone in the body

(Figure 6-23•). Distally, the femur articulates with the tibia of the leg at the knee joint. The rounded epiphysis, or head, of the femur articulates with the pelvis at the acetabulum. The **greater trochanter** arises lateral to the juncture of the neck and the shaft; the **lesser trochanter** originates along the crest near the medial surface of the

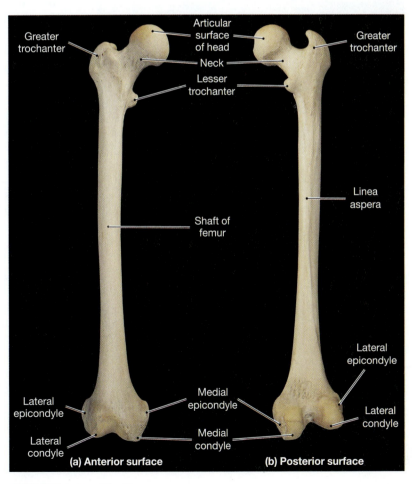

Greater trochanter

Articular surface of head

Neck

Lesser trochanter

Greater trochanter

Linea aspera

Shaft of femur

Lateral epicondyle

Lateral epicondyle

Medial epicondyle

Lateral condyle

Lateral condyle

Medial condyle

(a) Anterior surface

(b) Posterior surface

•**FIGURE 6-23   The Femur**
Bone markings on the right femur.

femur. Both trochanters develop where large tendons attach to the femoral shaft. On the posterior surface of the femur, a stout ridge, the **linea aspera**, marks the attachment of powerful muscles that pull the shaft of the femur toward the midline, a movement called *adduction* (*ad-*, toward + *duco*, to lead).

The proximal femoral shaft is round in cross section. Moving distally, the shaft becomes more flattened and ends in two large **epicondyles** (**lateral** and **medial**). The inferior surfaces of the epicondyles form the *lateral* and *medial condyles*. The articular condyles merge anteriorly to produce an articular surface with elevated lateral borders. This is the **patellar surface** over which the **patella** (*kneecap*) glides. The patella bone forms within the tendon of the *quadriceps femoris*, a group of muscles that straighten the knee.

The Tibia and Fibula

Figure 6-24● shows the structure of the tibia and fibula. The condyles of the femur articulate with the *lateral* and *medial condyles* of the **tibia**, or *shinbone*,

the large medial bone of the leg. A ligament from the patella attaches to the **tibial tuberosity** just below the knee joint.

A projecting **anterior crest** extends almost the entire length of the anterior surface. The tibia broadens at its distal end into a large process, the **medial malleolus** (ma-LĒ-ō-lus; *malleolus*, hammer). The inferior surface of the tibia forms a joint with the proximal bone of the ankle; the medial malleolus provides medial support for the ankle.

The slender **fibula** parallels the lateral border of the tibia. The fibular **head** articulates along the lateral margin of the tibia, inferior and slightly posterior to the lateral condyle. The fibula does not participate in the knee joint, and it does not bear weight. However, it is an important surface for muscle attachment, and the distal **lateral malleolus** provides lateral stability to the ankle. A fibrous membrane extending between the two bones helps stabilize their relative positions and provides additional surface area for muscle attachment.

The Ankle and Foot

The ankle, or *tarsus*, includes seven separate **tarsal bones**: (1) the *talus*, (2) the *calcaneus*, (3) the *navicular bone*, (4) the *cuboid bone*, and (5–7) the *first, second,* and *third cuneiform bones* (Figure 6-25●). Only the proximal tarsal bone, the **talus**, articulates with the tibia and fibula. The talus then passes the weight to the ground via other bones of the foot.

When you are standing normally, most of your weight is transmitted to the ground through the talus to the large **calcaneus** (kal-KĀ-nē-us), or *heel bone*. The posterior projection of the calcaneus receives the composite **calcanean tendon**, or *Achilles tendon*, of the calf muscles that raise the heel and depress the sole (plantar flexion). The rest of the body weight is passed through the cuboid bone and cuneiform bones to the **metatarsal bones**, which support the sole of the foot.

The basic organizational pattern at the metatarsals and phalanges of the foot resembles that of the hand. The metatarsals are numbered I to V from medial to lateral, and their distal ends form the ball of the foot. The same number of phalanges present in the thumb (2) and fingers (3 each) also make up the great toe, or **hallux**, and other toes.

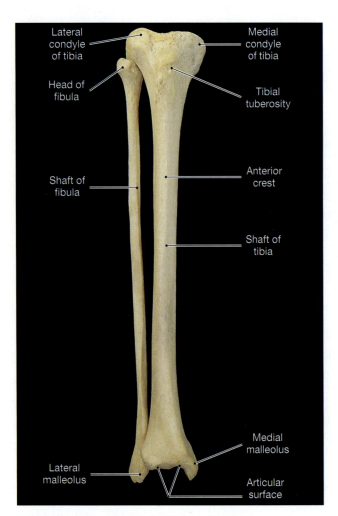

●**FIGURE 6-24   The Right Tibia and Fibula**
An anterior view.

✓ Which three bones make up the coxa?

✓ The fibula does not participate in the knee joint nor does it bear weight, but when it is fractured, walking is difficult. Why?

✓ While jumping off the back steps at his house, 10-year-old Joey lands on his right heel and breaks his foot. Which foot bone is most likely broken?

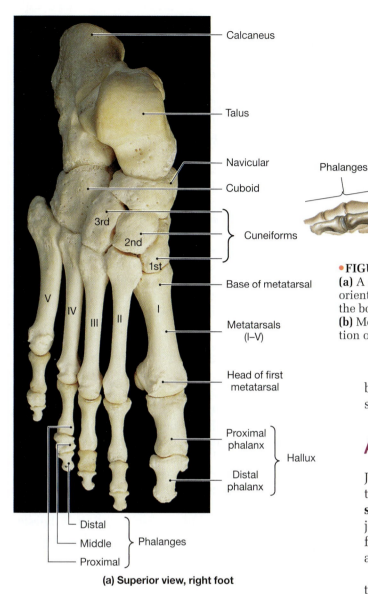

- Calcaneus
- Talus
- Navicular
- Cuboid
- 3rd
- 2nd
- 1st
- } Cuneiforms
- V
- IV
- III
- II
- I
- Base of metatarsal
- Metatarsals (I–V)
- Head of first metatarsal
- Proximal phalanx
- Distal phalanx
- } Hallux
- Distal
- Middle } Phalanges
- Proximal

(a) Superior view, right foot

Tarsal bones — Tibia
Cuneiform bone
Navicular — Talus
Metatarsal bones
Phalanges — 1st
Calcaneus

(b) Medial view, right foot

• **FIGURE 6-25   The Bones of the Ankle and Foot**
(a) A superior view of the bones of the right foot. Notice the orientation of the tarsal bones, which convey the weight of the body to the heel and the plantar surfaces of the foot. **(b)** Medial view, showing the relative positions and orientation of the tarsal and metatarsal bones.

ARTICULATIONS

Joints, or **articulations**, exist wherever two bones meet. The function of each joint depends on its anatomy. Each joint reflects a workable compromise between the need for strength and the need for mobility. When movement is not required, or when relative movement could actually be dangerous, joints can be very strong. For example, joints such as the sutures of the skull are so intricate and extensive that they lock the elements together as if they were a single bone. This rigidity is crucial because the sutures weld the cranium into a solid case that encloses and protects the delicate tissues of the brain. At other joints, movement is more important than strength. The interconnections can then be less extensive and the joint correspondingly weaker. For example, the articulation at the shoulder permits a range of arm movement that is limited more by the surrounding muscles than

by joint structure. The joint itself is relatively weak, and shoulder injuries are rather common.

A Classification of Joints

Joints can be classified according to the range of motion they permit (Table 6-2). An immovable joint is a **synarthrosis** (sin-ar-THRŌ-sis; *syn-*, together + *arthros*, joint); a slightly movable joint is an **amphiarthrosis** (am-fē-ar-THRŌ-sis; *amphi-*, on both sides); and a freely movable joint is a **diarthrosis** (dī-ar-THRŌ-sis; *dia-*, through).

Subdivisions are further recognized within each of these three major categories. Synarthrotic or amphiarthrotic joints are classified according to the type of connective tissue binding them together, such as *fibrous* or *cartilaginous*. Diarthrotic joints, however, are categorized according to the types, or ranges, of movement permitted.

Immovable Joints (Synarthroses)

At a synarthrosis, the bony edges are quite close together and may even interlock. A **suture** (*sutura*, a sewing together) is a synarthrotic joint between the bones of the skull. The edges of the bones are interlocked and bound together by dense connective tissue. In another synarthrosis, called a **gomphosis** (gom-FŌ-sis; *gomphosis*, a bolting together), a ligament binds each tooth in the mouth within a bony socket (*alveolus*).

An epiphyseal plate also represents an articulation between two bones, even though the two are part of the same skeletal element. ∞ *p. 125* Such a rigid, cartilaginous connection characterizes a **synchondrosis** (sin-kon-DRŌ-sis; *syn*, together + *chondros*, cartilage).

6

TABLE 6-2   A Functional Classification of Articulations

Functional Category	Structural Category	Description	Example
Synarthrosis (no movement)	**Fibrous**		
	Suture	Fibrous connections plus interdigitation	Between the bones of the skull
	Gomphosis	Fibrous connections plus insertion in alveolus	Between the teeth and jaws
	Cartilaginous		
	Synchondrosis	Interposition of cartilage plate	Epiphyseal plates
Amphiarthrosis (little movement)	**Fibrous**		
	Syndesmosis	Ligamentous connection	Between the tibia and fibula
	Cartilaginous		
	Symphysis	Connection by a fibrocartilage pad	Between right and left halves of pelvis; between adjacent vertebrae of spinal column
Diarthrosis (free movement)	**Synovial**	Complex joint bounded by joint capsule and containing synovial fluid	Numerous; subdivided by range of movement

Slightly Movable Joints (Amphiarthroses)

An amphiarthrosis permits very limited movement, and the bones are usually farther apart than they are at a synarthrosis. The bones may be connected by collagen fibers or cartilage. At a **syndesmosis** (sin-dez-MŌ-sis; *desmos*, a band or ligament), they are connected by a ligament. Examples are the articulations between the two bones of the leg, the tibia and fibula. At a **symphysis**, the bones are separated by a broad disc or pad of fibrocartilage. The articulations between the spinal vertebrae and the anterior connection between the two pelvic bones, or coxae, are examples of symphyses.

Freely Movable Joints (Diarthroses)

Diarthroses, or **synovial** (si-NŌ-vē-al) **joints**, permit a wide range of motion. The basic structure of a synovial joint was introduced in Chapter 4 in the discussion of synovial membranes. ∞ *p. 96* Figure 6-26a• shows the structure of a representative synovial joint.

Synovial joints are typically found at the ends of long bones, such as those of the arms and legs. Under normal conditions the bony surfaces do not contact one another, for they are covered with special **articular cartilages**. The joint is surrounded by a fibrous **joint capsule**, or *articular capsule*, and the inner surfaces of the joint cavity are lined with a synovial membrane. **Synovial fluid** diffuses across the synovial membrane and provides lubrication that reduces the friction between the moving surfaces in the joint.

In complex joints such as the knee, additional padding lies between the opposing articular surfaces. An example of such shock-absorbing, fibrocartilage pads are the **menisci** (men-IS-kē; *meniscus*, crescent), shown

in Figure 6-26b•. Also present in such joints are **fat pads**, which protect the articular cartilages and act as packing material. When the bones move, the fat pads fill in the spaces created as the joint cavity changes shape.

The joint capsule that surrounds the entire joint is continuous with the periostea of the articulating bones. In addition, **ligaments** joining bone to bone may be found on the outside or inside the joint capsule. Where a tendon or ligament rubs against other tissues, **bursae**, small pockets containing synovial fluid, form to reduce friction and act as shock absorbers. Bursae are characteristic of many synovial joints and may also appear around tendon sheaths, covering a bone, or within other connective tissues exposed to friction or pressure.

✳ DISLOCATIONS

The disruption or displacement of a joint due to trauma is a *dislocation*. In order for a joint to dislocate, the soft tissue of the joint capsule and ligaments must be stretched beyond the normal range of motion. Oftentimes, the ligaments are torn, allowing the bones of the joint to separate. Because of the associated soft tissue damage, dislocations can cause paralysis of the affected limb as the nerves and arteries leading to the extremity pass quite close to the joint and may be compressed or torn.

Dislocations are common in fingers, elbows, shoulders, hips, knees, and toes. Often, in addition to the dislocation, a fracture (broken bone) occurs at the time of injury.

The joints of the spine are at risk for dislocation, especially in high-energy accidents such as auto and motorcycle collisions, skiing injuries, and diving injuries. Spinal dislocations can be catastrophic as the spinal cord can be damaged when the dislocation occurs.

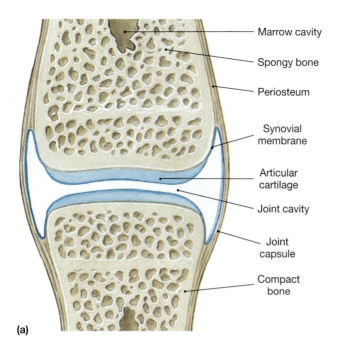

Marrow cavity

Spongy bone

Periosteum

Synovial membrane

Articular cartilage

Joint cavity

Joint capsule

Compact bone

(a)

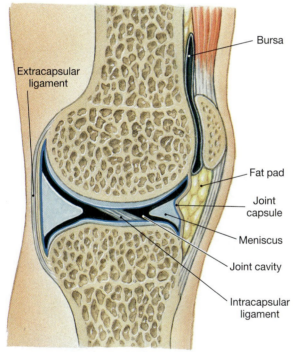

Extracapsular ligament

Bursa

Fat pad

Joint capsule

Meniscus

Joint cavity

Intracapsular ligament

(b)

•**FIGURE 6-26   The Structure of a Synovial Joint**
(a) A diagrammatic view of a simple articulation. **(b)** A sectional view of the knee joint.

It is essential for emergency personnel to carefully assess any potential dislocation to assure that the patient has an adequate pulse and neurological function distal to the injury. Also, some dislocations may result in the extremity's being deformed, making transporting the patient difficult. In these cases, it may be necessary to gently move the affected extremity back to its normal position. Dislocations, like broken bones, should be splinted to prevent undesired movement.

Articular Form and Function

In discussions of motion at synovial joints, phrases such as "bend the leg" or "raise the arm" are not sufficiently precise. Anatomists use descriptive terms that have specific meanings. We will consider these movements with regard to the basic categories of movement considered earlier.

Types of Movement

Gliding.   In **gliding**, two opposing surfaces slide past each other. Gliding occurs between articulating carpals and tarsals, and between the clavicles and sternum. The movement can occur in almost any direction, but the amount of movement is slight. Rotation is usually prevented by the capsule and associated ligaments.

Angular Motion.   Examples of angular motion are *flexion*, *extension*, *adduction*, and *abduction*. The description of each movement is based on reference to an individual in the anatomical position.

Flexion/Extension.   **Flexion** (FLEK-shun) can be defined as movement in the anterior-posterior plane that reduces the angle between the articulating elements. **Extension** occurs in the same plane, but it increases the angle between articulating elements (Figure 6-27a•). When you bring your head toward your chest, you flex the intervertebral joints of the neck. When you bend down to touch your toes, you flex the entire vertebral column. Extension reverses these movements.

Flexion at the shoulder or hip moves the limbs forward, whereas extension moves them back. Flexion of the wrist moves the palm forward, and extension moves it back. In each of these examples, extension can be continued past the anatomical position, in which case **hyperextension** occurs. You can also hyperextend the neck, a movement that enables you to gaze at the ceiling. Hyperextension of other joints is usually prevented by ligaments, bony processes, or soft tissues.

Abduction/Adduction.   **Abduction** (*ab-*, from) is movement *away from the midline of the body* in the frontal plane. For example, swinging the upper limb to the side is abduction of the limb (Figure 6-27b•). **Adduction** is movement *toward the midline of the body*. Adduction of the wrist moves the heel of the hand toward the body, whereas abduction moves it farther away. Spreading the fingers or toes apart abducts them, because they move *away* from a central digit (finger or toe), as in Figure 6-27c•. Bringing them together constitutes adduction. Abduction and adduction always refer to movements of the appendicular skeleton.

Circumduction.   A special type of angular motion, **circumduction** (*circum*, around), is shown in Figure 6-27d•. An example of circumduction is moving your arm in a loop, as when drawing a large circle on a chalkboard.

6

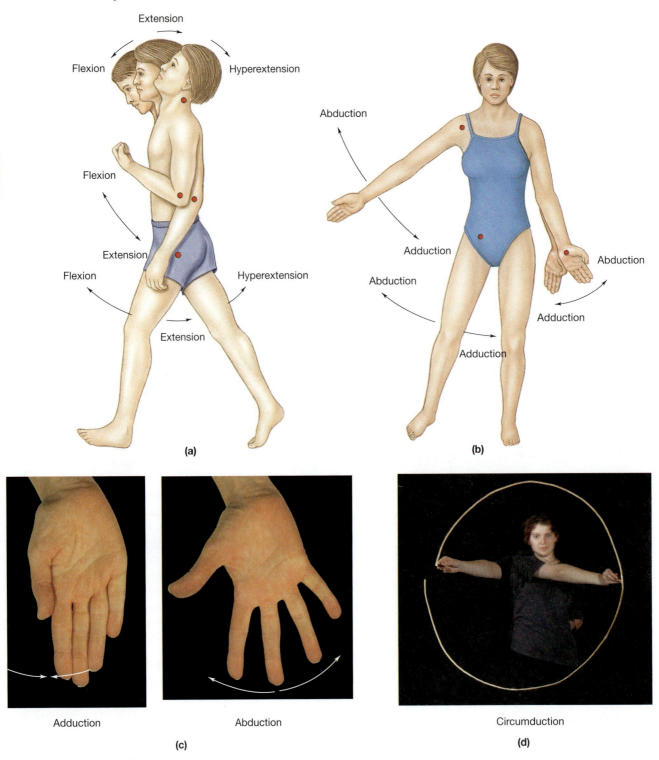

(a)

(b)

Adduction   Abduction

(c)

Circumduction

(d)

● **FIGURE 6-27   Angular Movements**
The red dots mark the locations of joints involved in the movements.

Rotation.   Rotational movements are also described with reference to a figure in the anatomical position. **Rotation** involves turning around the longitudinal axis of the body or limb. For example, you may rotate your head to look to one side, or rotate your arm to screw in a light bulb. Rotational movements are illustrated in Figure 6-28●.

Pronation/Supination.   The articulations between the radius and ulna permit the rotation of the distal end of the radius across the anterior surface of the ulna. This rotation moves the wrist and hand from palm-facing-front to palm-facing-back. This motion is called **pronation** (prō-NĀ-shun). The opposing movement, in which the palm is turned forward, is **supination** (su-pi-NĀ-shun).

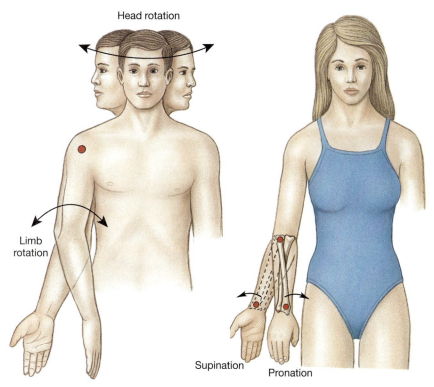

•FIGURE 6-28 Rotational Movements

Dorsiflexion/Plantar Flexion. These terms also refer to movements of the foot. **Dorsiflexion** is flexion of the ankle and elevation of the sole, as in "digging in the heels." **Plantar flexion** (*planta*, sole), the opposite movement, extends the ankle and elevates the heel, as in standing on tiptoes.

Opposition. Opposition is the special movement of the thumb that enables it to grasp and hold an object.

Protraction/Retraction. Protraction entails moving a part of the body anteriorly in the horizontal plane. **Retraction** is the reverse movement. You protract your jaw when you grasp your upper lip with your lower teeth, and you protract your clavicles when you cross your arms.

Elevation/Depression. These movements occur when a structure moves in a superior or inferior direction. You **depress** your mandible when you open your mouth, and **elevate** it as you close it.

A Functional Classification of Synovial Joints

Synovial joints can be described as *gliding, hinge, pivot, ellipsoidal, saddle,* or *ball-and-socket* joints on the basis of the shapes of the articulating surfaces (Figure 6-30•).

Special Movements. Special terms apply to specific articulations or to unusual types of movement (Figure 6-29•).

Inversion/Eversion. Inversion (*in-*, into + *vertere*, to turn) is a twisting motion of the foot that turns the sole inward. The opposite movement is called **eversion** (ē-VER-shun; *e-*, out).

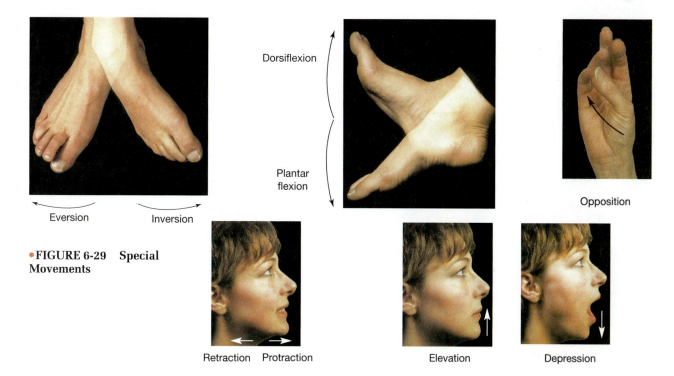

•FIGURE 6-29 Special Movements

•FIGURE 6-30   A Functional Classification of Synovial Joints

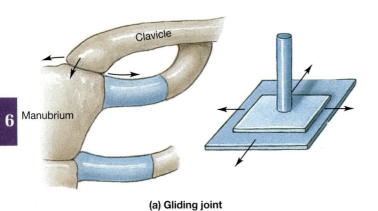

(a) Gliding joint

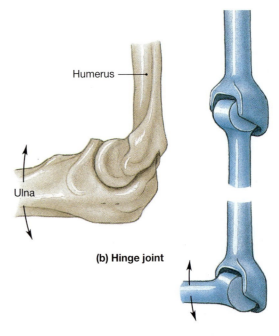

(b) Hinge joint

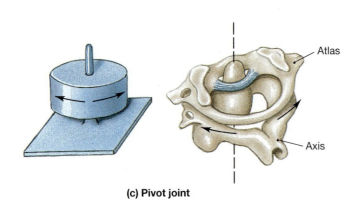

(c) Pivot joint

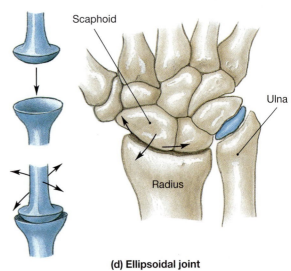

(d) Ellipsoidal joint

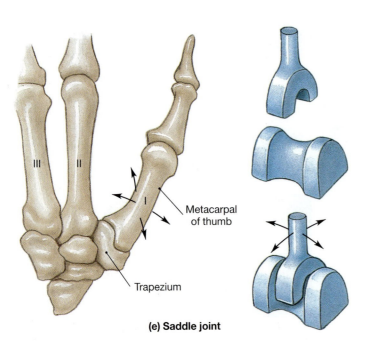

(e) Saddle joint

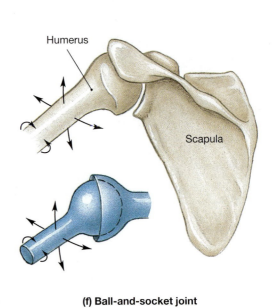

(f) Ball-and-socket joint

Each type of joint permits a different type and range of motion:

- **Gliding joints** have flattened or slightly curved faces (Figure 6-30a•). The relatively flat articular surfaces slide across one another, but the amount of movement is very slight. Although rotation is theoretically possible at such a joint, ligaments usually prevent or restrict such movement. Gliding joints are found at the ends of the clavicles, between the carpal bones, between the tarsal bones, and between the articular facets of adjacent vertebrae.

- **Hinge joints** permit angular movement in a single plane, like the opening and closing of a door (Figure 6-30b•). Examples are the joint between the occipital bone and atlas, in the axial skeleton, and the elbow, knee, ankle, and interphalangeal joints of the appendicular skeleton.

- **Pivot joints** permit only rotation (Figure 6-30c•). A pivot joint between the atlas and axis enables you to rotate your head to either side, and another between the head of the radius and the proximal shaft of the ulna permit pronation and supination of the palm.

- In an **ellipsoidal joint**, an oval articular face nestles within a depression on the opposing surface (Figure 6-30d•). With such an arrangement, angular motion occurs in two planes, along or across the length of the oval. Ellipsoidal joints connect the fingers and toes with the metacarpal bones and metatarsal bones, respectively.

- **Saddle joints** have articular faces that resemble saddles (Figure 6-29e•). Each face is concave on one axis and convex on the other, and the opposing faces nest together. This arrangement permits angular motion, including circumduction, but prevents rotation. The carpometacarpal joint at the base of the thumb is the best example of a saddle joint, and "twiddling your thumbs" will demonstrate the possible movements.

- In a **ball-and-socket joint**, the round head of one bone rests within a cup-shaped depression in another (Figure 6-29f•). All combinations of movements, including circumduction and rotation, can be performed at ball-and-socket joints. Examples are the shoulder and hip joints.

✓ In a newborn infant, the large bones of the skull are joined by fibrous connective tissue. Which type of joint is this?

✓ These bones later grow, interlock, and form immovable joints. Which type of joints are these?

✓ Give the proper term for each of the following types of motion: (a) moving your arm away from the midline of the body, (b) turning your palms so that they face forward, and (c) bending your elbow.

Representative Articulations

This section considers examples of articulations that demonstrate important functional principles. We will first consider the *intervertebral articulations* of the axial skeleton. We will then proceed to a discussion of the *synovial articulations* of the appendicular skeleton: the shoulder and elbow of the upper limb and the hip and knee of the lower limb.

Intervertebral Articulations

The vertebrae articulate with one another in one of two ways: (1) at gliding joints between the superior and inferior **articular processes**, and (2) at **symphyseal joints** between the vertebral bodies. Articulations between the superior and inferior articular processes of adjacent vertebrae permit small movements that are associated with flexion and rotation of the vertebral column. Little gliding occurs between adjacent vertebral bodies. Figure 6-31• illustrates the structure of these joints.

As noted earlier, the vertebrae are separated and cushioned by pads called *intervertebral discs*. Each intervertebral disc consists of a tough outer layer of fibrocartilage. The collagen fibers of that layer attach the discs to adjacent vertebrae. The fibrocartilage surrounds a soft, elastic and gelatinous core, which gives the disc resiliency and enables it to act as a shock absorber.

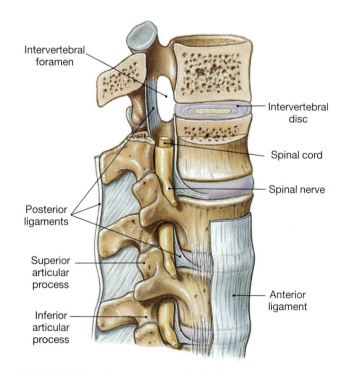

Intervertebral foramen

Intervertebral disc

Spinal cord

Spinal nerve

Posterior ligaments

Superior articular process

Inferior articular process

Anterior ligament

•**FIGURE 6-31 Intervertebral Articulations**

Articulations of the Upper Limb

The shoulder, elbow, and wrist are responsible for positioning the hand, which performs precise and controlled movements. The shoulder has great mobility, the elbow has great strength, and the wrist makes fine adjustments in the orientation of the palm and fingers.

The Shoulder Joint.   The shoulder joint permits the greatest range of motion of any joint in the body. Because it is also the most frequently dislocated joint, it provides an excellent demonstration of the principle that strength and stability must be sacrificed to obtain mobility.

Figure 6-32● shows the structure of the shoulder joint. The relatively loose joint capsule extends from the scapular neck to the humerus, and this oversized capsule permits an extensive range of motion. As at other joints, bursae at the shoulder reduce friction where large muscles and tendons pass across the joint capsule. The bursae of the shoulder are especially large and numerous. Several bursae are associated with the capsule, the processes of the scapula, and large shoulder muscles. Inflammation of any of these bursae, a condition called *bursitis*, can restrict motion and produce pain.

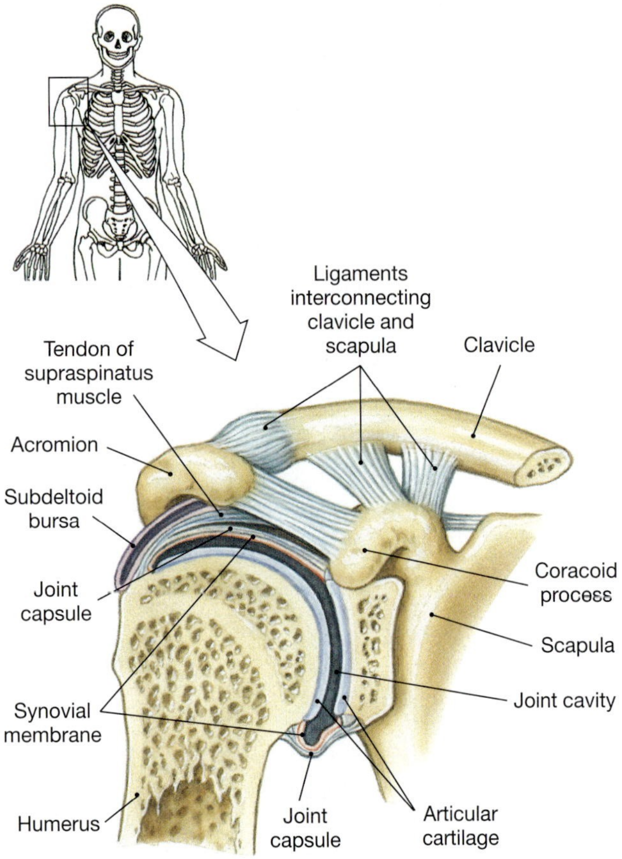

Muscles that move the humerus do more to stabilize the shoulder joint than all its ligaments and capsular fibers combined. Powerful muscles originating on the trunk, shoulder girdle, and humerus cover the anterior, superior, and posterior surfaces of the capsule. These muscles form the *rotator cuff*, a group of muscles that swing the arm through an impressive range of motion.

The Elbow Joint.   Figure 6-33● shows the structure of the elbow joint, which consists of two articulations: the humerus and ulna, and the humerus and radius. It is the articulation with the ulna that provides stability and limits movement at the elbow joint. The ulna is more important at the elbow than the radius. A large muscle that extends the elbow, the *triceps brachii*, attaches to the rough surface of the olecranon process. Arising on the front of the arm, the smaller *brachialis muscle* attaches to the ulnar tuberosity. Contraction of this muscle flexes the elbow.

The elbow joint is extremely stable because (1) the bony surfaces of the humerus and ulna interlock; (2) the joint capsule is very thick; and (3) the capsule is reinforced by stout ligaments. Nevertheless, the joint can be damaged by severe impacts or unusual stresses. When you fall on your hand with a partially flexed elbow, powerful contractions of the muscles that extend the elbow can break the ulna at the center of the trochlear notch.

✓ Would a tennis player or a jogger be more likely to develop inflammation of the subdeltoid bursa? Why?

✓ Mary falls on her hands with her elbows slightly flexed. After the fall, she can't move her left arm at the elbow. If a fracture exists, which bone is most likely broken?

●FIGURE 6-32   The Shoulder Joint
An anterior view of a section through the right shoulder.

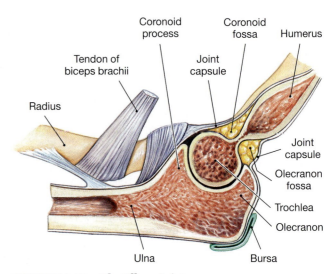

●FIGURE 6-33   The Elbow Joint
A longitudinal section through the right elbow.

Articulations of the Lower Limb

The joints of the hip, ankle, and foot are sturdier than those at corresponding locations in the upper limb, and they have smaller ranges of motion. The knee has a range of motion comparable to that of the elbow, but it is subjected to much greater forces and therefore is less stable.

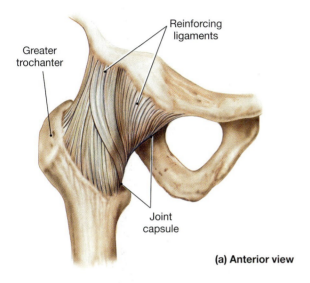

(a) Anterior view

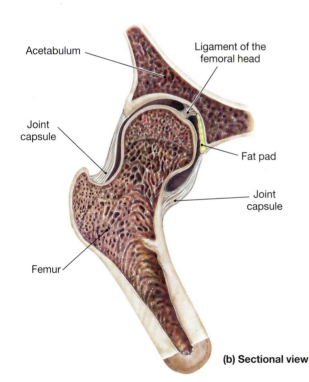

(b) Sectional view

•**FIGURE 6-34   The Hip Joint**
(a) The right hip joint, which is extremely strong and stable, in part because of the massive capsule and surrounding ligaments. **(b)** A sectional view of the right hip joint.

The Hip Joint.   Figure 6-34• shows the structure of the hip joint. The articulating surface of the acetabulum has a fibrocartilage pad along its edges, a fat pad covered by synovial membrane in its central portion, and a stout central ligament. This combination of coverings and membranes resists compression, absorbs shocks, and stretches and distorts without damage.

Compared with that of the shoulder, the joint capsule of the hip joint, a ball-and-socket diarthrosis, is denser and stronger. It extends from the lateral and inferior surfaces of the pelvic girdle to the femur and encloses both the femoral head and neck. This arrangement helps keep the head from moving away from the acetabulum. Three broad ligaments reinforce the joint capsule, while a fourth, the *ligament of the femoral head*, originates inside the acetabulum and attaches to the center of the femoral head. Additional stabilization comes from the bulk of the surrounding muscles.

The combination of an almost complete bony socket, a strong joint capsule, supporting ligaments, and muscular padding makes this an extremely stable joint. Fractures of the femoral neck or between the trochanters are actually more common than hip dislocations. Although flexion, extension, adduction, abduction, and rotation are permitted, the total range of motion is considerably less than that of the shoulder. Hip flexion is the most important normal movement, and the primary limits are imposed by the surrounding muscles. Other directions of movement are restricted by ligaments and capsular fibers.

✳ HIP FRACTURES

In the aged, simple falls can cause a *fractured* (broken) hip. These injuries are devastating, with most patients requiring ambulance transport to the hospital. Most hip fractures require surgical repair. Fractures that occur low on the femoral neck can often be treated with a specialized nail that retains the native ball-and-socket joint. Fractures higher up the femoral neck usually require a prosthesis that replaces the native ball-and-socket joint. Hip fractures can be extremely debilitating and are one of the most common reasons for nursing home placement.

The Knee Joint.   The hip joint passes weight to the femur, and at the knee joint, the femur transfers the weight to the tibia. Compared to the structure of other joints, that of the knee joint is quite complicated. Although the knee functions as a hinge joint, the articulation is far more complex than that of the elbow or even the ankle. The rounded femoral condyles roll across the top of the tibia, so the points of contact are constantly changing. Important features of the knee joint are shown in Figure 6-35•.

6

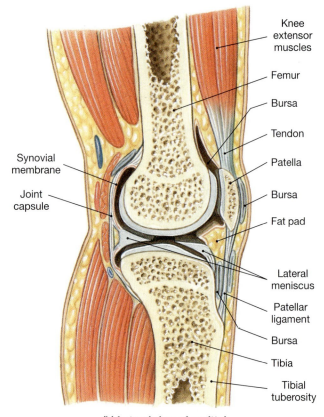

Lateral condyle

Anterior cruciate ligament

Patellar surface

Posterior cruciate ligament

Lateral ligament

Lateral meniscus

Medial condyle

Medial ligament

Cut tendon

Tibia

Medial meniscus

Fibula

(a) Anterior, flexed

Knee extensor muscles

Femur

Bursa

Tendon

Patella

Bursa

Fat pad

Synovial membrane

Joint capsule

Lateral meniscus

Patellar ligament

Bursa

Tibia

Tibial tuberosity

(b) Lateral view of sagittal section through right knee

•**FIGURE 6-35   The Knee Joint**
(a) The flexed right knee. **(b)** The extended knee.

Structurally, the knee combines three separate joints—two between the femur and tibia (medial to medial condyle and lateral to lateral condyle), and one between the patella and the femur. There is no single unified capsule, nor is there a common synovial cavity. A pair of fibrocartilage pads, the **medial** and **lateral menisci**, lie between the femoral and tibial surfaces. They act as cushions and conform to the shape of the articulating surfaces as the femur changes position. Prominent fat pads provide padding around the margins of the joint and assist the bursae in reducing friction between the patella and other tissues.

Ligaments stabilize the anterior, posterior, medial, and lateral surfaces of this joint, and a complete dislocation of the knee is an extremely rare event. The tendon from the muscles responsible for extending the knee passes over the anterior surface of the joint. The patella is embedded within this tendon, and the **patellar ligament** continues its attachment on the anterior surface of the tibia. This ligament provides support to the front of the knee joint. Posterior ligaments between the femur and the heads of the tibia and fibula reinforce the back of the knee joint. The lateral and medial surfaces of the knee joint are reinforced by another pair of ligaments. These ligaments stabilize the joint at full extension.

Additional ligaments are found inside the joint capsule (Figure 6-35b•). Inside the joint a pair of ligaments, the *anterior cruciate* and *posterior cruciate*, cross each other as they attach the tibia to the femur. (The term *cruciate* is derived from the Latin word *crucialis*, meaning a cross.) These ligaments limit the anterior and posterior movement of the femur.

✓ Why is a complete dislocation of the knee joint an infrequent event?

✓ What symptoms would you expect to see in an individual who has damaged the menisci of the knee joint?

INTEGRATION WITH OTHER SYSTEMS

Although the bones may seem inert, you should now realize that they are quite dynamic structures. The entire skeletal system is intimately associated with other systems. For example, bones are attached to the muscular system, extensively connected to the cardiovascular and lymphatic systems, and largely under the physiological control of the endocrine system. These functional relationships are diagrammed in Figure 6-36•.

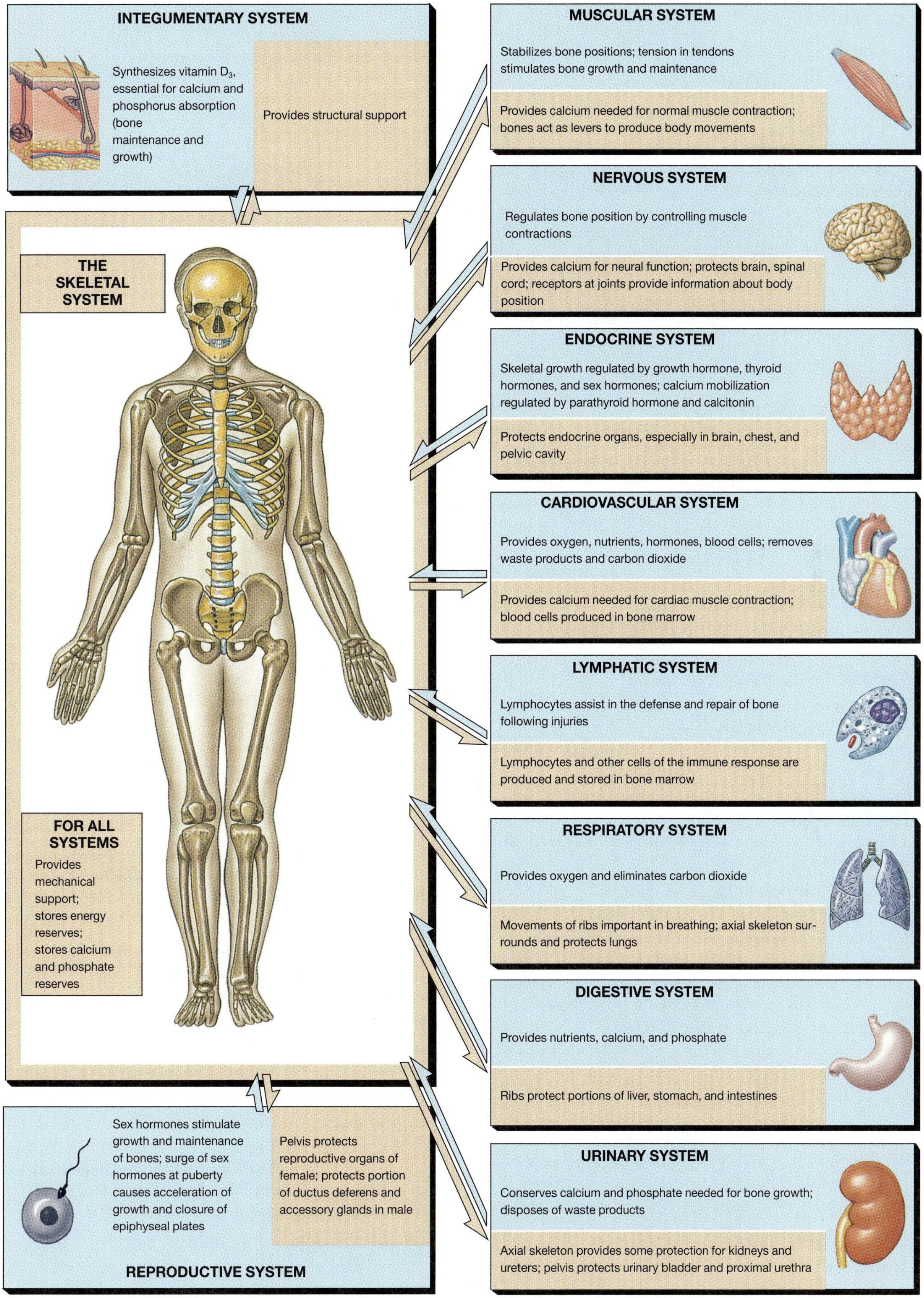

INTEGUMENTARY SYSTEM

Synthesizes vitamin D_3, essential for calcium and phosphorus absorption (bone maintenance and growth)

Provides structural support

MUSCULAR SYSTEM

Stabilizes bone positions; tension in tendons stimulates bone growth and maintenance

Provides calcium needed for normal muscle contraction; bones act as levers to produce body movements

NERVOUS SYSTEM

Regulates bone position by controlling muscle contractions

Provides calcium for neural function; protects brain, spinal cord; receptors at joints provide information about body position

ENDOCRINE SYSTEM

Skeletal growth regulated by growth hormone, thyroid hormones, and sex hormones; calcium mobilization regulated by parathyroid hormone and calcitonin

Protects endocrine organs, especially in brain, chest, and pelvic cavity

CARDIOVASCULAR SYSTEM

Provides oxygen, nutrients, hormones, blood cells; removes waste products and carbon dioxide

Provides calcium needed for cardiac muscle contraction; blood cells produced in bone marrow

LYMPHATIC SYSTEM

Lymphocytes assist in the defense and repair of bone following injuries

Lymphocytes and other cells of the immune response are produced and stored in bone marrow

RESPIRATORY SYSTEM

Provides oxygen and eliminates carbon dioxide

Movements of ribs important in breathing; axial skeleton surrounds and protects lungs

DIGESTIVE SYSTEM

Provides nutrients, calcium, and phosphate

Ribs protect portions of liver, stomach, and intestines

URINARY SYSTEM

Conserves calcium and phosphate needed for bone growth; disposes of waste products

Axial skeleton provides some protection for kidneys and ureters; pelvis protects urinary bladder and proximal urethra

THE SKELETAL SYSTEM

FOR ALL SYSTEMS

Provides mechanical support; stores energy reserves; stores calcium and phosphate reserves

Sex hormones stimulate growth and maintenance of bones; surge of sex hormones at puberty causes acceleration of growth and closure of epiphyseal plates

Pelvis protects reproductive organs of female; protects portion of ductus deferens and accessory glands in male

REPRODUCTIVE SYSTEM

•FIGURE 6-36   Functional Relationships Between the Skeletal System and Other Systems

6

Chapter Review

KEY TERMS

amphiarthrosis, *p. 149*	**epiphysis**, *p. 123*	**osteocyte**, *p. 123*
appendicular skeleton, *p. 130*	**fracture**, *p. 127*	**osteon**, *p. 123*
articulation, *p. 149*	**ligament**, *p. 150*	**periosteum**, *p. 123*
axial skeleton, *p. 130*	**marrow**, *p. 123*	**spongy bone**, *p. 123*
bursa, *p. 150*	**meniscus**, *p. 150*	**synarthrosis**, *p. 149*
compact bone, *p. 123*	**ossification**, *p. 125*	**synovial fluid**, *p. 150*
diaphysis, *p. 123*	**osteoblast**, *p. 124*	
diarthrosis, *p. 149*	**osteoclast**, *p. 124*	

SUMMARY OUTLINE

INTRODUCTION *p. 122*

1. The skeletal system includes the bones of the skeleton and the cartilages, ligaments, and other connective tissues that stabilize or interconnect bones. Its functions include structural support, storage, blood cell production, protection, and leverage.

THE STRUCTURE OF BONE *p. 122*

1. **Bone**, or **osseous tissue**, is a supporting connective tissue with a solid *matrix*.

Macroscopic Features of Bone *p. 122*

2. General categories of bones are **long bones**, **short bones**, **flat bones**, and **irregular bones**. *(Figure 6-1)*

3. The features of a long bone include a **diaphysis**, **epiphyses**, and a central *marrow cavity*. *(Figure 6-2)*

4. The two types of bone tissue are **compact**, or *dense*, **bone** and **spongy**, or *cancellous*, **bone**.

5. A bone is covered by a **periosteum** and lined with an **endosteum**.

Microscopic Features of Bone *p. 123*

6. Both types of bone contain **osteocytes** in **lacunae**. Layers of calcified matrix are **lamellae**, interconnected by **canaliculi**. *(Figure 6-3)*

7. The basic functional unit of compact bone is the **osteon**, containing osteocytes arranged around a **central canal**.

8. Spongy bone contains **trabeculae**, often in an open network.

9. Compact bone is located where stresses come from a limited range of directions; spongy bone is located where stresses are few or come from many different directions.

10. Cells other than osteocytes are also present in bone. **Osteoclasts** dissolve the bony matrix through the process of *osteolysis*. **Osteoblasts** synthesize the matrix in the process of *osteogenesis*.

BONE DEVELOPMENT AND GROWTH *p. 125*

1. **Ossification** is the process of converting other tissues to bone.

Intramembranous Ossification *p. 125*

2. **Intramembranous ossification** begins when stem cells in connective tissue differentiate into osteoblasts and can produce spongy or compact bone.

Endochondral Ossification *p. 125*

3. **Endochondral ossification** begins by the formation of a cartilage model of a bone that is gradually replaced by bone. *(Figure 6-4)*

Bone Growth and Body Proportions *p. 125*

4. There are differences between bones and between individuals regarding the timing of epiphyseal closure.

Requirements for Normal Bone Growth *p. 126*

5. Normal osteogenesis requires a reliable source of minerals, vitamins, and hormones.

REMODELING AND HOMEOSTATIC MECHANISMS *p. 127*

1. The organic and mineral components of bone are continuously recycled and renewed through the process of **remodeling**.

Remodeling and Support *p. 127*

2. The shapes and thicknesses of bones reflect the stresses applied to them. Mineral turnover allows bone to adapt to new stresses.

Homeostasis and Mineral Storage *p. 127*

3. Calcium is the most abundant mineral in the human body, with roughly 99 percent of it located in the skeleton. The skeleton acts as a calcium reserve.

Injury and Repair *p. 127*

4. A **fracture** is a crack or break in a bone. Repair of a fracture involves the formation of a **fracture hematoma**, an **external callus**, and an **internal callus**. *(Figure 6-5) (Focus: A Classification of Fractures)*

Aging and the Skeletal System *p. 128*

5. The effects of aging on the skeleton can include **osteopenia** and **osteoporosis**.

AN OVERVIEW OF THE SKELETON *p. 130*

Skeletal Terminology *p. 130*

1. **Bone markings** can be used to describe and identify specific bones. *(Table 6-1)*

Skeletal Divisions *p. 130*

2. The skeletal system consists of the axial skeleton and the appendicular skeleton. The **axial skeleton** can be subdivided into the **skull**, the **auditory ossicles** (ear bones), the **hyoid**, the **thoracic cage** (*rib cage*) composed of the **ribs** and **sternum**, and the **vertebral column**. *(Figure 6-6)*

3. The **appendicular skeleton** includes the upper and lower limbs and the **pectoral** and **pelvic girdles**.

THE AXIAL DIVISION *p. 131*

The Skull, *p. 131*

1. The **cranium** encloses the **cranial cavity**, a division of the dorsal body cavity that encloses the brain.

2. The **frontal bone** forms the forehead and superior surface of each **orbit**. *(Figures 6-7, 6-8, 6-9)*

3. The **parietal bones** form the upper sides and roof of the cranium. *(Figures 6-7, 6-9)*

4. The **occipital bone** surrounds the **foramen magnum** and articulates with the sphenoid, temporal, and parietal bones to form the back of the cranium. *(Figures 6-7, 6-8, 6-9)*

5. The **temporal bones** help form the sides and base of the cranium and fuse with the parietal bones along the *squamosal suture*. *(Figures 6-7, 6-8, 6-9)*

6. The **sphenoid bone** acts like a bridge, uniting the cranial and facial bones. *(Figures 6-7, 6-8, 6-9)*

7. The **ethmoid bone** stabilizes the brain and forms the roof and sides of the nasal cavity. Its **cribriform plate** contains perforations for olfactory nerves, and the **perpendicular plate** forms part of the bony *nasal septum*. *(Figures 6-7, 6-8, 6-9)*

8. The left and right **maxillary bones**, or *maxillae*, articulate with all the other facial bones except the *mandible*. *(Figures 6-7, 6-8, 6-9)*

9. The **palatine bones** form the posterior portions of the *hard palate* and contribute to the walls of the nasal cavity and to the floor of each orbit. *(Figures 6-8, 6-9)*

10. The **vomer** forms the inferior portion of the bony nasal septum. *(Figures 6-8, 6-9)*

11. The **zygomatic bones** help complete the orbit and together with the temporal bones form the **zygomatic arch** (*cheekbone*). *(Figures 6-7, 6-8)*

12. The **nasal bones** articulate with the frontal bone and maxillary bones. *(Figures 6-7, 6-8, 6-9)*

13. The **lacrimal bones** are within the orbit on its medial surface. *(Figures 6-7, 6-8)*

14. The **inferior nasal conchae** inside the nasal cavity aid the **superior** and **middle nasal conchae** of the ethmoid bone to slow incoming air. *(Figures 6-8a, 6-9c)*

15. The **nasal complex** includes the bones that form the superior and lateral walls of the nasal cavity and the sinuses that drain into them. The **nasal septum** divides the nasal cavities. Together the **frontal**, **sphenoidal**, **ethmoidal**, **palatine**, and **maxillary sinuses** make up the **paranasal sinuses**. *(Figures 6-8, 6-9)*

16. The **mandible** is the bone of the lower jaw. *(Figures 6-7, 6-8, 6-9)*

17. The hyoid bone is suspended below the skull by ligaments from the styloid processes of the temporal bones.

18. Fibrous connections of tissue called **fontanels** permit the skulls of infants and children to continue growing. *(Figure 6-10)*

The Neck and Trunk *p. 138*

19. There are 7 **cervical vertebrae**, 12 **thoracic vertebrae** (which articulate with ribs), and 5 **lumbar vertebrae** (which articulate with the sacrum). The **sacrum** and **coccyx** consist of fused vertebrae. *(Figure 6-11)*

20. The spinal column has four **spinal curves**, which accommodate the unequal distribution of body weight and keep it in line with the body axis. *(Figure 6-11)*

21. A typical vertebra has a **body** and a **vertebral arch**; it articulates with other vertebrae at the **articular processes**. Adjacent vertebrae are separated by an **intervertebral disc**. *(Figure 6-12)*

22. Cervical vertebrae are distinguished by the shape of the body and by **transverse foramina** on either side. *(Figures 6-12, 6-13)*

23. Thoracic vertebrae have distinctive heart-shaped bodies. *(Figure 6-12)*

24. The lumbar vertebrae are the most massive and least mobile; they are subjected to the greatest strains, and a *herniated disc* can occur. *(Figure 6-12)*

25. The sacrum protects reproductive, digestive, and excretory organs. At its **apex**, the sacrum articulates with the coccyx. At its **base**, the sacrum articulates with the last lumbar vertebra. *(Figure 6-14)*

26. The skeleton of the thorax consists of the thoracic vertebrae, the ribs, and the sternum. The ribs and sternum form the thoracic cage, or rib cage. *(Figure 6-15)*

27. Ribs 1 to 7 are **true ribs**. Ribs 8 to 12 lack direct connections to the sternum and are called **false ribs**; they include two pairs of **floating ribs**. The medial end of each rib articulates with a thoracic vertebra. *(Figure 6-15)*

28. The sternum consists of a **manubrium**, a **body**, and a **xiphoid process**. *(Figure 6-15)*

THE APPENDICULAR DIVISION *p. 142*

The Pectoral Girdle *p. 142*

1. Each arm articulates with the trunk at the pectoral girdle, or *shoulder girdle*, which consists of the **scapula** and **clavicle**. *(Figures 6-6, 6-16, 6-17)*

2. The clavicle and scapula position the shoulder joint, help move the arm, and provide a base for arm movement and muscle attachment. *(Figures 6-16, 6-17)*

3. Both the **coracoid process** and the **acromion** are attached to ligaments and tendons. The **scapular spine** crosses the posterior surface of the scapular body. *(Figure 6-17)*

6

The Upper Limb *p. 144*

4. The **humerus** articulates with the scapula at the shoulder joint. The **greater tubercle** and **lesser tubercle** of the humerus are important sites for muscle attachment. Other prominent landmarks include the **deltoid tuberosity**, the **medial** and **lateral epicondyles**, and the articular **condyle**. *(Figure 6-18)*

5. Distally, the humerus articulates with the radius and ulna. The medial **trochlea** extends from the **coronoid fossa** to the **olecranon fossa**. *(Figure 6-18)*

6. The **radius** and **ulna** are the bones of the forearm. The olecranon fossa accommodates the **olecranon process** during extension of the arm. The coronoid and radial fossae accommodate the **coronoid process** of the ulna. *(Figure 6-19)*

7. The bones of the wrist form two rows of **carpal bones**. The distal carpal bones articulate with the **metacarpal bones** of the palm. The metacarpal bones articulate with the proximal **phalanges**, or finger bones. Four of the fingers contain three phalanges; the **pollex**, or thumb, has only two. *(Figure 6-20)*

The Pelvic Girdle *p. 145*

8. The pelvic girdle consists of two **coxae**. *(Figure 6-21)*

9. The largest coxal bone, the **ilium**, fuses with the **ischium**, which in turn fuses with the **pubis**. The **pubic symphysis** limits movement between the pubic bones. *(Figure 6-21)*

10. The **pelvis** consists of the coxae, the sacrum, and the coccyx. *(Figures 6-21, 6-22)*

The Lower Limb *p. 147*

11. The **femur**, or *thighbone*, is the longest bone in the body. It articulates with the **tibia** at the knee joint. A ligament from the **patella**, the *kneecap*, attaches at the **tibial tuberosity**. *(Figures 6-23, 6-24)*

12. Other tibial landmarks include the **anterior crest** and the **medial malleolus**. The fibular **head** articulates with the tibia below the knee, and the **lateral malleolus** stabilizes the ankle. *(Figure 6-24)*

13. The ankle includes seven **tarsal bones**; only the **talus** articulates with the tibia and fibula. When we stand normally, most of our weight is transferred to the **calcaneus**, or *heel bone*, and the rest is passed on to the **metatarsal bones**. *(Figure 6-25)*

14. The basic organizational pattern of the metatarsals and phalanges of the foot resembles that of the hand.

ARTICULATIONS *p. 149*

A Classification of Joints *p. 149*

1. **Articulations** (joints) exist wherever two bones interact. Immovable joints are **synarthroses**, slightly movable joints are **amphiarthroses**, and those that are freely movable are called **diarthroses**. *(Table 6-2)*

2. Examples of synarthroses are a **suture**, a **gomphosis**, and a **synchondrosis**.

3. Examples of amphiarthroses are a **syndesmosis** and a **symphysis**.

4. The bony surfaces at diarthroses, or **synovial joints**, are covered by **articular cartilages**, lubricated by **synovial fluid**, and enclosed within a **joint capsule**. Other synovial structures include **menisci**, **fat pads**, **bursae**, and various **ligaments**. *(Figure 6-26)*

Articular Form and Function *p. 151*

5. Important terms that describe dynamic motion at synovial joints are **gliding**, **flexion**, **extension**, **hyperextension**, **abduction**, **adduction**, **circumduction**, and **rotation**. *(Figures 6-27, 6-28)*

6. The bones in the forearm permit **pronation** and **supination**. *(Figure 6-28)*

7. Movements of the foot include **inversion** and **eversion**. The ankle undergoes **dorsiflexion** and **plantar flexion**. **Opposition** is the thumb movement that enables us to grasp and hold objects. *(Figure 6-29)*

8. **Protraction** involves moving a part of the body forward; **retraction** involves moving it back. **Depression** and **elevation** occur when we move a structure inferiorly and superiorly, respectively. *(Figure 6-29)*

9. Major types of joints include **gliding joints**, **hinge joints**, **pivot joints**, **ellipsoidal joints**, **saddle joints**, and **ball-and-socket joints**. *(Figure 6-30)*

Representative Articulations *p. 155*

10. The articular processes form gliding joints with those of adjacent vertebrae. The vertebral bodies form **symphyseal joints**. They are separated by pads called *intervertebral discs*. *(Figure 6-31)*

11. The shoulder joint is formed by the **glenoid cavity** and the head of the humerus. This joint is extremely mobile and, for that reason, it is also unstable and easily dislocated. *(Figure 6-32)*

12. Bursae at the shoulder joint reduce friction from muscles and tendons during movement. *(Figure 6-32)*

13. The elbow joint permits only flexion and extension. It is extremely stable because of extensive ligaments and the shapes of the articulating elements. *(Figure 6-33)*

14. The hip joint is formed by the union of the **acetabulum** with the head of the femur. This ball-and-socket diarthrosis permits flexion and extension, adduction and abduction, circumduction, and rotation. *(Figure 6-34)*

15. The knee joint is a complicated hinge joint. The patella, or kneecap, is embedded within a tendon that supports the front of the joint. *(Figure 6-35)*

INTEGRATION WITH OTHER SYSTEMS *p. 158*

1. The skeletal system is dynamically associated with other systems. *(Figure 6-36)*

REVIEW QUESTIONS

LEVEL 1   Reviewing Facts and Terms

Match each item in column A with the most closely related item in column B. Use letters for answers in the spaces provided.

Column A

___ 1. osteocytes
___ 2. diaphysis
___ 3. auditory ossicles
___ 4. cribriform plate
___ 5. osteoblasts
___ 6. C_1
___ 7. C_2
___ 8. hip and shoulder
___ 9. patella
___10. calcaneus
___11. synarthrosis
___12. moving the hand into a palm-front position
___13. osteoclasts
___14. raising the arm laterally
___15. elbow and knee

Column B

a. abduction
b. heelbone
c. ball-and-socket joints
d. bone-dissolving cells
e. hinge joints
f. axis
g. immovable joint
h. bone shaft
i. mature bone cells
j. bone-producing cells
k. atlas
l. olfactory nerves
m. ear bones
n. supination
o. kneecap

16. Skeletal bones store energy reserves as lipids in areas of:
(a) red marrow
(b) yellow marrow
(c) the matrix of bone tissue
(d) the ground substance

17. The two types of osseous tissue are:
(a) compact bone and spongy bone
(b) dense bone and compact bone
(c) spongy bone and cancellous bone
(d) a, b, and c are correct

18. The basic functional units of mature compact bone are:
(a) lacunae
(b) osteocytes
(c) osteons
(d) canaliculi

19. The axial skeleton consists of the bones of the:
(a) pectoral and pelvic girdles
(b) skull, thorax, and vertebral column
(c) arm, legs, hand, and feet
(d) limbs, pectoral girdle, and pelvic girdle

20. The appendicular skeleton consists of the bones of the:
(a) pectoral and pelvic girdles
(b) skull, thorax, and vertebral column
(c) arm, legs, hand, and feet
(d) limbs, pectoral girdle, and pelvic girdle

21. Which of the following contains *only* bones of the cranium?
(a) frontal, parietal, occipital, sphenoid
(b) frontal, occipital, zygomatic, parietal
(c) occipital, sphenoid, temporal, parietal
(d) mandible, maxilla, nasal, zygomatic

22. Of the following bones, which one is unpaired?
(a) vomer
(b) maxilla
(c) palatine
(d) nasal

23. At the glenoid cavity, the scapula articulates with the proximal end of the:
(a) humerus
(b) radius
(c) ulna
(d) femur

24. While an individual is in the anatomical position, the ulna lies:
(a) medial to the radius
(b) lateral to the radius
(c) inferior to the radius
(d) superior to the radius

25. Each coxa of the pelvic girdle consists of three fused bones:
(a) ulna, radius, humerus
(b) ilium, ischium, pubis
(c) femur, tibia, fibula
(d) hamate, capitate, trapezium

26. Joints that are typically located at the end of long bones are:
(a) synarthroses
(b) amphiarthroses
(c) diarthroses
(d) sutures

27. The function of the synovial fluid is:
(a) to nourish chondrocytes
(b) to provide lubrication
(c) to absorb shock
(d) a, b, and c are correct

28. Abduction and adduction always refer to movements of the:
(a) axial skeleton
(b) appendicular skeleton
(c) skull
(d) vertebral column

29. Standing on tiptoe is an example of a movement called:
    (a) elevation
    (b) dorsiflexion
    (c) plantar flexion
    (d) retraction
30. What are the five primary functions of the skeletal system?
31. What is the primary difference between intramembranous ossification and endochondral ossification?

32. What unique characteristic of the hyoid bone makes it different from all the other bones in the body?
33. What two primary functions are performed by the thoracic cage?
34. Which two large scapular processes are associated with the shoulder joint?

6 LEVEL 2   Reviewing Concepts

35. Why are stresses or impacts to the side of the shaft in a long bone more dangerous than stress applied to the long axis of the shaft?
36. During the growth of a long bone, how is the epiphysis forced farther from the shaft?
37. Why are ruptured intervertebral discs more common in lumbar vertebrae, and dislocations and fractures more common in cervical vertebrae?

38. Why are clavicular injuries common?
39. What is the difference between the pelvic girdle and the pelvis?
40. How do articular cartilages differ from other cartilages in the body?
41. What is the significance of the fact that the pubic symphysis is a slightly movable joint?

LEVEL 3   Critical Thinking and Clinical Applications

42. While playing on her swingset, 10-year-old Sally falls and breaks her right leg. At the emergency room, the physician tells Sally's parents that the proximal end of the tibia, where the epiphysis meets the diaphysis, is fractured. The fracture is properly set and eventually heals. During a routine physical when she is 18, Sally learns that her right leg is 2 cm shorter than her left, probably because of her accident. What might account for this difference?
43. Tess is diagnosed with a disease that affects the membranes surrounding the brain. The physician tells Tess's family that the disease is caused by an airborne virus. Explain how this virus could have entered the cranium.
44. While working at an excavation, an archaeologist finds several small skull bones. She examines the frontal, parietal, and occipital bones and concludes that the skulls

are those of children not yet 1 year old. How can she tell their ages from examining the bones?
45. Frank Fireman is fighting a fire in a building when part of the ceiling collapses and a beam strikes him on his left shoulder. He is rescued by his friends, but he has a great deal of pain in his shoulder and cannot move his arm properly, especially in the anterior direction. His clavicle is not broken, and his humerus is intact. What is the probable nature of Frank's injury?
46. Ed "overturns" his ankle while playing tennis. He experiences swelling and pain, but after examination, he is told that there are no torn ligaments and the structure of the ankle is not affected. On the basis of the symptoms and the examination results, what do you think happened to Ed's ankle?

ANSWERS TO CONCEPT CHECK QUESTIONS

Page 125
1. If the ratio of collagen to calcium in a bone increased, the bone would be more flexible and less strong.   2. Concentric layers of bone around a central canal are indicative of an osteon (or Haversian system). Osteons make up compact bone. Since the ends (epiphyses) of long bones are primarily cancellous (spongy) bone, this sample most likely came from the shaft (diaphysis) of a long bone.   3. Since osteoclasts function in breaking down or demineralizing bone, the bone would have less mineral content and as a result would be weaker.

Page 126
1. Long bones of the body, such as the femur, have a plate of cartilage, called the epiphyseal plate, that separates the epiphysis from the diaphysis as long as the bone is still growing lengthwise. An X-ray would indicate whether the epiphyseal plate is still present. If it is, then growth is still occurring; if not, the bone has reached its adult length.   2. The increase in the male sex hormone testosterone that occurs at puberty contributes to an increased rate of bone growth and the closure of the epiphyseal plates. Since the source of testosterone, the testes, is removed in castration, we would expect these boys to have a longer, though slower, growth period and be taller than they would have been if they had not been castrated.   3. Women who are pregnant need large amounts of calcium to support the needs of the developing fetus for bone growth. If the expectant mother does not include enough calcium in her diet, her body will mobilize the calcium reserves of her own skeleton to provide for the needs of the fetus, resulting in weakened bones and an increased risk of fracture.

Page 128
1. The larger arm muscles of the weight lifter will apply more mechanical stress to the bones of the arms. In response to the stress, the bones will grow thicker. For similar reasons, we would expect the jogger to have heavier thigh bones.   2. The sex hormones known as estrogens play an important role in moving calcium into bones. After menopause, the level of these hormones decreases dramatically. As a result, it is difficult to replace the calcium in bones that is being lost due to normal aging. Males do not show a decrease in sex hormone levels (androgens).

Page 136
1. The mastoid and styloid processes are projections on the temporal bones of the skull.   2. The sella turcica contains the pituitary gland and is located in the sphenoid bone.   3. The occipital condyles of the occipital bone of the cranium articulate with the vertebral column.

Page 137

1. The bone that forms the superior portion of the orbit is the frontal bone, and the maxilla and the zygomatic bones form the inferior portion of the orbit. These would be the three bones fractured by the ball. **2.** The paranasal sinuses make some of the heavier skull bones lighter and provide sites of mucus production; the mucus formed there warms, moistens, and filters incoming air. **3.** The most powerful muscles that are involved in closing the mouth attach to the mandible at the coronoid process. A fracture of the coronoid process would make it difficult for these muscles to function properly and to close the mouth. **4.** Since many muscles that move the tongue and the larynx are attached to the hyoid bone, you would expect a person with a fractured hyoid bone to have difficulty moving the tongue, breathing, and swallowing.

Page 141

1. The odontoid process is located on the second cervical vertebra, or axis, which is in the neck. **2.** Improper compression of the chest during CPR could and frequently does result in a fracture of the sternum or ribs. **3.** In adults, the five sacral vertebrae fuse to form a single sacrum.

Page 145

1. The clavicle attaches the scapula to the sternum and thus restricts the scapula's range of movement. If the clavicle is broken, then the scapula will have a greater range of movement and will be less stable. **2.** The two rounded prominences on either side of the elbow are parts of the humerus (the lateral and medial epicondyles).

Page 148

1. The three bones that make up the coxa are the ilium, ischium, and the pubis. **2.** Although the fibula is not part of the knee joint and does not bear weight, it is an important point of attachment for many leg muscles. When the fibula is fractured, these muscles cannot function properly to move the leg and walking is difficult and painful. The fibula also helps stabilize the ankle joint. **3.** Joey has most likely fractured his calcaneus (heel bone).

Page 155

1. Originally, the joint is a type of syndesmosis. **2.** When the bones interlock, they form sutural joints. **3.** (a) abduction; (b) supination; (c) flexion.

Page 156

1. Since the subscapular bursa is located in the shoulder joint, the tennis player would have inflammation of this structure (bursitis). The condition is associated with the intensity of repetitive motion that occurs at the shoulder, such as swinging a tennis racket. The jogger would be more at risk for injuries to the knee joint. **2.** Mary has most likely fractured her ulna.

Page 158

1. Seven major ligaments stabilize the knee joint. As a result, a complete dislocation is rare. **2.** Damage to the menisci in the knee joint would result in a decrease in the joint's stability. The individual would have a harder time locking the knee in place while standing and would have to use muscle contractions to stabilize the joint. When the individual stands for long periods, the muscles would fatigue and the knee would "give out." We would also expect the individual to experience pain.

6

Emergency Care Applications

OVERVIEW

The skeletal system forms the underlying framework of the body. It consists of 206 or more bones and the associated ligaments and cartilage. Numerous emergencies can arise affecting the skeletal system. Most are due to trauma, although several disease processes also can lead to skeletal-system emergencies. The skeletal system's numerous important functions include support of the soft tissues, production of blood cells, storage of minerals and lipids, and movement of the body as a whole (in conjunction with the muscular system). Because of their integrated relationship, the skeletal system and the muscular system often are referred to jointly as the *musculoskeletal system.* Physicians who specialize in the treatment of bone-related problems are called *orthopedic surgeons. Rheumatologists* are physicians who specialize in the medical treatment of joint problems, especially those of autoimmune origin. The following is a discussion of common bone and related injuries encountered in the emergency setting.

SKELETAL INJURIES

There are four general types of skeletal and joint injuries: sprains, subluxations, dislocations, and fractures.

Sprains

The sprain is an injury that stretches or tears one or more ligaments within a joint. This tearing of ligaments weakens the joint. Stresses to a joint can extend the joint beyond its normal range of motion, causing ligamentous injury (Figure A6-1•). The injury results in acute pain at the site, followed shortly by inflammation and swelling. Sprains are classified, or graded, according to their severity, using the following criteria:
- *Grade I.* Minor and incomplete tear. The ligament is painful and tender, but there is no laxity. Swelling and ecchymosis are usually minimal. The joint is stable.

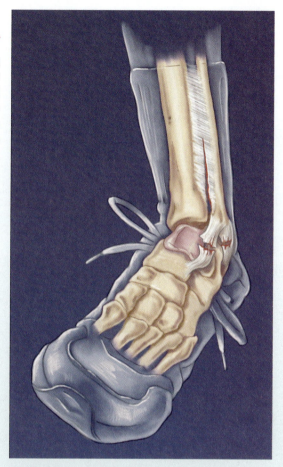

•FIGURE A6-1   Grade-2 Ankle Sprain Following Common Inversion Injury
The anterior tabofibular ligament appears completely torn, while the posterior tabofibular ligament is only partially torn. The vast majority of ankle sprains involve the lateral ligaments.

- *Grade II.* Significant but incomplete tear. There is laxity, but also an end-point beyond which no further opening of the joint occurs. Swelling and ecchymosis may be moderate to severe, and pain may range from moderate to severe. The joint is unstable but intact.
- *Grade III.* Complete tear and total failure of the ligament or ligaments involved. No end-point is felt when stress is applied to the ligament during examination of the joint. Pain and muscle spasm can often mask a grade III sprain, so the diagnosis is

easily missed. Due to severe pain and spasm, the injury may be mistaken for a fracture. A repeat examination several days later can help confirm the diagnosis. The joint is unstable.

Subluxation

A *subluxation,* also called a partial dislocation, is a partial displacement of a bone end from its position within a joint capsule. It occurs as the joint separates under stress, stretching the ligaments. A subluxation differs from a sprain in that it more significantly reduces the joint's integrity.

Dislocation

A *dislocation* is a complete displacement of bone ends from their normal position within a joint. The joint often fixes in an abnormal position with noticeable deformity (Figure A6-2●). This injury occurs when the bones of the joint move beyond their normal range of motion, usually with great force. It carries with it the danger of entrapping, compressing, or tearing nearby blood vessels and nerves. A dislocation should be suspected whenever a joint is deformed or does not move in a normal fashion.

Fracture

A *fracture* is an injury that interrupts the structural integrity of a bone. Most fractures are the result of significant trauma to a healthy bone. The bony cortex may be disrupted by many different forces including: a direct blow, angular (bending) forces, axial loading, twisting (torque) stress, or any combination of these.

Fractures also can occur in a bone that is diseased or otherwise abnormal. These pathological processes weaken the bone making it susceptible to fracture by forces that would, under normal circumstances, not typically disrupt the cortex. These fractures are called *pathological* fractures and can result from relatively minor trauma. Examples of pathological fractures include fractures through lytic metastatic (cancerous) lesions, fractures through benign bone cysts, and vertebral compression fractures in patients with advanced osteoporosis. Vertebral compression fractures are the most common type of pathological fracture.

Growth-Plate Injuries

Fractures can involve the epiphyseal growth plate in children. The cartilaginous epiphyseal plate, also called the physis, is readily injured because it is weaker than ossified bone or ligaments (Figure A6-3●). Damage to the epiphyseal plate during a child's growth may destroy all or part of the bone's ability to produce new bone, resulting in stunted or deformed growth thereafter. The potential for a growth disturbance from a growth-plate injury is re-

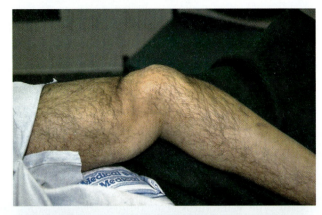
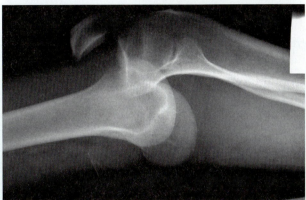

● **FIGURE A6-2   Anterior Dislocation of the Knee**
This rare injury poses a significant threat to blood vessels and nerves that transverse the knee. Immediate reduction is indicated.

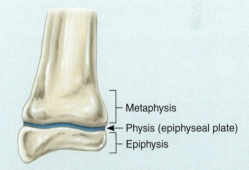

● **FIGURE A6-3   Growth Plate in a Child's Long Bone**
The growth plate is also called the physis or epiphyseal plate. The portion of bone proximal to the physis is the metaphysis; the segment distal to the physis is the epiphysis.

lated to the number of years the child has yet to grow. Thus, the older the child, the less time remains for a deformity to develop. The *Salter-Harris system* is often used to classify growth-plate injuries. The potential for growth disturbance increases as the classification number increases. The prognosis is best for type I fractures and

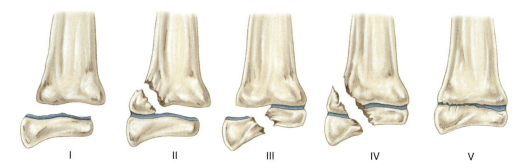

• **FIGURE A6-4 Salter-Harris System of Classifying Growth Plate Injuries**
The likelihood of a permanent growth plate deformity increases as the classification number increases.

I   II   III   IV   V

A6

worst for type V fractures. The Salter-Harris classifications for growth-plate injuries are (Figure A6-4•):

- *Salter-Harris Type I.* The fracture line runs through the physis. There is usually little, if any, separation of the epiphysis from the rest of the bone. It is often difficult to see the fracture line on X-ray, as the line is hidden within the growth plate. A type I injury is the least severe epiphyseal fracture type.
- *Salter-Harris Type II.* The entire epiphysis and a portion of the metaphysis are broken off. The fracture line runs through the physis and into the metaphysis.
- *Salter-Harris Type III.* A portion of the epiphysis is broken off. The fracture line runs through the physis, into the epiphysis, and into the joint.
- *Salter-Harris Type IV.* A portion of the epiphysis and a portion of the metaphysis are broken off. The fracture line runs through the metaphysis, the physis, the epiphysis, and into the joint.
- *Salter-Harris Type V.* The epiphyseal plate is compressed, usually through an axial loading type force. These injuries are difficult to diagnose and are sometimes only evident retrospectively when a growth disturbance develops.

Types of Fractures

There are many systems for classifying fractures. Generally, fractures are classified as either closed or open. In a *closed fracture,* the skin is not broken and there is no communication between the fracture site and the environment. In an *open fracture,* the skin is broken and a communication exists between the fracture site and the environment. The difference in these two classifications has significant emergency care considerations. Open fractures are usually taken to the operating room, where the fracture site is exposed, cleansed, and irrigated to prevent infection. Closed fractures can be splinted, placed in a cast, or otherwise immobilized (Figure A6-5•).

Fractures are also classified based upon the orientation of the fracture line as seen in radiographic (X-ray) studies (Figure A6-6•).

- *Greenstick fracture.* Greenstick fractures are seen almost exclusively in children. In a greenstick fracture, one side of the bone is broken and the other side bent.

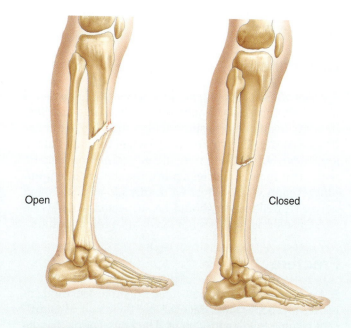

Open   Closed

• **FIGURE A6-5 Open and Closed Fractures**
Open fractures, also called compound fractures, have a direct communication with the environment. Closed fractures, also called simple fractures, do not have any communication with the environment.

This occurs due to the large amount of cartilage in the bones of children.

- *Torus fracture.* Torus fractures occur almost exclusively in children. In a torus fracture, there is localized buckling or swelling (or torus) of the cortex, with little or no displacement of the bone itself.
- *Transverse fracture.* A transverse fracture is a fracture line perpendicular to the long axis of the bone.
- *Oblique fracture.* In an oblique fracture, the break extends obliquely to the long axis of the bone.
- *Spiral fracture.* A spiral fracture, also called a *torsion fracture,* occurs when a twisting force is applied to a long bone.
- *Comminuted fracture.* Comminuted fractures are those where the bone at the fracture site has multiple bone fragments.
- *Segmental fracture.* A segmental fracture is an injury where there are multiple fracture sites along the axis

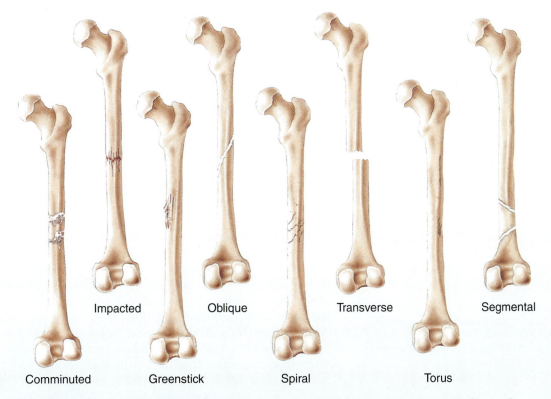

Impacted   Oblique   Transverse   Segmental

Comminuted   Greenstick   Spiral   Torus

• **FIGURE A6-6** Fracture Types Based on the Appearance of the Fracture Line on Radiographs

of the bone leaving a free-floating segment of bone between the two fracture sites. Segmental fractures are often mistakenly called comminuted fractures.

- *Impacted fracture.* An impacted fracture is an injury where an axial loading force is applied to the bone, resulting in the bone ends at the fracture site being driven together.

Specific Fractures

Several specific types of fractures are important to emergency medical care.

Upper Extremity Fractures.   Upper extremity fractures are common. Falls on an outstretched arm can result in fractures of the wrist, elbow, humerus, and clavicle. In fact, the clavicle is the most frequently fractured bone in the body. A common forearm fracture is the *Colle's fracture* (Figure A6-7•). It usually results from a fall on an outstretched arm. The deformity resembles that of a dinner fork. Supracondylar fractures are fractures of the distal humerus, just above the elbow. Fractures resulting from extension-type injuries usually cause posterior displacement of the distal segment. With flexion-type injuries, the distal fracture seg-

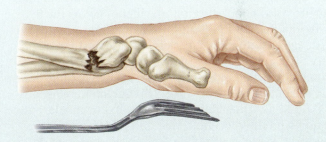

• **FIGURE A6-7** Colle's Fracture
In these common forearm fractures, the shape of the wrist after the injury often resembles a dinner fork.

ment is usually displaced anteriorly. Flexion-type injuries occur much less frequently than extension-type injuries. Most supracondylar fractures occur in children and are associated with a number of complications including nerve and vascular injuries due to these structures' close proximity to the fracture site (Figure A6-8•). Supracondylar fractures involving a growth plate can cause growth abnormalities often resulting

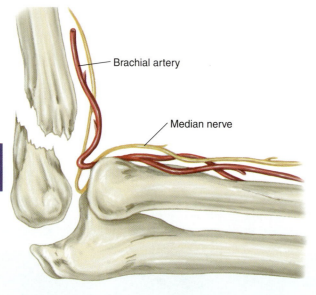

Brachial artery

Median nerve

● **FIGURE A6-8   Supracondylar Fracture**
Supracondylar fractures have a high incidence of associated nervous and vascular tissue injury. In children, some supracondylar fractures can involve the growth plate, possibly leading to permanent deformity or disability.

in permanent deformity. Because of the high complication rate, supracondylar fractures should be promptly evaluated and treated by an orthopaedic surgeon.

Hip Fractures.   Although the femur is the largest bone in the body, fractures of the proximal femur, or hip, are frequently seen, especially in the elderly. The hip is a ball-and-socket joint consisting of the acetabulum and the proximal femur, two to three inches below the lesser trochanter. The incidence of hip fracture increases with age and doubles for every decade past the age of fifty. The incidence is two to three times higher in women than men, primarily due to decreased bone density secondary to osteoporosis. Hip fractures are usually classified as either intracapsular or extracapsular, depending on their location. With intracapsular fractures, the blood vessels supplying the femoral head are often compromised, which can lead to necrosis of the femoral head. The four types of intracapsular hip fractures are capital, subcapital, transcervical, or basicervical (Figure A6-9●). Subcapital fractures are by far the most common type of intracapsular hip fracture. There are three types of extracapsular hip fractures: trochanteric, intertrochanteric, and subtrochanteric. Of these, intertrochanteric fractures are the most common. All hip fractures in ambulatory patients require open reduction and internal fixation in the operating room. Intracapsular fractures usually require replacement of the entire hip joint with a prosthetic hip and acetabulum. Most extracapsular fractures can be stabilized by placement of a surgical pin or nail to hold the bone segments together while healing. As a rule, early fixation of hip

fractures ($<$ 72 hours) in the elderly reduces morbidity and mortality.

Facial Fractures.   Fractures of the maxilla usually result from high-energy injuries. As a result, patients with facial fractures may also sustain other associated injuries such as spinal, chest, and abdominal injuries. There are several identifiable facial fracture patterns that were first described by LeFort. He developed a facial fracture classification system that bears his name (Figure A6-10●). A LeFort I fracture is limited to the maxilla at the level of the nares. In a LeFort I fracture, only the hard palate and upper teeth move with gentle palpation and mobilization. With a LeFort II injury, the triangular fracture line extends across the ridge of the cheeks and into the orbits. Mobilization of the fracture segment will move the nose but not the eyes. In a LeFort III fracture, the facial skeleton is separated from the skull. The entire face, including both orbits, shifts with palpation and gentle mobilization. This injury is also called a *cranial-facial disjunction.* Although not identified by LeFort, a LeFort IV facial fracture has been described. It is similar to a LeFort III fracture, but the fracture line extends upward into the frontal bones.

Fracture Healing

A fracture heals in three phases: inflammatory, reparative, and remodeling. Each phase of healing gradually blends into the next.

Immediately following a fracture, microscopic blood vessels that cross the fracture line are severed, thus interrupting blood supply to the injured bone ends. In the following days, these blood-deprived bone ends become necrotic. This triggers a classic inflammatory response with essential inflammatory cells migrating to the fracture site. Soon, granulation tissue begins to fill the affected area. Within the inflammatory response are cells capable of forming cartilage, collagen, and bone. Together, these three components form the bone callus that gradually surrounds the fractured bone ends and stabilizes them. There are both internal and external calluses. Over time, the external callus becomes harder as minerals, especially calcium, are laid down. Underneath the callus, the necrotic edges of bone at the fracture site are removed by osteoclasts, cells whose function is to resorb bone. Finally, following the reparative phase, the remodeling phase begins. Remodeling is the tendency of the bone to regain its original shape and contour. During this phase, the excess parts of the callus are removed and new bone is laid down along natural lines of stress. Remodeling can continue for years and is affected by such factors as the patient's age and health and the magnitude of the original fracture. Typically, within a year or so, all evidence that a fracture occurred has disappeared and the bone appears completely normal. Fractures heal most rapidly in young children and slowest in the elderly. A five-year-old child with an uncomplicated wrist fracture

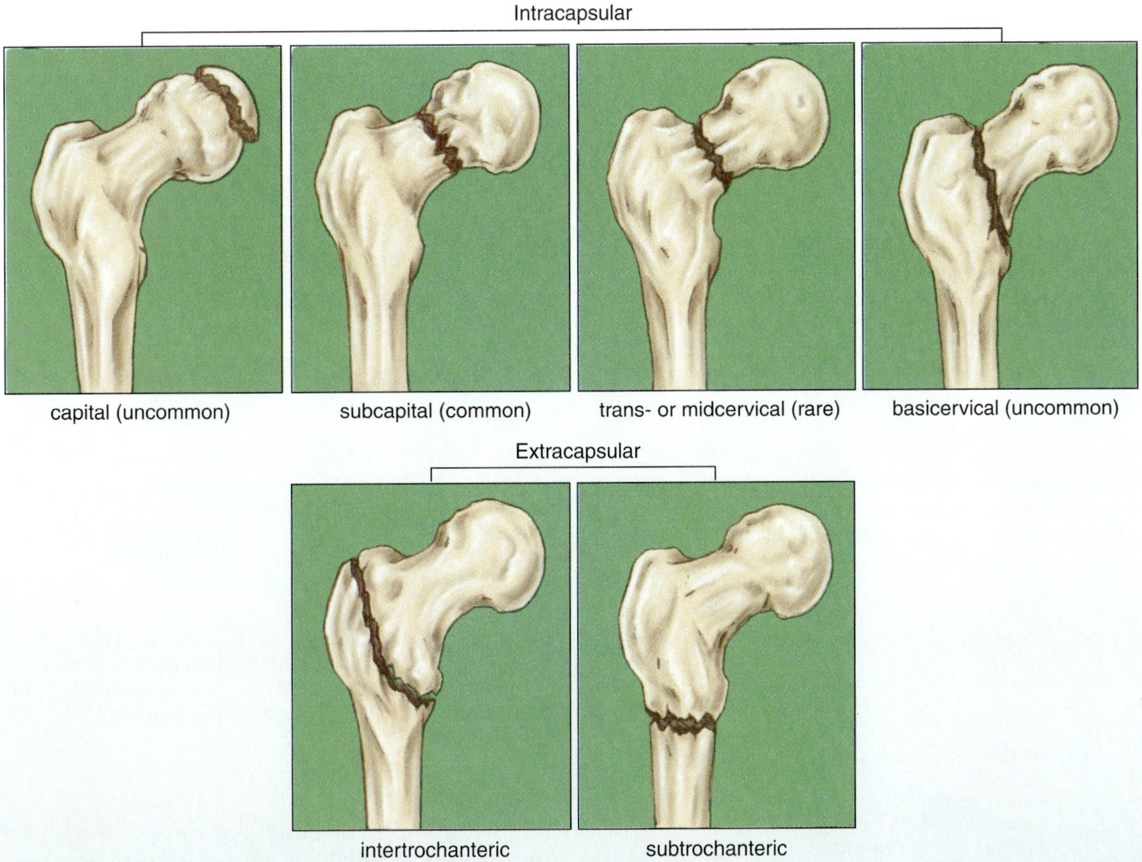

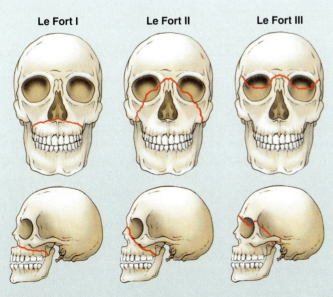

Intracapsular

capital (uncommon) subcapital (common) trans- or midcervical (rare) basicervical (uncommon)

Extracapsular

intertrochanteric subtrochanteric

● **FIGURE A6-9** **Types of Hip Fractures**
Subcapital and intertrochanteric fractures are the most common.

Le Fort I **Le Fort II** **Le Fort III**

● **FIGURE A6-10** **LeFort System of Classifying Facial Fractures**

may only need to be in a cast for three weeks while an elderly patient with the same injury can expect to be in a cast for six weeks or more.

Intraosseous Needle Placement

The bones are highly vascular, living tissues. By taking advantage of this characteristic, we can place a needle into the medullary cavity of the bone in order to provide emergency fluids and medications. This route should be considered when an IV cannot be placed and the patient is in need of rapid fluid resuscitation or drug therapy.

Placement of a needle into the bone marrow, referred to as intraosseous (IO) infusion, was described as early as 1922. However, the technique was all but abandoned until the mid-1980s when it was reintroduced in response to the need for vascular access during pediatric cardiopulmonary resuscitation. Since then, the technique has become widespread and has been accepted as an alternative to IV access for pediatric emergencies. Initially, IO therapy was limited to children. A device now available provides for rapid placement of a special intraosseous needle into the upper part of the sternum. This can be used for emergency vascular access for adults, including those needing cardiopulmonary resuscitation.

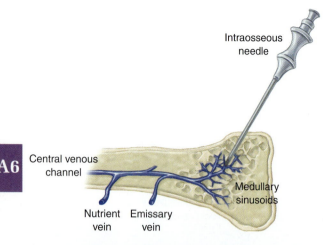

Intraosseous needle

Central venous channel

Nutrient vein   Emissary vein

Medullary sinusoids

• **FIGURE A6-11   Intraosseous Needle Properly Placed into Marrow Cavity and Medullar Sinusoids**
Fluid promptly drains from the sinusoids and exits via the emissary vein or nutrient vein and enters the central venous circulation.

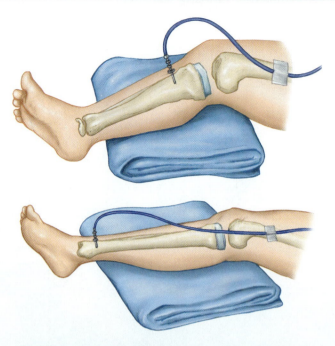

• **FIGURE A6-13   Proper Placement of an Intraosseous Needle in the Proximal Anterior Tibia (upper drawing) and Proximal to Medial Malleolus (lower drawing)**

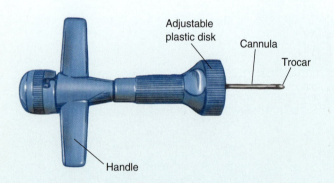

Adjustable plastic disk

Cannula

Trocar

Handle

• **FIGURE A6-12   Special Intraosseous Needle for Emergency Intraosseous Access**

Large bones, such as the tibia, are especially vascular and can accept large volumes of fluids and transfer them to the central circulation. The bone receives most of its blood supply through a nutrient artery, which enters the cortex of the bone and divides into ascending and descending branches. These branches further divide into arterioles and then capillaries. The capillaries drain into the medullary venous sinusoids throughout the medullary space of the bone (Figure A6-11•). Specially designed IO needles are available to pierce the cortex of the bone (Figure A6-12•). Fluids and medications administered through a properly placed IO needle enter the medullary sinusoids. The medullary cavity functions as a rigid, noncollapsable vein, even in the setting of cardiopulmonary arrest or shock. The medullary sinusoids act as a central venous channel that exits the bone

as either nutrient veins or emissary veins. Fluids and drugs administered through an IO needle enter the central circulation promptly, nearly as fast as through a central IV line. Virtually all emergency IV fluids and medications can be administered by the IO route.

In children less than six years of age, the preferred site for placement of an IO needle is the anterior proximal tibia, 1–3 centimeters distal to the tibial tuberosity. Alternate sites include the distal tibia just above the medial malleolus (Figure A6-13•). A less frequently used site is the distal femur, 2–3 centimeters above the external condyles.

SUMMARY

The skeletal system is an essential body system. Most emergencies involving the skeletal system are secondary to trauma. Common types of skeletal trauma include sprains, subluxations, dislocations, and fractures. As a member of the emergency medical team, you will encounter a significant number of skeletal emergencies in the course of your work. Remember that skeletal tissue is living, vascular tissue. Significant bleeding and hematoma formation may accompany fractures and sprains. Also, we can take advantage of this characteristic by placing an intraosseous needle into the marrow cavity in order to obtain emergency vascular access when traditional IV access cannot be obtained.

7

The Muscular System

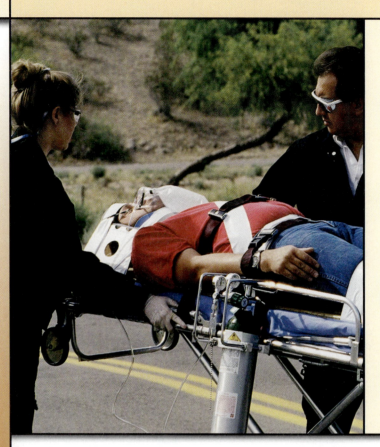

The muscular system consists of approximately 700 individual muscles. Injuries to muscles (strains) are quite common. Because of the interrelationship between the muscular and skeletal systems, determining the exact structures involved in an injury is often difficult. Also, it is not uncommon for both body systems to be involved. For example, an ankle sprain can result in tears to muscles of the lower leg and foot; stretching or tearing of the ligaments; and, in severe cases, fracture of one or more of the ankle bones.

Chapter Outline and Objectives

Vocabulary Development

aer, air; *aerobic*
an, not; *anaerobic*
bi, two; *biceps*
caput, head; *biceps*
clavius, clavicle; *clavicle*
di, two; *digastricus*
epi-, on; *epimysium*
ergon, work; *synergist*
fasciculus, a bundle; *fascicle*
galea, a helmet; *galea aponeurotica*
gaster, stomach; *gastrocnemius*
hyper, above; *hypertrophy*
iso-, equal; *isometric*
kneme, knee; *gastrocnemius*
lemma, husk; *sarcolemma*
meros, part; *sarcomere*
metron, measure; *isometric*
mys, muscle; *epimysium*
*osteo-, bone; *osteopathic*
peri-, around; *perimysium*
platys, flat; *platysma*
sarkos, flesh; *sarcolemma*
syn-, together; *synergist*
tetanos, convulsive tension; *tetanus*
tonos, tension; *isotonic*
trope, a turning; *tropomyosin*
-trophy, nourishing; *atrophy*

It is hard to imagine what life would be like without muscle tissue. We would be unable to sit, stand, walk, speak, or grasp objects. Blood would not circulate, because there would be no heartbeat to propel it through the vessels. The lungs could not rhythmically empty and fill, nor could food move through the digestive tract. Muscle tissue, one of the four primary tissue types, consists chiefly of elongated muscle cells that are highly specialized for contraction. The three types of muscle tissue—*skeletal muscle, cardiac muscle,* and *smooth muscle*—were introduced in Chapter 4. ∞ *p. 97* These muscle tissues share four basic properties:

1. **Excitability:** the ability to respond to stimulation. For example, skeletal muscles normally respond to stimulation by the nervous system, and some smooth muscles respond to circulating hormones.

2. **Contractility:** the ability to shorten actively and exert a pull, or tension, that can be harnessed by connective tissues.

3. **Extensibility:** the ability to continue to contract over a range of resting lengths. For example, a smooth muscle cell can be stretched to several times its original length and still contract on stimulation.

4. **Elasticity:** the ability of a muscle to rebound toward its original length after a contraction.

This chapter begins with the organization of skeletal muscle tissue. Although most of the muscle tissue in the body is skeletal muscle, this section will also consider cardiac and smooth muscle tissue. We will then proceed to a consideration of the functional organization of the muscular system.

FUNCTIONS OF SKELETAL MUSCLE

Skeletal muscle tissue, connective tissues, and neural tissue combine to form **skeletal muscles**, contractile organs that are directly or indirectly attached to bones. The muscular system includes approximately 700 skeletal muscles. These muscles perform the following functions:

1. *Produce movement.* Muscle contractions pull on tendons and move the bones of the skeleton.

2. *Maintain posture and body position.* Without constant muscular tension, you could not sit upright without collapsing or stand without toppling over.

3. *Support soft tissues.* The abdominal wall and the floor of the pelvic cavity consist of layers of muscle that support the weight of visceral organs and shield internal tissues from injury.

4. *Guard entrances and exits.* Skeletal muscles guard openings to the digestive and urinary tracts and provide voluntary control over swallowing, defecation, and urination.

5. *Maintain body temperature.* Muscle contractions require energy, and whenever energy is used in the body, some of it is converted to heat. The heat lost by working muscles keeps the body temperature in the normal range.

THE ANATOMY OF SKELETAL MUSCLES

When naming structural features of muscles and their components, anatomists often used the Greek words *sarkos* (flesh) and *mys* (muscle). These word roots will be encountered in the following discussions of the anatomy of skeletal muscle.

Gross Anatomy

Figure 7-1● illustrates the appearance and organization of a typical skeletal muscle. A skeletal muscle contains connective tissues, blood vessels, nerves, and skeletal muscle tissue.

Connective Tissue Organization

Three layers of connective tissue are part of each muscle: an outer epimysium, a central perimysium, and an inner endomysium (Figure 7-1●). The entire muscle is surrounded by the **epimysium** (ep-i-MIS-ē-um; *epi-,* on + *mys*, muscle), a layer of collagen fibers that separates the muscle from surrounding tissues and organs.

At each end of the muscle, the epimysial fibers come together to form **tendons**, bands of collagen fibers that attach skeletal muscles to bones. ∞ *p. 92* The tendon fibers are interwoven into the periosteum of the bone, providing a firm attachment. Any contraction of the muscle will exert a pull on its tendon and in turn on the attached bone.

The connective tissue fibers of the **perimysium** (per-i-MIS-ē-um; *peri-,* around) divide the skeletal muscle into a series of compartments, each containing a bundle of muscle fibers called a **fascicle** (FA-sik-ul; *fasciculus,* a bundle). In addition to collagen and elastic fibers, the perimysium contains blood vessels and nerves that supply the fascicles.

Within a fascicle, the **endomysium** (en-dō-MIS-ē-um; *endo-,* inside) surrounds each skeletal muscle fiber and ties adjacent muscle fibers together. Stem cells scattered among the fibers help repair damaged muscle tissue.

Nerves and Blood Vessels

Skeletal muscles are often called *voluntary muscles* because their contractions can occur under voluntary control. Many of these skeletal muscles may also be controlled involuntarily. For example, skeletal muscles involved with breathing, such as the *diaphragm,* usually work under involuntary control. Each skeletal muscle

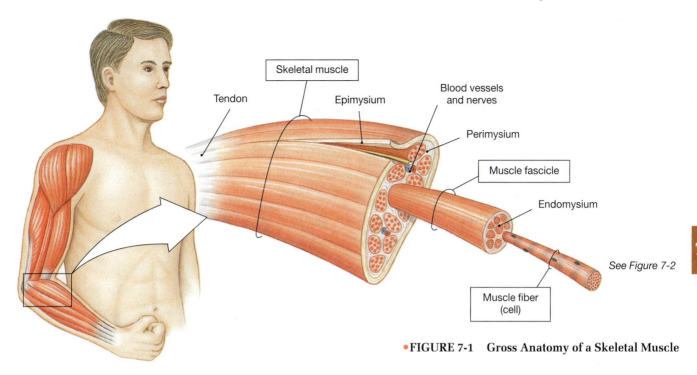

See Figure 7-2

•**FIGURE 7-1**   **Gross Anatomy of a Skeletal Muscle**

fiber is controlled by a *motor neuron* whose cell body lies within the central nervous system. *Axons*, or nerve fibers, of the motor neurons involved with a particular skeletal muscle penetrate the epimysium, branch through the perimysium, and enter the endomysium to control individual muscle fibers. Since muscle contraction requires a tremendous amount of energy, an extensive network of blood vessels delivers the oxygen and nutrients needed for the production of ATP in active skeletal muscles.

Microanatomy

Skeletal muscle fibers (Figures 7-1• and 7-2•) are quite different from the "typical" cell described in Chapter 3. One obvious difference is their enormous size. For example, a skeletal muscle fiber from a leg muscle could have a diameter of 100 μm and a length equal to that of the entire muscle (30–40 cm, or 10–16 in.). In addition, each skeletal muscle fiber is *multinucleate*, meaning it contains hundreds of nuclei just beneath the cell membrane. The genes contained in these nuclei direct the production of enzymes and structural proteins required for normal contraction, and the presence of multiple copies of these genes speeds up the process.

The cell membrane, or **sarcolemma** (sar-cō-LEM-a; *sarkos*, flesh + *lemma*, husk) of a muscle fiber surrounds the cytoplasm, or **sarcoplasm** (SAR-kō-plazm). Openings scattered across the surface of the sarcolemma lead into a network of narrow tubules called **transverse tubules**, or **T tubules**. Transverse tubules begin at the sarcolemma and extend into the sarcoplasm at right

angles to the membrane surface. They are filled with extracellular fluid, and they form passageways through the muscle fiber, like a series of tunnels through a mountain. The T tubules play a major role in coordinating the contraction of the muscle fiber.

Transverse Tubules and the Sarcoplasmic Reticulum

A muscle fiber contraction occurs through the orderly interaction of both electrical and chemical events. Electrical events at the sarcolemma trigger a contraction by altering the chemical environment everywhere inside the muscle fiber. The electrical "message" is distributed by the transverse tubules that extend deep into the sarcoplasm of the muscle fiber. There they encircle the individual **myofibrils**, cylindrical structures that are responsible for the contraction of the muscle fiber.

As a T tubule encircles a myofibril, it makes close contact with expanded chambers of the **sarcoplasmic reticulum**, a specialized form of endoplasmic reticulum. These chambers are called *cisternae*. As it encircles a myofibril, a transverse tubule lies sandwiched between a pair of cisternae, forming a *triad* (Figure 7-2a•).

These cisternae contain high concentrations of calcium ions. The calcium ion concentration in the cytoplasm of all cells is kept very low. Most cells, including skeletal muscle fibers, pump calcium ions across their cell membranes and into the extracellular fluid. Skeletal muscle fibers, however, also actively transport calcium ions into the cisternae of the sarcoplasmic reticulum. A muscle contraction begins when the stored calcium ions are released by the cisternae.

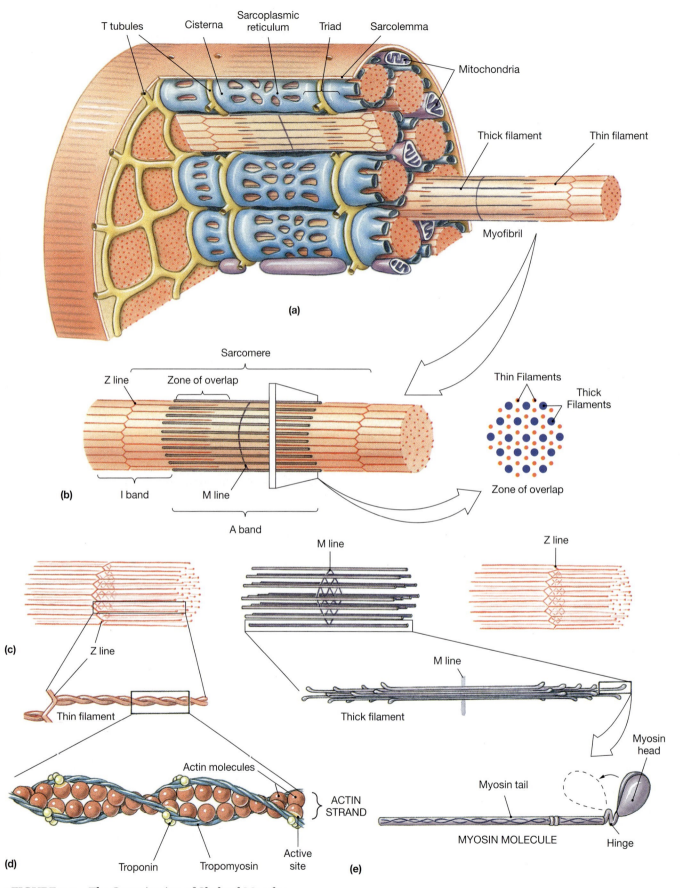

●**FIGURE 7-2   The Organization of Skeletal Muscles**
(a) The structure of a skeletal muscle fiber. **(b)** The organization of a sarcomere, part of a single myofibril. **(c)** The sarcomere in part c, stretched such that thick and thin filaments no longer overlap. (This cannot happen in an intact muscle fiber.) **(d)** The structure of a thin filament. **(e)** The structure of a thick filament.

Myofibrils and Myofilaments

The sarcoplasm contains hundreds to thousands of myofibrils. Each myofibril is a cylinder 1–2 μm in diameter and as long as the entire muscle fiber. Myofibrils are responsible for muscle fiber contraction. Because they are attached to the sarcolemma at each end of the cell, their contraction shortens the entire cell. Scattered between the myofibrils are mitochondria and glycogen granules. The breakdown of glycogen and the activity of mitochondria provide the ATP needed to power muscular contractions.

Myofibrils are bundles of **myofilaments**, protein filaments consisting primarily of the proteins *actin* and *myosin*. Actin molecules are found in **thin filaments**, and the myosin molecules are found in **thick filaments**. Myofilaments are organized in repeating functional units called **sarcomeres** (SAR-kō-mērz; *sarkos*, flesh + *meros*, part) (Figure 7-2b•).

Sarcomere Organization

The arrangement of thick and thin filaments within a sarcomere produces a banded appearance. All of the myofibrils are arranged parallel to the long axis of the cell, with their sarcomeres lying side by side. As a result, the entire muscle fiber has a banded, or striated, appearance corresponding to the bands of the individual sarcomeres (Figure 7-2a•).

Each myofibril consists of a linear series of approximately 10,000 sarcomeres. *The sarcomere is the smallest functional unit of the muscle fiber; interactions between the thick and thin filaments of sarcomeres are responsible for muscle contraction.*

Figure 7-2b• diagrams the external and internal structure of an individual sarcomere. Each sarcomere has a resting length of about 2.6 μm. The thick filaments lie in the center of the sarcomere. Thin filaments at either end of the sarcomere are attached to interconnecting proteins that make up the **Z lines**, the boundaries of each sarcomere. From the Z lines, the thin filaments extend toward the center of the sarcomere, passing among the thick filaments in the *zone of overlap*. The **M line** is made up of proteins that connect the central portions of each thick filament to its neighbors. The relationships of Z lines and M lines are shown in Figure 7-2c•.

The differences in the size and density of thick and thin filaments account for the banded appearance of the sarcomere. The **A band** is the area containing thick filaments. The region between two successive A bands—including the Z line—is the **I band**. (It may help you to remember that the A band appears d<u>A</u>rk and the I band l<u>I</u>ght in a light micrograph.)

Thin and Thick Filaments

Each thin filament consists of a twisted strand of actin molecules (Figure 7-2d•). Each actin molecule has an **active site** capable of interacting with myosin. In a rest-

ing muscle, the active sites along the thin filaments are covered by strands of the protein **tropomyosin** (trō-pō-MĪ-o-sin; *trope*, turning). The tropomyosin strands are held in position by molecules of **troponin** (TRŌ-pō-nin) that are bound to the actin strand.

Thick filaments are composed of myosin molecules, each with an attached *tail* and a free globular *head*. The myosin molecules are oriented away from the center of the sarcomere, with the heads projecting outward (Figure 7-2e•). The myosin heads interact with actin molecules during a contraction. This interaction cannot occur unless the troponin changes position, moving the tropomyosin and exposing the active sites.

Calcium is the key that unlocks the active sites and starts a contraction. When calcium ions bind to troponin, the protein changes shape, swinging the tropomyosin away from the active sites. Myosin-actin binding can then occur, and a contraction begins. The cisternae of the sarcoplasmic reticulum are the source of the calcium that triggers muscle contraction, and the effect on the sarcomere is almost instantaneous.

Sliding Filaments

When a sarcomere contracts, the Z lines move closer together as the thin filaments slide toward the center of the sarcomere, parallel to the thick filaments. Figure 7-3• presents a two-dimensional view of this process. The sliding occurs through interactions between the thick and thin filaments. It begins when the myosin heads of thick

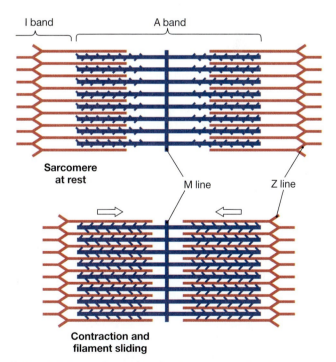

•**FIGURE 7-3   Changes in the Appearance of a Sarcomere During Contraction of a Skeletal Muscle Fiber**
During a contraction, the A band stays the same width, but the Z lines move closer together and the I band gets smaller.

filaments bind to active sites on thin filaments, in much the same way that a substrate molecule binds to the active site of an enzyme. When they connect thick filaments and thin filaments, the myosin heads are called **crossbridges**. When a cross-bridge binds to an active site, it pivots toward the center of the sarcomere, pulling the thin filament in that direction. The cross-bridge then detaches and returns to its original position, ready to repeat a cycle of "attach, pivot, detach, and return," like a person pulling in a rope one-handed.

✳ RHABDOMYOLYSIS

Patients who are unconscious or immobile for a prolonged time are at risk for developing rhabdomyolysis, a breakdown of muscle tissue where the patient has been lying. When this occurs, numerous substances, most notably myoglobin, muscle enzymes, and electrolytes, are released from the damaged muscle. Myoglobin concentrates in the urine (myoglobinuria), turning it dark reddish brown. In severe cases, the patient can develop kidney failure.

✓ How would severing the tendon that was attached to a muscle affect the ability of the muscle to move a body part?

✓ Why does skeletal muscle appear striated when viewed with a microscope?

✓ Where would you expect to find the greatest concentration of calcium ions in resting skeletal muscle?

THE CONTROL OF MUSCLE FIBER CONTRACTION

Chapter 8 examines neural physiology in detail, so our discussion here will focus on neural stimulation of skeletal muscles. Before proceeding, however, you should take a moment to review the details of neuron structure that were introduced in Chapter 4. ∞ *p. 99*

The Structure and Function of the Neuromuscular Junction

Communication between the nervous system and a skeletal muscle fiber occurs at a specialized intercellular connection known as a **neuromuscular junction** (Figure 7-4a•). Each skeletal muscle fiber is controlled by a motor neuron at a single neuromuscular junction midway along its length. Figure 7-4b• summarizes key features of this structure.

Each axon or branch of an axon ends at a **synaptic knob**. The cytoplasm of the synaptic knob contains mitochondria and vesicles filled with molecules of **acetylcholine** (as-ē-til-KŌ-lēn), or **ACh**. Acetylcholine is an example of a *neurotransmitter*, a chemical released by

a neuron to change the activities of other cells. The release of ACh from the synaptic knob results in changes in the sarcolemma that trigger the contraction of the muscle fiber.

A narrow space, the **synaptic cleft**, separates the synaptic knob from the sarcolemma. This portion of the membrane, which contains receptors that bind ACh, is known as the **motor end plate**. The motor end plate has deep creases that increase the membrane surface area and the number of ACh receptors. Both the synaptic cleft and the motor end plate contain the enzyme **acetylcholinesterase** (**AChE**, or *cholinesterase*), which breaks down molecules of ACh.

Neurons control skeletal muscle fibers by stimulating the production of an **action potential**, or electrical impulse, in the sarcolemma. The sequence of events shown in Figure 7-4c• can be summarized as follows:

Step 1: *The release of acetylcholine.* An action potential travels along the axon of a motor neuron. When this impulse reaches the synaptic knob, vesicles in the synaptic knob release acetylcholine into the synaptic cleft.

Step 2: *The binding of ACh at the motor end plate.* The ACh molecules diffuse across the synaptic cleft and bind to ACh receptors on the sarcolemma. This event changes the permeability of the membrane to sodium ions. It is this sudden rush of sodium ions into the sarcoplasm that produces an action potential in the sarcolemma. (We will examine the formation and conduction of action potentials more closely in Chapter 8.)

Step 3: *The conduction of action potentials by the sarcolemma.* The action potential spreads over the entire sarcolemma surface. It also travels down all of the transverse tubules toward the cisternae that encircle the sarcomeres of the muscle fiber. The passage of an action potential triggers a sudden, massive release of calcium ions by the cisternae.

As the calcium ion concentration rises, active sites are exposed on the thin filaments, cross-bridge interactions occur, and a contraction begins. Because all of the cisternae in the muscle fiber are affected, this contraction is a combined effort involving every sarcomere on every myofibril. While the contraction process gets under way, the acetylcholine is being broken down by acetylcholinesterase.

The Contraction Cycle

In the resting sarcomere, each cross-bridge is bound to a molecule of ADP and phosphate (PO_4^{3-}), the products released by the breakdown of a molecule of ATP. In addition to binding the breakdown products, the cross-

•**FIGURE 7-4   Neural Control of Muscle
Contraction**
(a) A colorized SEM of a neuromuscular
junction. **(b)** An action potential (in red)
arrives at the synaptic knob. **(c)** Steps in the
chemical communication between the
synaptic knob and motor end plate.

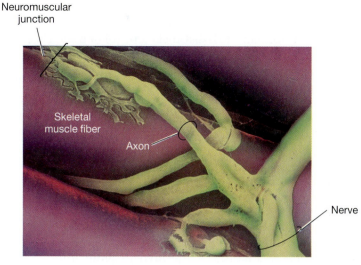

(a)

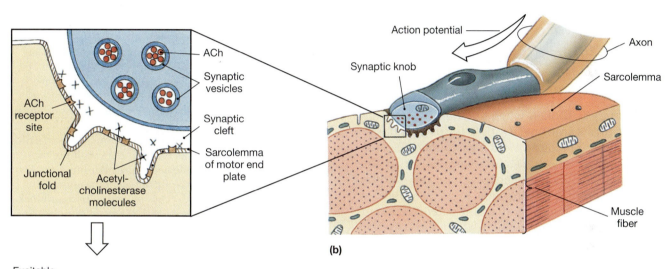

(b)

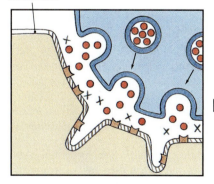

Step 1: Release of Acetylcholine.
Vesicles in the synaptic knob release their
contents into the synaptic cleft.

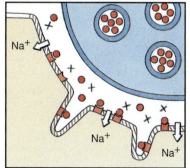

**Step 2: ACh Binding at the Motor End
Plate.**   The binding of ACh to
the receptors changes the membrane
permeability and induces an action
potential in the sarcolemma.

(c)

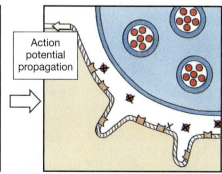

**Step 3: Action Potential Conduction
by the Sarcolemma.**   The action
potential spreads across the membrane
surface and travels down the
transverse tubules, triggering the
release of calcium ions at the cisternae.
While this occurs, AChE removes the
acetylcholine from the synaptic cleft.

7

bridge stores the energy released by the rupture of the high-energy bond. In effect, the resting cross-bridge is "primed" for a contraction, like a cocked pistol or a set mousetrap.

The contraction process involves the following five interlocking steps, which are shown schematically in Figure 7-5•:

Step 1: The exposure of the active site following the binding of calcium ions (Ca^{2+}) to troponin.

Step 2: The attachment of the myosin cross-bridge to the exposed active site on the thin filaments.

Step 3: The pivoting of the attached myosin head toward the center of the sarcomere and the release of ADP and a phosphate group. This step uses the energy that was stored in the myosin molecule at rest.

Step 4: The detachment of the cross-bridges when the myosin head binds another ATP molecule.

Step 5: The reactivation of the detached myosin head as it splits the ATP and captures the released energy. The entire cycle can now be repeated, beginning with step 2.

This cycle is broken when calcium ion concentrations return to normal resting levels, primarily through active transport into the sarcoplasmic reticulum. If a single action potential sweeps across the sarcolemma, calcium ion removal occurs very rapidly and the contraction will be very brief. A sustained contraction will occur only if action potentials occur one after another, and calcium loss from the cisternae continues.

RIGOR MORTIS

Dead human bodies suddenly sitting up in a morgue are a part of many urban legends. In actuality, this does not occur. Approximately 6 hours after death (the time varies depending on environmental temperature), the skeletal muscles have depleted all remaining glucose and ATP molecules. Waste products, primarily metabolic acids, accumulate. After the ATP is gone, the sarcoplasmic reticulum cannot remove calcium ions from the sarcoplasm. Then, myosin fibers cannot separate from actin fibers, and *rigor mortis,* a sustained contraction, sets in. The smaller muscles, usually those of the jaw, are affected first. Eventually, the entire body is affected. Finally, 12–24 hours later, lysosomal enzymes from the muscle cells break down the contracted myofilaments, and the muscles relax.

Muscle Contraction: A Summary

Table 7-1 (p. 176) provides a summary of the contraction process, from ACh release to the end of the contraction.

NEUROMUSCULAR BLOCKING DRUGS

Control of the airway is a paramount concern in any emergency. However, securing an airway can be difficult in combative patients with closed head injuries or drug overdoses. In these cases, it is often necessary to administer a drug that temporarily paralyzes the patient so that the airway can be controlled.

Drugs that cause paralysis of skeletal muscles are called neuromuscular blockers, as they interfere with nervous impulse transmission at the neuromuscular junction. They either mimic acetylcholine or compete for acetylcholine receptors. Regardless, both types of neuromuscular blockers cause reversible paralysis of the skeletal muscles, including the respiratory muscles. During neuromuscular blockade, the patient must receive mechanical ventilation.

✳ CLINICAL NOTE   LABORATORY TESTING IN HEART ATTACK

Diagnosing a heart attack is often difficult. A heart attack (*acute myocardial infarction*) occurs most commonly when an artery supplying blood to a part of the heart muscle is occluded. Initially, the area of the heart muscle supplied by that artery will become injured (*myocardial ischemia*). If this continues, the affected portion will die (*myocardial infarction*). Because of this, it is important for emergency personnel to recognize heart attacks early so that treatment can be provided to restore blood flow.

Several diagnostic tools are routinely used to determine whether a heart attack has occurred. These include the electrocardiogram (ECG), X-rays, laboratory tests, and others. Following injury to the heart muscle, chemical components of the heart muscle are released into the circulation. Laboratory assays of these chemicals can aid in the diagnosis of heart attack. Commonly assayed chemicals include creatine kinase (CK) and troponin, among others.

Creatine kinase (CK) is an enzyme found in muscle and brain tissue. There are subtle differences in CK structure (*isoenzymes*), depending on the source. CK-MM comes from skeletal muscle, CK-BB comes from brain tissue, and CK-MB comes from heart tissue. The amount of CK-MB in the blood should not exceed 2–4% of the total CK level. Any elevation in the percentage of CK-MB indicates myocardial injury. The CK-MB level begins to increase within 4 hours of injury, peaks at 18–24 hours, and remains elevated 3–4 days.

Troponin, an important contractile protein, is not normally present in the blood. Thus, the presence of troponin in the blood indicates heart muscle damage. Troponin (*troponin I*) can be detected within 3–6 hours following myocardial injury and remains elevated 14 days.

When myocardial ischemia is suspected, patients are usually admitted to the hospital and serial lab tests are performed, usually over a 24-hour period. The chance of detecting myocardial ischemia with a single sampling of CK-MB is only 34%. However, repeated sampling over 24-hours increases the accuracy to 90% or better.

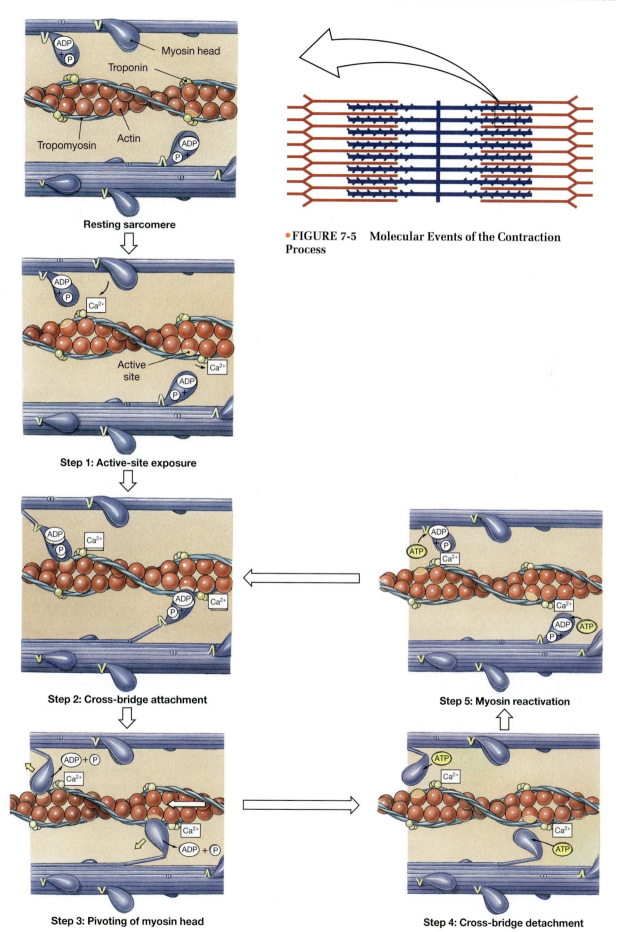

Resting sarcomere

Step 1: Active-site exposure

Step 2: Cross-bridge attachment

Step 3: Pivoting of myosin head

Step 4: Cross-bridge detachment

Step 5: Myosin reactivation

Myosin head
Troponin
Tropomyosin
Actin
Active site

• **FIGURE 7-5   Molecular Events of the Contraction Process**

7

TABLE 7-1   **A Summary of the Steps Involved in Skeletal Muscle Contraction**

Key steps in the initiation of a contraction include:

1. At the neuromuscular junction, ACh released by the synaptic knob binds to receptors on the sarcolemma.
2. The resulting change in the membrane potential of the muscle fiber leads to the production of an action potential that spreads across its entire surface and reaches the triads via the transverse tubules.
3. The sarcoplasmic reticulum releases stored calcium ions, increasing the calcium concentration of the sarcoplasm in and around the sarcomeres.
4. Calcium ions bind to troponin, resulting in the movement of tropomyosin and the exposure of active sites on the thin (actin) filaments.
5. Repeated cycles of cross-bridge binding, pivoting, and detachment occur, powered by the breakdown of ATP. These events produce filament sliding, and the muscle fiber shortens.

This process continues for a brief period, until:

6. Action potential generation ceases as ACh is removed by acetylcholinesterase.
7. The sarcoplasmic reticulum reabsorbs calcium ions, and the concentration of calcium ions in the sarcoplasm declines.
8. When calcium ion concentrations approach normal resting levels, the troponin and tropomyosin molecules return to their normal positions. These changes cover the active sites and prevent further cross-bridge interaction.
9. Without cross-bridge interactions, further sliding will not take place and the contraction will end.
10. Muscle relaxation occurs, muscle returns passively toward resting length.

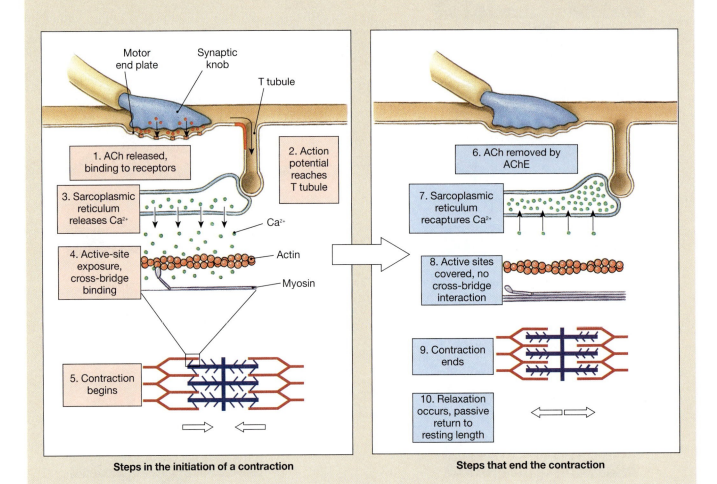

Steps in the initiation of a contraction   **Steps that end the contraction**

✓ How would a drug that interferes with cross-bridge formation affect muscle contraction?

✓ What would you expect to happen to a resting skeletal muscle if the sarcolemma suddenly became very permeable to calcium ions?

✓ Predict what would happen to a muscle if the motor end plate did not contain acetylcholinesterase.

MUSCLE MECHANICS

Now that we are familiar with muscle contraction of individual muscle fibers, we can examine the performance of skeletal muscles. In this section we will consider the coordinated contractions of an entire population of muscle fibers.

The amount of tension produced by an individual muscle fiber depends solely on the number of cross-bridge interactions. If a muscle fiber at a given resting length is stimulated to contract, it will always produce the same amount of tension. No mechanism regulates the amount of tension produced in that contraction: The muscle fiber is either "ON" (producing tension) or "OFF" (relaxed). This is the **all-or-none principle**.

An entire skeletal muscle contracts when its component muscle fibers are stimulated. The amount of tension produced in the skeletal muscle *as a whole* is determined by (1) the frequency of stimulation and (2) the number of muscle fibers activated.

The Frequency of Muscle Stimulation

A **twitch** is a single stimulus-contraction-relaxation sequence in a muscle fiber. Its duration can be as brief as 7.5 msec, as in an eye muscle fiber, or up to 100 msec, as in calf muscle fibers. Figure 7-6• is a graph, or *myogram*, of the phases of a twitch in the *gastrocnemius muscle*, a prominent calf muscle:

• The **latent period** begins at stimulation and typically lasts about 2 msec. Over this period the action potential sweeps across the sarcolemma, and calcium ions are released by the sarcoplasmic reticulum. No tension is produced by the muscle fiber, because the contractile mechanism is not yet activated.

• In the **contraction phase**, tension rises to a peak. Throughout this period the cross-bridges are interacting with the active sites on the actin filaments.

• During the **relaxation phase**, muscle tension falls to resting levels as the cross-bridges detach.

A single stimulation produces a single twitch, but twitches in a skeletal muscle do not accomplish anything useful. All normal activities involve more sustained muscle contractions. Such contractions result from repeated stimulations.

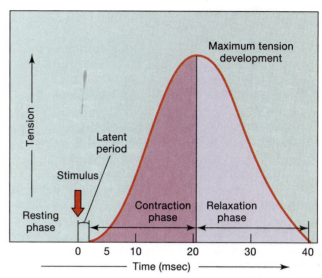

•**FIGURE 7-6**   **The Twitch and Development of Tension**
A myogram showing the time course of a single twitch contraction in the gastrocnemius muscle.

Incomplete Tetanus

If a second stimulus arrives before the relaxation phase has ended, a second, more powerful contraction occurs. The addition of one twitch to another in this way is called **summation** (Figure 7-7a•). If you continue to stimulate the muscle, never allowing it to relax completely, tension will peak, as illustrated in Figure 7-7b•. A muscle producing peak tension during rapid cycles of contraction and relaxation is said to be in **incomplete tetanus** (*tetanos*, convulsive tension).

Complete Tetanus

Complete tetanus occurs when the rate of stimulation is increased until the relaxation phase is completely eliminated (Figure 7-7c•). In complete tetanus, the action potentials are arriving so fast that the sarcoplasmic reticulum does not have time to reclaim the calcium ions. The high calcium ion concentration in the cytoplasm prolongs the state of contraction, making it continuous. Virtually all normal muscular contractions involve complete tetanus of the participating muscle units.

The Number of Muscle Fibers Involved

We have a remarkable ability to control the amount of tension exerted by our skeletal muscles. During a normal movement, our muscles contract smoothly, not jerkily, because activated muscle fibers are responding in complete tetanus. The *total force* exerted by the muscle as a whole depends on how many muscle fibers are activated.

A typical skeletal muscle contains thousands of muscle fibers. Although some motor neurons control a single muscle fiber, most control hundreds or thousands

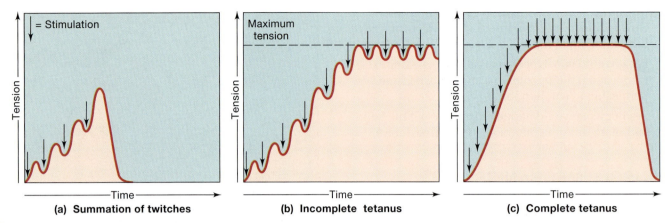

(a) Summation of twitches   **(b) Incomplete tetanus**   **(c) Complete tetanus**

• **FIGURE 7-7   The Effects of Repeated Stimulations**
(a) During summation, tension rises when successive stimuli arrive before relaxation has been completed. **(b)** Incomplete tetanus occurs if the rate of stimulation increases further. Tension production will rise to a peak, and the periods of relaxation will be very brief. **(c)** In complete tetanus, the frequency of stimulation is so high that the relaxation phase has been completely eliminated and tension plateaus at maximal levels.

of muscle fibers through multiple synaptic knobs. All of the muscle fibers controlled by a single motor neuron constitute a **motor unit**. The size of a motor unit indicates how fine the control of movement can be. In the muscles of the eye, where precise control is extremely important, a motor neuron may control two or three muscle fibers. We have much less precise control over our leg muscles, where up to 2000 muscle fibers may respond to the call of a single motor neuron.

When a decision is made to perform a specific movement, specific groups of motor neurons within the central nervous system (brain and spinal cord) are stimulated. The stimulated neurons do not respond spontaneously, and over time, the number of activated motor units gradually increases. The smooth but steady increase in muscular tension produced by increasing the number of active motor units is called **recruitment**.

Peak tension production occurs when all of the motor units in the muscle are contracting in complete tetanus. Such contractions do not last long, however, because the muscle fibers soon use up their available energy supplies. During a sustained **tetanic contraction**, motor units are activated on a rotating basis, so that some are resting while others are contracting.

Muscle Tone

Some of the motor units within any particular muscle are always active, even when the entire muscle is not contracting. Their contractions do not produce enough tension to cause movement, but they do tense and firm the muscle. This resting tension in a skeletal muscle is called **muscle tone**. A muscle with little muscle tone appears limp and flaccid, whereas one with moderate muscle tone is quite firm and solid.

A skeletal muscle that is not stimulated by a motor neuron on a regular basis will **atrophy** (AT-rō-fē; *a*, without + *-trophy*, nourishing): Its muscle fibers will become smaller and weaker. Individuals paralyzed by spinal injuries or other damage to the nervous system gradually lose muscle tone and volume in the areas affected. Even a temporary reduction in muscle use can lead to muscular atrophy, as is easily seen by comparing limb muscles before and after a cast has been worn. Muscle atrophy is initially reversible, but dying muscle fibers are not replaced, and in extreme atrophy the functional losses are permanent. That is why physical therapy is so important in cases where patients are temporarily unable to move normally.

Isotonic and Isometric Contractions

Muscle contractions may be classified as isotonic or isometric on the basis of the pattern of tension production and overall change in shape. In an **isotonic** (*iso-*, equal + *tonos*, tension) **contraction**, tension rises to a level that is maintained until relaxation occurs. During such contractions, the muscle shortens as the tension in the muscle remains constant. Lifting an object off a desk, walking, running, and so forth involve isotonic contractions of this kind.

In an **isometric** (*metron*, measure) **contraction**, tension continues to rise but the muscle as a whole does not change in length. Examples of isometric contractions are pushing against a wall and trying to pick up a large car. These are rather unusual movements, but many of the everyday reflexive muscle contractions that keep the body upright when standing or sitting involve isometric contractions of muscles that oppose gravity.

Normal daily activities involve a combination of isotonic and isometric muscular contractions. As you sit reading this text, isometric contractions of postural muscles stabilize your vertebrae and maintain your upright position. When you next turn a page, the movements of your arm, forearm, hand, and fingers are produced by isotonic contractions.

Muscle Elongation

Upon entering the relaxation phase, a muscle fiber is at its contracted length (see Figure 7-6•). How then does it return to its original (uncontracted) length? There is no active mechanism for muscle fiber elongation; contraction is active, but elongation is passive. After a contraction, a muscle fiber usually returns to its original length through a combination of (1) elastic forces and (2) the movements of opposing muscles.

Elastic Forces

Every time a muscle fiber contracts, its organelles are compressed and the extracellular fibers, such as those of the endomysium, are stretched. When the contraction ends, the intracellular and extracellular elements rebound to their original dimensions, gradually returning the muscle fiber to its original resting length.

Opposing Muscle Movements

Much more rapid returns to resting length result from the contraction of opposing muscles. For example, contraction of the *biceps brachii* muscle on the anterior part of the arm flexes the elbow; contraction of the *triceps brachii* muscle on the posterior surface of the arm extends the elbow. When the biceps brachii contracts, the triceps brachii is stretched; when the biceps brachii relaxes, contraction of the triceps brachii extends the elbow and stretches the muscle fibers of the biceps brachii to their original length.

✓ What factor is responsible for the amount of tension that a muscle fiber develops?

✓ A motor unit from a skeletal muscle contains 1500 muscle fibers. Would this muscle be involved in fine, delicate movements or powerful, gross movements? Explain.

✓ Is it possible for a muscle to contract without shortening? Explain.

THE ENERGETICS OF MUSCULAR ACTIVITY

Muscle contraction requires large amounts of energy. For example, an active skeletal muscle fiber may require some 600 trillion molecules of ATP each second, not including the energy needed to pump the calcium ions back into the sarcoplasmic reticulum. Although resting skeletal muscle cells contain large energy reserves in the form of ATP and other high-energy compounds, the reserves are only enough to sustain a contraction until additional ATP can be generated. Throughout the rest of the contraction, the muscle fiber will generate ATP at roughly the same rate as it is used.

ATP and CP Reserves

The primary function of ATP is the transfer of energy from one location to another, rather than the long-term storage of energy. At rest, a skeletal muscle fiber produces more ATP than it needs, and under these conditions ATP transfers energy to another high-energy compound, **creatine phosphate (CP)** (Figure 7-8a•). *Creatine* is a nitrogen-containing compound produced by the body that can bind a high-energy phosphate group. During a contraction, each cross-bridge breaks down ATP, producing ADP and a phosphate group. The energy stored in CP is then used to "recharge" the ADP back to ATP.

A resting skeletal muscle fiber contains about six times as much creatine phosphate as ATP. But when a muscle fiber is contracting repeatedly, both of these energy reserves will be exhausted in about 30 seconds. At such times, the muscle fiber must then rely on other mechanisms to convert ADP to ATP.

ATP Generation

As you may recall from Chapter 3, most cells in the body generate ATP through *aerobic* (oxygen-requiring) *metabolism* in mitochondria. ⚯ *p. 69*

Aerobic Metabolism

Aerobic metabolism normally provides 95 percent of the ATP needed by a resting cell. In this process, mitochondria absorb oxygen, ADP, phosphate ions, and organic substrates from the surrounding cytoplasm. The organic substrates are carbon chains produced by disassembling carbohydrates, lipids, or proteins. The absorbed molecules are then completely broken down in the *TCA cycle*, a series of chemical reactions described in Chapter 18. The carbon atoms and oxygen atoms are released as carbon dioxide (CO_2). The hydrogen atoms are shuttled to *respiratory enzymes* on the mitochondrial cristae, and they ultimately combine with oxygen to form water (H_2O). Along the way, large amounts of energy are released and used to make ATP.

The maximum rate of ATP generation within mitochondria is limited by the availability of oxygen. A sufficient supply of oxygen becomes a problem as the energy demands of the muscle fiber increase. Although oxygen consumption and energy production by mitochondria can increase to 40 times resting levels, the energy demands of the muscle fiber may increase by 120 times. Thus at peak levels of exertion, mitochondrial activity provides only around one-third of the required ATP. The rest is produced through *glycolysis*.

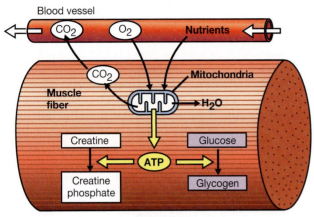

(a) Rest

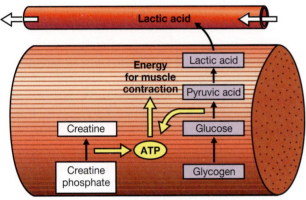

(b) Peak activity

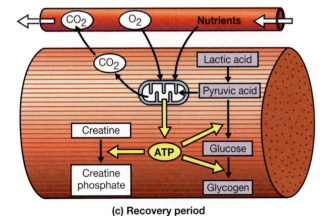

(c) Recovery period

•**FIGURE 7-8   Muscle Metabolism**
(a) A resting muscle, maintaining its energy reserves.
(b) A muscle at peak activity, using its energy reserves.
(c) The recovery period and the rebuilding of energy reserves.

Glycolysis

Glycolysis is the breakdown of glucose to pyruvic acid in the cytoplasm of the cell. It is called an **anaerobic** process because it does not require oxygen. This reaction provides a net gain of 2 molecules of ATP and generates 2 molecules of pyruvic acid. The ATP yield of glycolysis is much lower than that of aerobic metabolism; the breakdown of 2 pyruvic acid molecules in mitochondria would generate 34 ATP. However, *glycolysis can continue to provide ATP when the availability of oxygen limits mitochondrial activity.*

During periods of peak activity, glycolysis becomes the primary source of ATP (Figure 7-8b•). The glucose broken down under these conditions is obtained from glycogen reserves in the sarcoplasm. Glycogen is a polysaccharide chain of glucose molecules. ∞ *p. 39* Typical skeletal muscle fibers contain large glycogen reserves in the form of insoluble granules. When the muscle fiber begins to run short of ATP and CP, enzymes break the glycogen molecules apart, releasing glucose that can be used to generate more ATP.

The anaerobic process of glycolysis enables the cell to continue generating ATP when mitochondrial activity alone cannot meet the demand. However, this pathway has its drawbacks. For example, when glycolysis produces pyruvic acid faster than it can be used by the mitochondria, pyruvic acid levels in the sarcoplasm increase. Under these conditions, the pyruvic acid is converted to **lactic acid**, a related three-carbon molecule. The conversion of pyruvic acid to lactic acid poses a problem because lactic acid is an organic acid whose accumulation can cause dangerous changes in the pH inside and outside the muscle fiber. In addition, glycolysis is inefficient. Under anaerobic conditions, 18 molecules of glucose must be converted to lactic acid molecules to obtain the same amount of energy produced by the aerobic catabolism of a single glucose molecule.

Muscle Fatigue

A skeletal muscle fiber is said to be fatigued when it can no longer contract despite continued neural stimulation. **Muscle fatigue** is caused by the exhaustion of energy reserves or the buildup of lactic acid.

If the muscle contractions use ATP at or below the maximum rate of mitochondrial ATP generation, the muscle fiber can function aerobically. Under these conditions, fatigue will not occur until glycogen and other reserves such as lipids and amino acids are depleted. This type of fatigue affects the muscles of long-distance athletes, such as marathon runners, after hours of exertion.

When a muscle produces a sudden, intense burst of activity, the ATP is provided by glycolysis. After a relatively short time (seconds to minutes), the rising lactic acid levels lower the tissue pH, and the muscle can no longer function normally. Athletes running sprints, such as the 100-yard dash, suffer from this type of muscle fatigue.

The Recovery Period

When a muscle fiber contracts, the conditions in the sarcoplasm are changed. For example, energy reserves are consumed, heat is released, and lactic acid may be present. During the **recovery period**, conditions inside the muscle are returned to normal preexertion levels (Figure 7-8c•). The muscle's metabolic activity focuses on the removal of lactic acid and the replacement of intracellular energy reserves, and the body as a whole loses the heat generated during intense muscular contraction.

Lactic Acid Recycling

The reaction that converts pyruvic acid to lactic acid is freely reversible. During the recovery period, when lactic acid concentration is high, the lactic acid is converted back to pyruvic acid. This pyruvic acid can then be used (1) to synthesize glucose and (2) to generate ATP through mitochondrial activity. The ATP produced is used to convert creatine to creatine phosphate and to store the newly synthesized glucose as glycogen.

During the recovery period, the body's oxygen demand goes up considerably. The extra oxygen is consumed by liver cells, as they produce ATP for the conversion of lactic acid back to glucose, and by muscle cells, as they restore their reserves of ATP, creatine phosphate, and glycogen. The additional oxygen required during the recovery period is often called an *oxygen debt*. While that debt is being repaid, the breathing rate and depth are increased. That is why you continue to breathe heavily for some time even after you stop exercising.

Heat Loss

Muscular activity generates substantial amounts of heat that warms the sarcoplasm, interstitial fluid, and circulating blood. Since muscle makes up a large portion of the total mass of the body, muscle contractions play an important role in the maintenance of normal body temperature. For example, shivering can help keep you warm in a cold environment. But when skeletal muscles are contracting at peak levels, body temperature soon begins to climb. In response, blood flow to the skin increases, promoting heat loss through mechanisms described in Chapters 1 and 5. ∞ *pp. 14, 114*

MUSCLE PERFORMANCE

Muscle performance can be considered in terms of sheer **power**, the maximum amount of tension produced by a particular muscle or muscle group, and **endurance**, the amount of time for which the individual can perform a particular activity. Two major factors determine the capabilities of a particular skeletal muscle: (1) the types of muscle fibers within the muscle and (2) physical conditioning or training.

Types of Skeletal Muscle Fibers

There are two contrasting types of skeletal muscle fibers in the human body: fast fibers and slow fibers.

Fast Fibers

Most of the skeletal muscle fibers in the body are called **fast fibers** because they can contract in 0.01 second or less following stimulation. Fast fibers are large in diameter; they contain densely packed myofibrils, large glycogen reserves, and relatively few mitochondria. The tension produced by a muscle fiber is directly proportional to the number of sarcomeres, so fast-fiber muscles produce powerful contractions. However, because these contractions use ATP in massive amounts, prolonged activity is primarily supported by glycolysis, and fast fibers fatigue rapidly.

Slow Fibers

Slow fibers are only about half the diameter of fast fibers, and they take three times as long to contract after stimulation; however, they can continue contracting for extended periods, long after a fast muscle would have become fatigued. Three specializations related to the availability of oxygen and its use make this possible:

1. *Oxygen supply.* Slow muscle tissue contains a more extensive network of capillaries than does typical fast muscle tissue, so oxygen supply is dramatically increased.

2. *Oxygen storage.* Slow muscle fibers contain the red pigment **myoglobin** (MĪ-ō-glō-bin), a globular protein structurally related to hemoglobin, the oxygen-carrying pigment found in blood. ∞ *p. 43* Because myoglobin also binds oxygen molecules, resting slow muscle fibers contain oxygen reserves that can be mobilized during a contraction.

3. *Oxygen use.* Slow muscle fibers contain a relatively larger number of mitochondria than do fast muscle fibers.

The Distribution of Muscle Fibers and Muscle Performance

The percentage of fast and slow muscle fibers in a particular skeletal muscle can be quite variable. Muscles dominated by fast fibers appear pale, and they are often called **white muscles**. Chicken breasts contain "white meat" because chickens use their wings for only brief intervals, as when fleeing from a predator, and the power for flight comes from fast fibers in their breast muscles. The extensive blood vessels and myoglobin in slow muscle fibers give them a reddish color, and muscles dominated by slow fibers are therefore known as **red muscles**. Chickens walk around all day, and the movements are performed by the slow muscle fibers in the "dark meat" of their legs.

Most human muscles contain a mixture of both fiber types, and therefore appear pink. However, there are no slow fibers in muscles of the eye and hand, where swift but brief contractions are required. Many back and calf muscles are dominated by slow fibers; these muscles contract almost continuously to maintain an upright posture. The percentage of fast versus slow fibers in each muscle is genetically determined, but the fatigue resistance of fast muscle fibers can be increased through athletic training.

Physical Conditioning

Physical conditioning and training schedules enable athletes to improve both power and endurance. In practice, the training schedule varies depending on whether the activity is primarily supported by aerobic or anaerobic energy production.

Anaerobic endurance is the ability to support sustained, powerful muscle contractions through anaerobic mechanisms. Examples of activities that require anaerobic endurance are a 50-yard dash or swim, a pole vault, and a weight-lifting competition. Such activities are performed by fast muscle fibers. Athletes training to develop anaerobic endurance perform frequent, brief, intensive workouts. The net effect is an enlargement, or **hypertrophy** (hī-PER-trō-fē), of the stimulated muscle as seen in champion weight lifters or bodybuilders.

Aerobic endurance refers to the length of time for which a muscle can continue to contract while being supported by mitochondrial activities. Because mitochondrial activities yield relatively large quantities of ATP, muscle contractions can continue for an extended period. Training to improve aerobic endurance usually involves sustained low levels of muscular activity. Examples are jogging, distance swimming, and other exercises that do not require peak tension production. Because glucose is a preferred energy source, aerobic athletes, such as marathon runners, often "load" or "bulk up" on carbohydrates on the day before an event.

✓ Why would a sprinter experience muscle fatigue before a marathon runner would?

✓ Which activity would be more likely to create an oxygen debt, swimming laps or lifting weights?

✓ Which type of muscle fibers would you expect to predominate in the large leg muscles of someone who excels at endurance activities such as cycling or long-distance running?

CARDIAC AND SMOOTH MUSCLE TISSUES

Cardiac muscle tissue and smooth muscle tissue were introduced in Chapter 4. Table 7-2 compares skeletal, cardiac, and smooth muscle tissue in greater detail.

Cardiac Muscle Tissue

Cardiac muscle cells are relatively small and usually have a single, centrally placed nucleus. Cardiac muscle tissue is found only in the heart.

TABLE 7-2	A Comparison of Skeletal, Cardiac, and Smooth Muscle Tissues		
Property	*Skeletal Muscle Fiber*	*Cardiac Muscle Cell*	*Smooth Muscle Cell*
Fiber dimensions (diameter × length)	100 µm × up to 30 cm	15 µm × 100 µm	5–10 µm × 30–200 µm
Nuclei	Multiple, near sarcolemma	Usually single, centrally located	Single, centrally located
Filament organization	Sarcomeres along myofibrils	Sarcomeres along myofibrils	Scattered throughout sarcoplasm
Control mechanism	Neural, at single neuromuscular junction	Automaticity (pacemaker cells)	Automaticity (pacesetter cells), neural or hormonal control
Ca²⁺ source	Release from sarcoplasmic reticulum	Across sarcolemma and release from sarcoplasmic reticulum	Across sarcolemma
Contraction	Rapid onset; tetanus can occur; rapid fatigue	Slower onset; tetanus cannot occur; resistant to fatigue	Slow onset; tetanus can occur; resistant to fatigue
Energy source	Aerobic metabolism at moderate levels of activity; glycolysis (anaerobic) during peak activity	Aerobic metabolism, usually lipid or carbohydrate substrates	Primarily aerobic metabolism

Differences Between Cardiac Muscle and Skeletal Muscle

Figure 7-9a● shows cardiac muscle tissue. Like skeletal muscle fibers, cardiac muscle cells contain an orderly arrangement of myofibrils and are striated, but significant differences exist in their structure and function. The most obvious structural difference is that cardiac muscle cells are branched, and each cardiac cell contacts several others at specialized sites called **intercalated** (in-TER-ka-lā-ted) **discs** (see Figure 4-13b●, p. 98). These cellular connections contain gap junctions that provide a means for the movement of ions and small molecules and the rapid passage of action potentials from cell to cell, resulting in their simultaneous contraction. Because the myofibrils are

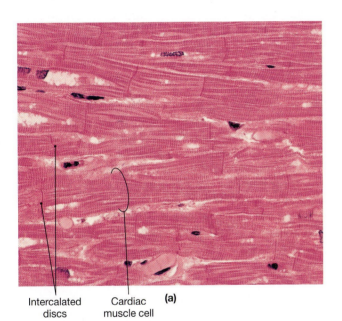

Intercalated   Cardiac   **(a)**
discs   muscle cell

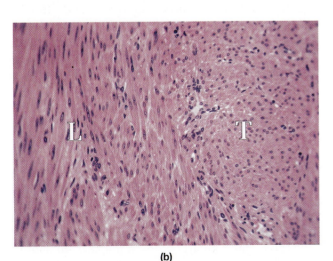

(b)

●**FIGURE 7-9   Cardiac and Smooth Muscle Tissues**
(a) An LM of cardiac muscle tissue. Notice the striations and the intercalated discs. **(b)** Many visceral organs contain layers or sheets of smooth muscle fibers. This view shows smooth muscle cells in longitudinal (L) and transverse (T) sections.

also attached to the intercalated discs, the cells "pull together" quite efficiently.

There are also several important functional differences between cardiac muscle and skeletal muscle:

- Cardiac muscle tissue contracts without neural stimulation, a property called *automaticity*. The timing of contractions is normally determined by specialized cardiac muscle cells called **pacemaker cells**.
- Cardiac muscle cell contractions last roughly 10 times as long as those of skeletal muscle fibers.
- The properties of cardiac muscle cell membranes differ from those of skeletal muscle fibers. As a result, cardiac muscle tissue cannot undergo tetanus, or sustained contraction. This property is important because a heart in tetany could not pump blood.
- Cardiac muscle cells rely on aerobic metabolism for the energy needed to continue contracting. Sarcoplasm thus contains large numbers of mitochondria and abundant myoglobin reserves (to store oxygen).

Smooth Muscle Tissue

Smooth muscle cells are similar in size to cardiac muscle cells; they also contain a single, centrally located nucleus within each spindle-shaped cell (Figure 7-9b●). Smooth muscle tissue is found within almost every organ, forming sheets, bundles, or sheaths around other tissues. In the skeletal, muscular, nervous, and endocrine systems, smooth muscles around blood vessels regulate blood flow through vital organs. In the digestive and urinary systems, rings of smooth muscles, called *sphincters*, regulate movement along internal passageways.

Differences Between Smooth Muscle and Other Muscle Tissues

Structural Differences.   Actin and myosin are present in all three muscle types. In skeletal and cardiac muscle cells, these proteins are organized into sarcomeres. The internal organization of a smooth muscle cell is very different from that of skeletal or cardiac muscle cells:

- There are no myofibrils, sarcomeres, or striations in smooth muscle tissue.
- The thin filaments of a smooth muscle cell are anchored within the cytoplasm and to the sarcolemma.
- Adjacent smooth muscle cells are bound together at these anchoring sites, thus transmitting the contractile forces throughout the tissue.

Functional Differences.   Smooth muscle tissue differs from other muscle types in several major ways:

- Calcium ions trigger contractions through a different mechanism than that found in other muscle types.

- Smooth muscle cells are able to contract over a greater range of lengths than skeletal or cardiac muscle because the actin and myosin filaments are not rigidly organized. This property is important because layers of smooth muscle are found in the walls of organs such as the urinary bladder and stomach, which undergo large changes in volume.

- Many smooth muscle cells are not innervated by motor neurons, and the muscle cells contract automatically, or in response to environmental or hormonal stimulation. When smooth muscle fibers are innervated by motor neurons, the neurons involved are not under voluntary control.

✓ How do intercalated discs enhance the functioning of cardiac muscle tissue?

✓ Why are cardiac and smooth muscle contractions more affected by changes in extracellular calcium ions than are skeletal muscle contractions?

✓ Smooth muscle can contract over a wider range of resting lengths than skeletal muscle. Why?

ANATOMY OF THE MUSCULAR SYSTEM

The **muscular system** includes all of the skeletal muscles that can be controlled voluntarily (Figure 7-10•). The general appearance of each of the nearly 700 skeletal muscles provides clues to its primary function. Muscles involved with locomotion and posture work across joints, producing skeletal movement. Those that support soft tissue form slings or sheets between relatively stable bony elements, whereas those that guard an entrance or exit completely encircle the opening.

Origins, Insertions, and Actions

Each muscle begins at an **origin**, ends at an **insertion**, and contracts to produce a specific **action**. In general, the origin end remains stationary while the insertion moves. For example, the *triceps brachii* muscle inserts on the olecranon process and originates closer to the shoulder. Such determinations are made during normal movement.

Almost all skeletal muscles either originate or insert on the skeleton. When they contract, they may produce *flexion, extension, adduction, abduction, protraction, retraction, elevation, depression, rotation, circumduction, pronation, supination, inversion,* or *eversion.* (You may wish to review Figures 6-27 to 6-29•, pp. 152–53.)

Muscles can be grouped by their **primary actions**:

- A **prime mover**, or **agonist** (AG-o-nist), is a muscle whose contraction is chiefly responsible for producing a particular movement. The *biceps brachii* muscle is a prime mover that flexes the elbow.

- **Antagonists** (an-TAG-o-nists) are prime movers whose actions oppose that of the agonist under consideration. The *triceps brachii* muscle is a prime mover that extends the elbow. It is therefore an antagonist of the biceps brachii, and the biceps brachii is an antagonist of the triceps brachii. Agonists and antagonists are functional opposites—if one produces flexion, the other has extension as its primary action.

- When a **synergist** (*syn-*, together + *ergon*, work) contracts, it assists the prime mover in performing that action. Synergists may provide additional pull near the insertion or stabilize the point of origin. In many cases, they are most useful at the start of a movement, when the prime mover is stretched and its power is relatively low. For example, the *deltoid* muscle acts to lift the arm away from the body (abduction). A smaller muscle, the *supraspinatus* muscle, assists the deltoid in starting this movement.

Names of Skeletal Muscles

The human body has approximately 700 skeletal muscles. You need not learn the name of every one of them, but you should become familiar with the most important ones. Fortunately, the names assigned to muscles provide clues to their identification. Table 7-3 (p. 187), which summarizes muscle terminology, will be a useful reference as you go through the rest of this chapter.

Some names, often with Greek or Latin roots, refer to the orientation of the muscle fibers. For example, *rectus* means "straight," and *rectus muscles* are parallel muscles whose fibers generally run along the long axis of the body, as in the *rectus abdominis* muscle. In a few cases, a muscle is such a prominent feature that the regional name alone can identify it, such as the *temporalis* muscle of the head. Other muscles are named after structural features. For example, a *biceps muscle* has two tendons of origin (*bi-*, two + *caput*, head), whereas the *triceps* has three. Table 7-3 also lists names reflecting shape, length, size, and whether a muscle is visible at the body surface (*externus, superficialis*) or lying beneath (*internus, profundus*). Superficial muscles that position or stabilize an organ are called *extrinsic muscles*; those that operate within an organ are called *intrinsic muscles*.

The first part of many names indicates the origin and the second part the insertion of the muscle. The *sternohyoid* muscle, for example, originates at the sternum and inserts on the hyoid bone. Other names may indicate the primary function of the muscle as well. For example, the *extensor carpi radialis* is a muscle found along the radial (lateral) border of the forearm, and its contraction produces extension at the wrist joint. With only two exceptions (the *platysma* and the *diaphragm*, the complete name of every muscle includes the word "muscle." For simplicity, we have not included it in figures and tables. You will thus find *tibialis anterior* rather than *tibialis anterior muscle*.

•**FIGURE 7-10   An Overview of the Major Skeletal Muscles**
(a) An anterior view.

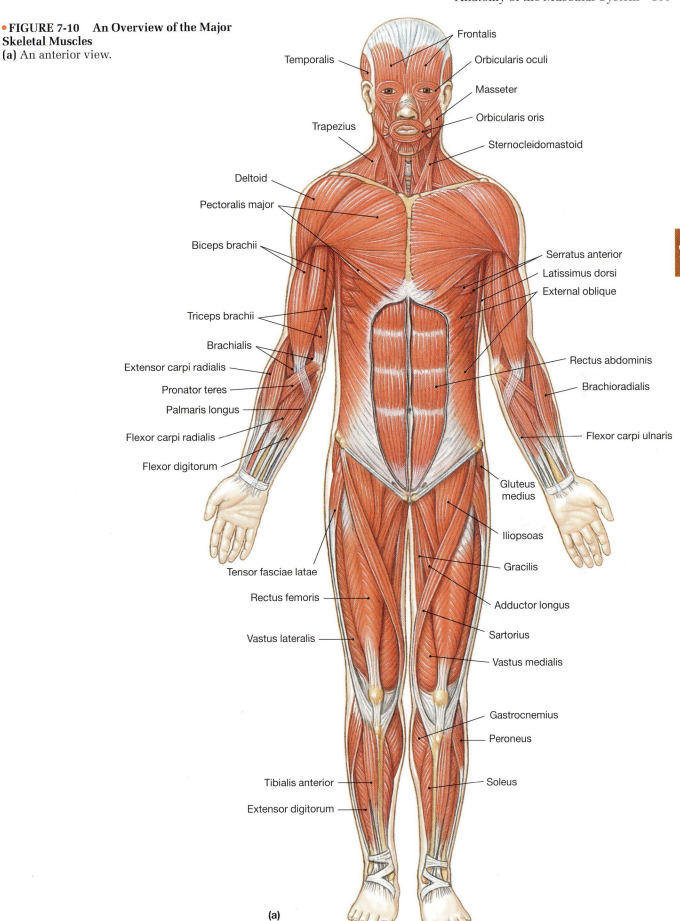

Frontalis

Temporalis

Orbicularis oculi

Masseter

Orbicularis oris

Sternocleidomastoid

Trapezius

Deltoid

Pectoralis major

Biceps brachii

Serratus anterior

Latissimus dorsi

External oblique

Triceps brachii

Brachialis

Extensor carpi radialis

Pronator teres

Palmaris longus

Flexor carpi radialis

Flexor digitorum

Rectus abdominis

Brachioradialis

Flexor carpi ulnaris

Gluteus medius

Iliopsoas

Tensor fasciae latae

Rectus femoris

Vastus lateralis

Gracilis

Adductor longus

Sartorius

Vastus medialis

Gastrocnemius

Peroneus

Tibialis anterior

Extensor digitorum

Soleus

7

(a)

7

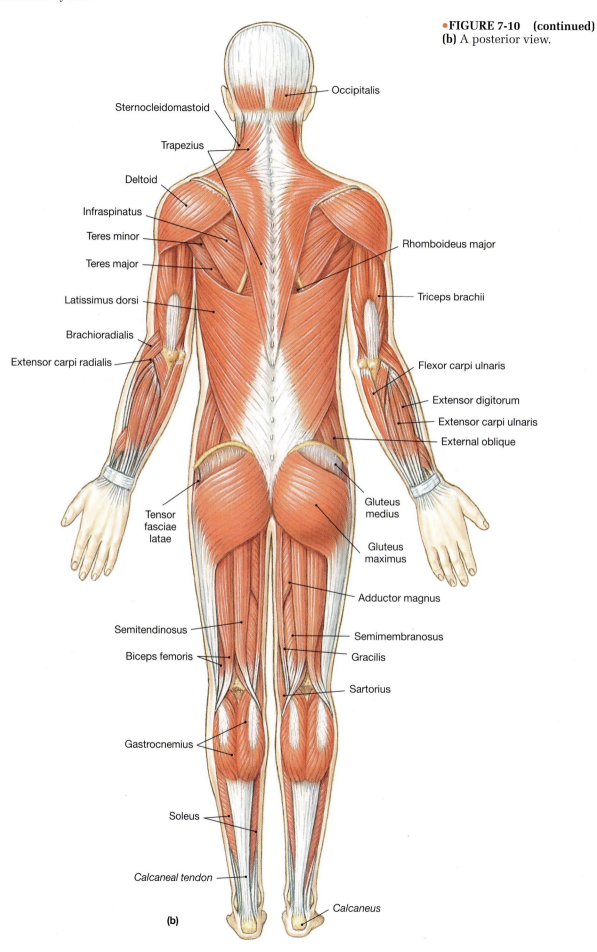

•FIGURE 7-10   (continued)
(b) A posterior view.

Occipitalis

Sternocleidomastoid

Trapezius

Deltoid

Infraspinatus

Teres minor

Teres major

Latissimus dorsi

Brachioradialis

Extensor carpi radialis

Rhomboideus major

Triceps brachii

Flexor carpi ulnaris

Extensor digitorum

Extensor carpi ulnaris

External oblique

Tensor fasciae latae

Gluteus medius

Gluteus maximus

Adductor magnus

Semitendinosus

Biceps femoris

Semimembranosus

Gracilis

Sartorius

Gastrocnemius

Soleus

Calcaneal tendon

Calcaneus

(b)

TABLE 7-3	Muscle Terminology		
Terms Indicating Direction Relative to Axes of the Body	**Terms Indicating Specific Regions of the Body***	**Terms Indicating Structural Characteristics of the Muscle**	**Terms Indicating Actions**
Anterior (front)	Abdominis (abdomen)	**Origin**	**General**
Externus (superficial)	Anconeus (elbow)	Biceps (two heads)	Abductor
Extrinsic (outside)	Auricularis (auricle of ear)	Triceps (three heads)	Adductor
Inferioris (inferior)	Brachialis (brachium)	Quadriceps (four heads)	Depressor
Internus (deep, internal)	Capitis (head)		Extensor
Intrinsic (inside)	Carpi (wrist)	**Shape**	Flexor
Lateralis (lateral)	Cervicis (neck)	Deltoid (triangle)	Levator
Medialis/medius (medial, middle)	Cleido/clavius (clavicle)	Orbicularis (circle)	Pronator
	Coccygeus (coccyx)	Pectinate (comblike)	Rotator
Obliquus (oblique)	Costalis (ribs)	Piriformis (pear-shaped)	Supinator
Posterior (back)	Cutaneous (skin)	Platys- (flat)	Tensor
Profundus (deep)	Femoris (femur)	Pyramidal (pyramid)	
Rectus (straight, parallel)	Genio- (chin)	Rhomboideus (rhomboid)	**Specific**
Superficialis (superficial)	Glosso/glossal (tongue)	Serratus (serrated)	Buccinator (trumpeter)
Superioris (superior)	Hallucis (great toe)	Splenius (bandage)	Risorius (laugher)
Transversus (transverse)	Ilio- (ilium)	Teres (long and round)	Sartorius (like a tailor)
	Inguinal (groin)	Trapezius (trapezoid)	
	Lumborum (lumbar region)		
	Nasalis (nose)	**Other Striking Features**	
	Nuchal (back of neck)	Alba (white)	
	Oculo- (eye)	Brevis (short)	
	Oris (mouth)	Gracilis (slender)	
	Palpebrae (eyelid)	Lata (wide)	
	Pollicis (thumb)	Latissimus (widest)	
	Popliteus (behind knee)	Longissimus (longest)	
	Psoas (loin)	Longus (long)	
	Radialis (radius)	Magnus (large)	
	Scapularis (scapula)	Major (larger)	
	Temporalis (temples)	Maximus (largest)	
	Thoracis (thoracic region)	Minimus (smallest)	
	Tibialis (tibia)	Minor (smaller)	
	Ulnaris (ulna)	-tendinosus (tendinous)	
	Uro- (urinary)	Vastus (great)	

*For other regional terms, refer to Figure 1-6, p. 17, which shows anatomical landmarks.

The separation of the skeletal system into axial and appendicular divisions provides a useful guideline for subdividing the muscular system as well:

- The **axial musculature** arises on the axial skeleton. It positions the head and spinal column and also moves the rib cage, assisting in the movements that make breathing possible. It does not play a role in movement or support of the pectoral or pelvic girdles or appendages. This category encompasses roughly 60 percent of the skeletal muscles in the body.

- The **appendicular musculature** stabilizes or moves components of the appendicular skeleton.

✓ Which type of muscle would you expect to find guarding the opening between the stomach and the small intestine?

✓ Which muscle would be the antagonist of the biceps brachii?

✓ What does the name *flexor carpi radialis* tell you about this muscle?

7

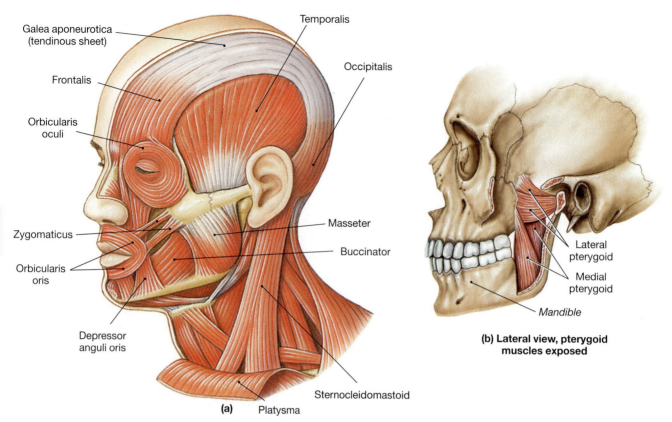

Galea aponeurotica
(tendinous sheet)

Temporalis

Frontalis

Occipitalis

Orbicularis
oculi

Zygomaticus

Masseter

Buccinator

Orbicularis
oris

Depressor
anguli oris

Sternocleidomastoid

(a)   Platysma

Lateral
pterygoid

Medial
pterygoid

Mandible

**(b) Lateral view, pterygoid
muscles exposed**

•**FIGURE 7-11   Muscles of the Head and Neck**
(a) An anterior and lateral view. **(b)** The pterygoid muscles.

The Axial Musculature

The axial muscles fall into four logical groups based on location, function, or both:

1. *The muscles of the head and neck.* These muscles include the muscles responsible for facial expression, chewing, and swallowing.
2. *The muscles of the spine.* This group includes flexors and extensors of the head, neck, and spinal column.
3. *The muscles of the trunk.* The *oblique* and *rectus muscles* form the muscular walls of the thoracic and abdominopelvic cavities.
4. *The muscles of the pelvic floor.* These muscles extend between the sacrum and pelvic girdle and form the muscular *perineum*, which closes the pelvic outlet.

Muscles of the Head and Neck

The muscles of the head and neck are shown in Figures 7-11• and 7-12• and detailed in Table 7-4 (pp. 190–191). The muscles of the face originate on the surface of the skull and insert into the dermis of the skin. When they contract, the skin moves. For example, the **frontalis** muscle of the forehead raises the eyebrows and pulls on the skin of the scalp. The largest group of facial muscles is associated with the mouth. The **orbicularis oris** constricts the opening, and other muscles move the lips or the corners of the mouth. The **buccinator** (BUK-si-nā-tor), one of the muscles associated with the mouth, compresses the cheeks, as when pursing the lips and blowing forcefully. (*Buccinator* translates as "trumpet player.") During chewing, contraction and relaxation of the buccinator move food back across the teeth from the space inside the cheeks. The chewing motions are primarily produced by contractions of the **masseter**, assisted by the **temporalis** and the **pterygoid** muscles used in various combinations.

Smaller groups of muscles control movements of the eyebrows and eyelids, the scalp, the nose, and the external ear. The scalp contains two muscles—the frontalis and the **occipitalis**. These muscles are separated by an *aponeurosis*, or tendinous sheet, called the **galea aponeurotica** (GĀ-lē-uh ap-ō-nū-RO-ti-kuh; *galea*, helmet). The **platysma** (pla-TIZ-ma; *platys*, flat) covers the ventral surface of the neck, extending from the base of the neck to the mandible and the corners of the mouth.

The muscles of the neck control the position of the larynx, depress the mandible, tense the floor of the mouth, and provide a stable foundation for muscles of the tongue and pharynx (Figure 7-12•). These muscles include the following:

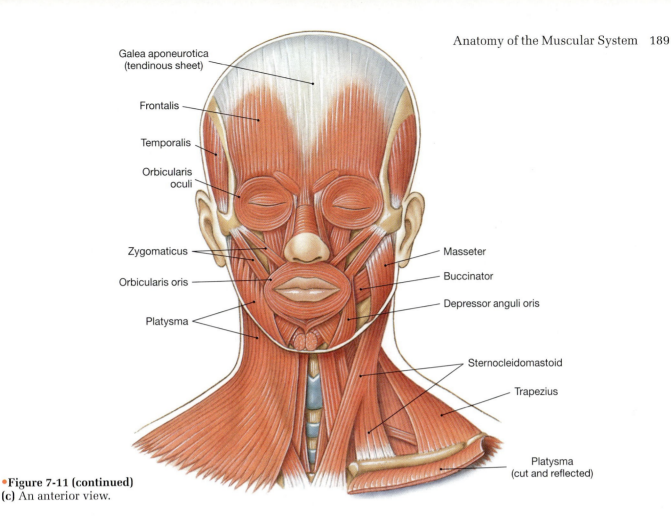

Galea aponeurotica
(tendinous sheet)

Frontalis

Temporalis

Orbicularis
oculi

Zygomaticus

Orbicularis oris

Platysma

Masseter

Buccinator

Depressor anguli oris

Sternocleidomastoid

Trapezius

Platysma
(cut and reflected)

•Figure 7-11 (continued)
(c) An anterior view.

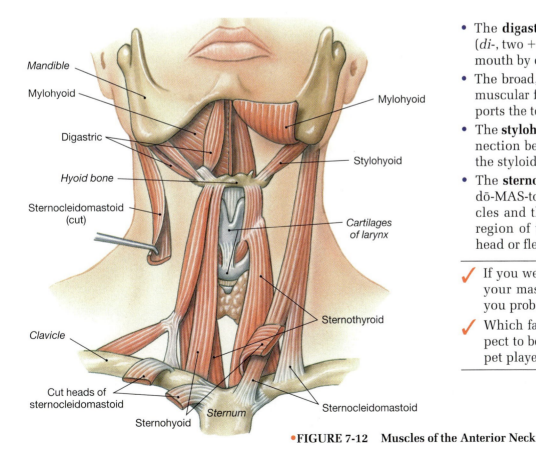

Mandible

Mylohyoid

Digastric

Hyoid bone

Sternocleidomastoid
(cut)

Clavicle

Cut heads of
sternocleidomastoid

Sternohyoid

Mylohyoid

Stylohyoid

Cartilages
of larynx

Sternothyroid

Sternocleidomastoid

Sternum

•FIGURE 7-12   Muscles of the Anterior Neck

- The **digastric**, which has two bellies (*di-*, two + *gaster*, stomach), opens the mouth by depressing the mandible.
- The broad, flat **mylohyoid** provides a muscular floor to the mouth and supports the tongue.
- The **stylohyoid** forms a muscular connection between the hyoid bone and the styloid process of the skull.
- The **sternocleidomastoid** (ster-nō-klī-dō-MAS-toyd) extends from the clavicles and the sternum to the mastoid region of the skull. It can rotate the head or flex the neck.

✓ If you were contracting and relaxing your masseter muscle, what would you probably be doing?

✓ Which facial muscle would you expect to be well developed in a trumpet player?

TABLE 7-4   **Muscles of the Head and Neck**

Region/Muscle	Origin	Insertion	Action
MOUTH			
Buccinator	Maxillary bone and mandible	Blends into fibers of orbicularis oris	Compresses cheeks
Orbicularis oris	Maxillary bone and mandible	Lips	Compresses, purses lips
Depressor anguli oris	Mandibular body	Skin at angle of mouth	Depresses corner of mouth
Zygomaticus	Zygomatic bone	Angle of mouth	Draws corner of mouth back and up
EYE			
Orbicularis oculi	Medial margin of orbit	Skin around eyelids	Closes eye
SCALP			
Frontalis	Galea aponeurotica	Skin of eyebrow and bridge of nose	Raises eyebrows, wrinkles forehead
Occipitalis	Occipital bone	Galea aponeurotica	Tenses, retracts scalp
LOWER JAW			
Masseter	Zygomatic arch	Lateral surface of mandible	Elevates mandible
Temporalis	Along temporal lines of skull	Coronoid process of mandible	Elevates mandible
Pterygoids	Inferior processes of sphenoid	Median surface of mandible	Elevate, protract, and/or move mandible to either side

Muscles of the Spine

The muscles of the spine are covered by more superficial back muscles, such as the trapezius and latissimus dorsi (see Figure 7-10b•). The most superior of the spinal muscles are the posterior neck muscles, the superficial **splenius capitis** and the deeper **semispinalis capitis** (Figure 7-13• and Table 7-5). These muscles assist each other in extending the head when their left and right pairs contract together. When they contract on one side, both assist in tilting the head. Because of its more lateral insertion, the contraction of the splenius capitis also acts to rotate the head. The *spinal extensors*, or **erector spinae**, act to maintain an erect spinal column and head. Moving laterally from the spine, these muscles can be subdivided into **spinalis, longissimus,** and **iliocostalis** divisions. In the lower lumbar and sacral regions, the border between the longissimus and iliocostalis muscles becomes indistinct, and they are sometimes known as the *sacrospinalis* muscles. When contracting together, these muscles extend the spinal column. When only the muscles on one side contract, the spine is bent laterally.

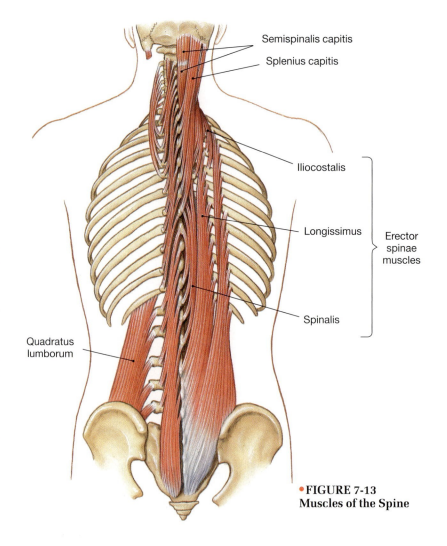

•**FIGURE 7-13**
Muscles of the Spine

Region/Muscle	Origin	Insertion	Action
NECK			
Platysma	From cartilage of second rib to acromion of scapula	Mandible and skin of cheek	Tenses skin of neck, depresses mandible
Digastric	Mastoid region of temporal and inferior surface of chin	Hyoid bone	Depresses mandible and/or elevates larynx
Mylohyoid	Medial surface of mandible	Median connective tissue band	Elevates floor of mouth and hyoid, and/or depresses mandible
Sternohyoid	Clavicle and sternum	Hyoid bone	As above
Sternothyroid	Dorsal surface of sternum and 1st rib	Thyroid cartilage of larynx	As above
Stylohyoid	Styloid process of temporal bone	Hyoid bone	Elevates larynx
Sternocleidomastoid	Superior margins of sternum and clavicle	Mastoid region of skull	Together they flex the neck; alone one side bends head toward shoulder and turns face to opposite side

7

| TABLE 7-5 | **Muscles of the Spine** |

Region/Muscle	Origin	Insertion	Action
SPINAL EXTENSORS			
Splenius capitis	Spinous processes of lower cervical and upper thoracic vertebrae	Mastoid process, base of the skull, and upper cervical vertebrae	The two sides act together to extend the neck; either alone rotates and tilts head to that side
Semispinalis capitis	Spinous processes of lower cervical and upper thoracic vertebrae	Base of skull, upper cervical vertebrae	The two sides act together to extend the neck; either alone tilts head to that side
Spinalis group	Spinous processes and transverse processes of cervical and thoracic vertebrae	Base of skull and spinous processes of cervical and upper thoracic vertebrae	The two sides act together to extend vertebral column; either alone extends neck and tilts head or rotates vertebral column to that side
Longissimus group	Processes of lower cervical, thoracic, and upper lumbar vertebrae	Mastoid processes of temporal bone, transverse processes of cervical vertebrae and inferior surfaces of ribs	The two sides act together to extend vertebral column; either alone rotates and tilts head or vertebral column to that side
Iliocostalis group	Superior borders of ribs and iliac crest	Transverse processes of cervical vertebrae and inferior surfaces of ribs	Extends vertebral column or bends to that side; moves ribs
SPINAL FLEXOR			
Quadratus lumborum	Iliac crest	Last rib and transverse processes of lumbar vertebrae	Together they depress ribs, flex vertebral column; one side acting alone produces lateral flexion

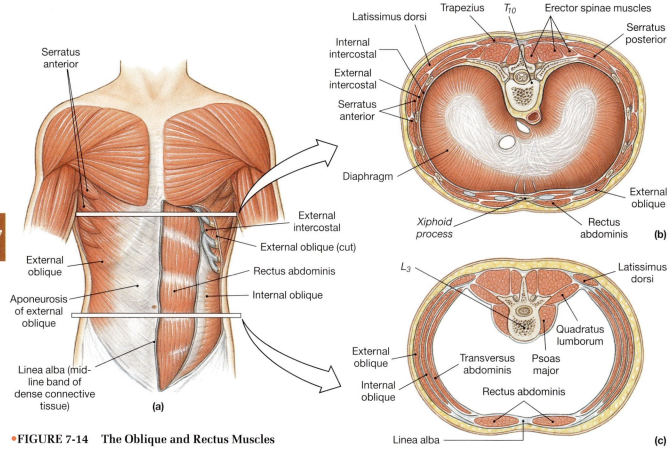

●**FIGURE 7-14**   **The Oblique and Rectus Muscles**

The Axial Muscles of the Trunk

The *oblique muscles* and the *rectus muscles* form the muscular walls of the thoracic and abdominopelvic cavities between the first thoracic vertebra and the pelvis. In the thoracic area, these muscles are partitioned by the ribs, but over the abdominal surface they form broad muscular sheets (Figure 7-14● and Table 7-6). The oblique muscles can compress underlying structures or rotate the spinal column, depending on whether one or both sides are contracting. The rectus muscles are important flexors of the spinal column, opposing the erector spinae.

The axial muscles of the trunk include (1) the external and internal **intercostals** and **obliques**, (2) the **transversus abdominis**, (3) the **rectus abdominis**, (4) the muscular **diaphragm** that separates the thoracic and abdominopelvic cavities, and (5) muscles that form the floor of the pelvic cavity.

Muscles of the Pelvic Floor

The floor of the pelvic cavity is called the **perineum** (Table 7-7 and Figure 7-15●, p. 194). It is formed by a broad sheet of muscles that connects the sacrum and coccyx to the ischium and pubis. These muscles support the organs of the pelvic cavity and control the movement of materials through the urethra and anus.

✳ LUMBAR STRAIN

Back injuries are one of the most frequent and debilitating problems in modern society. Because of the nature of their job, EMS personnel are at increased risk of sustaining a back injury. Emergency care providers often must lift heavy patients or equipment, sometimes while in awkward positions. This can cause excessive stress to the large muscles of the lower back, resulting in stretching or tearing of these muscles (lumbar strain). Signs and symptoms include pain, tenderness over the affected muscles, muscle spasm, and decreased range of motion. Because of its debilitating nature, EMS personnel who sustain a lumbar strain should receive immediate medical care. Fortunately, lumbar strains are the least severe type of low back injury, and most cases heal well with rest and ice, followed by heat and therapeutic exercise. Prevention of back injury should be a primary goal. Many EMS careers have been cut short by debilitating back injuries that could have been prevented.

✓ Damage to the external intercostal muscles would interfere with what important process?

✓ If someone were to hit you in your rectus abdominis muscle, how would your body position then change?

TABLE 7-6	Axial Muscles of the Trunk		
Region/Muscle	*Origin*	*Insertion*	*Action*
THORACIC REGION			
External intercostals	Inferior border of each rib	Superior border of next rib	Elevate ribs
Internal intercostals	Superior border of each rib	Inferior border of the previous rib	Depress ribs
Diaphragm	Xiphoid process, cartilages of ribs 4–10, and anterior surfaces of lumbar vertebrae	Central tendinous sheet	Contraction expands thoracic cavity, compresses abdominopelvic cavity
ABDOMINAL REGION			
External oblique	Lower eight ribs	Linea alba and iliac crest	Compresses abdomen, depresses ribs, flexes or laterally flexes vertebral column
Internal oblique	Iliac crest and adjacent connective tissues	Lower ribs, xiphoid of sternum, and linea alba	As above
Transversus abdominis	Cartilages of lower ribs, iliac crest, and adjacent connective tissues	Linea alba and pubis	Compresses abdomen
Rectus abdominis	Superior surface of pubis around symphysis	Inferior surfaces of costal cartilages (ribs 5–7) and xiphoid process	Depresses ribs, flexes vertebral column

7

TABLE 7-7	Muscles of the Perineum		
Muscle	*Origin*	*Insertion*	*Action*
Bulbospongiosus:			
male	Base of penis; fibers cross over urethra	Midline and central tendon of perineum	Compresses base, stiffens penis, ejects urine or semen
female	Base of clitoris; fibers run on either side of urethral and vaginal openings	Central tendon of perineum	Compresses and stiffens clitoris, narrows vaginal opening
Ischiocavernosus	Inferior medial surface of ischium	Symphysis pubis anterior to base of penis or clitoris	Compresses and stiffens penis or clitoris
Transverse perineus	Inferior, medial surface of ischium	Central tendon of perineum	Stabilizes central tendon of perineum
External urethral sphincter:			
male	Inferior, medial surfaces of ischium and pubis	Midline at base of penis; inner fibers encircle urethra	Closes urethra, compresses prostate and bulbourethral glands
female	As above	Midline; inner fibers encircle urethra	Closes urethra, compresses vagina and greater vestibular glands
External anal sphincter	Via tendon from coccyx	Encircles anal opening	Closes anal opening
Levator ani	Ischial spine and pubis	Coccyx	Tenses floor of pelvis, supports pelvic organs, flexes coccyx, elevates and retracts anus

7

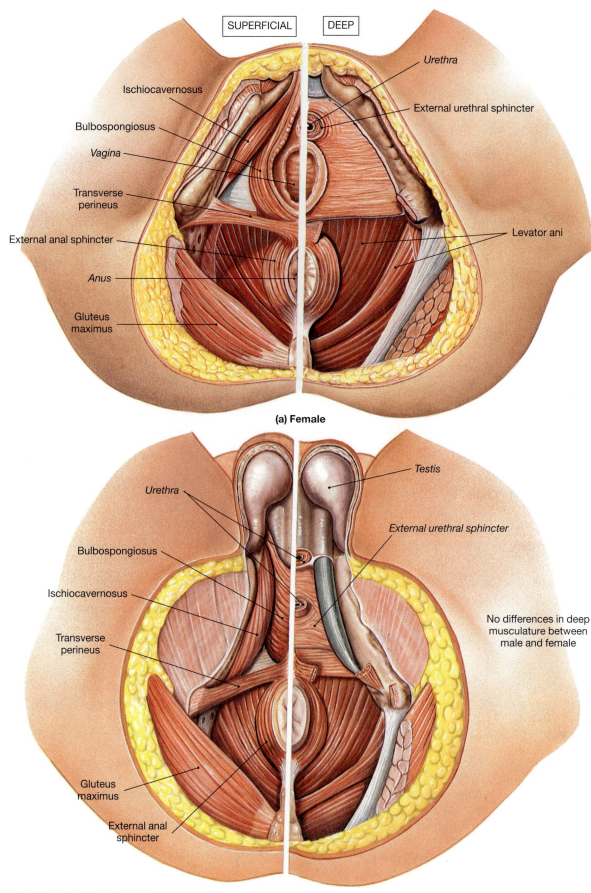

SUPERFICIAL   DEEP

Ischiocavernosus

Bulbospongiosus

Vagina

Transverse
perineus

External anal sphincter

Anus

Gluteus
maximus

Urethra

External urethral sphincter

Levator ani

(a) Female

Urethra

Bulbospongiosus

Ischiocavernosus

Transverse
perineus

Gluteus
maximus

External anal
sphincter

Testis

External urethral sphincter

No differences in deep
musculature between
male and female

(b) Male

•**FIGURE 7-15   Muscles of the Perineum**
(a) Female. **(b)** Male.

The Appendicular Musculature

The appendicular musculature includes (1) the muscles of the shoulders and upper limbs and (2) the muscles of the pelvic girdle and lower limbs. Because the functions and required ranges of motion are very different, few similarities exist between the two groups. In addition to increasing the mobility of the upper limb, the muscular connections between the pectoral girdle and the axial skeleton must act as shock absorbers. For example, people who are jogging can still perform delicate hand movements because the muscular connections between the axial and appendicular skeleton smooth out the bounces in their stride. In contrast, the pelvic girdle has evolved to transfer weight from the axial to the appendicular skeleton. A muscular connection would reduce the efficiency of the transfer, and the emphasis is on sheer power rather than versatility.

Muscles of the Shoulder and Upper Limb

The large, superficial **trapezius** muscles cover the back and portions of the neck, reaching to the base of the skull. These muscles form a broad diamond (Figure 7-16a● and Table 7-8). Its actions are quite varied because specific regions can be made to contract independently. The **rhomboideus** muscles and the **levator scapulae** are covered by the trapezius. Contraction of the rhomboids adducts the scapula, pulling it toward the center of the back. The levator scapulae elevates the scapula, as when you shrug your shoulders.

On the chest, the **serratus anterior** originates along the anterior surfaces of several ribs and inserts along the vertebral border of the scapula. When the serratus anterior contracts, it pulls the shoulder anteriorly. The **pectoralis minor** attaches to the coracoid process of the scapula. When it contracts, it depresses and protracts the scapula.

7

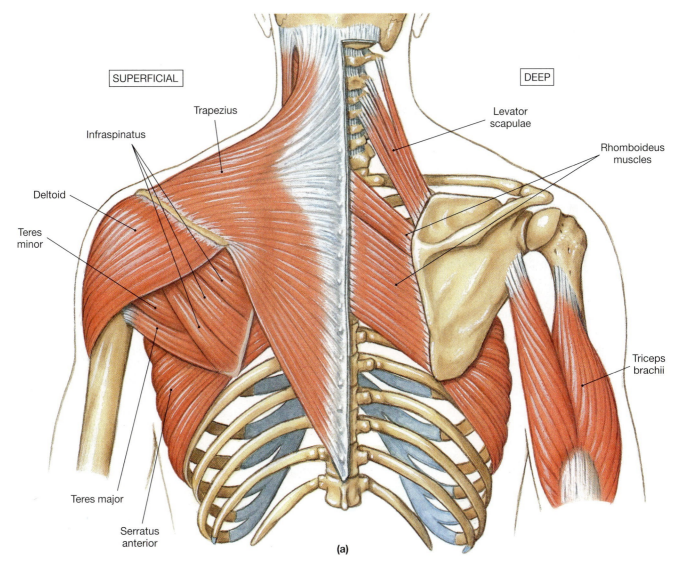

SUPERFICIAL

DEEP

Trapezius

Infraspinatus

Deltoid

Teres minor

Teres major

Serratus anterior

(a)

Levator scapulae

Rhomboideus muscles

Triceps brachii

●**FIGURE 7-16   Muscles of the Shoulder**
(a) A posterior view.

•Figure 7-16 (continued)
(b) An anterior view.

7

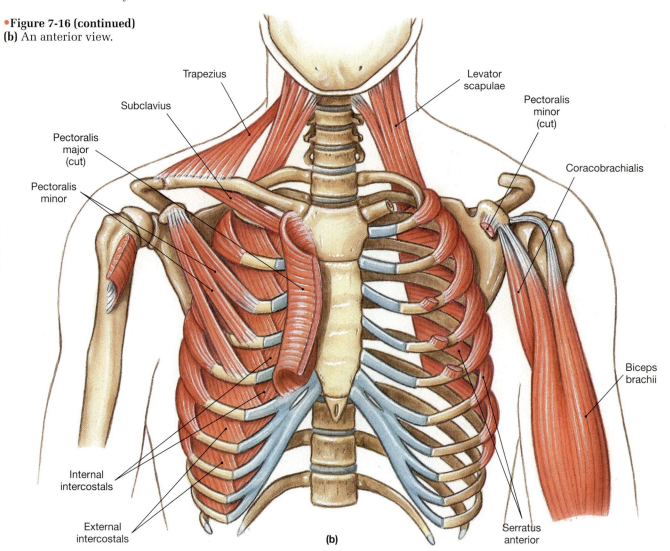

Trapezius

Subclavius

Pectoralis major (cut)

Pectoralis minor

Levator scapulae

Pectoralis minor (cut)

Coracobrachialis

Biceps brachii

Internal intercostals

External intercostals

Serratus anterior

(b)

TABLE 7-8	Muscles of the Shoulder		
Muscle	*Origin*	*Insertion*	*Action*
Levator scapulae	Posterior surface of first 4 cervical vertebrae	Vertebral border of scapula	Elevates scapula
Pectoralis minor	Anterior surfaces of ribs 3–5	Coracoid process of scapula	Depresses and protracts shoulder; rotates scapula laterally; elevates ribs if scapula is stationary
Rhomboideus muscles	Spinous processes of lower cervical and upper thoracic vertebrae	Vertebral border of scapula	Adducts and rotates scapula laterally
Serratus anterior	Anterior and superior margins of ribs 1–9	Anterior surface of vertebral border of scapula	Protracts shoulder, abducts and medially rotates scapula
Subclavius	First rib	Clavicle	Depresses and protracts shoulder
Trapezius	Occipital bone and spinous processes of thoracic vertebrae	Clavicle and scapula (acromion and scapular spine)	Depends on active region and state of other muscles; may elevate, adduct, depress, or rotate scapula and/or elevate clavicle; can also extend or hyperextend neck

Muscles That Move the Arm. The muscles that move the arm (Table 7-9 and Figure 7-17•) are easiest to remember when grouped by primary actions:

- The **deltoid** is the major abductor of the arm, and the **supraspinatus** assists at the start of this movement.
- The **subscapularis**, **teres major**, **infraspinatus**, and **teres minor** rotate the arm.
- The **pectoralis major** extends between the chest and the greater tubercle of the humerus; the **latissimus dorsi** extends between the thoracic vertebrae and the lesser tubercle of the humerus. The pectoralis major produces flexion at the shoulder joint, and the latissimus dorsi produces extension. The two muscles also work together to produce adduction and rotation.

These muscles provide substantial support for the shoulder joint. The tendons of the supraspinatus, infraspinatus, subscapularis, teres major, and teres minor blend with and support the capsular fibers that enclose the shoulder joint. They are the muscles of the *rotator cuff*, a frequent site of sports injuries. As noted in Chapter 6, these muscles must stabilize the shoulder joint while controlling an extensive range of movement. ∞ *p. 156* Powerful, repetitive arm movements, such as pitching a fastball at 96 mph for nine innings, can place intolerable strains on the muscles of the rotator cuff, leading to a muscle strain (a tear or break in the muscle), *bursitis*, and other painful injuries.

Muscles That Move the Forearm and Wrist. Although most of the muscles that insert upon the forearm and wrist (Figure 7-18•, p. 199, and Table 7-10, p. 200) originate on the humerus, there are two noteworthy exceptions. The **biceps brachii** and **triceps brachii**, which insert on the bones of the forearm, originate on the scapula. Although their contractions can have a secondary effect on the shoulder, their primary actions are at the elbow. The triceps brachii extends the elbow when, for example, you do push-ups. The biceps brachii both flexes the elbow and supinates the forearm. With the forearm pronated (palm facing back), the biceps brachii cannot function effectively. As a result, when picking up a heavy weight in the hand, you always turn the palm forward; the biceps brachii then makes a prominent bulge.

Other important muscles include the following:

- The **brachialis** and **brachioradialis** also flex the elbow, opposed by the triceps brachii.
- The **flexor carpi ulnaris**, the **flexor carpi radialis**, and the **palmaris longus** are superficial muscles that

TABLE 7-9	Muscles That Move the Arm		
Muscle	*Origin*	*Insertion*	*Action*
Coracobrachialis	Coracoid process	Medial margin of shaft of humerus	Adduction and flexeion at shoulder joint
Deltoid	Clavicle and scapula (acromion and adjacent scapular spine)	Deltoid tuberosity of humerus	Abduction at shoulder joint
Latissimus dorsi	Spinous processess of lower thoracic vertebrae, ribs, and lumbar vertebrae	Lesser tubercle, intertubercular groove of humerus	Extension, adduction, and medial rotation at shoulder joint
Pectoralis major	Cartilages of ribs 2–6, body of sternum, and clavicle	Greater tubercle of humerus	Flexion, adduction, and medial rotation at shoulder joint
ROTATOR CUFF MUSCLES			
Supraspinatus	Supraspinous fossa of scapula	Greater tubercle of humerus	Abduction at shoulder joint
Infraspinatus	Infraspinous fossa of scapula	Greater tubercle of humerus	Lateral rotation at shoulder joint
Subscapularis	Subscapular fossa of scapula	Lesser tubercle of humerus	Medial rotation at shoulder joint
Teres minor	Axillary border of scapula	Greater tubercle of humerus	Lateral rotation at shoulder joint
Teres major	Inferior angle of scapula	Intertubercular groove of humerus	Adduction and medial rotation at shoulder joint

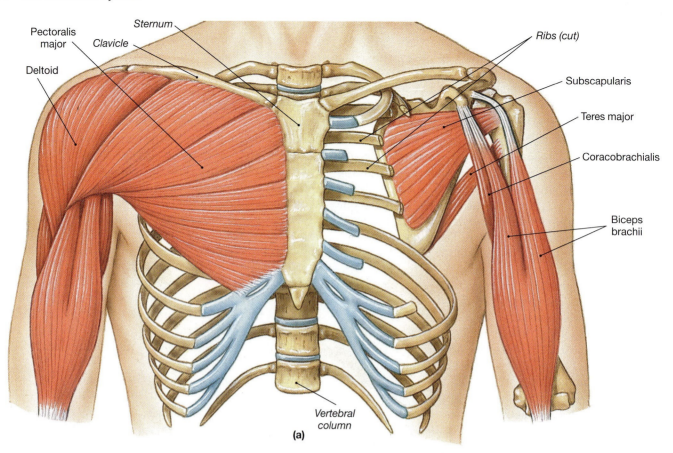

Pectoralis major

Clavicle

Sternum

Deltoid

Ribs (cut)

Subscapularis

Teres major

Coracobrachialis

Biceps brachii

Vertebral column

(a)

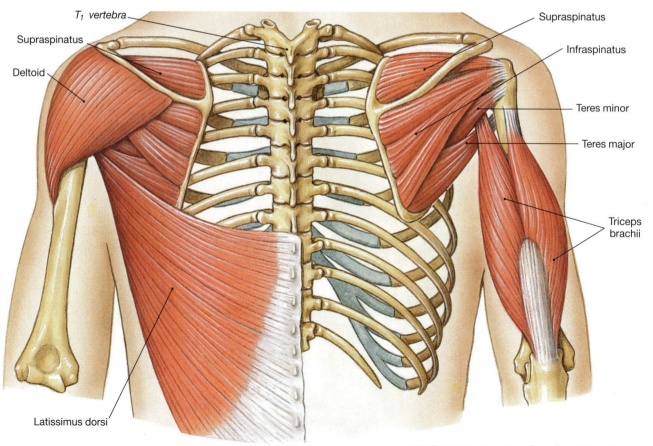

T_1 vertebra

Supraspinatus

Deltoid

Supraspinatus

Infraspinatus

Teres minor

Teres major

Triceps brachii

Latissimus dorsi

(b)

•**FIGURE 7-17   Muscles That Move the Arm**
(a) An anterior view. **(b)** A posterior view.

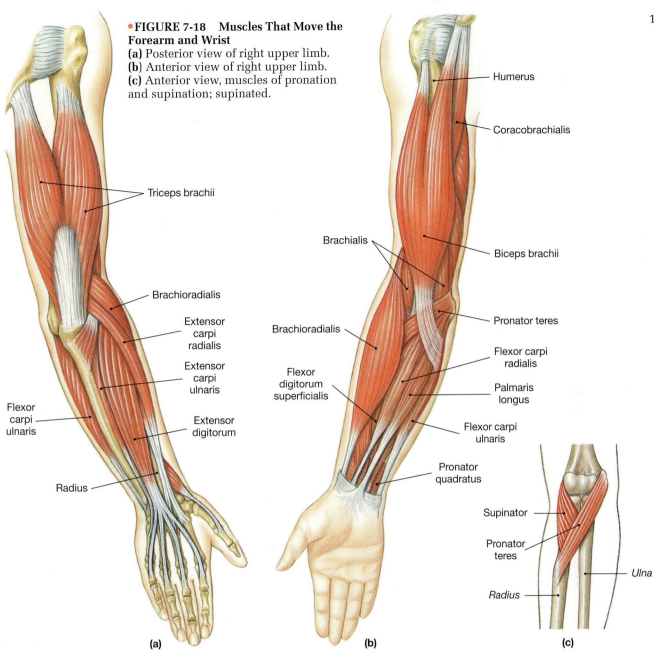

●FIGURE 7-18   **Muscles That Move the Forearm and Wrist**
(a) Posterior view of right upper limb.
(b) Anterior view of right upper limb.
(c) Anterior view, muscles of pronation and supination; supinated.

(a)

Triceps brachii

Brachioradialis

Extensor carpi radialis

Extensor carpi ulnaris

Flexor carpi ulnaris

Extensor digitorum

Radius

(b)

Humerus

Coracobrachialis

Brachialis

Biceps brachii

Brachioradialis

Pronator teres

Flexor digitorum superficialis

Flexor carpi radialis

Palmaris longus

Flexor carpi ulnaris

Pronator quadratus

(c)

Supinator

Pronator teres

Ulna

Radius

7

work together to produce flexion of the wrist. Because they originate on opposite sides of the humerus, the flexor carpi radialis flexes and abducts while the flexor carpi ulnaris flexes and adducts.

- The **extensor carpi radialis** muscles and the **extensor carpi ulnaris** have a similar relationship; the former produces extension and abduction at the wrist, the latter extension and adduction.

- The **pronators** and the **supinator** rotate the radius at its proximal and distal articulations with the ulna; the supinator may be assisted by the biceps brachii.

Muscles That Move the Palm and Fingers.   The muscles of the forearm perform flexion and extension at the finger joints (Table 7-10). These muscles stop before reaching the hand, and only their tendons cross the wrist. These are relatively large muscles, and keeping them clear of the joints ensures maximum mobility at both the wrist and hand. The tendons that cross the dorsal and ventral surfaces of the wrist pass through *tendon sheaths*, elongate bursae that reduce friction. Inflammation of tendon sheaths can restrict movement and irritate the *median nerve*, a nerve that innervates the palm of the hand. Chronic pain, often associated with weakness in the hand muscles, is the result. This condition is known as *carpal tunnel syndrome*.

✔ Which muscle do you use to shrug your shoulders?

✔ Sometimes baseball pitchers will suffer from rotator cuff injuries. Which muscles are involved in this type of injury?

✔ Injury to the flexor carpi ulnaris would impair which two movements?

TABLE 7-10   **Muscles That Move the Forearm, Wrist, and Hand**

Muscle	Origin	Insertion	Action
PRIMARY ACTION AT THE ELBOW			
Flexors			
Biceps brachii	From the coracoid process (short head) and body (long head) of scapula	Tuberosity of radius	Flexes elbow and supinates forearm by rotation at radioulnar joints
Brachialis	Anterior, distal surface of humerus	Tuberosity of ulna	Flexes elbow
Brachioradialis	Lateral epicondyle of humerus	Styloid process of radius	As above
Extensor			
Triceps brachii	Superior, posterior, and lateral margins of humerus, and the scapula	Olecranon process of ulna	Extends elbow
Pronators/Supinator			
Pronator quadratus	Medial surface of distal portion of ulna	Anterior and lateral surface of distal portion of radius	Pronates forearm by rotation at radioulnar joints
Pronator teres	Medial epicondyle of humerus and coronoid process of ulna	Distal lateral surface	As above
Supinator	Lateral epicondyle of humerus and ulna	Anterior and lateral surface of radius distal to the radial tuberosity	Supinates forearm by rotation at radioulnar joints
PRIMARY ACTION AT THE WRIST			
Flexors			
Flexor carpi radialis	Medial epicondyle of humerus	Bases of 2nd and 3rd metacarpal bones	Flexes and abducts wrist
Flexor carpi ulnaris	Medial epicondyle of humerus and adjacent surfaces of ulna	Pisiform bone, hamate bone, and base of 5th metacarpal bone	Flexes and adducts wrist
Palmaris longus	Medial epicondyle of humerus	A tendinous sheet on the palm	Flexes wrist
Extensors			
Extensor carpi radialis	Distal lateral surface and lateral epicondyle of humerus	Bases of 2nd and 3rd metacarpal bones	Extends and abducts wrist
Extensor carpi ulnaris	Lateral epicondyle of humerus and adjacent surface of ulna	Base of 5th metacarpal bone	Extends and adducts wrist
ACTION AT THE HAND			
Extensor digitorum	Lateral epicondyle of humerus	Posterior surfaces of the phalanges	Extends wrist and finger joints
Flexor digitorum	Proximal medial and anterior surface of ulna and radius; medial epicondyle of humerus	Distal phalanges	Flexes finger joints

7

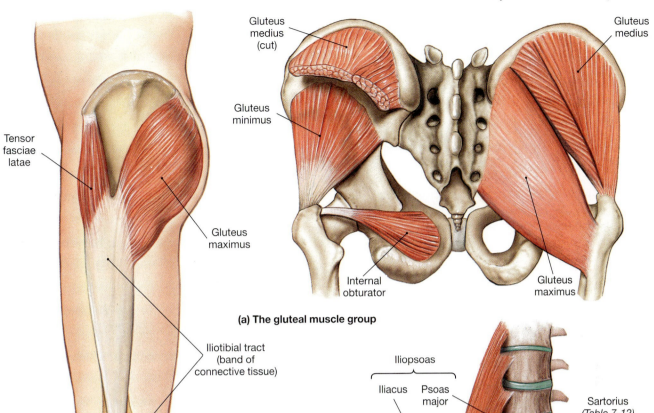

(a) The gluteal muscle group

•**FIGURE 7-19   Muscles That Move the Thigh**
(a) The gluteal muscle group (lateral and posterior views). **(b)** The iliopsoas muscle and the adductor group (anterior view).

Muscles of the Lower Limb

The muscles of the lower limb can be divided into three functional groups: (1) muscles that move the thigh, working across the hip joint; (2) muscles that move the leg, working across the knee joint; and (3) muscles that move the ankles, feet, and toes across the various joints of the foot.

Muscles That Move the Thigh.   The muscles that move the thigh are detailed in Figure 7-19• and Table 7-11.

• **Gluteal muscles** cover the lateral surfaces of the ilia (Figure 7-19a•). The **gluteus maximus** is the largest and most posterior of the gluteal muscles, which produce extension, rotation, and abduction at the hip.

• The adductors of the thigh include the **adductor magnus**, the **adductor brevis**, the **adductor longus**, the **pectineus** (pek-TIN-ē-us), and the **gracilis** (GRAS-i-lis) (Figure 7-19b•). When an athlete suffers a *pulled groin*, the problem is a strain in one of these adductor muscles.

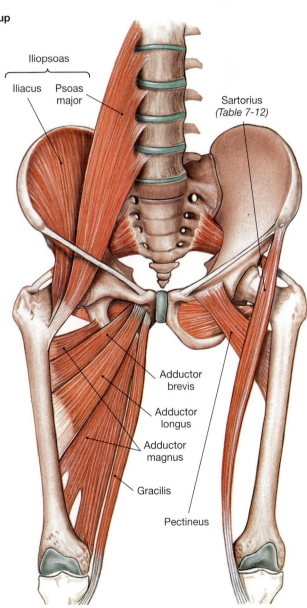

(b) The iliopsoas muscle and the adductor group

TABLE 7-11   Muscles That Move the Thigh

Group/Muscle	Origin	Insertion	Action
GLUTEAL GROUP			
Gluteus maximus	Iliac crest of ilium, sacrum, and coccyx	Iliotibial tract and gluteal tuberosity of femur	Extension and lateral rotation at hip joint
Gluteus medius	Anterior iliac crest and lateral surface of ilium	Greater trochanter of femur	Abduction and medial rotation at hip joint
Gluteus minimus	Lateral surface of ilium	Greater trochanter of femur	Abduction and medial rotation at hip joint
Tensor fasciae latae	Iliac crest and surface of ilium between anterior iliac spines	Iliotibial tract	Flexion, abduction, and medial rotation at hip joint; tenses fascia lata, which laterally supports the thigh
ADDUCTOR GROUP			
Adductor brevis	Ramus of pubis	Linea aspera of femur	Adduction at hip joint
Adductor longus	Ramus of pubis	As above	Adduction, flexion, and medial rotation at hip joint
Adductor magnus	Ramus of pubis	As above	Adduction at hip joint; anterior portion produces flexion; posterior portion produces extension
Pectineus	Ramus of pubis	Inferior to lesser trochanter of femur	Adduction, flexion, and medial rotation at hip joint
Gracilis	Inferior rami of pubis and ischium	Anterior surface of tibia inferior to medial condyle	Flexes knee and adducts hip
ILIOPSOAS			
Iliacus	Medial surface of ilium	Femur distal to lesser trochanter; tendon fused with that of psoas major	Flexes hip and/or lumbar spine
Psoas major	Anterior surfaces and transverse processes of lumbar vertebrae	Femur distal to lesser trochanter in company with iliacus	As above

- The largest hip flexor is the **iliopsoas** (il-ē-ō-SŌ-us) muscle. The iliopsoas is really two muscles, the **psoas major** and the **iliacus** (il-Ē-ah-kus), that share a common insertion at the greater trochanter.

Muscles That Move the Leg.   The general pattern of muscle distribution in the lower limb is that extensors are found along the anterior and lateral surfaces of the limb, and flexors lie along the posterior and medial surfaces.

- The flexors of the knee include three muscles collectively known as the *hamstrings*—(the **biceps femoris** (FEM-or-is), the **semimembranosus** (sem-ē-mem-bra-NŌ-sus), and the **semitendinosus** (sem-ē-ten-di-NŌ-sus)—and the **sartorius** (sar-TŌR-ē-us) (Figure 7-20a•).

- Collectively the *knee extensors* are known as the **quadriceps femoris**. The three **vastus** muscles and the **rectus femoris** insert on the patella, which is attached to the tibial tuberosity by the patellar ligament. (Because the vastus intermedius lies under the other quadriceps femoris muscles, it is not visible in Figure 7-20•.)

- The **popliteus** muscle medially rotates the tibia. When you stand, a slight lateral rotation of the tibia can lock the knee in the extended position. This enables you to stand for long periods with minimal muscular effort, but the locked knee cannot be flexed. The popliteus medially rotates the tibia back into its normal position, unlocking the joint.

The muscles that move the leg are detailed in Table 7-12, p. 204.

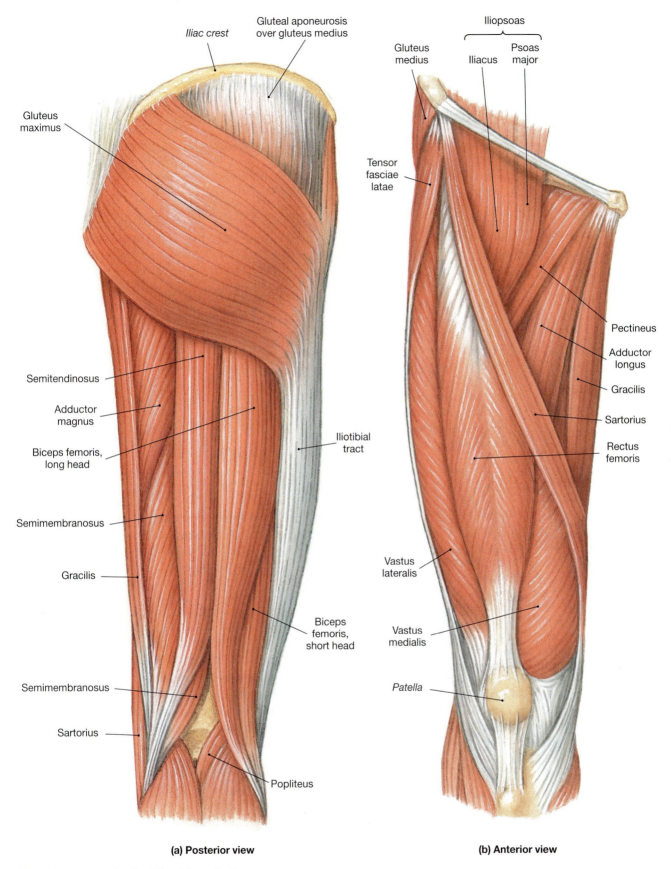

Iliac crest

Gluteal aponeurosis
over gluteus medius

Gluteus
maximus

Iliopsoas

Gluteus
medius

Iliacus   Psoas
major

Tensor
fasciae
latae

Semitendinosus

Adductor
magnus

Biceps femoris,
long head

Semimembranosus

Gracilis

Semimembranosus

Sartorius

Iliotibial
tract

Biceps
femoris,
short head

Popliteus

Pectineus

Adductor
longus

Gracilis

Sartorius

Rectus
femoris

Vastus
lateralis

Vastus
medialis

Patella

(a) Posterior view

(b) Anterior view

•FIGURE 7-20   Muscles That Move the Leg
(a) A posterior view of the thigh. (b) An anterior view of the thigh.

7

TABLE 7-12   Muscles That Move the Leg

Muscle	Origin	Insertion	Action
FLEXORS			
Biceps femoris	Inferior surface of ischium and linea aspera of femur	Head of fibula, lateral condyle of tibia	Flexes knee, extends and adducts hip
Semimembranous	Inferior surface of ischium	Posterior surface of medial condyle of tibia	Flexes knee; produces extension, adduction, and medial rotation at hip
Semitendinosus	Inferior surface of ischium	Proximal, posterior, and medial surface of tibia	As above
Sartorius	Anterior superior spine of ilium	Medial surface of tibia near tibial tuberosity	Flexes knee; produces flexion and lateral rotation at hip
Popliteus	Lateral condyle of femur	Posterior surface of proximal tibial shaft	Rotates tibia medially (or rotates femur laterally)
EXTENSORS			
Rectus femoris	Anterior inferior spine and superior acetabular rim of ilium	Tibial tuberosity via patellar ligament	Extends knee, flexes hip
Vastus intermedius	Anterior and lateral surface of femur along linea aspera	As above	Extends knee
Vastus lateralis	Anterior and inferior to greater trochanter of femur and along linea aspera	As above	As above
Vastus medialis	Entire length of linea aspera of femur	As above	As above

✳ INTRAMUSCULAR DRUG ADMINISTRATION

Injecting medications into muscle tissue *(intramuscular administration, IM)* is a safe, effective, simple, and relatively painless method of drug administration. The medication is absorbed into the network of blood vessels within the muscle and subsequently enters the circulatory system. The onset of action of medications administered by this route is typically 10–15 minutes. Drug absorption is steady and usually predictable and may continue for hours to days, depending upon the medication injected. In addition, drugs administered by this route, unlike those administered by the oral route, do not have to pass through the liver before arriving at their site of action.

The muscles most often used for IM injection are the deltoid muscle of the upper arm and the gluteus muscle in the buttock. These muscles are easy to access and large enough to handle large volumes of medication. Care must be taken to avoid nearby neurovascular structures. Typically, a 1½ inch needle is attached to a syringe containing the medication. The needle is inserted through the skin and subcutaneous tissue into the middle of the muscle. The plunger on the syringe is pulled back to assure that a blood vessel has not been inadvertently entered. Then, the plunger is depressed and the drug is deposited into the muscle tissue. The medication is then absorbed into the blood vessels and continues until all of the medication is gone. Second to the oral route, IM injection is the most frequently used method of drug administration.

Muscles That Move the Foot and Toes.   Muscles that move the foot and toes are shown in Figure 7-21● and detailed in Table 7-13, p. 206. Most of the muscles that move the ankle produce the plantar flexion involved with walking and running movements.

- The large **gastrocnemius** (gas-trok-NĒ-mē-us; *gaster*, stomach + *kneme*, knee) of the calf is assisted by the underlying **soleus** muscle. These muscles share a common tendon, the **calcanean tendon**, or *Achilles tendon*.
- A pair of deep **peroneus** muscles produce eversion of the foot as well as plantar flexion of the ankle.
- Inversion of the foot is caused by contraction of the **tibialis** muscles; the large **tibialis anterior** opposes the gastrocnemius and soleus, and dorsiflexes the ankle.

Important digital muscles originate on the surface of the tibia, the fibula, or both. Several smaller muscles originate on the bones of the tarsus and foot, and their contractions move the toes.

✓ You often hear of athletes suffering a "pulled hamstring." To what does this phrase refer?

✓ How would you expect a torn calcaneal tendon to affect movement of the foot?

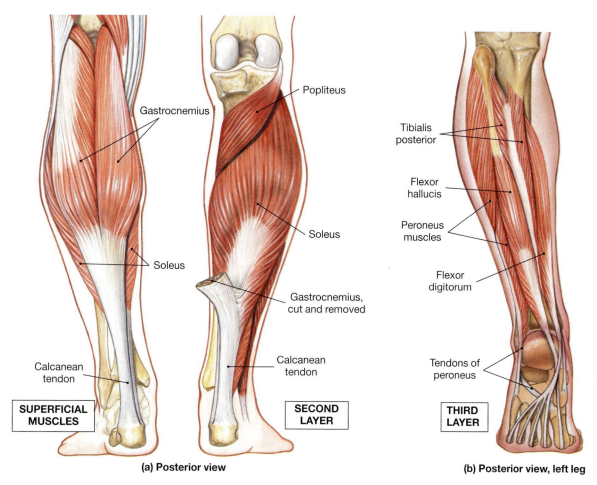

Gastrocnemius

Soleus

Calcanean
tendon

**SUPERFICIAL
MUSCLES**

Popliteus

Soleus

Gastrocnemius,
cut and removed

Calcanean
tendon

**SECOND
LAYER**

(a) Posterior view

Tibialis
posterior

Flexor
hallucis

Peroneus
muscles

Flexor
digitorum

Tendons of
peroneus

**THIRD
LAYER**

(b) Posterior view, left leg

7

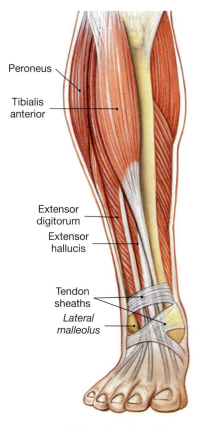

Peroneus

Tibialis
anterior

Extensor
digitorum

Extensor
hallucis

Tendon
sheaths

*Lateral
malleolus*

(c) Anterior view, right leg

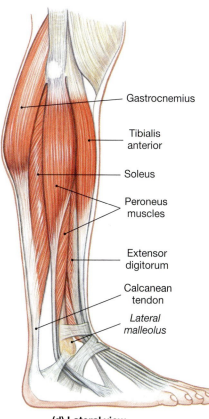

Gastrocnemius

Tibialis
anterior

Soleus

Peroneus
muscles

Extensor
digitorum

Calcanean
tendon

*Lateral
malleolus*

(d) Lateral view

● **FIGURE 7-21   Muscles
That Move the Foot and Toes**

TABLE 7-13 **Muscles That Move the Foot and Toes**

Muscle	Origin	Insertion	Action
Dorsiflexor			
Tibialis anterior	Lateral condyle and proximal shaft of tibia	Base of 1st metatarsal bone	Dorsiflexes ankle
Plantar flexors			
Gastrocnemius	Above femoral condyles	Calcaneus by way of calcanean tendon	Plantar flexes ankle; inverts knee and adducts foot; flexes knee
Peroneus	Fibula and lateral condyle of tibia	Bases of 1st and 5th metatarsal bones	Everts foot and plantar flexes ankle
Soleus	Head and proximal shaft of fibula, and adjacent shaft of tibia	Calcaneus by way of calcanean tendon	Plantar flexes ankle, inverts and adducts foot
Tibialis posterior	Connective tissue membrane and adjacent shafts of tibia and fibula	Tarsal and metatarsal bones	Adducts and inverts foot
ACTION AT THE TOES			
Flexors			
Flexor digitorum	Posterior and medial surface of tibia	Inferior surface of phalanges, toes 2–5	Flexion at joints of toes 2–5
Flexor hallucis	Posterior surface of fibula	Inferior surface, last phalanx of great toe	Flexion at joints of great toe
Extensors			
Extensor digitorum	Lateral condyle of tibia, anterior surface of fibula	Superior surfaces of phalanges, toes 2–5	Extension at joints of toes 2–5
Extensor hallucis	Anterior surface of fibula	Superior surface, terminal phalanx of great toe	Extension at joints of great toe

AGING AND THE MUSCULAR SYSTEM

As the body ages, a general reduction in the size and the power of all muscle tissues occurs. The effects of aging on the muscular system can be summarized as follows:

1. *Skeletal muscle fibers become smaller in diameter.* The overall effects are a reduction in muscle strength and endurance and a tendency to fatigue rapidly. Because cardiovascular performance also decreases with age, blood flow to active muscles does not increase with exercise as rapidly as it does in younger people.

2. *Skeletal muscles become smaller and less elastic.* Aging skeletal muscles develop increasing amounts of fibrous connective tissue, a process called *fibrosis*.

Fibrosis makes the muscle less flexible, and the collagen fibers can restrict movement and circulation.

3. *The tolerance for exercise decreases.* A lower tolerance for exercise as age increases results in part from the tendency for rapid fatigue, and in part from the reduction in thermoregulatory ability (described in Chapters 1 and 5, pp. 14 and 114), which leads to overheating.

4. *The ability to recover from muscular injuries decreases.* When an injury occurs, repair capabilities are limited, and scar tissue formation is the usual result.

The rate of decline in muscular performance is the same in all people, regardless of their exercise patterns or lifestyle. Therefore, to be in good shape late in life, an individual must be in very good shape early in life. Regular exercise helps control body weight, strengthens bones, and generally improves the quality of life at all ages. Extremely demanding exercise is not as important as regular exercise. In fact, extreme exercise in the elderly may lead to problems with tendons, bones, and joints. Although it has obvious effects on the quality of life, there is no clear evidence that exercise prolongs life expectancy.

INTEGRATION WITH OTHER SYSTEMS

To operate at maximum efficiency, the muscular system must be supported by many other systems. The changes that occur during exercise provide a good example of such interaction. As noted in earlier sections, active muscles consume oxygen and generate carbon dioxide and heat. Responses of other systems include the following:

- *Cardiovascular system.* The blood vessels dilate in the active muscles and the skin, and the heart rate increases. These adjustments accelerate the delivery of oxygen and the removal of carbon dioxide at the muscle and bring heat to the skin for radiation into the environment.

- *Respiratory system.* The rate and depth of respiration increase. Air moves into and out of the lungs more quickly, keeping pace with the increased rate of blood flow through the lungs.

- *Integumentary system.* Blood vessels dilate, and secretion by the sweat glands increases. This combination of changes helps promote evaporation at the skin surface and removes the excess heat generated by muscular activity.

- *Nervous system and endocrine system.* These systems direct the responses of other systems by controlling the heart rate, the respiratory rate, and sweat gland activity.

Even at rest, the muscular system has extensive interactions with other systems. Figure 7-22• summarizes the range of interactions between the muscular system and other systems of the body.

Chapter Review

KEY TERMS

anaerobic, *p. 180*	motor unit, *p. 178*	sarcoplasmic reticulum, *p. 169*
cross-bridges, *p. 172*	myofilaments, *p. 171*	synergist, *p. 184*
glycolysis, *p. 180*	myoglobin, *p. 181*	tendon, *p. 168*
insertion, *p. 184*	neuromuscular junction, *p. 172*	tetanic contraction, *p. 178*
isometric contraction, *p. 178*	origin, *p. 184*	transverse tubules, *p. 169*
isotonic contraction, *p. 178*	prime mover, *p. 184*	
lactic acid, *p. 180*	sarcomere, *p. 171*	

SUMMARY OUTLINE

INTRODUCTION *p. 168*

1. The three types of muscle tissue are *skeletal muscle, cardiac muscle,* and *smooth muscle.* The muscular system includes all the skeletal muscle tissue that can be controlled voluntarily.

FUNCTIONS OF SKELETAL MUSCLE *p. 168*

1. **Skeletal muscles** attach to bones directly or indirectly and perform the following functions: (1) produce skeletal movement, (2) maintain posture and body position, (3) support soft tissues, (4) guard entrances and exits, and (5) maintain body temperature.

THE ANATOMY OF SKELETAL MUSCLES *p. 168*

Gross Anatomy *p. 168*

1. Each muscle fiber is surrounded by an **endomysium.** Bundles of muscle fibers are sheathed by a **perimysium,** and the entire muscle is covered by an **epimysium.** At the end of the muscle is a **tendon.** *(Figure 7-1)*

Microanatomy *p. 169*

2. A muscle cell has a **sarcolemma** (cell membrane), **sarcoplasm** (cytoplasm), and a **sarcoplasmic reticulum,** similar to the smooth endoplasmic reticulum of other cells. **Trans-**

INTEGUMENTARY SYSTEM

Removes excess body heat; synthesizes vitamin D_3 for Ca^{2+} and PO_4^{3-} absorption; protects underlying muscles

Skeletal muscles pulling on skin of face produce facial expressions

SKELETAL SYSTEM

Maintains normal calcium and phosphate levels in body fluids; supports skeletal muscles; provides sites of attachment

Provides movement and support; stresses exerted by tendons maintain bone mass; stabilizes bones and joints

NERVOUS SYSTEM

Controls skeletal muscle contractions; adjusts activities of respiratory and cardiovascular systems during periods of muscular activity

Muscle spindles monitor body position; facial muscles express emotions; intrinsic laryngeal muscles permit speech

ENDOCRINE SYSTEM

Hormones adjust muscle metabolism and growth; parathyroid hormone and calcitonin regulate calcium and phosphate ion concentrations

Skeletal muscles provide protection for some endocrine organs

THE MUSCULAR SYSTEM

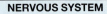

7

FOR ALL SYSTEMS

Generates heat that maintains normal body temperature

CARDIOVASCULAR SYSTEM

Delivers oxygen and nutrients; removes carbon dioxide, lactic acid, and heat

Skeletal muscle contractions assist in moving blood through veins; protects deep blood vessels

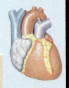

LYMPHATIC SYSTEM

Defends skeletal muscles against infection and assists in tissue repairs after injury

Protects superficial lymph nodes and the lymphatic vessels in the abdominopelvic cavity

RESPIRATORY SYSTEM

Provides oxygen and eliminates carbon dioxide

Muscles generate CO_2; control entrances to respiratory tract, fill and empty lungs, control airflow through larynx, and produce sounds

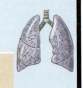

DIGESTIVE SYSTEM

Provides nutrients; liver regulates blood glucose and fatty acid levels and removes lactic acid from circulation

Protects and supports soft tissues in abdominal cavity; controls entrances to and exits from digestive tract

REPRODUCTIVE SYSTEM

Reproductive hormones accelerate skeletal muscle growth

Contractions of skeletal muscles eject semen from male reproductive tract; muscle contractions during sex act produce pleasurable sensations

URINARY SYSTEM

Removes waste products of protein metabolism; assists in regulation of calcium and phosphate concentrations

External sphincter controls urination by constricting urethra

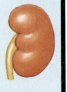

• **FIGURE 7-22**   **Functional Relationships Between the Muscular System and Other Systems**

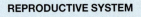

verse tubules (T tubules) and **myofibrils** aid in contraction. Filaments in a myofibril are organized into repeating functional units called **sarcomeres**. *(Figure 7-2a–c)*

3. **Myofilaments** consist of **thin filaments** (*actin*) and **thick filaments** (*myosin*). *(Figure 7-2d,e)*

4. The relationship between the thick and thin filaments changes as the muscle contracts and shortens. The **Z lines** move closer together as the thin filaments slide past the thick filaments. *(Figure 7-3)*

5. The contraction process involves **active sites** on thin filaments and **cross-bridges** of the thick filaments. For each cross-bridge, sliding involves repeated cycles of "attach, pivot, detach, and return." At rest, the necessary interactions are prevented by **tropomyosin** and **troponin** proteins on the thin filaments.

THE CONTROL OF MUSCLE FIBER CONTRACTION *p. 172*

1. Neural control of muscle function involves a link between electrical activity in the sarcolemma and the initiation of a contraction.

The Structure and Function of the Neuromuscular Junction *p. 172*

2. Each skeletal muscle fiber is controlled by a neuron at a **neuromuscular junction**; the junction includes the **synaptic knob**, the **synaptic cleft**, and the **motor end plate**. **Acetylcholine (ACh)** and **acetylcholinesterase (AChE)** play a role in the chemical communication between the synaptic knob and muscle fiber. *(Figure 7-4a,b)*

3. When an **action potential** arrives at the synaptic knob, acetylcholine is released into the synaptic cleft. The binding of ACh to receptors on the motor end plate leads to the generation of an action potential in the sarcolemma. The passage of an action potential along a transverse tubule triggers the release of calcium ions from the *cisternae* of the sarcoplasmic reticulum. *(Figure 7-4c)*

The Contraction Cycle *p. 172*

4. A contraction involves a repeated cycle of "attach, pivot, detach, and return." It begins when calcium ions are released by the sarcoplasmic reticulum. The calcium ions bind to troponin, which changes position and moves tropomyosin away from the active sites of actin. Cross-bridge binding of myosin heads to actin can now occur. After binding, each myosin head pivots at its base, pulling the actin filament toward the center of the sarcomere. *(Figure 7-5)*

Muscle Contraction: A Summary *p. 174*

5. A summary of the contraction process, from ACh release to the end of the contraction, is shown in *Table 7-1*.

MUSCLE MECHANICS *p. 177*

1. There is no mechanism to regulate the amount of tension produced in the contraction of an individual muscle fiber. It is either "ON" (producing tension) or "OFF" (relaxed). This is known as the **all-or-none principle**.

2. Both the number of activated muscle fibers and their rate of stimulation control the tension developed by an entire skeletal muscle.

The Frequency of Muscle Stimulation *p. 177*

3. A muscle fiber **twitch** (a single stimulus-contraction-relaxation sequence) consists of a **latent period**, a **contraction phase**, and a **relaxation phase**. *(Figure 7-6)*

4. Repeated stimulation before the relaxation phase ends can result in the addition of twitches (known as **summation**) and produce **incomplete tetanus** (in which tension will peak because the muscle is never allowed to relax completely), or **complete tetanus** (in which the relaxation phase is completely eliminated). Almost all normal muscular contractions involve the complete tetanus of the participating muscle units. *(Figure 7-7)*

The Number of Muscle Fibers Involved *p. 177*

5. The number and size of a muscle's **motor units** indicate how precisely controlled its movements are.

6. An increase in muscle tension is produced by increasing the number of motor units through **recruitment**.

7. Resting **muscle tone** stabilizes bones and joints. Inadequate stimulation causes muscles to undergo **atrophy**.

Isotonic and Isometric Contractions *p. 178*

8. Normal activities usually include both **isotonic contractions** (in which the tension in a muscle remains constant as the muscle shortens) and **isometric contractions** (in which the muscle's tension rises but the length of the muscle remains constant).

Muscle Elongation *p. 179*

9. Contraction is active, but elongation of a muscle fiber is a passive process that can occur either through elastic forces or through the contraction of opposing muscles.

THE ENERGETICS OF MUSCULAR ACTIVITY *p. 179*

1. Muscle contractions require large amounts of ATP energy.

ATP and CP Reserves *p. 179*

2. ATP is an energy-transfer molecule, not an energy-storage molecule. **Creatine phosphate (CP)** can release stored energy to convert ADP to ATP. A resting muscle cell contains many times more CP than ATP.

ATP Generation *p. 179*

3. At rest or moderate levels of activity, *aerobic metabolism* in mitochondria can provide most of the necessary ATP to support muscle contractions. *(Figure 7-8a)*

4. When a muscle fiber runs short of ATP and CP, enzymes can break down glycogen molecules to release glucose that can be broken down via **glycolysis**.

5. At peak levels of activity the cell relies heavily on the **anaerobic** process of glycolysis to generate ATP, because the mitochondria cannot obtain enough oxygen to meet the existing ATP demands. *(Figure 7-8b)*

Muscle Fatigue *p. 180*

6. **Muscle fatigue** occurs when a muscle can no longer contract, despite neural stimulation, due to pH changes, lack of energy, or other problems.

The Recovery Period *p. 180*

7. The **recovery period** begins immediately after a period of muscle activity and continues until conditions inside the muscle have returned to preexertion levels. The *oxygen debt* created during exercise is the amount of oxygen used in the recovery period to restore normal conditions. *(Figure 7-8c)*

MUSCLE PERFORMANCE *p. 181*

1. Muscle performance can be considered in terms of **power** (the maximum amount of tension produced by a particular muscle or muscle group) and **endurance** (the duration of muscular activity).

Types of Skeletal Muscle Fibers *p. 181*

2. The two types of human skeletal muscle fibers are **fast fibers** and **slow fibers**.

3. Fast fibers are large in diameter, contain densely packed myofibrils, large reserves of glycogen, and few mitochondria. They produce rapid and powerful contractions of relatively short duration.

4. Slow fibers are smaller in diameter and take three times as long to contract after stimulation. Specializations such as an extensive capillary supply, abundant mitochondria, and high concentrations of **myoglobin** enable them to contract for long periods of time.

Physical Conditioning *p. 182*

5. **Anaerobic endurance** is the ability to support sustained, powerful muscle contractions through anaerobic mechanisms. Training to develop anaerobic endurance can lead to **hypertrophy** (enlargement) of the stimulated muscles.

6. **Aerobic endurance** is the time over which a muscle can continue to contract while supported by mitochondrial activities.

CARDIAC AND SMOOTH MUSCLE TISSUES *p. 182*

Cardiac Muscle Tissue *p. 182*

1. Cardiac muscle cells and skeletal muscle fibers differ structurally in terms of (1) size, (2) the number and location of nuclei, (3) their relative dependence on aerobic metabolism when contracting at peak levels, and (4) the presence or absence of **intercalated discs**. *(Figure 7-9a; Table 7-2)*

2. Cardiac muscle cells have *automaticity* and do not require neural stimulation to contract. Their contractions last longer than those of skeletal muscles, and cardiac muscle cannot undergo tetanus.

Smooth Muscle Tissue *p. 183*

3. Smooth muscle is nonstriated, involuntary muscle tissue that can contract over a greater range of lengths than skeletal muscle cells. *(Figure 7-9b; Table 7-2)*

4. Many smooth muscle fibers lack direct connections to motor neurons; those that are innervated are not under voluntary control.

ANATOMY OF THE MUSCULAR SYSTEM *p. 184*

1. The **muscular system** includes approximately 700 skeletal muscles that can be voluntarily controlled. *(Figure 7-10)*

Origins, Insertions, and Actions *p. 184*

2. Each muscle can be identified by its **origin**, **insertion**, and **primary action**. A muscle can be classified by its primary action as a **prime mover**, or **agonist**; a **synergist**; or an **antagonist**.

Names of Skeletal Muscles *p. 184*

3. The names of muscles often provide clues to their location, orientation, or function. *(Table 7-3)*

4. The **axial musculature** arises on the axial skeleton; it positions the head and spinal column and moves the rib cage. The **appendicular musculature** stabilizes or moves components of the appendicular skeleton.

The Axial Musculature *p. 188*

5. The axial muscles fall into four logical groups based on location and/or function: muscles of (a) the head and neck, (b) the spine, (c) the trunk, and (d) the pelvic floor.

6. The muscles of the head include the **frontalis, orbicularis oris, buccinator, masseter, temporalis, pterygoids,** and **platysma**. *(Figure 7-11; Table 7-4)*

7. The muscles of the neck include the **digastric, mylohyoid, stylohyoid,** and **sternocleidomastoid**. *(Figures 7-11, 7-12; Table 7-4)*

8. The **splenius capitis** and **semispinalis capitis** are the most superior muscles of the spine. The extensor muscles of the spine, or **erector spinae**, can be classified into the **spinalis, longissimus,** and **iliocostalis** divisions. In the lower lumbar and sacral regions, the longissimus and iliocostalis are sometimes called the *sacrospinalis* muscles. *(Figure 7-13; Table 7-5)*

9. The muscles of the trunk include the **oblique** and **rectus** muscles. The thoracic region muscles include the **intercostal** and **transversus** muscles. Also important to respiration is the **diaphragm**. *(Figure 7-14; Table 7-6)*

10. The muscular floor of the pelvic cavity is called the **perineum**. These muscles support the organs of the pelvic cavity and control the movement of materials through the urethra and anus. *(Figure 7-15; Table 7-7)*

The Appendicular Musculature *p. 195*

11. Together, the **trapezius** and the sternocleidomastoid affect the position of the shoulder, head, and neck. Other muscles inserting on the scapula include the **rhomboideus**, the **levator scapulae**, the **serratus anterior**, and the **pectoralis minor**. *(Figure 7-16; Table 7-8)*

12. The **deltoid** and the **supraspinatus** produce abduction of the arm at the shoulder abductors. The **subscapularis, teres major, infraspinatus,** and **teres minor** rotate the arm at the shoulder. *(Figure 7-17; Table 7-9)*

13. The **pectoralis major** flexes the elbow, and the **latissimus dorsi** extends the elbow. Both of these muscles adduct and rotate the arm at the shoulder joint. *(Figure 7-17; Table 7-9)*

14. The primary actions of the **biceps brachii** and the **triceps brachii** (long head) affect the elbow. The **brachialis** and **brachioradialis** flex the elbow. The **flexor carpi ulnaris**, the **flexor carpi radialis**, and the **palmaris longus** cooperate to flex the wrist. They are opposed by the **extensor carpi radialis** and the **extensor carpi ulnaris**. The **pronator** muscles pronate the forearm, opposed by the **supinator** and the biceps brachii. *(Figure 7-18; Table 7-10)*

15. **Gluteal muscles** cover the lateral surfaces of the ilia. They produce extension, abduction, and rotation at the hip. *(Figure 7-19a; Table 7-11)*

16. Adductors of the thigh work across the hip joint; these muscles include the **adductor magnus**, **adductor brevis**, **adductor longus**, **pectineus**, and **gracilis**. *(Figure 7-19b; Table 7-11)*

17. The **psoas major** and the **iliacus** merge to form the **iliopsoas** muscle, a powerful flexor of the hip. *(Figure 7-19b; Table 7-11)*

18. The flexors of the knee, include the hamstrings (**biceps femoris**, **semimembranosus**, and **semitendinosus**) and **sartorius**. The **popliteus** aids flexion by unlocking the knee. *(Figure 7-20; Table 7-12)*

19. The *knee extensors* are known as the **quadriceps femoris**. This group includes the three **vastus** muscles and the **rectus femoris**. *(Figure 7-20; Table 7-12)*

20. The **gastrocnemius** and **soleus** muscles produce plantar flexion. A pair of **peroneus** muscles produce eversion as well as plantar flexion. The **tibialis anterior** performs dorsiflexion. *(Figure 7-21; Table 7-13)*

21. Control of the phalanges is provided by muscles originating at the tarsal bones and at the metatarsal bones. *(Table 7-13)*

AGING AND THE MUSCULAR SYSTEM
p. 206

1. The aging process reduces the size, elasticity, and power of all muscle tissues. Both exercise tolerance and the ability to recover from muscular injuries decrease.

INTEGRATION WITH OTHER SYSTEMS
p. 207

1. To operate at maximum efficiency, the muscular system must be supported by many other systems. Even at rest, it interacts extensively with other systems. *(Figure 7-22)*

7

REVIEW QUESTIONS

LEVEL 1   Reviewing Facts and Terms

Match each item in column A with the most closely related item in column B. Use letters for answers in the spaces provided.

Column A

___ 1. epimysium
___ 2. fascicle
___ 3. endomysium
___ 4. motor end plate
___ 5. transverse tubule
___ 6. actin
___ 7. myosin
___ 8. extensor of the knee
___ 9. sarcomeres
___10. tropomyosin
___11. recruitment
___12. muscle tone
___13. white muscles
___14. flexor of the leg
___15. red muscles
___16. hypertrophy

Column B

a. resting tension
b. contractile units
c. thin filaments
d. surrounds muscle fiber
e. enlargement
f. surrounds muscle
g. slow fibers
h. thick filaments
i. muscle bundle
j. hamstring muscles
k. covers active sites
l. conducts action potentials
m. fast fibers
n. quadriceps muscles
o. multiple motor units
p. binds ACh

17. A skeletal muscle contains:
   (a) connective tissues
   (b) blood vessels and nerves
   (c) skeletal muscle tissue
   (d) a, b, and c are correct

18. The type of contraction in which the tension rises but the resistance does not move is called:
   (a) a wave summation
   (b) a twitch
   (c) an isotonic contraction
   (d) an isometric contraction

19. What are the five functions of skeletal muscle?

20. What five interlocking steps are involved in the contraction process?

21. What forms of energy reserves are found in resting skeletal muscle cells?

22. What two mechanisms are used to generate ATP from glucose in muscle cells?

23. What is the functional difference between the axial musculature and the appendicular musculature?

LEVEL 2   Reviewing Concepts

24. Areas of the body where no slow fibers would be found include the:
    (a) back and calf muscles
    (b) eye and hand
    (c) chest and abdomen
    (d) a, b, and c are correct

25. Describe the basic sequence of events that occurs at a neuromuscular junction.

26. Why is the multinucleate condition important in skeletal muscle fibers?

27. The muscles of the spine include many dorsal extensors but few ventral flexors. Why?

28. What specific structural characteristic makes voluntary control of urination and defecation possible?

29. What types of movements are affected when the hamstrings are injured?

LEVEL 3   Critical Thinking and Clinical Applications

30. Many potent insecticides contain toxins called *organophosphates* that interfere with the action of the enzyme acetylcholinesterase. Terry is using an insecticide containing organophosphates and is very careless. He does not use gloves or a dust mask and absorbs some of the chemical through his skin. He inhales a large amount as well. What symptoms would you expect to observe in Terry as a result of the organophosphate poisoning?

31. The time of a murder victim's death is commonly estimated by the flexibility of the body. Explain why this is possible.

32. Jeff is interested in building up his leg muscles, specifically the quadriceps group. What exercises would you recommend to help Jeff accomplish his goal?

ANSWERS TO CONCEPT CHECK QUESTIONS

Page 172
1. Since tendons attach muscles to bones, severing the tendon would disconnect the muscle from the bone. When the muscle contracted, nothing would happen.   **2.** Skeletal muscle appears striated when viewed under the microscope because this muscle is composed of the myofilaments actin and myosin, which have an arrangement that produces a banded appearance in the muscle.   **3.** You would expect to find the greatest concentration of calcium ions in the cisternae of the sarcoplasmic reticulum of the muscle.

Page 177
1. Since the ability of a muscle to contract depends on the formation of cross-bridges between the myosin and actin myofilaments, a drug that would interfere with cross-bridge formation would prevent the muscle from contracting.   **2.** Because the amount of cross-bridge formation is proportional to the amount of available calcium ions, increased permeability of the sarcolemma to calcium ions would lead to an increased intracellular concentration of calcium and a greater degree of contraction. In addition, since relaxation depends on decreasing the amount of calcium in the sarcoplasm, an increase in the permeability of the sarcolemma to calcium could result in a situation in which the muscle would not be able to relax completely.   **3.** Without acetylcholinesterase, the motor end plate would be continuously stimulated by the acetylcholine, and the muscle would be locked into contraction.

Page 179
1. The ability of the muscle to contract depends on the ability to form cross-bridges between the actin and myosin. If the myofilaments overlap very little, then very few cross-bridges are formed and the contraction is weak. If the myofilaments do not overlap at all, then no cross-bridges form and the muscle cannot contract.   **2.** A motor unit with 1500 fibers is most likely from a large muscle involved in powerful, gross body movement. Muscles that control fine or precise movements, such as movement of the eye or the fingers, have only a few fibers per motor unit, whereas muscles of the legs, for instance, that are involved in powerful contractions have hundreds of fibers per motor unit.   **3.** There are two types of muscle contractions, iso-

metric and isotonic. In an isotonic contraction, tension remains constant and the muscle shortens. In isometric contractions, however, the same events of contraction occur, but instead of the muscle's shortening, the tension in the muscle increases.

Page 182
1. The sprinter requires large amounts of energy for a relatively short burst of activity. To supply this demand for energy, the muscles switch to anaerobic metabolism. Anaerobic metabolism is not as efficient in producing energy as is aerobic metabolism, and the process also produces acidic waste products. The lower energy and the waste products contribute to fatigue. Marathon runners, conversely, derive most of their energy from aerobic metabolism, which is more efficient and does not produce the level of waste products that anaerobic respiration does.   **2.** We would expect activities that require short periods of strenuous activity to produce a greater oxygen debt because this type of activity relies heavily on energy production by anaerobic respiration. Since lifting weights is more strenuous over the short term, we would expect this type of exercise to produce a greater oxygen debt than would swimming laps, which is an aerobic activity.   **3.** Individuals who are naturally better at endurance activities, such as cycling and marathon running, have a higher percentage of slow muscle fibers, which are physiologically better adapted to this type of activity than are fast fibers, which are less vascular and fatigue faster.

Page 184
1. The cell membranes of cardiac muscle cells are extensively interwoven and are bound tightly to each other at intercalated discs, allowing these muscles to "pull together" efficiently. The intercalated discs also contain gap junctions, which allow ions and small molecules to flow directly from one cell to another. This flow results in the rapid passage of action potentials from cell to cell, so their contraction is simultaneous.   **2.** Cardiac muscle and smooth muscle are more affected by changes in the concentration of calcium ions in the extracellular fluid than is skeletal muscle because in cardiac and smooth muscles, the majority of the calcium ions that trigger a contraction come from the extracellular fluid. In skeletal muscle, most of the calcium ions come from the sarcoplasmic reticulum.   **3.** The

actin and myosin filaments of smooth muscle are not as rigidly organized as they are in skeletal muscle. This organization allows smooth muscle to contract over a relatively large range of resting lengths.

Page 187

1. The opening between the stomach and the small intestine is guarded by a circular muscle known as a sphincter muscle. The concentric circles of muscle fibers in sphincter muscles are ideally suited for opening and closing holes and for acting as valves in the body. **2.** The *triceps brachii* extends the forearm and is an antagonist of the biceps brachii. **3.** The name *flexor carpi radialis longus* tells you that this muscle is a long muscle that lies next to the radius and functions to flex the hand.

Page 189

1. Contraction of the masseter muscle raises the mandible, whereas relaxation of this muscle depresses the mandible. These movements are important in the process of chewing, or mastication. **2.** You would expect the buccinator muscle, which forms the mouth for blowing, to be well-developed in a trumpet player.

Page 192

1. Damage to the external intercostal muscles would interfere with the process of breathing. **2.** A blow to the rectus abdominis would cause the muscle to contract forcefully, resulting in flexion of the torso. In other words, you would "double up."

Page 199

1. When you shrug your shoulders, you are contracting your levator scapulae muscles. **2.** The rotator cuff muscles include the supraspinatus, infraspinatus, subscapularis, teres major, and teres minor. The tendons of these muscles help enclose and stabilize the shoulder joint. **3.** Injury to the flexor carpi ulnaris would impair the ability to flex and adduct the hand.

Page 204

1. The hamstring is a group of three muscles that collectively function in flexing the leg: the biceps femoris, the semimembranous, and the semitendinosus. **2.** The Achilles (calcaneal) tendon attaches the soleus and gastrocnemius muscles to the calcaneus (heel bone). When these muscles contract, they extend the foot. A torn Achilles tendon would make extension of the foot difficult and the opposite action, flexion, would be more pronounced as a result of less antagonism from the soleus and gastrocnemius.

7

OVERVIEW

The most abundant type of muscle tissue in the body is skeletal muscle. Skeletal muscle is also called *voluntary muscle* because it is primarily under control of the voluntary nervous system. Skeletal muscle tissue, connective tissue, and neural tissue combine to form the skeletal muscle system—a system of approximately 700 individual muscles. Skeletal muscles are either directly or indirectly attached to the bones of the skeleton. The skeletal muscular system has numerous functions including movement, maintenance of posture and body position, support of soft tissues, protection of body entrances and exits, and maintenance of body temperature.

Various physician specialties concentrate on the muscular system. *Physiatrists* specialize in physical medicine and rehabilitation, focusing on the diagnosis and treatment of muscle injuries and diseases. They also plan and supervise musculoskeletal rehabilitation regimens. *Osteopathic physicians* recognize the importance of the musculoskeletal system in health and disease and emphasize the musculoskeletal system in their diagnosis and treatment of injuries and illness.

Skeletal muscle injuries are common. Although these injuries are usually self-limited, emergency personnel must be familiar with the anatomy, physiology, and pathophysiology of the skeletal muscle system.

SKELETAL MUSCLE INJURIES

Skeletal muscle injuries are common and rarely require medical care. The most common skeletal muscle injury is the *strain.* A strain is an abnormal stretching or tearing of a muscle, tendon, or both. Following a strain, a small amount of bleeding may occur at the site of the injury leading to the formation of a hematoma. This can cause pain or deformity that may last until the hematoma is resorbed and the injury healed. Rest and immobilization are usually all that is required in the treatment of a strain.

MUSCULOSKELETAL BACK DISORDERS

Back pain is one of the most common complaints encountered in modern emergency medical practice. In fact, low back pain is secondary only to the common cold as a cause of missed time from work. It is also the primary cause of reduced work capacity. Between 60 and 90 percent of the population will experience back pain in their lifetime. EMS is a physically demanding occupation (Figure A7-1•). EMS personnel are particularly vulnerable to back injury and should take precautions to minimize the chances of injury. This includes proper lifting techniques and requesting assistance when needed (Figure A7-2•).

• **FIGURE A7-1   Physical Demands of EMS**
Lifting and moving patients and equipment can cause low back injury if not performed correctly.

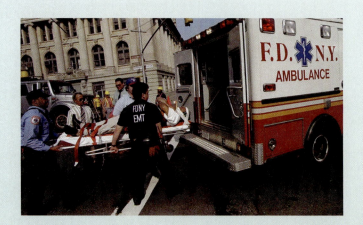

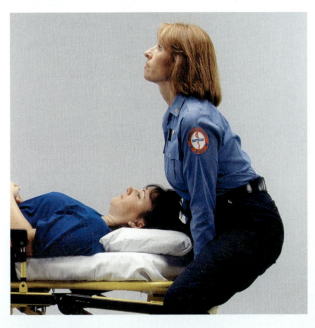

• FIGURE A7-2 **Proper Lifting Technique**
By lifting with the legs, the large paraspinous muscles of
the back are not overstressed.

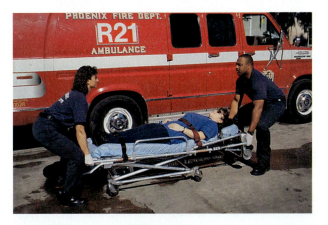

• FIGURE A7-3   **Lifting in Unison**
Back strains in EMS personnel usually occur when a team
member moves awkwardly during a lift. Twisting, turning, or
other movements can place stress on the large back muscles,
resulting in a back strain.

There are numerous causes of back pain, ranging
from a simple muscle strain to a ruptured aortic
aneurysm. Back strains usually occur when an abnormal
or exaggerated movement stretches or tears a muscle or
group of muscles in the back (Figure A7-3•). Carrying
heavy loads can also stress or tear back muscles resulting
in a strain. Back strains, especially those that involve a
group of muscles, initially causes localized bleeding at
the injury site. This is followed by the formation of a
hematoma. Hematoma formation is often accompanied
by pain. Often, the affected muscles, and other muscles
in the area, will spasm. This causes increased irritation
of the previously injured muscle and increased pain. Occasionally, the spasm can be so severe that pressure is
placed on nerve roots that exit the spine at each level. Irritation of the nerve roots can cause pain along the distribution of the affected spinal nerve.

There are three layers of muscles along the spine,
collectively referred to as the *paraspinous muscles.* The
superficial layer, consisting of the *spinalis,* the *longissimus,* and the *iliocostalis* is palpable during physical
examination. Tenderness or spasm can usually be pal-
pated. Occasionally, spasm is limited to one side and an
obvious lateral curvature of the spine can be seen.

A lumbar muscle strain can be quite painful. It is not
uncommon for these patients to be in such severe pain
that they must be medicated before they can lie down on
the ambulance stretcher for transport. The definitive treatment of a lumbar strain is to rest the affected muscles
and minimize inflammation. Initially, this should include
the application of ice and rest. Later, moist heat can be ap-

plied to the affected muscles. Anti-inflammatory medications are also helpful. Moderate to severe pain may
require a short course of narcotic pain medicine. Muscle
relaxant medications are somewhat controversial. Their
effectiveness in the treatment of lumbar muscle strains
varies significantly from patient to patient. Most of the
muscle relaxants have sedating side effects that may help
a patient to sleep. The application of physical therapy
modalities, osteopathic manipulation, or chiropractic adjustment can sometimes help to alleviate acute pain and
shorten the recovery period.

SPASMODIC TORTICOLLIS

Spasmodic torticollis is an intermittent or continuous
spasm of the muscles of the neck, most commonly the
sternocleidomastoid and *trapezius* muscles. It is usually
more pronounced on one side resulting in turning or tip-
ping of the head toward the affected muscles. Torticollis
is involuntary and cannot be inhibited. It tends to be
worse when the patient sits, stands, or walks. Torticollis
affects women twice as often as men.

Torticollis should not be confused with a cervical
muscle strain or spasm. Torticollis belongs to a class of
diseases referred to as focal dystonias. Dystonias are an
abnormal state of muscle tone. Focal dystonias affect a
single area of the body. They occur more frequently in
adults than in children, remain stable, and rarely spread
to other body parts. Spasmodic torticollis is the most
common focal dystonia. It is always important to exclude
an extrapyramidal system reaction as a cause of spasmodic torticollis. Many of the antipsychotic drugs can
cause focal dystonias, including torticollis, especially
when administered in higher doses.

A simple neck muscle spasm, generally referred to as
a "crick in the neck," often results from overuse, awkward positioning, or sleeping in an unusual position. The

spasm can be quite intense and painful and can last for several days. The initial "injury" can slightly tear or stretch the affected muscle causing pain and spasm. Most cases respond to local ice or heat, immobilization, and anti-inflammatory drugs. In severe cases, narcotics may be required for pain control, and intravenous diazepam (Valium) may be needed to help alleviate the muscle spasm.

HERNIAS

Contraction of the abdominal muscles can significantly increase the pressure within the abdominal cavity. During forceful exercise or lifting, the pressures within the abdominopelvic cavity can increase even more. If a weakness exists in the wall of the abdominal cavity, this increased pressure can force a portion of a visceral organ into the weakened area. The presence of a visceral organ in a weakened area of the abdominal wall is referred to as a *hernia*. Hernias can develop virtually anywhere in the abdominal wall. However, the inguinal region is particularly vulnerable to hernia development.

During development of the male, the testes descend from the abdominal cavity into the scrotum. They pass through the abdominal wall at the inguinal canals and carry remnants of the abdominal wall and membranes with them. In the adult male, the spermatic ducts and associated blood vessels penetrate the abdominal wall at the inguinal canals on their way to the testicles. The inguinal canal is weaker than other portions of the muscular abdominal wall. With age and increased intra-abdominal pressure, the inguinal canal slowly enlarges. On occasion, the inguinal canal enlarges and allows some of the abdominal contents, usually a portion of the small intestine, to enter. The presence of abdominal viscera in the inguinal canal is referred to as an *inguinal hernia*. Usually, the affected small intestine is forced into the canal when pressure within the abdomen increases; it returns to the abdomen when pressure is relieved. If the affected portion of the hernial site becomes trapped, and cannot return to the abdominal cavity, the hernia is said to be *incarcerated*. If blood supply to the hernia is compromised, the hernia is said to be *strangulated*. Emergency surgery is necessary to remove the hernia sac from the inguinal canal before bowel ischemia and necrosis occurs (Figure A7-4●).

In addition to inguinal hernias, several other types of hernias can occur. Patients who have had abdominal surgery may have a weakness in the abdominal wall along the scar of the incision. When intra-abdominal pressure increases, a visceral organ can be forced through this weakness to form an *incisional hernia*. This situation is more common in obese patients. Often, a piece of surgical mesh must be placed in the abdominal wall in order to prevent hernia formation. Females tend to develop *femoral hernias,* which develop in the femoral ring underneath the inguinal ligament. The incidence of femoral hernias is much lower than that of inguinal hernias.

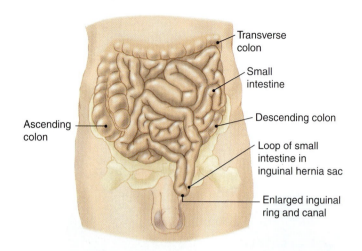

Transverse colon

Small intestine

Descending colon

Ascending colon

Loop of small intestine in inguinal hernia sac

Enlarged inguinal ring and canal

● **FIGURE A7-4   Inguinal Hernia**
An inguinal hernia occurs when a loop of abdominal viscera, usually the small intestine, enters a weakened and dilated inguinal canal. In severe cases, the loop of small intestine can be entrapped within the canal, often cutting off the blood supply. This situation, referred to as a strangulated inguinal hernia, is a surgical emergency.

A weakness in the diaphragm can result in some of the abdominal contents being forced into the chest cavity. A *hiatal hernia* is common. In these, the proximal portion of the stomach is forced upward through the esophageal hiatus (the point where the esophagus enters the abdomen). Hiatal hernias are usually managed with diet, weight loss, and medication. Surgery is rarely indicated.

FIBROMYALGIA

Fibromyalgia is a chronic inflammatory disorder of the muscular system. It is classified by the American Academy of Rheumatology as the presence of 11 of 18 specific tender points, nonrestorative sleep, muscle stiffness, and generalized aching pain, with symptoms present for more than 3 months' duration. Furthermore, the pains and stiffness cannot be explained by other mechanisms. Fibromyalgia can be quite debilitating. It commonly affects women under 40 years of age and is almost always associated with chronic fatigue. Many of the problems associated with fibromyalgia can be attributed to other conditions, such as depression. However, the presence of the tender points is the diagnostic key to fibromyalgia.

MYASTHENIA GRAVIS

Myasthenia gravis is an autoimmune disease characterized by muscle weakness and fatigue. It is particularly evident with repetitive use of voluntary muscles. Antibodies against acetylcholine receptors impair the function of the acetylcholine receptor at the neuromuscular

A7

junction causing varying degrees of motor weakness. The muscle weakness is most pronounced in the proximal muscles and is generally relieved by rest.

The signs and symptoms of myasthenia gravis can be quite varied. The first symptom is usually weakness of the eye muscles and drooping eyelids. The facial muscles are also often weak and can result in a peculiar smile known as the myasthenic snarl. As the illness progresses, the patient develops trouble swallowing and has difficulty holding his head upright. The weakness then spreads to the muscles of the trunk.

The diagnosis of myasthenia gravis can usually be made by performing a Tensilon test. Prior to administering Tensilon, a patient is given an apple to bite and chew. Then, a dose of the cholinesterase inhibitor *edrophonium chloride (Tensilon)* is administered. The patient is then asked to bite and chew the apple. A marked increase in muscle strength and the ability to eat the apple after administration of Tensilon helps establish the diagnosis. In myasthenia gravis, edrophonium causes a dramatic difference in the patient's ability to eat the apple. Cholinesterase inhibitors, such as edrophonium or neostigmine, inhibit the enzyme cholinesterase. Cholinesterase breaks down acetylcholine at the neuromuscular junction. Inhibition of cholinesterase allows acetylcholine to accumulate in the neuromuscular junction and overcome the effects of the acetylcholine receptor antibodies. For chronic treatment of myasthenia gravis, long-acting cholinesterase agents can be used to prevent skeletal muscle weakness.

NEUROMUSCULAR BLOCKADE

Certain emergency situations require chemically paralyzing a patient so that an endotracheal tube can be placed to assist or manage breathing. This procedure, referred to as *rapid sequence intubation (RSI),* involves the use of medications that act on the neuromuscular junction, the connection between the peripheral nerves and the skeletal muscle. Nerve impulses travel down the nerve and release a chemical neurotransmitter that stimulates (depolarizes) the associated skeletal muscle fibers resulting in contraction. Acetylcholine is the principle neurotransmitter in the neuromuscular junction. Blocking its action results in relaxation of skeletal (voluntary) muscles.

There are two ways to block the neuromuscular junction. One is by the administration of depolarizing agents that substitute for acetylcholine. Unlike acetylcholine, these depolarizing agents act over a prolonged time resulting in continued muscle depolarization and muscle paralysis. Because they have a stimulating effect, they often produce fasiculations (generalized, involuntary muscle twitching), especially in children, immediately after administration. The prototypical depolarizing neuromuscular blocker is succinylcholine (Anectine). It is the most commonly used neuromuscular blocker for rapid sequence intubation.

The other way to block the neuromuscular junction is to administer a drug that blocks the reuptake of acetylcholine into the nerve terminal. This produces an excess of acetylcholine in the neuromuscular junction, thus inhibiting the stimulation of the muscle. Because these drugs do not depolarize the affected muscle fibers, they are referred to as nondepolarizing blockers. They do not cause muscle fasiculations. Drugs in this class are similar in action to curare and include vecuronium, atracurium, and pancuronium.

Chemically paralyzing a patient causes complete voluntary muscle relaxation, including the muscles of respiration. This allows caregivers to take control of the airway and provide unimpeded mechanical ventilation. Esophageal and stomach muscles, and therefore sphincter tone, also relax, increasing the risk of vomiting and aspiration. Because neuromuscular blocking agents do not affect mental status or pain sensation, patients should be sedated or put to sleep before administration of neuromuscular blockers. If pain is present or expected, an analgesic should be administered.

SUMMARY

The muscular system consists of the skeletal muscles, tendons, and associated soft tissue and nerves. It is a vital body system responsible for movement, posture, support and maintenance of body temperature. Emergencies involving the muscular system are usually minor. However, emergency personnel should be familiar with several illnesses and injuries that involve the muscular system. Of these, the most frequently encountered will be strains of the back muscles.

8 Neural Tissue and the Central Nervous System

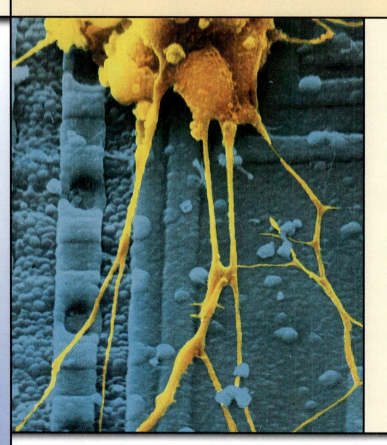

Science is constantly pushing the envelope of neurobiology. This scanning electron photomicrograph shows a human neuron growing on the surface of a silicon computer chip. Are androids really that distant in our future?

Chapter Outline and Objectives

Vocabulary Development

a-, without; *aphasia*
af, to; *afferent*
amygdale, almond; *amygdaloid bodies*
arachne, spider; *arachnoid membrane*
astro-, star; *astrocyte*
ataxia, a lack of order; *ataxia*
axon, axis; *axon*
cauda, tail; *cauda equina*
cephalo-, head; *diencephalon*
*cerebro-, brain; *cerebrovascular*
choroid, a vascular coat; *choroid plexus*
colliculus, a small hill; *superior colliculus*
commissura, a joining together; *commissure*
cortex, rind; *neural cortex*
cyte, cell; *astrocyte*
dia, through; *diencephalon*
dura, hard; *dura mater*
equus, horse; *cauda equina*
ef-, ex-, from; *efferent*
*encephalo-, brain; *encephalitis*
extero-, outside; *exteroceptor*
ferre, to carry; *afferent*
ganglio, knot; *ganglion*
glia, glue; *neuroglia*
hypo-, below; *hypothalamus*
inter-, between; *interneurons*
lexis, diction; *dyslexia*
limbus, a border; *limbic system*
mamilla, a little breast; *mamillary bodies*
mater, mother; *dura mater*
meninx, membrane; *meninges*
meso-, middle; *mesencephalon*
neuro-, nerve; *neuron*
nigra, black; *substantia nigra*
oligo-, few; *oligodendrocytes*
phasia, speech; *aphasia*
pia, delicate; *pia mater*
plexus, a network; *choroid plexus*
saltare, to leap; *saltatory*
vas, vessel; *vasomotor*

Two organ systems, the *nervous system* and the *endocrine system*, coordinate organ system activities in response to changing environmental conditions. The nervous system controls relatively swift but brief responses to stimuli, whereas the endocrine system usually controls processes that are slower but longer-lasting. For example, the nervous system adjusts body position and moves your eyes across this page, while the endocrine system is regulating the daily rate of energy use by the entire body. We will consider the mechanics of endocrine regulation in Chapter 11.

The nervous system is complex and versatile. As you read these words and think about them, at the involuntary level your nervous system is also monitoring the external environment and internal systems, and issuing appropriate commands as needed to maintain homeostasis. In a few hours, at mealtime or while you are sleeping, the pattern of nervous system activity will be very different. The change from one pattern of activity to another can be almost instantaneous because neural function relies on electrical events that proceed at great speed.

This chapter first examines neurons and other cells of the nervous system and then discusses the basic organization of the *central nervous system*—the brain and the spinal cord.

THE NERVOUS SYSTEM

The **nervous system** (1) monitors the internal and external environments, (2) integrates sensory information, and (3) coordinates voluntary and involuntary responses of many other organ systems. These functions are performed by neurons, which are supported and protected by surrounding neuroglia.

The two major anatomical subdivisions of the nervous system are detailed in Figure 8-1●. The **central nervous system (CNS)**, consisting of the *brain* and the *spinal cord*, integrates and coordinates sensory data and motor commands. The CNS is also the seat of higher functions, such as intelligence, memory, and emotion. All communication between the CNS and the rest of the body occurs over the **peripheral nervous system (PNS)**. The peripheral nervous system includes all the neural tissue *outside* the CNS. Its **afferent division** (*af-*, to + *ferre*, to carry) brings sensory information to the CNS, and its **efferent division** (*ef-*, from) carries motor commands to muscles and glands. Within the efferent division, the **somatic nervous system (SNS)** provides voluntary

control over skeletal muscles, and the *visceral motor system*, or **autonomic nervous system (ANS)**, provides automatic, involuntary regulation of smooth muscle, cardiac muscle, and glandular activity or secretions.

CELLULAR ORGANIZATION IN NEURAL TISSUE

The nervous system includes all the neural tissue in the body. Neural tissue, introduced in Chapter 4, consists of two kinds of cells, *neurons* and *neuroglia*. ∞ *p. 99* **Neurons** (*neuro-*, nerve) are the basic units of the nervous system. All neural functions involve the communication of neurons with one another and with other cells. The **neuroglia** (noo-RŌG-lē-a; *glia*, glue) regulate the environment around the neurons, provide a supporting framework for neural tissue, and act as phagocytes. Although they are much smaller cells, neuroglia, also called *glial cells*, far outnumber neurons.

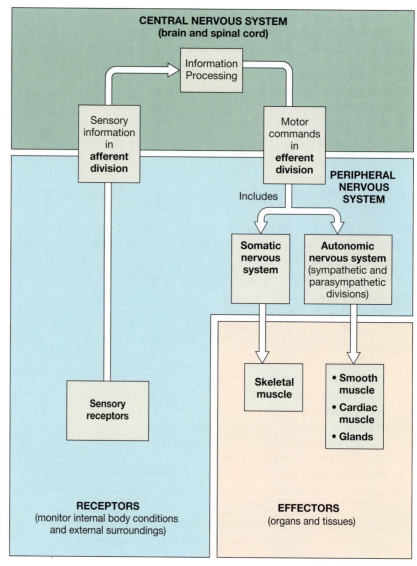

●**FIGURE 8-1**   **A Functional Overview of the Nervous System**

Neurons

Functional Classification of Neurons

Neurons are sorted into three functional groups: (1) *sensory neurons*, (2) *motor neurons*, and (3) *interneurons*.

Sensory Neurons. Sensory neurons of the afferent division convey information from both the external and internal environments to other neurons inside the CNS. Sensory neurons form the afferent division of the PNS, and there are approximately 10 million sensory neurons in the human body. These neurons connect a *sensory receptor* in peripheral tissues with the spinal cord or brain. Stimulation of a receptor usually leads to the stimulation of the sensory neuron. The receptor itself may be a process of a sensory neuron or a specialized cell that communicates with the sensory neuron. Receptors are broadly categorized as exteroceptors, proprioceptors, and interoceptors. **Exteroceptors** (*extero-*, outside) provide information about the external environment in the form of touch, temperature, and pressure sensations and the more complex senses of sight, smell, hearing, and touch. **Proprioceptors** (prō-prē-ō-SEP-torz; *proprius,* one's own + *capio,* to take) monitor the position of skeletal muscles and joints. **Interoceptors** monitor the activities of the digestive, respiratory, cardiovascular, urinary, and reproductive systems and provide sensations of taste, deep pressure, and pain.

Motor Neurons. The half million **motor neurons** of the efferent division carry instructions from the CNS to other tissues, organs, or organ systems. The peripheral targets are called *effectors* because they change their activities in response to the commands issued by the motor neurons. For example, a skeletal muscle is an effector that contracts on neural stimulation. There are two efferent divisions in the PNS, each targeting a separate class of effectors. The **somatic motor neurons** of the somatic nervous system innervate skeletal muscles, and the **visceral motor neurons** of the autonomic nervous system innervate other peripheral effectors, such as cardiac muscle, smooth muscle, and glands.

Interneurons. The 20 billion **interneurons**, or *association neurons,* are located entirely within the brain and the spinal cord. Interneurons, as the name implies (*inter-*, between), interconnect other neurons. Interneurons are responsible for the analysis of sensory inputs and the coordination of motor outputs. The more complex the response to a given stimulus, the greater the number of interneurons involved.

The General Structure of Neurons

As shown in Figure 8-2•, a representative neuron has (1) a cell body, or **soma;** (2) several branching, sensitive **dendrites,** which receive incoming signals; and (3) an elongate **axon,** which carries outgoing signals toward (4) one or more **synaptic terminals**. At each synaptic terminal, the neuron communicates with another cell. (Because the synaptic terminals between neurons are rounded, they are also called **synaptic knobs**.) Neurons can have a variety of shapes; Figure 8-2• shows a very common type of neuron in the CNS.

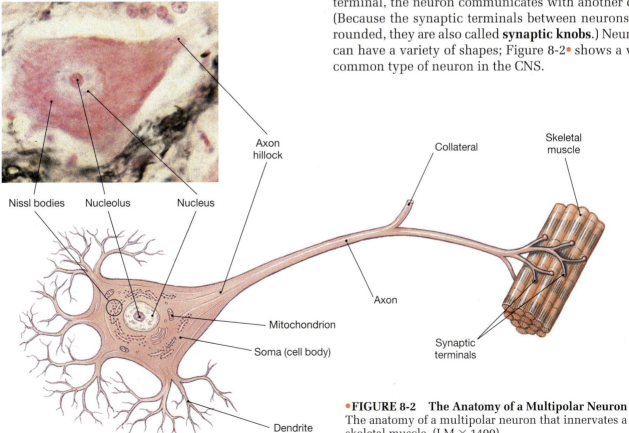

•**FIGURE 8-2   The Anatomy of a Multipolar Neuron**
The anatomy of a multipolar neuron that innervates a skeletal muscle. (LM × 1400)

The soma of a typical neuron contains a relatively large, round nucleus with a prominent nucleolus. There are usually no centrioles, organelles that in other cells form the spindle fibers that move chromosomes during cell division. Most neurons lose their centrioles during differentiation and become incapable of undergoing mitosis. As a result, most neurons lost to injury or disease cannot be replaced.

The soma also contains the organelles that provide energy and synthesize organic compounds. The numerous mitochondria, free and fixed ribosomes, and membranes of the rough endoplasmic reticulum (RER) give the cytoplasm a coarse, grainy appearance. The soma contains clusters of rough ER and free ribosomes. These dense clusters, known as **Nissl bodies**, give a gray color to areas containing neuron cell bodies.

Projecting from the soma are a variable number of dendrites and a single large axon. The cell membrane of the dendrites and soma is sensitive to chemical, mechanical, or electrical stimulation. In a process described later, such stimulation often leads to the generation of an electrical impulse, or *action potential*, that is conducted along the axon. The base of the axon is attached to the soma at a thickened region known as the *axon hillock*. Action potentials begin at the axon hillock. The axon may branch along its length, producing branches called *collaterals*. Synaptic terminals are found at the tips of each branch. A synaptic terminal is part of a **synapse**, a site where a neuron communicates with another cell. How signals are transmitted from cell to cell across the synapse will be the focus of a later section.

Structural Classification of Neurons

The neuron described above is called a **multipolar neuron** because there are multiple processes extending away from the cell body. Multipolar neurons are very common within the CNS (Figure 8-3a●). For example, all of the motor neurons that control skeletal muscles are multipolar.

Other types of neurons may have fewer extensions from the cell body. In a **unipolar neuron**, the dendritic and axonal processes are continuous, and the cell body lies off to one side (Figure 8-3b●). In a unipolar neuron, the action potential begins at the base of the dendrites, and the rest of the process is considered an axon on both structural and functional grounds. Sensory neurons of the peripheral nervous system are usually unipolar. **Bipolar neurons** have two processes, one dendrite and one axon, with the soma between them (Figure 8-3c●). Bipolar neurons are important components of special sense organs such as the eye and ear.

Neuroglia

Neuroglia are found in both the CNS and PNS, but the CNS has the greatest diversity of glial cells. There are four types of glial cells in the central nervous system (Figure 8-4●):

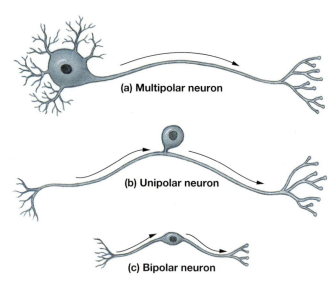

(a) Multipolar neuron

(b) Unipolar neuron

(c) Bipolar neuron

●**FIGURE 8-3   A Structural Classification of Neurons**
The neurons are not drawn to scale; bipolar neurons are many times smaller than typical unipolar and multipolar neurons.

1. **Astrocytes** (AS-trō-sīts; *astro-*, star + *cyte*, cell) are the largest and most numerous neuroglia. Astrocytes secrete chemicals vital to the maintenance of the *blood-brain barrier*, which isolates the CNS from chemicals in the general circulation. Astrocytes also create a structural framework for the CNS and perform repairs in damaged neural tissues.

2. **Oligodendrocytes** (o-li-gō-DEN-drō-sīts; *oligo-*, few) have cytoplasmic extensions that can wrap around axons, creating a membranous sheath called **myelin**. Myelin improves the speed of impulse conduction along the axon, by a mechanism detailed later in the chapter. Many oligodendrocytes are needed to coat an entire axon with myelin. The gaps between adjacent cell processes are called *nodes*, or the *nodes of Ranvier* (RAHN-vē-ā). The areas covered in myelin are called *internodes*. An axon coated with myelin is said to be **myelinated**. Not every axon in the CNS is myelinated, and those without a myelin coating are said to be **unmyelinated**. Myelin is lipid-rich, and on dissection areas of the CNS containing myelinated axons appear glossy white. These areas constitute the **white matter** of the CNS, whereas areas of **gray matter** are dominated by neuron cell bodies.

3. **Microglia** (mī-KRŌG-lē-a) are the smallest and rarest of the neuroglia in the CNS. Microglia are phagocytic cells derived from white blood cells that have migrated across capillary walls in the CNS. They perform protective functions similar to those of white blood cells.

4. **Ependymal cells** line the *central canal* of the spinal cord and the chambers, or *ventricles*, of the brain. This lining is called the **ependyma** (ep-EN-di-mah). In some regions of the brain, the ependyma produces *cerebrospinal fluid (CSF)*, and the cilia on ependy-

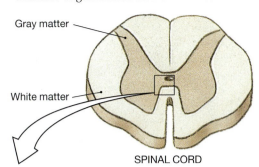

Gray matter

White matter

SPINAL CORD

•**FIGURE 8-4   Neuroglia in the CNS**
A diagrammatic view of neural tissue in the CNS, showing relationships between neuroglia and neurons.

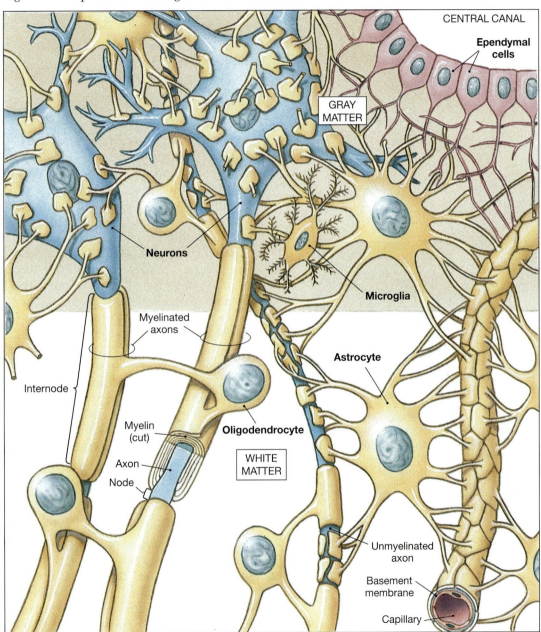

CENTRAL CANAL

**Ependymal
cells**

GRAY
MATTER

Neurons

Microglia

Myelinated
axons

Astrocyte

Internode

Myelin
(cut)

Oligodendrocyte

Axon

WHITE
MATTER

Node

Unmyelinated
axon

Basement
membrane

Capillary

8

mal surfaces in other locations help circulate this
fluid within and around the CNS.

Schwann cells are the most important glial cells in
the peripheral nervous system. Schwann cells cover every
axon outside the CNS, whether it is myelinated or un-

myelinated. In creating a myelin sheath, a Schwann cell
wraps itself around a segment of a single axon (Figure
8-5a•). Although the mechanism of myelination differs between the CNS and PNS, myelination in both divisions
creates nodes and internodes, and the presence of
myelin—however formed—increases the rate of impulse

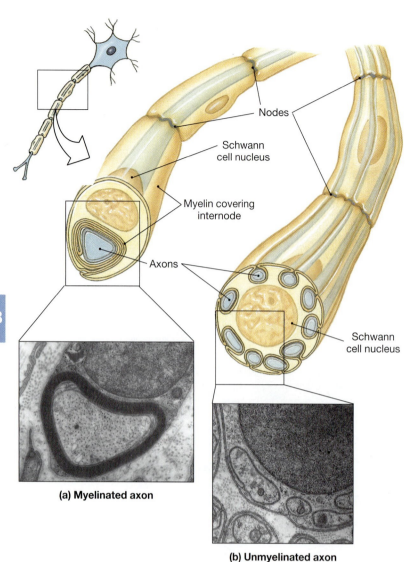

•FIGURE 8-5   Schwann Cells and Peripheral Axons
(a) A single Schwann cell forms the myelin sheath around a portion of a single axon. This arrangement differs from the way myelin forms in the CNS; compare with Figure 8-4 (TEM × 14,048). **(b)** A single Schwann cell can encircle several unmyelinated axons. Unlike the situation in the CNS (Figure 8-4), every axon in the PNS is completely enclosed by glial cells.

conduction. A Schwann cell may surround portions of several different unmyelinated axons (Figure 8-5b•).

✓ What would damage to the afferent division of the nervous system affect?

✓ Examination of a tissue sample shows unipolar neurons. Are these more likely to be sensory neurons or motor neurons?

✓ Which type of glial cell would you expect to be present in large numbers in brain tissue from a person suffering from an infection of the central nervous system?

NEUROPHYSIOLOGY

The sensory, integrative, and motor functions of the nervous system are dynamic and ever-changing. All of the important communications between neurons and other cells occur at membrane surfaces, through changes in the membrane potential. These membrane changes are electrical events that proceed at great speed.

The Membrane Potential

The cell membrane of an undisturbed cell has an excess of positive charges on the outside and an excess of negative charges on the inside. Such an uneven distribution of charges is known as a *potential difference*, and the size of the potential difference is measured in *volts*. Because the charges are separated by a cell membrane, the potential difference across the cell membrane of a living cell is called a **membrane potential**, or *transmembrane potential*. The **resting potential**, or membrane potential of an undisturbed cell, is very small. For example, the resting potential of a neuron averages about 0.070 volts, versus around 1.5 volts for a flashlight battery. Because they are so small, membrane potentials are usually reported in *millivolts* (mV, thousandths of volts) rather than volts. The resting potential of a neuron is −70 mV, with the minus sign indicating that the inside of the cell membrane contains an excess of negative charges as compared with the outside.

Factors Responsible for the Membrane Potential

As noted in earlier chapters, the intracellular and extracellular fluids differ markedly in ionic composition. For example, the extracellular fluid contains relatively high concentrations of sodium ions (Na^+) and chloride ions (Cl^-), whereas the intracellular fluid contains high concentrations of potassium ions (K^+) and negatively charged proteins (Pr^-).

The intracellular and extracellular fluids are separated by the cell membrane. The proteins cannot cross the membrane, and the ions can enter or leave the cell only by passing through membrane channels. ∞*p. 59* There are many different types of channels in the membrane; some are always open (leak channels), and others open or close under specific circumstances (gated channels).

Because the intracellular concentration of potassium ions is relatively high, potassium ions tend to diffuse out of the cell. This movement is driven by the concentration gradient for potassium ions. Similarly, the concentration gradient for sodium ions tends to promote their movement into the cell. However, the cell membrane is significantly more permeable to potassium ions than to sodium ions. As a result, potassium ions diffuse out of the cell faster than sodium ions enter the cytoplasm. The cell therefore experiences a net loss of positive charges, and as a result, the interior of the cell membrane contains an excess of negative charges, primarily from negatively charged proteins.

The resting potential remains stable over time because the cell membrane contains the sodium-potassium exchange pump, an ion pump introduced in Chapter 3. ∞ *p. 62* At a membrane potential of −70 mV, the rate of sodium entry to potassium loss can be precisely balanced by the sodium-potassium exchange pump. Figure 8-6• presents a diagrammatic view of the cell membrane at the resting potential.

Changes in the Membrane Potential

Every living cell has a resting potential. Any stimulus that (1) alters membrane permeability to sodium or potassium or (2) alters the activity of the exchange pump will disturb the resting potential of a cell. Examples of stimuli that can affect the membrane potential include exposure to specific chemicals, mechanical pressure, changes in temperature, or shifts in the extracellular ion concentrations. Any change in the resting potential can have an immediate effect on the cell. For example, in a skeletal muscle fiber, permeability changes in the sarcolemma trigger a contraction. ∞ *p. 172*

In most cases, a stimulus opens gated ion channels that are closed when the cell membrane is at the normal resting potential. The opening of these channels accelerates the movement of ions across the cell membrane, and this movement changes the membrane potential. For example, the opening of gated sodium channels will accelerate sodium entry into the cell. As the number of positively charged ions increases on the inner surface of the cell membrane, the membrane potential will shift toward 0 mV. A shift in this direction is called a *depolarization* of the membrane. A stimulus that opens gated potassium ion channels will shift the membrane potential away from 0 mV, because additional potassium ions will leave the cell. Such a change, which may take the membrane potential from −70 mV to −80 mV, is called a *hyperpolarization*.

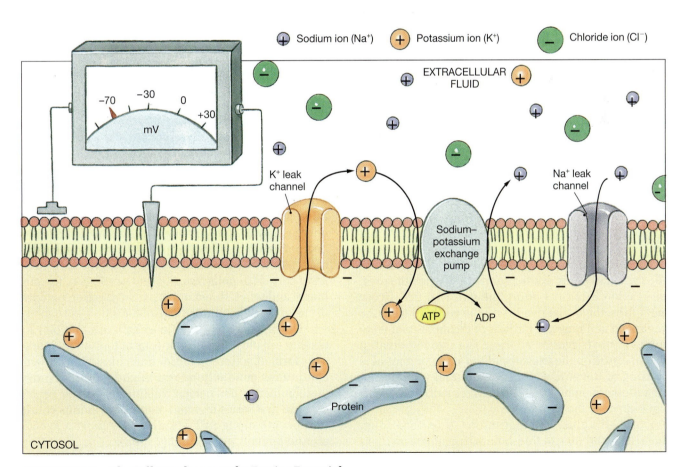

•FIGURE 8-6   The Cell Membrane at the Resting Potential

Information transfer between neurons and other cells involves graded potentials and action potentials. **Graded potentials** affect only a limited portion of the cell membrane. For example, if a chemical stimulus applied to the cell membrane of a neuron opens gated sodium ion channels at a single site, the sodium ions entering the cell will depolarize the membrane at that location. The sodium ions will then diffuse along the inner surface of the membrane in all directions. Because the sodium ions are spreading out, the degree of depolarization decreases with distance away from the point of entry.

Graded potentials occur in the membranes of all cells in response to environmental stimuli. These changes can trigger shifts in cellular function, and motor neurons control other cells by producing graded potentials in their cell membranes. For example, chemicals released by motor neurons produce graded potentials in the membranes of gland cells, and these potential changes can stimulate or inhibit glandular secretion. However, graded potentials affect too small an area to have an effect on the activities of relatively enormous cells, such as skeletal muscle fibers or neurons. In these cells, graded potentials can influence operations in distant portions of the cell only if they lead to the production of an *action potential*, an electrical signal that affects the entire membrane surface.

An **action potential** is a conducted change in the permeability of the cell membrane. Skeletal muscle fibers and axons have membranes that will conduct action potentials. In a skeletal muscle fiber, the action potential begins at the neuromuscular junction and travels across the entire membrane surface, including the T tubules. ∞ *p. 172* The resulting ion movements trigger a contraction. In an axon, an action potential usually begins near the axon hillock and travels along the length of the axon toward the synaptic terminals, where its arrival activates the synapses.

Action potentials are created by the opening and closing of sodium and potassium channels in response to a local depolarization. The graded depolarization acts like pressure on the trigger of a gun. A gun fires only after a certain minimum pressure has been applied to the trigger. It does not matter whether the pressure builds gradually or is exerted suddenly—when the pressure reaches a critical point, the gun will fire. Every time it fires, the bullet that leaves the gun will have the same speed and range, regardless of the forces that were applied to the trigger. In an axon, the graded potential is the pressure on the trigger, and the action potential is the firing of the gun. An action potential will not appear unless the membrane depolarizes sufficiently to a level known as the **threshold**.

Every stimulus, whether minor or extreme, that brings the membrane to threshold will generate an identical action potential. This is called the **all-or-none principle**: A given stimulus either triggers a typical action potential or does not produce one at all. The all-or-none principle applies to all excitable membranes.

The Generation of an Action Potential

An action potential begins when the cell membrane depolarizes to threshold. Figure 8-7• diagrams the steps involved in the generation of an action potential, beginning with a graded depolarization to threshold (from -70 to -60 mV) and ending with a return to the resting potential (-70 mV).

From the moment that the sodium channels open at threshold until *repolarization* (the return to the resting potential) is completed, the membrane cannot respond normally to further stimulation. This is the **refractory period**. The refractory period limits the number of action potentials that can be generated in an excitable membrane. (The maximum rate of action potential generation is 500–1000 per second.)

Potentially deadly forms of human poisoning result from eating seafood containing *neurotoxins*, poisons that primarily affect neurons. Several neurotoxins, such as *tetrodotoxin* (TTX) from puffer fish, either block open sodium channels or prevent their opening. Motor neurons cannot function under these conditions, and death may result from paralysis of the respiratory muscles.

Conduction of an Action Potential

An action potential initially involves a relatively small segment of the total membrane surface. But unlike graded potentials, which diminish rapidly with distance, action potentials affect the entire membrane surface. The basic mechanism of action potential conduction along unmyelinated and myelinated axons is shown in Figure 8-8•. (The areas of the membrane that are in the refractory period are shaded.)

At a given site, for a brief moment at the peak of the action potential, the inside of the cell membrane contains an excess of positive ions. Because opposite charges attract one another, these ions immediately begin spreading along the inner surface of the membrane, drawn to the surrounding negative charges. This *local current* depolarizes adjacent portions of the membrane, and when threshold is reached, action potentials occur at these locations (Figure 8-8a•).

The process continues in a chain reaction that soon reaches the most distant portions of the cell membrane. This form of action potential transmission is known as **continuous conduction**. You might compare continuous conduction to a person walking heel-to-toe; progress is made in a series of small steps. Continuous conduction occurs along unmyelinated axons at a speed of around 1 meter per second (2 mph).

In a myelinated fiber, the axon is wrapped in layers of myelin. This wrapping is complete except at the

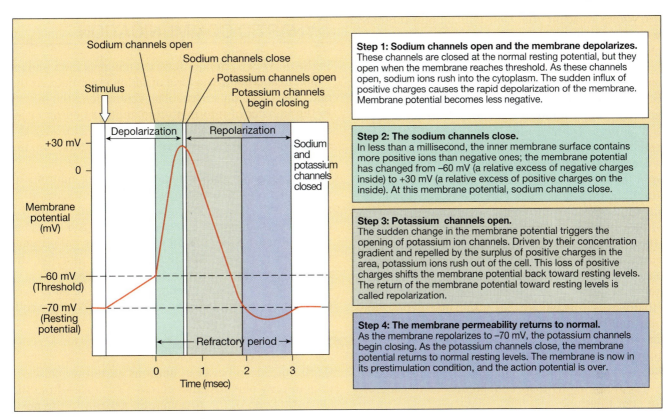

•**FIGURE 8-7   An Action Potential**
A sufficiently strong depolarizing stimulus will bring the membrane potential to threshold and trigger an action potential.

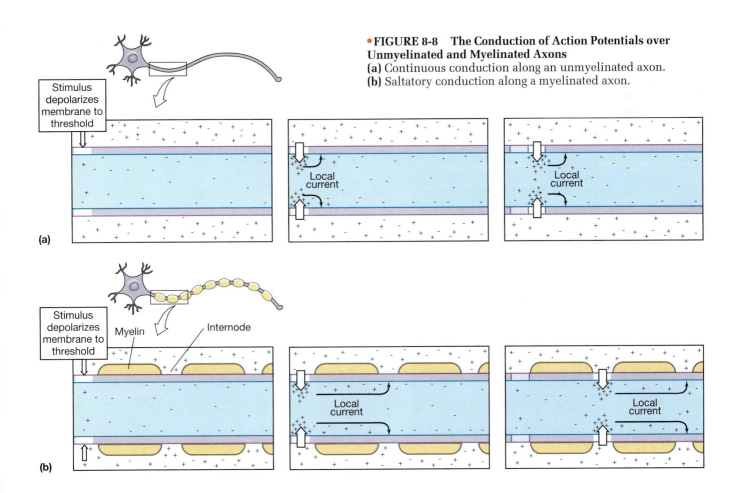

•**FIGURE 8-8   The Conduction of Action Potentials over Unmyelinated and Myelinated Axons**
(**a**) Continuous conduction along an unmyelinated axon.
(**b**) Saltatory conduction along a myelinated axon.

nodes, where adjacent glial cells contact one another. Between the nodes, the lipids of the myelin sheath block the flow of ions across the membrane. As a result, continuous conduction cannot occur. Instead, when an action potential occurs at the base of the axon, the local current skips the internode and depolarizes the closest node to threshold. The action potential jumps from node to node, rather than proceeding in a series of small steps. This process is called **saltatory conduction**, taking its name from *saltare*, the Latin word meaning "to leap." Saltatory conduction, illustrated in Figure 8-8b•, carries nerve impulses along an axon roughly seven times as fast as continuous conduction.

Demyelination is the progressive destruction of myelin sheaths, accompanied by inflammation, axon damage, and scarring of neural tissue. In most cases, the result is a gradual loss of sensation and motor control that leaves affected regions numb and paralyzed. In one demyelination disorder, **multiple sclerosis** (skler-Ō-sis; *sklerosis*, hardness), or **MS**, axons in the optic nerve, brain, and/or spinal cord are affected. Common symptoms of MS include partial loss of vision and problems with speech, balance, and general motor coordination.

✓ How would a chemical that blocks the sodium channels in a neuron's cell membrane affect the neuron's ability to depolarize?

✓ Two axons are tested for propagation velocities. One carries action potentials at 10 meters per second, the other at 1 meter per second. Which axon is myelinated?

SYNAPTIC COMMUNICATION

In the nervous system, information moves from one location to another in the form of action potentials. At the end of an axon, the arrival of an action potential results in the transfer of information to another neuron or effector cell. The information transfer occurs through the release of chemicals called **neurotransmitters** from the synaptic knob.

Neurons can communicate with other neurons or other cell types. When one neuron communicates with another, the synapse may occur on a dendrite, on the cell body, or along the length of the axon. Synapses between a neuron and another cell type are called **neuroeffector junctions**. At a *neuromuscular junction*, the neuron communicates with a muscle cell, as we saw in Chapter 7. ∞ *p. 172* At a *neuroglandular junction*, a neuron controls or regulates the activity of a secretory cell.

Structure of a Synapse

Communication between neurons and other cells occurs in only one direction across a synapse—from the synaptic knob of the **presynaptic neuron** to the **postsynaptic neuron** (Figure 8-9•) or other cell type. The opposing cell membranes are separated by a narrow space called the **synaptic cleft**.

Each synaptic knob contains mitochondria, synaptic vesicles, and endoplasmic reticulum. Every synaptic vesicle contains several thousand molecules of a specific neurotransmitter, and on stimulation many of these vesicles release their contents into the synaptic cleft. The neurotransmitter then diffuses across the synaptic cleft and binds to receptors on the postsynaptic membrane.

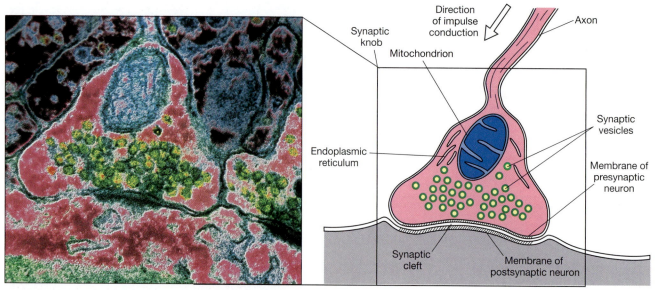

•**FIGURE 8-9   The Structure of a Cholinergic Synapse** (TEM × 222,000)

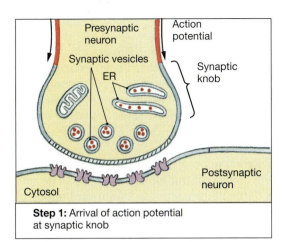

Step 1: Arrival of action potential at synaptic knob

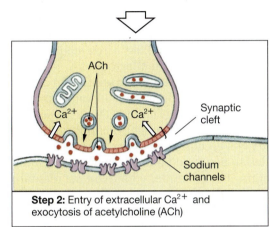

Step 2: Entry of extracellular Ca^{2+} and exocytosis of acetylcholine (ACh)

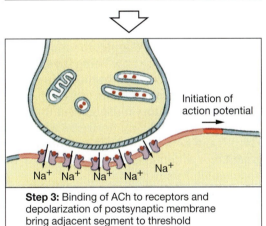

Step 3: Binding of ACh to receptors and depolarization of postsynaptic membrane bring adjacent segment to threshold

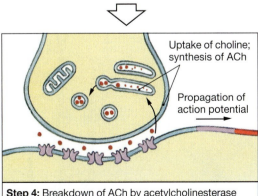

Step 4: Breakdown of ACh by acetylcholinesterase (AChE); reabsorption of choline by synaptic knob

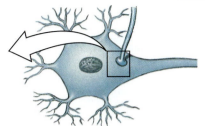

•**FIGURE 8-10   The Function of a Cholinergic Synapse**

Synaptic Events and Neurotransmitters

There are many different neurotransmitters. The neurotransmitter **acetylcholine**, or **ACh**, is released at **cholinergic synapses**. Cholinergic synapses are widespread inside and outside of the CNS; the neuromuscular junction described in Chapter 7 is one example. Figure 8-10• shows the major events that occur at a cholinergic synapse following the arrival of an action potential at the presynaptic neuron:

Step 1: *The arrival of action potential at the synaptic knob.* The arriving action potential depolarizes the presynaptic membrane.

Step 2: *The release of neurotransmitter.* Depolarization of the presynaptic membrane causes the brief opening of calcium channels that allows extracellular calcium ions to enter the synaptic knob. Their arrival triggers the release of ACh through exocytosis.

Step 3: *The binding of ACh and depolarization of the postsynaptic membrane.* The binding of ACh to sodium channels causes them to open and allows sodium ions to enter. If the resulting depolarization of the postsynaptic membrane reaches threshold, an action potential is produced.

Step 4: *The removal of ACh by AChE.* The effects on the postsynaptic membrane are temporary because the synaptic cleft and postsynaptic membrane contain the enzyme acetylcholinesterase (AChE). The AChE breaks down ACh into acetate and choline.

Table 8-1 summarizes the sequence of events that occur at a cholinergic synapse.

Another common neurotransmitter, **norepinephrine** (nōr-ep-i-NEF-rin), or **NE**, is important in the brain and in portions of the autonomic nervous system. It is also called *noradrenaline*, and synapses releasing NE are described as **adrenergic**. Both ACh and NE usually have an excitatory effect due to the depolarization of postsynaptic neurons. Like ACh, NE's effect is temporary; it is broken down by an enzyme called *monoamine oxidase*.

Dopamine (DŌ-pah-mēn), **gamma aminobutyric** (GAM-ma a-MĒ-nō-bū-TIR-ik) **acid**, also known as **GABA**, and **serotonin** (ser-ō-TŌ-nin) are CNS neurotransmitters whose effects are usually inhibitory due to the hyperpolarization of postsynaptic neurons. There are at least 50 other neurotransmitters whose functions aren't well understood.

TABLE 8-1   Sequence of Events at a Typical Cholinergic Synapse

Step 1:
- An arriving action potential depolarizes the synaptic knob and the presynaptic membrane.

Step 2:
- Calcium ions enter the cytoplasm of the synaptic knob.
- ACh release occurs through diffusion and exocytosis of neurotransmitter vesicles.

Step 3:
- ACh diffuses across the synaptic cleft and binds to receptors on the postsynaptic membrane.
- Chemically regulated sodium channels on the postsynaptic surface are activated, producing a graded depolarization.
- ACh release ceases because calcium ions are removed from the cytoplasm of the synaptic knob.

Step 4:
- The depolarization ends as ACh is broken down into acetate and choline by AChE.
- The synaptic knob reabsorbs choline from the synaptic cleft and uses it to resynthesize ACh.

NEURONAL POOLS

As noted previously, the neurotransmitters released at a synapse may have excitatory or inhibitory effects. Whether an action potential appears in the postsynaptic neuron depends on the balance between the depolarizing and hyperpolarizing stimuli arriving at any moment. For example, suppose that a neuron will generate an action potential if it receives 10 depolarizing stimuli. That could mean 10 active synapses if all release excitatory neurotransmitters. But if, at the same moment, 10 other synapses release inhibitory neurotransmitters, the excitatory and inhibitory effects will cancel one another, and no action potential will develop. The activity of a neuron thus depends on the balance between excitation and inhibition. The interactions are extremely complex—synapses at the cell body and dendrites may involve tens of thousands of other neurons, some releasing excitatory neurotransmitters and others releasing inhibitory neurotransmitters.

An individual neuron is the simplest level of organization within the central nervous system. The next level is that of the neuronal pool. A **neuronal pool** consists of a group of interneurons with one or more specific functions. Each neuronal pool has a limited number of input sources and output destinations, and each may contain excitatory and inhibitory neurons. The output of one pool may (1) stimulate or depress the activity of other pools or (2) exert direct control over motor neurons and peripheral effectors.

Neurons communicate with one another in several patterns. In **divergence**, information spreads from one neuron to several neurons (Figure 8-11a●). Divergence usually occurs when sensory neurons bring information into the CNS, because the sensory information must be distributed to neuronal pools throughout the spinal cord and brain. For example, when you accidentally touch a hot stove, divergence is what allows you to feel the pain and flex your arm at the same time.

In **convergence** (Figure 8-11b●), several neurons synapse on the same postsynaptic neuron. Convergence makes possible both voluntary and involuntary control of some body processes. For example, the movements of your diaphragm and ribs are now being involuntarily controlled by respiratory centers in the brain. These centers activate or inhibit motor neurons in the spinal cord that control the respiratory muscles. But the same movements can be controlled voluntarily, as when you take a deep breath and hold it. Although voluntary commands originate in a different neuronal pool, they influence the same motor neurons.

Parallel processing (Figure 8-11c●) occurs when several neuronal pools receive the same information at

●**FIGURE 8-11   The Organization of Neuronal Pools**
(a) Divergence, a mechanism for spreading stimulation to multiple neurons or neuronal pools in the CNS. **(b)** Convergence, a mechanism providing input to a single neuron from multiple sources. **(c)** Parallel processing, in which neurons or pools process information simultaneously.

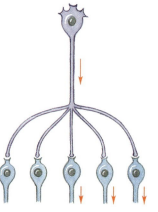

(a) Divergence

(b) Convergence

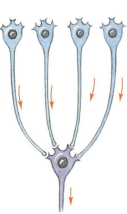

(c) Parallel processing

the same time. Thanks to parallel processing, many different responses occur simultaneously. For example, stepping on a tack stimulates sensory neurons that distribute the information to a number of neuronal pools. As a result, within a heartbeat you can feel the pain, withdraw your foot, shift your weight, move your arms, cry "ouch," and remember the last time you stepped on a tack, all at the same time.

AN INTRODUCTION TO REFLEXES

Conditions inside or outside the body can change rapidly and unexpectedly. **Reflexes** are automatic motor responses, triggered by specific stimuli, that help us preserve homeostasis by making rapid adjustments in the function of our organs or organ systems. Such involuntary responses include the control of heart rate, blood pressure, swallowing, and sneezing. The response shows little variability—when a particular reflex is activated it always produces the same motor response. *Spinal reflexes* are processed within the spinal cord; reflexes processed in the brain are called *cranial reflexes*. Specific examples of these reflexes will be considered in Chapter 9.

The Reflex Arc

The "wiring" of a single reflex is called a **reflex arc**. A reflex arc begins at a receptor and ends at an effector, such as a muscle or gland. Figure 8-12• diagrams the five steps involved in a neural reflex: (1) *arrival of a stimulus and activation of a receptor*, (2) *activation of a sensory neuron*, (3) *information processing*, (4) *activation of a motor neuron*, and (5) *response by an effector* (muscle or gland).

A reflex response usually removes or opposes the original stimulus. In Figure 8-12•, the contracting muscle pulls the hand away from the painful stimulus. This reflex arc is therefore an example of a negative feedback control mechanism. ∞ *p. 14* By opposing potentially harmful changes in the internal or external environment, reflexes play an important role in homeostatic maintenance.

✓ A neurotransmitter causes potassium channels but not sodium channels to open. What effect would this neurotransmitter produce at the postsynaptic membane?

✓ How would synapse function be affected if the uptake of calcium were blocked at the presynaptic membrane of a cholinergic synapse?

✓ What is the minimum number of neurons needed for a reflex arc?

AN INTRODUCTION TO THE ANATOMY OF THE NERVOUS SYSTEM

The basic functioning of the nervous system depends on the action potentials generated at the level of the individual neuron. More complex functions of the nervous system depend on the interactions between neurons in neuronal pools, and the most complex interactions occur in the spinal cord and brain. Neurons and their axons are not randomly scattered in the CNS and PNS. Instead, they form masses or bundles with distinct anatomical boundaries and are identified by specific

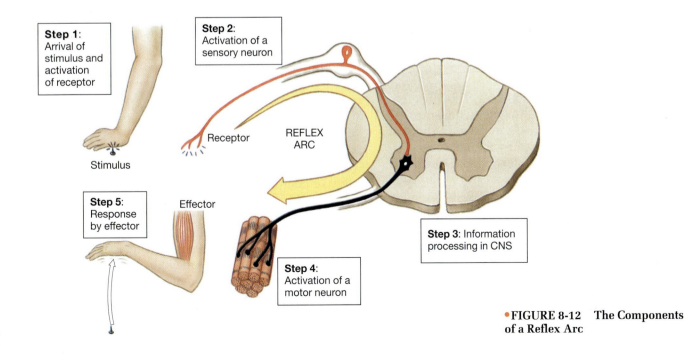

Step 1: Arrival of stimulus and activation of receptor

Step 2: Activation of a sensory neuron

Receptor   REFLEX ARC

Stimulus

Step 5: Response by effector

Effector

Step 3: Information processing in CNS

Step 4: Activation of a motor neuron

•FIGURE 8-12   The Components of a Reflex Arc

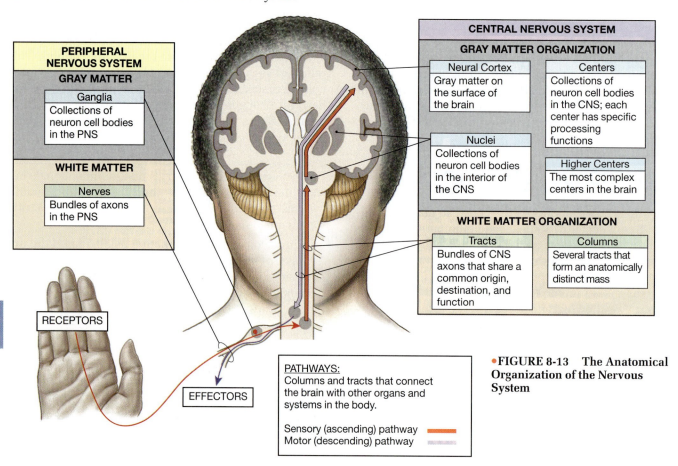

PERIPHERAL NERVOUS SYSTEM

GRAY MATTER

Ganglia
Collections of neuron cell bodies in the PNS

WHITE MATTER

Nerves
Bundles of axons in the PNS

RECEPTORS

EFFECTORS

CENTRAL NERVOUS SYSTEM

GRAY MATTER ORGANIZATION

Neural Cortex
Gray matter on the surface of the brain

Centers
Collections of neuron cell bodies in the CNS; each center has specific processing functions

Nuclei
Collections of neuron cell bodies in the interior of the CNS

Higher Centers
The most complex centers in the brain

WHITE MATTER ORGANIZATION

Tracts
Bundles of CNS axons that share a common origin, destination, and function

Columns
Several tracts that form an anatomically distinct mass

PATHWAYS:
Columns and tracts that connect the brain with other organs and systems in the body.

Sensory (ascending) pathway
Motor (descending) pathway

•FIGURE 8-13   The Anatomical Organization of the Nervous System

terms. We shall use these terms again and again, so a brief overview here will prove helpful.

In the PNS:

- **Ganglia** are groups of neuron cell bodies.
- **Nerves** are bundles of axons, with *spinal nerves* connected to the spinal cord and *cranial nerves* connected to the brain.

In the CNS:

- **Centers** are collections of neuron cell bodies that share a particular function. A center with a discrete anatomical boundary is called a **nucleus**. Portions of the brain surface are covered by a thick blanket of gray matter called **neural cortex** (*cortex*, rind). The term *higher centers* refers to the most complex integration centers, nuclei, and cortical areas in the brain.
- **Tracts** are bundles of axons inside the CNS that share common origins, destinations, and functions. Tracts in the spinal cord form larger groups, called **columns**.
- **Pathways** link the centers of the brain with the rest of the body. For example, **sensory** (*ascending*) **pathways** distribute information from sensory receptors to processing centers in the brain, and **motor** (*descending*) **pathways** begin at motor centers in the

CNS and end at the skeletal muscles they control. These relationships are diagrammed in Figure 8-13•.

The central nervous system consists of the spinal cord and brain. These masses of neural tissue are extremely delicate and must be protected against shocks, infection, and other dangers. In addition to glial cells within the neural tissue, the CNS is protected by a series of covering layers, the *meninges*, and by the special properties of the *blood-brain barrier*.

The Meninges

Neural tissue has a very high metabolic rate and requires abundant nutrients and a constant supply of oxygen. At the same time, the CNS must be isolated from a variety of compounds in the blood that could interfere with its complex operations. Delicate neural tissues must also be defended against damaging contact with the surrounding bones. These diverse needs have resulted in special adaptations for the protection and support of the brain. One such adaptation is provided by a series of specialized membranes, the **meninges** (men-IN-jēz) (Figure 8-14•). Blood vessels branching within these layers also deliver oxygen and nutrients to the CNS. At the foramen magnum of the skull, the meninges

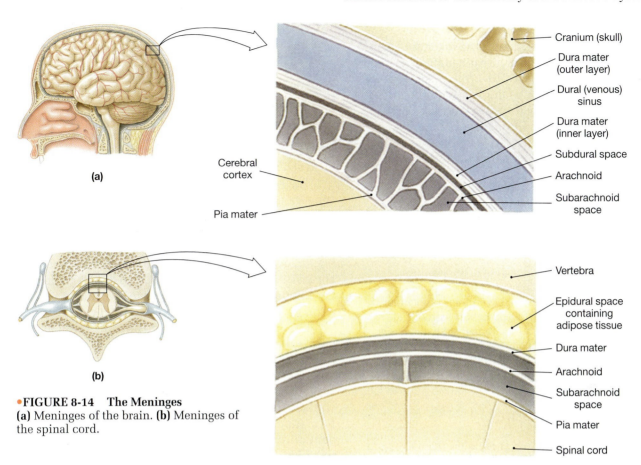

•FIGURE 8-14   The Meninges
(a) Meninges of the brain. **(b)** Meninges of
the spinal cord.

covering the brain are continuous with the meninges
that surround the spinal cord. There are three meningeal
layers: the *dura mater*, the *arachnoid*, and the *pia
mater*. The meninges cover the cranial and spinal nerves
as they penetrate the skull or pass through the intervertebral foramina, becoming continuous with the connective tissues surrounding the peripheral nerves.

The Dura Mater

The tough, fibrous **dura mater** (DOO-ra MĀ-ter; *dura*,
hard + *mater*, mother) forms the outermost covering of
the central nervous system. The dura mater surrounding the brain consists of two fibrous layers, with the
outermost fused to the periosteum of the skull. The
inner and outer layers are separated by a slender gap
that contains tissue fluids and blood vessels, including
the large veins known as *dural sinuses*. At several locations, the innermost layer of the dura mater extends
deep into the cranial cavity, providing additional stabilization and support to the brain.

Between the dura mater of the spinal cord and the
walls of the vertebral canal lies the **epidural space**, which
contains loose connective tissue, blood vessels, and adipose tissue. Injecting an anesthetic into the epidural space
produces a temporary sensory and motor paralysis known
as an *epidural block*. This technique has the advantage of

affecting only the spinal nerves in the immediate area of
the injection. Epidural blocks in the lower lumbar or sacral
regions may be used to control pain during childbirth.

The Arachnoid

A narrow **subdural space** separates the inner surface of
the dura mater from the second meningeal layer, the
arachnoid (a-RAK-noyd; *arachne*, spider). This intervening space contains a small quantity of lymphatic
fluid, which reduces friction between the opposing surfaces. The arachnoid is a layer of squamous cells; deep
to this epithelial layer lies the **subarachnoid space**,
which contains a delicate web of collagen and elastic
fibers. The subarachnoid space is filled with *cerebrospinal fluid*, which acts as a shock absorber and
transports dissolved gases, nutrients, chemical messengers, and waste products.

BURR HOLES

Bleeding in the epidural space, called an *epidural
hematoma,* usually results from laceration of an artery during
blunt head trauma. This causes rapid swelling and compression of the brain. Lifesaving emergency treatment may require drilling *burr holes* through the skull over the hematoma
to relieve the pressure. Although burr holes are usually performed by neurosurgeons, the emergency physician may
have to place them if a neurosurgeon is unavailable.

The Pia Mater

The subarachnoid space separates the arachnoid from the innermost meningeal layer, the **pia mater** (*pia*, delicate + *mater*, mother). Unlike more superficial meninges, the pia mater is bound firmly to the underlying neural tissue. The blood vessels servicing the brain and spinal cord are found in this layer. The pia mater of the brain is highly vascular, and large vessels branch over the surface of the brain, supplying the superficial areas of neural cortex. This extensive circulatory supply is extremely important, for the brain has a very high rate of metabolism; at rest, the 1.4 kg (3.1 lb) brain uses as much oxygen as 28 kg (61.6 lb) of skeletal muscle.

✴ MENINGITIS

Meningitis is an inflammation of the meninges. Usually caused by a bacterial or viral infection, meningitis can be life threatening. Signs and symptoms of meningitis include headache, fever, stiff neck, light sensitivity, altered mental status, and seizures. To make the diagnosis, spinal fluid is withdrawn in a procedure called *lumbar puncture*. Permanent disability or death can result if appropriate treatment is not promptly administered.

The Blood-Brain Barrier

The neural tissue in the CNS is isolated from the general circulation by the **blood-brain barrier**. This barrier is maintained by astrocytes, whose secretions cause the capillaries of the CNS to become impermeable to many compounds. In general, only lipid-soluble compounds can diffuse into the interstitial fluid of the brain and spinal cord. Water-soluble compounds cannot cross the endothelial lining without the assistance of specific carriers. For example, there are separate transport systems for glucose, large amino acids, and glycine (the smallest amino acid). Most of the transport mechanisms of the blood-brain barrier involve facilitated diffusion and so occur down concentration gradients. ∞ *p. 62*

We will now take a closer look at the organization of the central nervous system. Here we will examine the relatively simple structure of the spinal cord and then proceed to the brain. Chapter 9 will examine the peripheral nervous system and the ways the CNS and PNS interact to control body functions.

THE SPINAL CORD

The spinal cord serves as the major highway for the passage of sensory impulses to the brain and motor impulses from the brain. In addition, the spinal cord integrates information on its own and controls spinal reflexes, ranging from withdrawal from pain (Figure 8-12•, p. 227) to complex reflex patterns involved with sitting, standing, walking, and running.

Gross Anatomy

The spinal cord, detailed in Figure 8-15•, is approximately 45 cm (18 in.) long. It has a **central canal**, a narrow internal passageway filled with cerebrospinal fluid. The posterior surface of the spinal cord has a shallow groove, the *posterior median sulcus*, and the anterior surface has a deeper crease, the *anterior median fissure*. With two exceptions, the diameter of the cord decreases in size as it extends toward the sacral region.

The two exceptions are regions concerned with the sensory and motor control of the limbs. The *cervical enlargement* supplies nerves to the shoulder girdle and upper limbs, and the *lumbar enlargement* provides innervation to the pelvis and lower limbs. Below the lumbar enlargement, the spinal cord becomes tapered and conical. A slender strand of fibrous tissue extends from the inferior tip of the spinal cord to the coccyx, serving as an anchor that prevents superior movement.

The entire spinal cord consists of 31 segments, each identified by a letter and number designation. Every spinal segment is associated with a pair of **dorsal root ganglia**, which contain the cell bodies of sensory neurons (Figure 8-15b•). The **dorsal roots**, which contain the axons of these neurons, bring sensory information to the spinal cord. A pair of **ventral roots** contain the axons of CNS motor neurons that control muscles and glands. On either side, the dorsal and ventral roots from each segment leave the vertebral column between adjacent vertebrae at the *intervertebral foramen*.

Distal to each dorsal root ganglion, the sensory (dorsal) and motor (ventral) roots are bound together into a single *spinal nerve*. All spinal nerves are classified as *mixed nerves*, because they contain both sensory and motor fibers. The spinal nerves on either side form outside the vertebral canal, where the ventral and dorsal roots unite, so that the dorsal root ganglion lies between the pedicles of succeeding vertebra. (You may wish to review the description of vertebral anatomy in Chapter 6.) ∞ *p. 138*

The adult spinal cord extends only to the level of the first or second lumbar vertebrae. When seen in gross dissection, the long ventral and dorsal roots inferior to the tip of the spinal cord reminded early anatomists of a horse's tail. With that in mind, they called this complex of nerve roots the *cauda equina* (KAW-da ek-WĪ-na; *cauda*, tail + *equus*, horse).

Sectional Anatomy

The anterior median fissure and the posterior median sulcus mark the division between left and right sides of the spinal cord (Figure 8-15b•). The *gray matter* is dominated by the cell bodies of neurons and glial cells. It forms a rough H, or butterfly shape, around the narrow

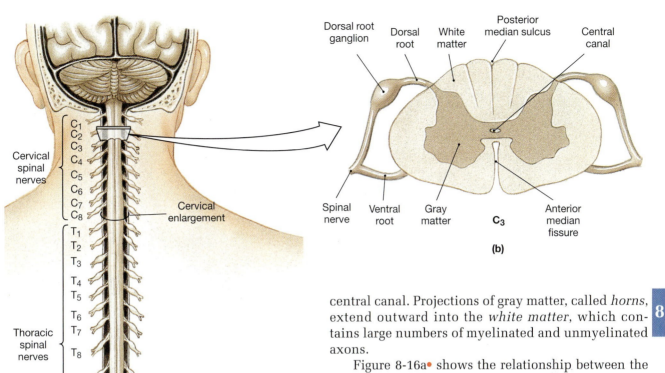

(b)

central canal. Projections of gray matter, called *horns*, extend outward into the *white matter*, which contains large numbers of myelinated and unmyelinated axons.

Figure 8-16a• shows the relationship between the function of a particular nucleus (sensory or motor) and its relative position within the gray matter of the spinal cord. The *posterior gray horns* contain sensory nuclei, whereas the *anterior gray horns* deal with the motor control of skeletal muscles. Nuclei in the *lateral gray horns* contain the visceral motor neurons that control smooth muscle, cardiac muscle, and glands. The *gray commissures* above and below the central canal interconnect the horns on either side of the spinal cord.

The white matter can be divided into a half-dozen regions, or *columns* (Figure 8-16b•). The *posterior white columns* extend between the posterior gray horns and the posterior median sulcus. The *anterior white columns* lie between the anterior gray horns and the anterior median fissure; they are interconnected by the *anterior white commissure*. The white matter between the anterior and posterior columns makes up the *lateral white columns*.

Each column contains tracts whose axons carry either sensory data or motor commands. Small tracts carry sensory or motor signals between segments of the spinal cord, and larger tracts connect the spinal cord with the brain. **Ascending tracts** carry sensory information toward the brain, and **descending tracts** convey motor commands into the spinal cord.

Injuries affecting the spinal cord or cauda equina produce symptoms of sensory loss or motor paralysis that reflect the specific nuclei, tracts, or spinal nerves involved. A general paralysis can result from severe damage to the spinal cord in an auto crash or other accident, and the damaged tracts seldom undergo even partial repairs. Extensive damage at the fourth or fifth cervical vertebra will eliminate sensation and motor control of the upper and lower limbs. The extensive

•**FIGURE 8-15   Gross Anatomy of the Spinal Cord**
(a) The superficial anatomy and orientation of the adult spinal cord. The numbers to the left identify the spinal nerves. **(b)** A cross section through the cervical region of the spinal cord, showing the arrangement of gray matter and white matter.

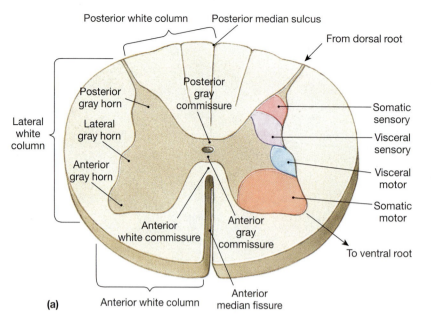

Posterior white column   Posterior median sulcus
From dorsal root
Posterior gray horn
Posterior gray commissure
Lateral gray horn
Lateral white column
Anterior gray horn
Somatic sensory
Visceral sensory
Visceral motor
Somatic motor
Anterior white commissure
Anterior gray commissure
To ventral root
Anterior white column
Anterior median fissure

(a)

•FIGURE 8-16   Sectional Anatomy of the Spinal Cord (a) The left half of this sectional view shows important anatomical landmarks and the major regions of white matter and gray matter. The right half indicates the functional organization of the gray matter in the anterior, lateral, and posterior gray horns. (b) A micrograph of a section through the spinal cord, showing major landmarks. Compare with (a).

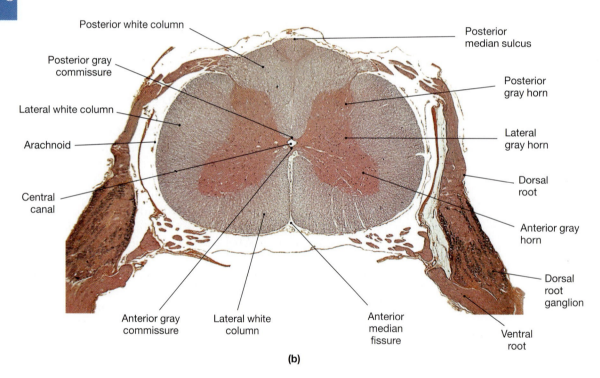

Posterior white column
Posterior median sulcus
Posterior gray commissure
Posterior gray horn
Lateral white column
Lateral gray horn
Arachnoid
Dorsal root
Central canal
Anterior gray horn
Dorsal root ganglion
Anterior gray commissure
Lateral white column
Anterior median fissure
Ventral root

(b)

paralysis produced is called *quadriplegia. Paraplegia,* the loss of motor control of the lower limbs, may follow damage to the thoracic vertebrae.

✓ Damage to which root of a spinal nerve would interfere with motor function?

✓ A man with polio has lost the use of his leg muscles. In what area of the spinal cord would you expect to locate his virus-infected motor neurons?

✓ Why are spinal nerves also called mixed nerves?

THE BRAIN

The brain is far larger and more complex than the spinal cord, and its responses to stimuli are more versatile. It contains roughly 35 billion neurons organized into hundreds of neuronal pools; it has a complex three-dimensional structure and performs a bewildering array of functions. All of our dreams, passions, plans, and memories are the result of brain activity.

The adult human brain contains almost 98 percent of the neural tissue in the body. A representative adult brain weighs 1.4 kg (3 lb) and has a volume of 1200 cc (71 in.^{3}). There is considerable individual variation, and the brains of males are generally about 10 percent larger than those of females, because of differences in average body size. There is no correlation between brain size intelligence, and people with either the smallest (750 cc) or largest (2100 cc) brains are functionally normal.

Major Divisions of the Brain

The adult brain has six major regions: (1) the *cerebrum*, (2) the *diencephalon*, (3) the *midbrain*, (4) the *pons*, (5) the *medulla oblongata*, and (6) the *cerebellum*. Major landmarks are indicated in Figure 8-17●.

Viewed from the superior surface, the **cerebrum** (SER-e-brum or se-RĒ-brum) can be divided into large,

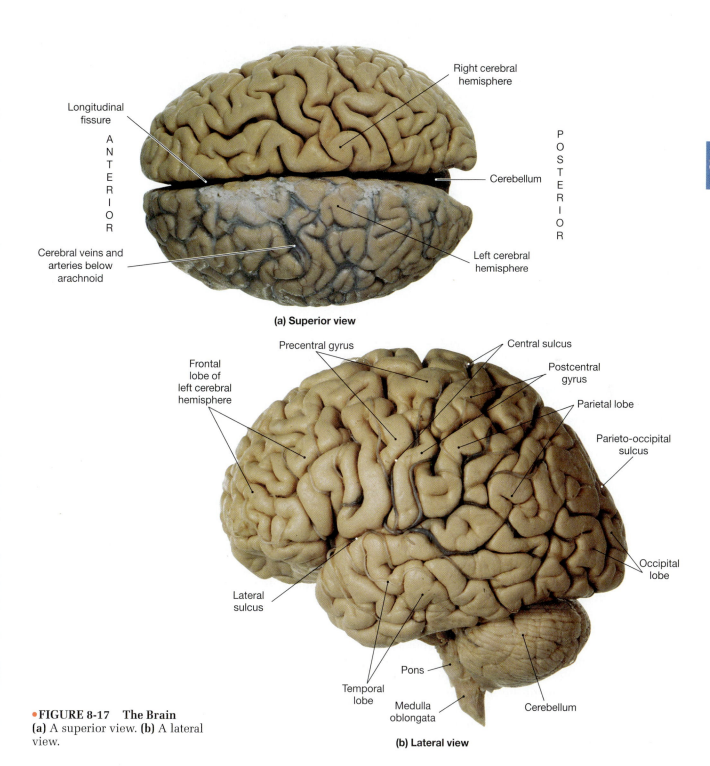

(a) Superior view

(b) Lateral view

●**FIGURE 8-17   The Brain**
(a) A superior view. **(b)** A lateral view.

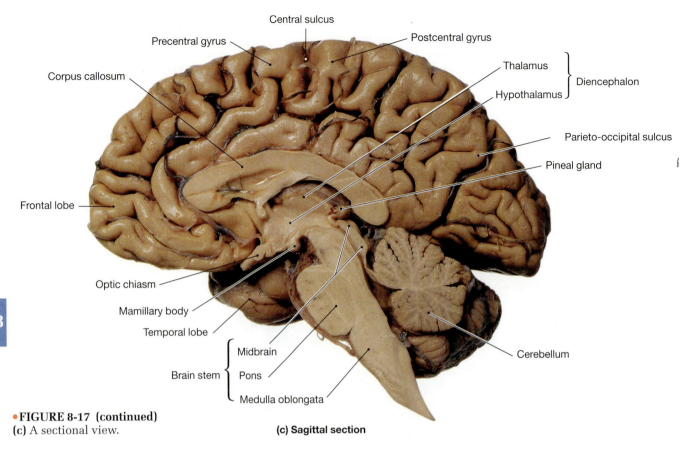

Central sulcus

Precentral gyrus

Postcentral gyrus

Corpus callosum

Thalamus

Diencephalon

Hypothalamus

Parieto-occipital sulcus

Pineal gland

Frontal lobe

Optic chiasm

Mamillary body

Temporal lobe

Brain stem { Midbrain
Pons
Medulla oblongata

Cerebellum

8

• **FIGURE 8-17 (continued)**
(c) A sectional view.

(c) Sagittal section

paired **cerebral hemispheres**. Conscious thought processes, sensations, intellectual functions, memory storage and retrieval, and complex motor patterns originate in the cerebral hemispheres. The hollow **diencephalon** (dī-en-SEF-a-lon; *dia-*, through + *cephalo*, head) is connected to the cerebrum. Its sides form the **thalamus**, which contains relay and processing centers for sensory information. A narrow stalk connects the **hypothalamus** (*hypo-*, below), or floor of the diencephalon, to the *pituitary gland*. The hypothalamus contains centers involved with emotions, autonomic function, and hormone production. The pituitary gland, the primary link between the nervous and endocrine systems, is discussed in Chapter 11.

The midbrain, pons, and medulla oblongata form the **brain stem**. The brain stem contains important processing centers and relay stations for information headed to or from the cerebrum or cerebellum. Nuclei in the **midbrain**, or *mesencephalon* (mez-en-SEF-a-lon; *meso-*, middle), process visual and auditory information and generate involuntary motor responses. This region also contains centers involved with the maintenance of consciousness. The term **pons** refers to a bridge, and the pons of the brain connects the cerebellum to the brain stem. In addition to tracts and relay centers, this region of the brain also contains nuclei involved with somatic and visceral motor control. The pons is also connected to the **medulla**

oblongata, the segment of the brain that is attached to the spinal cord. The medulla oblongata relays sensory information to the thalamus and other brain stem centers; it also contains major centers for the regulation of autonomic function, such as heart rate, blood pressure, respiration, and digestive activities.

The large cerebral hemispheres and the smaller hemispheres of the **cerebellum** (ser-e-BEL-um) almost completely cover the brain stem. The cerebellum adjusts voluntary and involuntary motor activities on the basis of sensory information and stored memories of previous movements.

✓ Describe one major function of each of the six regions of the brain.

✓ The pituitary gland links the nervous and endocrine systems. To which portion of the diencephalon is it attached?

The Ventricles of the Brain

Like the spinal cord, the brain is hollow; it contains internal cavities filled with cerebrospinal fluid. The brain has a central passageway that expands to form four chambers, called **ventricles** (VEN-tri-kls) (Figure 8-18•). The largest of these, the two lateral ventri-

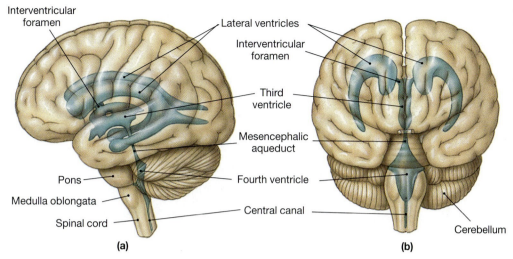

Interventricular foramen

Lateral ventricles

Interventricular foramen

Third ventricle

Mesencephalic aqueduct

Pons

Fourth ventricle

Medulla oblongata

Central canal

Spinal cord

Cerebellum

(a)

(b)

•FIGURE 8-18 **The Ventricles of the Brain** (a) The orientation and extent of the ventricles as seen through a transparent brain in lateral view. (b) An anterior view of the ventricles, showing the relationships between the lateral ventricles and the third ventricle.

cles, are located in each cerebral hemisphere. There is no direct connection between the lateral ventricles, but an opening, the *interventricular foramen*, allows each of them to communicate with the **third ventricle** of the diencephalon. Instead of a ventricle, the midbrain has a slender canal known as the *mesencephalic aqueduct* (*cerebral aqueduct*), which connects the third ventricle with the **fourth ventricle** of the pons and upper portion of the medulla oblongata. Within the medulla oblongata the fourth ventricle narrows and becomes continuous with the central canal of the spinal cord.

Cerebrospinal Fluid

Cerebrospinal fluid, or **CSF**, provides cushioning for delicate neural structures. It also provides support, because the brain essentially floats in the cerebrospinal fluid. A human brain weighs about 1400 g (3.1 lb) in air, but only about 50 g (1.76 oz.) when supported by the cerebrospinal fluid. Finally, the CSF transports nutrients, chemical messengers, and waste products. Except at the *choroid plexus*, the ependymal lining is freely permeable, and the CSF is in constant chemical communication with the interstitial fluid of the CNS.

Cerebrospinal fluid is produced at the **choroid plexus** (*choroid*, a vascular coat + *plexus*, a network), a vascular network that extends into each of the four ventricles (Figure 8-19a•). The capillaries of the choroid plexus are covered by large ependymal cells that secrete cerebrospinal fluid at a rate of about 500 ml/day. The total volume of CSF at any given moment is approximately 150 ml; this means that the entire volume of CSF is replaced roughly every 8 hours. Despite this rapid turnover, the composition of CSF is closely regulated, and the rate of removal normally keeps pace with the rate of production. If it does not, a variety of clinical problems may appear.

Figure 8-19• diagrams the circulation of cerebrospinal fluid. CSF forms at the choroid plexus and circulates between the different ventricles, passes along the central canal, and enters the subarachnoid space. Once inside the subarachnoid space, the CSF circulates around the spinal cord and cauda equina and across the surfaces of the brain. Between the cerebral hemispheres, slender extensions of the arachnoid penetrate the inner layer of the dura mater. These **arachnoid granulations** (Figure 8-19b•) project into the *superior sagittal sinus*, a large cerebral vein. Diffusion across the arachnoid granulations returns excess cerebrospinal fluid to the venous circulation.

Because free exchange occurs between the interstitial fluid and CSF, changes in CNS function may produce changes in the composition of the CSF. Samples of the CSF can be obtained through a *lumbar puncture*, or *spinal tap*, providing useful clinical information concerning CNS injury, infection, or disease.

The Cerebrum

The cerebrum, the largest region of the brain, is the site where conscious thought and intellectual functions originate. Much of the cerebrum is involved in receiving somatic sensory information and then exerting voluntary or involuntary control over somatic motor neurons. In general, we are aware of these events. However, most sensory processing and all visceral motor (autonomic) control occur elsewhere in the brain, usually outside our conscious awareness.

The cerebrum includes gray matter and white matter. Gray matter is found in a superficial layer of neural cortex and in deeper *cerebral nuclei*. The *central white matter*, composed of myelinated axons, lies beneath the neural cortex and surrounds the cerebral nuclei.

8

Extension of choroid plexus into right lateral ventricle

Arachnoid granulations

Choroid plexus of third ventricle

Mesencephalic aqueduct

Choroid plexus of fourth ventricle

Arachnoid

Subarachnoid space

Spinal cord

Dura mater

Central canal

• FIGURE 8-19   The Circulation of Cerebrospinal Fluid
(a) A sagittal section indicating the routes of formation and circulation of cerebrospinal fluid.
(b) The orientation of the arachnoid granulations.

(a)

Dura mater (outer layer)   Cranium   Endothelial lining

Fluid movement

Superior sagittal sinus

Arachnoid granulation

Dura mater (inner layer)

Subdural space

Cerebral cortex   Subarachnoid space   Arachnoid

Pia mater

Superior sagittal sinus

(b)

and 8-20•). Extending laterally from the longitudinal fissure is a deep groove, the **central sulcus**. Anterior to this is the **frontal lobe**, bordered inferiorly by the **lateral sulcus**. The cortex inferior to the lateral sulcus is the **temporal lobe**, which overlaps the **insula** (IN-su-la), an "island" of cortex that is otherwise hidden. The **parietal lobe** extends between the central sulcus and the **parieto-occipital sulcus**. What remains is the **occipital lobe**.

In each lobe, some regions are concerned with sensory information and others with motor commands. Each cerebral hemisphere is connected to the opposite side of the body. For example, the left cerebral hemisphere controls the right side of the body, and the right cerebral hemisphere controls the left side.

Motor and Sensory Areas of the Cortex

Figure 8-20• details the major motor and sensory regions of the cerebral cortex. The central sulcus separates the motor and sensory portions of the cortex. The **precentral gyrus** of the frontal lobe forms the anterior margin of the central sulcus, and its surface is the **primary motor cortex**. Neurons of the primary motor cortex direct voluntary movements by controlling somatic motor neurons in the brain stem and spinal cord.

The **postcentral gyrus** of the parietal lobe forms the posterior margin of the central sulcus, and its surface contains the **primary sensory cortex**. Neurons in this region receive somatic sensory information from touch, pressure, pain, and temperature receptors. We are consciously aware of these sensations because the brain stem nuclei relay sensory information to the primary sensory cortex.

Sensory information concerning sensations of sight, taste, sound, and smell arrive at other portions of the

Structure of the Cerebral Hemispheres

Figure 8-20• presents a diagrammatic superficial view of the cerebrum. A thick blanket of neural cortex known as the **cerebral cortex** covers the paired *cerebral hemispheres*, which form the superior surface of the cerebrum. This outer surface forms a series of elevated ridges, or **gyri** (JĪ-rī), separated by shallow depressions, called **sulci** (SUL-sī), or deeper grooves, called **fissures**. Gyri increase the surface area of the cerebral hemispheres and the number of neurons in the cortex.

The two cerebral hemispheres are separated by a deep **longitudinal fissure**. Each hemisphere can be divided into well-defined regions, or **lobes**, named after the overlying bones of the skull (Figures 8-17, pp. 233–234,

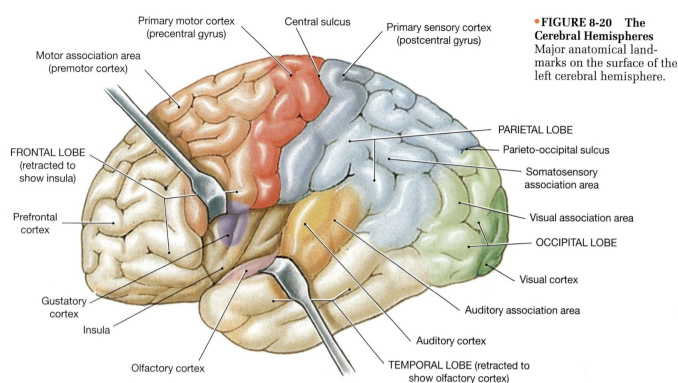

Motor association area
(premotor cortex)

Primary motor cortex
(precentral gyrus)

Central sulcus

Primary sensory cortex
(postcentral gyrus)

FRONTAL LOBE
(retracted to
show insula)

Prefrontal
cortex

Gustatory
cortex

Insula

Olfactory cortex

PARIETAL LOBE

Parieto-occipital sulcus

Somatosensory
association area

Visual association area

OCCIPITAL LOBE

Visual cortex

Auditory association area

Auditory cortex

TEMPORAL LOBE (retracted to
show olfactory cortex)

•FIGURE 8-20   The
Cerebral Hemispheres
Major anatomical land-
marks on the surface of the
left cerebral hemisphere.

8

cerebral cortex. The **visual cortex** of the occipital lobe receives visual information, the **gustatory cortex** of the frontal lobe receives taste sensations, and the **auditory cortex** and **olfactory cortex** of the temporal lobe receive information about hearing and smell, respectively.

Association Areas

The sensory and motor regions of the cortex are connected to nearby **association areas**, regions that interpret incoming data or coordinate a motor response. For example, the **premotor cortex**, or *motor association area*, is responsible for coordinating learned movements, such as the eye movements involved in following the lines on this page. The functional distinctions between the motor and sensory association areas are most evident after localized brain damage has occurred. For example, someone with damage to the premotor cortex might understand written letters and words but be unable to read owing to an inability to track along the lines on a printed page. In contrast, someone with a damaged **visual association area** can scan the lines of a printed page but cannot figure out what the letters mean.

Cortical Connections

The various regions of the cerebral cortex are interconnected by the white matter that lies beneath the cerebral cortex. This white matter interconnects areas within a single cerebral hemisphere and links the two hemispheres across the **corpus callosum** (Figure 8-17c•, p. 234). Other bundles of axons link the cerebral cortex

with the diencephalon, brain stem, cerebellum, and spinal cord.

Cerebral Processing Centers

There are also "higher-order" integrative centers that receive information through axons from many different association areas. These regions, shown in Figure 8-21•, control extremely complex motor activities and perform complicated analytical functions. They may be found in the lobes and cortical areas of both cerebral hemispheres, or they may be restricted to either the left or the right side.

The General Interpretive Area. The *general interpretive area* receives information from all the sensory association areas. This center is present in only one hemisphere, usually the left. Damage to this area affects the ability to interpret what is read or heard, even though the words are understood as individual entities. For example, an individual might understand the meaning of the words "sit" and "here" but be totally bewildered by the instruction "Sit here."

The Speech Center. The general interpretive area is connected to the *speech center* (*Broca's area*), which lies along the edge of the premotor cortex in the same hemisphere as the general interpretive area. The speech center regulates the patterns of breathing and vocalization needed for normal speech. The corresponding regions on the opposite hemisphere are not inactive, but their functions are less well defined. Damage to the speech

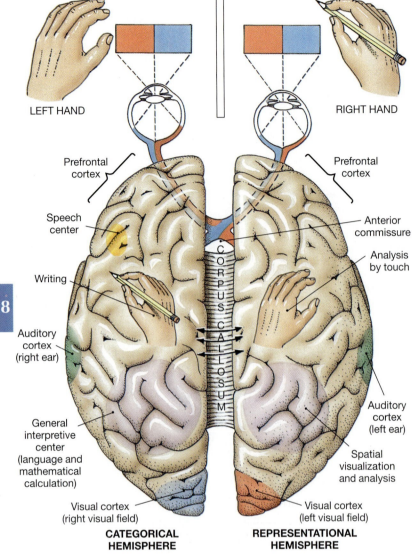

LEFT HAND

RIGHT HAND

Prefrontal cortex

Prefrontal cortex

Speech center

Anterior commissure

Writing

Analysis by touch

8

Auditory cortex (right ear)

General interpretive center (language and mathematical calculation)

Auditory cortex (left ear)

Spatial visualization and analysis

Visual cortex (right visual field)

Visual cortex (left visual field)

CATEGORICAL HEMISPHERE

REPRESENTATIONAL HEMISPHERE

CORPUS CALLOSUM

•FIGURE 8-21   Hemispheric Specialization
Functional differences between the left and right cerebral hemispheres.

center can manifest itself in various ways. Some people have difficulty speaking even when they know exactly what words to use; others talk constantly but use all the wrong words.

The Prefrontal Cortex. The **prefrontal cortex** of the frontal lobe coordinates information from the secondary and special association areas of the entire cortex. In doing so, it performs such abstract intellectual functions as predicting the future consequences of events or actions. The prefrontal cortex also has connections with other portions of the brain, such as the limbic system, discussed later. Feelings of frustration, tension, and anxiety are generated at the prefrontal cortex as it interprets ongoing events and predicts future situations or consequences. If the connections between the prefrontal cortex and other brain regions are severed, the tensions, frustrations, and anxieties are removed. Early

in the 1900s this rather drastic procedure, called a *prefrontal lobotomy*, was used to "cure" a variety of mental illnesses, especially those associated with violent or antisocial behavior.

✳ BRAIN ATTACK

A *brain attack* is death or injury of brain tissue due to deprivation of oxygen. Also called *stroke* or *cerebrovascular accident (CVA),* brain attack is caused by blockage of an artery that supplies blood to a part of the brain or by hemorrhage from a ruptured blood vessel in the brain. A stroke caused by blockage is an *ischemic stroke* and occurs when a blood clot from another part of the body occludes a cerebral artery (*embolic stroke*). Alternatively, ischemic stroke can occur when the blockage forms within the cerebral artery itself.

A brain attack caused by bleeding is termed a *hemorrhagic stroke* and is often due to long-standing, poorly controlled high blood pressure. It can also occur when an *aneurysm,* a weak area within one of the cerebral arteries, ruptures.

The signs and symptoms of brain attack can vary based upon the amount of brain tissue affected. They include one-sided weakness or numbness, altered mental status, difficulty speaking (*aphasia*), and others. Early treatment with "clot-busting" drugs can oftentimes reduce the severity of a stroke.

Memory

What was the topic of the last sentence you read? What do your parents look like? What is your Social Security number? What does a red traffic light mean? What does a hot dog taste like? Answering these questions involves accessing *memories,* stored bits of information gathered through prior experience. **Fact memories** are specific bits of information, such as the color of a stop sign or the smell of a certain perfume. **Skill memories** are learned motor behaviors. For example, you can probably remember how to light a match or open a screw-top jar. With repetition, skill memories become incorporated at the unconscious level. Examples would include the complex motor patterns involved in skiing, playing the violin, and similar activities. Skill memories related to programmed behaviors, such as eating, are stored in appropriate portions of the brain stem. Complex skill memories involve an interplay between the cerebullum and the cerebral cortex.

Two classes of memories exist. **Short-term memories**, or *primary memories*, do not last long, but while they persist, the information can be recalled immediately. Primary memories contain small bits of information, such as a person's name or a telephone number. Repeating a phone number or other bit of information reinforces the original short-term memory and helps ensure its conversion to a long-term memory. **Long-term memories** remain for much longer periods, in some cases for an entire lifetime. Some long-term memories fade with time and may require considerable effort to recall. Other long-term memories seem to be part of consciousness, such as your name or the contours of your own body.

The conversion from short-term to long-term memory is called *memory consolidation*. Although much remains to be learned about this process, it is clear that anatomical and physiological changes occur at the cellular level. For example, the rates of neurotransmitter production and release in the stimulated neurons. Efficient conversion from short-term to long-term memory storage takes time, usually at least an hour and often longer. Whether or not that conversion occurs depends on several factors, including the nature, intensity, and frequency of the original stimulus. Very strong, repeated, or exceedingly pleasant (or unpleasant) events are excellent candidates for conversion to long-term memories. Drugs that stimulate the CNS, such as caffeine and nicotine, may enhance memory consolidation.

Most long-term memories are stored in the cerebral cortex. Conscious motor and sensory memories are referred to the appropriate association areas. For example, visual memories are stored in the visual association area, and memories of voluntary motor activity are kept in the premotor cortex. Special portions of the occipital and temporal lobes retain the memories of faces, voices, and words. In at least some cases, a specific memory probably reflects the activity of a single neuron. For example, in one portion of the temporal lobe an individual neuron responds to the sound of one word and ignores others.

Amnesia refers to the loss of memory from disease or trauma. The type of memory loss depends on the specific regions of the brain affected. For example, damage to the auditory association areas may make it difficult to remember sounds. Damage to thalamic and limbic structures, especially the *hippocampus*, will affect memory storage and consolidation.

Hemispheric Specialization

Although the two hemispheres are very similar in appearance, there are significant functional differences between them. The assignment of a specific function to a region of the cerebral cortex is not always straightforward. Not only can one region have several different functions, but also some aspects of cortical function, such as consciousness, cannot easily be assigned to any single region.

Figure 8-21• indicates the major functional differences between the hemispheres. Higher-order centers in the left and right hemispheres have different but complementary functions. In most people, the left hemisphere contains the general interpretive and speech centers, and this is the hemisphere responsible for reading, writing, and speaking. The left hemisphere is also important in performing analytical tasks, such as mathematical calculations and logical decision making. Although the left hemisphere was formerly called the *dominant hemisphere*, a more appropriate term is the *categorical hemisphere*, because the right hemisphere also has many important functions.

The right cerebral hemisphere analyzes sensory information and relates the body to the sensory environment. Interpretive centers in this hemisphere permit the identification of familiar objects by touch, smell, taste, or feel. Because it deals with spatial relationships and analyses, the term *representational hemisphere* is used to refer to the right hemisphere. Interestingly, there may be a link between handedness and sensory/spatial abilities. An unusually high percentage of musicians and artists are left-handed; the complex motor activities performed by these individuals are directed by the primary motor cortex and association areas on the right hemisphere.

Hemispheric specialization does not mean that the two hemispheres function independently of each other. As noted above, the white fibers of the corpus callosum link the two hemispheres, including their sensory information and motor commands. The corpus callosum alone contains over 200 million axons, carrying an estimated 4 billion impulses per second!

The Electroencephalogram

The specific areas just described were mapped by direct stimulation in patients undergoing brain surgery. Noninvasive methods are also used to correlate the activity of different cortical regions with function. One of the most common noninvasive methods involves monitoring the electrical activity of the brain.

Neural function depends on electrical events within the cell membrane. The brain contains billions of nerve cells, and their activity generates an electrical field that can be measured by placing electrodes on the brain or the outer surface of the skull. The electrical activity changes constantly as nuclei and cortical areas are stimulated or quiet down. An **electroencephalogram (EEG)** is a printed record of this electrical activity over time. The electrical patterns are called **brain waves**, and these can be correlated with the individual's level of consciousness. Electroencephalograms can also provide useful diagnostic information regarding brain disorders. Four types of brain wave patterns are shown in Figure 8-22•.

The Cerebral Nuclei

The **cerebral nuclei** are masses of gray matter that lie beneath the lateral ventricles and within the central white matter of each cerebral hemisphere as diagrammed in

(a) Alpha waves	Alpha waves are characteristic of normal resting adults 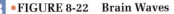
(b) Beta waves	Beta waves typically accompany intense concentration
(c) Theta waves	Theta waves are seen in children and in frustrated adults
(d) Delta waves	Delta waves occur in deep sleep and in certain pathological states

1 sec

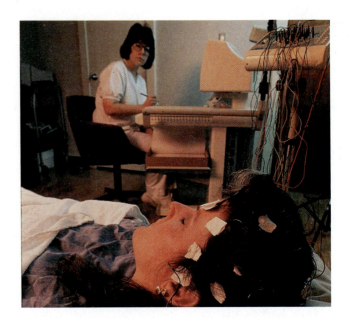

8 •**FIGURE 8-22**   **Brain Waves**

Figure 8-23a•. The **caudate nucleus** has a massive head and slender, curving tail that follows the curve of the lateral ventricle (Figure 8-23b•). Inferior to the head of the caudate nucleus is the **lentiform** (*lens-shaped*) **nucleus**, which consists of a **global pallidus** (GLŌ-bus PAL-i-dus; pale globe) and **putamen** (pū-TĀ-men). Together, the caudate and lentiform nuclei are also called the *corpus striatum* (striated body). Inferior to the caudate and lentiform nuclei is another nucleus, the **amygdaloid** (ah-MIG-da-loyd; *amygdale*, almond) **body**. It is a component of the *limbic system* and is discussed in the next section.

By inhibiting excessive movement, the cerebral nuclei play an important roll in the involuntary control of skeletal muscle tone and the coordination of learned movement patterns. These nuclei do not start a movement—that decision is a voluntary one—but once a movement is under way, the cerebral nuclei provide pattern and rhythm. For example, during a simple walk the cerebral nuclei control the cycles of arm and thigh movements that occur between the time the decision is made to "start walking" and the time the "stop" order is given.

✳ SEIZURES

An alteration in the electrical activity of the brain is called a *seizure*. A seizure is not a disease itself, but rather a sign of some underlying problem. Seizures can vary significantly depending on the part of the brain affected. They may be as minor as a brief period of unresponsiveness *(petit mal seizure)* to generalized tonic-clonic contraction of the skeletal muscles *(grand mal seizure)*. The causes of seizures include drug or alcohol use, brain tumor, congenital brain defects, infection, trauma, or problems with the body's chemistry. In many cases, the cause cannot be determined *(idiopathic)*. Most seizure disorders can be controlled with medication allowing the patients to live normal lives.

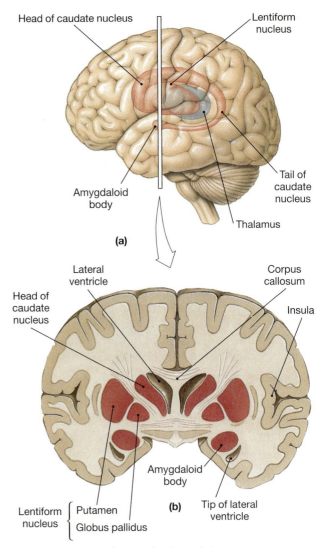

•**FIGURE 8-23**   **The Cerebral Nuclei**
(a) The relative positions of the cerebral nuclei in the intact brain. **(b)** The cerebral nuclei in frontal section.

The Limbic System

The **limbic system** (LIM-bik; *limbus*, a border), shown in Figure 8-24•, includes the olfactory cortex, several cerebral nuclei, gyri, and tracts along the border between the cerebrum and diencephalon. This system is a functional grouping rather than an anatomical one. The functions of the limbic system include (1) establishing emotional states and related behavioral drives; (2) linking the conscious, intellectual functions of the cerebral cortex with the unconscious, autonomic functions of the brain stem; and (3) long-term memory storage and retrieval. The amygdaloid bodies and the hippocampus, for example, play a vital role in learning and in the storage of long-term memories. Damage to the hippocampus that occurs in Alzheimer's disease interferes with memory storage and retrieval.

The limbic system also includes hypothalamic centers that control (1) emotional states, such as rage, fear, and sexual arousal, and (2) reflex movements that can be consciously activated. For example, the limbic system includes the *mamillary bodies* (MAM-i-lar-ē; *mamilla*, or *mammilla*, a little breast) of the hypothalamus. These nuclei control reflex movements associated with eating, such as chewing, licking, and swallowing.

✓ How would decreased diffusion across the arachnoid granulations affect the volume of cerebrospinal fluid in the ventricles?

✓ Mary suffers a head injury that damages her primary motor cortex. Where is this area located?

✓ What senses would be affected by damage to the temporal lobes of the cerebrum?

The Diencephalon

The diencephalon (Figure 8-25•) provides switching and relay centers that integrate the conscious and unconscious sensory and motor pathways. The diencephalon contains the *third ventricle*, a central chamber filled with cerebrospinal fluid. The diencephalic roof contains (1) an extensive area of *choroid plexus* and (2) the *pineal gland*, an endocrine structure that secretes the hormone *melatonin*. Among other functions, melatonin is important in regulating day-night cycles.

The Thalamus

The thalamus (Figure 8-25•) is the final relay point for all ascending sensory information, other than olfactory, that will reach our conscious awareness. It acts as a filter, passing on to the primary sensory cortex only a small

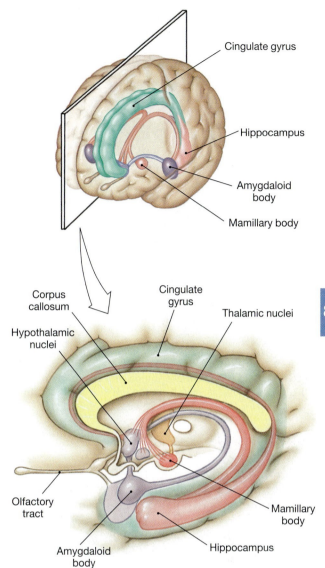

Cingulate gyrus

Hippocampus

Amygdaloid body

Mamillary body

Corpus callosum

Cingulate gyrus

Hypothalamic nuclei

Thalamic nuclei

Olfactory tract

Mamillary body

Amygdaloid body

Hippocampus

8

•**FIGURE 8-24 The Limbic System**
A three-dimensional reconstruction of the limbic system, showing the relationships among the system's major components.

portion of the arriving sensory information. The rest is relayed to the cerebral nuclei and centers in the brain stem. The thalamus also plays a role in the coordination of voluntary and involuntary motor commands.

The Hypothalamus

The hypothalamus (1) contains centers associated with the emotions of rage, pleasure, pain, thirst, hunger, and sexual arousal; (2) adjusts and coordinates the activities of autonomic centers in the pons and medulla oblongata; (3) coordinates neural and endocrine activities; (4) produces a variety of hormones, including *antidiuretic hormone (ADH)* and *oxytocin*; (5) coordinates voluntary and autonomic functions; and (6) maintains normal body temperature.

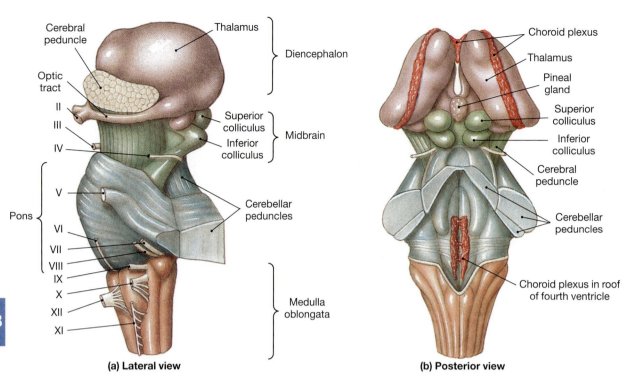

(a) Lateral view

(b) Posterior view

•**FIGURE 8-25   The Diencephalon and Brain Stem**
(a) A lateral view, as seen from the left side. Roman numerals indicate the positions of cranial nerves. **(b)** A posterior view.

The Midbrain

The midbrain (Figure 8-25•) contains various nuclei and bundles of ascending and descending nerve fibers. It includes two pairs of sensory nuclei, or *col-liculi* (kol-IK-ū-lī; singular colliculus, a small hill), dealing with the processing of visual and auditory sensations. These midbrain nuclei direct the involuntary motor reflexes to sudden visual and auditory stimuli (such as a blinding flash of light or a loud noise). The midbrain also contains motor nuclei for two of the cranial nerves (N III, IV) involved in the control of eye movements. Descending bundles of nerve fibers on the ventrolateral surface of the midbrain make up the **cerebral peduncles** (*peduncles*, little feet). Some of the descending fibers go to the cerebellum by way of the pons, and others carry voluntary motor commands from the primary motor cortex of each cerebral hemisphere.

The midbrain is also headquarters to one of the most important brain stem components, the **reticular formation**, which is involved in the regulation of many involuntary functions. The reticular formation is a network of interconnected nuclei that extends the length of the brain stem. The reticular formation of the midbrain contains the *reticular activating system (RAS)*. The output of this system directly affects the activity of the cerebral cortex. When the RAS is inactive, so are we; when the RAS is stimulated, so is our state of attention or wakefulness.

The maintenance of muscle tone and posture is due to midbrain nuclei that integrate information from the cerebrum and cerebellum and issue the appropriate involuntary motor commands. Other midbrain nuclei play an important role in regulating the motor output of the cerebral nuclei. For example, the *substantia nigra* (NĪ-grah; black) inhibit the activity of the cerebral nuclei by releasing the neurotransmitter dopamine. ∞ *p. 225* If the substantia nigra are damaged or the neurons secrete less dopamine, the cerebral nuclei become more active. The result is a gradual increase in muscle tone and the appearance of symptoms characteristic of *Parkinson's disease*. Persons with Parkinson's disease have difficulty starting voluntary movements, because opposing muscle groups do not relax—they must be overpowered. Once a movement is under way, every aspect must be voluntarily controlled through intense effort and concentration.

The Pons

The pons (Figure 8-25•) links the cerebellum with the midbrain, diencephalon, cerebrum, and spinal cord. One group of nuclei within the pons includes the sensory and motor nuclei for four of the cranial nerves (N V–VIII). Other nuclei are concerned with the involuntary control of the pace and depth of respiration. Tracts passing through the pons link the cerebellum with the brain stem, cerebrum, and spinal cord.

The Cerebellum

The cerebellum (Figure 8-17b,c•, pp. 233–234) performs two important functions: (1) It makes rapid adjustments in muscle tone and position to maintain balance and equilibrium by modifying the activity of nuclei in the brain stem; and (2) it programs and fine-tunes voluntary and involuntary movements. These functions are performed indirectly, by regulating activity along motor pathways at the cerebrum and brain stem. The tracts that link the cerebellum with these different regions are the **cerebellar peduncles** (Figure 8-25•). Like the cerebral hemispheres, the cerebellar hemispheres are composed of white matter covered by a layer of neural cortex called the *cerebellar cortex.*

The cerebellum can be permanently damaged by trauma or stroke or temporarily affected by drugs such as alcohol. These alterations can produce *ataxia* (a-TAK-sē-a; *ataxia,* a lack of order), a disturbance in balance.

The Medulla Oblongata

The medulla oblongata (Figure 8-25•) physically connects the brain with the spinal cord, and many of its functions are directly related to this fact. All communication between the brain and spinal cord involves tracts that ascend or descend through the medulla oblongata. These tracts often synapse in the medulla oblongata, in sensory or motor nuclei that act as relay stations and processing centers. In addition to these nuclei, the medulla oblongata contains sensory and motor nuclei associated with cranial nerves N VIII–XII.

Within the medulla oblongata, a variety of nuclei and centers representing the reticular formation regulate vital autonomic functions. These reflex centers receive inputs from cranial nerves, the cerebral cortex, and the brain stem, and their output controls or adjusts the activities of one or more peripheral systems. The *cardiovascular centers* adjust heart rate, the strength of cardiac contractions, and the flow of blood through peripheral tissues. On functional grounds, the cardiovascular centers may be subdivided into a *cardiac center* regulating the heart rate and a *vasomotor center* controlling peripheral blood flow. The *respiratory rhythmicity center* sets the basic pace for respiratory movements, and its activity is adjusted by the respiratory centers of the pons.

✓ The thalamus acts as a relay point to all but what type of sensory information?

✓ Which area of the diencephalon would be stimulated by changes in body temperature?

✓ The medulla oblongata is one of the smallest sections of the brain, yet damage there can cause death, whereas similar damage in the cerebrum might go unnoticed. Why?

AGING AND THE NERVOUS SYSTEM

Age-related anatomical and physiological changes in the nervous system begin shortly after maturity (probably by age 30) and accumulate over time. Although an estimated 85 percent of individuals above age 65 lead relatively normal lives, there are noticeable changes in mental performance and CNS functioning. These include:

- *A reduction in brain size and weight, primarily from a decrease in the volume of the cerebral cortex.* The brains of elderly individuals have narrower gyri and wider sulci than those of young persons, and the subarachnoid space is larger.

- *A reduction in the number of neurons.* Brain shrinkage has been linked to a loss of cortical neurons, although evidence exists that neuronal loss does not occur (at least to the same degree) in brain stem nuclei.

- *A decrease in blood flow to the brain.* With age, fatty deposits gradually accumulate in the walls of blood vessels. Like a kink in a garden hose or a clog in a drain, these deposits reduce the rate of blood flow through arteries. (This process, called *arteriosclerosis,* affects arteries throughout the body; it is discussed further in Chapter 14.) The reduction in blood flow does not cause a cerebral crisis, but it does increase the chances that the individual will suffer a stroke.

- *Changes in synaptic organization of the brain.* The number of dendritic branchings and interconnections appears to decrease. Synaptic connections are lost, and the rate of neurotransmitter production declines.

- *Intracellular and extracellular changes in CNS neurons.* Many neurons in the brain begin accumulating abnormal intracellular deposits, such as pigments or abnormal proteins that have no known function. The significance of these abnormalities remains to be determined. There is evidence that these changes occur in all aging brains, but when present in excess they seem to be associated with clinical abnormalities.

As a result of these anatomical changes, neural function is impaired. Memory consolidation, the conversion of short-term memory to long-term memory (such as repeating a telephone number), often becomes more difficult. Other memories, especially those of the recent past, also become harder to access. The sensory systems, notably hearing, balance, vision, smell, and taste, become less acute. Light must be brighter, sounds louder, and smells stronger before they are perceived. Reaction times are slowed, and reflexes—even some withdrawal reflexes—become weaker or disappear. The precision of motor control decreases, so it takes longer to perform a given motor pattern than it did 20 years earlier.

For roughly 85 percent of the elderly, these changes do not interfere with their abilities to function. But for as yet unknown reasons, many individuals become incapacitated by progressive CNS changes.

✳ CLINICAL NOTE   ALZHEIMER'S DISEASE

Alzheimer's disease is a particular form of dementia that affects over 4 million Americans and accounts for more than half of all forms of dementia in the elderly. Alzheimer's disease is not a normal part of the aging process. It is a chronic degenerative disorder of the brain resulting in impaired memory, thinking, and behavior. It is caused by the development of tangled plaques of nerve fibers within the brain. The onset of Alzheimer's disease is usually insidious and subtle. The disease generally occurs in three stages, each with different signs and symptoms. These include:

• *Early stage.* Characterized by loss of recent memory, inability to learn new material, mood swings, and personality changes. Aggression or hostility is common. Poor judgment is evident.

• *Intermediate stage.* Characterized by a complete inability to learn new material; wandering, particularly at night; increased falls; and loss of ability for self-care, including bathing and use of the toilet.

• *Terminal stage.* Characterized by an inability to walk and regression to infant stage, including the loss of bowel and bladder function. Eventually, the patient loses the ability to eat and swallow.

There is increasing evidence that Alzheimer's disease may be inherited. Treatment, at the present time, is limited primarily to controlling symptoms and providing supportive care.

---

8 Chapter Review

KEY TERMS

action potential, *p. 222*	limbic system, *p. 241*	neuroglia, *p. 216*
axon, *p. 217*	medulla oblongata, *p. 234*	neurotransmitter, *p. 224*
cerebellum, *p. 234*	membrane potential, *p. 220*	pons, *p. 234*
cerebrospinal fluid, *p. 235*	meninges, *p. 228*	reflex, *p. 227*
cerebrum, *p. 233*	midbrain, *p. 234*	somatic nervous system, *p. 216*
diencephalon, *p. 234*	multipolar neuron, *p. 218*	synapse, *p. 218*
hypothalamus, *p. 234*	myelin, *p. 218*	thalamus, *p. 234*

SUMMARY OUTLINE

INTRODUCTION *p. 216*

1. Two organ systems, the nervous and endocrine systems, coordinate organ system activity. The nervous system provides swift but brief responses to stimuli; the endocrine system adjusts metabolic operations and directs long-term changes.

THE NERVOUS SYSTEM *p. 216*

1. The **nervous system** includes all the neural tissue in the body. Its anatomical divisions include the **central nervous system (CNS)** (the brain and spinal cord) and the **peripheral nervous system (PNS)** (all of the neural tissue outside the CNS).

2. Functionally, it can be divided into an **afferent division**, which brings sensory information to the CNS, and an **efferent division**, which carries motor commands to muscles and glands. The efferent division includes the **somatic nervous system (SNS)** (voluntary control over skeletal muscle contractions) and the **autonomic nervous system (ANS)** (automatic, involuntary regulation of smooth muscle, cardiac muscle, and glandular activity). *(Figure 8-1)*

CELLULAR ORGANIZATION IN NEURAL TISSUE *p. 216*

1. There are two types of cells in neural tissue: **neurons**, which are responsible for information transfer and processing, and **neuroglia**, or *glial cells*, which provide a supporting framework and act as phagocytes.

Neurons *p. 217*

2. **Sensory neurons** form the afferent division of the PNS and deliver information to the CNS. **Motor neurons** stimulate or modify the activity of a peripheral tissue, organ, or organ system. **Interneurons (association neurons)** may be located between sensory and motor neurons; they analyze sensory inputs and coordinate motor outputs.

3. Sensory receptors are classified according to their source of stimuli: (1) **exteroceptors** provide information about the external environment; (2) **proprioceptors** monitor the position of the body's skeletal muscles and joints; and (3) **interoceptors** monitor activities of various organ systems of the body.

4. A typical neuron has a **soma** (cell body), an **axon**, and several branching, sensitive **dendrites**. *(Figure 8-2)*

5. Synaptic terminals occur at the end of axons. A synaptic knob is a synaptic terminal. *(Figure 8-2)*

6. Neurons may be described as **unipolar**, **bipolar**, or **multipolar**. *(Figure 8-3)*

Neuroglia *p. 218*

7. The four types of neuroglia in the CNS are (1) **astrocytes**, which are the largest and most numerous; (2) **oligodendro-**

cytes, which are responsible for the **myelination** of CNS axons; (3) **microglia**, phagocytic white blood cells; and (4) **ependymal cells**, with functions related to the *cerebrospinal fluid (CSF)*. *(Figure 8-4)*

8. Nerve cell bodies in the PNS are clustered into *ganglia* (singular *ganglion*). Their axons are covered by myelin wrappings of **Schwann cells**. *(Figure 8-5)*

NEUROPHYSIOLOGY *p. 220*

The Membrane Potential *p. 220*

1. The **resting potential**, or **membrane potential** of an undisturbed nerve cell, is due to a balance between the rate of sodium ion entry and potassium ion loss and to the sodium-potassium exchange pump. Any stimulus that affects this balance will alter the resting potential of the cell. *(Figure 8-6)*

2. An **action potential** appears when the membrane depolarizes to a level known as the **threshold**. The steps involved include: opening of sodium channels and membrane depolarization; the closing of sodium channels and opening of potassium channels; and the return to normal permeability. *(Figure 8-7)*

Conduction of an Action Potential, *p. 222*

3. In **continuous conduction**, an action potential spreads across the entire excitable membrane surface in a series of small steps. *(Figure 8-8a)*

4. During **saltatory conduction**, the action potential appears to leap from node to node, skipping the intervening membrane surface. *(Figure 8-8b)*

SYNAPTIC COMMUNICATION *p. 224*

1. A **synapse** is a site where intercellular communication occurs through the release of chemicals called **neurotransmitters**. A synapse where neurons communicate with other cell types is a **neuroeffector junction**.

Structure of a Synapse *p. 224*

2. Neural communication moves from the **presynaptic neuron** to the **postsynaptic neuron** over the **synaptic cleft**. *(Figure 8-9)*

Synaptic Events and Neurotransmitters *p. 225*

3. *Cholinergic synapses* release the neurotransmitter **acetylcholine (ACh)**. ACh is broken down in the synaptic cleft by the enzyme **acetylcholinesterase (AChE)**. *(Figure 8-10; Table 8-1)*

4. Other neurotransmitters include **norepinephrine (NE)**, **dopamine, gamma aminobutyric acid (GABA)**, and **serotonin**. ACh and NE usually have an excitatory effect on postsynaptic membranes; dopamine, GABA, and serotonin are typically inhibitory.

NEURONAL POOLS *p. 226*

1. The roughly 20 billion interneurons are organized into **neuronal pools** (groups of interconnected neurons with specific functions).

2. **Divergence** is the spread of information from one neuron to several neurons or from one neuronal pool to several pools. In **convergence**, several neurons synapse on the same postsynaptic neuron. In **parallel processing**, several neuronal pools process the same information simultaneously. *(Figure 8-11)*

AN INTRODUCTION TO REFLEXES *p. 227*

1. A **reflex** is an automatic, involuntary motor response that helps preserve homeostasis by rapidly adjusting the functions of organs or organ systems.

The Reflex Arc *p. 227*

2. A **reflex arc** is the "wiring" of a single reflex. It begins at a receptor and ends at an effector (such as a muscle or gland).

3. There are five steps involved in a neural reflex: (1) arrival of a stimulus and activation of a receptor, (2) activation of a sensory neuron, (3) information processing, (4) activation of a motor neuron, and (5) response by an effector. *(Figure 8-12)*

AN INTRODUCTION TO THE ANATOMY OF THE NERVOUS SYSTEM *p. 227*

1. The functions of the nervous system as a whole depend on interactions between neurons in neuronal pools. In the PNS, *spinal nerves* communicate with the spinal cord, and *cranial nerves* are connected to the brain.

2. In the CNS, a collection of neuron cell bodies that share a particular function is called a **center**. A center with a discrete anatomical boundary is called a **nucleus**. Portions of the brain surface are covered by a thick layer of gray matter called the **neural cortex**. *(Figure 8-13)*

3. The white matter of the CNS contains bundles of axons, or **tracts**, that share common origins, destinations, and functions. Tracts in the spinal cord form larger group, called *columns*. *(Figure 8-13)*

4. **Sensory** (*ascending*) **pathways** carry information from peripheral sensory receptors to processing centers in the brain; **motor** (*descending*) **pathways** extend from CNS centers concerned with motor control to the associated skeletal muscles. *(Figure 8-13)*

The Meninges *p. 228*

5. Special covering membranes, the **meninges**, protect and support the spinal cord and delicate brain. The cranial meninges (the dura mater, arachnoid, and pia mater) are continuous with those of the spinal cord, the spinal meninges. *(Figure 8-14)*

6. The **dura mater** covers the brain and spinal cord. The **epidural space** separates the spinal dura mater from the walls of the vertebral canal.

7. Inferior to the inner surface of the dura mater lies the **arachnoid** (the second meningeal layer) and the **subarachnoid space**. The subarachnoid space contains **cerebrospinal fluid** (the CSF), which acts as a shock absorber and a diffusion medium for dissolved gases, nutrients, chemical messengers, and waste products.

8. The **pia mater**, the innermost meningeal layer, is bound to the underlying neural tissue.

The Blood-Brain Barrier *p. 230*

9. The **blood-brain barrier** isolates neural tissue from the general circulation.

THE SPINAL CORD *p. 230*

1. In addition to relaying information to and from the brain, the spinal cord integrates and processes information on its own.

Gross Anatomy *p. 230*

2. The adult spinal cord includes localized enlargements that provide innervation to the limbs. *(Figure 8-15a)*

3. The spinal cord has 31 segments, each associated with a pair of **dorsal root ganglia** and their **dorsal roots** and a pair of **ventral roots**. *(Figures 8-15b; 8-16b)*

Sectional Anatomy *p. 230*

4. The white matter contains myelinated and unmyelinated axons; the gray matter contains cell bodies of neurons and glial cells. The projections of gray matter toward the outer surface of the spinal cord are called *horns*. *(Figure 8-16a)*

THE BRAIN *p. 232*

Major Divisions of the Brain *p. 233*

1. There are six regions in the adult brain: cerebrum, diencephalon, midbrain, cerebellum, pons, and medulla oblongata. *(Figure 8-17)*

2. Conscious thought, intellectual functions, memory, and complex involuntary motor patterns originate in the **cerebrum**. The **cerebellum** adjusts voluntary and involuntary motor activities on the basis of sensory data and stored memories. *(Figure 8-17)*

3. The walls of the **diencephalon** form the **thalamus**, which contains relay and processing centers for sensory information. The **hypothalamus** contains centers involved with emotions, autonomic function, and hormone production. *(Figure 8-17c)*

4. Three regions make up the **brain stem**. (1) The **midbrain** processes visual and auditory information and generates involuntary somatic motor responses. (2) The **pons** connects the cerebellum to the brain stem and is involved with somatic and visceral motor control. (3) The spinal cord connects to the brain at the **medulla oblongata**, which relays sensory information and regulates autonomic functions. *(Figure 8-17c)*

The Ventricles of the Brain *p. 234*

5. The central passageway of the brain expands to form four chambers called **ventricles**. Cerebrospinal fluid continuously circulates from the ventricles and central canal of the spinal cord into the subarachnoid space of the meninges that surround the CNS. *(Figures 8-18, 8-19)*

The Cerebrum *p. 235*

6. The cortical surface contains **gyri** (elevated ridges) separated by **sulci** (shallow depressions) or deeper grooves (**fissures**). The **longitudinal fissure** separates the two **cerebral hemispheres**. The **central sulcus** marks the boundary between the **frontal lobe** and the **parietal lobe**. Other sulci form the boundaries of the **temporal lobe** and the **occipital lobe**. *(Figures 8-17; 8-20)*

7. Each cerebral hemisphere receives sensory information and generates motor commands that concern the opposite side of the body.

8. The **primary motor cortex** of the **precentral gyrus** directs voluntary movements. The **primary sensory cortex** of the **postcentral gyrus** receives somatic sensory information from touch, pressure, pain, and temperature receptors. *(Figure 8-20)*

9. **Association areas**, such as the **visual association area** and **premotor cortex** (motor association area), control our ability to understand sensory information and coordinate a motor response. *(Figure 8-20)*

10. "Higher-order" integrative centers receive sensory information from many different association areas and then direct complex motor activities and analytical functions. *(Figure 8-21)*

11. The left hemisphere is usually the *categorical hemisphere*, which contains the general interpretive and speech centers and is responsible for language-based skills. The right hemisphere, or *representational hemisphere*, is concerned with spatial relationships and analyses. *(Figure 8-21)*

12. An **electroencephalogram (EEG)** is a printed record of **brain waves**. *(Figure 8-22)*

The Cerebral Nuclei *p. 239*

13. The **cerebral nuclei** lie within the central white matter and aid in the coordination of learned movement patterns and other somatic motor activities. *(Figure 8-23)*

The Limbic System *p. 241*

14. The **limbic system** includes the *hippocampus*, which is involved in memory and learning, and the *mamillary bodies*, which control reflex movements associated with eating. The functions of the limbic system involve emotional states and related behavioral drives. *(Figure 8-24)*

The Diencephalon *p. 241*

15. The diencephalon provides the switching and relay centers necessary to integrate the conscious and unconscious sensory and motor pathways. The diencephalic roof contains the *pineal gland* and a vascular network that produces cerebrospinal fluid. *(Figure 8-25)*

16. The thalamus is the final relay point for ascending sensory information. It acts as a filter, passing on only a small portion of the arriving sensory information to the cerebral cortex, relaying the rest to the cerebral nuclei and centers in the brain stem. *(Figure 8-25)*

17. The hypothalamus contains important control and integrative centers. It can (1) produce emotions and behavioral drives, (2) control autonomic function, (3) coordinate activities of the nervous and endocrine systems, (4) secrete hormones, (5) coordinate voluntary and autonomic functions, and (6) regulate body temperature.

The Midbrain *p. 242*

18. The midbrain contains two pairs of sensory nuclei, the *colliculi*, which receive visual and auditory information. It is also the center of the **reticular formation**, nuclei that affect cerebral activity. *(Figure 8-25)*

The Pons *p. 242*

19. The pons contains (1) sensory and motor nuclei for four cranial nerves, (2) nuclei concerned with involuntary control of respiration, and (3) ascending and descending tracts. *(Figure 8-25)*

The Cerebellum *p. 243*

20. The cerebellum oversees the body's postural muscles and programs and tunes voluntary and involuntary movements. The **cerebellar peduncles** are tracts that link the cerebellum with the brain stem, cerebrum, and spinal cord. *(Figures 8-17; 8-25)*

The Medulla Oblongata *p. 243*

21. The medulla oblongata connects the brain to the spinal cord. Its nuclei relay information from the spinal cord and brain stem to the cerebral cortex. Its reflex centers, including the *cardiovascular centers* and the *respiratory rhythmicity center*, control or adjust the activities of one or more peripheral systems. *(Figure 8-25)*

AGING AND THE NERVOUS SYSTEM *p. 243*

1. Age-related changes in the nervous system include (1) a reduction of brain size and weight, (2) a reduction of the number of neurons, (3) decreased blood flow to the brain, (4) changes in synaptic organization of the brain, and (5) intracellular and extracellular changes in CNS neurons.

REVIEW QUESTIONS

LEVEL 1   Reviewing Facts and Terms

Match each item in column A with the most closely related item in column B. Use letters for answers in the spaces provided.

Column A

___ 1. neuroglia
___ 2. microglia
___ 3. sensory neurons
___ 4. motor neurons
___ 5. ganglia
___ 6. oligodendrocytes
___ 7. ascending tracts
___ 8. descending tracts
___ 9. saltatory conduction
___10. continuous conduction
___11. dura mater
___12. pia mater
___13. choroid plexus
___14. cerebellum
___15. Nissl bodies
___16. hypothalamus
___17. medulla oblongata

Column B

a. coat CNS axons with myelin
b. carry sensory information to the brain
c. occurs along unmyelinated axons
d. outermost covering of brain and spinal cord
e. production of CSF
f. supporting cells
g. phagocytic white blood cells
h. occurs along myelinated axons
i. link between nervous and endocrine systems
j. carry motor commands to spinal cord
k. efferent division of the PNS
l. aggregations of RER and ribosomes
m. masses of neuron cell bodies
n. connects the brain to the spinal cord
o. innermost meningeal layer
p. afferent division of the PNS
q. maintains muscle tone and posture

18. Regulation by the nervous system provides:
    (a) relatively slow but long-lasting responses to stimuli
    (b) swift, long-lasting responses to stimuli
    (c) swift but brief responses to stimuli
    (d) relatively slow, short-lived responses to stimuli

19. All the motor neurons that control skeletal muscles are:
    (a) multipolar neurons
    (b) myelinated bipolar neurons
    (c) unipolar, unmyelinated sensory neurons
    (d) proprioceptors

20. Depolarization of a neuron cell membrane will shift the membrane potential toward:
    (a) 0 mV
    (b) −70 mV
    (c) −90 mV
    (d) a, b, and c are correct

21. The primary determinant of the resting membrane potential is the:
    (a) membrane permeability to sodium
    (b) membrane permeability to potassium
    (c) intracellular negatively charged proteins
    (d) negatively charged chloride ions in the extracellular fluid

22. The structural and functional link between the cerebral hemispheres and the components of the brain stem is the:
    (a) neural cortex
    (b) medulla oblongata
    (c) mesencephalon
    (d) diencephalon

23. The ventricles in the brain are filled with:
    (a) blood   (b) cerebrospinal fluid
    (c) air   (d) neural tissue

24. Reading, writing, and speaking are dependent on processing in the:
    (a) right cerebral hemisphere
    (b) left cerebral hemisphere
    (c) prefrontal cortex
    (d) postcentral gyrus

25. Establishment of emotional states and related behavioral drives are functions of the:
    (a) limbic system
    (b) pineal gland
    (c) mamillary bodies
    (d) thalamus

26. The final relay point for ascending sensory information that will be projected to the primary sensory cortex is the:
    (a) hypothalamus
    (b) thalamus
    (c) spinal cord
    (d) medulla oblongata

27. What two integrated steps are necessary for the transfer of nerve impulses from neuron to neuron?

28. State the all-or-none principle of action potentials.

29. What are the primary functions of the cerebrum?

LEVEL 2   Reviewing Concepts

30. A graded potential:
    (a) decreases with distance from the point of stimulation
    (b) spreads passively because of local currents
    (c) may involve either depolarization or hyperpolarization
    (d) a, b, and c are correct

31. The loss of positive ions from the interior of a neuron produces:
    (a) depolarization
    (b) threshold
    (c) hyperpolarization
    (d) an action potential

32. What purpose do axon collaterals serve in the nervous system?

33. What would happen if the ventral root of a spinal nerve was damaged or transected?

34. Stimulation of which part of the brain would produce sensations of hunger and thirst?

35. Which major part of the brain is associated with respiratory and cardiac activity?

36. Multiple sclerosis (MS) is a demyelination disorder. How does this condition produce muscular paralysis and sensory losses?

LEVEL 3   Critical Thinking and Clinical Applications

37. If neurons in the central nervous system lack centrioles and are unable to divide, how can a person develop brain cancer?

38. Myelination of peripheral neurons occurs rapidly through the first year of life. How can this process explain the increased abilities of infants during their first year?

39. A police officer has just stopped Bill on suspicion of driving while intoxicated. The officer asks Bill to walk the yellow line on the road and then asks him to place the tip of his index finger on the tip of his nose. How would these activities indicate Bill's level of sobriety? Which part of the brain is being tested by these activities?

ANSWERS TO CONCEPT CHECK QUESTIONS

Page 220
1. The afferent division of the nervous system is composed of nerves that carry sensory information to the brain and spinal cord. Damage to this division would interfere with a person's ability to experience a variety of sensory stimuli.   2. Sensory neurons of the peripheral nervous system are usually unipolar; thus this tissue is most likely associated with a sensory organ.   3. Microglial cells are small phagocytic cells that are found in increased number in damaged and diseased areas of the CNS.

Page 224
1. Depolarization of the neuron membrane involves the opening of the sodium channels and the rapid influx of sodium ions into the cell. If the sodium channels were blocked, a neuron would not be able to depolarize and conduct an action potential.   2. Action potentials are propagated along myelinated axons by saltatory propagation at speeds much higher than those along unmyelinated axons. An axon with a propagation speed of 10 m/sec must be myelinated.

Page 227
1. A neurotransmitter that opens the potassium channels but not the sodium channels would cause a hyperpolarization at the postsynaptic membrane. The transmembrane potential would be greater and it would be more difficult to bring the membrane to threshold.   2. When an action potential reaches the presynaptic terminal of a cholinergic synapse, calcium channels are opened and the influx of calcium triggers the release of acetylcholine into the synapse to stimulate the next neuron. If the calcium channels were blocked, the acetylcholine would not be released and transmission across the synapse would cease.   3. The minimum number of neurons required for a reflex arc is two. One must be a sensory neuron to bring impulses to the central nervous system, and the other a motor neuron that can bring about a response to the sensory input.

Page 232
1. The ventral root of spinal nerves is composed of visceral and somatic motor fibers. Damage to this root would interfere with motor function.

2. Since the polio virus would be located in the somatic motor neurons, we would find it in the anterior gray horns of the spinal cord, where the cell bodies of these neurons are located.   3. All spinal nerves are classified as mixed nerves because they contain both sensory and motor fibers.

Page 234

1. The six regions in the adult brain and their major functions are (1) the *cerebrum*: conscious thought processes; (2) the *diencephalon*: the thalamic portion contains relay and processing centers for sensory information, and the hypothalamic portion contain centers involved with emotions, autonomic function, and hormone production; (3) the *midbrain*: processes visual and auditory information and generates involuntary motor responses; (4) the *pons*: contains tracts and relay centers that connect the brain stem to the cerebellum; (5) the *medulla oblongata*: contains major centers concerned with the regulation of autonomic function, such as heart rate, blood pressure, respiration, and digestive activities; and (6) the *cerebellum*: adjusts voluntary and involuntary motor activities.   2. The pituitary gland is attached to the floor of the diencephalon, or hypothalamus.

Page 241

1. Diffusion across the arachnoid granulations is the means by which cerebrospinal fluid reenters the bloodstream. If this process decreased, then excess fluid would start to accumulate in the ventricles and the volume of fluid in the ventricles would increase.   2. The primary motor cortex is located in the precentral gyrus of the frontal lobe of the cerebrum.   3. Damage to the temporal lobes of the cerebrum would interfere with the processing of olfactory (smell) and auditory (sound) impulses.

Page 243

1. All ascending sensory information other than olfactory passes through the thalamus before reaching our conscious awareness. 2. Changes in body temperature would stimulate the hypothalamus, a division of the diencephalon.   3. Even though the medulla oblongata is small, it contains many vital reflex centers, including those that control breathing and regulate the heart and blood pressure. Damage to the medulla oblongata can result in a cessation of breathing or life-threatening changes in heart rate and blood pressure.

8

8 Emergency Care Applications

OVERVIEW

The nervous system and the endocrine system are the body's two control systems. The nervous system controls relatively swift but brief responses to stimuli as the body strives to maintain homeostasis. The endocrine system usually controls processes that are slower and somewhat longer lasting.

The nervous system is extremely complex. It is typically divided into the *central nervous system (CNS)* and the *peripheral nervous system (PNS).* The CNS consists of the brain and the spinal cord. The PNS includes all of the structures outside the CNS and serves as the link between the CNS and the rest of the body.

The study and treatment of diseases of the nervous system is called *neurology.* Physicians who specialize in medical disorders of the nervous system are called *neurologists.* Those who treat the surgical diseases of the nervous system are called *neurosurgeons.* Because the field of neurology is so complex, some physicians specialize in certain areas of neurology such as pediatric neurology, pediatric neurosurgery, neuro-oncology, vascular neurosurgery, neuroelectrophysiology, and others.

MEDICAL DISORDERS OF THE NERVOUS SYSTEM

Cerebrovascular Accident (Brain Attack)

Cerebrovascular accident (CVA), also called *stroke,* is a general term that describes injury or death of brain tissue. CVA usually results from an interruption of blood supply to the affected area of the brain. The term *"brain attack"* is used because it compares the physiology of a stroke with that of a heart attack. Strokes are the third most common cause of death and the leading cause of disability.

A stroke results from any disease process that interrupts the blood flow to parts of the brain. The two general categories of stroke are ischemic and hemorrhagic. *Ischemic* strokes are due to blockage of a blood vessel that supplies a part of the brain. *Hemorrhagic strokes* occur due to rupture of a blood vessel that supplies a part of the brain (Figure A8-1•). Approximately 80–85 percent of strokes are ischemic, whereas 15–20 percent are hemorrhagic.

Ischemic strokes can be divided into two general categories: thrombotic and embolic.

• FIGURE A8-1   Postmortem **Specimen Illustrating Massive Hemorrhagic Stroke Affecting the Vast Majority of One Hemisphere of the Brain**

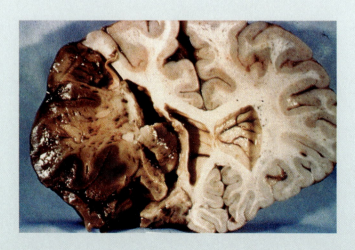

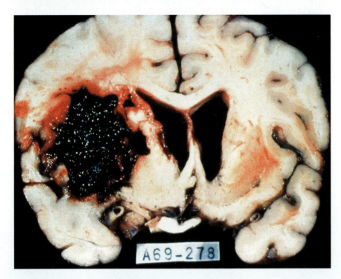

• **FIGURE A8-2   Hemorrhagic Stroke Involving the Tissues Adjoining the Lateral Ventricle (Periventricular Hemorrhage)**
Massive brain injury is evident.

In *thrombotic strokes* a clot forms at the site of the blockage. Often, the artery is narrowed or irregular due to atherosclerosis, which promotes clot formation. In *embolic strokes,* the blood clot forms elsewhere in the body, usually in the heart or great vessels, travels through the circulatory system, and ultimately lodges in a cerebral artery causing occlusion. Unlike thrombotic strokes, embolic strokes tend to occur in blood vessels that are relatively free of disease or narrowing.

Hemorrhagic strokes tend to occur in younger patients than do ischemic strokes. Most hemorrhagic strokes occur within the substance of the brain (intracerebral hemorrhage) (Figure A8-2•). Some hemorrhagic strokes, however, will cause bleeding into the subarachnoid space (subarachnoid hemorrhage). In *subarachnoid hemorrhage,* the sudden release of blood under high pressure and the subsequent rise in intracranial pressure (ICP) causes direct cellular injury. Most subarachnoid hemorrhages are due to rupture of *berry aneurysms.* Berry aneurysms are sac-like dilations of blood vessels that supply a part of the brain. They are usually congenital and produce weakened areas of the blood vessel. The highest incidence of berry-aneurysm rupture or bleeding occurs in patients from 20 to 50 years of age.

The signs and symptoms of a stroke depend upon the part or parts of the brain affected. Blockage of one of the smaller cerebral vessels may cause minimal, if any, symptoms. Blockage of a larger cerebral vessel can cause catastrophic symptoms and even death. Blood supply to the brain is derived from two sources: the anterior and posterior circulation. The *anterior circulation* is supplied by the carotid arteries and provides blood to 80 percent of the brain. The *posterior circulation* receives blood from the vertebral arteries. Although the posterior circulation provides only 20 percent of the brain's

blood, it supplies critical structures such as the brainstem, which is essential for movement, sensation, and normal consciousness.

Because each hemisphere of the brain controls the opposite side of the body, weakness and sensory loss will be noted on the side of the body opposite the stroke. If the dominant hemisphere of the brain is affected, there may be a loss of the ability to speak (*aphasia*). In right-handed patients and in up to 80 percent of left-handed patients, the left hemisphere is the dominant hemisphere.

Diagnosis of stroke is based on the history, physical examination, and computed tomography (CT). With CT, hemorrhagic strokes are readily identified. Ischemic strokes are more difficult to see in the acute phase. As time progresses, scar tissue replaces the parts of the brain affected, and ischemic lesions become more visible.

Treatment of strokes has changed significantly over the last decade. If treated promptly (usually within 3 hours), patients with ischemic strokes may be candidates for thrombolytic therapy. A thrombolytic agent, such as *tissue plasminogen activator (tPA),* can be administered and may dissolve the clot causing the ischemia. If blood flow can be restored to the affected parts of the brain in time, then the patient may not suffer any permanent injury. Because of this, the concept of "brain attack" has been promoted so that the public will recognize the signs and symptoms of stroke early and get the patient to an appropriate treatment facility.

A8

Transient Ischemic Attacks

Some patients will develop stroke-like symptoms that spontaneously resolve. This is referred to as a *transient ischemic attack (TIA)* and is often a precursor to a full-blown stroke. In most cases of TIA, the symptoms resolve in a few hours, although some may last for 24 hours or more. The occurrence of TIAs prompts a detailed investigation to determine the cause.

Seizure Disorders

A *seizure* is an episode of abnormal neurological function caused by an abnormal electrical discharge of brain neurons. The seizure is the clinical event experienced by the patient following the abnormal electrical discharge. *Epilepsy* is a clinical syndrome in which an individual is subject to recurrent seizures. The occurrence of one or more seizures indicates an abnormal function of cerebral neurons. Where a cause for attacks in patients who are otherwise normal cannot be determined, seizures are referred to as *primary,* or *idiopathic.* Seizures that result from some identifiable condition, such as brain tumor or brain trauma, are referred to as *secondary* seizures.

Seizures are common and are a frequent reason that EMS is summoned. Most are self-limited and last less than a minute. Seizures can be categorized as generalized or partial, depending upon the part of the brain involved. Generalized seizures involve the entire cerebral cortex, and usually begin with a loss of consciousness. This may be the only symptom, or it may be followed by motor activity. *Generalized tonic-clonic seizures* are the most familiar and dramatic seizure type. Often referred to as *grand mal seizures,* generalized tonic-clonic seizures cause the patient to become stiff and fall to the ground. This is followed by alternating contraction and relaxation of the skeletal muscles. Urinary and fecal incontinence is common. A seizure usually lasts 6–90 seconds, and as it ends, the patient is left flaccid and unconscious. The patient may be confused for up to an hour following the attack (*postictal confusion*). Fatigue is common and may last for hours after the event.

Absence seizures, also called *petit mal seizures,* are very brief, often lasting only a few seconds. Absence seizures are generalized seizures in which the patient suddenly loses consciousness without any loss of postural tone. These attacks end abruptly and the patients resume their activities. Often the patient and bystanders are unaware that anything has happened.

Focal seizures are due to electrical discharges that are limited to a portion of the cerebral cortex and are often secondary seizures resulting from a lesion in the brain. The effects of focal seizure depend upon the part of the brain involved. If the seizure's focus is in the motor cortex, tonic or clonic muscle contractions involving a single extremity may result. Sensory hallucinations suggest a focus in the sensory cortex. Visual symptoms, such as flashing lights, suggest a focus in the occipital lobe. Focal seizures isolated in the temporal lobe can cause altered thinking or behavior. Commonly referred to as *psychomotor seizures,* they can be mistakenly diagnosed as psychiatric disease.

Most seizure disorders can be controlled with medication. Modern anticonvulsant medications have minimal side effects and are highly effective. In fact, most seizures seen in the emergency setting occur because patients fail to take their medication or take it improperly.

NERVOUS SYSTEM INFECTIONS

Infections of the nervous system can be life threatening. The most common nervous system infection is meningitis. Its causes include viruses, bacteria, fungi, parasites, and prions. Less common CNS infections include encephalitis and brain abscess. CNS infections are classified as acute, subacute, or chronic depending upon the duration of the disease.

Meningitis

Meningitis is an infection of the meninges. Bacterial meningitis is a medical emergency that begins when the causative organisms enter the subarachnoid space. The three principi-

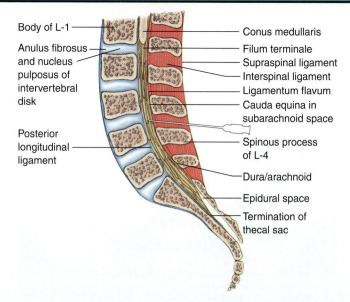

Body of L-1
Anulus fibrosus and nucleus pulposus of intervertebral disk
Posterior longitudinal ligament

Conus medullaris
Filum terminale
Supraspinal ligament
Interspinal ligament
Ligamentum flavum
Cauda equina in subarachnoid space
Spinous process of L-4
Dura/arachnoid
Epidural space
Termination of thecal sac

• **FIGURE A8-3   Cross-Section of the Distal Spine and Spinal Cord Showing Proper Positioning of a Spinal Needle During Lumbar Puncture**
Note that the puncture site is several segments below the terminal end of the spinal cord.

ple organisms are *Streptococcal pneumoniae, Haemophilus influenza (type b),* and *Neissiera meningitidis.* They enter the subarachnoid space, usually through the upper airway, and trigger infection and inflammation. The signs and symptoms of meningitis are fever, headache, altered mental status, photophobia, and stiffness of the neck (*meningismus*). With meningismus, passive flexion of the neck causes flexion of the hips and knees. This finding, referred to as *Brudzin-ski's sign,* is due to inflammation of the meninges. *Kernig's sign,* an inability to extend the legs when the knees are flexed is also due to meningeal inflammation. Brudzinski's sign and Kernig's sign are seen in approximately 50 percent of patients with bacterial meningitis. The diagnosis of meningitis is based on the history, physical examination, and lumbar puncture (spinal tap).

A *lumbar puncture* is an important diagnostic procedure that obtains *cerebrospinal fluid (CSF)* for laboratory analysis. The puncture is usually made between the third and fourth lumbar vertebrae, well below the terminal end of the spinal cord (Figure A8-3•). The patient is placed in a seated or a lateral recumbent position. The skin is cleansed and a sterile spinal needle is slowly inserted through the skin of the lower back into the subarachnoid space. Often, a "pop" can be felt as the needle penetrates the tough dura mater. Once the needle is properly placed, the CSF pressure is measured. Then, approximately 3–4 milliliters of CSF are removed. Spinal fluid is normally clear and does not contain cells. In meningitis, the spinal fluid becomes cloudy due to the presence of white blood cells (*pleocytosis*) and bacteria.

Bacterial meningitis can be rapidly fatal. As soon as the diagnosis is suspected, empiric antibiotics are administered. In adults, *N. meningitidis* and *S. pneumoniae* are the most common organisms. The incidence of *H. influen-*

zae has steadily declined with the introduction of a vaccine. Infection with *N. meningitidis,* referred to as *meningiococcemia,* is particularly severe. Emergency personnel who have been in close contact with a patient who has meningiococcemia may require prophylactic antibiotics.

Viral Meningitis

The signs and symptoms of viral meningitis are typically less severe than those of bacterial forms. The CSF fluid will typically contain white blood cells, but an infectious organism cannot be seen or cultured. Because of this, viral meningitis is often called *aseptic meningitis.* Viral meningitis often occurs in winter, and outbreaks are not uncommon. Treatment is supportive.

Unusual Forms of Meningitis

Although viral and bacterial meningitis are by far the most common, some other types of meningitis can be life threatening. The incidence of some infections is increasing due to increasing numbers of patients with incompetent immune systems. These include AIDS patients, patients who have received an organ transplant, and patients who are undergoing chemotherapy treatment for cancer. Often, the causative agent is not infectious and may actually be a part of the body's normal flora, but in patients with immunosuppression from drugs or disease, it can cause infection. Because of this, these types of meningitis are referred to as *opportunistic infections.*

Fungal meningitis is uncommon and, when present, tends to be chronic. Treatment is difficult and often requires long periods of therapy with antifungal drugs. It is most commonly seen in AIDS patients or in others who are immunocompromised.

Tubercular (TB) meningitis is being seen with increasing frequency, primarily in AIDS patients. The symptoms include headache, low-grade fever, nausea, vomiting, irritability, difficulty sleeping, and fatigue. As the disease progresses, confusion, stiff neck, behavioral changes, and seizures can occur. Despite the severity, the recovery rate approaches 90 percent if therapy is initiated in time.

Occasionally, meningitis can result from infection with free-living amoebas, particularly *Naegleria.* These organisms are found in both fresh and brackish water including that from lakes, swimming pools, hot springs, and heating and air conditioning units. Infection occurs when persons swimming in, or exposed to, the water inhale the organism. It invades the olfactory nervous tissue from the nasal cavity. After an incubation period or 2–15 days, the patient develops high fever, severe headache, nausea, vomiting, and meningismus. Rapid progression to seizures and coma occurs, and most patients die within a week. Only four survivors have been reported.

Parasitic Brain Infections

Cestodes are flatworms commonly referred to as tapeworms. The most commonly encountered member of

this group is the pork tapeworm (*Taenia solium).* It is a significant problem in developing countries and is occasionally encountered in the United States, especially in immigrants and visitors from Central America and the Middle East.

The larval stage of *T. solium* can cause clinical disease referred to as *cysticercosis,* which can be serious and often fatal. *Taenia* cysts can enter the subcutaneous tissue, the eye, the brain, and the heart and cause seizures and hydrocephalus. Cysticercosis should be considered a possible cause of new-onset seizures in recent immigrants from Central America. It can be identified through CT scanning of the brain and by isolation of cysts in the stool. Treatment with antiparasitic medications is usually effective if administered in time.

Brain Abscess

Brain abscesses are localized collections of pus within the parenchyma of the brain or spinal cord (Figure A8-4●). They tend to occur most frequently in men between the ages of 30 and 40 years. They can be caused by open trauma or neurosurgical procedures, by infection that has spread from the middle ear or nose, or by spreading from abscesses elsewhere in the body. AIDS patients are particularly susceptible to brain abscesses caused by the protozoan *Toxoplasma gondii* (*toxoplasmosis).* Treatment of brain abscess generally requires surgical drainage.

Encephalitis

Encephalitis is an acute infection, usually of viral origin, with CNS involvement. Most cases of encephalitis are due to viruses carried by mosquitoes. Outbreaks of encephalitis usually occur in summer. Causative

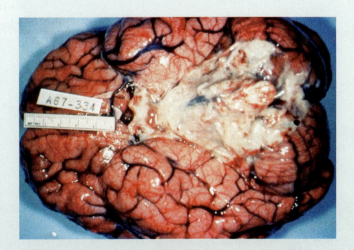

● **FIGURE A8-4   Large Brain Abscess Secondary to Intravenous Injection of Narcotics**
Bacteria are introduced to the brain resulting in abscess formation.

viruses include: *Eastern equine encephalitis, Western equine encephalitis, St. Louis encephalitis,* and *California encephalitis.* Encephalitis can also occur as a complication of viral diseases that usually affect other body systems, such as rabies or mononucleosis. Encephalitis is also seen in AIDS patients. Common causative viruses in this population include *herpes virus* and *cytomegalovirus (CMV).* The most common signs and symptoms of encephalitis are headache and fever. Delirium, confusion, seizures, and unconsciousness can occur in severe cases. Treatment for epidemic encephalitis is usually supportive. Opportunistic viral infections in AIDS patients are often treated with antiviral drugs.

Prion Diseases

A8

Until recently, scientists thought the smallest particle capable of transmitting disease was a virus. However, researchers have demonstrated that a protein alone is capable of transmitting disease. Protein particles, referred to as *prions,* have been identified as the causative agent of a group of diseases called *spongiform encephalopathies.* These diseases cause the brain to develop large vacuoles in the cortex and cerebellum adversely affecting central nervous system (CNS) function. It appears that traditional sterilization methods do not inactivate prions and they can remain communicable for long periods of time.

Previously, prion diseases have been rare. However, with the outbreak of mad cow disease in Europe, considerable attention has been focused on them. Mad cow disease, also known as *bovine spongiform encephalopathy (BSE),* initially appeared in the United Kingdom and has spread to parts of Europe. BSE apparently is transmitted through cattle feed. In the cattle industry, it is not uncommon for cattle feed to contain the by-products of other cattle. Apparently, parts of infected cattle were unknowingly ground up and mixed in cattle feed and fed to cattle in commercial feedlots. Some cattle that ate the tainted feed developed BSE.

Several human diseases are known to be caused by prions, the most common being *Creutzfeldt-Jakob Disease (CJD).* Prior to the outbreak of BSE, the incidence of CJD was only one person per million per year. However, the incidence has increased since the outbreak of BSE. Now, there appears to be a direct link between BSE and a form of CJD.

Early symptoms of CJD include failing memory, changes in behavior, lack of coordination, and visual disturbances. These are followed by a rapid, progressive dementia, involuntary jerking movements, and progressive motor dysfunction. The duration of CJD from the onset of symptoms to death is usually less than a year. Death is typically caused by secondary pneumonia. There is no treatment or cure for CJD.

Two interesting prion diseases are *fatal familial insomnia (FFI)* and *kuru.* FFI presents with untreatable insomnia, autonomic nervous system dysfunction, and eventually death. It is associated with severe, selective atrophy of the thalamus. Kuru occurs only in isolated tribes in the Fore highlands of New Guinea. In these tribes, the brains of dead relatives were removed and eaten as part of a religious ritual honoring the dead relative. Tribal members ground the brain up into a pale, gray soup, heated it, and ate it. The disease clinically resembles CJD, and some scientists have speculated that the brain tissue was highly infectious, with the causative prion being transmitted through ingestion. An effort by the New Guinea government to curtail cannibalism has caused the incidence of kuru to rapidly decline, and the disease is now almost unknown.

HEADACHE

Headache is a common complaint and usually a benign symptom. However, it can be associated with serious disease processes such as meningitis, brain tumor, and uncontrolled hypertension. The several *benign primary headache syndromes* include migraine headache, cluster headaches, and tension headaches.

Migraine Headache

Migraine headache is a common benign primary headache syndrome. It usually begins in the early teenage years and is more common in women than men. Migraine headaches appear to be caused by a particular trigger that sets a chain of events into motion. This complex chain of events includes neurological, vascular, hormonal, and neurotransmitter components. The phases of migraine headache are: (1) initial trigger phase initiated by external factors; (2) an aura with inhibition of neuronal activity in the cortex and a reduction in blood flow; (3) release of chemical substances that affect the blood vessels including serotonin and histamine; and (4) activation of fibers in the fifth cranial nerve (trigeminal nerve) causing dilation of the dural arteries. These vascular changes cause the typical migraine headache.

Migraine headaches are usually classified as classic migraine or common migraine. In *classic migraine,* the headache is often preceded by an aura that is due to a slowly expanding area of reduced blood flow. These auras vary from patient to patient but commonly include blurred vision and flashing lights (scotoma). Some patients may report a strange taste or smell. The aura always occurs before the headache begins. In *common migraine,* the headache develops without a preceding aura.

Migraine headache generally develops slowly and lasts from 4 to 72 hours. It is typically located on one side of the head and pulsates. Physical activity usually worsens migraine headache, causing the patient to lie motionless. Nausea and vomiting are very common. Sensitivity to light (photophobia) and sound (phonophobia) commonly accompany migraine headache. In rare cases, (complex migraine) migraines can cause total blindness, weakness or paralysis of one side of the body, and speech difficulties.

Migraine headaches are a common reason people seek emergency care. Due to a better understanding of the mechanism of migraine, several medications have been developed that will actually abort the headache if administered in time. These medications are most effective if administered as soon as possible following the onset of the aura or the headache. Once the headache has developed, medications for nausea and vomiting and for pain are often required.

Cluster Headache

Cluster headache is characterized by very severe, unilateral pain in the orbit, forehead, or temple. These headaches usually occur in men, with onset typically after age 20. The pain of cluster headache is usually so severe that patients cannot lie still. Generally, they pace and are very restless. Often there will be tearing of the eye or redness of the conjunctiva on the affected side. The headaches usually last from 15 to 180 minutes and generally occur in "clusters" occurring daily on the same side of the face for several weeks. Oxygen is an effective treatment in up to 70 percent of patients, and some of the medications developed for migraine headaches also have proven effective in cluster headaches.

Tension Headache

Tension headache is a common type of headache occurring in 40–60 percent of the population. The average age of onset is from 25 to 30 years. Tension headache is usually located on both sides of the head and is nonpulsating. Unlike migraine headaches, tension headaches are not associated with nausea and vomiting and are not worsened by physical exertion. Treatment is aimed at alleviating the symptoms.

NEUROLOGICAL TRAUMA

Although well protected by bony structures, the brain and spinal cord are susceptible to injury. Injuries are the leading cause of death in persons less than 45 years of age, with approximately half being due to head trauma. *Traumatic brain injury (TBI)* can be devastating, causing permanent disability. Young male adults are at greatest risk of neurological trauma, although children and the elderly are at increased risk due to underlying anatomical and physiological factors.

Neurological trauma is usually classified as penetrating or blunt. *Blunt trauma* is more common and results from motor vehicle collisions (MVCs), assaults, and

sporting injuries. *Penetrating trauma* is most often due to gunshot or stab wounds. Neurological trauma can also be described as primary or secondary. In *primary injury,* neuronal damage occurs immediately at impact. In *secondary injury,* neuronal damage occurs from minutes to days after the event and results from indirect causes such as brain swelling, lack of oxygen, or inadequate perfusion.

Blunt Trauma

Blunt trauma can cause focal injuries or diffuse injuries, depending upon the location of the force. *Focal injuries* occur at a specific location in the brain, whereas *diffuse injuries* are generalized. Head trauma can cause injury immediately under the point of impact *(coup injury)* or on the opposite side of the brain *(contrecoup injury).* Contrecoup injury results from the forceful movement of the brain away from the impact, which causes it to impact the interior of the skull opposite the injury. Contrecoup injuries can occur with trauma to the front or back of the head, as well as on either side (Figure A8-5●).

Diffuse Injuries

During head impact, a shearing, tearing, or stretching force is applied to the nerve fibers and causes damage to the axons. Referred to as *diffuse axonal injury (DAI),* the damage can range from mild to severe. A *concussion* is a mild to moderate form of DAI and the most common result of blunt head trauma. In a concussion, there is neuronal dysfunction without underlying anatomical damage. This is characterized by a transient episode of confusion, disorientation, or event amnesia, followed by a rapid return to normal. A brief loss of consciousness can occur. Usually there is no permanent neurological impairment.

Bruising of brain tissue following injury causes moderate DAI. If the cerebral cortex or the reticular activating system is affected, the patient may be rendered

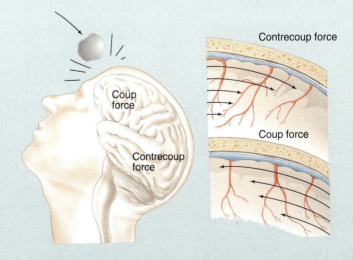

● **FIGURE A8-5   Coup and Contrecoup Injuries Following Blunt Trauma to the Head**

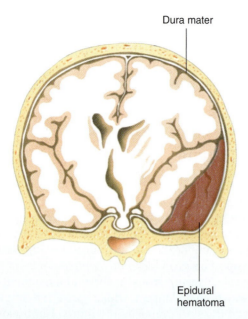

Dura mater

Epidural
hematoma

● **FIGURE A8-6   Epidural Hematoma**
The bleeding usually results from arterial bleeding and can
develop rapidly.

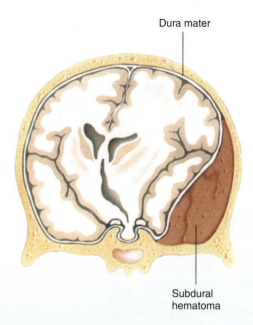

Dura mater

Subdural
hematoma

● **FIGURE A8-7   Subdural Hematoma**
The bleeding usually is venous and develops much slower
than in epidural hematomas.

unconscious. This injury is more severe than a mild concussion and can cause both short- and long-term signs
and symptoms. These include immediate unconsciousness, followed by persistent confusion, inability to concentrate, disorientation, and amnesia.

Severe DAI is caused by mechanical disruption of
many axons in both cerebral hemispheres with extension into the brainstem. This injury usually results in
coma and causes an increase in intracranial pressure
(ICP). Many patients do not survive severe DAI, and those
who do survive usually have some degree of permanent
neurological impairment.

Focal Injuries

Focal injuries occur at a specific location in the brain and
include contusions and intracranial hemorrhages. A *cerebral contusion* is due to capillary bleeding into the substance of the brain at the location of the impact. It can
cause confusion and other types of neurological deficits
depending upon the location involved. For example, injury to the frontal lobe can cause personality changes.

Blunt trauma can cause bleeding at several locations
within the brain. Bleeding between the dura mater and
the interior surface of the skull is an *epidural hematoma*
(Figure A8-6●). This usually is caused by damage to the
middle meningeal arteries from a skull fracture. Because
the bleeding is arterial, epidural hematomas develop
quickly and can cause herniation of the brainstem if not
treated expeditiously. The classic history of an epidural
hematoma is for the patient to experience an immediate
loss of consciousness after blunt head trauma. The patient then awakens and has a *lucent period* before again

falling unconscious as the hematoma expands. However,
the classic syndrome occurs in only about 20 percent of
patients with epidural hematoma. Treatment is neurosurgical evacuation of the hematoma as soon as possible.
Rarely, when neurosurgical care is unavailable, emergency
physicians may be required to place burr holes in the skull
above the hematoma to prevent brainstem herniation.

Bleeding beneath the dura mater and within the
subarachnoid space is a *subdural hematoma*. This type
of bleeding occurs very slowly and is usually due to
rupture of venous vessels, such as the bridging veins of
the dural sinus. Subdural hematoma usually causes few
initial signs and symptoms unless the hematoma is large
(Figure A8-7●). Treatment of subdural hematoma is
based on its severity. Small hematomas may be monitored with the blood being resorbed over a few days.
Large hematomas may require surgical decompression.
Associated brain injury is common.

Intracerebral hemorrhage (ICH) results from a ruptured blood vessel within the substance of the brain.
Blood loss is usually minimal but particularly damaging. It causes inflammation and swelling of the brain.
The signs and symptoms of ICH, which are similar to
those of a stroke, depend upon the portion of the brain involved. Treatment is directed at controlling ICP in order
to minimize secondary injury.

Penetrating Trauma

Penetrating trauma to the brain or spinal cord is potentially devastating. Penetrating injuries are usually due to
gunshots or stab wounds or to sharp objects encountered

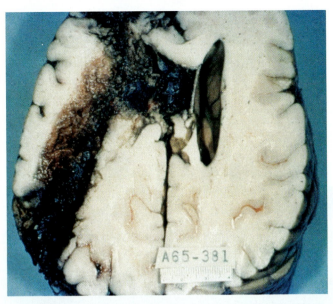

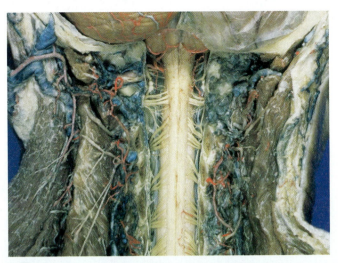

• **FIGURE A8-9** Detailed Dissection of the Proximal Spinal Cord Illustrating Essential Structures and Spinal Nerve Roots

• **FIGURE A8-8** Postmortem Specimen Showing Massive Missile Tract Through the Substance of the Brain Following a High-Velocity, High-Energy Gunshot

in an MVC. Often, as the penetrating object enters the head, it fractures the skull and carries bone fragments into the substance of the brain. Penetrating injuries can also cause bleeding if a blood vessel is struck during entry. As the brain is exposed to the environment, the possibility of infection exists.

The velocity and energy associated with the penetrating object are major factors in the type of injury encountered. Stab wounds are generally low velocity and low energy. Their damage is limited primarily to the point of entry. Small-caliber bullets may not have enough energy to both enter and exit the skull. Instead, after the bullet enters the skull, it strikes the interior surface of the skull on the opposite side and ricochets throughout the brain, often causing significant tissue damage. High-energy, large caliber bullets usually have enough energy to penetrate and exit the skull. Because of the tremendous energy associated with these missiles, damage to the brain is significant, with the exit wound destroying a significant part of the skull (Figure A8-8•). Increased ICP is usually not a concern in penetrating trauma due to the open wound. Penetrating injuries are often fatal. Those who survive often have serious permanent neurological damage.

Spinal Cord Injuries

The spinal cord is well protected by the vertebral bodies (Figure A8-9•). Spinal cord injuries usually are due to vertebral injuries that usually result from the extremes of normal motion such as flexion, extension, rotation, and lateral bending. Damaging mechanisms also include forces transmitted along the axis of the spine:

axial loading and *distraction*. Finally, spinal injury can result either directly from blunt or penetrating trauma or indirectly when an expanding mass (edema or hematoma) compresses the cord or a disruption of blood supply damages it (Figure A8-10•). It is possible to have spinal cord injury without any spinal column injury.

The bones, ligaments, and joints of the vertebral column may be damaged by hyperflexion or hyperextension. This most frequently occurs in the cervical and lumbar regions. These motions can cause the vertebral column to fracture or dislocate. With fractures, bone fragments can damage the spinal cord. With dislocations, abnormal movement of the vertebrae can compress or even shear the spinal cord.

Spinal cord injury varies in severity; its classifications include the following:

- *Cord concussion.* A temporary interruption in cord-mediated functions.
- *Cord contusion.* Bruising of the neural tissue resulting in swelling and temporary loss of cord-mediated functions.
- *Cord compression.* Results from pressure on the cord causing ischemia. Surgery to decompress the cord is often required to prevent permanent damage.
- *Cord lacerations.* Tearing of the neural tissues from bone fragments or shearing forces. Slight damage may be reversible, but permanent damage can occur if spinal tracts are disrupted.
- *Complete transection.* Severing of the spinal cord causing permanent loss of function.
- *Incomplete transection.* Part of the spinal cord is severed, but some tracts are spared.
- *Cord hemorrhage.* Bleeding into the neural tissues secondary to blood vessel damage following injury.

• **FIGURE A8-10   Mechanisms Associated with Cervical Spine Vertebral and Spinal Cord Injury**

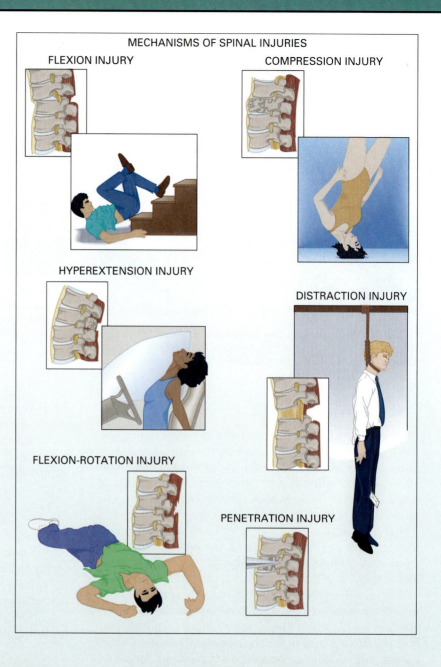

MECHANISMS OF SPINAL INJURIES

FLEXION INJURY

COMPRESSION INJURY

HYPEREXTENSION INJURY

DISTRACTION INJURY

FLEXION-ROTATION INJURY

PENETRATION INJURY

Several syndromes can develop with spinal cord injury. These result from partial cord injuries where some spinal tracts are destroyed while others are spared. These syndromes include:

- *Anterior-cord syndrome.* Results from compression of the anterior part of the spinal cord, often from hyperflexion of the cervical spine. It causes complete paralysis below the lesion with loss of pain and temperature sensation. Vibratory and light touch ability are spared in this injury.
- *Central-cord syndrome.* Results from disruption of blood supply to the spinal cord, often due to hyperextension injuries. It causes quadriparesis that is greater in the upper extremities than in the lower extremities. There may be some loss of pain and temperature sensation.

- *Brown-Séquard syndrome.* Results from transection of half of the spinal cord or from unilateral cord compression. It causes spastic paresis and loss of position and vibratory sensation on the affected side and loss of temperature and pain sensation on the opposite side.
- *Cauda equina syndrome.* Results from injury to the cauda equina from lumbar vertebral fractures of herniated discs. It can cause weakness and sensory loss in the lower extremities, sciatica, and possible bowel or bladder dysfunction.
- *Spinal shock.* Results from partial or complete spinal cord injury at T6 or above. It causes loss of reflexes, sensation, and flaccid paralysis below the level of the lesion. In addition, there is a flaccid bladder, loss of rectal sphincter tone, bradycardia, and hypotension.

A8

As central nervous system tissues cannot regenerate, spinal cord injuries are usually permanent. Occasionally, if treated in time, the injury can be minimized by the administration of extremely high doses of corticosteroids. This appears to limit the inflammation associated with the injury and prevent secondary injury from swelling.

Significant research is directed at the biochemical control of nerve growth and regeneration. In addition, electronic devices and computers are being used to stimulate specific muscles and muscle groups. This has allowed persons with spinal cord injuries to walk short distances.

SUMMARY

The nervous system is the body's major control system. Because of this, injuries and illnesses affecting the nervous system can be devastating. Emergency personnel must have a good understanding of the normal anatomy and physiology of the nervous system as well as common disease and injury patterns. Early recognition of serious neurological emergencies is essential. Treatment for many nervous system emergencies can minimize permanent disability or even avoid it altogether. To route patients with nervous system emergencies to the correct facilities, emergency personnel must be familiar with the capabilities of local medical centers.

A8

The Peripheral Nervous System and Integrated Neural Functions

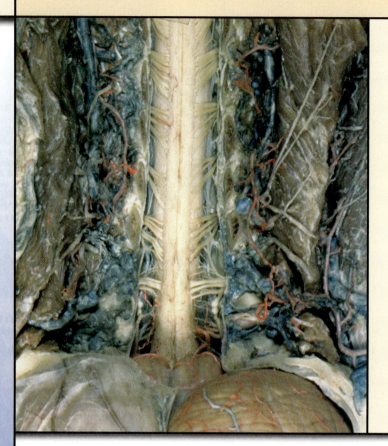

This prosection of the posterior neck illustrates the complexity of the proximal spinal cord and associated structures. The nerve rootlets supply sensory and motor function to the peripheral tissues. Injuries to the spinal cord in this region are devastating and, in many cases, fatal.

Chapter Outline and Objectives

Vocabulary Development

chiasm, a crossing; *optic chiasm*
cochlea, snail shell; *cochlear nerve*
glossus, tongue; *glossopharyngeal nerve*
mono-, one; *monosynaptic*
murus, wall; *intramural ganglia*
*neuro-, nerve; *neurotransmitter*
poly-, many; *polysynaptic*
trochlea, a pulley; *trochlear nerve*
vagus, wandering; *vagus nerve*
vestibulum, a cavity; *vestibular nerve*

The peripheral nervous system (PNS) is the link between the neurons of the central nervous system (CNS) and the rest of the body; all sensory information and motor commands are carried by axons of the PNS (see Figure 8-1•). ∞ *p. 216* As a result, although the PNS contains less than 2 percent of the neural tissue in the body, it is absolutely vital to the function of the nervous system. The essential communication between the CNS and PNS occurs over tracts and nuclei that relay sensory information and motor commands. *Pathways* consist of the nuclei and tracts that link the brain with the rest of the body. Sensory and motor pathways involve a series of synapses, one after the other. For example, a sensation carried by a sensory (ascending) pathway may be relayed across synapses in the medulla oblongata and the thalamus before reaching the cerebral cortex and our conscious awareness. At each synapse there are opportunities for divergence and for the distribution of information to neuronal pools operating at an involuntary level. For example, while you are consciously planning a response to a stumble, centers in the brain stem and cerebellum may already be issuing the motor commands necessary to prevent a fall.

This chapter begins with a consideration of the structure of the peripheral nervous system. We will then examine the integrated functioning of the nervous system, beginning with simple spinal reflexes and proceeding to the organization of representative sensory and motor pathways that produce conscious sensations and control skeletal muscles. We will conclude with an overview of the autonomic nervous system, which coordinates cardiovascular, respiratory, digestive, excretory, and reproductive functions, usually without instructions or interference from the conscious mind.

THE PERIPHERAL NERVOUS SYSTEM

The PNS is dominated by axons heading to or from the CNS. These axons, bundled together and wrapped in connective tissue, form **peripheral nerves**, or simply *nerves*. The PNS also contains both the cell bodies and the axons of sensory neurons and motor neurons of the autonomic nervous system. The cell bodies are clustered together in masses called **ganglia** (singular *ganglion*) (see Figure 8-13•). ∞ *p. 228* The peripheral nervous system includes *cranial nerves* and *spinal nerves*.

The Cranial Nerves

The **cranial nerves** are components of the peripheral nervous system that connect to the brain rather than to the spinal cord. The 12 pairs of cranial nerves, shown in Figure 9-1•, are numbered according to their posi-

tion along the longitudinal axis of the brain. The letter N designates a cranial nerve, and Roman numerals are used to distinguish the individual nerves. For example, N I refers to the first pair of cranial nerves, the *olfactory nerves*.

Distribution and Function

Functionally, each nerve can be classified as primarily sensory, motor, or mixed (sensory and motor). Many cranial nerves, however, have secondary functions. For example, several cranial nerves (N III, VII, IX, and X) also distribute autonomic fibers to PNS ganglia, just as spinal nerves deliver them to ganglia along the spinal cord. The distribution and functions of the cranial nerves are described below and summarized in Table 9-1 (p. 254).

Few people are able to remember the names, numbers, and functions of the cranial nerves without a struggle. Many people use mnemonic phrases, such as Oh, Once One Takes The Anatomy Final, Very Good Vacations Are Heavenly, in which the first letter of each word represents the cranial nerves.

The Olfactory Nerves (N I).   The first pair of cranial nerves, the **olfactory nerves**, are the only cranial nerves attached to the cerebrum. The rest originate or terminate within nuclei of the brain stem. These nerves carry special sensory information responsible for the sense of smell. The olfactory nerves originate in the epithelium of the upper nasal cavity and penetrate the cribriform plate of the ethmoid bone to synapse in the olfactory bulbs of the brain. From the olfactory bulbs, the axons of postsynaptic neurons travel within the *olfactory tracts* to the olfactory centers of the brain.

The Optic Nerves (N II).   The **optic nerves** carry visual information from the eyes. After passing through the **optic foramina** of the orbits, these nerves intersect at the **optic chiasm** ("crossing") (Figure 9-1a•) before they continue to the *lateral geniculate nuclei* of the thalamus.

The Oculomotor Nerves (N III).   The motor nuclei controlling the third cranial nerves are in the midbrain. Each **oculomotor nerve** innervates four of the six muscles that move an eyeball (the *superior*, *medial*, and *inferior rectus* muscles and the *inferior oblique* muscle). These nerves also carry autonomic (parasympathetic) fibers to intrinsic eye muscles that control (1) the amount of light entering the eye and (2) the shape of the lens.

The Trochlear Nerves (N IV).   The **trochlear** (TRŌK-lē-ar; *trochlea*, a pulley) **nerves**, the smallest of the cranial nerves, innervate the *superior oblique* muscles of the eyes. The motor nuclei that control these nerves lie in the midbrain. The name "trochlear" refers to the ligamentous sling, or pulley, through which the tendon of the superior oblique muscle passes to reach its attachment on the eyeball (see Figure 10-8•, p. 280).

The Trigeminal Nerves (N V).　The pons contains the nuclei associated with cranial nerve N V. The **trigeminal** (trī-JEM-i-nal) **nerves** are the largest of the cranial nerves. These nerves provide sensory information from the head and face and motor control over the chewing muscles, such as the *temporalis* and *masseter*. As the name implies, the trigeminal has three major branches. The *ophthalmic branch* provides sensory information from the orbit of the eye, the nasal cavity and sinuses, and the skin of the forehead, eyebrows, eyelids, and nose. The *maxillary branch* provides sensory information from the lower eyelid, upper lip, cheek, nose, upper gums and teeth, palate, and portions of the pharynx. The *mandibular branch*, the largest of the three, provides sensory information from the skin of the temples, the lower gums and teeth, the salivary glands, and the an-

terior portions of the tongue. It also provides motor control over the chewing muscles (the *temporalis*, *masseter*, and *pterygoid* muscles). ∞ *p. 188*

The Abducens Nerves (N VI).　The **abducens** (ab-DOO-senz) **nerves** innervate only the *lateral rectus*, the sixth of the extrinsic eye muscles. Their nuclei are in the pons. The nerves emerge at the border between the pons and the medulla oblongata and reach the orbit of the eye along with the oculomotor and trochlear nerves. The

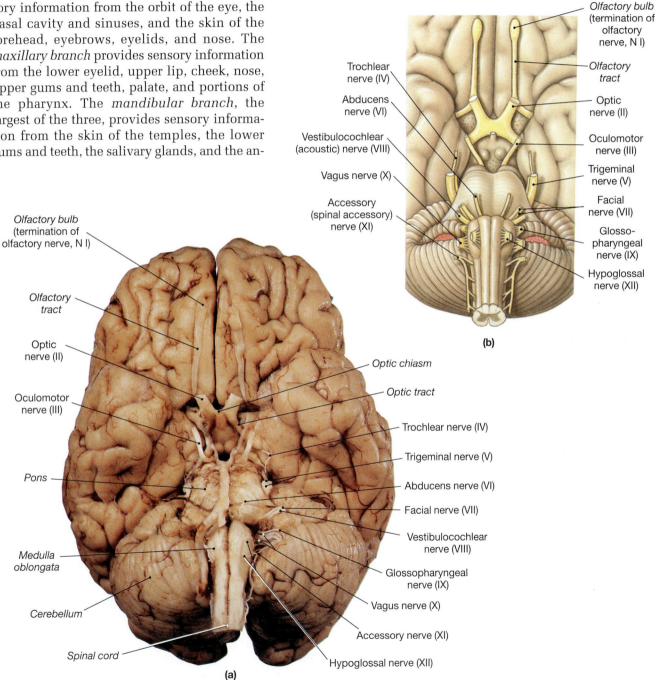

(b)

(a)

•**FIGURE 9-1　The Cranial Nerves**
(a) An inferior view of the brain. **(b)** A diagrammatic view, showing the attachment of the 12 pairs of cranial nerves.

TABLE 9-1	**The Cranial Nerves**	
Cranial Nerves (Number)	Primary Function	Innervation
Olfactory (I)	Special sensory	Olfactory epithelium
Optic (II)	Special sensory	Retina of eye
Oculomotor (III)	Motor	Inferior, medial, superior rectus and intrinsic muscles of eye
Trochlear (IV)	Motor	Superior oblique muscle of eye
Trigeminal (V)	Mixed	Areas associated with the jaws: *Sensory* from orbital structures, nasal cavity, skin of forehead, upper eyelid, eyebrows, nose, lips, gums and teeth; cheek, palate, pharynx, and tongue
		Motor to chewing (temporalis, masseter, pterygoids) muscles
Abducens (VI)	Motor	Lateral rectus muscle of eye
Facial (VII)	Mixed	*Sensory* to taste receptors on the anterior 2/3 of tongue
		Motor to muscles of facial expression, lacrimal gland, submandibular gland, sublingual salivary glands
Vestibulocochlear (Acoustic) (VIII)	Special sensory	Cochlea (receptors for hearing) Vestibule (receptors for motion and balance)
Glossopharyngeal (IX)	Mixed	*Sensory* from posterior 1/3 of tongue; pharynx and palate (part); blood pressure and composition
		Motor to pharyngeal muscles, parotid salivary gland
Vagus (X)	Mixed	*Sensory* from pharynx; pinna and external meatus; diaphragm; visceral organs in thoracic and abdominopelvic cavities
		Motor to palatal and pharyngeal muscles and visceral organs in thoracic and abdominopelvic cavities
Accessory (Spinal Accessory) (XI)	Motor	Voluntary muscles of palate, pharynx, and larynx; sternocleidomastoid and trapezius muscles
Hypoglossal (XII)	Motor	Tongue muscles

name "abducens" is based on the action of this nerve's innervated muscle, which abducts the eyeball, causing it to rotate laterally, away from the midline of the body.

The Facial Nerves (N VII).   The **facial nerves** are mixed nerves of the face whose sensory and motor roots emerge from the side of the pons. The motor fibers produce facial expressions by controlling the superficial muscles of the scalp and face and muscles near the ear. The sensory fibers monitor proprioceptors in the facial muscles, provide deep pressure sensations over the face, and taste information from receptors along the anterior two-thirds of the tongue.

The Vestibulocochlear Nerves (N VIII).   The **vestibulocochlear nerves**, also called *acoustic nerves*, monitor the sensory receptors of the inner ear. The pons and medulla oblongata contain nuclei associated with these nerves. Each vestibulocochlear nerve has two components: (1) a **vestibular nerve** (*vestibulum*, a cavity), which originates at the *vestibule*, the portion of the inner ear concerned with balance sensations, conveys information on position, movement, and balance; and (2) the **cochlear** (KOK-lē-ar; *cochlea*, snail shell) **nerve**, which monitors the receptors of the *cochlea*,

the portion of the inner ear responsible for the sense of hearing.

The Glossopharyngeal Nerves (N IX).   The **glossopharyngeal** (glos-ō-fah-RIN-jē-al; *glossus*, tongue) **nerves** are mixed nerves innervating the tongue and pharynx. The associated sensory and motor nuclei are in the medulla oblongata. The sensory portion of this nerve provides taste sensations from the posterior third of the tongue and monitors blood pressure and dissolved gas concentrations in major blood vessels. The motor portion controls the pharyngeal muscles involved in swallowing.

The Vagus Nerves (N X).   The **vagus** (VĀ-gus; *vagus*, wandering) **nerves** provide sensory information from the ear canals, the diaphragm, and taste receptors in the pharynx and from visceral receptors along the esophagus, respiratory tract, and abdominal organs as far away as the last portions of the large intestine. The associated sensory and motor nuclei of the vagus are located in the medulla oblongata. The sensory information provided by N X is vital to the autonomic control of visceral function, but we are not consciously aware of these sensations, because they are seldom relayed to the cerebral cortex. The motor components of the vagus nerves control skeletal muscles of the soft palate, pharynx, and esophagus and affect cardiac muscle, smooth muscle, and glands of the esophagus, stomach, intestines, and gallbladder.

The Accessory Nerves (N XI).   The **accessory nerves**, sometimes called the *spinal accessory nerves*, are mixed nerves that innervate structures in the neck and back. These nerves differ from other cranial nerves in that some of their motor fibers originate in the lateral gray horns of the first five cervical vertebrae as well as in the medulla oblongata. The *medullary branch* innervates the voluntary swallowing muscles of the soft palate and pharynx and the laryngeal muscles that control the vocal cords and produce speech. The *spinal branch* controls the *sternocleidomastoid* and *trapezius* muscles associated with the pectoral girdle. ∞ *pp. 189, 195*

The Hypoglossal Nerves (N XII).   The **hypoglossal** (hī-pō-GLOS-al) **nerves** provide voluntary control over the skeletal muscles of the tongue. The nuclei for these motor nerves are located in the medulla oblongata.

✓ What symptoms would you associate with damage to the abducens nerve (N VI)?

✓ John is having trouble moving his tongue. His physician tells him it is due to pressure on a cranial nerve. Which cranial nerve is involved?

The Spinal Nerves

The 31 pairs of **spinal nerves** can be grouped according to the region of the vertebral column from which they originate (Figure 9-2•). They include 8 pairs of cervical nerves (C_1–C_8), 12 pairs of thoracic nerves (T_1–T_{12}), 5 pairs of lumbar nerves (L_1–L_5), 5 pairs of sacral nerves (S_1–S_5), and 1 pair of coccygeal nerves (Co_1). Each pair of spinal nerves monitors a specific region of the body surface, and damage or infection of a spinal nerve will produce a characteristic loss of sensation in specific parts of the skin. For example, in *shingles*, a virus that infects dorsal root ganglia causes a painful rash whose distribution corresponds to that of the affected sensory nerves.

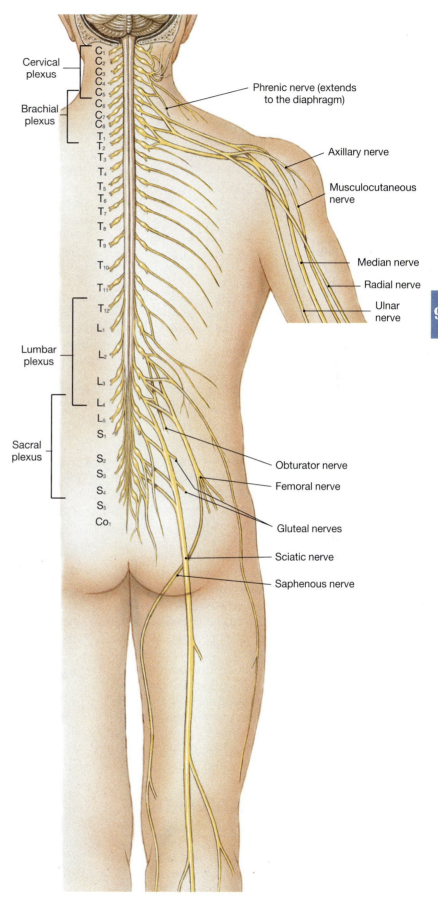

•**FIGURE 9-2   Peripheral Nerves and Nerve Plexuses**

TABLE 9-2	Nerve Plexuses and Major Nerves	
Plexus	*Major Nerve*	*Distribution*
Cervical Plexus **(C₁–C₅)**	Phrenic nerve	Diaphragm
	Other branches	Muscles of the neck; skin of upper chest, neck, and ears
Brachial Plexus **(C₅–T₁)**	Axillary nerve	Deltoid and teres minor muscles; skin of shoulder
	Musculocutaneous nerve	Flexor muscles of the arm and forearm; skin on lateral surface of forearm
	Median nerve	Flexor muscles of forearm and hand; skin over lateral surface of hand
	Radial nerve	Extensor muscles of the arm, forearm, and hand; skin on posterolateral surface of the arm
	Ulnar nerve	Flexor muscles of forearm and small digital muscles; skin of medial surface of hand
Lumbosacral Plexus **Lumbar Plexus (T₁₂–L₄)** **Sacral Plexus (L₄–S₄)**	Obturator nerve	Adductors of hip; skin over medial surface of thigh
	Femoral nerve	Adductors of hip, extensors of knee; skin over medial surfaces of thigh and leg
	Gluteal nerve	Adductors and extensors of hip; skin over posterior surface of thigh
	Sciatic nerve	Flexors of knee and ankle, flexors and extensors of toes; skin over anterior and posterior surfaces of leg and foot
	Saphenous nerve	Skin over medial surface of leg

Nerve Plexuses

During development, skeletal muscles commonly fuse, forming larger muscles innervated by nerve trunks containing axons derived from several spinal nerves. These compound nerve trunks originate at networks called **nerve plexuses**. The plexuses and major peripheral nerves are shown in Figure 9-2●.

The **cervical plexus** innervates the muscles of the neck and extends into the thoracic cavity to control the diaphragm. The **brachial plexus** innervates the shoulder girdle and upper limb. The **lumbosacral plexus** supplies the pelvic girdle and lower limb. It can be further subdivided into a *lumbar plexus* and a *sacral plexus*. Table 9-2 lists the spinal nerve plexuses and describes some of the major nerves and their distribution.

Peripheral *nerve palsies*, also known as *peripheral neuropathies*, are characterized by regional losses of sensory and motor function as the result of nerve trauma or compression. You have experienced a mild, temporary palsy if your arm or leg has ever "fallen asleep."

THE CNS AND PNS: INTEGRATED FUNCTIONS

The central nervous system and peripheral nervous system can be studied separately, but they function together. To consider the ways the CNS and PNS interact, we begin with simple reflex responses to stimulation.

Simple Reflexes

As we learned in Chapter 8, a **reflex** is an automatic motor response triggered by a specific stimulus. ∞ *p. 227* A reflex arc includes a receptor, a sensory neuron, a motor neuron, and an effector; interneurons may be found between the sensory neuron and the motor neuron. In the simplest reflex arc, a sensory neuron synapses directly on a motor neuron. ∞ *p. 217* Such a reflex is called a **monosynaptic reflex**. Because there is only one synapse, monosynaptic reflexes control the most rapid, stereotyped motor responses of the nervous system. The best-known example is the *stretch reflex*.

The Stretch Reflex

The **stretch reflex** provides automatic regulation of skeletal muscle length. The sensory receptors in the stretch reflex are called **muscle spindles**, bundles of small, specialized skeletal muscle fibers scattered throughout the skeletal muscles. The stimulus (increasing muscle length) activates a sensory neuron that triggers an immediate motor response (contraction of the stretched muscle) that counteracts the stimulus.

Stretch reflexes are important in the maintenance of normal posture and balance and in making automatic adjustments in muscle tone. Physicians can use the sensitivity of the stretch reflex to test the general condition of the spinal cord, peripheral nerves, and muscles. For example, in the **knee jerk**, or *patellar reflex*, a sharp rap

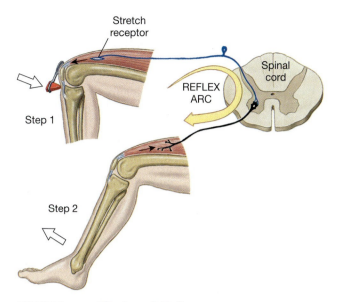

•FIGURE 9-3   The Stretch Reflex
The patellar reflex is a stretch reflex controlled by stretch receptors (muscle spindles) in the muscles that straighten the knee. Step 1: A reflex hammer strikes the muscle tendon, stretching the muscle spindles. This stretching results in a sudden increase in the activity of the sensory neurons. These neurons synapse on motor neurons in the spinal cord. Step 2: The activation of spinal motor neurons produces an immediate muscle contraction and a reflexive kick.

on the patellar ligament stretches muscle spindles in the quadriceps muscles (Figure 9-3•). With so brief a stimulus, the reflexive contraction occurs unopposed and produces a noticeable kick. If this contraction shortens the muscle spindles below their original resting lengths, the sensory nerve endings are compressed, the sensory neuron is inhibited, and the leg drops back.

Complex Reflexes

Many spinal reflexes have at least one interneuron between the sensory (afferent) neuron and the motor (efferent) neuron. Because there are more synapses, these **polysynaptic reflexes** have a longer delay between a stimulus and response. But they can produce far more complicated responses because the interneurons can control several muscle groups simultaneously.

Withdrawal Reflexes

Withdrawal reflexes move stimulated parts of the body away from a source of stimulation. The strongest withdrawal reflexes are triggered by painful stimuli, but these reflexes are also initiated by the stimulation of touch or pressure receptors. The **flexor reflex** is a withdrawal reflex affecting the muscles of a limb. Stepping on a tack produces a dramatic flexor reflex in the affected limb (Figure 9-4•). When the pain receptors in the foot are stimulated, the sensory neurons activate interneurons in the spinal cord that stimulate motor neurons in the anterior gray horns. The result is a contraction of flexor muscles that yanks the foot off the ground.

When a specific muscle contracts, opposing, or *antagonistic*, muscles are stretched. For example, the flexor muscles that bend the knee are opposed by *extensor muscles*, which straighten it out. A potential conflict exists here: Contraction of a flexor muscle should trigger a stretch reflex in the extensors that would cause them to contract, opposing the movement that is under way. Interneurons in the spinal cord prevent such competition through **reciprocal inhibition**. When one set of motor neurons is stimulated, those controlling antagonistic muscles are inhibited.

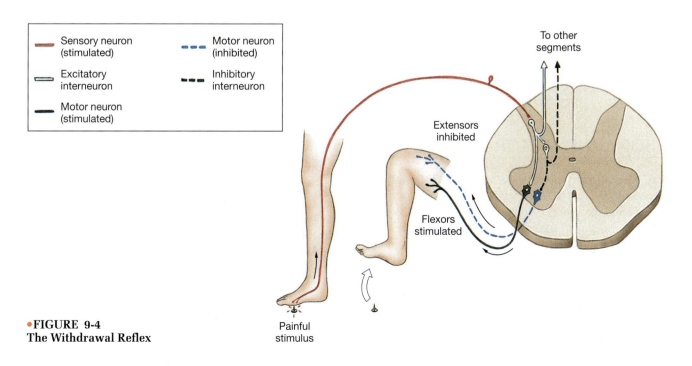

——	Sensory neuron (stimulated)	- - -	Motor neuron (inhibited)
——	Excitatory interneuron	■■■	Inhibitory interneuron
——	Motor neuron (stimulated)		

•FIGURE 9-4
The Withdrawal Reflex

Integration and Control of Spinal Reflexes

Although reflexes are automatic, higher centers in the brain influence these responses by stimulating or inhibiting the interneurons and motor neurons involved. The sensitivity of a reflex can thus be modified. For example, an effort to pull apart clasped hands elevates the general state of stimulation along the spinal cord, leading to the exaggeration of spinal reflexes.

Other descending fibers have an inhibitory effect on spinal reflexes. Stroking an infant's foot on the side of the sole produces a fanning of the toes known as the **Babinski sign**, or *positive Babinski reflex*. This response disappears as descending inhibitory synapses develop, so in adults the same stimulus produces a curling of the toes, called a **plantar reflex**, or *negative Babinski reflex*, after about a one-second delay. If either the higher centers or the descending tracts are damaged, the Babinski sign will reappear. As a result, this reflex is often tested if CNS injury is suspected.

When higher centers issue motor commands, they can activate the complex motor patterns already programmed into the spinal cord. The use of preexisting patterns allows a relatively small number of descending fibers to control complex motor functions. For example, the motor patterns for walking, running, and jumping are primarily directed by neuronal pools in the spinal cord. The descending pathways facilitate, inhibit, or fine-tune the established patterns.

✓ Which common reflex is used by physicians to test the general condition of the spinal cord, peripheral nerves, and muscles?

✓ Polysynaptic reflexes can produce more complicated responses than can monosynaptic reflexes. Why?

✓ After suffering an injury to his back, Tom exhibits a positive Babinski reflex. What does this reaction imply about Tom's injury?

SENSORY AND MOTOR PATHWAYS

As already mentioned, the communication between the central nervous system (CNS), the peripheral nervous system (PNS), and organs and systems occurs over pathways, nerve tracts, and nuclei that relay sensory and motor information. The major sensory (ascending) and motor (descending) tracts of the spinal cord are named with regard to the destinations of the axons. If the name of a tract begins with *spino-*, the tract *starts* in the spinal cord and ends in the brain, and it therefore carries sensory information. If the name of a tract ends in *-spinal*, its axons *start* in the higher centers and *end* in the spinal cord, bear-

TABLE 9-3	Sensory and Motor Pathways
Pathway	*Function*
SENSORY	
Posterior column pathway	Delivers highly localized sensations of fine touch, pressure, vibration, and proprioception to the primary sensory cortex
Spinothalamic pathway	Delivers poorly localized sensations of touch, pressure, pain, and temperature to the primary sensory cortex
Spinocerebellar pathway	Delivers proprioceptive information concerning the positions of muscles, bones, and joints to the cerebellar cortex
MOTOR	
Pyramidal system	Conscious control of skeletal muscles throughout the body
Extrapyramidal system	Subconscious regulation of skeletal muscle tone, controls reflexive skeletal muscle responses to equilibrium sensations and to sudden or strong visual and auditory stimuli

ing motor commands. The rest of the tract name indicates the associated nucleus or cortical area of the brain.

Table 9-3 lists examples of sensory and motor pathways and their functions.

Sensory Pathways

Sensory receptors monitor conditions in the body or the external environment. A **sensation**, the information gathered by a sensory receptor, arrives in the form of action potentials in an afferent (sensory) fiber. Most of the processing of arriving sensations occurs in centers along the sensory pathways in the spinal cord or brain stem; only about 1 percent of the information provided by afferent fibers reaches the cerebral cortex and our conscious awareness. For example, we usually do not feel the clothes we wear or hear the hum of the engine in our car.

The Posterior Column Pathway

One ascending, sensory pathway is the **posterior column pathway** (Figure 9-5•). It sends highly localized ("fine") touch, pressure, vibration, and proprioceptive (position) sensations to the cerebral cortex. In the

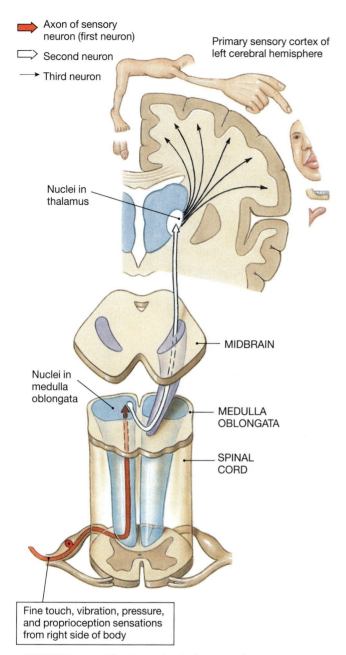

Axon of sensory neuron (first neuron)

Second neuron

Third neuron

Primary sensory cortex of left cerebral hemisphere

Nuclei in thalamus

MIDBRAIN

Nuclei in medulla oblongata

MEDULLA OBLONGATA

SPINAL CORD

Fine touch, vibration, pressure, and proprioception sensations from right side of body

•FIGURE 9-5 **The Posterior Column Pathway**
The posterior column pathway delivers fine touch, vibration, and proprioception information to the primary sensory cortex of the cerebral hemisphere on the opposite side of the body. (For clarity, this figure shows only the pathway for sensations originating on the right side of the body.)

process, the information is relayed from one neuron to another.

Step 1: The sensations reach the CNS through the dorsal roots of spinal nerves. (Recall from Chapter 8 that the dorsal roots contain the axons of sensory neurons.) ∞ *p. 230* Once inside the spinal cord, the axons ascend within the posterior column pathway to synapse in a sensory nucleus of the medulla oblongata.

Step 2: The axons of the neurons in this ganglion cross over to the opposite side of the brain stem before continuing to the thalamus.

Step 3: The location of the synapse in the thalamus depends on the region of the body involved. The thalamic neuron then relays the information to an appropriate primary sensory cortex.

The sensations arrive organized such that sensory information from the toes reaches one end of the primary sensory cortex and information from the head reaches the other. As a result, the sensory cortex contains a miniature map of the body surface. That map is distorted because the area of sensory cortex devoted to a particular region is proportional not to its size, but to the number of sensory receptors it contains. In other words, it takes many more cortical neurons to process sensory information arriving from the tongue, which has tens of thousands of taste and touch receptors, than it does to analyze sensations originating on the back, where touch receptors are few and far between.

Motor Pathways

In response to information provided by sensory systems, the CNS issues motor commands that are distributed by the *somatic nervous system* (*SNS*) and the *autonomic nervous system* (*ANS*). The SNS, under voluntary control, issues somatic motor commands that direct the contractions of skeletal muscles. The motor commands of the ANS, which are issued outside our conscious awareness, controls the smooth and cardiac muscles, glands, and fat cells.

Two integrated motor pathways, the *pyramidal system* and the *extrapyramidal system*, provide control over skeletal muscles. Refer to Table 9-3 for examples and functions of these motor pathways. We will focus on the pyramidal system, which provides conscious control.

The Pyramidal System

The **pyramidal system** provides conscious, voluntary control of skeletal muscles. Figure 9-6• shows the motor pathway providing voluntary control over the right side of the body. The neurons of the primary motor cortex are organized into a miniature map of the body. It is just as distorted as the sensory map on the primary sensory cortex; the proportions indicate the number of motor units present in that portion of the body. For example, the grossly oversized hands provide an indication of how many different muscles and motor units are involved in writing, grasping, and manipulating objects in our environment.

The pyramidal system begins at the **pyramidal cells** of the cerebral cortex. (In section, their cell bodies

9

resemble upside-down pyramids.) The axons of these cells extend into the brain stem and spinal cord to synapse on somatic motor neurons. For example, the *corticospinal tracts* (Figure 9-6•) synapse with motor neurons in the anterior gray horns of the spinal cord. All axons of the corticospinal tracts cross over to reach motor neurons on the opposite side of the body. As a result, the left side of the body is controlled by the right cerebral hemisphere, and the right side is controlled by the left cerebral hemisphere.

The Extrapyramidal System

The **extrapyramidal system** provides subconscious, involuntary control of skeletal tone. It coordinates learned movement patterns and other voluntary motor activities (Table 9-3).

The components of the extrapyramidal motor system are spread throughout the brain. They include nuclei in the brain stem (midbrain, pons, and medulla oblongata); relay stations in the thalamus; the cerebral nuclei (basal ganglia) of the cerebrum; and the cerebellum. Output from the cerebral nuclei and cerebellum exerts the highest level of control. For example, they can (1) stimulate or inhibit other extrapyramidal nuclei or (2) stimulate or inhibit the activities of pyramidal cells in the primary motor cortex. Axons from the brain stem's extrapyramidal motor nuclei synapse on the same motor neurons innervated by the pyramidal system.

✳ EXTRAPYRAMIDAL MOTOR SYNDROMES

Several of the drugs used in emergency medicine can cause side effects involving the *extrapyramidal system (EPS)*. The drugs most frequently implicated are those used in the treatment of nausea and vomiting and in the treatment of acute psychotic disorders. Most belong to a class of medications called *phenothiazines.* These drugs block the neurotransmitter *dopamine* in the brain and can affect the parts of the brain that control the EPS.

EPS side effects are similar to the effects of Parkinson's disease but are reversible. They are usually seen in the first few days of treatment and can be misdiagnosed as anxiety. EPS signs and symptoms include muscle spasms of the neck, face, tongue, and back *(dystonia);* a sensation of restlessness *(akathisia);* a shuffling gait; rigidity of the extremities; and drooling. These symptoms can be quite disconcerting for patients and their families.

Treatment usually results in prompt, and often dramatic, reversal of symptoms. Drugs used in the treatment of Parkinson's disease (benztropine) or antihistamines (diphenhydramine) are highly effective.

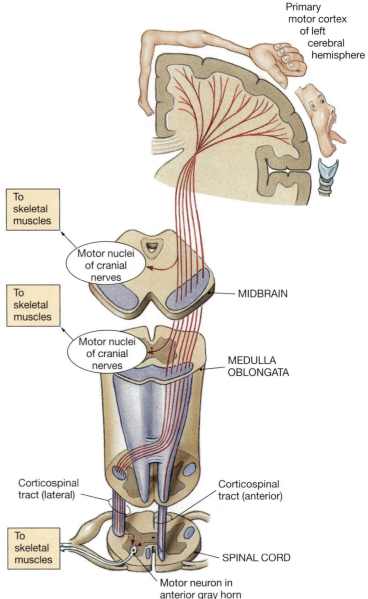

•FIGURE 9-6   The Pyramidal System
The pyramidal system originates at the primary motor cortex. Axons of the pyramidal cells descend to reach motor nuclei in the brain stem and spinal cord. Most of the pyramidal fibers cross over in the medulla oblongata before descending into the spinal cord as the corticospinal tracts.

✓ As a result of pressure on her spinal cord, Jill cannot feel touch or pressure on her legs. What sensory pathway is being compressed?

✓ The primary motor cortex of the right cerebral hemisphere controls motor function on which side of the body?

✓ An injury to the superior portion of the motor cortex would affect which part of the body?

THE AUTONOMIC NERVOUS SYSTEM

Using the pathways already discussed, we can respond to sensory information and exert voluntary control over the activities of our skeletal muscles. Yet our conscious sensations, plans, and responses represent only a tiny fraction of the activities of the nervous system. In practical terms, conscious activities have little to do with our immediate or long-term survival, and the adjustments made by the **autonomic nervous system** are much more important. Without the ANS, a simple night's sleep would be a life-threatening event.

Chapter 8 introduced the two efferent divisions of the nervous system, the **somatic nervous system** (SNS) and the autonomic nervous system. The SNS controls skeletal muscles over the pyramidal and extrapyramidal motor pathways. The ANS controls the involuntary regulation of smooth muscle, cardiac muscle, and glands. There are clear anatomical differences between the SNS and ANS (Figure 9-7•). In the ANS, there is always a synapse be-

tween the central nervous system and the peripheral effector. The motor neurons in the CNS, known as **preganglionic neurons**, send their axons, called *preganglionic fibers*, to *autonomic ganglia* outside the CNS. In these ganglia, the axons of the preganglionic neurons synapse on **ganglionic neurons**. The axons of these neurons leave the ganglia, and these **postganglionic fibers** innervate cardiac muscle, smooth muscles, glands, and adipocytes.

The ANS consists of two divisions: (1) the sympathetic division and (2) the parasympathetic division. Preganglionic fibers from the thoracic and lumbar spinal segments synapse in ganglia near the spinal cord; these axons and ganglia are part of the **sympathetic division** of the ANS. The sympathetic division is often called the "fight or flight" system because it usually stimulates tissue metabolism, increases alertness, and prepares the body to deal with emergencies.

Preganglionic fibers originating in the brain and the sacral spinal segments synapse on neurons of **intramural ganglia** (*murus*, wall), located near or within the tissues of visceral organs. These components are part of the **parasympathetic division** of the ANS, often

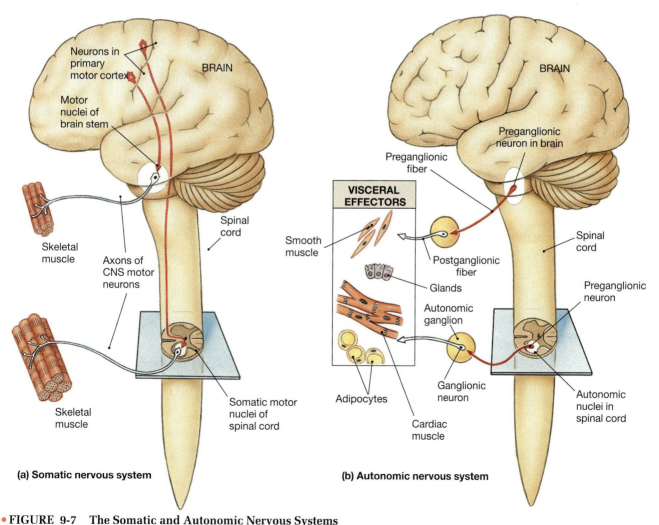

(a) Somatic nervous system

Neurons in primary motor cortex

BRAIN

Motor nuclei of brain stem

Skeletal muscle

Axons of CNS motor neurons

Spinal cord

Skeletal muscle

Somatic motor nuclei of spinal cord

(b) Autonomic nervous system

BRAIN

Preganglionic neuron in brain

Preganglionic fiber

VISCERAL EFFECTORS

Smooth muscle

Glands

Autonomic ganglion

Adipocytes

Cardiac muscle

Postganglionic fiber

Ganglionic neuron

Spinal cord

Preganglionic neuron

Autonomic nuclei in spinal cord

•**FIGURE 9-7   The Somatic and Autonomic Nervous Systems**
(a) In the SNS, a motor neuron in the CNS has direct control over skeletal muscle fibers. **(b)** In the ANS, preganglionic neurons synapse on ganglionic neurons that innervate effectors, such as smooth and cardiac muscles, glands, and fat cells.

regarded as the "rest and repose" or "rest and digest" system because it conserves energy and promotes sedentary activities, such as digestion.

The sympathetic and parasympathetic divisions affect target organs through the controlled release of specific neurotransmitters by the postganglionic fibers. Whether the result is a stimulation or an inhibition of activity depends on the response of the membrane receptor to the presence of the neurotransmitter. Some general patterns are worth noting:

- All preganglionic autonomic fibers are *cholinergic*: They release acetylcholine (ACh) at their synaptic terminals. ∞ *p. 225* The effects are always excitatory.
- Postganglionic parasympathetic fibers are also cholinergic, but the effects are excitatory or inhibitory, depending on the nature of the target cell receptor.
- Most postganglionic sympathetic terminals are *adrenergic*: They release norepinephrine (NE). ∞ *p. 225* The effects are usually excitatory.

The Sympathetic Division

The sympathetic division (Figure 9-8●) consists of:

- *Preganglionic neurons located between segments T_1 and L_2 of the spinal cord.* These neurons are situated in the lateral gray horns, and their short axons enter the ventral roots of these segments.
- *Ganglionic neurons located in ganglia near the vertebral column.* Two types of sympathetic ganglia exist. Paired *sympathetic chain ganglia* on either side of the vertebral column contain neurons that control effectors in the body wall and inside the thoracic cavity. Unpaired *collateral ganglia*, anterior to the vertebral column, contain ganglionic neurons that innervate tissues and organs in the abdominopelvic cavity.
- *Specialized neurons in a modified ganglion in the interior of each adrenal gland*, a region known as the *adrenal medulla*. The ganglionic neurons of the medullae have very short axons—when stimulated, they release the neurotransmitters norepinephrine and epinephrine into the general circulation.

The sympathetic division shows extensive divergence, and a single sympathetic motor neuron inside the CNS can produce a complex and coordinated response.

The Sympathetic Chain

From spinal segments T_1 to L_2, sympathetic preganglionic fibers join the ventral root of each spinal nerve. All of these fibers then exit the spinal nerve to enter the sympathetic chain ganglia. For motor commands to the body wall, a synapse occurs at the chain ganglia, and then the postganglionic fibers return to the spinal nerve for distribution. For the thoracic cavity, a synapse also occurs at the chain ganglia, but the postganglionic fibers then form nerves that go directly to their targets (Figure 9-8●).

Sympathetic innervation distributed by the spinal nerves stimulates sweat gland activity and arrector pili muscles (producing "goose bumps"), reduces circulation to the skin and body wall, accelerates blood flow to skeletal muscles, releases stored lipids from adipose tissue, and dilates the pupils. The activation of the autonomic nerves accelerates the heart rate, increases the force of cardiac contractions, and dilates the respiratory passageways. All of these changes prepare the individual for sudden, intense physical activity.

The Collateral Ganglia

The abdominopelvic viscera receive sympathetic innervation over preganglionic fibers from lower thoracic and upper lumbar segments that pass through the sympathetic chain without synapsing, and instead synapse within separate, unpaired **collateral ganglia**. The nerves traveling to the collateral ganglia are known as *splanchnic nerves*. The three collateral ganglia and the organs their postganglionic fibers innervate are diagrammed in Figure 9-8●.

The fibers leaving the collateral ganglia extend throughout the abdominopelvic cavity. In general, they reduce the blood flow and energy use by visceral organs that are not important to short-term survival, such as the digestive tract, and they stimulate the release of stored carbohydrate and lipid reserves.

The Adrenal Medullae

Preganglionic fibers entering each adrenal gland proceed to its center, to the region called the **adrenal medulla**. There they synapse on modified neurons that perform an endocrine function. When stimulated, these cells release the neurotransmitters norepinephrine and epinephrine into surrounding capillaries, which carry them throughout the body. In general, the effects of these neurotransmitters resemble those produced by the stimulation of sympathetic postganglionic fibers. However, (1) they also affect cells not innervated by sympathetic postganglionic fibers, and (2) their effects last much longer than those produced by direct sympathetic innervation.

The Parasympathetic Division

The parasympathetic division of the ANS includes:

- *Preganglionic neurons in the brain stem (midbrain, pons, and medulla oblongata) and in the lateral gray horns of sacral segments S_2 to S_4.*
- *Ganglionic neurons in peripheral ganglia or adjacent to the target organs.* Preganglionic fibers of the parasympathetic division do not diverge as extensively as those of the sympathetic division. Thus, the effects of parasympathetic stimulation are more specific and localized than those of the sympathetic division.

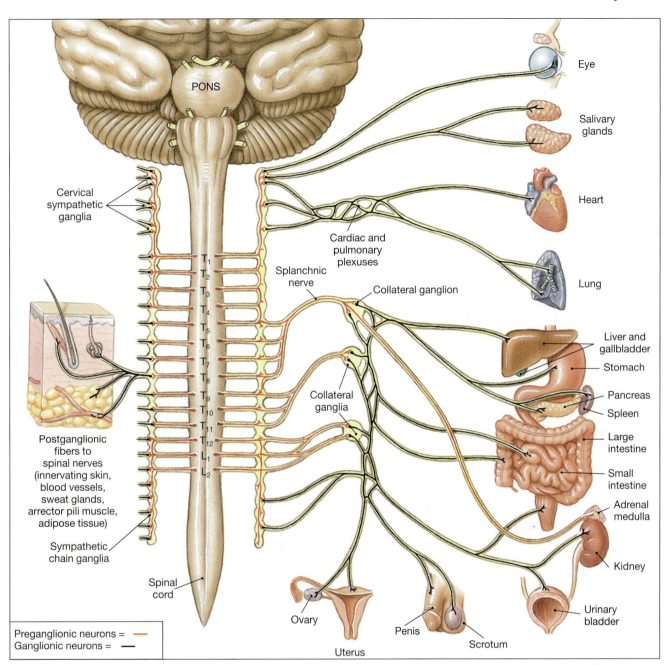

●**FIGURE 9-8   The Sympathetic Division**
The distribution of sympathetic fibers is the same on both sides of the body. For clarity, the innervation of somatic structures is shown to the left and the innervation of visceral structures to the right.

Organization

Figure 9-9● diagrams the pattern of parasympathetic innervation. Preganglionic fibers leaving the brain travel within cranial nerves III (oculomotor), VII (facial), IX (glossopharyngeal), and X (vagus). These fibers synapse in ganglia located in peripheral tissues, and short postganglionic fibers then continue to their targets. The vagus nerves provide preganglionic parasympathetic innervation to ganglia in organs of the thoracic and abdominopelvic cavities as distant as the last segments of the large intestine. The vagus nerves provide roughly 75 percent of all parasympathetic outflow and innervate most of those organs.

The sacral parasympathetic outflow leaves the sacral segments of the spinal cord, and the preganglionic fibers form distinct **pelvic nerves**, which innervate intramural ganglia in the kidney and urinary bladder, the last segments of the large intestine, and the sex organs.

General Functions

Among other things, the parasympathetic division constricts the pupils, increases secretions by the digestive glands, increases smooth muscle activity of the digestive tract, stimulates defecation and urination, constricts respiratory passageways, and reduces the heart rate and

9

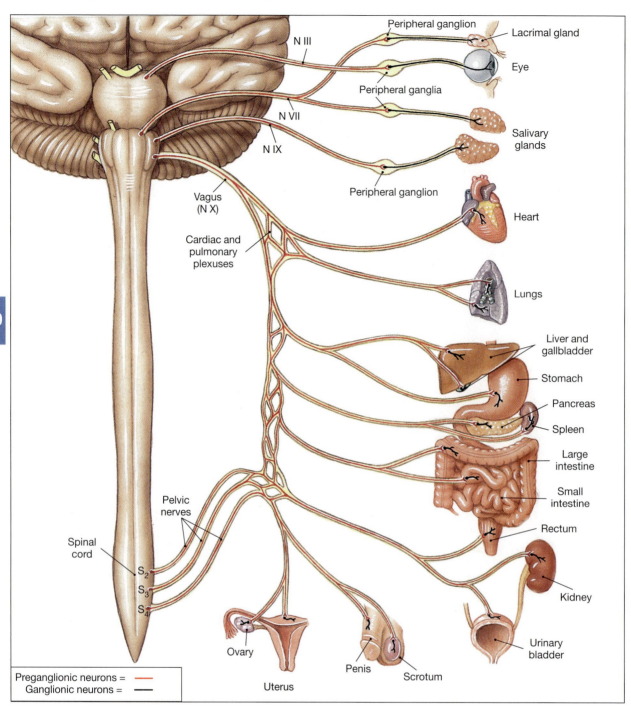

Peripheral ganglion
Lacrimal gland
N III
Eye
Peripheral ganglia
Peripheral ganglion
Salivary glands
N VII
N IX
Vagus (N X)
Heart
Cardiac and pulmonary plexuses
Lungs
Liver and gallbladder
Stomach
Pancreas
Spleen
Large intestine
Small intestine
Pelvic nerves
Rectum
Spinal cord
Kidney
S_2
S_3
S_4
Urinary bladder
Ovary
Penis
Scrotum
Uterus

Preganglionic neurons = ——
Ganglionic neurons = ——

•**FIGURE 9-9   The Parasympathetic Division**
The distribution of parasympathetic fibers is the same on both sides of the body.

the force of cardiac contractions. These functions center on relaxation, food processing, and energy absorption. Stimulation of the parasympathetic division leads to a general increase in the nutrient content of the blood. Cells throughout the body respond to this increase by absorbing nutrients and using them to support growth and the storage of energy reserves. The effects of parasympathetic stimulation are usually brief and are restricted to specific organs and sites.

Relationships between the Sympathetic and Parasympathetic Divisions

The sympathetic division has widespread impact, reaching visceral and somatic structures throughout the body, whereas the parasympathetic division innervates only visceral structures serviced by the cranial nerves or lying within the abdominopelvic cavity. Although some or-

TABLE 9-4	The Effects of the Sympathetic and Parasympathetic Divisions of the ANS on Various Organs	
Structure	*Sympathetic Innervation Effect*	*Parasympathetic Innervation Effect*
EYE	Dilation of pupil Focusing for distance vision	Constriction of pupil Focusing for near vision
SKIN **Sweat glands** **Arrector pili muscles**	 Increases secretion Contraction, erection of hairs	 None (not innervated) None (not innervated)
TEAR GLANDS	None (not innervated)	Secretion

CARDIOVASCULAR SYSTEM
Blood vessels
Heart
	
	Vasoconstriction and vasodilation
	Increases heart rate, force of
	  contraction, and blood pressure
		
		None (not innervated)
		Decreases heart rate, force of
		  contraction, and blood pressure

ADRENAL GLANDS	Secretion of epinephrine and norepinephrine by adrenal medullae	None (not innervated)
RESPIRATORY SYSTEM **Airways** **Respiratory rate**	 Increases diameter Increases rate	 Decreases diameter Decreases rate
DIGESTIVE SYSTEM **General level of activity** **Liver**	 Decreases activity Glycogen breakdown, glucose synthesis and release	 Increases activity Glycogen synthesis
SKELETAL MUSCLES	Increases force of contraction, glycogen breakdown	None (not innervated)

URINARY SYSTEM
Kidneys
Urinary bladder
	
	Decreases urine production
	Constricts sphincter, relaxes
	  urinary bladder
		
		Increases urine production
		Tenses urinary bladder, relaxes
		  sphincter to eliminate urine

REPRODUCTIVE SYSTEM	Increased glandular secretions;
	  ejaculation in males
		Erection of penis (males)
		  or clitoris (females)

9

gans are innervated by one division or the other, most vital organs receive **dual innervation**—that is, instructions from both autonomic divisions. Where dual innervation exists, the two divisions often have opposing effects. Table 9-4 provides examples of different organs and the effects of either single or dual innervation.

✓ While out for a brisk walk, Megan is suddenly confronted by an angry dog. Which division of the ANS is responsible for the physiological changes that occur as she turns and runs from the animal?

✓ Why is the parasympathetic division of the ANS sometimes referred to as the anabolic system?

✓ What effect would loss of sympathetic stimulation have on blood flow to a tissue?

✓ What physiological changes would you expect to observe in a patient who is about to undergo a root canal procedure and who is quite anxious about it?

INTEGRATION WITH OTHER SYSTEMS

The relationships between the nervous system and other organ systems are shown in Figure 9-10•. Many of these interactions will be explored in detail in later chapters.

Chapter Review

KEY TERMS

adrenal medulla, *p. 262*	**ganglion/ganglia**, *p. 252*	**preganglionic neuron**, *p. 261*
autonomic nervous system (ANS), *p. 261*	**nerve plexus**, *p. 256* **parasympathetic division**, *p. 261*	**reflex**, *p. 256* **somatic nervous system**, *p. 261*
cranial nerves, *p. 252*	**polysynaptic reflex**, *p. 257*	**spinal nerves**, *p. 255*
dual innervation, *p. 265*	**postganglionic fiber**, *p. 261*	**sympathetic division**, *p. 261*

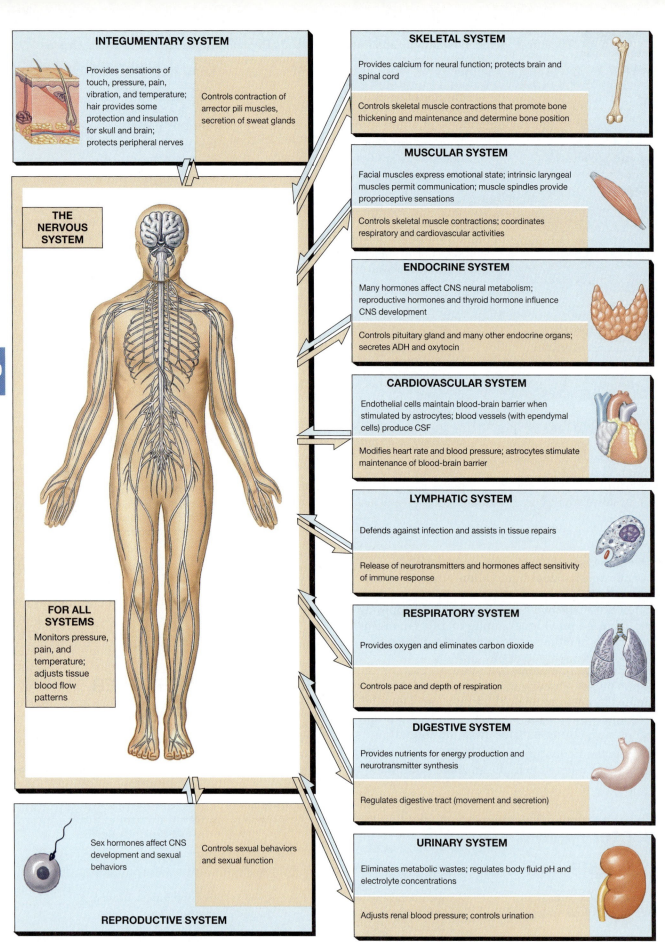

INTEGUMENTARY SYSTEM

Provides sensations of touch, pressure, pain, vibration, and temperature; hair provides some protection and insulation for skull and brain; protects peripheral nerves

Controls contraction of arrector pili muscles, secretion of sweat glands

SKELETAL SYSTEM

Provides calcium for neural function; protects brain and spinal cord

Controls skeletal muscle contractions that promote bone thickening and maintenance and determine bone position

MUSCULAR SYSTEM

Facial muscles express emotional state; intrinsic laryngeal muscles permit communication; muscle spindles provide proprioceptive sensations

Controls skeletal muscle contractions; coordinates respiratory and cardiovascular activities

ENDOCRINE SYSTEM

Many hormones affect CNS neural metabolism; reproductive hormones and thyroid hormone influence CNS development

Controls pituitary gland and many other endocrine organs; secretes ADH and oxytocin

CARDIOVASCULAR SYSTEM

Endothelial cells maintain blood-brain barrier when stimulated by astrocytes; blood vessels (with ependymal cells) produce CSF

Modifies heart rate and blood pressure; astrocytes stimulate maintenance of blood-brain barrier

LYMPHATIC SYSTEM

Defends against infection and assists in tissue repairs

Release of neurotransmitters and hormones affect sensitivity of immune response

RESPIRATORY SYSTEM

Provides oxygen and eliminates carbon dioxide

Controls pace and depth of respiration

DIGESTIVE SYSTEM

Provides nutrients for energy production and neurotransmitter synthesis

Regulates digestive tract (movement and secretion)

URINARY SYSTEM

Eliminates metabolic wastes; regulates body fluid pH and electrolyte concentrations

Adjusts renal blood pressure; controls urination

THE NERVOUS SYSTEM

FOR ALL SYSTEMS

Monitors pressure, pain, and temperature; adjusts tissue blood flow patterns

Sex hormones affect CNS development and sexual behaviors

Controls sexual behaviors and sexual function

REPRODUCTIVE SYSTEM

9

•FIGURE 9-10   Functional Relationships Between the Nervous System and Other Systems

SUMMARY OUTLINE

INTRODUCTION *p. 252*

1. The **peripheral nervous system (PNS)** links the central nervous system (CNS) with the rest of the body; all sensory information and motor commands are carried by axons of the PNS.

THE PERIPHERAL NERVOUS SYSTEM *p. 252*

1. Structures of the PNS include sensory and motor axons bundled together into **peripheral nerves**, or nerves, and clusters of cell bodies, or **ganglia**.

2. The PNS includes cranial nerves and spinal nerves.

The Cranial Nerves *p. 252*

3. There are 12 pairs of **cranial nerves**, which connect to the brain, not to the spinal cord. *(Figure 9-1; Table 9-1)*

4. The **olfactory nerves (N I)** carry sensory information responsible for the sense of smell.

5. The **optic nerves (N II)** carry visual information from special sensory receptors in the eyes.

6. The **oculomotor nerves (N III)** are the primary sources of innervation for four of the six muscles that move the eyeball.

7. The **trochlear nerves (N IV)**, the smallest cranial nerves, innervate the superior oblique muscles of the eyes.

8. The **trigeminal nerves (N V)**, the largest cranial nerves, are mixed nerves with ophthalmic, maxillary, and mandibular branches.

9. The **abducens nerves (N VI)** innervate the sixth extrinsic eye muscle, the lateral rectus.

10. The **facial nerves (N VII)** are mixed nerves that control muscles of the scalp and face. They provide pressure sensations over the face and receive taste information from the tongue.

11. The **vestibulocochlear nerves (N VIII)** contain the vestibular nerves, which monitor sensations of balance, position, and movement, and the cochlear nerves, which monitor hearing receptors.

12. The **glossopharyngeal nerves (N IX)** are mixed nerves that innervate the tongue and pharynx and control swallowing.

13. The **vagus nerves (N X)** are mixed nerves that are vital to the autonomic control of visceral function and have a variety of motor components.

14. The **accessory nerves (N XI)** have a medullary branch, which innervates voluntary swallowing muscles of the soft palate and pharynx, and a spinal branch, which controls muscles associated with the pectoral girdle.

15. The **hypoglossal nerves (N XII)** provide voluntary control over tongue movements.

The Spinal Nerves *p. 255*

16. There are 31 pairs of **spinal nerves**: 8 cervical, 12 thoracic, 5 lumbar, 5 sacral, and, 1 coccygeal. *(Figure 9-2)*

Nerve Plexuses *p. 256*

17. A complex, interwoven network of nerves is called a **nerve plexus**. The three large plexuses are the **cervical plexus**, the **brachial plexus**, and the **lumbosacral plexus**. The latter can be divided into the *lumbar plexus* and the *sacral plexus*. *(Figure 9-2; Table 9-2)*

THE CNS AND PNS: INTEGRATED FUNCTIONS *p. 256*

Simple Reflexes *p. 256*

1. A **monosynaptic reflex** is the simplest reflex arc, in which a sensory neuron synapses directly on a motor neuron that acts as the processing center.

2. The **stretch reflex** is a monosynaptic reflex that automatically regulates skeletal muscle length and muscle tone. The sensory receptors involved are **muscle spindles**. *(Figure 9-3)*

Complex Reflexes *p. 257*

3. **Polysynaptic reflexes**, which have at least one interneuron between the sensory afferent and the motor efferent, have a longer delay between stimulus and response than does a monosynaptic synapse.

4. Polysynaptic reflexes can also produce more complicated responses. Examples include the **withdrawal reflexes**, which move affected portions of the body away from a source of stimulation. The **flexor reflex** is a withdrawal reflex affecting the muscles of a limb. *(Figure 9-4)*

Integration and Control of Spinal Reflexes *p. 258*

5. The brain can facilitate or inhibit reflex motor patterns based in the spinal cord.

6. Motor control involves a series of interacting levels. Monosynaptic reflexes form the lowest level, while at the highest level are the centers in the brain that can enhance, inhibit, or build on programmed reflexes.

SENSORY AND MOTOR PATHWAYS *p. 258*

1. The essential communication between the CNS and PNS occurs over pathways that relay sensory information and motor commands. *(Table 9-3)*

Sensory Pathways *p. 258*

2. A **sensation** arrives in the form of an action potential in an afferent fiber. The **posterior column pathway** carries fine touch, pressure, and proprioceptive sensations. The axons ascend within this pathway and synapse with neurons in the medulla oblongata. These axons then cross over and travel on to the thalamus. The thalamus sorts the sensations according to the region of the body involved and projects them to specific regions of the primary sensory cortex. *(Figure 9-5; Table 9-3)*

Motor Pathways *p. 259*

3. The neurons of the primary motor cortex are **pyramidal cells**. The **pyramidal system** provides conscious skeletal muscle control. The pyramidal system provides a rapid, direct mechanism for controlling skeletal muscles. *(Figure 9-6; Table 9-3)*

4. The **extrapyramidal system** exerts subconscious control over skeletal muscles.

THE AUTONOMIC NERVOUS SYSTEM *p. 261*

1. The autonomic nervous system (ANS) coordinates cardiovascular, respiratory, digestive, excretory, and reproductive functions.

2. **Preganglionic neurons** in the CNS send axons to synapse on **ganglionic neurons** in **autonomic ganglia** outside the CNS. The axons of the ganglionic neurons (postganglionic fibers)

9

innervate cardiac muscle, smooth muscles, glands, and adipose tissues. *(Figure 9-7)*

3. Preganglionic fibers from the thoracic and lumbar segments form the **sympathetic division** ("fight or flight" system) of the ANS. Preganglionic fibers leaving the brain and sacral segments form the **parasympathetic division** ("rest and repose" or "rest and digest" system).

The Sympathetic Division *p. 262*

4. The sympathetic division consists of preganglionic neurons between segments T_1 and L_2, ganglionic neurons in ganglia near the vertebral column, and specialized neurons in the adrenal gland. Sympathetic ganglia are paired **sympathetic chain ganglia** or unpaired **collateral ganglia**. *(Figure 9-8)*

5. Some postganglionic fibers enter each spinal nerve to innervate the body wall and limbs. Postganglionic fibers targeting thoracic cavity structures form nerves that go directly to their visceral destination. Preganglionic fibers running between the sympathetic chain ganglia interconnect them to form an elongated sympathetic chain. *(Figure 9-8)*

6. The abdominopelvic viscera receive sympathetic innervation via preganglionic fibers that synapse within collateral ganglia. The preganglionic fibers that innervate the three collateral ganglia form the *splanchnic nerves. (Figure 9-8)*

7. Preganglionic fibers entering the adrenal glands synapse within the **adrenal medullae**. During sympathetic activation these endocrine organs secrete epinephrine and norepinephrine into the bloodstream.

8. In crises, the entire division responds, producing increased alertness, a feeling of energy and euphoria, increased cardiovascular and respiratory activity, and elevation in muscle tone.

The Parasympathetic Division *p. 262*

9. The parasympathetic division includes preganglionic neurons in the brain stem and sacral segments of the spinal cord and ganglionic neurons in peripheral ganglia located within or next to target organs. *(Figure 9-9)*

10. Preganglionic fibers leaving the sacral segments form **pelvic nerves**. *(Figure 9-9)*

11. The effects produced by the parasympathetic division center on relaxation, food processing, and energy absorption.

12. The effects of stimulation are usually brief and restricted to specific sites.

Relationships between the Sympathetic and Parasympathetic Divisions *p. 264*

13. The sympathetic division has widespread impact, reaching visceral and somatic structures throughout the body.

14. The parasympathetic division innervates only visceral structures serviced by cranial nerves or lying within the abdominopelvic cavity. Organs with **dual innervation** receive instructions from both divisions. *(Table 9-4)*

INTEGRATION WITH OTHER SYSTEMS *p. 265*

1. The nervous system monitors pressure, pain, and temperature and adjusts tissue blood flow for all systems. *(Figure 9-10)*

REVIEW QUESTIONS

LEVEL 1   Reviewing Facts and Terms

Match each item in column A with the most closely related item in column B. Use letters for answers in the spaces provided.

Column A

___ 1. olfactory nerve
___ 2. optic nerve
___ 3. vestibulocochlear nerve
___ 4. hypoglossal nerve
___ 5. sympathetic division
___ 6. parasympathetic division
___ 7. somatic nervous system
___ 8. autonomic nervous system
___ 9. monosynaptic reflex
___10. polysynaptic reflex
___11. negative Babinski reflex
___12. dual innervation
___13. Babinski sign

Column B

a. "fight or flight"
b. controls smooth and cardiac muscle and glands
c. sensory, vision
d. stretch reflex
e. opposing effects
f. motor, tongue movements
g. equilibrium, hearing
h. controls contractions of skeletal muscles
i. sensory, smell
j. "rest and repose"
k. plantar reflex
l. flexor reflex
m. fanning of toes on infant's foot

14. Spinal nerves are called mixed nerves because they:
    (a) contain sensory and motor fibers
    (b) exit at intervertebral foramina
    (c) are associated with a pair of dorsal root ganglia
    (d) are associated with a pair of dorsal and ventral roots

15. If a tract name begins with *spino-*, it:
    (a) starts in the brain and ends in the spinal cord
    (b) carries motor commands from brain to spinal cord
    (c) carries sensory information from brain to spinal cord
    (d) starts in the spinal cord and ends in the brain

16. The contraction of flexor muscles and the relaxation of extensor muscles illustrates the principle of:
    (a) reverberating circuitry
    (b) generalized facilitation
    (c) reciprocal inhibition
    (d) reinforcement

17. There is always a synapse between the CNS and the peripheral effector in the:
    (a) ANS   (b) SNS
    (c) reflex arc   (d) a, b, and c are correct

18. All preganglionic autonomic fibers release _____ at their synaptic terminals, and the effects are always _____.
    (a) NE; inhibitory   (b) NE; excitatory
    (c) ACh; excitatory   (d) ACh; inhibitory

19. Approximately 75 percent of parasympathetic outflow is provided by the:
    (a) vagus nerve   (b) sciatic nerve
    (c) glossopharyngeal nerves   (d) pelvic nerves

20. Using the mnemonic device "Oh, Once One Takes The Anatomy Final, Very Good Vacations Are Heavenly," list the 12 pairs of cranial nerves and their functions.

21. What are pyramidal cells, and what is their function?

22. How does the emergence of sympathetic fibers from the spinal cord differ from the emergence of parasympathetic fibers?

LEVEL 2   Reviewing Concepts

23. Dual innervation refers to situations in which:
    (a) vital organs receive instructions from sympathetic and parasympathetic fibers
    (b) the atria and ventricles of the heart receive autonomic stimulation from the same nerves
    (c) sympathetic and parasympathetic fibers have similar effects
    (d) a, b, and c are correct

24. Why is response time in a monosynaptic reflex much faster than response time in a polysynaptic reflex?

25. Compare the general effects of the sympathetic and parasympathetic divisions of the ANS.

26. Why is the adrenal medulla considered to be a modified sympathetic ganglion?

27. You are alone in your home late at night when you hear what sounds like breaking glass. What physiological effects would this experience probably produce, and what would be their cause?

9

LEVEL 3   Critical-Thinking and Clinical Applications

28. In some severe cases of stomach ulcers, the branches of the vagus nerve (N X) that lead to the stomach are surgically severed. How might this procedure control the ulcers?

29. Improper use of crutches can produce a condition known as crutch paralysis, which is characterized by a lack of response by the extensor muscles of the arm and a condition known as wrist drop. Which nerve is involved?

30. While playing football, Ramon is tackled hard and suffers an injury to his left leg. As he tries to get up, he finds that he cannot flex his left hip or extend the knee. Which nerve is damaged, and how would this damage affect sensory perception in the left leg?

ANSWERS TO CONCEPT CHECK QUESTIONS

Page 255
1. The abducens nerve (N VI) controls lateral movements of the eyes via the lateral rectus muscles. An individual with damage to this nerve would be unable to move his or her eyes laterally, or to the side. **2.** The hypoglossal nerve (N XII) controls the voluntary muscles of the tongue.

Page 258
1. Physicians use the sensitivity of stretch reflexes, such as the knee jerk, or *patellar reflex,* to test the general condition of the spinal cord, peripheral nerves, and muscles. **2.** In a monosynaptic reflex, a sensory neuron synapses directly on a motor neuron and produces a rapid, stereotyped movement. More complicated responses occur with polysynaptic reflexes because the interneurons between the sensory and motor neurons may control several muscle groups simultaneously. In addition, some interneurons may stimulate a muscle group or groups, while others may inhibit other muscle groups. **3.** A positive Babinski reflex is abnormal for an adult and indicates possible damage of descending tracts in the spinal cord.

Page 260
1. A tract within the posterior column of the spinal cord is responsible for carrying information about touch and pressure from the lower part of the body to the brain. **2.** The anatomical basis of opposite-side motor control is that crossing-over occurs, so the pyramidal motor fibers innervate lower motor neurons on the opposite side of the body.

Most of the axons of the pyramidal cells cross over to opposite sides in the medulla oblongata. **3.** The superior portion of the motor cortex exercises control over the hand, arm, and upper portion of the leg. An injury to this area would affect the ability to control the muscles in those regions of the body.

Page 265
1. The sympathetic division of the autonomic nervous system is responsible for the physiological changes that occur in response to stress and increased activity. **2.** The parasympathetic division is sometimes referred to as the anabolic system because parasympathetic stimulation leads to a general increase in the nutrient content of the blood. Cells throughout the body respond to the increase by absorbing the nutrients and using them to support growth and other anabolic activities. **3.** Since most blood vessels receive sympathetic stimulation, a decrease in sympathetic stimulation would lead to a relaxation of the muscles in the walls of the vessels and vasodilation (an increase in vessel diameter). These in turn would result in increased blood flow to the tissue. **4.** A patient who is anxious about an impending root canal would probably exhibit some or all of the following changes: a dry mouth, increased heart rate, increased blood pressure, increased rate of breathing, cold sweats, an urge to urinate or defecate, change in motility of the digestive tract ("butterflies" in the stomach), and dilated pupils. These changes would be the result of anxiety or stress causing an increase in sympathetic stimulation.

OVERVIEW

Most of the autonomic nervous system (ANS) is located within the peripheral nervous system. The autonomic nervous system controls all involuntary (automatic) functions. The sympathetic and parasympathetic components of the ANS are in constant opposition. During periods of stress, the effects of the sympathetic nervous system predominate. During periods of rest, the effects of the parasympathetic nervous system predominate.

The sympathetic nervous system arises from the thoracic and lumbar segments of the spinal cord. Sympathetic preganglionic fibers are short and terminate in the sympathetic chain ganglia adjacent to the spinal column. Long postganglionic fibers exit the sympathetic chain and innervate the target organs.

The parasympathetic nervous system arises from four cranial nerves and the sacral region of the spinal cord. Cranial nerves III, VII, IX, and X contain parasympathetic fibers. Parasympathetic preganglionic fibers from these four cranial nerves and from sacral segments of the spinal cord are long, terminating in ganglia that are located near the target organs. The postganglionic fibers exit the parasympathetic ganglia and innervate the target organs.

Because several of the common emergency medications affect various components of the autonomic nervous system, emergency personnel should have a good understanding of the autonomic nervous system and of the emergencies that involve its components.

NEUROTRANSMITTERS

No actual physical connection exists between two nerve cells or between a nerve cell and the organ it innervates. Instead, there is a space or *synapse,* between nerve cells. Specialized chemicals called *neurotransmitters* conduct the nervous impulse between nerve cells or between a nerve cell and its target organ.

The two neurotransmitters of the autonomic nervous system are *acetylcholine* and *norepinephrine.* Acetylcholine is utilized in the preganglionic nerves of the sympathetic nervous system and in both the preganglionic and postganglionic nerves of the parasympathetic nervous system. Norepinephrine is the postganglionic neurotransmitter of the sympathetic nervous system. Synapses that use acetylcholine as the neurotransmitter are *cholinergic synapses.* Synapses that use norepinephrine as the neurotransmitter are *adrenergic synapses.*

PARASYMPATHETIC NERVOUS SYSTEM

Acetylcholine, which is present in the neuromuscular junction, is the neurotransmitter for the somatic nervous system as well as for the parasympathetic nervous system. Acetylcholine is very short-lived. Within a fraction of a second after its release, it is deactivated by another chemical called *acetylcholinesterase.* Acetylcholinesterase, commonly called *cholinesterase,* breaks acetylcholine into *acetic acid* and *choline.* These two substances are taken back up by the presynaptic neuron and recycled for future use (Figure A9-1●).

The parasympathetic nervous system has two types of acetylcholine receptors, *nicotinic* and *muscarinic.* Understanding these receptors will significantly aid in understanding the function of many emergency medications. *Nicotinic$_N$* (neuron) receptors are found in all autonomic ganglia, both parasympathetic and sympathetic, where acetylcholine serves as the neurotransmitter. *Nicotinic$_M$* (muscle) receptors are found on the neuromuscular junction and initiate muscle contraction as part of somatic nervous system function. *Muscarinic* receptors are found in many organs throughout the body and are primarily responsible for promoting the parasympathetic response. Table *A9-1* summarizes the locations and actions of muscarinic receptors. Because both nicotinic and muscarinic receptors are specific for acetylcholine, they are collectively referred to as cholinergic receptors.

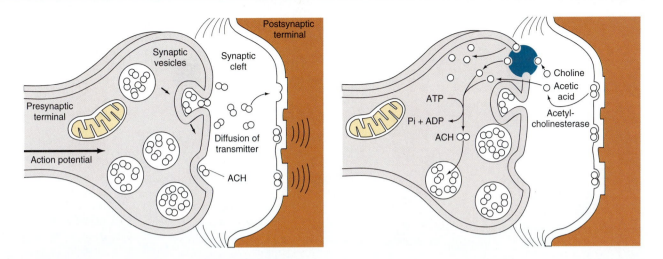

• **FIGURE A9-1   Acetylcholine Neurotransmission**
Acetylcholine is the neurotransmitter of the parasympathetic nervous system, the ganglia of the sympathetic nervous system, and the somatic nervous system. It is promptly degraded into acetic acid and choline by the enzyme acetylcholinesterase and those components are taken up by the presynaptic membrane.

TABLE A9-1	Location and Effect of Muscarinic Receptors	
Organ	*Functions*	*Location*
Heart	Decreased heart rate	Sinoatrial node
	Decreased conduction rate	Atrioventricular node
Arterioles	Dilation	Coronary
	Dilation	Skin and mucosa
	Dilation	Cerebral
GI Tract	Relaxed	Sphincters
	Increased	Motility
	Increased salivation	Salivary glands
	Increased secretion	Exocrine glands
Lungs	Bronchoconstriction	Bronchiole smooth muscle
	Increased mucus production	Bronchial glands
Gallbladder	Contraction	
Urinary bladder	Relaxation	Urinary sphincter
	Contraction	Detrusor muscle
Liver	Glycogen synthesis	
Lacrimal glands	Secretion (increased tearing)	Eye
Eye	Contraction for near vision	Ciliary muscle
	Constriction	Pupil
Penis	Erection	

SYMPATHETIC NERVOUS SYSTEM

Sympathetic stimulation ultimately results in the release of norepinephrine from postganglionic sympathetic nerves. The norepinephrine crosses the synaptic cleft and interacts with adrenergic receptors on the postsynaptic nerves or target organ. Shortly thereafter, the norepinephrine is either taken up whole by the presynaptic neuron for reuse or broken down by enzyme systems within the synapse. The two most common of these enzyme systems are *monamine oxidase (MAO)* and *catechol-O-methyltransferase (COMT)* (Figure A9-2•). Sympathetic stimulation also results in the release of epinephrine and

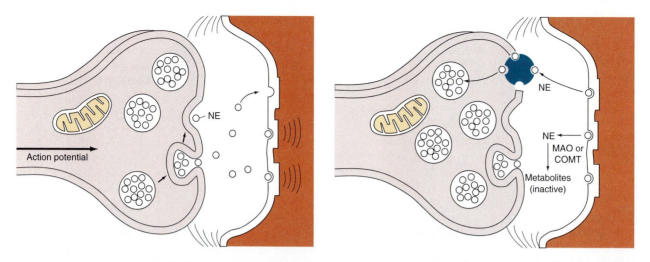

● **FIGURE A9-2** **Norepinephrine Neurotransmission**
Norepinephrine is the neurotransmitter of the postganglionic sympathetic nervous system. It is taken up into the presynaptic membrane or broken down by the enzymes monamine oxidase or catechol-O-methyltransferase.

TABLE A9-2	Location of Adrenergic Receptors and Effects of Stimulation	
Receptor	*Response to Stimulation*	*Location*
Alpha 1 (α_1)	Constriction	Arterioles
	Constriction	Veins
	Mydriasis	Eye
	Ejaculation	Penis
Alpha 2 (α_2)	Presynaptic terminals inhibition*	
Beta 1 (β_1)	Increased heart rate	Heart
	Increased conductivity	
	Increased automaticity	
	Increased contractility	
	Renin release	Kidney
Beta 2 (β_2)	Bronchodilation	Lungs
	Dilation	Arterioles
	Inhibition of contractions	Uterus
	Tremors	Skeletal muscle
Dopaminergic	Vasodilation (increased blood flow)	Kidney, Heart, Brain

Stimulation of α_2 adrenergic receptors inhibits the continued release of norepinephrine from the presynaptic terminal. It is a feedback mechanism that limits the adrenergic response at the synapse. These receptors have no other identified peripheral effects.

norepinephrine from the adrenal medulla. These hormones interact with other adrenergic receptors on the membranes of target organs. This action effectively amplifies the magnitude of the sympathetic response.

The two known types of sympathetic receptors are the adrenergic receptors and the dopaminergic receptors. The adrenergic receptors are generally divided into four types. These four receptors are designated alpha 1 (α_1), alpha 2 (α_2), beta 1 (β_1), and beta 2 (β_2). The α_1 receptors cause peripheral vasoconstriction, mild bronchoconstriction, and stimulation of metabolism. The α_2 receptors are found on the presynaptic surfaces of sympathetic neuroeffector junctions. Stimulation of α_2 receptors is inhibitory. These receptors serve to prevent overrelease of norepinephrine in the synapse. When the level of norepinephrine in the synapse gets high enough, the α_2 receptors are stimulated and norepinephrine release is inhibited. Stimulation of the β_1 receptors causes an increase in heart rate, cardiac contractile force, and cardiac automaticity and conduction. Stimulation of β_2 receptors causes vasodilation and bronchodilation. Dopaminergic receptors, although not fully understood, evidently cause dilation of the renal, coronary, and cerebral arteries. This helps maintain circulation to critical organs during periods of intense stress. Table *A9-2* describes the chief locations and primary actions of each receptor.

ORGANOPHOSPHATE POISONINGS

Organophosphates are a class of insecticides used widely in agriculture. Examples of organophosphates include Diazinon, orthene, malathion, parathion, and others. In addition, organophosphates have been used as chemical warfare agents since World War II. Most recently, the organophosphate sarin was used in the terrorist attack on a Japanese subway in 1995. The potency of organophosphate compounds varies significantly.

The principle action of the organophosphates is deactivation of the enzyme acetylcholinesterase (cholinesterase) in the nervous system. This leads to the accumulation of acetylcholine at nerve synapses and at the neuromuscular junctions, resulting in overstimulation of the acetylcholine receptors. This is followed by paralysis of cholinergic synaptic transmission.

Organophosphates bind irreversibly to cholinesterase, thus inactivating the enzyme. Organophosphates can enter the body through the skin or through the respiratory tract. Acute systemic organophosphate poisoning results in a variety of CNS, muscarinic, nicotinic, and somatic motor manifestations.

CNS symptoms include anxiety, restlessness, tremor, headache, dizziness, mental confusion, and seizures. Muscarinic receptor stimulation causes increased salivation, lacrimation, sweating, urinary incontinence, diarrhea, gastrointestinal system distress, vomiting, and bradycardia. Nicotinic receptor stimulation causes pallor, dilated pupils (mydriasis), and hypertension. Nicotinic stimulation at the neuromuscular junction also causes muscle fasiculations, cramps, and muscle weakness. This can progress to paralysis and a loss of reflexes.

The diagnosis of organophosphate poisoning is made by recognition of the signs and symptoms. Treatment is directed at support of essential functions such as maintenance of the airway and support of respirations. Initially, the drug atropine sulfate is administered. Atropine competes with acetylcholine for the acetylcholine receptors. In severe poisonings, exceedingly large doses of atropine may be required. This helps to reverse muscarinic and CNS symptoms. The antidote for organophosphate poisoning is *pralidoxime (2-PAM),* which restores cholinesterase activity by regenerating cholinesterase. Pralidoxime also appears to prevent toxicity by detoxifying the remaining organophosphate molecules.

REFLEXES

Reflex testing can be a useful physical examination tool. A reflex is an automatic motor response triggered

TABLE A9-3	Reflex Scale
Grade	*Description*
0	No response
+	Diminished, below normal
++	Average, normal
+++	Brisker than normal
++++	Hyperactive, associated with clonus

by a particular stimulus. A reflex arc includes a receptor, a sensory neuron, a motor neuron, and an effector. In simple reflex arcs, a sensory neuron interacts directly with a motor neuron. These simple monosynaptic reflexes are quite rapid. They protect parts of the body from injury by withdrawing the affected part when it is exposed to a noxious stimulus, such as heat. The best example of this is the stretch reflex, which provides automatic regulation of skeletal muscle length.

Stretch reflexes can be evaluated by tapping on a part of the muscle with a reflex hammer. The brief stimulus of a hammer tap results in a noticeable contraction in the affected muscle. This response is considered the reflex and is generally graded on a scale of 0–4. Table *A9-3* illustrates the reflex grading scale. Reflexes on one side of the body are usually compared to their corresponding reflexes on the other side of the body. Asymmetry of the reflexes may indicate an abnormality. Testing reflexes provides information about the corresponding spinal segment. The four most commonly examined reflexes are the ankle jerk, biceps reflex, patellar reflex, and abdominal reflex. The ankle jerk reflex evaluates sacral spinal segments S1 and S2. The biceps reflex evaluates spinal nerves C5 and C6. The patellar reflex examines spinal nerves L2, L3, and L4. The abdominal reflex is a contraction of the abdominal muscles that moves the umbilicus (navel) toward the stimulus. The portion of the abdomen above the umbilicus corresponds to thoracic spinal segments T8, T9, and T10, while the portion of the abdomen below the umbilicus corresponds the thoracic spinal segments T10, T11, and T12 (Figure A9-3●).

A decreased reflex (hyporeflexia), or an absent reflex (areflexia), may be due to temporary or permanent damage to skeletal muscles, dorsal or ventral nerve roots, spinal nerves, the spinal cord, or the brain. An increased reflex (hyperreflexia) usually results from diseases that affect higher centers or descending tracts. In certain patients, a tap on a tendon with a reflex hammer can cause a sustained contraction or several successive contractions, referred to as clonus.

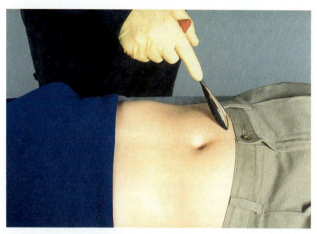

• FIGURE A9-3   Abdominal Reflex
Gently stroking the skin of the abdomen should cause contraction of the underlying muscles moving the umbilicus toward the location of the stimulus.

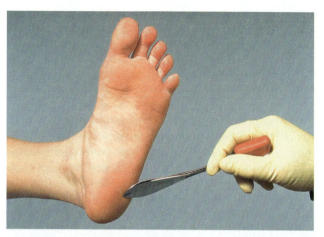

• FIGURE A9-4   Plantar Reflex
Stroking the aspect of the plantar surface of the foot should cause plantar flexion of the toes. Dorsiflexion of the great toe and fanning of the other toes following stimulation is a positive Babinski reflex, which suggests problems with higher centers in the brain.

In a pronounced type of hyperreflexia that occurs following severe spinal injury, the motor neurons of the spinal cord lose contact with higher centers in the brain. Initially following the injury will be a period of areflexia known as spinal shock. When the reflexes return, they respond in an exaggerated fashion, even to mild stimuli.

Stroking the bottom of the feet along the lateral aspect of the sole should cause plantar flexion of the toes (Figure A9-4•). If the big toe dorsiflexes and the other toes fan out, this indicates a central nervous system lesion. Known as a *Babinski response,* this reflex should be assessed in all critically ill or critically injured patients.

SUMMARY

The peripheral nervous system is an important consideration in emergency medical care. The autonomic nervous system is primarily a part of the peripheral nervous system and an important control system. Many of the medications used in emergency care either directly or indirectly affect the autonomic nervous system. Because of this, emergency personnel must have a good understanding of the autonomic nervous system and the drugs that affect it. Emergency personnel also must understand the regions of the spinal cord and the spinal nerves. Testing peripheral reflexes can provide information about the status of the spinal cord above the segment in question.

Sensory Function

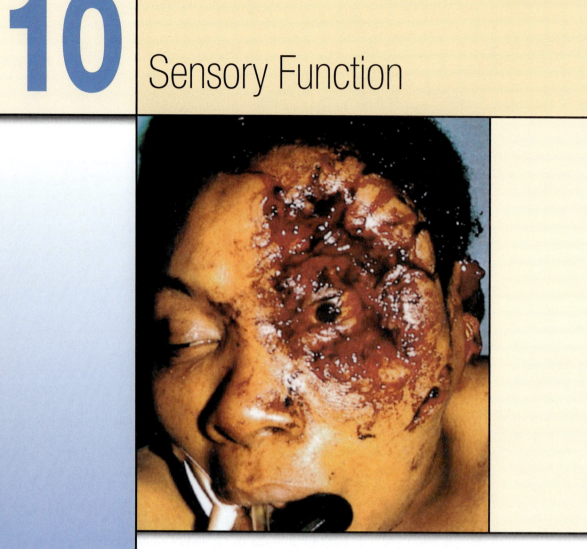

The structure of the globe of the eye makes it amazingly resilient to injury. In this case, the patient sustained massive trauma to the face. Although the bony orbit and adjoining structures are damaged, the globe remains intact. This is primarily due to the strength and integrity of the fibrous tunic and the resiliency of the vitreous humor and the aqueous humor. Proper prehospital emergency care, followed by rapid surgical care, often can salvage the eye and the patient's sight.

Chapter Outline and Objectives

Vocabulary Development

akousis, hearing; *acoustic*
baro-, pressure; *baroreceptors*
circa, about; *circadian*
circum-, around; *circumvallate papillae*
cochlea, snail shell; *cochlea*
dies, day; *circadian*
emmetro-, proper measure; *emmetropia*
incus, anvil; *incus* (auditory ossicle)
iris, colored circle; *iris*
labyrinthos, network of canals; *labyrinth*
lacrima, tear; *lacrimal gland*
lithos, a stone; *otolith*
macula, spot; *macula lutea*
malleus, a hammer; *malleus* (auditory ossicle)
myein, to shut; *myopia*
noceo, hurt; *nociceptor*
olfacere, to smell; *olfaction*
ops, eye; *myopia*
oto-, ear; *otolith*
presbys, old man; *presbyopia*
skleros, hard; *sclera*
stapes, stirrup; *stapes* (auditory ossicle)
tectum, roof; *tectorial membrane*
tympanon, drum; *tympanum*
vallum, wall; *circumvallate papillae*
vitreus, glassy; *vitreous body*

Our knowledge of the world around us is limited to those characteristics that stimulate our sensory receptors. Although we may not realize it, our picture of the environment is incomplete. Colors invisible to us guide insects to flowers, and sounds and smells we cannot detect are regular information to dogs, cats, and dolphins. Moreover, our senses are sometimes deceptive: In phantom limb pain, a person "feels" pain in a missing limb, and during an epileptic seizure, an individual may experience sights, sounds, or smells that have no physical basis.

All sensory information is picked up by *sensory receptors*, specialized cells that monitor internal and external conditions. The simplest receptors are the dendritic processes of sensory neurons. A dendritic array of this kind is called a **free nerve ending**. Free nerve endings are not protected by accessory structures, and they are sensitive to many types of stimuli. For example, the same free nerve endings in the skin may provide the sensation of pain in response to crushing, heat, or a cut. Other receptors are especially sensitive to one kind of stimulus. For example, a touch receptor is very sensitive to pressure but relatively insensitive to chemical stimuli; a taste receptor is sensitive to dissolved chemicals but insensitive to pressure. The most complex receptors, such as the visual receptors of the eye, are protected by accessory cells and layers of connective tissue. Not only are these receptor cells specialized to detect light, they are seldom exposed to any stimulus *except* light.

All sensory information arrives at the CNS in the form of action potentials in a sensory (afferent) fiber. In general, the stronger the stimulus, the higher the frequency of action potentials. When sensory information arrives at the CNS, it is routed according to the location and nature of the stimulus. For example, touch, pressure, pain, temperature, and taste sensations arrive at the primary sensory cortex; visual, auditory, and olfactory information reach the visual, auditory, and olfactory regions of the cortex, respectively. Because the CNS interprets the nature of sensory information entirely on the basis of the area of the brain stimulated, it cannot tell the difference between a "true" sensation and a "false" one. For instance, when rubbing your eyes, you may "see" flashes of light. Although the stimulus is mechanical rather than visual, any activity along the optic nerve is projected to the visual cortex and experienced as a visual perception.

Adaptation is a reduction in sensitivity in the presence of a constant stimulus. Familiar examples are stepping into a hot bath or jumping into a cold lake. Shortly afterward, neither temperature seems as extreme as it did initially. Adaptation reduces the amount of information arriving at the cerebral cortex. Most sensory information is routed to centers along the spinal cord or brain stem, potentially triggering involuntary reflexes, such as the withdrawal reflex. Only about 1 percent of the information provided by afferent fibers reaches the cerebral cortex and our conscious awareness.

Output from higher centers, however, can increase receptor sensitivity or facilitate transmission along a sensory pathway. For example, the *reticular activating system* in the midbrain helps focus attention and thus heightens or reduces awareness of arriving sensations. ∞ p. 242 This adjustment of sensitivity can occur under conscious or unconscious direction. When we "listen carefully," our sensitivity to and awareness of auditory stimuli increase. The reverse occurs when we enter a noisy factory or walk along a crowded city street, as we automatically "tune out" the high level of background noise.

The **general senses** are senses of temperature, pain, touch, pressure, vibration, and **proprioception** (body position). The receptors for the general senses are scattered throughout the body. The **special senses** are smell (**olfaction**), taste (**gustation**), vision, balance (**equilibrium**), and hearing. The receptors for the five special senses are concentrated within specific structures, the sense organs. This chapter explores both the general senses and the special senses.

THE GENERAL SENSES

Receptors for the general senses are scattered throughout the body and are relatively simple in structure. These receptors are classified according to the nature of the stimulus that excites them; important classes include receptors sensitive to pain (*nociceptors*); temperature (*thermoreceptors*); touch, pressure, and position (*mechanoreceptors*); and chemical stimuli (*chemoreceptors*).

Pain

Pain receptors, or **nociceptors** (nō-sē-SEP-tōrz; *noceo*, hurt), are especially common in the superficial portions of the skin, in joint capsules, within the periostea of bones, and around the walls of blood vessels. There are few nociceptors in other deep tissues or in most visceral organs.

Once pain receptors in a region are stimulated, two types of axons carry the painful sensations. Myelinated fibers carry very localized sensations of **fast pain**, or *prickling pain*, such as that caused by an injection or deep cut. These sensations reach the CNS quickly, leading to somatic reflexes and stimulation of the primary sensory cortex. Slower, unmyelinated fibers carry sensations of **slow pain**, or *burning and aching pain*. Unlike fast pain sensations, slow pain sensations enable you to determine only the general area involved.

Pain sensations from visceral organs are often perceived as originating in more superficial regions, generally regions innervated by the same spinal nerves. The perception of pain coming from parts of the body that are not actually stimulated is called **referred pain**. The precise mechanism responsible for referred pain remains to be determined, but several clinical examples are shown in Figure 10-1•. Cardiac pain, for example, is often perceived as originating in the upper chest and left arm.

Pain receptors continue to respond as long as the painful stimulus remains. However, the *awareness* of the pain can decrease over time because of the inhibition of pain centers in the thalamus, reticular formation, lower brain stem, and spinal cord.

Temperature

Temperature receptors, or **thermoreceptors**, are free nerve endings scattered immediately beneath the surface of the skin. They are also located in skeletal muscles, in the liver, and in the hypothalamus. Cold receptors are three or four times as numerous as warm

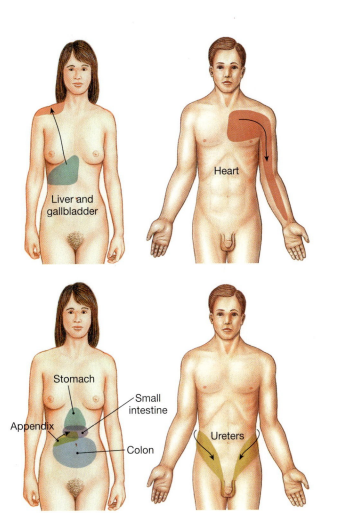

•**FIGURE 10-1   Referred Pain**
Pain sensations originating in visceral organs are often perceived as involving specific regions of the body surface innervated by the same spinal nerves.

receptors. There are no known structural differences between warm and cold thermoreceptors.

Temperature sensations are relayed along the same pathways that carry pain sensations. They are distributed to the reticular formation, the thalamus, and, to a lesser extent, the primary sensory cortex. Thermoreceptors are very active when the temperature is changing, but they quickly adapt to a stable temperature. When we enter an air-conditioned classroom on a hot summer day or a toasty lecture hall on a brisk fall evening, the temperature seems unpleasant at first, but the discomfort fades as adaptation occurs.

Touch, Pressure, and Position

Mechanoreceptors are receptors sensitive to stimuli that distort their cell membranes. They contain *mechanically regulated ion channels*, which open or close in response to stretching, compression, twisting, or other distortions of the membrane. There are three classes of mechanoreceptors: (1) *tactile (touch) receptors*, (2) *baroreceptors (pressure)*, and (3) *proprioceptors (position)*.

Tactile Receptors

Tactile receptors provide sensations of touch, pressure, and vibration. The distinctions between these are hazy, for a touch also represents a pressure, and a vibration consists of an oscillating touch/pressure stimulus. **Fine touch and pressure receptors** provide detailed information about a source of stimulation, including its exact location, shape, size, texture, and movement. **Crude touch and pressure receptors** provide poor localization and little additional information about the stimulus.

Tactile receptors range in complexity from free nerve endings to specialized sensory complexes with accessory cells and supporting structures. Figure 10-2• shows six types of tactile receptors in the skin:

1. Free nerve endings are sensitive to touch and pressure and are situated between epidermal cells. No structural differences have been found between these receptors and the free nerve endings that provide temperature or pain sensations.

2. The **root hair plexus** is made up of free nerve endings that monitor the distortion and movement of hairs.

3. **Merkel's** (MER-kelz) **discs** are fine touch and pressure receptors. They are neurons whose dendrites contact large epithelial cells (*Merkel's cells*) in the lower epidermal layer of the skin.

4. **Meissner's** (MĪS-nerz) **corpuscles** are fine touch and pressure receptors. They are abundant in the eyelids, lips, fingertips, nipples, and external genitalia.

5. **Pacinian** (pa-SIN-ē-an) **corpuscles** are large receptors sensitive to deep pressure and to pulsing or high-frequency vibrations. They are common in the

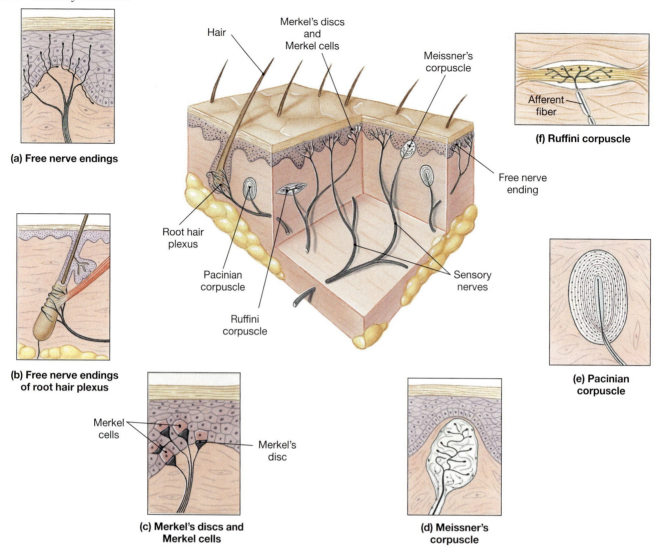

(a) Free nerve endings

(b) Free nerve endings of root hair plexus

(c) Merkel's discs and Merkel cells

Merkel cells

Merkel's disc

(d) Meissner's corpuscle

(e) Pacinian corpuscle

(f) Ruffini corpuscle

Afferent fiber

Hair

Merkel's discs and Merkel cells

Meissner's corpuscle

Free nerve ending

Root hair plexus

Pacinian corpuscle

Ruffini corpuscle

Sensory nerves

•**FIGURE 10-2   Tactile Receptors in the Skin**
(a) Free nerve endings. **(b)** A root hair plexus. **(c)** Merkel's discs and Merkel cells. **(d)** A Meissner's corpuscle. **(e)** A Pacinian corpuscle. **(f)** A Ruffini corpuscle.

skin of the fingers, breasts, and external genitalia. They are also present in joint capsules, mesenteries, the pancreas, and the wall of the urinary bladder.

6. **Ruffini** (roo-FĒ-nē) **corpuscles** are also sensitive to pressure and distortion of the skin, but they are located in its deeper layer, the dermis.

Tactile sensations travel through the posterior column and spinothalamic pathways. ∞ *pp. 258–259* Our sensitivity to tactile sensations can be altered by peripheral infection, disease processes, and damage to sensory neurons or pathways. Several clinical tests can be used to evaluate tactile sensitivity.

Baroreceptors

Baroreceptors (bar-ō-rē-SEP-tōrz; *baro-*, pressure) monitor changes in pressure. These receptors consist of free nerve endings that branch within the elastic tissues in the wall of a distensible organ, such as a blood vessel or a portion of the respiratory, digestive, or urinary tract. When the pressure inside the vessel or tract changes, the elastic walls of these vessels or tracts stretch or recoil. This movement distorts the dendritic branches and alters the rate of action potential generation. Baroreceptors respond immediately to a change in pressure, but they adapt rapidly, and the output along the afferent fibers gradually returns to "normal."

Figure 10-3• gives examples of important baroreceptor functions. Baroreceptors monitor blood pressure in the walls of major blood vessels, including the carotid artery (at the *carotid sinus*) and the aorta (at the *aortic sinus*). The information plays a major role in regulating cardiac function and adjusting blood flow to vital tissues. Baroreceptors in the lungs

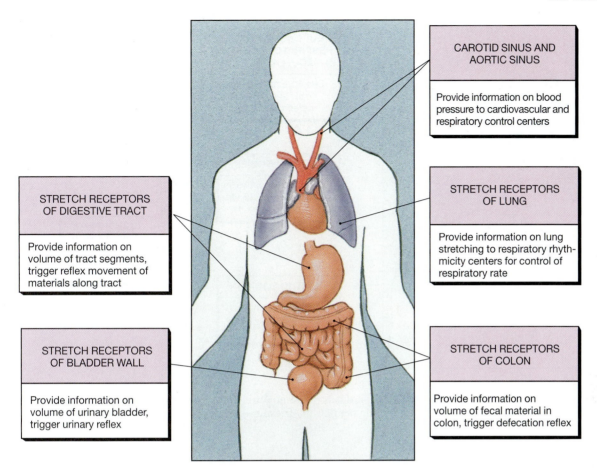

CAROTID SINUS AND
AORTIC SINUS

Provide information on blood
pressure to cardiovascular and
respiratory control centers

STRETCH RECEPTORS
OF LUNG

Provide information on lung
stretching to respiratory rhythmicity centers for control of
respiratory rate

STRETCH RECEPTORS
OF DIGESTIVE TRACT

Provide information on
volume of tract segments,
trigger reflex movement of
materials along tract

STRETCH RECEPTORS
OF BLADDER WALL

Provide information on
volume of urinary bladder,
trigger urinary reflex

STRETCH RECEPTORS
OF COLON

Provide information on
volume of fecal material in
colon, trigger defecation reflex

• **FIGURE 10-3 Baroreceptors and the Regulation of Autonomic Functions**
Baroreceptors provide information essential to the regulation of autonomic activities, including digestion,
urination, blood pressure monitoring, respiration, and defecation.

monitor the degree of lung expansion. This information is relayed to respiratory rhythmicity centers in
the brain, which set the pace of respiration. Baroreceptors in the digestive and urinary tracts trigger various visceral reflexes, including those of urination
and defecation.

Proprioceptors

Proprioceptors monitor the position of joints, the tension in tendons and ligaments, and the state of muscular contraction. Of all the general sensory receptors,
the proprioceptors are the most structurally and functionally complex. Two representative examples are
tendon organs, which monitor the strain on a tendon,
and *muscle spindles*, which monitor the length of a
skeletal muscle. ∞ *p. 256* In general, proprioceptors
do not adapt to constant stimulation, and each receptor continuously sends information to the CNS. Most
of this information is processed subconsciously, and
only a small proportion of it reaches your conscience
awareness.

Chemical Detection

In general, **chemoreceptors** respond only to water-soluble
and lipid-soluble substances that are dissolved in the surrounding fluid. Adaptation usually occurs over a few seconds following stimulation. Except for the special senses
of taste and smell, there are no well-defined chemosensory
pathways in the brain or spinal cord. The locations of important chemoreceptors are shown in Figure 10-4•. Neurons within the respiratory centers of the brain respond to
the concentration of hydrogen ions (pH) and carbon dioxide molecules in the cerebrospinal fluid. Other receptors
in the periphery monitor the oxygen concentration of arterial blood. These chemoreceptive neurons are found in
the **carotid bodies**, near the origin of the internal carotid
arteries on each side of the neck, and in the **aortic bodies**,
between the major branches of the aortic arch. The afferent fibers leaving the carotid and aortic bodies reach the
respiratory centers by traveling along the ninth (glossopharyngeal) and tenth (vagus) cranial nerves. These
chemoreceptors play an important role in the reflexive
control of respiration and cardiovascular function.

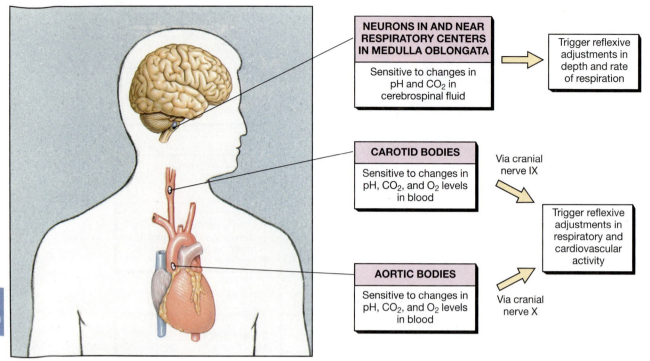

•FIGURE 10-4   Chemoreceptors
Chemoreceptors are located in the CNS, on the ventrolateral surfaces of the medulla oblongata, and in the aortic and carotid bodies. These receptors are involved in the autonomic regulation of respiratory and cardiovascular function.

SMELL

The sense of smell, or *olfaction*, is provided by paired **olfactory organs**. These organs, shown in Figure 10-5•, are located in the nasal cavity on either side of the nasal septum just inferior to the cribriform plate of the ethmoid bone. Each olfactory organ consists of an **olfactory epithelium**, which contains the **olfactory receptors**, supporting cells, and *basal cells* (stem cells). Beneath this basement membrane, large **olfactory glands** produce a pigmented mucus that covers the epithelium. The olfactory glands produce a continuous stream of mucus that passes across the surface of the olfactory organ, preventing the buildup of potentially dangerous or overpowering stimuli and keeping the area moist and free from dust or other debris. Once the dissolved chemicals have reached the olfactory organs, they must diffuse into the mucus before they can stimulate the olfactory receptors.

The olfactory receptors are highly modified neurons. The exposed tip of each receptor forms a prominent knob that provides a base for elongate cilia. All together, between 10 and 20 million olfactory receptors are packed into an area of roughly 5 cm^2. Nevertheless, our olfactory sensitivities cannot compare to those of other vertebrates such as dogs, cats, or [a] German shepherd sniffing for smuggled [ex]plosives has an olfactory receptor surface

72 times greater than that of the nearby customs inspector.

Olfactory reception occurs as dissolved chemicals interact with receptors on the surfaces of the cilia. This interaction changes the permeability of the receptor membrane, producing action potentials. This information is relayed to the central nervous system, which interprets the smell on the basis of the particular pattern of receptor activity.

The Olfactory Pathways

The axons leaving the olfactory epithelium collect into 20 or more bundles that penetrate the cribriform plate of the ethmoid bone to reach the **olfactory bulbs**. Axons leaving each olfactory bulb travel along the *olfactory tract* to reach the olfactory cortex of the cerebrum, the hypothalamus, and portions of the limbic system.

Olfactory stimuli are the only type of sensory information that reaches the cerebral cortex without first synapsing in the thalamus. The extensive limbic and hypothalamic connections help explain the profound emotional and behavioral responses that certain smells can produce. The perfume industry, which understands the practical implications of these connections, spends billions of dollars to develop odors that trigger sexual responses.

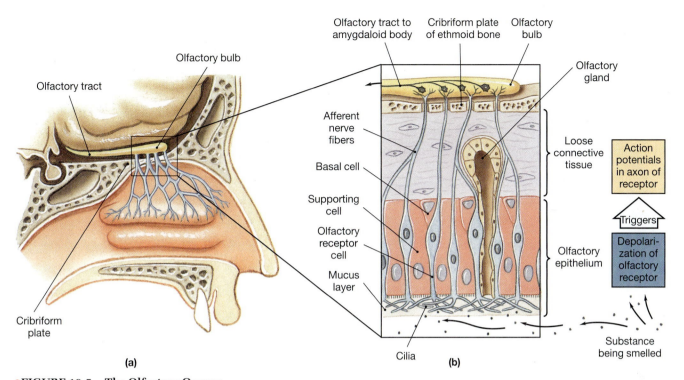

•FIGURE 10-5   The Olfactory Organs
(a) The structure of the olfactory organ on the left side of the nasal septum. **(b)** An olfactory receptor is a modified neuron with multiple cilia extending from its free surface.

TASTE

The **gustatory** (GUS-ta-tōr-ē), or **taste**, **receptors** are distributed over the surface of the tongue and adjacent portions of the pharynx and larynx in individual organs called **taste buds**. The taste buds are particularly well protected from the excessive mechanical stress due to chewing, for they lie along the sides of epithelial projections called **papillae** (pa-PIL-lē). The greatest number of taste buds are associated with the large *circumvallate papillae*, which form a V that points toward the attached base of the tongue (Figure 10-6•).

Each taste bud contains slender sensory receptors, known as **gustatory cells**, and supporting cells. Each gustatory cell extends slender microvilli, sometimes called *taste hairs*, into the surrounding fluids through a narrow opening, the **taste pore**. The mechanism behind gustatory reception seems to parallel that of olfaction. Dissolved chemicals contacting the taste hairs stimulate a change in the membrane potential of the taste cell, which leads to action potentials in the sensory neuron.

The four **primary taste sensations** are sweet, salt, sour, and bitter. Each taste bud shows a particular sensitivity to one of these tastes, and a sensory map of the tongue indicates that each is concentrated in a different area (Figure 10-6•). The threshold for receptor stimulation varies for each of the primary taste sensations, and the taste receptors respond most readily to unpleasant rather than pleasant stimuli.

The Taste Pathways

Taste buds are monitored by the facial (N VII), glossopharyngeal (N IX), and vagus (N X) cranial nerves (Figure 10-6a•). The sensory afferents of the different nerves synapse within a nucleus in the medulla oblongata, and the axons of the postsynaptic neurons synapse in the thalamus. The information is then projected to the appropriate portions of the primary sensory cortex.

The information received from the taste buds is correlated with other sensory data to assemble a conscious perception of taste. Our perception of the general texture of the food, together with the taste-related sensations of "peppery" or "burning," result from the stimulation of general sensory afferents in the trigeminal nerve (N V). In addition, information from the olfactory receptors plays an overwhelming role in taste perception. We are several thousand times more sensitive to "tastes" when our olfactory organs are fully functional. If you have a cold and airborne molecules cannot reach your olfactory receptors, meals taste dull and unappealing even when your taste buds are responding normally.

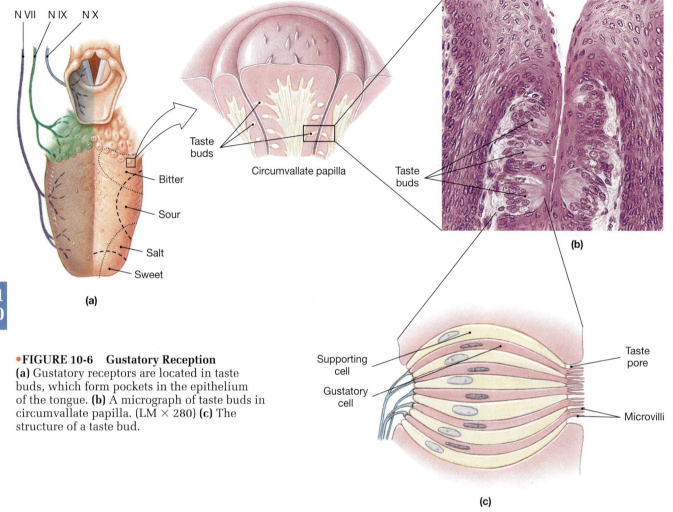

●**FIGURE 10-6   Gustatory Reception**
(a) Gustatory receptors are located in taste buds, which form pockets in the epithelium of the tongue. **(b)** A micrograph of taste buds in circumvallate papilla. (LM × 280) **(c)** The structure of a taste bud.

✓ When you first enter the anatomy and physiology laboratory for dissection, you are very aware of the odor of the preservative, but by the end of the lab period the smell doesn't seem nearly as strong. Why?

✓ When the nociceptors in your hand are stimulated, what sensation do you perceive?

✓ What would happen to an individual if the information from proprioceptors in the legs was blocked from reaching the CNS?

✓ If you completely dry the surface of the tongue and then place salt or sugar crystals on it, you cannot taste them. Why not?

VISION

Humans rely more on vision than on any other sense. Our visual receptors are contained in elaborate structures, the eyes, which enable us not only to detect light but to create detailed visual images. We will begin our discussion of these complex organs by considering the accessory structures of the eye, which provide protection, lubrication, and support.

The Accessory Structures of the Eye

The **accessory structures** of the eye include the (1) eyelids and associated exocrine glands, (2) the superficial epithelium of the eye, (3) structures associated with the production, secretion, and removal of tears, and (4) the extrinsic eye muscles.

The **eyelids**, or **palpebrae** (pal-PĒ-brē), are a continuation of the skin. They act like windshield wipers: Their blinking movements keep the surface of the eye lubricated and free from dust and debris. They can also close firmly to protect the delicate surface of the eye. The medial and lateral points of attachment of the upper and lower eyelids are called the **medial canthus** (KAN-thus) and the **lateral canthus**, respectively (Figure 10-7a●). The eyelashes are very robust hairs that help prevent foreign particles such as dirt and insects from reaching the surface of the eye.

Several types of exocrine glands protect the eye and its accessory structures. Large sebaceous glands are as-

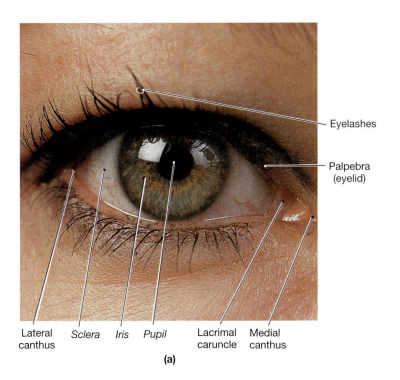

Eyelashes

Palpebra
(eyelid)

Lateral
canthus | *Sclera* | *Iris* | *Pupil* | Lacrimal
caruncle | Medial
canthus

(a)

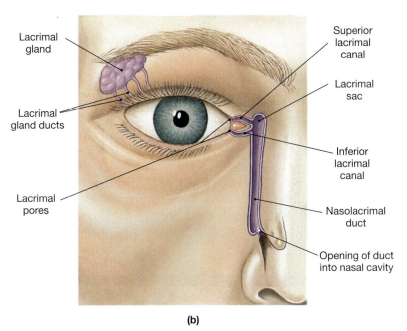

Lacrimal
gland

Lacrimal
gland ducts

Lacrimal
pores

Superior
lacrimal
canal

Lacrimal
sac

Inferior
lacrimal
canal

Nasolacrimal
duct

Opening of duct
into nasal cavity

(b)

•**FIGURE 10-7   The Accessory Structures of the Eye**
(a) The gross and superficial anatomies of the accessory structures.
(b) The details of the lacrimal apparatus.

sociated with the eyelashes, as they are with other hairs and hair follicles. ⚭ *p. 113* Modified sebaceous glands along the inner margins of the eyelids secrete a lipid-rich substance that keeps them from sticking together. At the medial canthus, the **lacrimal caruncle** (KAR-unk-ul), a soft mass of tissue, contains glands that produce thick secretions that contribute to the gritty deposits occasionally found after a night's sleep. The accessory glands of the eye sometimes become infected by bacte-

ria. An infection in a sebaceous gland of one of the eyelashes, or in one of the adjacent sweat glands, produces a painful localized swelling known as a **sty**.

The anterior surface of the eye is covered by the **conjunctiva** (kon-junk-TĪ-va), a distinctive epithelium continuous with the inner lining of the eyelids. The conjunctiva extends to the delicate *corneal epithelium*, which covers the transparent **cornea** (KŌR-nē-a). The conjunctiva contains many free nerve endings and is very sensitive. The painful condition of **conjunctivitis**, or "pink-eye," results from damage to and irritation of the conjunctival surface. The most obvious symptom results from dilation of the blood vessels beneath the conjunctival epithelium.

A constant flow of tears keeps the surfaces of the conjunctiva moist and clean. Tears reduce friction, remove debris, prevent bacterial infection, and provide nutrients and oxygen to the conjunctival epithelium. The **lacrimal apparatus** produces, distributes, and removes tears (Figure 10-7b•). Above the eyeball is the **lacrimal gland**, or *tear gland*, which has a dozen or more ducts that empty into the pocket between the eyelid and the eye. This gland nestles within a depression in the frontal bone, just inside the orbit and superior and lateral to the eyeball. The lacrimal gland normally provides the key ingredients and most of the volume of the tears. Its secretions are watery, slightly alkaline, and contain *lysozyme*, an enzyme that attacks bacteria. The blinking of the eye sweeps the tears across the surface of the eye to the medial canthus. Two small pores direct the tears into the **lacrimal canals**, passageways that end at the lacrimal sac. From this sac, the **nasolacrimal duct** carries the tears to the nasal cavity.

Six **extrinsic eye muscles**, or *oculomotor* (ok-ū-lō-MŌ-ter) *muscles*, originate on the surface of the orbit and control the position of the eye. These muscles are the **inferior rectus**, **lateral rectus**, **medial rectus**, **superior rectus**, **inferior oblique**, and **superior oblique** (Figure 10-8• and Table 10-1).

The Anatomy of the Eye

The eyes are extremely specialized visual organs, more versatile and adaptable than the most expensive cameras, yet light, compact, and durable. Each eye is roughly spherical, with a diameter of nearly 2.5 cm (1 in.), and weighs around 8 g (0.28 oz). The eyeball shares

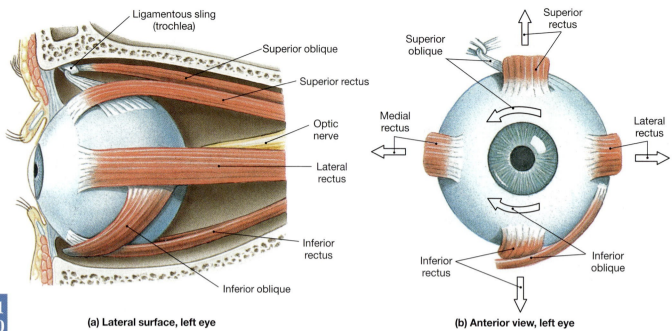

(a) Lateral surface, left eye

(b) Anterior view, left eye

•FIGURE 10-8   The Extrinsic Eye Muscles

space within the orbit with the extrinsic eye muscles, the lacrimal gland, and the various cranial nerves and blood vessels that service the eye and adjacent areas of the orbit and face. A mass of *orbital fat* provides padding and insulation.

The eyeball is hollow, and its interior can be divided into two cavities: the posterior cavity and the anterior cavity (Figure 10-9•). The large **posterior cavity** is also called the *vitreous chamber*, because it contains the gelatinous *vitreous body*. The smaller **anterior cavity** is subdivided into the *anterior chamber* and the *posterior chamber*. The shape of the eye is stabilized in part by the vitreous body and the **aqueous humor**, which fills the anterior cavity. The wall of the eye contains

three distinct layers, or *tunics*: an outer *fibrous tunic*, an intermediate *vascular tunic*, and an inner *neural tunic*.

The Fibrous Tunic

The **fibrous tunic**, the outermost layer covering the eye, (1) provides mechanical support and some degree of physical protection, (2) serves as an attachment site for the extrinsic eye muscles, and (3) assists in the focusing process. This layer consists of the sclera and cornea. The **sclera** (SKLER-a), or "white" of the eye, is a layer of dense fibrous connective tissue containing both collagen and elastic fibers (Figure 10-9•). It is thickest over the posterior surface of the eye and thinnest over the

TABLE 10-1	Extrinsic Eye Muscles *(Figure 10-8)*			
Muscle	*Origin*	*Insertion*	*Action*	*Innervation*
Inferior rectus	Sphenoid bone around optic canal	Inferior, medial surface of eyeball	Eye looks down	Oculomotor nerve (N III)
Medial rectus	As above	Medial surface of eyeball	Eye rotates medially	As above
Superior rectus	As above	Superior surface of eyeball	Eye looks up	As above
Inferior oblique	Maxillary bone at anterior portion of orbit	Inferior, lateral surface of eyeball	Eye rolls, looks up and to the side	As above
Superior oblique	Sphenoid bone around optic canal	Superior, lateral surface of eyeball	Eye rolls, looks down and to the side	Trochlear nerve (N IV)
Lateral rectus	As above	Lateral surface of eyeball	Eye rotates laterally	Abducens nerve (N VI)

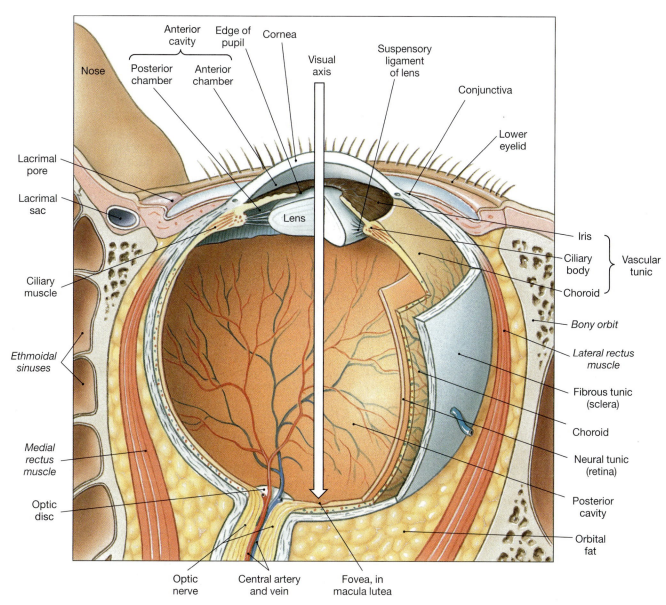

•FIGURE 10-9 The Sectional Anatomy of the Eye
Landmarks and features of the eye in a horizontal section through the right eye.

anterior surface. The six extrinsic eye muscles insert on the sclera.

The posterior surface of the sclera contains small blood vessels and nerves that penetrate the sclera to reach internal structures. On the anterior surface of the eye, however, these blood vessels lie under the conjunctiva. Because this network of small capillaries does not carry enough blood to lend an obvious color to the sclera, the white color of the collagen fibers is visible.

The transparent **cornea** is continuous with the sclera, but the collagen fibers of the cornea are organized into a series of layers that do not interfere with the passage of light. Because the cornea has only a limited ability to repair itself, corneal injuries must be treated immediately to prevent serious vision losses. Restoration of vision after corneal scarring usually re-

quires replacement of the cornea through a *corneal transplant*.

The Vascular Tunic

The **vascular tunic** contains numerous blood vessels, lymphatics, and all of the *intrinsic eye muscles*. The functions of this layer include (1) providing a route for blood vessels and lymphatics that supply tissues of the eye, (2) regulating the amount of light entering the eye, (3) secreting and reabsorbing the aqueous humor that circulates within the eye, and (4) controlling the shape of the lens, an essential part of the focusing process.

The vascular tunic includes the *iris*, the *ciliary body*, and the *choroid* (Figure 10-9•). Visible through the transparent corneal surface, the **iris** contains blood vessels, pigment cells, and two layers of smooth muscle fibers. When these muscles contract, they change the diameter of the central opening, or **pupil**, of the iris. Dilation and constriction are controlled by the autonomic nervous system in response to sudden changes in light intensity. Exposure to bright light produces a rapid reflexive decrease in pupil diameter, under parasympathetic stimulation. A sudden reduction in light levels produces a much slower pupillary dilation, under the control of the sympathetic division.

The thickness of the iris and the number and distribution of pigment cells determine its apparent color. When there are no pigment cells in the iris, light passes through it and bounces off its inner surface of pigmented epithelium. The eye then appears blue. In order, individuals with gray, brown, or black eyes have increasing numbers of pigment cells in the body and surface of the iris.

Along its outer edge, the iris attaches to the anterior portion of the **ciliary body**, the bulk of which consists of the *ciliary muscle*, a muscular ring that projects into the interior of the eye. The ciliary body begins at the junction between the cornea and sclera and extends to the scalloped border that also marks the anterior edge of the *retina*. Posterior to the iris, the surface of the ciliary body is thrown into folds called *ciliary processes*. The **suspensory ligaments** of the lens attach to these processes. These fibers position the lens so that light passing through the pupil passes through the center of the lens.

The **choroid** is a layer that separates the fibrous and neural tunics posterior to the ciliary body (Figure 10-9•). The choroid contains a capillary network that delivers oxygen and nutrients to the retina.

The Neural Tunic

The **neural tunic**, or **retina**, consists of a thin outer pigment layer and a thick inner layer, the *neural retina*. The pigment layer absorbs light after it passes through the receptor layer. The neural retina contains (1) the photoreceptors that respond to light, (2) supporting cells and neurons that perform preliminary processing and integration of visual information, and (3) blood vessels supplying tissues that line the posterior cavity. The neural retina forms a cup that establishes the posterior and lateral boundaries of the posterior cavity (Figure 10-9•).

Retinal Organization. The retina contains several layers of cells (Figure 10-10a•). The outermost layer, closest to the pigment layer, contains the photoreceptors. The two types of photoreceptors are **rods** and **cones**. Rods do not discriminate among colors of light. These receptors are very light-sensitive and enable us to see in dimly lit rooms, at twilight, or in pale moonlight. Cones provide us with color vision. The stimulation of three types of cones in various combinations provides the perception of different colors. Cones give us sharper, clearer images, but they require more intense light than do rods. If you

sit outside at sunset (or sunrise), you will probably be able to tell when your visual system shifts from cone-based vision (clear images in full color) to rod-based vision (relatively grainy images in black and white).

Rods and cones are not evenly distributed across the retina. If you think of the retina as a cup, the approximately 125 million rods are found on the sides and the roughly 6 million cones dominate the bottom. There are no rods in the region where the visual image arrives after passing through the cornea and lens. This area is the **macula lutea** (LOO-tē-a; yellow spot). The highest concentration of cones is found in the central portion of the macula lutea, an area called the **fovea** (FŌ-vē-a; shallow depression), or *fovea centralis* (Figure 10-10c•). The fovea is the center of color vision and the site of sharpest vision. When you look directly at an object, its image falls on this portion of the retina.

You are probably already aware of the visual consequences of this distribution. During the day, when there is enough light to stimulate the cones, you see a very good image. In very dim light, cones cannot function. For example, when you try to stare at a dim star, you are unable to see it. But if you look a little to one side rather than directly at the star, you will see it quite clearly. Shifting your gaze moves the image of the star from the fovea, where it does not provide enough light to stimulate the cones, to the edges of the retina, where it stimulates the more sensitive rods.

The rods and cones synapse with roughly 6 million **bipolar cells**. Bipolar cells in turn synapse within the layer of **ganglion cells** that faces the posterior cavity. The axons of the ganglion cells deliver the sensory information to the brain. *Horizontal cells* and *amacrine* (AM-a-krīn) *cells* can regulate communication between photoreceptors and ganglion cells, adjusting the sensitivity of the retina. The effect can be compared to adjusting the contrast setting on a television. These cells play an important role in the eye's adjustment to dim or brightly lit environments.

The Optic Disc. Axons from an estimated 1 million ganglion cells converge on the **optic disc**, a circular region just medial to the fovea. The optic disc is the origin of the optic nerve (N II) (Figure 10-10b•). From this point, the axons turn, penetrate the wall of the eye, and proceed toward the diencephalon. Blood vessels that supply the retina pass through the center of the optic nerve and emerge on the surface of the optic disc (Figure 10-10b,c•). The optic disc has no photoreceptors or other retinal structures. Because light striking this area goes unnoticed, it is commonly called the **blind spot**. You do not notice a blank spot in your visual field, because involuntary eye movements keep the visual image moving and allow your brain to fill in the missing information. A simple experiment, shown in Figure 10-11•, will demonstrate the presence and location of the blind spot.

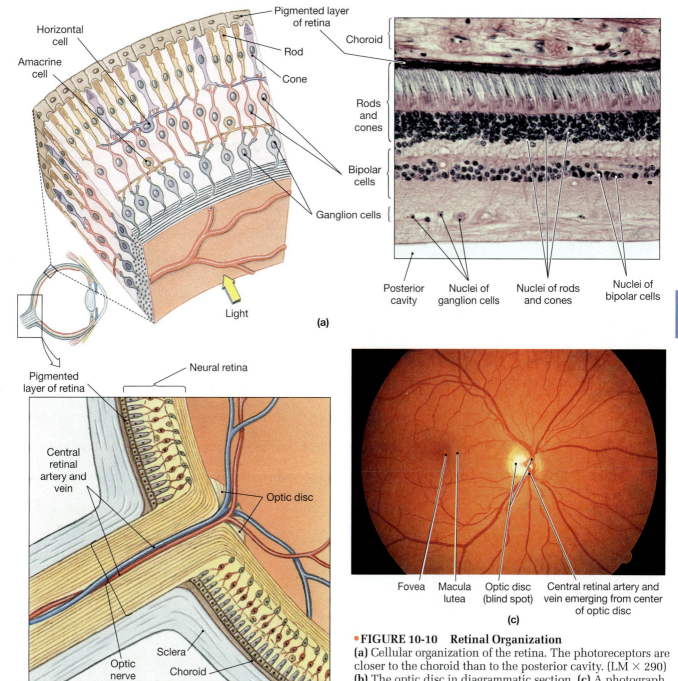

●FIGURE 10-10   Retinal Organization
(a) Cellular organization of the retina. The photoreceptors are closer to the choroid than to the posterior cavity. (LM × 290) **(b)** The optic disc in diagrammatic section. **(c)** A photograph of the retina as seen through the pupil of the eye.

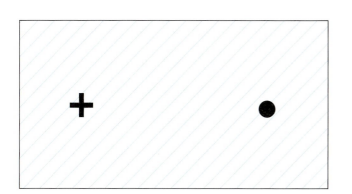

●FIGURE 10-11   The Optic Disc
Close your left eye and stare at the cross with your right eye, keeping the cross in the center of your field of vision. Begin with the page a few inches away from your eye and gradually increase the distance. The dot will disappear when its image falls on the blind spot. To check the blind spot in your left eye, close your right eye, stare at the dot, and repeat this sequence.

The Chambers of the Eye

The ciliary body and lens divide the interior of the eye into the small anterior cavity and the larger posterior cavity. The anterior cavity is further subdivided into the anterior chamber, which extends from the cornea to the iris, and the posterior chamber, between the iris and the ciliary body and lens. The anterior and posterior chambers are filled with aqueous humor. This fluid circulates within the anterior cavity, passing from the posterior to the anterior chamber via the pupil of the eye (Figure 10-12•). The posterior cavity is filled with a gelatinous substance known as the *vitreous body*. The vitreous body helps maintain the shape of the eye and also holds the retina against the choroid.

Aqueous Humor.   Aqueous humor forms at the ciliary processes through active secretion into the posterior chamber (Figure 10-12•). Pressure exerted by this fluid helps maintain the shape of the eye, and the circulation of aqueous humor transports nutrients and wastes. In the anterior chamber near the edge of the iris, the aqueous humor enters a passageway, known as the *canal of Schlemm*, that returns this fluid to the venous system.

Interference with the normal circulation and reabsorption of the aqueous humor leads to an elevation in the pressure inside the eye. If this condition, called **glaucoma**, is left untreated, it can eventually produce blindness by distortion of the retina and the optic disc.

The Lens

The **lens** lies behind the cornea and is held in place by suspensory ligaments. The primary function of the lens is to focus the visual image on the retinal receptors. It does so by changing its shape.

The Structure of the Lens.   The transparent lens consists of organized concentric layers of cells wrapped in a dense fibrous capsule. The capsule is elastic; unless an outside force is applied, it will contract and make the lens spherical. However, tension in the suspensory ligaments can overpower the elastic capsule and pull the lens into the shape of a flattened oval.

✳ HYPHEMA

Blunt trauma to the eye can rupture one of the blood vessels within the iris, causing blood to enter the anterior chamber of the eye. Blood in the anterior chamber, called a hyphema, is a serious emergency. The amount of blood in the chamber can range from microscopic to the so-called eight-ball hyphema, where blood fills the entire anterior chamber. Up to one-third of patients will suffer a rebleed within 3–5 days, and these rebleeds are often worse than the original bleeds. Complications of hyphema include reduced vision, secondary glaucoma, and staining of the cornea.

Treatment of hyphema includes use of medications that reduce pressure within the anterior chamber and anti-inflammatory medicines. Some patients require hospitalization and complete bed rest for up to 5 days to prevent clot dislodgement and rebleeding. Patients suffering a hyphema have the best outcome when the injury is promptly recognized and ophthalmologic care is given.

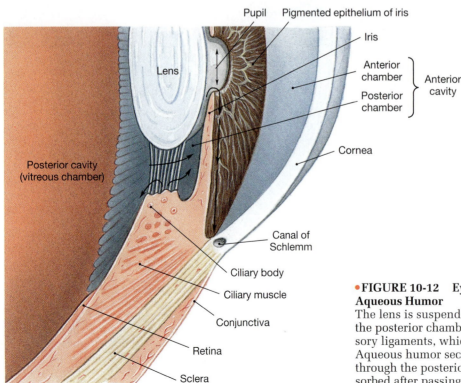

•**FIGURE 10-12   Eye Chambers and the Circulation of Aqueous Humor**
The lens is suspended between the vitreous chamber and the posterior chamber. Its position is maintained by suspensory ligaments, which attach the lens to the ciliary body. Aqueous humor secreted at the ciliary body circulates through the posterior and anterior chambers and is reabsorbed after passing along the canal of Schlemm.

Accommodation. As in a camera, in the eye the arriving image must be in focus if it is to provide useful information. "In focus" means that the rays of light arriving from the object strike the sensitive surface of the film (the retina) precisely ordered so as to form a miniature image of a viewed original. If the rays are not perfectly focused, the image will be blurry. Focusing normally occurs in two steps as light passes through the cornea and lens.

Light is bent, or *refracted*, when it passes between media of different densities. In the human eye, the greatest amount of refraction occurs when light passes from the air into the cornea. When the light enters the relatively dense lens, the lens provides the additional refraction needed to focus the light rays from an object toward a specific *focal point*. The distance between the center of the lens and the focal point is the *focal distance*. This distance is determined by (1) *the distance of the object from the lens* (the closer the object, the longer the focal distance) and (2) *the shape of the lens*

(the rounder the lens, the shorter the focal distance). In the eye, the lens changes shape to keep the focal distance constant, thereby keeping the image focused on the retina. **Accommodation** (Figure 10-13•) is the process of focusing an image on the retina by changing the shape of the lens. During accommodation, the lens either becomes rounder to focus the image of a nearby object on the retina or flattens to focus the image of a distant object.

The suspensory ligaments that hold the lens in place originate at the ciliary body. Smooth muscle fibers in the ciliary body encircle the lens. As you view a nearby object, your ciliary muscles contract and the ciliary body moves toward the lens (Figure 10-13c•). This movement reduces the tension in the suspensory ligaments, and the elastic capsule pulls the lens into a more spherical shape. When you view a distant object, your ciliary muscles relax, the suspensory ligaments pull at the circumference of the lens, and the lens becomes relatively flat (Figure 10-13d•).

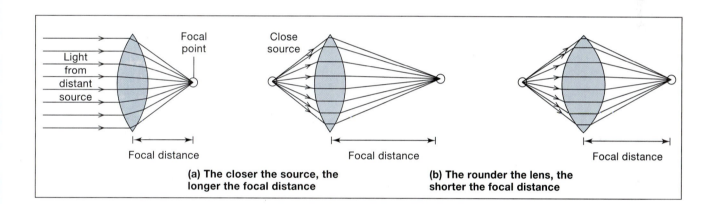

Focal point

Light from distant source

Focal distance

(a) The closer the source, the longer the focal distance

Close source

Focal distance

(b) The rounder the lens, the shorter the focal distance

Focal distance

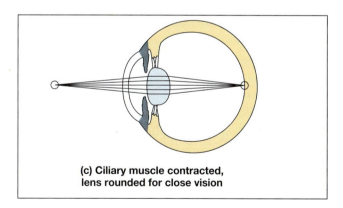

(c) Ciliary muscle contracted, lens rounded for close vision

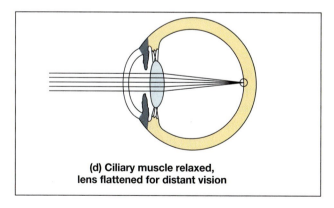

(d) Ciliary muscle relaxed, lens flattened for distant vision

• **FIGURE 10-13 Image Formation and Visual Accommodation**
(a) A lens refracts light toward a specific point. The distance from the center of the lens to that point is the focal distance of the lens. Light from a distant source arrives with all of the light waves traveling parallel to one another. Light from a nearby source, however, will still be diverging or spreading out from its source when it strikes the lens. Note the difference in focal distance after refraction. **(b)** For the eye to form a sharp image, the focal distance must equal the distance between the center of the lens and the retina. The lens compensates for variations in the distance between the eye and the object in view by changing its shape. The rounder the lens, the shorter the focal distance. **(c)** When the ciliary muscle contracts, the suspensory ligaments allow the lens to round up. **(d)** When the ciliary muscle relaxes, the ligaments pull against the margins of the lens and flatten it.

In the normal eye, when the ciliary muscles are relaxed and the lens is flattened, a distant image will be focused on the retinal surface (Figure 10-14a●), a condition called *emmetropia* (*emmetro-*, proper measure). However, irregularities in the shape of the lens or cornea can affect the clarity of the visual image. This condition, called *astigmatism*, can usually be corrected by glasses or special contact lenses.

Figure 10-14● diagrams two other common problems with the accommo-

dation mechanism. If the eyeball is too deep, the image of a distant object will form in front of the retina, and the retinal picture will be blurry and out of focus (Figure 10-14b●). Vision at close range will be normal, because the lens will be able to round up as needed to focus the image on the retina. As a result, such individuals are said to be "nearsighted." Their condition is more formally termed *myopia* (*myein*, to shut + *ops*, eye). Myopia can be corrected by placing a diverging lens in front of the eye (Figure 10-14c●).

If the eyeball is too shallow, hyperopia results (Figure 10-14d●). The ciliary muscles must contract to focus even a distant object on the retina, and at close range the lens cannot provide enough refraction. These individuals are said to be "farsighted" because they can see distant objects most clearly. Older individuals become farsighted as their lenses lose elasticity; this form of hyperopia is called *presbyopia* (*presbys*, old man). Hyperopia can be treated by placing a converging lens in front of the eye (Figure 10-14e●).

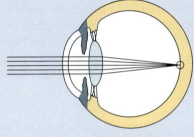

(a) Emmetropia

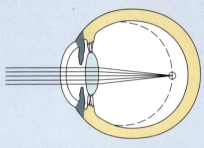

(b) Myopia

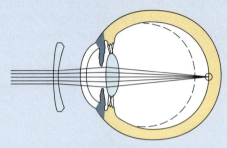

(c) Myopia (corrected)

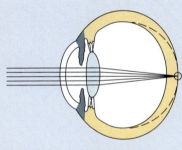

(d) Hyperopia

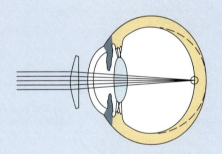

(e) Hyperopia (corrected)

●**FIGURE 10-14   Visual Abnormalities**
(a) In normal vision, the lens focuses the visual image on the retina. One common problem of accommodation involves **(b)** an inability to lengthen the focal distance enough to focus the image of a distant object on the retina—myopia. **(c)** A diverging lens is used to correct myopia. **(d)** Another accommodation problem is an inability to shorten the focal distance adequately for near objects—hyperopia. **(e)** A converging lens is used to correct hyperopia.

VISUAL ACUITY

How well the eye discriminates small details is determined by measuring the patient's visual acuity. Visual acuity testing is standardized and involves placing the patient exactly 20 feet from a Snellen eye chart. Eyes are individually tested by having the patient read the smallest line on the chart while covering the opposite eye. Then both eyes are tested together. Visual acuity is recorded as a fraction in which the numerator (top number) indicates the distance of the patient from the chart and the denominator (bottom number) indicates the distance at which the normal eye can read the line. A visual acuity of 20/20 or better is considered normal. Patients who cannot read any letter on the chart should be asked to count the number of fingers the examiner holds up. If the patient can accomplish this, then *CF* (counts fingers) is recorded. Patients who cannot count fingers should be examined to determine whether they are able to detect light. If they can detect light, then *LO* (light only) is recorded.

Visual Physiology

The rods and cones of the retina are called **photoreceptors** because they detect *photons*, basic units of visible light. Our eyes are sensitive to the spectrum of **visible light**. This spectrum, seen in a rainbow, can be remembered by the acronym ROY G. BIV (red, orange, yellow, green, blue, indigo, violet). Color depends on the wavelength of the light. The longer the wavelength, the lower the energy content of the light. Photons of red light have the longest wavelength and carry the least energy. Photons from the violet portion of the spectrum have the shortest wavelength and carry the most energy.

Rods and Cones

Rods provide the CNS with information about the presence or absence of photons, without regard to wavelength. As a result, they do not discriminate among colors of light.

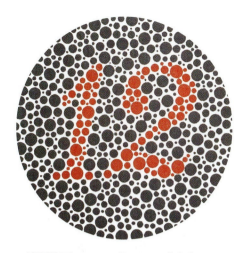

•FIGURE 10-15   Cones and Color Vision
Part of a standard test for color vision. The lack of one or more populations of cones will produce an inability to distinguish the patterned images.

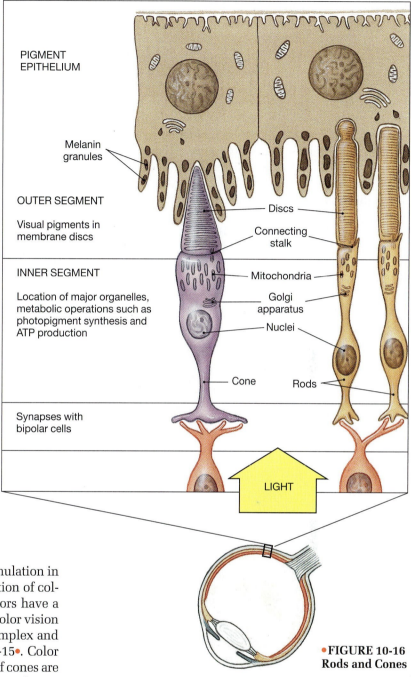

PIGMENT EPITHELIUM

Melanin granules

OUTER SEGMENT

Visual pigments in membrane discs

INNER SEGMENT

Location of major organelles, metabolic operations such as photopigment synthesis and ATP production

Synapses with bipolar cells

Discs

Connecting stalk

Mitochondria

Golgi apparatus

Nuclei

Cone   Rods

LIGHT

•FIGURE 10-16
Rods and Cones

They are very sensitive, however, and enable us to see in dimly lit rooms, at twilight, and in pale moonlight.

Cones provide information about the wavelength of photons. Because cones are less sensitive than rods, they function only in relatively bright light. We have three types of cones: blue cones, green cones, and red cones. Each type is sensitive to a different range of wavelengths of light, and their stimulation in various combinations accounts for our perception of colors. Persons unable to distinguish certain colors have a form of *color blindness*. The standard tests for color vision involve picking numbers or letters out of a complex and colorful picture, such as the one in Figure 10-15•. Color blindness occurs because one or more classes of cones are absent or nonfunctional. In the most common condition, the red cones are missing and the individual cannot distinguish red light from green light. Ten percent of men have some color blindness, whereas the incidence among women is only around 0.67 percent. Total color blindness is extremely rare; only 1 person in 300,000 has no cone pigments of any kind.

Photoreceptor Function

Figure 10-16• compares the structure of rods and cones. The outer portion of a photoreceptor contains hundreds to thousands of flattened membranous discs. The inner portion of a photoreceptor communicates with a bipolar cell. In the dark, each photoreceptor continually re-

leases neurotransmitters across these synapses. The arrival of a photon initiates a chain of events that alters the membrane potential of the photoreceptor and changes the rate of neurotransmitter release.

Visual Pigments

Light absorption, the first key step in the process of photoreception, requires special organic compounds called **visual pigments**. These compounds, located in the outer segments of all photoreceptors, are derivatives of the compound **rhodopsin** (rō-DOP-sin). Rhodopsin consists of a protein, the enzyme **opsin**, bound to the pigment **retinal** (RET-i-nal), synthesized from **vitamin A**. Retinal is identical in both rods and cones, but a different form of opsin is found in the rods and each of the three types of cones (red, blue, and green).

Photoreception begins when a photon strikes a rhodopsin molecule in the outer segment of a photoreceptor. When the photon is absorbed, a change in the shape of the retinal component activates opsin, starting a chain of enzymatic events that alters the rate of neurotransmitter release. This change is the signal that light has struck a photoreceptor at that particular location on the retina.

Shortly after the conformational change occurs, the rhodopsin molecule begins to break down into retinal and opsin, a process known as *bleaching* (Figure 10-17●). The retinal must be converted back to its former shape before it can recombine with opsin. This conversion requires energy in the form of ATP, and it takes time. Bleaching contributes to the lingering visual impression that you have after a camera flash goes off. After an intense exposure to light, a photoreceptor cannot respond to further stimulation until its rhodopsin molecules have been regenerated. As a result, a "ghost" image remains on the retina.

Anisocoria, or unequal pupils, is always a concern in the emergency patient. Pupillary constriction is controlled by the *oculomotor nerve (CN III)*. An expanding lesion in the brain can compress the nerve, causing pupillary dilation on the affected side. In a trauma patient, this may indicate an intracranial injury. In a medical patient, anisocoria may indicate intracranial bleeding or tumor. Because of this, the presence of anisocoria requires further investigation.

Anisocoria can be a normal finding. In fact, 20 percent of the general population has some degree of anisocoria. The difference is typically 1 millimeter or less and is not accompanied by other findings (such as drooping eyelids or extraocular muscle paralysis). Anisocoria may vary from day to day in the same person. Also, many medications, such as decongestants, can cause anisocoria. If necessary, old photographs, such as those on a driver's license, can help determine whether anisocoria is old or new.

The Visual Pathway

The visual pathway begins at the photoreceptors and ends at the visual cortex of the cerebral hemispheres. In other sensory pathways we have examined, there is at most one synapse between a receptor and a sensory neuron that delivers information to the CNS. In the visual pathway, the message must cross two synapses (photoreceptor to bipolar cell, and bipolar cell to ganglion cell) before it heads toward the brain. Axons from the entire population of ganglion cells converge on the optic disc, penetrate the wall of the eye, and proceed toward the diencephalon as the optic nerve (N II). The two optic nerves, one from each eye, reach the diencephalon at the optic chiasm (Figure 10-18●). From this point, approximately half of the fibers proceed toward the thalamus on the same side of the brain, while the other half cross over to reach the thalamus on the opposite side. Nuclei in the thalamus act as switching and processing centers that relay visual information to reflex centers in the brain stem as well as to the cerebral cortex. The visual information received by the superior colliculi (midbrain nuclei in the brain stem) controls pupil reflexes and reflexes that control eye movement. ∞ *p. 242*

The sensation of vision arises from the integration of information arriving at the visual cortex of the cerebrum. The visual cortex of each occipital lobe contains a sensory map of the entire field of vision. As with the primary sensory cortex, the map does not faith-

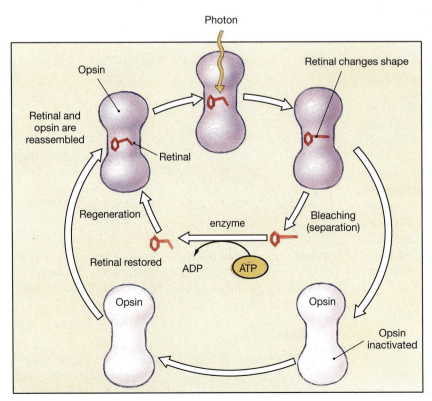

●**FIGURE 10-17　The Bleaching and Recovery of Visual Pigments**

fully duplicate the relative areas within the sensory field. For example, the area assigned to the fovea covers about 35 times the surface it would cover if the map were proportionally accurate.

Many centers in the brain stem receive visual information, from the thalamic nuclei or over collateral branches from the optic tracts. ∞ *p. 234* For example, some collaterals that bypass the thalamic nuclei synapse in the hypothalamus. Visual inputs there and at the pineal gland establish a daily pattern of activity that is tied to the day-night cycle. This *circadian* (*circa*, about + *dies*, day) *rhythm* affects metabolic rate, endocrine function, blood pressure, digestive activities, the awake-sleep cycle, and other processes. ∞ *p. 241*

✓ Which layer of the eye would be the first to be affected by inadequate tear production?

✓ When the lens is very round, are you looking at an object that is close to you or far from you?

✓ If a person is born without cones in her eyes, will she be able to see? Explain.

✓ How can a diet deficient in vitamin A affect vision?

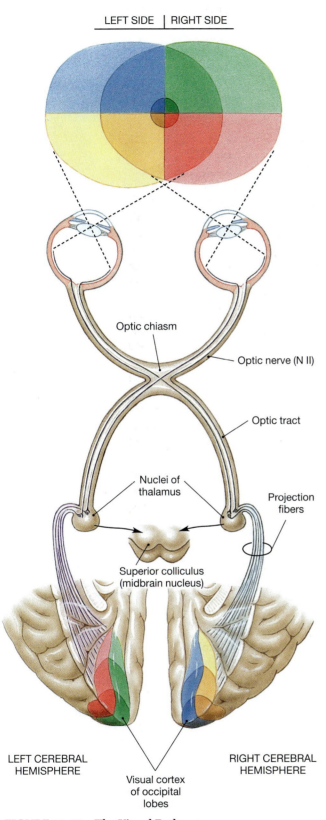

Optic chiasm

Optic nerve (N II)

Optic tract

Nuclei of thalamus

Projection fibers

Superior colliculus (midbrain nucleus)

LEFT CEREBRAL HEMISPHERE

RIGHT CEREBRAL HEMISPHERE

Visual cortex of occipital lobes

• **FIGURE 10-18   The Visual Pathway**
At the optic chiasm, a partial crossover of nerve fibers occurs. As a result, each hemisphere receives visual information from the lateral half of the retina on that side and from the medial half of the retina on the opposite side. Visual association areas integrate this information to develop a composite picture of the entire visual field.

LEFT SIDE   RIGHT SIDE

EQUILIBRIUM AND HEARING

The senses of equilibrium and hearing are provided by the *inner ear*, a receptor complex located in the temporal bone of the skull. ∞ *p. 133* The basic receptor mechanism for these senses is the same. The receptors, or *hair cells*, are simple mechanoreceptors. The complex structure of the inner ear and the different arrangements of accessory structures account for the abilities of the hair cells to respond to different stimuli and thus to provide the input for two senses:

1. Equilibrium, which informs us of the position of the body in space by monitoring gravity, linear acceleration, and rotation.

2. Hearing, which enables us to detect and interpret sound waves.

The Anatomy of the Ear

The ear is divided into three anatomical regions: the *external ear*, the *middle ear*, and the *inner ear* (Figure 10-19•). The external ear, which is the visible portion of the ear, collects and directs sound waves to the eardrum. The middle ear is a chamber located in a thickened portion of the temporal bone. Structures in the middle ear collect and amplify sound waves and transmit them to a portion of the inner ear concerned with hearing. The inner ear also contains the sensory organs responsible for equilibrium sensations.

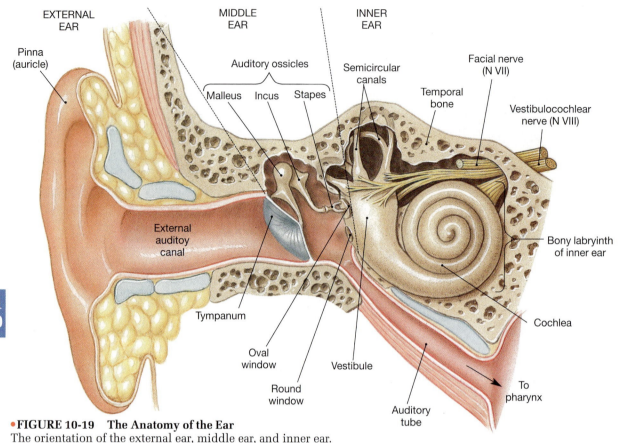

EXTERNAL EAR   MIDDLE EAR   INNER EAR

Pinna (auricle)

Auditory ossicles

Malleus   Incus   Stapes

Semicircular canals

Facial nerve (N VII)

Temporal bone

Vestibulocochlear nerve (N VIII)

External auditoy canal

Bony labryinth of inner ear

Tympanum

Cochlea

Oval window

Vestibule

Round window

To pharynx

Auditory tube

•FIGURE 10-19   The Anatomy of the Ear
The orientation of the external ear, middle ear, and inner ear.

The External Ear

The **external ear** includes the fleshy **pinna**, or *auricle*, which surrounds the entrance to the **external auditory canal**. The pinna, which is supported by elastic cartilage, protects the opening of the canal. It also provides directional sensitivity to the ear: Sounds coming from behind the head are partially blocked by the pinna; sounds coming from the side are collected and channeled into the external auditory canal. (When you "cup your ear" with your hand to hear a faint sound more clearly, you are exaggerating this effect.) **Ceruminous (se-ROO-mi-nus) glands** along the external auditory canal secrete a waxy material (*cerumen*) that slows the growth of microorganisms and reduces the chances of infection. In addition, small, outwardly projecting hairs help prevent the entry of foreign objects and insects. The external auditory canal ends at the **tympanum**, also called the *tympanic membrane* or *eardrum*. The tympanum is a thin sheet that separates the external ear from the middle ear (Figure 10-19•).

The Middle Ear

The **middle ear**, or *tympanic cavity*, is filled with air. It is separated from the external auditory canal by the tympanum, but it communicates with the superior portion of the pharynx, a region known as the *nasopharynx*, and with *air cells* in the mastoid process of the temporal bone. The connection with the nasopharynx is the **auditory tube**, also called the *pharyngotympanic tube* or the *Eustachian tube* (Figure 10-19•). The auditory tube permits the equalization of pressure on either side of the eardrum. Unfortunately, it can also allow microorganisms to travel from the nasopharynx into the tympanic cavity, leading to an unpleasant middle ear infection known as *otitis media*.

The Auditory Ossicles.   The middle ear contains three tiny ear bones, collectively called **auditory ossicles**. The ear bones connect the tympanum with the receptor complex of the inner ear (Figure 10-20•). The three auditory ossicles are the malleus, the incus, and the stapes. The **malleus** (*malleus*, hammer) attaches at three points to the interior surface of the tympanum. The middle bone, the **incus** (*incus*, anvil), attaches the malleus to the inner bone, the **stapes** (*stapes*, stirrup). The base of the stapes almost completely fills the *oval window*, a small opening in the bone enclosing the inner ear.

Vibration of the tympanum converts arriving sound energy into mechanical movements of the auditory ossicles. The ossicles act as levers that conduct the in-out vibrations to the inner ear's fluid-filled inner chamber. The tympanum is larger and heavier than the delicate membrane spanning the oval window, so the amount

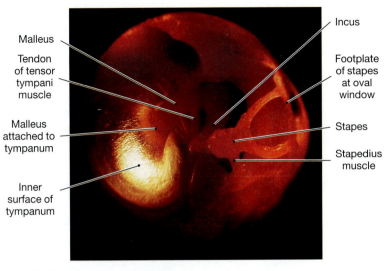

Malleus

Tendon
of tensor
tympani
muscle

Malleus
attached to
tympanum

Inner
surface of
tympanum

Incus

Footplate
of stapes
at oval
window

Stapes

Stapedius
muscle

•FIGURE 10-20   The Middle Ear
The tympanum and auditory ossicles.

of movement increases markedly from tympanum to oval window.

This magnification in movement allows us to hear very faint sounds. It can also be a problem, however, when we are exposed to very loud noises. Within the tympanic cavity, two small muscles protect the eardrum and ossicles from violent movements under noisy conditions. The *tensor tympani* (TEN-sor tim-PAN-ē) *muscle* increases the tension, or stiffness, of the tympanum and reduces the amount of possible movement. The *stapedius* (stā-PĒ-dē-us) *muscle* pulls on the stapes, thereby reducing its movement at the oval window.

The Inner Ear

The senses of equilibrium and hearing are provided by the receptors of the **inner ear**. The receptors lie within the **membranous labyrinth** (*labyrinthos*, network of canals), a collection of tubes and chambers filled with a fluid called **endolymph** (EN-dō-limf). The **bony labyrinth** is a shell of dense bone that surrounds and protects the membranous labyrinth. Its inner contours closely follow the contours of the membranous labyrinth (Figure 10-21a•), while its outer walls are fused with the surrounding temporal bone (see Figure 10-19•). Between the bony and membranous labyrinths flows another fluid, the **perilymph** (PER-i-limf).

The bony labyrinth can be subdivided into three parts as seen in Figure 10-21a•.

1. *Vestibule.* The **vestibule** (VES-ti-būl) includes a pair of membranous sacs, the **saccule** (SAK-ūl) and the **utricle** (Ū-tre-kl). Receptors in these sacs provide sensations of gravity and linear acceleration.

2. *Semicircular canals.* The **semicircular canals** enclose slender *semicircular ducts*. Receptors in the semicircular ducts are stimulated by rotation of the

head. The combination of vestibule and semicircular canals is called the **vestibular complex**, because the fluid-filled chambers within the vestibule are broadly continuous with those of the semicircular canals.

3. *Cochlea.* The bony **cochlea** (KOK-lē-a; *cochlea*, snail shell) contains the **cochlear duct** of the membranous labyrinth. Receptors in the cochlear duct provide the sense of hearing. The cochlear duct is sandwiched between a pair of perilymph-filled chambers, and the entire complex is coiled around a central bony hub.

The bony labyrinth's walls consist of dense bone everywhere except at two small areas near the base of the cochlea. (1) The *round window* is an opening in the bone of the cochlea. A thin, membranous partition spans the opening and separates perilymph in the cochlea from the air in the middle ear. (2) The membrane spanning the oval window is firmly attached to the base of the stapes. When a sound vibrates the tympanum, the movements are conducted over the malleus and incus to the stapes. Movement of the stapes ultimately leads to the stimulation of receptors in the cochlear duct, and we hear the sound.

Receptor Function in the Inner Ear.   The receptors of the inner ear are called **hair cells** (Figure 10-21b•). Each hair cell communicates with a sensory neuron by continually releasing small quantities of neurotransmitter. The free surface of this receptor supports 80–100 long microvilli called stereocilia. ∞ *p. 84* Hair cells do not actively move their stereocilia. However, when an external force pushes the stereocilia, their movement distorts the cell surface and alters its rate of neurotransmitter release. Displacement of the stereocilia in one direction stimulates the hair cells (and increases neurotransmitter release); displacement in the opposite direction inhibits the hair cells (and decreases neurotransmitter release).

Equilibrium

There are two aspects of equilibrium: (1) **dynamic equilibrium**, which aids us in maintaining our balance when the head and body are moved suddenly, and (2) **static equilibrium**, which maintains our posture and stability when the body is motionless. All equilibrium sensations are provided by hair cells of the vestibular complex. The receptors of dynamic equilibrium, the semicircular ducts, provide information about rotational movements of the head. For example, when you turn your head to the left, receptors in the semicircular ducts tell you how rapid the movement is and in which direction. The receptors of static equilibrium, the saccule and the utricle, provide information

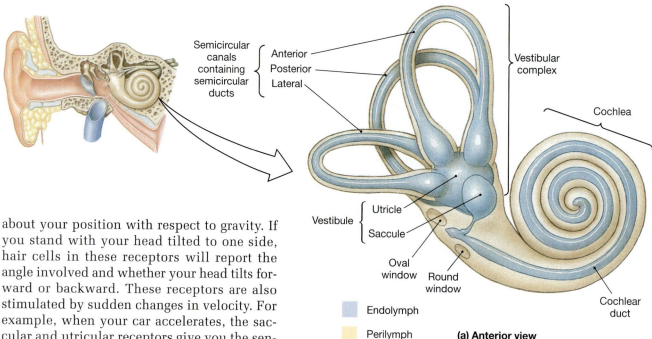

Semicircular
canals
containing
semicircular
ducts

Anterior
Posterior
Lateral

Vestibular
complex

Cochlea

Vestibule

Utricle

Saccule

Oval
window   Round
window

Cochlear
duct

■ Endolymph

■ Perilymph   **(a) Anterior view**

about your position with respect to gravity. If you stand with your head tilted to one side, hair cells in these receptors will report the angle involved and whether your head tilts forward or backward. These receptors are also stimulated by sudden changes in velocity. For example, when your car accelerates, the saccular and utricular receptors give you the sensation of increasing speed.

The Semicircular Ducts: Rotational Motion

Receptors in the semicircular ducts respond to rotational movements. Figure 10-21a● illustrates the **anterior**, **posterior**, and **lateral semicircular ducts** and their continuity with the utricle. Each semicircular duct contains a swollen region, the *ampulla*, which contains the sensory receptors (Figure 10-22a●). Hair cells are attached to the wall of the ampulla, with their stereocilia embedded in a gelatinous structure called the *cupula* (KŪ-pū-luh), which nearly fills the ampulla (Figure 10-22b●). When the head rotates in the plane of the canal, movement of the endolymph pushes against this structure and stimulates the hair cells (Figure 10-22c●).

Each semicircular duct responds to one of three possible rotational movements. To distort the cupula and stimulate the receptors, endolymph must flow along the axis of the duct; that flow will occur only when there is rotation in that plane. A horizontal rotation, as in shaking the head "no," stimulates the hair cells of the lateral semicircular duct. Nodding "yes" excites receptors of the anterior duct, and tilting the head from side to side activates receptors in the posterior duct. The three planes monitored by the semicircular ducts correspond to the three dimensions in the world around us, and they can provide accurate information about even the most complex movements.

The Vestibule: Gravity and Linear Acceleration

Receptors in the utricle and saccule respond to gravity and linear acceleration. As depicted in Figure 10-22a●, the hair cells of the utricle and saccule are clustered in oval **maculae** (MAK-ū-lē; *macula*, spot). As in the ampullae, the hair cell processes in the maculae are embedded in a gelatinous mass, but the macular receptors lie under a thin layer of densely

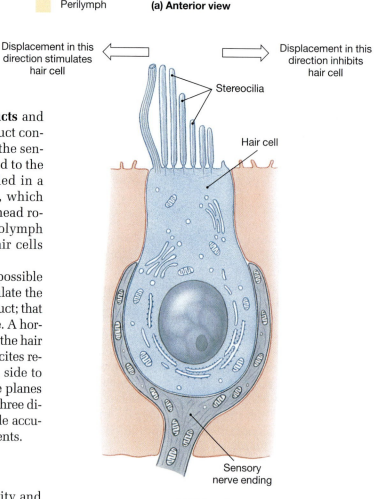

Displacement in this
direction stimulates
hair cell

Displacement in this
direction inhibits
hair cell

Stereocilia

Hair cell

Sensory
nerve ending

(b) Hair cell

●**FIGURE 10-21   The Inner Ear**
(a) An anterior view of the bony labyrinth, showing the outline of the enclosed membranous labyrinth. **(b)** A representative hair cell (receptor) from the vestibular complex.

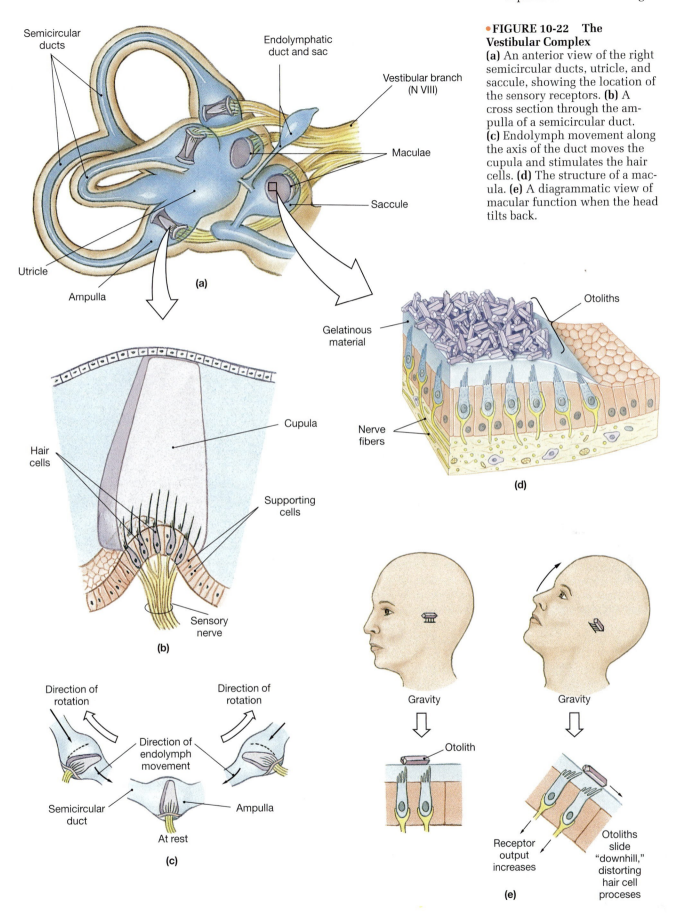

•FIGURE 10-22 The Vestibular Complex
(a) An anterior view of the right semicircular ducts, utricle, and saccule, showing the location of the sensory receptors. (b) A cross section through the ampulla of a semicircular duct. (c) Endolymph movement along the axis of the duct moves the cupula and stimulates the hair cells. (d) The structure of a macula. (e) A diagrammatic view of macular function when the head tilts back.

packed mineral crystals. One of these *otoliths* (*oto-*, ear + *lithos*, a stone) can be seen in Figure 10-22d•. When the head is in the normal, upright position, the otolith sits atop the macula. Its weight presses down on the macular surface, pushing the sensory hairs downward rather than to one side or another. When the head is tilted, the pull of gravity on the otolith shifts its weight to the side, distorting the sensory hairs. The change in receptor activity tells the CNS that the head is no longer level (Figure 10-22e•).

Otoliths are relatively dense and heavy, and they are connected to the rest of the body only by the sensory processes of the macular cells. So whenever the rest of the body makes a sudden movement, the otoliths lag behind. For example, when an elevator starts downward, we are immediately aware of it because the otoliths no longer push so forcefully against the surfaces of the receptor cells. Once they catch up and the elevator has reached a constant speed, we are no longer aware of any movement until the elevator brakes to a halt. As the body slows down, the otoliths press harder against the hair cells and we "feel" the force of gravity increase.

A similar mechanism accounts for our perception of linear acceleration in a car that speeds up suddenly. The otoliths lag behind, distorting the sensory hairs and changing the activity in the sensory neurons. A comparable otolith movement occurs when the chin is raised and gravity pulls the otoliths backward. On the basis of visual information, the brain decides whether the arriving sensations indicate acceleration or a change in head position. Flight simulators and some new arcade games take advantage of this mechanism; they provide visual images that make the brain interpret a tilt as an acceleration.

Central Processing of Vestibular Sensations

Hair cells of the vestibule and of the semicircular canals are monitored by sensory neurons whose fibers form the **vestibular branch** of the vestibulocochlear nerve, N VIII. These fibers synapse on neurons in the *vestibular nuclei* located at the boundary between the pons and the medulla oblongata. The two vestibular nuclei (1) integrate the sensory information arriving from each side of the head; (2) relay information to the cerebellum; (3) relay information to the cerebral cortex, providing a conscious sense of position and movement; and (4) send commands to motor nuclei in the brain stem and in the spinal cord. These reflexive motor commands are distributed to the motor nuclei for cranial nerves involved with eye, head, and neck movements (N III, IV, VI, and XI). Descending instructions along the *vestibulospinal tracts* of the spinal cord adjust peripheral muscle tone to complement the reflexive movements of the head or neck.

Hearing

The receptors of the cochlear duct provide us with a sense of hearing that enables us to detect the quietest whisper yet remain functional in a crowded, noisy room. The receptors responsible for auditory sensations are hair cells similar to those of the vestibular complex. However, their placement within the cochlear duct and the organization of the surrounding accessory structures shield them from stimuli other than sound. In conveying vibrations from the tympanum to the membrane spanning the oval window, the auditory ossicles convert sound energy (pressure waves) in air to pressure pulses in the perilymph of the cochlea. These pressure pulses stimulate hair cells along the cochlear spiral. The *frequency* of the perceived sound is determined by the part of the cochlear duct that is stimulated. The *intensity* (volume) of the perceived sound is determined by the number of hair cells stimulated at that part of the cochlear duct.

The Cochlear Duct

In sectional view, the cochlear duct, or *scala media*, lies between the **vestibular duct** (*scala vestibuli*) and the **tympanic duct** (*scala tympani*), a pair of perilymphatic chambers (Figure 10-23a•). The vestibular and tympanic ducts are interconnected at the tip of the cochlear spiral. The outer surfaces of these ducts are encased by the bony labyrinth everywhere except at the oval window (base of the vestibular duct) and the round window (base of the tympanic duct).

The Organ of Corti.   The hair cells of the cochlear duct are located in the **organ of Corti**, or *spiral organ* (Figure 10-23b•). This sensory structure sits above the **basilar membrane**, which separates the cochlear duct from the tympanic duct. The hair cells are arranged in a series of longitudinal rows, with their stereocilia in contact with the overlying **tectorial membrane** (tek-TŌR-ē-al; *tectum*, roof). This membrane is firmly attached to the inner wall of the cochlear duct. When a portion of the basilar membrane bounces up and down, the stereocilia of the hair cells are distorted as they are pushed up against the tectorial membrane. The basilar membrane moves in response to pressure waves in the perilymph. These waves are produced when sounds arrive at the tympanum. To understand how pressure waves develop, we must consider the basic properties of sound.

The Hearing Process

Hearing is the detection of sound, which consists of pressure waves conducted through air, water, and solids. Physicists use the term **cycles** rather than waves, and the number of cycles per second (cps), or **hertz** (**Hz**), represents the **frequency** of the sound. What we per-

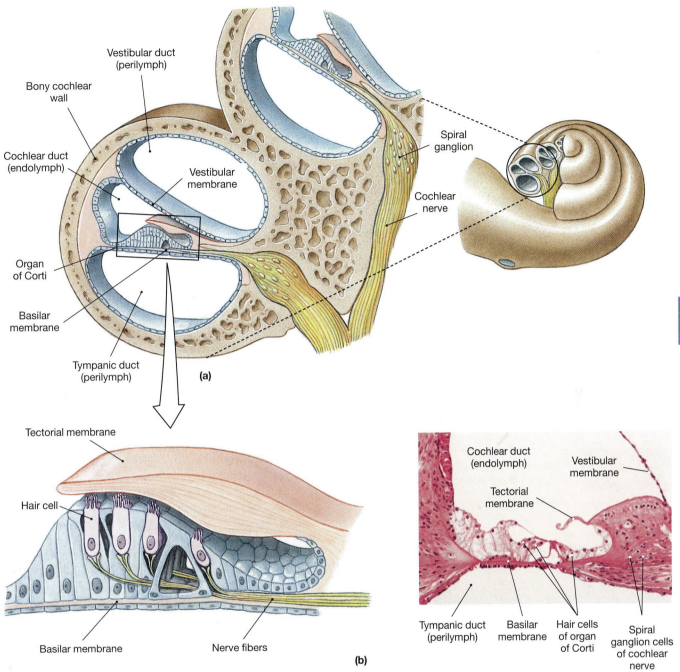

Vestibular duct (perilymph)

Bony cochlear wall

Cochlear duct (endolymph)

Vestibular membrane

Spiral ganglion

Cochlear nerve

Organ of Corti

Basilar membrane

Tympanic duct (perilymph)

(a)

Tectorial membrane

Hair cell

Basilar membrane

Nerve fibers

(b)

Cochlear duct (endolymph)

Vestibular membrane

Tectorial membrane

Tympanic duct (perilymph)

Basilar membrane

Hair cells of organ of Corti

Spiral ganglion cells of cochlear nerve

•**FIGURE 10-23   The Cochlea and Organ of Corti**
(a) A section of the cochlea. **(b)** The three-dimensional structure of the tectorial membrane and hair cell complex of the organ of Corti.

ceive as the **pitch** of a sound (how high or low it is) is our sensory response to its frequency. A sound of high frequency (high pitch) might have a frequency of 15,000 Hz or more; a sound of low frequency (low pitch) could have a frequency of 100 Hz or less.

Hearing can be divided into six basic steps, diagrammed in Figure 10-24• and summarized in Table 10-2.

Step 1: *Sound waves arrive at the tympanum.* Sound waves enter the external auditory canal and travel toward the tympanum. Sound waves approaching

the side of the head have direct access to the tympanum on that side, whereas sounds arriving from another direction must bend around corners or pass through the pinna or other body tissues.

Step 2: *The vibration of the tympanum causes movement of the auditory ossicles.* The tympanum provides the surface for sound collection. It vibrates to sound waves with frequencies between approximately 20 and 20,000 Hz (in a young child). When the tympanum vibrates, so does the malleus and, via their articulations, so do the incus and stapes.

10

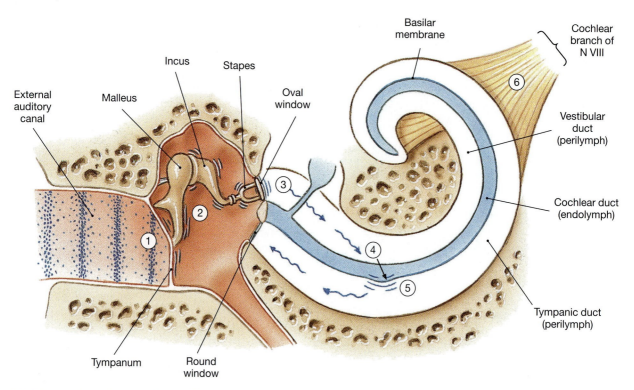

• FIGURE 10-24 Sound Reception and Hearing
The steps in the reception of sound and the process of hearing (see Table 10-2).

TABLE 10-2	**Steps in the Production of an Auditory Sensation**

1. Sound waves arrive at the tympanum.
2. The vibration of the tympanum causes movement of the auditory ossicles.
3. The movement of the stapes at the oval window establishes pressure waves in the perilymph of the vestibular duct.
4. The pressure waves distort the basilar membrane on their way to the round window of the tympanic duct.
5. The vibration of the basilar membrane causes the vibration of hair cells against the tectorial membrane.
6. Information about the region and intensity of stimulation is relayed to the CNS over the cochlear branch of N VIII.

Step 3: *The movement of the stapes at the oval window establishes pressure waves in the perilymph of the vestibular duct.* When it moves, the stapes applies pressure to the perilymph of the vestibular duct. Because the rest of the cochlea is sheathed in bone, pressure applied at the oval window can be relieved only at the round window. When the stapes moves inward, the membrane spanning the round window bulges outward.

Step 4: *The pressure waves distort the basilar membrane on their way to the round window of the tympanic duct.* These pressure waves cause movement in the basilar membrane. The basilar membrane does not have the same structure throughout its length. Near the oval window, it is narrow and stiff, and at its terminal end, it is wider and more flexible. As a result, the location of maximum stimulation varies with the frequency of the sound. High-frequency sounds vibrate the basilar membrane near the oval window. The lower the frequency of the sound, the farther from the oval window the area of maximum distortion will be. The actual *amount* of movement at a given location will depend on the amount of force applied by the stapes. The louder the sound, the greater the movement of the basilar membrane.

Step 5: *The vibration of the basilar membrane causes the vibration of hair cells against the tectorial membrane.* The vibration of the affected region of the basilar membrane moves hair cells against the tectorial membrane. The resulting displacement of the hair cells' stereocilia stimulates sensory neurons. The hair cells are arranged in several rows; a very soft sound may stimulate only a few hair cells in a portion of one row. As the volume of a sound increases, not only do these hair cells become more active but additional hair cells—at first in the same row, and then in adjacent rows—are stimulated as well. The number of hair cells responding in a given region of the organ of Corti thus provides information about the volume of the sound.

Step 6: *Information about the region and intensity of stimulation is relayed to the CNS over the cochlear branch of N VIII.* The cell bodies of the sensory neurons that monitor the cochlear hair cells are located at the center of the bony cochlea (Figure 10-23a•) in the *spiral ganglion.* The information is carried to the cochlear nuclei of the medulla oblongata for subsequent distribution to other centers in the brain.

Auditory Pathways

Hair cell stimulation activates sensory neurons whose cell bodies are in the adjacent spiral ganglion. Their afferent fibers form the **cochlear branch** (Figure 10-25•) of the vestibulocochlear nerve (N VIII). These axons enter the medulla oblongata and synapse at the *cochlear nucleus.* From here the information crosses to the opposite side of the brain and ascends to the *inferior colliculus* of the midbrain. This processing center coordinates a number of responses to acoustic stimuli, including auditory reflexes involving skeletal muscles of the head, face, and trunk. For example, these reflexes automatically change the position of the head in response to a sudden loud noise.

Before reaching the cerebral cortex and our conscious awareness, ascending auditory sensations synapse in the thalamus. Thalamic fibers then deliver the information to the auditory cortex of the temporal lobe. In effect, the auditory cortex contains a map of the organ of Corti. High-frequency sounds activate one portion of the cortex and low-frequency sounds affect another. If the auditory cortex is damaged, the individual will respond to sounds and have normal acoustic reflexes, but sound interpretation and pattern recognition will be difficult or impossible. Damage to the adjacent association area leaves the ability to detect the tones and patterns, but produces an inability to comprehend their meaning.

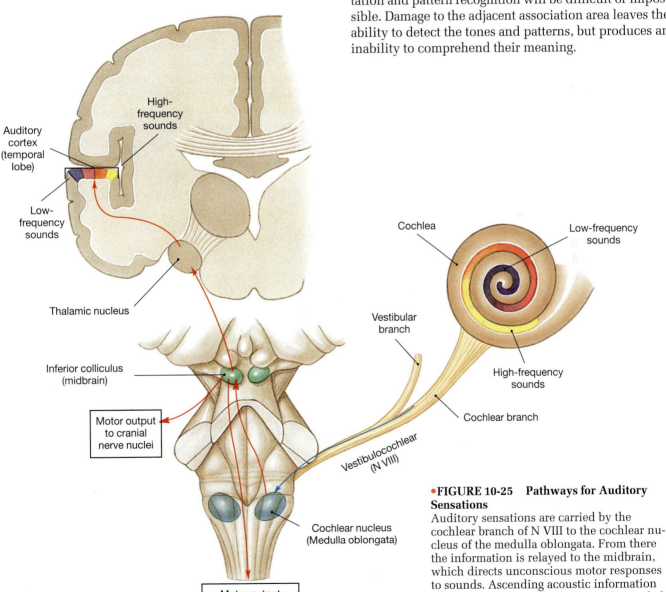

•**FIGURE 10-25 Pathways for Auditory Sensations**
Auditory sensations are carried by the cochlear branch of N VIII to the cochlear nucleus of the medulla oblongata. From there the information is relayed to the midbrain, which directs unconscious motor responses to sounds. Ascending acoustic information goes to the thalamus before being forwarded to the auditory cortex of the temporal lobe.

Auditory Sensitivity

Our hearing abilities are remarkable, though it is difficult to assess the absolute sensitivity of the system. From the softest audible sound to the loudest tolerable blast represents a trillionfold increase in power. Theoretically, if we were to remove the stapes, the receptor mechanism is so sensitive that we could hear the sound of air molecules bouncing off the oval window, responding to displacements as small as one-tenth the diameter of a hydrogen atom. We never utilize the full potential of this system, because body movements and our internal organs produce squeaks, groans, thumps, and other sounds that are tuned out by adaptation. When other environmental noises fade away, the level of adaptation drops and the system becomes increasingly sensitive. If we relax in a quiet room, our heartbeat seems to get louder and louder as the auditory system adjusts to the level of background noise.

✱ HEARING LOSS

Hearing occurs by air conduction and bone conduction. Hearing loss is a common problem, affecting 5–10 percent of the general population. Problems in the external auditory canal and the middle ear cause *conductive hearing losses,* while problems in the inner ear or *vestibulocochlear nerve (CN VIII)* cause *sensorineural hearing loss.*

Conductive hearing loss results from blockage of the external auditory canal, damage to the tympanic membrane, disruption of the auditory ossicles, or from fluid or scarring within the middle ear. Sensorineural hearing loss is primarily due to damage to the hair cells of the organ of Corti. Causes include intense noise, infections, ototoxic drugs, fracture of the temporal bone, Ménière's disease, and aging.

The type of hearing loss can be differentiated by comparing the threshold of hearing by air conduction to that of bone conduction *(Rinne's test).* For this, a tuning fork is struck and placed near the ear. Then the tuning fork is struck and the stem placed on the mastoid process. Normally, air conduction is louder than bone conduction. When bone conduction is louder than air conduction, a conductive loss is suspected. With a sensorineural hearing loss, both are reduced.

Sensorineural loss can be detected with *Weber's test.* For this, a tuning fork is struck and the stem placed on the head in the midline. The tone should be heard equally in both ears. With unilateral conductive hearing loss, the tone is perceived in the affected ear. With unilateral sensorineural loss, the tone is perceived in the unaffected ear.

AGING AND THE SENSES

The general lack of replacement of neurons in the nervous system leads to an inevitable decline in sensory function with age. Although part of this decline can be compensated by an increase in stimuli strength or concentration, the loss of axons to conduct sensory action potentials cannot be increased in a like manner. Other effects of aging also take their toll on the senses:

Olfactory Sensitivity

Unlike populations of other neurons, the population of olfactory receptor cells is regularly replaced by the division of basal stem cells in the olfactory epithelium. Despite this process, the total number of receptors declines with age, and the remaining receptors become less sensitive. As a result, elderly individuals have difficulty detecting odors in low concentrations. This drop in the number receptors accounts for "Grandmother's" tendency to apply perfume in excessive quantities and explains why "Grandfather's" aftershave lotion seems so overdone. They must apply more to be able to smell it.

Gustatory Sensitivity

Tasting abilities change with age due to the thinning of mucous membranes and a reduction in the number and sensitivity of taste buds. We begin life with more than 10,000 taste buds, but that number begins declining dramatically by age 50. The sensory loss becomes especially significant because aging individuals also experience a decline in the number of olfactory receptors. As a result, many of the elderly find that their food tastes bland and unappetizing. Children, however, find the same food too spicy.

Vision

Various disorders of vision are associated with normal aging; the most common involve the lens and the neural retina. With age, the lens loses its elasticity and stiffens. As a result, it becomes more difficult to see objects up close, and older individuals become farsighted—a condition called *presbyopia.* ∞ *p. 286* For example, the inner limit of clear vision, known as the *near point of vision,* changes from 7–9 cm in children to 15–20 cm in young adults and typically reaches 83 cm by age 60. As noted earlier, the most common cause of the development of a cataract (the loss of transparency in the lens) is advancing age. Such cataracts are called senile cataracts. ∞ *p. 284* In addition to changes in the near point of vision and some changes in lens transparency, there is a gradual loss of rods with age. This reduction explains why individuals over age 60 need almost twice as much light to read by than those of age 40.

Another contributor to the loss of vision with age is *macular degeneration,* the leading cause of blindness in persons over 50. It is typically associated with the growth and proliferation of blood vessels in the retina. The leakage of blood and plasma from these abnormal vessels causes retinal scarring and a loss of photoreceptors. The vascular growth begins in the macula lutea, the area of the retina correlated with acute vision. Color vision is affected as the cones deteriorate.

Hearing

Hearing is generally affected less by aging than are the other senses. However, because the tympanum loses some of its elasticity, it becomes more difficult to hear high-pitched sounds. The progressive loss of hearing that occurs with aging is called *presbycusis* (prez-bē-KŪ-sis; *presbys*, old man + *akousis*, hearing).

✓ If the round window were not able to bulge out with increased pressure in the perilymph, how would sound perception be affected?

✓ How would the loss of stereocilia from the hair cells of the organ of Corti affect hearing?

Chapter Review

KEY TERMS

accommodation, *p. 285*	**iris**, *p. 281*	**proprioception**, *p. 272*
cochlea, *p. 291*	**macula**, *p. 292*	**pupil**, *p. 282*
fovea, *p. 282*	**nociceptors**, *p. 272*	**retina**, *p. 282*
gustation, *p. 272*	**olfaction**, *p. 272*	**sclera**, *p. 280*

10

SUMMARY OUTLINE

INTRODUCTION *p. 272*

1. The **general senses** are temperature, pain, touch, pressure, vibration, and proprioception; receptors for these sensations are distributed throughout the body. Receptors for the **special senses** (smell, taste, vision, balance, and hearing) are located in specialized areas or in sense organs.

2. A *sensory receptor* is a specialized cell that, when stimulated, sends a sensation to the CNS. The simplest receptors are **free nerve endings**; the most complex have specialized accessory structures that isolate them from most all but specific types of stimuli.

3. Sensory information is relayed in the form of action potentials in a sensory (afferent) fiber. In general, the larger the stimulus, the greater the frequency of action potentials. The CNS interprets the nature of the arriving sensory information on the basis of the area of the brain stimulated.

4. **Adaptation** (a reduction in sensitivity in the presence of a constant stimulus) involves changes in receptor sensitivity or inhibition along the sensory pathways.

THE GENERAL SENSES *p. 272*

Pain *p. 272*

1. **Nociceptors** respond to a variety of stimuli usually associated with tissue damage. The two types of these painful sensations are **fast pain**, or *prickling pain*, and **slow pain**, or *burning and aching pain*.

2. The perception of pain coming from parts of the body that are not actually stimulated is called **referred pain**. *(Figure 10-1)*

Temperature *p. 273*

3. **Thermoreceptors** respond to changes in temperature.

Touch, Pressure, and Position *p. 273*

4. **Mechanoreceptors** respond to physical distortion, contact, or pressure on their cell membranes; **tactile receptors** to touch, pressure, and vibration; **baroreceptors** to pressure changes in the walls of blood vessels, the digestive and urinary tracts, and the lungs; and **proprioceptors** to positions of joints and muscles.

5. **Fine touch and pressure receptors** provide detailed information about a source of stimulation; **crude touch and pressure receptors** are poorly localized. Important tactile receptors include the *root hair plexus*, *Merkel's discs*, *Meissner's corpuscles*, *Pacinian corpuscles*, and *Ruffini corpuscles*. *(Figure 10-2)*

6. Baroreceptors monitor changes in pressure; they respond immediately but adapt rapidly. Baroreceptors in the walls of major arteries and veins respond to changes in blood pressure. Receptors along the digestive tract help coordinate reflex activities of digestion. *(Figure 10-3)*

7. Proprioceptors monitor the position of joints, tension in tendons and ligaments, and the state of muscular contraction. Proprioceptors include *tendon organs* and *muscle spindles*.

Chemical Detection *p. 275*

8. In general, **chemoreceptors** respond to water-soluble and lipid-soluble substances dissolved in the surrounding fluid. They monitor the chemical composition of body fluids. *(Figure 10-4)*

SMELL *p. 276*

1. The **olfactory organs** contain the **olfactory epithelium** with **olfactory receptors** (neurons sensitive to chemicals dissolved in the overlying mucus), supporting cells, and *basal (stem) cells*. Their surfaces are coated with the secretions of the **olfactory glands**. *(Figure 10-5)*

2. The olfactory receptors are modified neurons. Our olfactory sensitivities are much lower than those of many other vertebrates.

The Olfactory Pathways *p. 276*

3. The olfactory system is very sensitive; its extensive limbic and hypothalamic connections help explain the emotional and behavioral responses that can be produced by certain smells.

TASTE *p. 277*

1. Gustatory (taste) receptors are clustered in **taste buds**, each of which contains **gustatory cells**, which extend *taste hairs* through a narrow **taste pore**. *(Figure 10-6)*

2. Taste buds are associated with **papillae**, epithelial projections on the superior surface of the tongue. *(Figure 10-6)*

3. The **primary taste sensations** are sweet, salt, sour, and bitter.

The Taste Pathways *p. 277*

4. The taste buds are monitored by cranial nerves that synapse within a nucleus of the medulla oblongata.

VISION *p. 278*

The Accessory Structures of the Eye *p. 278*

1. The **accessory structures** of the eye include the eyelids, the eyelashes, various exocrine glands, and the extrinsic eye muscles.

2. An epithelium called the **conjunctiva** covers the exposed surface of the eye except over the transparent **cornea**.

3. The slightly alkaline secretions of the **lacrimal gland** bathe the conjunctiva; these secretions contain a *lysozyme* (an enzyme that attacks bacteria). Tears reach the nasal cavity after passing through the **lacrimal canals**, the **lacrimal sac**, and the **nasolacrimal duct**. *(Figure 10-7)*

4. Six **extrinsic eye muscles** control external eye movements: the **inferior** and **superior rectus**, **lateral** and **medial rectus**, and **superior** and **inferior obliques**. *(Figure 10-8; Table 10-1)*

The Anatomy of the Eye *p. 279*

5. The eye has three layers: an outer fibrous tunic, a vascular tunic, and an inner neural tunic. Most of the ocular surface is covered by the **sclera** (a dense fibrous connective tissue), which is continuous with the cornea, both part of the **fibrous tunic**. *(Figure 10-9)*

6. The **vascular tunic** includes the **iris**, the **ciliary body**, and the **choroid**. The iris forms the boundary between the eye's anterior and posterior chambers. The ciliary body contains the *ciliary muscle* and the *ciliary processes*, which attach to the **suspensory ligaments** of the **lens**. *(Figure 10-9)*

7. The **neural tunic** consists of an outer **pigment layer** and an inner *neural retina*; the latter contains visual receptors and associated neurons. *(Figures 10-9, 10-10)*

8. From the photoreceptors, the information is relayed to **bipolar cells**, then to **ganglion cells**, and to the brain via the optic nerve. Horizontal cells and amacrine cells modify the signals passed between other retinal components. *(Figure 10-10)*

9. The ciliary body and lens divide the interior of the eye into a large **posterior cavity** and a smaller **anterior cavity**. The anterior cavity is subdivided into the **anterior chamber**, which extends from the cornea to the iris, and a **posterior chamber** between the iris and the ciliary body and lens. The posterior chamber contains the *vitreous body*, a gelatinous mass that helps stabilize the shape of the eye and supports the retina. *(Figure 10-12)*

10. Aqueous humor circulates within the eye and reenters the circulation after diffusing through the walls of the anterior chamber and into veins of the sclera through the *canal of Schlemm*. *(Figure 10-12)*

11. The lens, held in place by the suspensory ligaments, focuses a visual image on the retinal receptors. Light is refracted (bent) when it passes through the cornea and lens. During **accommodation**, the shape of the lens changes to focus an image on the retina. *(Figures 10-13, 10-14)*

Visual Physiology *p. 286*

12. Light is radiated in waves with a characteristic wavelength. A *photon* is a single energy packet of visible light. The two types of **photoreceptors** (visual receptors of the retina) are **rods** and **cones**. Rods respond to almost any photon, regardless of its energy content; cones have characteristic ranges of sensitivity. Many cones are densely packed within the **fovea** (the central portion of the **macula lutea**), the site of sharpest vision. *(Figures 10-15, 10-16)*

13. Each photoreceptor contains membranous **discs** containing **visual pigments**. Light absorption occurs in the visual pigments, which are derivatives of **rhodopsin** (opsin plus the pigment **retinal**, which is synthesized from **vitamin A**). A photoreceptor responds to light by changing its rate of neurotransmitter release and thereby altering the activity of a bipolar cell. *(Figure 10-17)*

The Visual Pathway *p. 288*

14. The message is relayed from photoreceptors to bipolar cells to ganglion cells within the retina. The axons of ganglion cells converge at the optic disc and leave the eye as the optic nerve. A partial crossover occurs at the optic chiasm before the information reaches a nucleus in the thalamus on each side of the brain. From these nuclei, visual information is relayed to the visual cortex of the occipital lobe, which contains a sensory map of the field of vision. *(Figure 10-18)*

EQUILIBRIUM AND HEARING *p. 289*

1. The senses of equilibrium (**dynamic equilibrium and static equilibrium**) and hearing are provided by the receptors of the **inner ear** (also known as the **membranous labyrinth**). Its chambers and canals contain the fluid **endolymph**. The **bony labyrinth** surrounds and protects the membranous labyrinth, and the space between them contains the fluid **perilymph**. The bony labyrinth consists of the **vestibule**, the **semicircular canals** (receptors in the vestibule and semicircular canals provide the sense of equilibrium) and the **cochlea** (these receptors provide the sense of hearing). The structures and air spaces of the **external ear** and **middle ear** help capture and transmit sound to the cochlea. *(Figures 10-19, 10-21)*

The Anatomy of the Ear *p. 289*

2. The external ear includes the **pinna** (*auricle*), which surrounds the entrance to the **external auditory canal**, which ends at the **tympanum**, or *tympanic membrane* (*eardrum*). *(Figure 10-19)*

3. The middle ear communicates with the nasopharynx via the **auditory tube** (*pharyngotympanic tube* or *Eustachian tube*). The middle ear encloses and protects the **auditory os-**

sicles, which connect the tympanum with the receptor complex of the inner ear. *(Figures 10-19, 10-20)*

4. The vestibule includes a pair of membranous sacs, the **saccule** and **utricle**, whose receptors provide sensations of gravity and linear acceleration. The semicircular canals contain the **semicircular ducts**, whose receptors provide sensations of rotation. The cochlea contains the **cochlear duct**, an elongated portion of the membranous labyrinth. *(Figure 10-21a)*

5. The basic receptors of the inner ear are **hair cells**, whose surfaces support *stereocilia*. Hair cells provide information about the direction and strength of mechanical stimuli. *(Figure 10-21b)*

Equilibrium *p. 291*

6. The **anterior**, **posterior**, and **lateral semicircular ducts** are attached to the utricle. Each semicircular duct contains an *ampulla* with sensory receptors. There the stereocilia contact the *cupula*, a gelatinous mass that is distorted when endolymph flows along the axis of the duct. *(Figures 10-21, 10-22a,b,c)*

7. In the saccule and utricle, hair cells cluster within **maculae**, where their cilia contact *otoliths* (densely packed mineral crystals). When the head tilts, the mass of otoliths shifts, and the resulting distortion in the sensory hairs signals the CNS. *(Figure 10-22d,e)*

8. The vestibular receptors activate sensory neurons whose axons form the **vestibular branch** of the vestibulocochlear nerve (N VIII), synapsing within the vestibular nuclei.

Hearing *p. 294*

9. Sound waves travel toward the tympanum, which vibrates; the auditory ossicles conduct the vibrations to the inner ear. Movement at the oval window applies pressure to the perilymph of the **vestibular duct**. *(Figures 10-23, 10-24; Table 10-2)*

10. Pressure waves distort the **basilar membrane** and push the hair cells of the **organ of Corti** against the **tectorial membrane**. The *tensor tympani* and *stapedius muscles* contract to reduce the amount of motion when very loud sounds arrive. *(Figure 10-24 and Table 10-2)*

11. The sensory neurons are located in the **spiral ganglion** of the cochlea. Afferent fibers of sensory neurons form the **cochlear branch** of the vestibulocochlear nerve (N VIII), synapsing at the cochlear nucleus. *(Figure 10-25)*

AGING AND THE SENSES *p. 298*

1. As part of the aging process, there are (1) gradual reductions in olfactory and gustatory sensitivity, (2) a tendency toward *presbyopia* and cataract formation in the eyes, and (3) a progressive loss of hearing (*presbycusis*).

REVIEW QUESTIONS

LEVEL 1   Reviewing Facts and Terms

Match each item in column A with the most closely related item in column B. Use letters for answers in the spaces provided.

Column A

___ 1. myopia
___ 2. fibrous tunic
___ 3. nociceptors
___ 4. proprioceptors
___ 5. cones
___ 6. accommodation
___ 7. tympanum
___ 8. thermoreceptors
___ 9. rods
___10. olfaction
___11. fovea
___12. hyperopia
___13. maculae
___14. semicircular ducts

Column B

a. pain receptors
b. free nerve endings
c. sclera and cornea
d. rotational movements
e. provide information on joint position
f. color vision
g. site of sharpest vision
h. active in dim light
i. eardrum
j. change in lens shape to focus retinal image
k. nearsighted
l. farsighted
m. smell
n. gravity and acceleration receptors

15. Regardless of the nature of a stimulus, sensory information must be sent to the central nervous system in the form of:
(a) dendritic processes
(b) action potentials
(c) neurotransmitter molecules
(d) generator potentials

16. A reduction in sensitivity in the presence of constant stimulus is called:
(a) transduction   (b) sensory coding
(c) line labeling   (d) adaptation

17. Mechanoreceptors that detect pressure changes in the walls of blood vessels and in portions of the digestive, reproductive, and urinary tracts are:
(a) tactile receptors   (b) baroreceptors
(c) proprioceptors   (d) free nerve endings

18. Examples of proprioceptors that monitor the position of joints and the state of muscular contraction are:
(a) Pacinian and Meissner's corpuscles
(b) carotid and aortic sinuses
(c) Merkel's discs and Ruffini corpuscles
(d) tendon organs and muscle spindles

19. When chemicals dissolve in the nasal cavity, they stimulate:
    (a) gustatory cells   (b) olfactory hairs
    (c) rod cells   (d) tactile receptors

20. The taste sensation of sweetness is experienced on the:
    (a) posterior part of the tongue
    (b) anterior part of the tongue
    (c) right and left lateral sides of the tongue
    (d) the middle part of the tongue

21. The purpose of tears produced by the lacrimal apparatus is to:
    (a) keep conjunctival surfaces moist and clean
    (b) reduce friction and remove debris from the eye
    (c) provide nutrients and oxygen to the conjunctival epithelium
    (d) a, b, and c are correct

22. The thickened gel-like fluid that helps support the structure of the eyeball is the:
    (a) vitreous humor
    (b) aqueous humor
    (c) cupula
    (d) perilymph

23. The retina is considered to be a component of the:
    (a) vascular tunic   (b) fibrous tunic
    (c) neural tunic   (d) a, b, and c are correct

24. At sunset or sunrise your visual system adapts to:
    (a) fovea vision
    (b) rod-based vision
    (c) macular vision
    (d) cone-based vision

25. The malleus, incus, and stapes are the tiny ear bones located in the:
    (a) outer ear
    (b) middle ear
    (c) inner ear
    (d) membranous labyrinth

26. Receptors in the saccule and utricle provide sensations of:
    (a) balance and equilibrium
    (b) hearing
    (c) vibration
    (d) gravity and linear acceleration

27. The organ of Corti is located within the _____ of the inner ear.
    (a) utricle
    (b) bony labyrinth
    (c) vestibule
    (d) cochlea

28. What three types of mechanoreceptors respond to stretching, compression, twisting, or other distortions of the cell membrane?

29. Identify six types of tactile receptors found in the skin and their sensitivities.

30. (a) What structures make up the fibrous tunic of the eye?
    (b) What are the functions of the fibrous tunic?

31. What structures are part of the vascular tunic of the eye?

32. What six basic steps are involved in the process of hearing?

LEVEL 2   Reviewing Concepts

33. The CNS interprets sensory information entirely on the basis of the:
    (a) strength of the action potential
    (b) number of generator potentials
    (c) area of brain stimulated
    (d) a, b, and c are correct

34. If the auditory cortex is damaged, the individual will respond to sounds and have normal acoustic reflexes, but:
    (a) the sounds may produce nerve deafness
    (b) the auditory ossicle may be immobilized
    (c) sound interpretation and pattern recognition may be impossible
    (d) normal transfer of vibration to the oval window is inhibited

35. Distinguish between the general senses and the special senses in the human body.

36. In what form does the CNS receive a stimulus detected by a sensory receptor?

37. Why are olfactory sensations long-lasting and an important part of our memories and emotions?

38. Jane makes an appointment with the optometrist for a vision test. Her test results are reported as 20/15. What does this test result mean? Is a rating of 20/20 better or worse?

LEVEL 3   Critical Thinking and Clinical Applications

39. You are at a park watching some deer 35 feet away from you. Your friend taps you on the shoulder to ask a question. As you turn to look at your friend, who is standing 2 feet away, what changes will occur regarding your eyes?

40. After attending a Fourth of July fireworks extravaganza, Millie finds it difficult to hear normal conversation, and her ears keep "ringing." What is causing her hearing problems?

41. After riding the express elevator from the twentieth floor to the ground floor, for a few seconds you still feel as if you are descending, even though you have obviously come to a stop. Why?

ANSWERS TO CONCEPT CHECK QUESTIONS

Page 278

1. By the end of the lab period, adaptation has occurred. In response to the constant level of stimulation, the receptor neurons have become less active, partially as the result of synaptic fatigue.   **2.** Since nociceptors are pain receptors, if they are stimulated, you would perceive a painful sensation in your affected hand.   **3.** Proprioceptors relay information about limb position and movement to the central nervous system, especially the cerebellum. Lack of this information would result in uncoordinated movements, and the individual probably would not be able to walk.   **4.** The taste receptors (taste buds) are sensitive only to molecules and ions that are in solution. If you dry the surface of the tongue, there is no moisture for the sugar molecules or salt ions to dissolve in and they will not stimulate the taste receptors.

Page 289

1. The first layer of the eye to be affected by inadequate tear production would be the conjunctiva. Drying of this layer would produce an irritated, scratchy feeling.   **2.** When the lens is round, you are looking at something close to you.   **3.** A person with a congenital lack of cone cells in the eye would be able to see as long as he or she had functioning rod cells. Since cone cells function in color vision, such a person would see only black and white.   **4.** A deficiency or lack of vitamin A in the diet would affect the quantity of retinal the body could produce and thus would interfere with night vision.

Page 299

1. Without the movement of the round window, the perilymph would not be moved by the vibration of the stapes at the oval window, and there would be little or no perception of sound.   **2.** Loss of stereocilia (as a result of constant exposure to loud noises for instance) would reduce hearing sensitivity and could eventually result in deafness.

10

Emergency Care Applications

OVERVIEW

Sensation is an important component of nervous system function. Nervous system receptors constantly monitor the body for pain (nociceptors); temperature (thermoreceptors); touch, pressure, position (mechanoreceptors); and chemical stimuli (chemoreceptors). The receptors often signal the occurrence of a problem that can lead to a medical emergency. Emergency personnel must understand the various components of sensory function.

PAIN

Pain is an important symptom in medicine. In fact, over 60 percent of people who present to hospital emergency departments do so because of pain. Despite this, inadequate analgesia continues to be a problem in emergency care, especially in children. Emergency pain management should include pain relief when possible and management of associated anxiety. This must be provided while continu-ously monitoring the patient's airway, vital signs, and mental status (Figure A10-1•).

The pathophysiology of the pain response is very complex. There are both peripheral and central mediators of pain. The peripheral pain system is activated when nociceptors and free nerve endings register the original noxious stimulus in the peripheral tissues and transmit it to the central nervous system. Several neurotransmitters are involved in the pain response including the excitatory amino acid *glutamate* and the neuropeptides *neurokinin-A, calcitonin-gene related peptide,* and *substance P.* Pain signals are integrated in the dorsal horn of the spinal cord. These are relayed to higher centers in the brain including the hypothalamus, thalamus, and the limbic and reticular activating systems. These centers integrate and process pain information allowing the detection of and perception of pain. Interpretation, identification, and localization of pain also occur at these sites.

Because pain is subjective, it is often difficult to assess. In the emergency setting, it is common to use a pain scale to determine the

• **FIGURE A10-1 Pain Control in Emergency Care**
All patients should be assessed for pain. When possible, analgesics should be administered, especially for injuries, such as fractures, that may be worsened by ambulance transport.

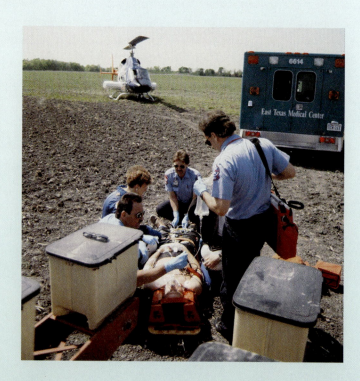

severity of a patient's pain. The most popular pain scale asks patients to rate their pain on a numeric scale that ranges from 0 to 10, with 0 indicating no pain and 10 indicating the worst possible pain. Pain scale ratings can be monitored to determine the effectiveness of medications and other treatments.

Analgesics are medications that help to alleviate pain. They may work on peripheral pain mediators, central pain mediators, or both. Nonsteroidal anti-inflammatory (NSAID) agents are commonly used for mild to moderate pain. NSAIDs primarily act on peripheral pain mediators and include aspirin, ibuprofen, naproxen, ketoprofen, and many others. These drugs decrease levels of inflammatory mediators, such as prostaglandins, generated at the site of tissue injury. Because they act peripherally, they do not cause sedation or respiratory depression and they do not interfere with bowel or bladder function. Acetaminophen (Tylenol) is also a peripherally acting analgesic. However, unlike the NSAIDs, it does not have anti-inflammatory properties and does not affect platelet aggregation (as does aspirin). Most peripherally acting analgesics must be administered orally or by topical application. The exception is ketorolac (Toradol), which is available for intramuscular or intravenous injection.

Moderate to severe pain usually requires opioid analgesics. Opioid analgesics include morphine, codeine, hydromorphone, meperidine, fentanyl, and others. They are most effective when they are administered parenterally (outside of the digestive system). Common routes of opioid injection are subcutaneous, intramuscular, and intravenous. Several opioids referred to as endorphins and enkephalins occur naturally in the body. These substances serve as natural painkillers. The opiate medications act on the same receptors as the endorphins and enkephalins. Opiate receptors' different shapes influence the fit of the corresponding opiate/opioid molecules. The principle opioid receptors, referred to as mu (μ) receptors, produce analgesia, euphoria, and respiratory depression. The mu receptors can be further classified as mu-1 and mu-2. Mu-1 (μ1) receptors cause analgesia, while mu-2 (μ2) receptors produce constipation, euphoria, physical dependence, and respiratory depression. Several other receptors involved in the central pain response include the delta, sigma, kappa, and epsilon receptors. The delta (δ) receptors also produce analgesia. The sigma (ζ) receptors stimulate respiratory and vasomotor activity as well as hallucinations and dysphoria. The kappa (κ) receptors influence spinal analgesia, sedation, and pupillary constriction. Finally, the epsilon (ε) receptors produce analgesia. Morphine and the other opiate derivatives have an affinity for the mu and kappa receptors.

Peripherally acting and centrally acting analgesics are often mixed to provide highly effective pain control. Usually, these are a combination of an opioid and acetaminophen or an opioid and ibuprofen. In addition, long-term pain control can be provided with delayed-release medications or skin patches that deliver a standard amount of opioid analgesia over 72-hours. Patient comfort and pain control are an important aspect of emergency care. Emergency personnel should assess the severity of a patient's pain and expeditiously provide adequate analgesia when possible.

EYE EMERGENCIES

Vision is one of our most important senses. The eyes are the principle sensory organs of vision, and emergencies involving the eye can threaten sight. Because of this, detailed evaluation and treatment of emergent eye illnesses and emergencies is essential. Two types of doctors specialize in treating eye disorders: ophthalmologists and optometrists. *Ophthalmologists* are physicians (M.D. or D.O.) who have graduated from medical school and completed a residency in ophthalmology. They specialize in the medical and surgical management of eye disorders. Optometrists are doctors of optometry (O.D.) who have completed four years of optometry school. They primarily perform refractive examinations and prescribe glasses and contact lenses. Optometrists do not perform surgery and, in many states, do not prescribe medication.

Conjunctival Injuries

Acute eye pain or a red eye are the most common initial complaints of patients with an ocular emergency. Injuries to the eye are common. One of the most striking eye injuries is a subconjunctival hemorrhage. Trauma can cause the fragile blood vessels within the conjunctiva to rupture. The bleeding is evident as it occurs over the white of the eye. In addition to trauma, sneezing, coughing, vomiting, and straining can cause a subconjunctival hemorrhage. High blood pressure also can cause a conjunctival hemorrhage. In many cases, a specific cause cannot be identified. Subconjunctival hemorrhages are painless, do not affect vision, and generally do not require treatment, resolving completely within a week or two. Abrasions of the conjunctival membranes, which are also common, heal completely within 2 to 3 days (Figure A10-2●).

Corneal Injuries

Trauma to the cornea can cause an abrasion. In addition to trauma, corneal abrasions can develop from contact lens wear. Pain, redness, tearing, and light sensitivity usually accompany a corneal abrasion. Assessment of corneal abrasions is often difficult because of the patient's discomfort. Often, these patients feel as though a foreign body is embedded in the eye, and they often worsen the abrasion by trying to remove the perceived foreign body. Usually, a drop or two of topical ophthalmic anesthetic will provide rapid pain relief so that an adequate examination can be carried out. Under magnification, a defect

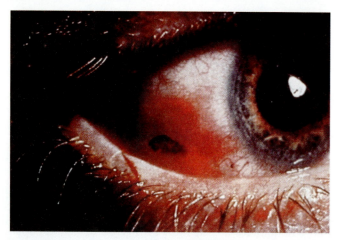

● FIGURE A10-2 Conjunctival Abrasion
A conjunctival foreign body and abrasion overlie a large subconjunctival hemorrhage.

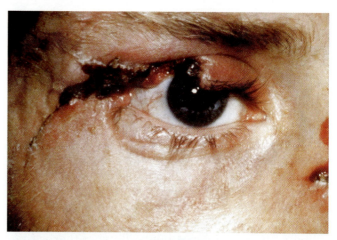

● FIGURE A10-3 Trauma to Right Eye
Significant trauma, such as this upper lid laceration, necessitates a detailed examination for other injuries such as a blowout fracture.

in the cornea can usually be seen. Corneal abrasions can be visualized by staining the eye with fluorescein. The injured cornea takes up the fluorescein, and examination under an ultraviolet light will clearly demonstrate the injury. Corneal abrasions usually heal within a matter of days. Treatment includes analgesics and placement of antibiotic drops or ointment.

Small particles, such as dust or metal fragments, can become embedded in the cornea. These corneal foreign bodies cause an underlying abrasion. Most foreign bodies are superficial and can be removed in the emergency department. A ring of rust may develop around metallic foreign bodies that are embedded more than 24 hours. The rust must be removed or it will permanently scar the cornea. Following removal of a corneal foreign body, it is important to evert the eyelid to make sure a second foreign body is not present.

Blunt Eye Trauma

Blunt trauma to the eye can cause swelling of the lids and the periorbital tissues. A direct blow to the eye can result in a *hyphema,* bleeding into the anterior chamber. A hyphema is a serious injury that can result in permanent blindness and should always be evaluated by an ophthalmologist. Hyphemas can cause increased pressures within the eye and permanent injury. The patient's head should be elevated to help decrease intraocular pressure. Spontaneous rebleeding is not uncommon with hyphemas.

Blunt trauma to the eye can sometimes result in a blowout fracture, a fracture of the wall or walls of the orbit. Most frequently, the inferior wall of the orbit is fractured into the maxillary sinus. Occasionally, the inferior rectus muscle may be entrapped in the fracture, preventing the eye from moving superiorly (looking up). The patient may report double vision on upward gaze. Blowout fractures require surgical treatment (Figure A10-3●).

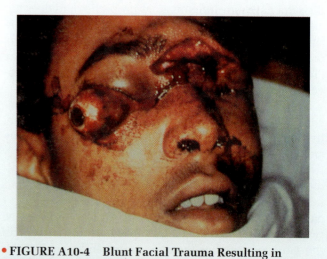

● FIGURE A10-4 Blunt Facial Trauma Resulting in Enucleation of the Right Eye
The globe should be carefully protected and the patient transported to a facility with ophthalmological surgery capabilities.

Penetrating Eye Injury

Any injury that penetrates the globe or ruptures the globe is extremely serious. Common causes include BB pellets, lawn mower projectiles, particles from hammering, grinding injuries, knife wounds, and gunshot wounds. Any penetrating injury has the potential for entering the eye. If a ruptured globe is suspected, a protective shield should be immediately placed over the affected eye, and the patient should be kept calm to prevent exacerbating the injury (Figure A10-4●).

Chemical Injuries

Chemical injuries to the eye are common. The severity of a chemical injury is directly related to the chemical agent involved. Immediately following a chemical injury, the eye should be irrigated with copious amounts of water for 10 minutes (if the chemical was an alkali, irrigation is carried out longer until pH of tears returns to normal) to help remove the offending agent. Following this, a detailed examination of the affected eye, including possible fluorescein staining, should be carried out to determine the severity of tissue injury.

Ultraviolet Keratitis

Ultraviolet keratitis is severe pain, tearing, light sensitivity, and foreign-body sensation that occurs from 6 to 12 hours after ocular exposure to a welding arc, tanning lights, or bright snow. Often, the patient is awakened with severe eye pain and tearing. This injury can be extremely painful but responds readily to topical anesthetics. It usually resolves in 24 to 48 hours.

Acute Glaucoma

Failure of the aqueous humor to enter the canal of Schlemm leads to glaucoma. Although drainage is im-

paired, the production of aqueous humor continues, and the intraocular pressure begins to rise. As this progresses, the soft tissues within the eye become distorted. *Acute angle-closure glaucoma* is a serious medical emergency. The patient often complains of cloudy vision, eye ache, headache, and frequently nausea and vomiting. Usually, there is no history of glaucoma. Acute angle-closure glaucoma requires hospitalization and treatment with medications that decrease intraocular pressure.

SUMMARY

The sensory functions of the nervous system are important. Pain and other sensory perceptions are the principle reasons people seek emergency health care. Emergency personnel should be familiar with the common problems that arise related to sensory function.

A10

11

The Endocrine System

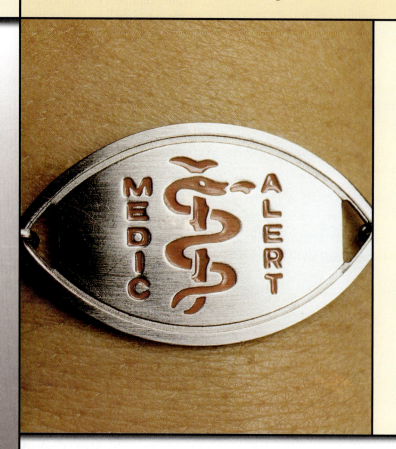

Diabetes is a common disease. Diabetics, especially those who are insulin-dependent, can rapidly develop hypoglycemia and coma. Oftentimes, by-standers may not know that the patient is diabetic. Emergency personnel should always look for identification, such as the Medic-Alert bracelet, to help establish the cause of the coma so proper treatment can be provided promptly.

Chapter Outline and Objectives

Vocabulary Development

ad-, to or toward; *adrenal*
andros, man; *androgen*
angeion, vessel; *angiotensin*
corpus, body; *corpus luteum*
diourein, to urinate; *diuresis*
diabetes, to pass through; *diabetes*
*endo-, inside; *endocrine*
erythros, red; *erythropoietin*
*-glyco; sugar; *hypoglycemia*
*hyper-, above; *hyperthyroidism*
*hypo-, under; *hypoglycemia*
infundibulum, funnel; *infundibulum*
insipidus, tasteless; *diabetes insipidus*
krinein, to secrete; *endocrine*
lac, milk; *prolactin*
mellitum, honey; *diabetes mellitus*
natrium, sodium; *natriuretic*
ouresis, making water; *polyuria*
oxy-, quick; *oxytocin*
para, beyond; *parathyroid*
poiesis, making; *erythropoietin*
pro-, before; *prolactin*
renes, kidneys; *adrenal*
synairesis, a drawing together; *synergistic*
teinein, to stretch; *angiotensin*
thyreos, an oblong shield; *thyroid*
tokos, childbirth; *oxytocin*
tropos, turning; *gonadotropins*

To function effectively, every cell in the body must communicate with its neighbors and with cells and tissues in distant regions of the body. Most of the communication involves the release and receipt of chemical messages. Each living cell is continually "talking" to its neighbors by releasing chemicals into the extracellular fluid. These chemicals let cells know what their neighbors are doing at any given moment, and the result is the coordination of tissue function at the local level.

The nervous system acts like a telephone company, carrying specific "messages" from one location to another inside the body. The source and the destination are quite specific, and the effects are short-lived. This form of communication is ideal for crisis management; if you are in danger of being hit by a speeding bus, the nervous system can coordinate and direct your leap to safety. Once the crisis is over and the neural circuit quiets down, things soon return to normal.

In cellular communication, hormones are like addressed letters, and the circulatory system is the postal service. A hormone released into the circulation will be distributed throughout the body. Each hormone has specific *target cells* that will respond to its presence. These cells possess the receptors needed to bind and "read" the hormonal message. Although a cell may be exposed to the mixture of hormones in circulation at any given moment, it will respond only to those hormones it can bind and read. The other hormones will be treated like junk mail, and ignored.

Because target cells can be anywhere in the body, a single hormone can alter the metabolic activities of multiple tissues and organs simultaneously. These effects may be slow to appear, but they often persist for days. This persistence makes hormones effective in coordinating cell, tissue, and organ activities on a sustained, long-term basis. For example, circulating hormones keep body water content and levels of electrolytes and organic nutrients within normal limits 24 hours a day throughout our entire lives.

While the effects of a single hormone persist, a cell may receive additional instructions from other hormones. The result will be a further modification in cellular operations. Gradual changes in the quantities and identities of circulating hormones can produce complex changes in physical structure and physiological capabilities. Examples are the processes of embryological and fetal development, growth, and puberty.

When viewed from a general perspective, the differences between the nervous and endocrine systems seem relatively clear. In fact, these broad organizational and functional distinctions are the basis for treating them as two separate systems. Yet when considered in detail, the two systems are organized along parallel lines. For example:

- Both systems rely on the release of chemicals that bind to specific receptors on their target cells.
- Both systems use many of the same chemical messengers; for example, norepinephrine and epinephrine are called *hormones* when released into the general circulation, and *neurotransmitters* when released across synapses.
- Both systems are primarily regulated by negative feedback control mechanisms.
- Both systems share a common goal: to coordinate and regulate the activities of other cells, tissues, organs, and systems and to maintain homeostasis.

This chapter introduces the components and functions of the endocrine system and explores the interactions between the nervous and endocrine systems. Later chapters will consider specific endocrine organs, hormones, and functions in greater detail.

An OVERVIEW OF THE ENDOCRINE SYSTEM

The endocrine system includes all of the endocrine cells and tissues of the body. As noted in Chapter 4, **endocrine cells** are glandular secretory cells that release their secretions internally rather than onto an epithelial surface. This feature distinguishes them from *exocrine cells*, which secrete onto epithelial surfaces. ∞ *p. 83* The chemicals released by endocrine cells may affect only adjacent cells, as in the case of the "local hormones" known as *prostaglandins*, or they may affect cells throughout the body. **Hormones** are chemical messengers that are released in one tissue and transported by the bloodstream to reach target cells in other tissues.

The components of the endocrine system are introduced in Figure 11-1•. This figure also lists the major hormones produced in each endocrine tissue and organ. Some of these organs, such as the pituitary gland, have endocrine secretion as a primary function; others, such as the pancreas, have many other functions besides endocrine secretion.

The Structure of Hormones

Hormones can be divided into three groups on the basis of chemical structure: amino acid derivatives, peptide hormones, and lipid derivatives.

1. *Amino acid derivatives.* Some hormones are relatively small molecules that are structurally similar to amino acids. (Amino acids, the building blocks of

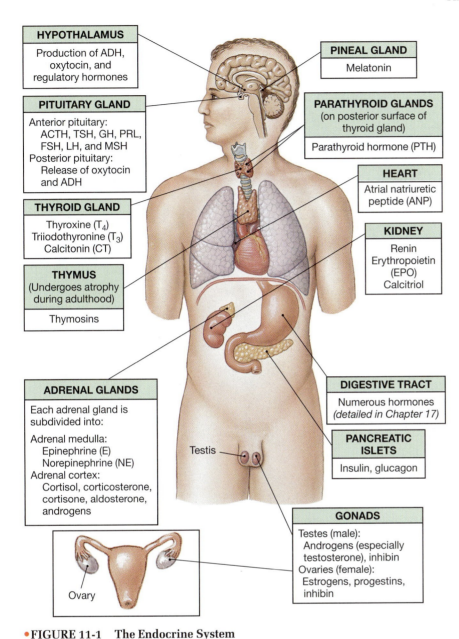

HYPOTHALAMUS
Production of ADH, oxytocin, and regulatory hormones

PINEAL GLAND
Melatonin

PITUITARY GLAND
Anterior pituitary:
    ACTH, TSH, GH, PRL, FSH, LH, and MSH
Posterior pituitary:
    Release of oxytocin and ADH

PARATHYROID GLANDS
(on posterior surface of thyroid gland)
Parathyroid hormone (PTH)

HEART
Atrial natriuretic peptide (ANP)

THYROID GLAND
Thyroxine (T_4)
Triiodothyronine (T_3)
Calcitonin (CT)

KIDNEY
Renin
Erythropoietin (EPO)
Calcitriol

THYMUS
(Undergoes atrophy during adulthood)
Thymosins

ADRENAL GLANDS
Each adrenal gland is subdivided into:
Adrenal medulla:
    Epinephrine (E)
    Norepinephrine (NE)
Adrenal cortex:
    Cortisol, corticosterone, cortisone, aldosterone, androgens

Testis

Ovary

DIGESTIVE TRACT
Numerous hormones
(detailed in Chapter 17)

PANCREATIC ISLETS
Insulin, glucagon

GONADS
Testes (male):
    Androgens (especially testosterone), inhibin
Ovaries (female):
    Estrogens, progestins, inhibin

•**FIGURE 11-1   The Endocrine System**

3. *Lipid derivatives.* There are two classes of lipid-based hormones: steroid hormones, derived from cholesterol; and those derived from *arachidonic acid*, a 20-carbon fatty acid. **Steroid hormones** are lipids structurally similar to cholesterol, a lipid introduced in Chapter 2. *p. 41* Steroid hormones are released by the reproductive organs and the adrenal glands. The fatty acid-based compounds, which include the **prostaglandins**, coordinate local cellular activities and affect enzymatic processes, such as blood clotting, that occur in extracellular fluids.

The Mechanisms of Hormonal Action

All cellular structures and functions are determined by proteins. Structural proteins determine the general shape and internal structure of a cell, and enzymes direct its metabolic activities. Hormones alter cellular operations by changing the *identities*, *activities*, or *quantities* of important enzymes and structural proteins in various **target cells**. The sensitivity of a target cell is determined by the presence or absence of a specific **receptor** with which the hormone interacts, either on the cell membrane or in the cytoplasm (Figure 11-2•).

proteins, were introduced in Chapter 2.) *p. 42* This group includes *epinephrine, norepinephrine,* the *thyroid hormones,* and the pineal hormone *melatonin.*

2. *Peptide hormones.* **Peptide hormones** consist of chains of amino acids. These molecules range from short amino acid chains, such as *ADH* and *oxytocin,* to small proteins such as *growth hormone* and *prolactin.* This is the largest class of hormones and includes all of the hormones secreted by the hypothalamus, pituitary gland, heart, kidneys, thymus, digestive tract, and pancreas.

Hormones and the Cell Membrane

Epinephrine, norepinephrine, and peptide hormones cannot diffuse through a cell membrane, because they are not lipid soluble; they are also too large to fit through membrane channels. Instead, these hormones, called **first messengers**, target receptors on the cell membrane. When a first messenger binds to an appropriate receptor, it triggers the appearance of a **second messenger** in the cytoplasm. The second messenger may function as an enzyme activator or inhibitor, but the net result will be a change in the cell's metabolic activities.

1
1

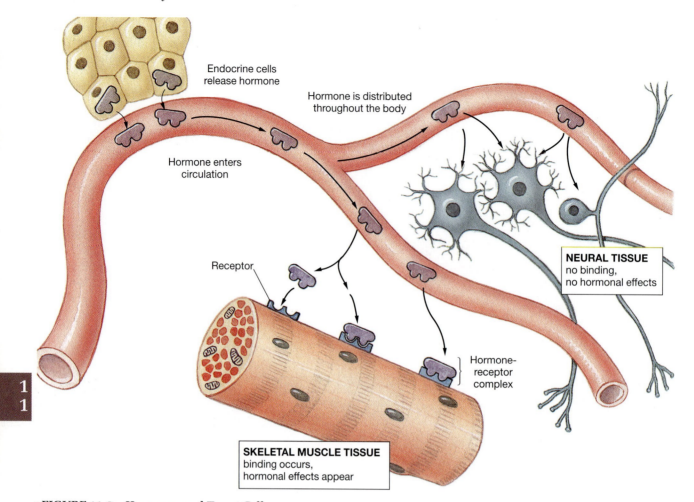

•FIGURE 11-2   Hormones and Target Cells
For a hormone to affect a target cell, that cell must have receptors that can bind the hormone and initiate a change in cellular activity. This hormone affects skeletal muscle tissue but not neural tissue because only the muscle tissue has the appropriate receptors.

One of the most important second messengers is **cyclic-AMP (cAMP)** (Figure 11-3a•). Its appearance depends on the activation of an enzyme called **adenylate cyclase,** in response to hormone binding. When activated, adenylate cyclase converts ATP to cyclic-AMP. The specific response of the target cell to cAMP depends on the nature of the enzymes already present in the cytoplasm. As a result, a single hormone can have one effect in one target tissue and quite different effects in other target tissues. The effects of cAMP are usually very short-lived, because another enzyme present in the cell, *phosphodiesterase*, quickly breaks down cAMP.

Cyclic-AMP is one of the most common second messengers, but there are many others. Important examples are calcium ions and the high-energy compound *cyclic-GMP*.

Hormones and Intracellular Receptors

The steroid hormones and thyroid hormones cross the cell membrane and bind to intracellular receptors (Figure 11-3b•). Steroid hormones diffuse rapidly through the lipid portion of the cell membrane and bind to receptors in the cytoplasm or nucleus. The resulting *hormone-receptor complex* then binds to DNA segments and triggers the activation or inactivation of specific genes. By altering the rate of mRNA transcription in the nucleus, steroid hormones can change the structure or function of the cell. For example, the hormone *testosterone* stimulates the production of enzymes and proteins in skeletal muscle fibers, increasing muscle size and strength.

Thyroid hormones cross the cell membrane through diffusion or carrier-mediated transport. Once within the cell, these hormones bind to receptors within the nucleus and on mitochondria. The hormone-receptor complexes in the nucleus activate specific genes. The result is an increase in metabolic activity due to changes in the nature or number of enzymes in the cytoplasm. Thyroid hormones bound to mitochondria increase the mitochondria's rates of ATP production.

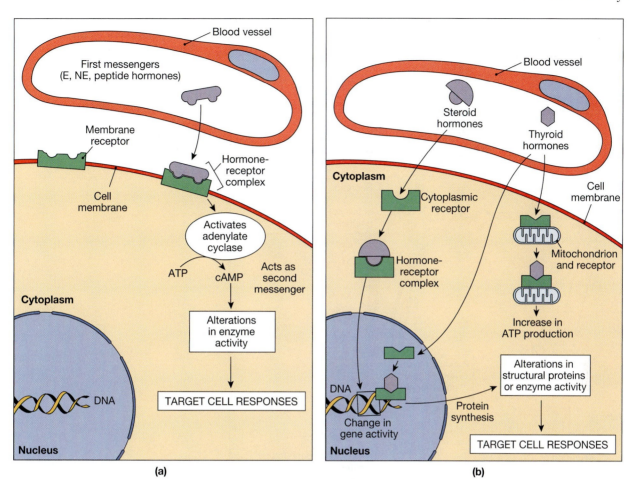

●FIGURE 11-3   Mechanisms of Hormone Action
(a) Nonsteroidal hormones, such as epinephrine, norepinephrine, and the peptide hormones, bind to cell membrane receptors. They exert their effects on target cells through a second messenger, such as cAMP, which alters the activity of enzymes present in the cell. (b) Both steroid hormones and thyroid hormones pass directly through target cell membranes. Steroid hormones bind to receptors in the cytoplasm that then enter the nucleus. Thyroid hormones proceed directly to the nucleus to reach hormonal receptors and/or mitochondria in the cytoplasm. In the nucleus, both steroid and thyroid hormone-receptor complexes directly affect gene activity and protein synthesis. Thyroid hormones also increase the rate of ATP production in the cell.

The Control of Endocrine Activity

Endocrine activity may be controlled directly, by a change in the composition of the extracellular fluid, or indirectly, by the hypothalamus. Negative feedback mechanisms provide the basis for the control of endocrine activity. ∞ *p. 14*

Direct Negative Feedback Control

In direct negative feedback control, endocrine cells respond to a change in the composition of the extracellular fluid by releasing their hormone into the bloodstream. The released hormone stimulates target cells to restore homeostasis. For example, consider the control of calcium levels by *parathyroid hormone* and *calcitonin*. When circulating calcium levels decline, parathyroid hormone is released, and the responses of target cells elevate blood calcium levels. When calci-

um levels rise, calcitonin is released, and responses of target cells lower blood calcium levels.

The Hypothalamus and Endocrine Regulation

Coordinating centers in the hypothalamus regulate the activities of the nervous and endocrine systems in three ways (Figure 11-4●):

1. The hypothalamus contains autonomic centers that control the endocrine cells of the adrenal medullae (the interior of the adrenal glands) through sympathetic innervation. ∞ *p. 262* When the sympathetic division is activated, the adrenal medullae release hormones into the bloodstream.

2. The hypothalamus itself acts as an endocrine organ, releasing the hormones ADH and oxytocin into the circulation at the posterior pituitary.

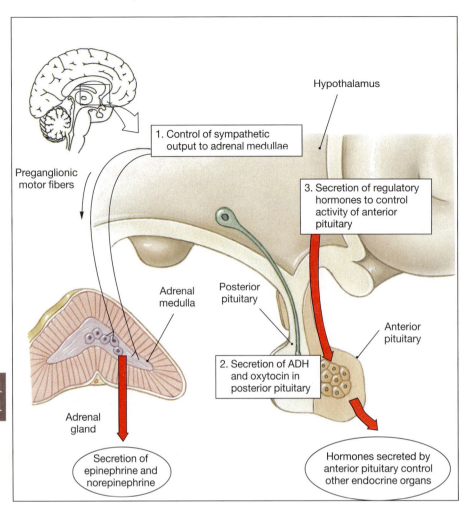

Hypothalamus

1. Control of sympathetic output to adrenal medullae

3. Secretion of regulatory hormones to control activity of anterior pituitary

Preganglionic motor fibers

Adrenal medulla

Posterior pituitary

Anterior pituitary

2. Secretion of ADH and oxytocin in posterior pituitary

Adrenal gland

Secretion of epinephrine and norepinephrine

Hormones secreted by anterior pituitary control other endocrine organs

3. The hypothalamus secretes **regulatory hormones**, special hormones that regulate the activities of endocrine cells in the anterior pituitary gland. There are two classes of regulatory hormones: **releasing hormones (RH)** stimulate the production of one or more hormones in the anterior pituitary, and **inhibiting hormones (IH)** prevent the synthesis and secretion of pituitary hormones.

THE PITUITARY GLAND

The **pituitary gland**, or **hypophysis** (hī-POF-i-sis), secretes nine different hormones. All are peptide hormones that bind to membrane receptors and use cyclic-AMP as a second messenger. This small, oval gland lies nestled within the *sella turcica*, a depression in the sphenoid bone of the skull (Figure 11-5●). ∞ *p. 136* The pituitary gland hangs beneath the hypothalamus, connected by a slender stalk, the **infundibulum** (in-fun-DIB-ū-lum; funnel). The pituitary gland has a complex structure, with distinct anterior and posterior regions.

The Anterior Pituitary Gland

The **anterior pituitary gland** contains endocrine cells surrounded by an extensive capillary network. The capillary network, part of the *hypophyseal portal system*, provides an entry into the circulatory system for the endocrine secretions of the anterior pituitary.

The Hypophyseal Portal System

The regulatory hormones produced by the hypothalamus regulate the activities of the anterior pituitary. These hormones, released by hypothalamic neurons near the attachment of the infundibulum, enter a network of highly permeable capillaries. Before leaving the hypothalamus, this capillary network unites to form a series of larger vessels that descend to the anterior pituitary and form a second capillary network.

This circulatory arrangement, illustrated in Figure 11-6●, is very unusual. A typical artery usually conducts blood from the heart to a capillary network, and a typical vein carries blood from a capillary net-

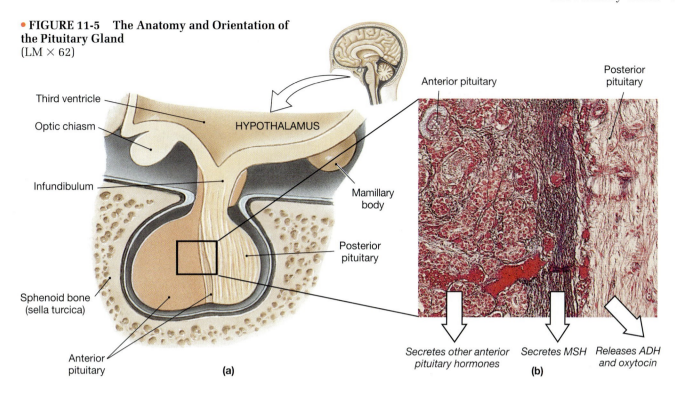

● FIGURE 11-5   The Anatomy and Orientation of the Pituitary Gland (LM × 62)

(a)

Third ventricle

Optic chiasm

HYPOTHALAMUS

Infundibulum

Mamillary body

Posterior pituitary

Sphenoid bone (sella turcica)

Anterior pituitary

Anterior pituitary

Posterior pituitary

Secretes other anterior pituitary hormones

Secretes MSH

Releases ADH and oxytocin

(b)

1 1

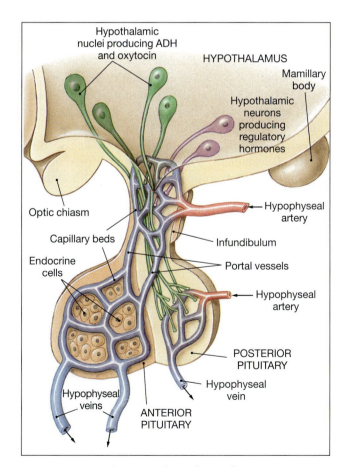

● FIGURE 11-6   The Hypophyseal Portal System

Hypothalamic nuclei producing ADH and oxytocin

HYPOTHALAMUS

Mamillary body

Hypothalamic neurons producing regulatory hormones

Optic chiasm

Hypophyseal artery

Capillary beds

Infundibulum

Endocrine cells

Portal vessels

Hypophyseal artery

POSTERIOR PITUITARY

Hypophyseal vein

Hypophyseal veins

ANTERIOR PITUITARY

work back to the heart. The vessels between the hypothalamus and the anterior pituitary, by contrast, carry blood from one capillary network to another. Blood vessels that link two capillary networks are called *portal vessels*, and the entire complex is termed a **portal system**.

Portal systems ensure that all of the blood entering the portal vessels will reach the intended target cells before returning to the general circulation. Portal vessels are named after their destinations, so this particular network of vessels represents the **hypophyseal portal system**.

Hypothalamic Control of the Anterior Pituitary

An endocrine cell in the anterior pituitary may be controlled by releasing hormones, inhibiting hormones, or some combination of the two. The regulatory hormones released at the hypothalamus are transported directly to the anterior pituitary via the hypophyseal system.

The rate of regulatory hormone secretion by the hypothalamus is regulated through negative feedback mechanisms. The basic regulatory patterns are diagrammed in Figure 11-7●; these will be referenced in the following description of pituitary hormones. Many of these hormones are called *tropins*, from the Greek word *tropos* (turning), because they turn on (activate) other tissues and organs.

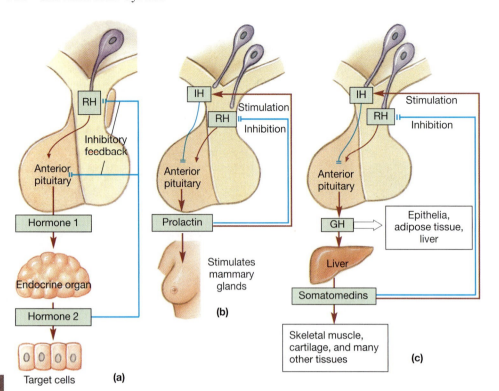

•FIGURE 11-7   Feedback Control of Endocrine Secretion (a) The typical pattern of regulation when multiple endocrine organs are involved. In these cases, the hypothalamus produces a releasing hormone to stimulate hormone production by other glands, and control is through negative feedback. (b) In some cases, both a releasing hormone and an inhibiting hormone are produced by the hypothalamus; when one is stimulated, the other is inhibited. This diagram summarizes the control of prolactin production by the anterior pituitary. (c) The regulation of growth hormone follows the basic pattern shown in part b, but intermediate steps are involved.

Hormones of the Anterior Pituitary

Seven hormones are produced by the anterior pituitary gland. Of those, four regulate the production of hormones by other endocrine glands.

1. **Thyroid-stimulating hormone (TSH)** targets the thyroid gland and triggers the release of thyroid hormones. The thyroid hormones released inhibit the pituitary production of TSH and the hypothalamic centers producing the associated releasing hormone. This pattern of regulatory control is shown in Figure 11-7a•.

2. **Adrenocorticotropic hormone (ACTH)** stimulates the release of steroid hormones by the adrenal glands. ACTH specifically targets cells producing hormones called *glucocorticoids* (gloo-kō-KOR-ti-koyds), which affect glucose metabolism. The feedback control mechanism is comparable to that for TSH (Figure 11-7a•).

3. **Follicle-stimulating hormone (FSH)** promotes egg development in women and stimulates the secretion of *estrogens*, steroid hormones produced by ovarian cells. In men, FSH production supports sperm production in the testes. The feedback control mechanism is comparable to that for TSH (Figure 11-7a•).

4. **Luteinizing** (LOO-tē-in-ī-zing) **hormone (LH)** induces ovulation in women and promotes the ovarian secretion of estrogens and the **progestins** (such as *progesterone*), which prepare the body for possible pregnancy. In men, the same hormone was once called

interstitial cell-stimulating hormone (ICSH) because it stimulates the *interstitial cells* of the testes to produce sex hormones. These hormones are called **androgens** (AN-drō-jenz; *andros*, man); the most important of them is *testosterone*. The feedback control mechanism is comparable to that of TSH (Figure 11-7a•).

FSH and LH are called **gonadotropins** (gō-nad-ō-TRŌ-pinz) because they regulate the activities of the male and female sex organs, or gonads.

5. **Prolactin** (prō-LAK-tin; *pro-*, before + *lac*, milk), or **PRL**, stimulates the development of the mammary glands and the production of milk. Although PRL exerts the dominant effect on the glandular cells, normal development of the mammary glands is regulated by the interaction of a number of hormones. Prolactin has no known effects in the human male. The regulation of prolactin release involves interactions between releasing and inhibiting hormones from the hypothalamus. The regulatory pattern is diagrammed in Figure 11-7b•.

6. **Growth hormone (GH)**, also called *human growth hormone (hGH)* or *somatotropin* (*soma*, body), stimulates cell growth and replication by accelerating the rate of protein synthesis. Although virtually every tissue responds to some degree, skeletal muscle cells and chondrocytes (cartilage cells) are particularly sensitive to levels of growth hormone.

The stimulation of growth by GH involves two different mechanisms. The primary mechanism, which is indirect, is best understood. Liver cells respond to the presence of growth hormone by synthesizing and releasing **somatomedins**, or *insulin-like growth factors (IGF)*, hormones that bind to receptor sites on a variety of cell membranes. Somatomedins increase the rate of amino acid uptake and their incorporation into new proteins. These effects develop almost immediately after GH release occurs, and they are particularly important after a meal, when the blood contains high concentrations of glucose and amino acids. The regulatory mechanism involved in controlling GH production is summarized in Figure 11-7c●.

The direct actions of GH usually do not appear until after blood glucose and amino acid concentrations have returned to normal levels. In epithelia and connective tissues, GH stimulates stem cell divisions and the differentiation of daughter cells. GH also has metabolic effects in adipose tissue and in the liver. In adipose tissue, it stimulates the breakdown of stored fats and the release of fatty acids into the blood. In the liver, GH stimulates the breakdown of glycogen reserves and the release of glucose into the circulation. GH thus plays a role in mobilizing energy reserves. The interactions between growth hormone and other hormones during normal development and maturation will be discussed in a later section.

7. **Melanocyte-stimulating hormone (MSH)** stimulates the melanocytes of the skin, increasing their production of melanin. MSH is important in the control of skin and hair pigmentation in fishes, amphibians, reptiles, and many mammals. The MSH-producing cells of the pituitary gland in adult humans are virtually nonfunctional, and the circulating blood usually does not contain MSH. However, MSH is secreted by the human pituitary (1) during fetal development, (2) in very young children, (3) in pregnant women, and (4) in some disease states. The functions of MSH under these circumstances are not known. Administration of a synthetic form of MSH causes darkening of the skin, and it has been suggested as a means of obtaining a "sunless tan."

The Posterior Pituitary Gland

The **posterior pituitary gland** contains the axons from two different groups of hypothalamic neurons. One group manufactures ADH, and the other oxytocin; both groups are located within the hypothalamus. Their products are transported within axons along the infundibulum to the posterior pituitary, as indicated in Figure 11-6●.

Antidiuretic hormone (ADH) is released in response to such stimuli as a rise in the concentration of electrolytes in the blood or a fall in blood volume or pressure. The primary function of ADH is to decrease the amount of water lost at the kidneys. With losses minimized, any water absorbed from the digestive tract will be retained, reducing the concentration of electrolytes. ADH also causes the constriction of peripheral blood vessels, which helps to increase blood pressure. The production of ADH is inhibited by alcohol, which explains the increased fluid excretion that follows the consumption of alcoholic beverages.

In women, **oxytocin** (*oxy-*, quick + *tokos*, childbirth) stimulates smooth muscle cells in the uterus and special contractile cells surrounding the secretory cells of the mammary glands. Until the last stages of pregnancy, the uterine muscles are insensitive to oxytocin, but they become more sensitive as the time of delivery approaches. (The mechanism behind this change of sensitivity is not fully understood.) The stimulation of uterine muscles by oxytocin helps maintain and complete normal labor and childbirth (discussed in Chapter 21). After delivery, oxytocin functions in the "milk letdown" reflex. In this reflex, oxytocin secreted in response to suckling triggers the release of milk into large collecting chambers.

In the male, oxytocin stimulates the smooth muscle contraction in the walls of the prostate gland. This action may be important in *emission*, the ejection of prostatic secretions, spermatozoa, and the secretions of other glands into the male reproductive tract before ejaculation occurs.

VASOPRESSIN

Antidiuretic hormone (ADH), also called *vasopressin,* is one of two hormones secreted by the posterior pituitary. It decreases the amount of water lost through the kidney and causes constriction of peripheral blood vessels (vasoconstriction). Both mechanisms serve to increase the blood pressure.

When vasopressin is given in unnaturally high doses, much higher than those needed for its antidiuretic hormone effects, its vasoconstrictive properties are enhanced. Because of this, vasopressin can be used to treat certain types of cardiac arrest and gastrointestinal bleeding (particularly bleeding esophageal varices). The side effects include nausea, intestinal cramps, the urge to defecate, bronchial constriction, and pallor of the skin. In women, it can also cause uterine contractions.

Studies have shown that circulating levels of natural vasopressin in patients who receive CPR are higher in those who survive than in those who do not. This appears to result from increased blood flow to vital organs including the heart and brain. Because vasopressin increases blood flow to vital organs, it appears to be a suitable alternative to epinephrine (adrenalin) in treating certain types of cardiac arrest.

Figure 11-8● and Table 11-1 (p. 315) summarize important information concerning the hormonal products of the pituitary gland.

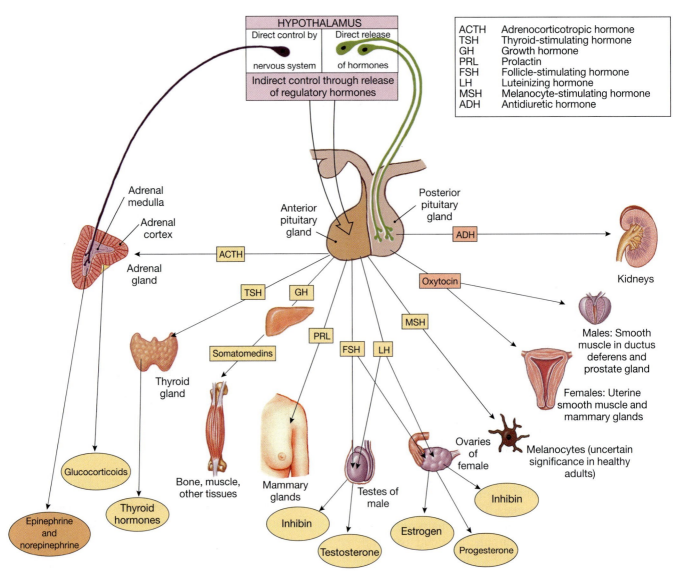

ACTH	Adrenocorticotropic hormone
TSH	Thyroid-stimulating hormone
GH	Growth hormone
PRL	Prolactin
FSH	Follicle-stimulating hormone
LH	Luteinizing hormone
MSH	Melanocyte-stimulating hormone
ADH	Antidiuretic hormone

•FIGURE 11-8   Pituitary Hormones and Their Targets

✓ Why is cyclic-AMP described as a second messenger?

✓ If a person was suffering from dehydration, how would this condition affect the level of ADH released by the posterior pituitary?

✓ A blood sample shows elevated levels of somatomedins. Which pituitary hormone would you expect to be elevated as well?

✓ What effect would elevated levels of cortisol, a hormone from the adrenal gland, have on the level of ACTH?

THE THYROID GLAND

The **thyroid gland** is located just below the **thyroid** ("shield-shaped") **cartilage**, which dominates the anterior surface of the larynx (Figure 11-9a•). The thyroid gland has a deep red coloration because of the large number of blood vessels servicing the glandular cells.

Thyroid Follicles and Thyroid Hormones

The thyroid gland contains large numbers of spherical **thyroid follicles**, shown in sectional view in Figure 11-9b•. Individual follicles are spheres lined by a simple cuboidal epithelium. The cavity within each follicle contains a viscous *colloid*, a fluid containing large amounts of suspended proteins. A network of capillaries surrounds each follicle, delivering nutrients and regulatory hormones to the glandular cells and accepting their secretory products and metabolic wastes.

Thyroid hormones are stored within the follicles. Under TSH stimulation, the epithelial cells take hormones from the follicles and release them into the

TABLE 11-1	The Pituitary Hormones		
Region	*Hormone*	*Target*	*Hormonal Effects*
Anterior pituitary	Thyroid-stimulating hormone (TSH)	Thyroid gland	Secretion of thyroid hormones
	Adrenocorticotropic hormone (ACTH)	Adrenal cortex	Glucocorticoid secretion
	Gonadotropic hormones: Follicle-stimulating hormone (FSH)	Follicle cells of ovaries in female	Estrogen secretion, follicle development
		Sustentacular cells of testes in male	Sperm maturation
	Luteinizing hormone (LH) or interstitial cell-stimulating hormone (ICSH)	Follicle cells of ovaries in female	Ovulation, formation of corpus luteum, and progesterone secretion
		Interstitial cells of testes in male	Testosterone secretion
	Prolactin (PRL)	Mammary glands	Production of milk
	Growth hormone (GH)	All cells	Growth, protein synthesis, lipid mobilization and catabolism
	Melanocyte-stimulating hormone (MSH)	Melanocytes of skin	Increased melanin synthesis in epidermis
Posterior pituitary	Antidiuretic hormone (ADH)	Kidneys	Reabsorption of water, elevation of blood volume and pressure
	Oxytocin	Uterus, mammary glands in female	Labor contractions, milk ejection
		Prostate gland in male	Smooth muscle contractions, ejection of secretions

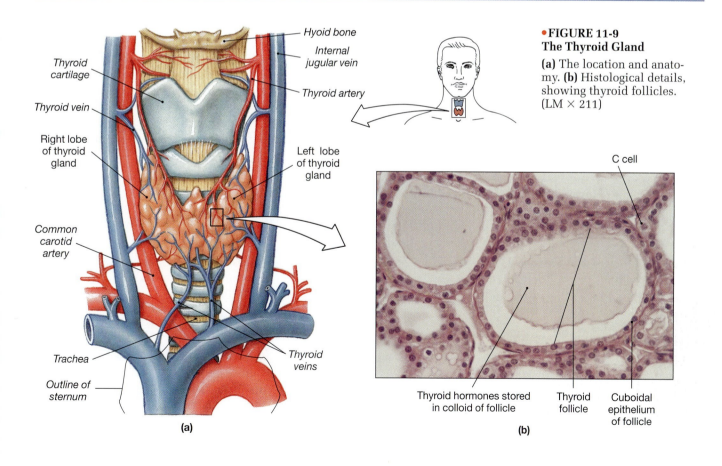

• **FIGURE 11-9**
The Thyroid Gland

(a) The location and anatomy. **(b)** Histological details, showing thyroid follicles. (LM × 211)

Hyoid bone
Internal jugular vein
Thyroid artery

Thyroid cartilage
Thyroid vein
Right lobe of thyroid gland
Left lobe of thyroid gland
Common carotid artery
Thyroid veins
Trachea
Outline of sternum

C cell
Thyroid hormones stored in colloid of follicle
Thyroid follicle
Cuboidal epithelium of follicle

(a)

(b)

circulation. However, almost all of the released thyroid hormones are unavailable because they become attached to carrier proteins in the bloodstream. Only the remaining small percentage of unbound thyroid hormones are free to diffuse into the target cells of body tissues. As the unbound hormones decrease in concentration, the carrier proteins release additional bound hormone. The bound thyroid hormones are a substantial reserve; in fact, the bloodstream normally contains more than a week's supply of thyroid hormones.

The thyroid hormones are structural derivatives of the amino acid *tyrosine*, to which three or four iodine atoms have been attached. The hormone **thyroxine** (thī-ROKS-ēn), or **TX**, contains four atoms of iodine; it is also known as *tetraiodothyronine* (tet-ra-ī-ō-dō-THĪ-rō-nēn), or **T$_4$**. Thyroxine accounts for roughly 90 percent of all thyroid secretions. **Triiodothyronine**, or **T$_3$**, is a related, more potent molecule containing three iodine atoms.

Thyroid hormones affect almost every cell in the body because they diffuse through the cytoplasm to reach receptor sites on mitochondria and in the nucleus (see Figure 11-3b•). The binding of thyroid hormones to mitochondria increases the rate of ATP production. Thyroid hormone-receptor complexes in the nucleus activate genes coding for the synthesis of enzymes involved in glycolysis and energy production, resulting in an increase in cellular rates of metabolism and oxygen consumption. Because the cell consumes more energy, and energy use is measured in *calories*, this is called the **calorigenic effect**. When the metabolic rate increases, more heat is generated and body temperature rises. In growing children, thyroid hormones are also essential to normal development of the skeletal, muscular, and nervous systems.

Normal production of thyroid hormones establishes the background rates of cellular metabolism. These hormones exert their primary effects on active tissues and organs, including skeletal muscles, the liver, the heart, and the kidneys. Overproduction or underproduction of thyroid hormones can therefore cause very serious metabolic problems. In many parts of the world, inadequate dietary iodine leads to an inability to synthesize thyroid hormones. Under these conditions, TSH stimulation continues, and the thyroid follicles become distended with nonfunctional secretions. The result is a swollen and enlarged thyroid gland, or *goiter*. This is seldom a problem in the United States because the typical American diet provides roughly three times the minimum daily requirement of iodine, thanks to the addition of iodine to table salt ("iodized salt").

Table 11-2 summarizes the effects of thyroid hormones on major organs and systems.

The C Cells of the Thyroid Gland: Calcitonin

C cells, which produce the hormone **calcitonin (CT)**, are a second population of endocrine cells sandwiched between the cuboidal follicle cells and their basement membrane. Calcitonin helps regulate calcium ion concentrations in body fluids. As Figure 11-10• illustrates, the C cells release calcitonin when the calcium ion concentration of the blood rises above normal. The target organs are the bones and the kidneys. Calcitonin reduces calcium levels by inhibiting osteoclasts and stimulating calcium excretion at the kidneys. The resulting reduction in the calcium ion concentrations eliminates the stimulus and "turns off" the C cells.

Several chapters have dealt with the importance of calcium ions in controlling muscle and nerve cell activities. Calcium ion concentrations also affect the sodium permeabilities of excitable membranes. At high calcium ion concentrations, sodium permeability decreases and membranes become less responsive. Such problems are prevented by the secretion of calcitonin under appropriate conditions. However, under normal

TABLE 11-2	Hormones of the Thyroid Gland, Parathyroid Glands, and Thymus		
Gland/Cells	*Hormone(s)*	*Targets*	*Hormonal Effects*
THYROID			
Follicular epithelium	Thyroxine (T$_4$), triiodothyronine (T$_3$)	Most cells	Increase energy utilization, oxygen consumption, growth, and development
C cells	Calcitonin (CT)	Bone, kidneys	Decreases Ca^{2+} concentrations in body fluids (see Figure 11-10)
PARATHYROIDS			
Chief cells	Parathyroid hormone (PTH)	Bone, kidneys	Increases Ca^{2+} concentrations in body fluids (see Figure 11-10)
THYMUS	Thymosins	Lymphocytes	Stimulate development and maturation of immune response

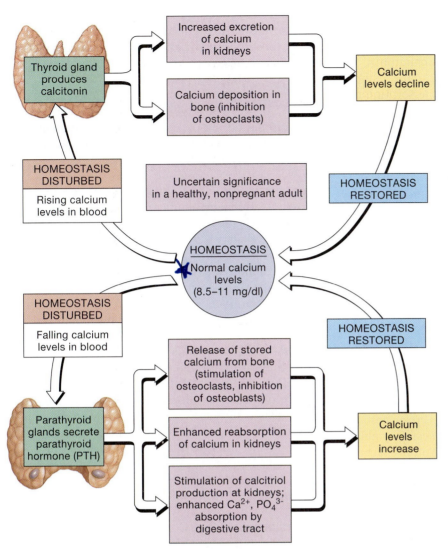

conditions, calcium ion levels seldom rise enough to trigger calcitonin secretion. Most homeostatic adjustments are intended to prevent lower than normal calcium ion concentrations. Low calcium concentrations are dangerous because sodium permeabilities then increase, and muscle cells and neurons become extremely excitable. If calcium levels fall too far, convulsions or muscular spasms will occur. The parathyroid glands and their hormone secretions are responsible for preventing such disastrous events.

THE PARATHYROID GLANDS

Two tiny pairs of **parathyroid glands** are embedded in the posterior surfaces of the thyroid gland (Figure 11-11a●). The gland cells are separated by the dense capsular fibers of the thyroid. The histological appearance of a parathyroid gland is shown in Figure 11-11b●. At least two different cell populations are found in the parathyroid gland. The **chief cells** produce parathyroid hormone; the functions of the other cell type are unknown.

Like the C cells of the thyroid, the chief cells monitor the circulating concentration of calcium ions. When

●FIGURE 11-10   The Homeostatic Regulation of Calcium Ion Concentrations

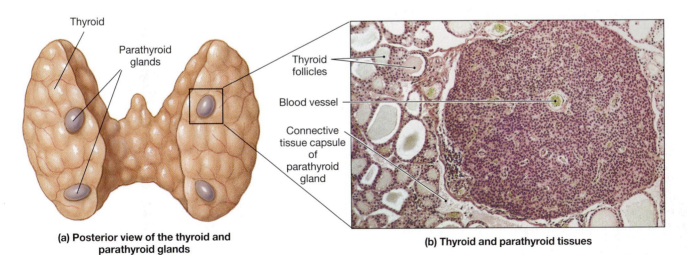

(a) Posterior view of the thyroid and parathyroid glands

(b) Thyroid and parathyroid tissues

● **FIGURE 11-11   The Parathyroid Glands**
(a) The location of the parathyroids on the posterior surface of the thyroid lobes. **(b)** A photomicrograph showing both parathyroid and thyroid tissues. (LM × 94)

the calcium concentration falls below normal, the chief cells secrete **parathyroid hormone (PTH)**, or *parathormone* (see Figure 11-10●). Although parathyroid hormone acts on the same target organs as calcitonin, it produces the opposite effects. PTH stimulates osteoclasts, inhibits osteoblasts, promotes the absorption of calcium by the intestines, and reduces urinary excretion of calcium ions until blood concentrations return to normal.

THE THYMUS

The **thymus** is embedded in a mass of connective tissue inside the thoracic cavity, usually just behind the sternum. In a newborn infant, the thymus is relatively enormous, often extending from the base of the neck to the superior border of the heart. As the child grows, the thymus continues to enlarge slowly, reaching its maximum size just before puberty, at a weight of around 40 g (1.4 oz.). After puberty, it gradually diminishes in size; by age 50, the thymus may weigh less than 12 g (0.4 oz.).

The thymus produces several hormones, collectively known as the **thymosins** (thī-MŌ-sinz), which play a key role in the development and maintenance of normal immunological defenses. It has been suggested that the gradual decrease in the size and secretory abilities of the thymus may make the elderly more susceptible to disease.

Information concerning the hormones of the thyroid and parathyroid glands and the thymus is summarized in Table 11-2. The histological organization of the thymus and the functions of the thymosins will be further considered in Chapter 15.

THE ADRENAL GLANDS

A single **adrenal gland** caps the superior border of each kidney (Figure 11-12●). Because of their location, the adrenals are also called the *suprarenal glands* (soo-pra-RĒ-nal; *supra-*, above + *renes*, kidneys). Each adrenal gland has two parts: a superficial *adrenal cortex* and an inner *adrenal medulla*.

The Adrenal Cortex

The **adrenal cortex** has a grayish yellow coloration because of the presence of stored lipids, especially cholesterol and various fatty acids. The adrenal cortex produces more than two dozen different steroid hormones, collectively called *adrenocortical steroids*, or simply **corticosteroids**. These hormones are vital; if the adrenal glands are destroyed or removed, corticosteroids must be administered or the individual will not survive. Overproduction or underproduction of any of the corticosteroids will have severe consequences because these hormones affect the metabolism of many different tissues.

Corticosteroids

The adrenal cortex produces the following classes of hormones (summarized in Table 11-3): *glucocorticoids*, *mineralocorticoids*, and *androgens*.

Glucocorticoids.   The steroid hormones collectively known as **glucocorticoids** affect glucose metabolism. **Cortisol** (KŌR-ti-sol; also called *hydrocortisone*), **corticosterone** (kor-ti-KOS-te-rōn), and **cortisone** are the three most important glucocorticoids. These hormones, secreted under ACTH stimulation, accelerate the rates of glucose synthesis and glycogen formation, especially within the liver. Simultaneously, adipose tissue responds by releasing fatty acids into the blood, and other tissues begin to break down fatty acids instead of glucose. Glucocorticoids also have *anti-inflammatory* effects; they suppress the activities of white blood cells and other components of the immune system. Glucocorticoid creams are often used to control irritating allergic rashes, such as those produced by poison ivy, and injections of glucocorticoids may be used to control more severe allergic reactions. Because they slow wound healing and suppress immune defenses, topical steroids are used to treat superficial rashes but are never applied to open wounds.

Mineralocorticoids.   Corticosteroids known as **mineralocorticoids** affect the electrolyte composition of bodily fluids. **Aldosterone** (al-DOS-ter-ōn), the principal mineralocorticoid, targets kidney cells that regulate the ionic composition of the urine. It causes the retention of sodium ions and water, reducing fluid losses in the urine. Aldosterone also reduces sodium and water losses at sweat glands, salivary glands, and along the digestive tract. The sodium ions recovered are exchanged for potassium ions, so aldosterone also lowers potassium ion concentrations in the extracellular fluid. Aldosterone secretion occurs in response to (1) stimulation by the hormone *angiotensin II* (*angeion*, vessel + *teinein*, to stretch) and (2) high extracellular potassium levels. The appearance of angiotensin II in the circulation involves a series of steps that begins with the secretion of an enzyme, *renin*, by kidney cells. The mechanism will be detailed further in Chapters 14 and 19.

Androgens.   The adrenal cortex in both sexes produces small quantities of sex hormones called androgens. Androgens are produced in large quantities by the testes of males, and the importance of the small adrenal production in both sexes remains uncertain.

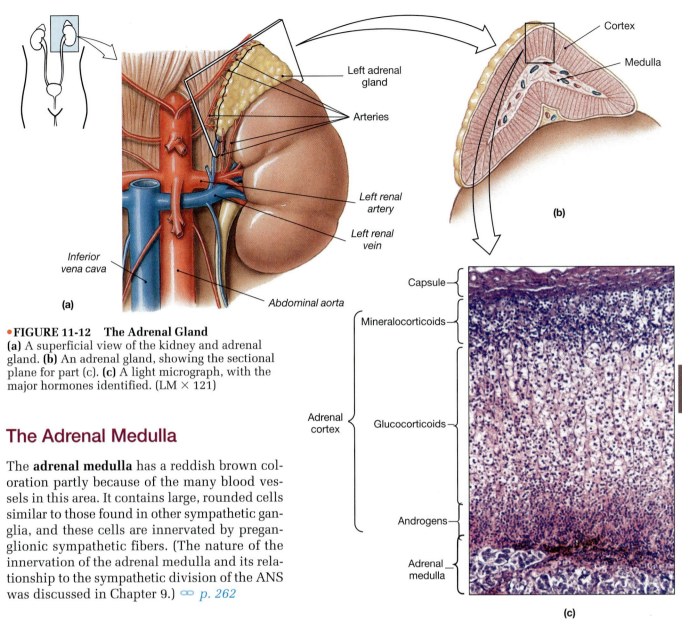

FIGURE 11-12   The Adrenal Gland
(a) A superficial view of the kidney and adrenal gland. (b) An adrenal gland, showing the sectional plane for part (c). (c) A light micrograph, with the major hormones identified. (LM × 121)

The Adrenal Medulla

The **adrenal medulla** has a reddish brown coloration partly because of the many blood vessels in this area. It contains large, rounded cells similar to those found in other sympathetic ganglia, and these cells are innervated by preganglionic sympathetic fibers. (The nature of the innervation of the adrenal medulla and its relationship to the sympathetic division of the ANS was discussed in Chapter 9.) p. 262

TABLE 11-3	The Adrenal Hormones		
Region	*Hormone*	*Target*	*Effects*
Adrenal cortex	Mineralocorticoids, primarily aldosterone	Kidneys	Increases reabsorption of sodium ions and water from the urine; accelerates urinary loss of potassium ions
	Glucocorticoids: cortisol (hydrocortisone), corticosterone, cortisone	Most cells	Releases amino acids from skeletal muscles, lipids from adipose tissues; promotes liver glycogen and glucose formation; promotes peripheral utilization of lipids; anti-inflammatory effects
	Androgens		Uncertain significance under normal conditions
Adrenal medulla	Epinephrine (E, adrenaline), norepinephrine (NE, noradrenaline)	Most cells	Increased cardiac activity, blood pressure, glycogen breakdown, blood glucose; release of lipids by adipose tissue (see Chapter 9)

The adrenal medulla contains two populations of secretory cells, one producing **epinephrine (E**, or *adrenaline*) and the other **norepinephrine (NE**, or *noradrenaline*). These hormones are normally released at a low rate, but sympathetic stimulation accelerates the rate of discharge dramatically.

Epinephrine makes up 75–80 percent of the secretions from the medulla; the rest is norepinephrine. These hormones accelerate cellular energy utilization and mobilize energy reserves. Receptors for epinephrine and norepinephrine are found on skeletal muscle fibers, in adipose tissues, and in the liver. Secretion by the medulla triggers a mobilization of glycogen reserves in skeletal muscles and accelerates the breakdown of glucose to provide ATP. This combination increases muscular power and endurance. In adipose tissue, stored fats are broken down to fatty acids, and in the liver, glycogen molecules are converted to glucose. The fatty acids and glucose are then released into the circulation for use by peripheral tissues. The heart also responds to adrenal medulla hormones with an increase in the rate and force of cardiac contractions.

The metabolic changes that follow epinephrine and norepinephrine release peak 30 seconds after adrenal stimulation and linger for several minutes thereafter. As a result, the effects produced by stimulation of the adrenal medulla outlast other signs of sympathetic activation.

✓ What symptoms would you expect to see in an individual whose diet lacks iodine?

✓ When a person's thyroid gland is removed, signs of decreased thyroid hormone concentration do not appear until about one week later. Why?

✓ Removal of the parathyroid glands would result in a decrease in the blood of what important mineral?

✓ What effect would elevated cortisol levels have on the level of glucose in the blood?

THE KIDNEYS

The kidneys are not primarily endocrine organs, but they release three hormones: *calcitriol, erythropoietin,* and *renin.* Calcitriol is important to calcium ion homeostasis. Erythropoietin and renin are involved in the regulation of blood pressure and blood volume.

Calcitriol is a steroid hormone secreted by the kidney in response to the presence of parathyroid hormone (PTH). Its synthesis is dependent on the availability of vitamin D_3, which may be synthesized in the skin or absorbed from the diet. Vitamin D_3 is absorbed by the liver and converted to an intermediary product that is released into the circulation and absorbed by the kidneys. Calcitriol stimulates the absorption of calcium and phosphate ions along the digestive tract.

Erythropoietin (e-rith-rō-poi-Ē-tin; *erythros,* red + *poiesis,* making), or EPO, is a peptide hormone released by the kidneys in response to low oxygen levels in kidney tissues. EPO stimulates the production of red blood cells by the bone marrow. The increase in the number of erythrocytes elevates blood volume to some degree, and because these cells transport oxygen, the increase in their number improves oxygen delivery to peripheral tissues. EPO will be considered in greater detail when we discuss the formation of blood cells in Chapter 12.

Renin (RĒ-nin) is released by kidney cells in response to a decline in blood volume, blood pressure, or both. Once in the bloodstream, renin functions as an enzyme that starts an enzymatic chain reaction that leads to the formation of **angiotensin II**. This hormone has several functions, including the stimulation of aldosterone production by the adrenal cortex. The renin-angiotensin system will be detailed in Chapters 14 and 19.

THE HEART

The endocrine cells in the heart are cardiac muscle cells in the walls of the *right atrium,* the chamber that receives venous blood. If the blood volume becomes too great, these cardiac muscle cells are excessively stretched. Under these conditions, they release *atrial natriuretic peptide (ANP)* (nā-trē-ū-RET-ik; *natrium,* sodium + *ouresis,* making water). This hormone lowers blood volume and reduces the stretching of the cardiac muscle cells in the atrial walls. We will consider the actions of this hormone in detail when we discuss the control of blood pressure and volume in Chapter 14.

ENDOCRINE TISSUES OF THE DIGESTIVE SYSTEM

The linings of the digestive tract, the liver, and the pancreas produce a variety of exocrine secretions that are essential to the normal breakdown and absorption of food. Although the pace of digestive activities can be affected by the autonomic nervous system, most digestive processes are controlled locally. The various components of the digestive tract communicate with one another by means of hormones that will be considered in Chapter 17. One digestive organ, the pancreas, produces two hormones with widespread effects.

The Pancreas

The **pancreas** lies in the J-shaped loop between the stomach and small intestine (Figure 11-13•). It is a slender, usually pink organ with a nodular (lumpy) consistency, and it contains both exocrine and endocrine cells. The **exocrine pancreas**, discussed further in Chapter 17, pro-

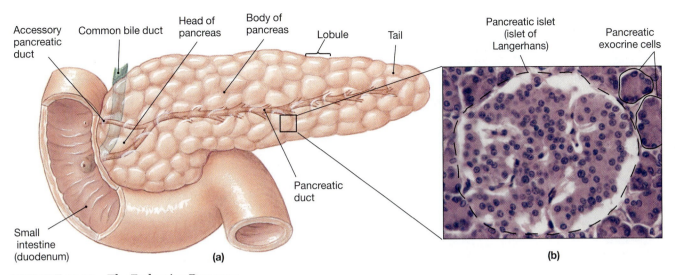

• **FIGURE 11-13   The Endocrine Pancreas**
(a) The gross anatomy of the pancreas. **(b)** A pancreatic islet surrounded by exocrine-secreting cells. (LM × 276)

duces large quantities of an alkaline, enzyme-rich fluid that is secreted into the digestive tract.

Cells of the **endocrine pancreas** form clusters known as **pancreatic islets**, or the *islets of Langerhans* (LAN-ger-hanz). The islets are scattered among the exocrine cells and account for only about 1 percent of all pancreatic cells. Each islet contains several cell types. The two most important are **alpha cells**, which produce the hormone **glucagon** (GLOO-ka-gon), and **beta cells**, which secrete **insulin** (IN-su-lin). Glucagon and insulin regulate blood glucose concentrations in the same way parathyroid hormone and calcitonin control blood calcium levels.

✳ DIABETES MELLITUS

Diabetes mellitus is the most common endocrine disease. In fact, it is not a single disease, but a group of disorders characterized by disturbed glucose tolerance. The disease is recognized in two forms.

Type I diabetes, formerly called *insulin-dependent diabetes mellitus,* usually begins in childhood. It is more common in males than females and accounts for 10 percent of all cases of diabetes mellitus. In Type I diabetes, antibodies destroy the islet cells of the pancreas. This causes circulating insulin levels to fall. The exact reason this occurs is unclear. Type I diabetics require insulin. In addition, they may develop ketoacidosis if supplemental insulin is not available.

Type II diabetes, formerly called *non-insulin dependent diabetes mellitus,* begins later in life and is associated with obesity. In Type II diabetes, the number and weight of beta cells decrease. In addition, the body's cells become resistant to insulin. Both result in rising blood-glucose levels. However, unlike Type II diabetes, patients with Type II diabetes do not usually require insulin. Instead, oral medications that reduce blood glucose levels can be used.

Regulation of Blood Glucose Concentrations

Figure 11-14• diagrams the mechanism of hormonal regulation of blood glucose levels. Glucose is the preferred energy source for most cells in the body, and under normal conditions, it is the only energy source for neurons. When blood glucose levels rise, beta cells of the pancreas release insulin, and this hormone stimulates glucose transport into its target cells. Almost all cells in the body are affected; the only exceptions are (1) neurons and red blood cells, which cannot metabolize other nutrients, and (2) epithelial cells of the kidney tubules and intestinal lining, where glucose is reabsorbed (in the kidneys) or obtained from the diet (in the intestines). When glucose is abundant, all cells use it as an energy source and stop breaking down amino acids and lipids.

The ATP generated by the breakdown of glucose molecules is used to build proteins and to increase energy reserves, and most cells increase their rates of protein synthesis in response to insulin. A secondary effect is an increase in the rate of amino acid transport across cell membranes. Insulin also stimulates fat cells to increase their rates of triglyceride (fat) synthesis and storage. In the liver and in skeletal muscles, insulin also accelerates the formation of glycogen. In summary, when glucose is abundant, insulin secretion stimulates glucose utilization to support growth and to establish glycogen and fat reserves.

When glucose levels decline, insulin secretion is suppressed, and so is glucose transport into its target cells. These cells now shift over to other energy sources, such as fatty acids. At the same time, the alpha cells of the pancreas release glucagon, and energy reserves are mobilized. Skeletal muscles and liver cells break down glycogen, adipose tissue releases fatty acids, and proteins are broken down into their component amino acids. The liver takes in the lipids and amino acids and converts them to

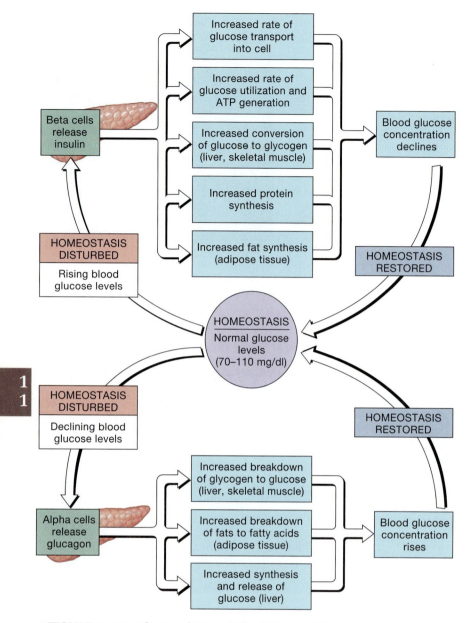

• **FIGURE 11-14** **The Regulation of Blood Glucose Concentrations**

ENDOCRINE TISSUES OF THE REPRODUCTIVE SYSTEM

The endocrine tissues of the reproductive system are primarily restricted to the male and female reproductive organs, the testes and ovaries. Details of the anatomy of the reproductive organs and the endocrinological control of reproductive function will be considered in Chapter 20.

The Testes

In the male, the **interstitial cells** of the paired testes produce the steroid hormones known as androgens. Testosterone (tes-TOS-ter-ōn) is the most important androgen. This hormone promotes the production of functional sperm, maintains the secretory glands of the male reproductive tract, and determines secondary sex characteristics such as the distribution of facial hair and body fat. Testosterone also affects metabolic operations throughout the body, notably stimulating protein synthesis and muscle growth, and produces aggressive behavioral responses. During embryonic development, the production of testosterone affects the development of male reproductive ducts, external genitalia, and CNS structures, including hypothalamic nuclei, that will later affect sexual behaviors.

Sustentacular cells are directly associated with the formation of functional sperm in the testes. These cells also secrete a hormone called **inhibin**. Inhibin production, which occurs under FSH stimulation, depresses the secretion of FSH by the anterior pituitary. Throughout adult life, these two hormones interact to maintain sperm production at normal levels.

The Ovaries

In the ovaries, female sex cells, or *ova*, develop in specialized structures called **follicles**, under stimulation by FSH. Follicle cells surrounding the ova produce **estrogens** (ES-trō-jenz). These steroid hormones support the maturation of the eggs and stimulate the growth of the uterine lining. Under FSH stimulation, follicular cells secrete inhibin, which suppresses FSH release

glucose that can be released into the circulation. As a result, blood glucose concentrations rise toward normal levels. The interplay between insulin and glucagon both stabilizes blood glucose levels and prevents competition between neural tissue and other tissues for limited glucose supplies.

Pancreatic alpha and beta cells are sensitive to blood glucose concentrations, and their regulatory activities are not under the direct control of other endocrine or nervous components. Yet because the islet cells are extremely sensitive to variations in blood glucose levels, any hormone that affects blood glucose concentrations will indirectly affect the production of insulin and glucagon.

through a feedback mechanism comparable to that in males. After ovulation has occurred, the follicular cells reorganize into a **corpus luteum**. The luteal cells then begin to release a mixture of estrogens and progestins, especially **progesterone** (prō-JES-ter-ōn). Progesterone accelerates the movement of fertilized eggs along the uterine tubes and prepares the uterus for the arrival of a developing embryo. Progesterone, along with other hormones, also causes an enlargement of the mammary glands.

The production of androgens, estrogens, and progestins is controlled by regulatory hormones released by the anterior pituitary gland. During pregnancy, the placenta itself functions as an endocrine organ, working together with the ovaries and the pituitary gland to promote normal fetal development and delivery.

Table 11-4 summarizes information concerning the reproductive hormones.

✳ ESTROGEN REPLACEMENT THERAPY

Estrogen protects women against heart disease and vaginal atrophy and conserves calcium and phosphorus, which helps prevent the bone loss of osteoporosis. Estrogen levels begin to slowly fall when a woman enters menopause, and although the incidence of heart disease in women is significantly lower than in men, women quickly catch up with men once menopause occurs.

Estrogen replacement therapy (ERT) has become common practice. In addition to preventing heart disease and osteoporosis, estrogen helps to minimize some of the uncomfortable side effects of menopause including "hot flashes" and vaginal atrophy. Most patients receiving ERT take estrogen on a cyclical basis unless they have had a hysterectomy, in which case they usually take it daily.

THE PINEAL GLAND

The **pineal gland** lies in the roof of the thalamus. It contains neurons, glial cells, and secretory cells that synthesize the hormone **melatonin** (mel-a-TŌ-nin). Collaterals (axonal branches of neurons) from the visual pathways enter the pineal gland and affect the rate of melatonin production. Melatonin production is lowest during daylight hours and highest in the dark of night.

Several functions have been suggested for melatonin secretion in humans:

- *Slows the timing of sexual maturity.* In a variety of other mammals, melatonin slows the maturation of sperm, eggs, and reproductive organs. The significance of this effect remains uncertain, but there is circumstantial evidence that melatonin may play a role in the timing of human sexual maturation. For example, melatonin levels in the blood decline at puberty, and pineal tumors that eliminate melatonin production will cause premature puberty in young children.

- *Acts as an antioxidant.* Melatonin is a very effective *antioxidant* that may protect CNS neurons from *free radicals*, such as nitric oxide (NO) or hydrogen peroxide (H_2O_2), that may be generated in active neural tissue. (Free radicals are highly reactive atoms or molecules that contain unpaired electrons in their outer electron shell.)

- *Establishes day-night cycles of activity.* Because of the cyclical nature of its rate of secretion, the pineal gland may also be involved with the establishment or maintenance of basic *circadian rhythms*, daily

TABLE 11-4	Hormones of the Reproductive System		
Structure/Cells	*Hormone*	*Primary Target*	*Effects*
TESTES **Interstitial cells**	Androgens	Most cells	Support functional maturation of sperm, protein synthesis in skeletal muscles, male secondary sexual characteristics, and associated behaviors
Sustentacular cells	Inhibin	Anterior pituitary	Inhibits secretion of FSH
OVARIES **Follicular cells**	Estrogens	Most cells	Support follicle maturation, female secondary sexual characteristics, and associated behaviors
	Inhibin	Anterior pituitary	Inhibits secretion of FSH
Corpus luteum	Progestins	Uterus, mammary glands	Prepare uterus for implantation; prepare mammary glands for secretory functions

changes in physiological processes that follow a regular day-night pattern. Increased melatonin secretion in darkness has been suggested as a primary cause for *seasonal affective disorder* (*SAD*). This condition, characterized by changes in mood, eating habits, and sleeping patterns, can develop during the winter in high latitudes, where sunshine is meager or lacking altogether.

✓ Which pancreatic hormone would cause skeletal muscle and liver cells to convert glucose to glycogen?

✓ What effect would increased levels of glucagon have on the amount of glycogen stored in the liver?

✓ Increased amounts of light would inhibit the production of which hormone?

PATTERNS OF HORMONAL INTERACTION

Although hormones are usually studied individually, the extracellular fluids contain a mixture of hormones whose concentrations change daily and even hourly. When a cell receives instructions from two different hormones at the same time, several results are possible:

- The two hormones may have opposing, or **antagonistic**, effects, as in the case of parathyroid hormone and calcitonin or insulin and glucagon.
- The two hormones may have additive, or **synergistic** (sin-er-JIS-tik; *synairesis*, a drawing together), effects. Sometimes the net result is not only greater than the effect that each would produce acting alone but is actually greater than the *sum* of their individual effects. An example is the stimulation of mammary gland development by prolactin, estrogens, progestins, and growth hormone.
- One hormone can have a **permissive** effect on another. In such cases, the first hormone is needed for the second to produce its effect. For example, epinephrine by itself has no apparent effect on energy production. It will exert its effect only if thyroid hormones are present in normal concentrations.
- Hormones may also produce different but complementary results in specific tissues and organs. These **integrative** effects are important in coordinating the activities of diverse physiological systems.

This section will discuss how hormones interact to control normal growth, reactions to stress, alterations of behavior, and the effects of aging. More detailed discussions will be found in chapters on cardiovascular function, metabolism, excretion, and reproduction.

Hormones and Growth

Normal growth requires the cooperation of several endocrine organs. Five hormones are especially important, although many others have secondary effects on growth rates and patterns:

1. *Growth hormone.* Growth hormone helps maintain normal blood glucose concentrations and mobilizes lipid reserves stored in adipose tissues. It is not the primary hormone involved, however, and an adult with a growth hormone deficiency but normal levels of thyroxine, insulin, and glucocorticoids will have no physiological problems. The effects of GH on protein synthesis and cellular growth are most apparent in children, in whom GH supports muscular and skeletal development. Undersecretion or oversecretion of GH can lead to *pituitary dwarfism* or *gigantism.*

2. *Thyroid hormones.* Normal growth also requires appropriate levels of thyroid hormones. If these hormones are absent for the first year after birth, the nervous system fails to develop normally, producing mental retardation. If thyroxine concentrations decline later in life but before puberty, normal skeletal development will not continue.

3. *Insulin.* Growing cells need adequate supplies of energy and nutrients. Without insulin, produced by the pancreas, the passage of glucose and amino acids across cell membranes will be drastically reduced or eliminated.

4. *Parathyroid hormone.* Parathyroid hormone promotes the absorption of calcium salts across the lining of the digestive tract, thereby maintaining normal calcium levels in the circulation, a requirement for normal bone growth.

5. *Gonadal hormones.* The activity of osteoblasts in key locations and the growth of specific cell populations are affected by the presence or absence of sex hormones. The differential growth induced by these hormones changes skeletal proportions and triggers the development of secondary sex characteristics.

Hormones and Behavior

As we have seen, many endocrine functions are regulated by the hypothalamus, and hypothalamic neurons monitor the levels of many circulating hormones. Other portions of the central nervous system are also quite sensitive to hormonal stimulation.

The clearest demonstrations of the effects of specific hormones involve individuals whose endocrine glands are oversecreting or undersecreting. Normal changes in circulating hormone levels can also cause behavioral changes. Chapter 6 noted that one of the

CLINICAL NOTE   THE PHYSIOLOGICAL RESPONSE TO STRESS

EMS is an inherently stressful profession. *Stress* can be defined as any condition within the body that threatens *homeostasis.* The word stress also refers to a "hardship or strain," or a "physical or emotional response to a stimulus." A person's reactions to stress are individual and varied. They are affected by previous exposure to the *stressor* (a stimulus that causes stress), the perception of the event, general life events, and personal coping skills.

Adapting to stress is a dynamic and evolving process. The body has a general physiological response to stress. In fact, all stressors produce the same basic pattern of hormonal and physiological adjustments. The stress response is called the *general adaptation syndrome (GAS)* and consists of three basic phases: *alarm, resistance,* and *exhaustion* (Figure 11-15). At the end comes a period of rest and recovery.

- *Stage I: Alarm.* The alarm phase is the "fight-or-flight" response. It occurs when the body physically and rapidly prepares to defend itself against a threat, whether real or imagined. Hormones begin to flood the body via the sympathetic nervous system under the control of the hypothalamus. *Epinephrine* and *norepinephrine* from the adrenal medulla increase the heart rate and blood pressure, dilate the pupils, increase the blood-sugar level, slow digestion, and dilate the bronchial tree. In addition, the pituitary gland begins releasing *adrenocorticotropic (ACTH)* hormones that stimulate the adrenal cortex.
- *Stage II: Resistance.* If the stress lasts longer than a few hours, the individual will enter the resistance phase. The glucocorticoid hormones dominate this stage, although other hormones are involved. Energy demands remain higher because of increased production of the glucocorticoids, epinephrine, growth hormone, and thyroid hormone. These serve to maintain an elevated level of blood glucose, which facilitates the mobilization of lipid and protein, the conservation of glucose for the brain and neural tissues, and the synthesis and release of glucose by the liver. In this stage, the individual begins to cope with the stress. Over time, the individual may become desensitized or adapted to stressors. Late in this stage, physiological parameters, such as blood pressure and pulse rate, may return to normal.
- *Stage III: Exhaustion.* When the resistance phase ends, the homeostatic regulatory mechanisms break down and the exhaustion phase begins. Prolonged exposure to the same stressors leads to exhaustion of an individual's ability to resist and adapt. Resistance to all stressors declines, and susceptibility to physical and psychological ailments increases. A period of rest and recovery is necessary for a healthy outcome. Unless corrective actions are taken, organ system failure will begin.

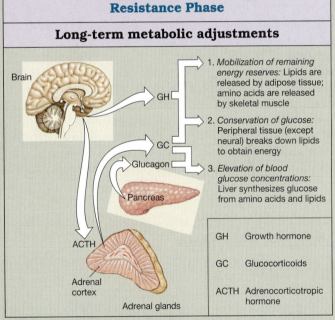

Alarm Phase

"Fight or Flight"
Immediate short-term responses to crises

Brain

General sympathetic activation

Sympathetic stimulation

Epinephrine Norepinephrine

Adrenal medullae

1. Mobilization of glucose reserves

2. Changes in circulation

3. Increases in heart and respiratory rates

4. Increased energy use by all cells

Resistance Phase

Long-term metabolic adjustments

Brain

GH

GC

Glucagon

Pancreas

ACTH

Adrenal cortex

Adrenal glands

1. *Mobilization of remaining energy reserves:* Lipids are released by adipose tissue; amino acids are released by skeletal muscle

2. *Conservation of glucose:* Peripheral tissue (except neural) breaks down lipids to obtain energy

3. *Elevation of blood glucose concentrations:* Liver synthesizes glucose from amino acids and lipids

GH	Growth hormone
GC	Glucocorticoids
ACTH	Adrenocorticotropic hormone

Exhaustion Phase

Collapse of vital systems

Causes may include:
— Exhaustion of lipid reserves
— Inability to produce glucocorticoids
— Failure of electrolyte balance
— Cumulative structural or functional damage to vital organs

•**FIGURE 11-15   The General Adaptation Syndrome**

triggers for closure of the epiphyses is the increase in sex hormone production at the time of puberty. ∞ *p. 125* In *precocious* (premature) *puberty*, sex hormones are produced at an inappropriate time, perhaps as early as 5 or 6 years of age. The affected children not only begin to develop adult secondary sex characteristics but also undergo significant behavioral changes. The "nice little kid" disappears, and the child becomes aggressive and assertive. These behavioral alterations represent the effects of sex hormones on CNS function. Thus, behaviors that in normal teenagers are usually attributed to external factors, such as peer pressure, actually have some physiological basis as well. In the adult, changes in the mixture of hormones reaching the CNS can have significant effects on intellectual capabilities, memory, learning, and emotional states.

Hormones and Aging

The endocrine system shows relatively few functional changes with age. The most dramatic exception is the decline in the concentration of reproductive hormones. Effects of these hormonal changes on the skeletal system were noted in Chapter 6; further discussion will be found in Chapter 21. ∞ *p. 128*

Blood and tissue concentrations of many other hormones, including TSH, thyroid hormones, ADH, PTH, prolactin, and glucocorticoids, remain unchanged with increasing age. But while hormone levels may remain within normal limits, some endocrine tissues become less responsive to stimulation. For example, in elderly people, less GH and insulin are secreted after a carbohydrate-rich meal is eaten or in a glucose tolerance test.

Finally, it should be noted that age-related changes in other tissues affect their abilities to respond to hormonal stimulation. As a result, peripheral tissues may become less responsive to some hormones. This loss of sensitivity has been documented for glucocorticoids and ADH.

ENDOCRINE DISORDERS

The symptoms of endocrine disorders can usually be assigned to one of two basic categories: symptoms of underproduction (inadequate hormonal effects) or symptoms of overproduction (excessive hormonal effects). The observed symptoms may reflect either abnormal hormone production (hyposecretion or hypersecretion) or abnormal cellular sensitivity. These conditions are interesting because they highlight the significance of normally "silent" hormonal contributions.

INTEGRATION WITH OTHER SYSTEMS

The relationships between the endocrine system and other systems are summarized in Figure 11-16•. This overview does not consider all of the hormones associated with the digestive system and the control of digestive functions. These hormones will be detailed in Chapter 17.

✓ Insulin lowers the level of glucose in the blood, and glucagon causes glucose levels to rise. What is this type of hormonal interaction called?

✓ The lack of which hormones would inhibit skeletal formation?

Chapter Review

KEY TERMS

adrenal cortex, *p. 318*	**glucagon**, *p. 321*	**pancreas**, *p. 320*
adrenal medulla, *p. 319*	**hormone**, *p. 306*	**peptide hormone**, *p. 307*
endocrine cell, *p. 306*	**hypophyseal portal system**, *p. 311*	**pituitary gland**, *p. 310*
first messenger, *p. 307*	**hypophysis**, *p. 310*	**second messenger**, *p. 307*
general adaptation syndrome, *p. 325*	**insulin**, *p. 321*	**steroid hormone**, *p. 307*

SUMMARY OUTLINE

INTRODUCTION *p. 306*

1. In general, the nervous system performs short-term "crisis management," while the endocrine system regulates longer-term, ongoing metabolic processes. Endocrine cells release chemicals called **hormones** that alter the metabolic activities of many different tissues and organs simultaneously. *(Figure 11-1)*

AN OVERVIEW OF THE ENDOCRINE SYSTEM *p. 306*

The Structure of Hormones *p. 306*

1. Hormones can be divided into three groups based on chemical structure: amino acid derivatives, peptide hormones, and lipid derivatives.

INTEGUMENTARY SYSTEM

Protects superficial endocrine organs; epidermis synthesizes cholecalciferol

Sex hormones stimulate sebaceous gland activity, influence hair growth, fat distribution, and apocrine sweat gland activity; PRL stimulates development of mammary glands; adrenal hormones alter dermal blood flow, stimulate release of lipids from adipocytes; MSH stimulates melanocyte activity

THE ENDOCRINE SYSTEM

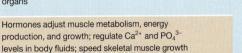

Male

FOR ALL SYSTEMS

Adjusts metabolic rates and substrate utilization; regulates growth and development

SKELETAL SYSTEM

Protects endocrine organs, especially in brain, chest, and pelvic cavity

Skeletal growth regulated by several hormones; calcium mobilization regulated by parathyroid hormone and calcitonin; sex hormones speed growth and closure of epiphyseal plates at puberty and help maintain bone mass in adults

MUSCULAR SYSTEM

Skeletal muscles provide protection for some endocrine organs

Hormones adjust muscle metabolism, energy production, and growth; regulate Ca^{2+} and PO_4^{3-} levels in body fluids; speed skeletal muscle growth

NERVOUS SYSTEM

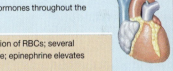

Hypothalamic hormones directly control pituitary and indirectly control secretions of other endocrine organs; controls adrenal medullae; secretes ADH and oxytocin

Several hormones affect neural metabolism; hormones help regulate fluid and electrolyte balance; reproductive hormones influence CNS development and behaviors

CARDIOVASCULAR SYSTEM

Circulatory system distributes hormones throughout the body; heart secretes ANP

Erythropoietin regulates production of RBCs; several hormones elevate blood pressure; epinephrine elevates heart rate and contractile force

LYMPHATIC SYSTEM

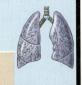

Lymphocytes provide defense against infection and, with other WBCs, assist in repair after injury

Glucocorticoids have anti-inflammatory effects; thymosins stimulate development of lymphocytes; many hormones affect immune function

RESPIRATORY SYSTEM

Provides O_2 and eliminates CO_2 generated by endocrine cells

Epinephrine and norepinephrine stimulate respiratory activity and dilate respiratory passageways

DIGESTIVE SYSTEM

Provides nutrients and substrates to endocrine cells; endocrine cells of pancreas secrete insulin and glucagon; liver produces and releases angiotensinogen

E and NE stimulate constriction of sphincters and depress activity along digestive tract; digestive tract hormones coordinate secretory activities along tract

Steroid sex hormones and inhibin suppress secretory activities in hypothalamus and pituitary

Hypothalamic factors and pituitary hormones regulate sexual development and function; oxytocin stimulates uterine and mammary gland smooth muscle contractions

REPRODUCTIVE SYSTEM

URINARY SYSTEM

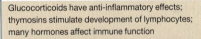

Kidney cells (1) release renin and erythropoietin when local blood pressure declines and (2) produce calcitriol

Aldosterone, ADH, and ANP adjust rates of fluid and electrolyte reabsorption in kidneys

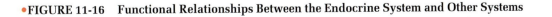

•FIGURE 11-16   Functional Relationships Between the Endocrine System and Other Systems

2. *Amino acid derivatives* are structurally similar to amino acids; they include *epinephrine*, *norepinephrine*, *thyroid hormones*, and *melatonin*.

3. **Peptide hormones** are chains of amino acids.

4. There are two classes of lipid derivatives. **Steroid hormones** are lipids structurally similar to cholesterol, and **prostaglandins** are fatty acid-based.

The Mechanisms of Hormonal Action *p. 307*

5. Hormones exert their effects by modifying the activities of **target cells** (peripheral cells that are sensitive to that particular hormone). *(Figure 11-2)*

6. Receptors for amino acid-derived and peptide hormones are located on the cell membranes of target cells; in this case, the hormone acts as a **first messenger** that causes a **second messenger** to appear in the cytoplasm. Thyroid and steroid hormones cross the cell membrane and bind to receptors in the cytoplasm or nucleus. Thyroid hormones also bind to mitochondria, where they increase the rate of ATP production. *(Figure 11-3)*

The Control of Endocrine Activity *p. 309*

7. The simplest patterns of endocrine control involve the direct negative feedback of changes in the extracellular fluid on the endocrine cells.

8. The most complex endocrine responses involve the hypothalamus. The hypothalamus regulates the activities of the nervous and endocrine systems via three mechanisms: (1) Its autonomic centers exert direct neural control over the endocrine cells of the adrenal medullae; (2) it acts as an endocrine organ itself by releasing hormones into the circulation; (3) it secretes **regulatory hormones** that control the activities of endocrine cells in the pituitary gland. *(Figure 11-4)*

†HE PITUITARY GLAND *p. 310*

1. The **pituitary gland** *(hypopohysis)* releases nine important peptide hormones; all bind to membrane receptors and use cyclic-AMP as a second messenger. *(Figure 11-5)*

The Anterior Pituitary Gland *p. 310*

2. Hypothalamic neurons release regulatory factors into the surrounding interstitial fluids. Their secretions then enter highly permeable capillaries.

3. The **hypophyseal portal system** ensures that all of the blood entering the *portal vessels* will reach target cells in the anterior pituitary before returning to the general circulation. *(Figure 11-6)*

4. The rate of regulatory hormone secretion by the hypothalamus is regulated through negative feedback mechanisms. *(Figure 11-7)*

5. The seven hormones of the **anterior pituitary gland** are: (1) **thyroid-stimulating hormone (TSH)**, which triggers the release of thyroid hormones; (2) **adrenocorticotropic hormone (ACTH)**, which stimulates the release of **glucocorticoids** by the adrenal gland; (3) **follicle-stimulating hor-**mone **(FSH)**, which stimulates *estrogen* secretion and egg development in women and sperm production in men; (4) **luteinizing hormone (LH)**, which causes ovulation and **progestin** production in women and **androgen** production in men; (5) **prolactin (PRL)**, which stimulates the development of the mammary glands and the production of milk; (6) **growth hormone (GH)**, which stimulates cell growth and replication by triggering the release of **somatomedins** from liver cells; and (7) **melanocyte-stimulating hormone (MSH)**, which stimulates melanocytes to produce melanin in other species but is not normally secreted by the nonpregnant human adult.

The Posterior Pituitary Gland *p. 313*

6. The **posterior pituitary gland** contains the axons of hypothalamic neurons that manufacture **antidiuretic hormone (ADH)** and **oxytocin**. ADH decreases the amount of water lost at the kidneys. In women, oxytocin stimulates smooth muscle cells in the uterus and contractile cells in the mammary glands. In men, it stimulates prostatic smooth muscle contractions. *(Figure 11-8; Table 11-1)*

†HE THYROID GLAND *p. 314*

1. The **thyroid gland** lies near the **thyroid cartilage** of the larynx and consists of two lobes. *(Figure 11-9)*

Thyroid Follicles and Thyroid Hormones *p. 314*

2. The thyroid gland contains numerous **thyroid follicles**. Thyroid follicles release several hormones, including **thyroxine (TX or T_4)** and **triiodothyronine (T_3)**. *(Table 11-2)*

3. Thyroid hormones exert a **calorigenic effect**, which enables us to adapt to cold temperatures.

The C Cells of the Thyroid Gland: Calcitonin *p. 316*

4. The **C cells** of the follicles produce **calcitonin (CT)**, which helps regulate calcium ion concentrations in body fluids. *(Table 11-2)*

†HE PARATHYROID GLANDS *p. 317*

1. Four **parathyroid glands** are embedded in the posterior surface of the thyroid gland. The **chief cells** of the parathyroid produce **parathyroid hormone (PTH)** in response to lower than normal concentrations of calcium ions. These and the C cells of the thyroid gland maintain calcium ion levels within relatively narrow limits. *(Figures 11-10, 11-11; Table 11-2)*

†HE THYMUS *p. 318*

1. The **thymus** produces several hormones, called **thymosins**, which play a role in developing and maintaining normal immunological defenses *(Table 11-2)*.

†HE ADRENAL GLANDS *p. 318*

1. A single **adrenal gland** lies along the superior border of each kidney. Each gland, surrounded by a fibrous capsule, can be subdivided into the superficial *adrenal cortex* and the inner *adrenal medulla*. *(Figure 11-12)*

The Adrenal Cortex, *p. 318*

2. The **adrenal cortex** manufactures steroid hormones called *adrenocortical steroids* (**corticosteroids**). The cortex produces (1) **glucocorticoids**—notably, **cortisol**, **corticosterone**, and **cortisone**, which, in response to ACTH, affect glucose metabolism; (2) **mineralocorticoids**—principally **aldosterone**, which, in response to *angiotensin II*, restricts sodium and water losses at the kidneys, sweat glands, digestive tract, and salivary glands; and (3) androgens of uncertain significance. *(Figure 11-12; Table 11-3)*

The Adrenal Medulla *p. 319*

3. The **adrenal medulla** produces **epinephrine** and **norepinephrine**. *(Figure 11-12; Table 11-3)*

THE KIDNEYS *p. 320*

1. Endocrine cells in the kidneys produce hormones important for calcium metabolism, blood volume, and blood pressure.

2. **Calcitriol** stimulates calcium and phosphate ion absorption along the digestive tract.

3. **Erythropoietin (EPO)** stimulates red blood cell production by the bone marrow.

4. On its release, **renin** functions as an enzyme whose activity leads to the formation of angiotensin II, the hormone that stimulates the adrenal production of aldosterone.

THE HEART *p. 320*

1. Specialized muscle cells in the heart produce *atrial natriuretic peptide* (ANP) when blood pressure and/or blood volume becomes excessive.

ENDOCRINE TISSUES OF THE DIGESTIVE SYSTEM *p. 320*

1. The linings of the digestive tract, the liver, and the pancreas produce exocrine secretions that are essential to the normal breakdown and absorption of food. These organs also produce a variety of hormones that coordinate digestive and metabolic activities.

The Pancreas *p. 320*

2. The **pancreas** contains both exocrine and endocrine cells. The **exocrine pancreas** secretes an enzyme-rich fluid that travels to the digestive tract. Cells of the **endocrine pancreas** form clusters called **pancreatic islets** (*islets of Langerhans*), containing **alpha cells** (which produce the hormone **glucagon**) and **beta cells** (which secrete **insulin**). *(Figure 11-13)*

3. Insulin lowers blood glucose by increasing the rate of glucose uptake and utilization; glucagon raises blood glucose by increasing the rates of glycogen breakdown and glucose synthesis in the liver. *(Figure 11-14)*

ENDOCRINE TISSUES OF THE REPRODUCTIVE SYSTEM *p. 322*

The Testes *p. 322*

1. The **interstitial cells** of the paired male testes produce androgens and **inhibin**. The androgen testosterone is the most important sex hormone in the male. (Table 11-4)

The Ovaries *p. 322*

2. In women, ova (eggs) develop in **follicles**; follicle cells surrounding the eggs produce **estrogens** and inhibin. After ovulation, the cells reorganize into a **corpus luteum** that releases a mixture of estrogens and progestins, especially **progesterone**. If pregnancy occurs, the placenta functions as an endocrine organ. *(Table 11-4)*

THE PINEAL GLAND *p. 323*

1. The **pineal gland** synthesizes **melatonin**. Melatonin appears to (1) slow the maturation of sperm, eggs, and reproductive organs, (2) protect neural tissue from *free radicals*, and (3) establish daily circadian rhythms.

PATTERNS OF HORMONAL INTERACTION *p. 324*

1. The endocrine system functions as an integrated unit, and hormones often interact. These interactions may have (1) **antagonistic** (opposing) effects, (2) **synergistic** (additive) effects, (3) **permissive** effects, or (4) **integrative** effects, in which hormones produce different but complementary results.

Hormones and Growth *p. 324*

2. Normal growth requires the cooperation of several endocrine organs. Five hormones are especially important: growth hormone, thyroid hormones, insulin, parathyroid hormone, and gonadal hormones.

Hormones and Behavior *p. 324*

3. Many hormones affect the functional state of the nervous system, producing changes in mood, emotional states, and various behaviors.

Hormones and Aging *p. 326*

4. The endocrine system shows relatively few functional changes with advanced age. The most dramatic endocrine change is the decline in the concentration of reproductive hormones.

INTEGRATION WITH OTHER SYSTEMS *p. 326*

1. The endocrine system affects all systems by adjusting metabolic rates and regulating growth and development. *(Figure 11-16)*

REVIEW QUESTIONS

LEVEL 1   Reviewing Facts and Terms _____

Match each item in column A with the most closely related item in column B. Use letters for answers in the spaces provided.

Column A

___ 1. thyroid gland

___ 2. pineal gland

___ 3. polyuria

___ 4. parathyroid gland

___ 5. thymus gland

___ 6. adrenal cortex

___ 7. heart

___ 8. endocrine pancreas

___ 9. gonadotropins

___ 10. hypothalamus

___ 11. pituitary gland

___ 12. growth hormone

Column B

a. islets of Langerhans

b. atrophies by adulthood

c. atrial natriuretic peptide

d. cell growth

e. melatonin

f. hypophysis

g. excessive urine production

h. calcitonin

i. secretes regulatory hormones

j. FSH and LH

k. secretes androgens, mineralocorticoids, and glucocorticoids

l. stimulated by low calcium levels

13. Adrenocorticotropic hormone (ACTH) stimulates the release of:
    (a) thyroid hormones by the hypothalamus
    (b) gonadotropins by the adrenal glands
    (c) somatotropins by the hypothalamus
    (d) steroid hormones by the adrenal glands

14. FSH production in males supports:
    (a) maturation of sperm by stimulating sustentacular cells
    (b) development of muscles and strength
    (c) production of male sex hormones
    (d) increased desire for sexual activity

15. The hormone that induces ovulation in women and promotes the ovarian secretion of progesterone is:
    (a) interstitial cell-stimulating hormone
    (b) estradiol
    (c) luteinizing hormone
    (d) prolactin

16. The two hormones released by the posterior pituitary are:
    (a) somatotropin and gonadotropin
    (b) estrogen and progesterone
    (c) growth hormone and prolactin
    (d) antidiuretic hormone and oxytocin

17. The primary function of antidiuretic hormone (ADH) is to:
    (a) increase the amount of water lost at the kidneys
    (b) decrease the amount of water lost at the kidneys
    (c) dilate peripheral blood vessels to decrease blood pressure
    (d) increase absorption along the digestive tract

18. The element required for normal thyroid function is:
    (a) magnesium
    (b) calcium
    (c) potassium
    (d) iodine

19. Reduced fluid losses in the urine due to retention of sodium ions and water is a result of the action of:
    (a) antidiuretic hormone
    (b) calcitonin
    (c) aldosterone
    (d) cortisone

20. The adrenal medullae produce the hormones:
    (a) cortisol and cortisone
    (b) epinephrine and norepinephrine
    (c) corticosterone and testosterone
    (d) androgens and progesterone

21. What seven hormones are released by the anterior pituitary gland?

22. What effects do calcitonin and parathyroid hormone have on blood calcium levels?

23. (a) What three phases of the general adaptation syndrome (GAS) constitute the body's response to stress?
    (b) What endocrine secretions play dominant roles in the alarm and resistance phases?

LEVEL 2   Reviewing Concepts

24. What is the primary difference in the way the nervous and endocrine systems communicate with their target cells?

25. How can a hormone modify the activities of its target cells?

26. What possible results occur when a cell receives instructions from two different hormones at the same time?

27. How would blocking the activity of phosphodiesterase affect a cell that responds to hormonal stimulation by the cAMP second messenger system?

LEVEL 3   Critical Thinking and Clinical Applications

28. Roger M. has been suffering from extreme thirst; he drinks numerous glasses of water every day and urinates a great deal. Name two disorders that could produce these symptoms. What test could a clinician perform to determine which disorder is present?

29. Julie is pregnant and is not receiving any prenatal care. She has a poor diet consisting mostly of fast food. She drinks no milk, preferring colas instead. How will this situation affect Julie's level of parathyroid hormone?

ANSWERS TO CONCEPT CHECK QUESTIONS

Page 314

1. Epinephrine, norepinephrine, and peptide hormones are the first messengers from the endocrine glands. Since these hormones cannot enter their target cells, intracellular cyclic-AMP acts as the second messenger from the endocrine glands.   **2.** Dehydration increases the osmotic pressure of the blood. The increase in blood osmotic pressure would stimulate the posterior pituitary gland to release more ADH.   **3.** Somatomedins are the mediators of growth hormone action. If the level of somatomedins is elevated, we would expect the level of growth hormone to be elevated as well.   **4.** Increased levels of cortisol would inhibit the cells that control ACTH release from the pituitary gland; therefore the level of ACTH would decrease. This is a negative feedback mechanism.

Page 320

1. An individual who lacked iodine would not be able to form the hormone thyroxine. As a result, we would expect to see the symptoms associated with thyroxine deficiency, such as decreased rate of metabolism, decreased body temperature, poor response to physiological stress, and an increase in the size of the thyroid gland (goiter).   **2.** Most of the thyroid hormone in the blood is bound to carrier proteins. This represents a large reservoir of thyroxine that guards against rapid fluctuations in the level of this important hormone. Because such a large amount is stored, it takes several days to deplete the supply of hormone, even after the thyroid gland has been removed.

3. The removal of the parathyroid glands would result in a decrease in the blood levels of calcium ion. This decrease could be counteracted by increasing the amount of vitamin D_3 and calcium in the diet.   **4.** One of the functions of cortisol is to decrease the cellular use of glucose while increasing the available glucose by promoting the breakdown of glycogen and the conversion of amino acids to carbohydrates. The net result would be an elevation in the level of glucose in the blood.

Page 324

1. Insulin increases the rate of conversion of glucose to glycogen in skeletal muscle and liver cells.   **2.** Glucagon stimulates the conversion of glycogen to glucose in the liver. Increased amounts of glucagon would then lead to decreased amounts of liver glycogen.   **3.** The pineal gland receives neural input from the optic tracts, and its secretion, melatonin, is influenced by light-dark cycles. Increased amounts of light inhibit the production and release of melatonin from the pineal gland.

Page 326

1. The hormonal interaction exemplified by the insulin and glucagon is antagonistic. In this type of hormonal interaction, two hormones have opposite effects on their target tissues.   **2.** Growth hormone, thyroid hormone, parathyroid hormone, and the gonadal hormones all play a role in the formation and development of the skeletal system.

11

OVERVIEW

The *endocrine system* is an important body system. Closely linked to the nervous system, it controls numerous physiological processes. Unlike the nervous system, which exerts its control through nervous impulses, the endocrine system controls the body through specialized chemical messengers called hormones. The term *hormone* comes from the Greek meaning "to set in motion," and hormones do just that, keeping in motion, or regulating, numerous vital cell processes. Hormones such as growth hormone and thyroid hormone regulate *metabolism*. Metabolism encompasses all of the cellular processes that produce the energy and molecules needed for growth or repair (Figure A11-1●). Physicians who specialize in the treatment of endocrine disorders are *endocrinologists*. They have completed a residency in internal medicine and fellowship training in endocrinology.

Many people have endocrine disorders involving excessive or deficient hormone production or function. Some common conditions, such as hypothyroidism, are readily controlled with hormone replacement medication. Other hormonal disorders may have a more difficult course. You will find that the hormonal disorder diabetes mellitus commonly results in prehospital medical emergencies.

DIABETES MELLITUS

The disease diabetes mellitus is marked by inadequate insulin activity in the body. Insulin is critical to maintaining normal blood glucose levels. Glucose is important for all cells, but it is especially critical for brain cells. In fact, glucose is the only substance that brain cells can readily and efficiently use as an energy source. In addition, insulin enables the body to store energy as glycogen, protein, and fat.

Diabetes mellitus, or sugar diabetes, is a common and ancient serious disease. Over 8 million Americans have been diagnosed with diabetes, and U.S. health experts believe nearly the same number of the populace may be living with undiagnosed diabetes. The disease was named in ancient times by Greek physicians who noted that affected persons produced large volumes of urine that attracted bees and other insects, hence *diabetes* (meaning "to siphon," or "to pass through") for excessive urine production and *mellitus* (meaning "honey sweet") for the presence of sugar in the urine.

Diabetes mellitus is typically categorized as Type I diabetes or Type II diabetes. In addition, diabetes can also be classified as primary or secondary. Secondary diabetes is due to another cause and is uncommon, affecting only about 1 percent of diabetics. Causes include drugs, infections, genetic disorders, other endocrine disorders, and immune-mediated diseases. Gestational diabetes, which occurs only during pregnancy, affects about 4 percent of pregnancies. Careful control of blood glucose levels in gestational diabetes is essential in preventing fetal cardiac and nervous system abnormalities. Untreated gestational diabetes is a major cause of large birth weight infants (macrosomia). Gestational diabetes must be treated with insulin, as oral hypoglycemic medications cross the placental barrier and adversely affect the developing fetus.

Type I Diabetes Mellitus

Type I diabetes mellitus is characterized by the destruction of the beta (β) cells of the pancreas, usually leading to absolute insulin deficiency. Type I diabetes is commonly called juvenile-onset diabetes because of the average age at diagnosis. The term *insulin-dependent diabetes mellitus (IDDM)* also is used because patients require regular insulin injections to maintain glucose homeostasis. This type of diabetes is less common than Type II diabetes, but it is more serious. Diabetes is regularly among the ten leading causes of death in the United States, and Type I diabetes accounts for most diabetes-related deaths.

Heredity is important in determining who will be predisposed to develop Type I diabetes. Although the cause of Type I diabetes is often unclear, viral infection, production of autoantibodies directed against beta cells, and genetically determined early deterioration of

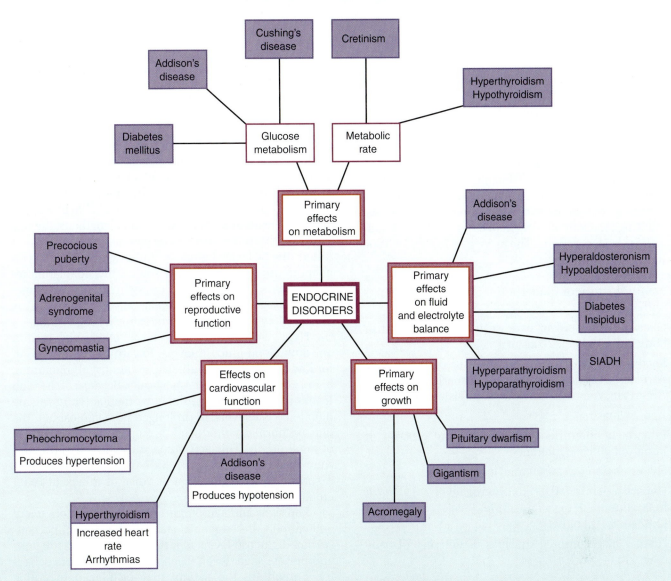

• **FIGURE A11-1**   **Overview of the Many Facets of Endocrine System Disorders**

beta cells are all possible causes. Regardless, the immediate cause of the disease is destruction of beta cells in the islets of Langerhans in the pancreas.

In untreated Type I diabetes, blood-glucose levels rise because, without adequate insulin, cells cannot take up the circulating glucose. Hyperglycemia in the range of 300 to 500 milligrams per deciliter is not uncommon. As glucose spills into the urine, large amounts of water are lost through osmotic diuresis. Catabolism of fat becomes significant as the body switches to fatty acids as the primary energy source. Overall, this pathophysiology accounts for the constant thirst (polydipsia), excessive urination (polyuria), ravenous appetite (polyphagia), weakness, and weight loss associated with untreated Type I diabetes. Ketosis can occur as the result of fat catabolism, and it may proceed to frank diabetic ketoacidosis, a medical emergency that you will encounter in the field.

Treatment of Type I diabetes requires the administration of insulin. Tight control of blood glucose levels minimizes many of the long-term complications of diabetes mellitus. To achieve this, insulin dosing must be individualized based upon the patient's activities of daily living. Frequent dosing of short- and medium-acting insulin provides tighter control of blood-glucose levels than a single daily dose of long-term or mixed insulin. Selected patients can benefit from an insulin pump that slowly administers insulin over a 24-hour period as programmed based on the patient's daily activities.

Type II Diabetes Mellitus

Type II diabetes mellitus, also called adult-onset diabetes or non-insulin-dependent diabetes (NIDDM), is associated with a moderate decline in insulin production accompanied by a markedly deficient response to the insulin present in the body. Some Type II patients will predominantly have insulin resistance with relative insulin deficiency, while others will have a predominantly secretory defect with insulin resistance.

Heredity may also play a role in predisposition to Type II diabetes. In addition, obese persons are more likely to develop Type II diabetes, and obesity probably plays a role in development of the disease. Increased weight (and increased size of fat cells) causes a relative deficiency in the number of insulin receptors per cell, which makes fat cells less responsive to insulin. This type of diabetes is far more common than Type I diabetes, accounting for about 90 percent of cases of diabetes mellitus. It is also less serious. The major risk factors for Type II diabetes mellitus are:

- Family history of diabetes (i.e., parents or siblings with diabetes)
- Obesity (≥20 percent over desired body weight or body mass index ≥27 kg/m²)
- Race or ethnicity with high risk of diabetes (e.g., African American, Hispanic American, Native American, Asian American, Pacific Islander)
- Age ≥45 years
- Previously identified impaired fasting glucose or impaired glucose tolerance
- Hypertension (≥140/90 mmHg)
- Hyperlipidemia (HDL cholesterol level ≤35 mg/dl [0.90 mmol/L] or triglyceride level ≥250 mg/dl [2.82 mmol/L] or both)
- History of gestational diabetes or delivery of baby over 9 lb (4.1 kg)

Untreated Type II diabetes typically presents with a lower level of hyperglycemia and fewer major signs of metabolic disruption than Type I diabetes. For instance, limited glucose use is usually sufficient to keep the body from switching to fats as the primary energy source. Thus, diabetic ketoacidosis (DKA) is uncommon in these patients. However, a complication called nonketotic hyperosmolar coma can occur, and you may see it as a medical emergency.

Medical treatment of Type II diabetes is less intensive than for Type I diabetes. Initial therapy often consists of dietary change and increased exercise in an attempt to improve body weight. If nonpharmacological therapy is insufficient to bring blood glucose levels down to the normal range, oral hypoglycemic agents may be prescribed. These drugs stimulate insulin secretion by beta cells and promote an increase in the number of insulin receptors per cell. In some cases, however, control may eventually require use of insulin.

Emergency Complications of Diabetes

Some of the complications of diabetes mellitus are medical emergencies and require prompt intervention. These include diabetic hypoglycemia (insulin shock), ketoacidosis (diabetic coma), and nonketotic hyperosmolar coma.

Hypoglycemia (Insulin Shock)

Hypoglycemia, or low blood glucose, is a medical emergency. It can occur when a patient takes too much insulin, eats too little to match an insulin dose, or physically overexerts and uses almost all of the available blood glucose. As the duration of hypoglycemia lengthens, the risk increases that brain cells will be permanently damaged or killed due to lack of glucose. Although brain cells can adapt to use fats as an energy source, this adaptation requires hours to develop, and the switch to fat-based metabolism cannot correct any damage already incurred. This is why every second counts in treating hypoglycemia.

Hypoglycemia, or insulin shock, reflects high insulin and low blood-glucose levels. Regardless of the reason for low blood sugar, insulin causes almost all remaining blood glucose to be taken up by cells. Because of the high level of insulin, glucagon may be ineffective in raising blood-glucose levels. In prolonged fasts, almost half the glucose normally produced through gluconeogenesis is of renal origin. This activity is stimulated by epinephrine. Diabetic patients with kidney failure may be predisposed to hypoglycemia because of a lack of renal gluconeogenesis.

The signs and symptoms of hypoglycemia are many and varied. Altered mental status is the most important. As blood-glucose levels fall, the patient may display inappropriate anger (even rage) or display a bizarre behavior. Sometimes the patient may be placed in police custody for such behavior or be involved in an automobile accident. Physical signs may include diaphoresis and tachycardia. If the blood glucose falls to a critically low level, the patient may have a hypoglycemic seizure or become comatose. In contrast to diabetic ketoacidosis, hypoglycemia can develop quickly. A clear change in mental status can occur without warning. Always consider hypoglycemia when encountering a patient with bizarre behavior. Additionally, hypoglycemia can cause symptoms resembling a CVA (hypoglycemic hemiparesis), which is why blood sugar evaluation is mandatory prior to treating for stroke.

In suspected cases of hypoglycemia, perform the initial assessment quickly. Look for a Medic-Alert bracelet. If possible, determine blood-glucose level. Because of the urgency of this emergency, most paramedic units must be able to perform this task or to rush a blood sample along with the patient. If the blood-glucose level is less that 60 mg/dL, 50 percent dextrose solution should be adminis-

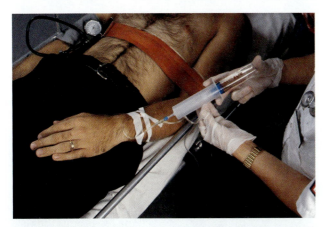

• **FIGURE A11-2   Intravenous Glucose Administration**
Patients with confirmed or suspected hypoglycemia must receive glucose before brain cells are destroyed.

tered intravenously (Figure A11-2•). If the patient is conscious and able to swallow, glucose administration may be provided orally with orange juice, sugared soft drinks, or commercially available glucose pastes.

When an IV cannot be started, hypoglycemic patients may improve following the administration of glucagon, which can be administered intramuscularly. This is a much slower process and will work only if adequate stores of glycogen are available. Glucagon must be reconstituted immediately prior to administration.

Diabetic Ketoacidosis (Diabetic Coma)

Diabetic ketoacidosis (DKA) is a serious, potentially life-threatening complication associated with Type I diabetes. It occurs when profound insulin deficiency is coupled with increased glucagon and stress hormone activity. It may occur as the initial presentation of severe diabetes, as a result of patient noncompliance with insulin injections, or as the result of physiologic stress, such as surgery, a myocardial infarction or serious infection.

Diabetic ketoacidosis reflects amplification of the same physiological mechanisms as ketosis. In the initial phase of diabetic ketoacidosis, profound hyperglycemia develops because of lack of insulin. Body cells cannot take in glucose for normal metabolic processes. Gluconeogenesis, the compensatory mechanism for low glucose levels within cells, only contributes more blood glucose. The consequent loss of glucose in the urine, accompanied by loss of water through osmotic diuresis, produces significant dehydration.

As the body switches to fat-based metabolism, the blood levels of ketones rise. The ketone load accounts for the observed acidosis. By the time the characteristic decrease in pH from about 7.4 to about 6.9 has occurred, the patient is within hours of death if left untreated. The onset of clinically obvious diabetic ketoacidosis is slow, lasting from 12 to 24 hours. In the initial phase, signs of osmotic diuresis appear, including increased urine production and dry, warm skin and mucous membranes. The individual often has excessive hunger and thirst coupled with a progressive sense of general malaise. Volume depletion induces tachycardia and feelings of physical weakness.

As ketoacidosis develops, a rapid deep breathing pattern termed Kussmaul's respirations appears. This major compensatory mechanism for acidosis helps expel carbon dioxide (CO_2) from the body. The breath itself may have a fruity or acetone-like smell as some blood acetone is expelled through the lungs. The blood profile includes not only hyperglycemia and acidic pH but also multiple electrolyte abnormalities. Low bicarbonate levels (HCO_3^-) reflect loss of acid-base buffer via Kussmaul's respirations. Low potassium levels may be found secondary to diuresis, with marked hypokalemia increasing the risk for cardiac dysrhythmias or death. Over time, mental function declines and frank coma may occur. A fever is not characteristic of ketoacidosis. If present, it is a sign of infection.

The treatment for a patient suffering from diabetic ketoacidosis is essentially the same as for any other patient who has mental impairment or is unconscious. The sweet, fruity odor of ketones occasionally can be detected in the breath. If possible, the blood glucose level should be determined. It is not uncommon for patients with ketoacidosis to have blood-glucose levels well in excess of 300 mg/dL. Prehospital treatment of DKA includes airway maintenance and fluid resuscitation to counteract dehydration. Often, the DKA patient will require several liters of an isotonic fluid. Definitive treatment includes insulin administration and correction of electrolyte deficiencies.

Nonketotic Hyperosmolar Coma

Nonketotic hyperosmolar coma (NKHC) is a serious complication associated with Type II diabetes. Typically, both insulin and glucagon activity are present. NKHC develops when two conditions occur: sustained hyperglycemia causes osmotic diuresis sufficient to produce marked dehydration, and water intake is inadequate to replace lost fluids. Renal or peritoneal dialysis, high-osmolarity feeding supplements, infection, and certain drugs also can be associated with development of NKHC.

As sustained hyperglycemia develops, glucose spills into the urine, causing osmotic diuresis and resultant dehydration. The level of hyperglycemia is often much higher than is seen in diabetic ketoacidosis (up to 1000 mg/dL). However, insulin activity in patients with NKHC is usually sufficient to prevent significant production of ketone bodies. Inadequate fluid replacement results in characteristic signs and symptoms.

The mortality rate for NKHC coma is higher than for ketoacidosis, ranging from 40 to 70 percent. The higher mortality rate may be due to the lack of early signs and symptoms that would bring patients with ketoacidosis to the attention of family or health care professionals.

The onset of NKHC is even slower than that of ketoacidosis, with development often occurring over several days. Early signs include increased urination and increased thirst. Subsequent volume depletion can result in orthostatic hypotension when the patient gets out of bed, along with other signs such as dry skin and mucous membranes, as well as tachycardia. The patient may become lethargic, confused, or enter frank coma. Kussmaul's respirations are rarely seen because of the lack of ketoacidosis.

Prehospital treatment of the patient suffering from NKHC is essentially the same as of any other patient who has mental impairment or is unconscious. Distinguishing diabetic ketoacidosis from NKHC is often difficult in the field. Therefore, the prehospital treatment of both emergencies is identical, and transportation should be expedited.

DISORDERS OF THE THYROID GLAND

A11 1

Disorders of the thyroid gland are typically chronic conditions. However, you may see patients with acute complications of thyroid disorders. The most common of these are:

- *Hyperthyroidism.* The presence of excess thyroid hormones in the blood.
- *Thyrotoxic crisis.* A condition that reflects prolonged exposure of body organs to excess thyroid hormones, with resultant changes in structure and function. Thyrotoxicosis is generally caused by Graves' disease.
- *Hypothyroidism.* The presence of inadequate thyroid hormones in the blood.
- *Myxedema.* A condition that reflects long-term exposure to inadequate levels of thyroid hormones, with resultant changes in structure and function.

The risk factors for developing thyroid dysfunction include:

- Female sex
- Older age
- Personal history:
  —Goiter
  —Previous surgery or radiotherapy affecting the thyroid gland
  —Other autoimmune diseases, including diabetes mellitus, vitiligo, pernicious anemia, and leukotrichia
  —Use of lithium or iodine-containing compounds
- Family history:
  —Thyroid disease
  —Pernicious anemia
  —Diabetes mellitus
  —Primary adrenal insufficiency

A11-5   The Endocrine System

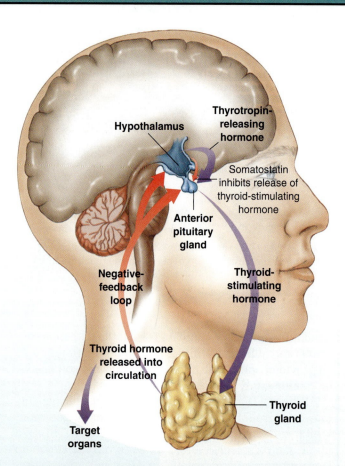

• FIGURE A11-3   The Thyroid Loop
The hypothalamus controls the anterior pituitary, which in turn controls the thyroid gland. Negative feedback loops prevent the oversecretion of thyroid hormones.

The thyroid gland is controlled by the anterior pituitary gland through the release of thyroid-stimulating hormone (TSH). The anterior pituitary, in turn, is controlled by the hypothalamus through the release of thyrotropin-releasing hormone (TRH). An increased level of TSH results in increased thyroid function, while a decreased level results in a decline. A negative feedback loop exists between the thyroid gland and the anterior pituitary gland and hypothalamus (Figure A11-3•). Table A11-1 compares common signs and symptoms of hypothyroidism and hyperthyroidism.

Graves' Disease

Excess circulating thyroid hormones result from Graves' disease. Roughly 15 percent of Graves' patients have a close relative with the disease, which suggests a strong hereditary role in predisposition to the disorder. In addition, Graves' disease is about six times more common in women than in men, with onset typically in young adulthood (20s and 30s).

Graves' disease has an autoimmune origin. Autoantibodies are generated that stimulate thyroid tissue to

TABLE A11-1	Common Signs and Symptoms of Thyroid Disease	
Hypothyroidism	*Hyperthyroidism*	
Fatigue	Fatigue	
Weight gain	Weight loss	
Cold intolerance	Heat intolerance	
Skin dry	Skin moist (hyperhidrous)	
Hair dryness and/or loss	Hair fine and silky	
Depression	Nervousness	
Dementia	Insomnia	
	Tremor	
Muscle cramps and myalgias	Muscle weakness	
	Dyspnea	
Bradycardia	Tachycardia	
	Palpitations	
Constipation	Hyperdefecation	
Infertility		
Edema		
Menstrual irregularity (hypermenorrhea common)	Menstrual irregularity (hypermenorrhea common)	

Source: Arch Intern Med. 2000:160:1573-75.

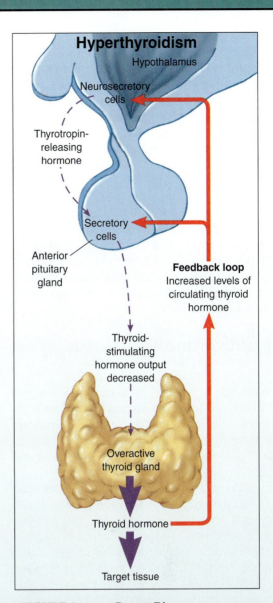

• FIGURE A11-4 **Graves Disease**
Hyperthyroidism results in an increase in the levels of circulating thyroid hormones.

produce excessive amounts of thyroid hormones (Figure A11-4•). The resultant changes in organ function are responses to either excess thyroid hormones or to the autoantibodies themselves.

The signs and symptoms of Graves' disease include agitation, emotional lability, insomnia, poor heat tolerance, weight loss despite increased appetite, weakness, dyspnea, and tachycardia or new-onset atrial fibrillation in the absence of a cardiac history. Nervous system symptoms tend to be more common in younger adults, whereas serious cardiovascular symptoms tend to predominate in older individuals. Prolonged exposure of orbital tissues to the pathological thyroid-stimulating autoantibodies can cause exophthalmos (protrusion of the eyeballs), whereas interaction of autoantibodies with thyroid tissue often produces diffuse goiter (a generally enlarged thyroid gland).

Cardiac dysfunction is probably the most likely context in which an emergency call may arise from thyrotoxicosis, usually caused by Graves' disease. Use of β-adrenergic blockers such as propranolol may temporarily reduce cardiac stress, but make sure the patient does not have heart failure or asthma before considering use. Glucocorticoid therapy (namely, dexamethasone) is sometimes helpful in quickly reducing the level of circulating T4.

Thyrotoxic Crisis (Thyroid Storm)

Thyrotoxic crisis, or thyroid storm, is a life-threatening emergency that can be fatal within as few as 48 hours if untreated. It is usually associated with severe physiological stress (e.g., trauma, infection), less often with psychological stress. You may also encounter thyroid storm secondary to overdose of thyroid hormone medication in a hypothyroid individual.

The mechanisms underlying thyrotoxic crisis are poorly understood. An acute increase in the levels of thyroid hormones does not appear to be the cause. More likely, thyroid storm is caused by a shift of thyroid hormone in the blood from the protein-bound (biologically inactive) to the free (biologically active) state. This significantly increases the amount of active hormone in the circulation, thus stimulating the thyroid gland.

The signs and symptoms associated with thyrotoxic crisis reflect the patient's extreme hypermetabolic state and increased activity of the sympathetic nervous system. The syndrome is characterized by high fever (106°F/41°C or higher), irritability, delirium or coma, tachycardia, hypotension, vomiting, and diarrhea. A less severe presentation may also occur, with slight fever and marked lethargy.

In the presence of the signs and symptoms of thyrotoxic crisis, field management is largely focused on supportive care: oxygenation, ventilatory assistance, fluid resuscitation, and cardiac monitoring. Glucocorticoids and β-adrenergic blockers may be helpful, especially if transport times are long. Transport should be expedited for definitive therapy that blocks the high blood levels of thyroid hormones.

Hypothyroidism and Myxedema

Hypothyroidism can be congenital or acquired and can affect both sexes. The recent increase in incidence of hypothyroidism in middle-aged women may reflect better diagnostics, a true rise in incidence, or both. Advanced myxedema in middle-aged and elderly individuals is the condition you are most likely to see in the emergency setting.

Hypothyroidism creates a low metabolic state, and early signs reflect poor organ function and poor response to challenges such as exercise or infection (Figure A11-5●). Over time, untreated severe hypothyroidism causes the additional sign of myxedema, a thickening of connective tissue in the skin and other tissues, including the heart. Patients with myxedema may progress into a hypothermic, stuporous state called myxedema coma, which can be fatal if respiratory depression occurs. Triggers for progression to myxedema coma include infection, trauma, a cold environment, or exposure to central nervous system depressants such as alcohol or certain drugs.

Early signs of hypothyroidism may be subtle. Symptoms may be as slight as fatigue and slowed mental function attributed falsely to aging. Typically, patients with hypothyroidism or myxedema show lethargy, cold intolerance, constipation, decreased mental function, or decreased appetite with increased weight. In addition, the relaxation stage of deep tendon reflexes (DTRs) is slowed. The classic appearance of myxedema is an unemotional, puffy-faced, and pale individual with thinned hair, enlarged tongue, and cool skin that looks and feels like dough. Myxedema coma may be difficult to identify. Note if the history is consistent with hypothyroidism and look for the physical appearance of myxedema. Other signs include profound hypothermia (temperatures as low as 75°F/24°C are not uncommon), low amplitude bradycardia, and carbon dioxide retention.

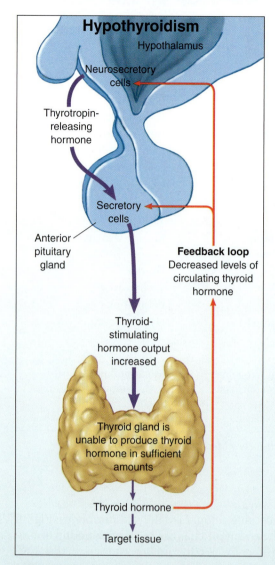

● FIGURE A11-5   Hypothyroidism
Hypothyroidism results in a decrease in the levels of circulating thyroid hormones.

These signs and symptoms may alert you to the possible presence of myxedema. Keep in mind that heart failure due to the combination of age, atherosclerosis, and myxedematous enlargement is not uncommon, so focus on maintaining the ABCs and closely monitoring cardiac and pulmonary status. Most patients with myxedema coma require intubation and ventilatory assistance. Active rewarming is contraindicated due to the risk of cardiac dysrhythmias and cardiovascular collapse secondary to vasodilatation. Although IV access is important, limit fluids because fluid and electrolyte imbalance is common and cardiac function is compromised. IV therapy should be guided by appropriate laboratory studies. Expedite transport to an appropriate facility for definitive treatment.

DISORDERS OF THE ADRENAL GLANDS

Two disorders of the adrenal cortex, Cushing's syndrome and Addison's disease, can play a part in medical emergencies or complicate responses to trauma. Cushing's syndrome is caused by excessive adrenocortical activity, while Addison's disease is caused by deficient adrenocortical activity.

Hyperadrenalism (Cushing's Syndrome)

Cushing's syndrome is a relatively common disorder of the adrenal glands. It usually affects middle-aged persons and is more common in women than in men. It results from excess glucocorticoids, primarily cortisol, which can be due to abnormalities in the anterior pituitary gland or in the adrenal cortex. It also can be due to treatment with glucocorticoids, such as prednisone. Check the history to note any recent steroid treatment for nonendocrine conditions such as cancer or rheumatologic disorders.

Long-term exposure to excess glucocorticoids produces numerous changes. Metabolically, cortisol is an antagonist to insulin. Gluconeogenesis is prominent, with profound protein catabolism. The body's handling of fats is altered: atherosclerosis and hypercholesterolemia are common. Over time, diabetes mellitus also may develop. Cortisol's mineralocorticoid activity causes sodium retention and increased blood volume. Increased vascular sensitivity to catecholamines occurs, and this may also contribute to hypertension. Potassium loss through the kidneys may cause hypokalemia. Cortisol's anti-inflammatory and immunosuppressive properties predispose the patient to infection.

Regardless of its cause, hyperadrenalism's presenting signs and symptoms are the same. The earliest sign is weight gain, particularly through the trunk of the body, face, and neck. A "moon-faced" appearance often develops (Figure A11-6•). The accumulation of fat on the upper back is occasionally referred to as a buffalo hump. Skin changes are also very common and may be an early clue to potential problems. These include the skin's thinning to an almost transparent appearance, a tendency to bruise easily, delayed healing from even minor wounds, and development of facial hair among women (hirsutism). Mood swings and impaired memory or concentration are also common.

Although you probably will not see patients with acute hyperadrenal crisis, you are likely to encounter patients with signs and symptoms of Cushing's syndrome. Remember that these patients have a higher incidence of cardiovascular disease, including hypertension and stroke. Pay particular attention to skin preparation when

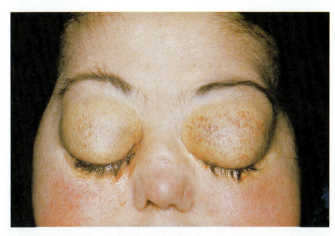

• **FIGURE A11-6   Facial Features of Cushing's Syndrome**

starting IV lines because of the patient's fragile skin and susceptibility to infection. Note any observations indicative of Cushing's syndrome in your report and relay them to hospital staff.

Adrenal Insufficiency (Addison's Disease)

Addison's disease is due to cortical destruction. Addison's has become less common as its former leading causes, such as tuberculosis, have come under control. Currently, over 90 percent of Addison's disease cases are due to autoimmune disease. As with Graves' disease, another autoimmune disorder, heredity plays a prominent role in an individual's predisposition for Addison's disease. In fact, patients with Addison's are more likely than average to have other autoimmune disorders, including Graves' disease.

Destruction of the adrenal cortex results in minimal production of all three classes of hormones: glucocorticoids, mineralocorticoids, and androgens. Low mineralocorticoid activity is key to the changes of Addison's, causing major disturbances in water and electrolyte balance. Increased sodium excretion in urine results in low blood volume, and potassium retention can cause hyperkalemia and ECG changes. Many cases of adrenal insufficiency are due to therapy with steroids such as prednisone, which can completely suppress normal adrenal function. Sudden cessation of the drug may trigger symptoms of Addison's disease or even an Addisonian crisis, with cardiovascular collapse.

Addison's disease is characterized by changes related to low corticosteroid activity: progressive weakness, fatigue, decreased appetite, and weight loss. Hyperpigmentation of the skin and mucous membranes, particularly in sun-exposed areas, is also characteristic.

Acute stresses, such as infection or trauma, may tip Addison's patients into a metabolic failure called Addisonian crisis, which is characterized by profound hypotension and electrolyte imbalances. Many patients will have gastrointestinal problems such as vomiting or diarrhea, which will exacerbate electrolyte imbalances, low blood volume, and hypotension and increase the potential for cardiac dysrhythmias. Be alert for this potentially life-threatening emergency, and include it in your list of possible causes of unexplained cardiovascular collapse, particularly if the history suggests primary Addison's disease or Addison's disease secondary to drug therapy.

The patient may reveal the presence of Addison's disease during the history, or the disease's signs and symptoms may lead you to suspect its presence. Focus emergency management on maintaining the ABCs and on closely monitoring cardiac and oxygenation status as well as blood-glucose level. Hypoglycemia poses its own threat. Assess blood-glucose levels and administer 25–50 grams of 50 percent dextrose to patients with blood glu-cose levels less than 50 mg/dL or those with altered mental status. Obtain a baseline 12-lead ECG to check for dysrhythmias related to electrolyte imbalance. Be aggressive in fluid resuscitation. Follow your local protocol or contact medical direction for specific orders based on your patient's presentation. Expedite transport to an appropriate facility for definitive treatment.

SUMMARY

Endocrine disorders are usually chronic conditions that can be effectively managed with medication and diet. With the exception of diabetes mellitus, endocrine disorders rarely cause medical emergencies. However, diabetes mellitus is common, and the failure to promptly treat hypoglycemia can result in permanent brain damage or even death.

12

Blood

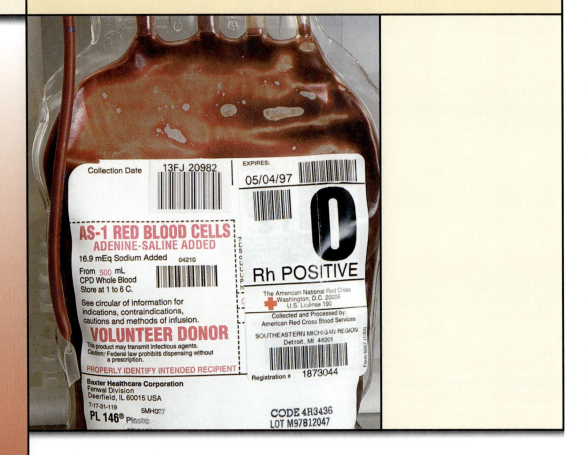

Blood is a living tissue that serves as the body's principal transport medium. Developments in the twentieth century made it possible to collect blood and place it into storage until needed. Prior to that, blood had to be collected from a donor and used immediately. Techniques that preserve blood have allowed for the development of blood banks. The immediate availability of banked blood has made the practice of medicine and surgery a much safer undertaking.

Chapter Outline and Objectives

Vocabulary Development

agglutinins, gluing; *agglutinization*
embolos, plug; *embolus*
erythros, red; *erythrocytes*
haima, blood; *hemostasis*
hypo-, below; *hypoxia*
karyon, nucleus; *megakaryocyte*
leukos, white; *leukocyte*
megas, big; *megakaryocyte*
myelos, marrow; *myeloid*
-osis, condition; *leukocytosis*
ox-, presence of oxygen; *hypoxia*
penia, poverty; *leukopenia*
poiesis, making; *hemopoiesis*
punctura, a piercing; *venipuncture*
stasis, halt; *hemostasis*
thrombos, clot; *thrombocytes*
vena, vein; *venipuncture*

The living body is in constant chemical communication with its external environment. Nutrients are absorbed through the lining of the digestive tract, gases move across the delicate epithelium of the lungs, and wastes are excreted in the feces and urine. These chemical exchanges occur at specialized sites or organs, but all parts of the body are linked by the **cardiovascular system**, an internal transport network.

Small embryos don't need cardiovascular systems, because diffusion across their exposed surfaces can exchange materials rapidly enough to meet their demands. By the time the embryo has reached a few millimeters in length, however, developing tissues will consume oxygen and nutrients and generate waste products faster than they can be provided or removed by simple diffusion. At that stage, the cardiovascular system must begin functioning to provide a rapid-transport system for oxygen, nutrients, and waste products. It is the first organ system to become fully operational: The heart begins beating by the end of the third week of embryonic life, when most other systems have barely started their development. When the heart starts beating, the blood begins circulating. The embryo can now make more efficient use of the nutrients obtained from the maternal bloodstream, and its size doubles in the next week.

The cardiovascular system can be compared to the cooling system of a car. The basic components are a circulating fluid (blood), a pump (the heart), and conducting pipes (the arteries, capillaries, and veins of the circulatory system). Although the cardiovascular system is far more complicated and versatile, both mechanical and biological systems can suffer from fluid losses, pump failures, or damaged pipes. This chapter considers the nature of the circulating blood. Chapter 13 focuses on the structure and function of the heart, and Chapter 14 examines the organization of blood vessels and the integrated functioning of the cardiovascular system. Chapter 15 considers the lymphatic system, a defense system intimately connected to the cardiovascular system.

THE FUNCTIONS OF BLOOD

The circulating fluid of the body is **blood**, a specialized connective tissue introduced in Chapter 4. ∞ *p. 92* Blood provides essential homeostatic services to each of the roughly 75 trillion individual cells in the human body. The five major functions of blood are:

1. *The transportation of dissolved gases, nutrients, hormones, and metabolic wastes.* Blood carries oxygen from the lungs to the tissues, and carbon dioxide from the tissues to the lungs. It distributes nutrients that are absorbed at the digestive tract or released from storage in adipose tissue or in the liver. Blood carries hormones from endocrine glands toward their target tissues. It also absorbs the wastes produced by tissue cells and carries these wastes to the kidneys for excretion.

2. *The regulation of the pH and electrolyte composition of interstitial fluids throughout the body.* Blood absorbs and neutralizes the acids generated by active tissues, such as the lactic acid produced by skeletal muscles.

3. *The restriction of fluid losses through damaged vessels or at other injury sites.* Blood contains enzymes and factors that respond to breaks in the vessel walls by initiating the process of blood clotting. The blood clot that develops acts as a temporary patch and prevents further changes in blood volume.

4. *Defense against toxins and pathogens.* Blood transports white blood cells, specialized cells that migrate into peripheral tissues to fight infections or remove debris. It also delivers antibodies, special proteins that attack invading organisms or foreign compounds.

5. *The stabilization of body temperature.* Blood absorbs the heat generated by active skeletal muscles and redistributes it to other tissues. When body temperature is already high, that heat can be lost across the surface of the skin. When body temperature is too low, the warm blood can be directed to the brain and to other temperature-sensitive organs.

THE COMPOSITION OF BLOOD

Blood is normally confined to the circulatory system, and it has a characteristic and unique composition (Figure 12-1•). It consists of plasma and formed elements. **Plasma** (PLAZ-mah), the ground substance of blood, is only slightly denser than water. It contains dissolved proteins rather than the network of insoluble fibers in loose connective tissue or cartilage. **Formed elements** are blood cells (red or white) and cell fragments (platelets) that are suspended in the plasma. **Red blood cells (RBCs)** transport oxygen and carbon dioxide. The less numerous **white blood cells (WBCs)** are components of the immune system. **Platelets** are small, membrane-enclosed packets of cytoplasm that contain enzymes and factors important to blood clotting.

Together the plasma and formed elements constitute **whole blood**. The volume of whole blood varies from 5 to 6 liters in the cardiovascular system of an adult man and from 4 to 5 liters in that of an adult woman. Whole blood components may be separated, or **fractionated**, for analytical or clinical purposes.

Blood Collection and Analysis

Fresh whole blood is usually collected from a superficial vein, such as the median cubital vein on the anterior surface of the elbow (Figure 12-1a•). This procedure

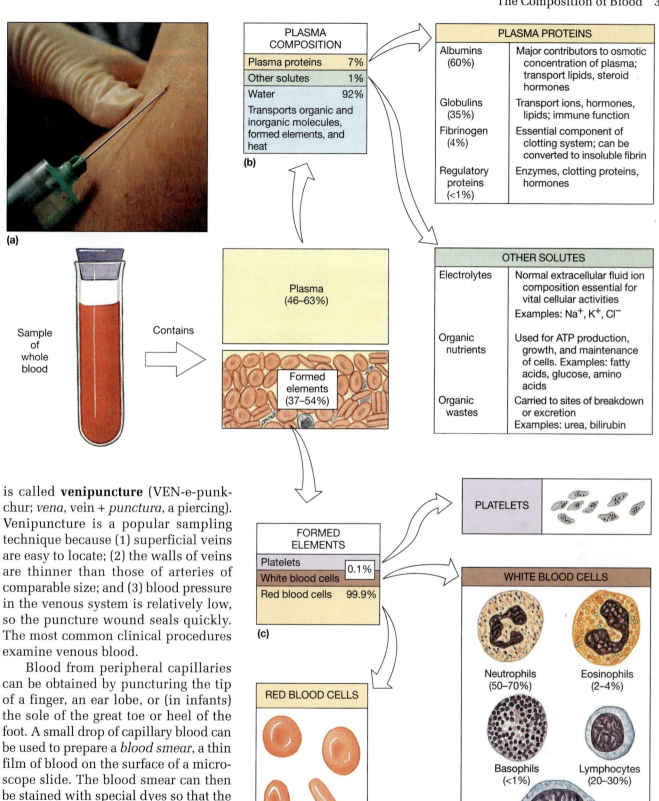

(a)

PLASMA COMPOSITION	
Plasma proteins	7%
Other solutes	1%
Water	92%
Transports organic and inorganic molecules, formed elements, and heat	

(b)

PLASMA PROTEINS	
Albumins (60%)	Major contributors to osmotic concentration of plasma; transport lipids, steroid hormones
Globulins (35%)	Transport ions, hormones, lipids; immune function
Fibrinogen (4%)	Essential component of clotting system; can be converted to insoluble fibrin
Regulatory proteins (<1%)	Enzymes, clotting proteins, hormones

Sample of whole blood

Contains

Plasma (46–63%)

Formed elements (37–54%)

OTHER SOLUTES	
Electrolytes	Normal extracellular fluid ion composition essential for vital cellular activities. Examples: Na^+, K^+, Cl^-
Organic nutrients	Used for ATP production, growth, and maintenance of cells. Examples: fatty acids, glucose, amino acids
Organic wastes	Carried to sites of breakdown or excretion. Examples: urea, bilirubin

is called **venipuncture** (VEN-e-punk-chur; *vena*, vein + *punctura*, a piercing). Venipuncture is a popular sampling technique because (1) superficial veins are easy to locate; (2) the walls of veins are thinner than those of arteries of comparable size; and (3) blood pressure in the venous system is relatively low, so the puncture wound seals quickly. The most common clinical procedures examine venous blood.

Blood from peripheral capillaries can be obtained by puncturing the tip of a finger, an ear lobe, or (in infants) the sole of the great toe or heel of the foot. A small drop of capillary blood can be used to prepare a *blood smear*, a thin film of blood on the surface of a microscope slide. The blood smear can then be stained with special dyes so that the different types of formed elements are easily distinguishable.

An **arterial puncture**, or "arterial stick," may be required for checking the efficiency of gas exchange at the lungs. Samples are usually drawn from the radial artery at the wrist or the brachial artery at the elbow.

PLATELETS

FORMED ELEMENTS	
Platelets	0.1%
White blood cells	
Red blood cells	99.9%

(c)

WHITE BLOOD CELLS

Neutrophils (50–70%)　Eosinophils (2–4%)

Basophils (<1%)　Lymphocytes (20–30%)

Monocytes (2–8%)

RED BLOOD CELLS

μm 0 5 10 15

•**FIGURE 12-1   The Composition of Whole Blood**
(a) Drawing blood. **(b)** The composition of plasma, the liquid portion of blood. **(c)** Formed elements include red blood cells, white blood cells, and platelets.

Whole blood from all of these sources has the same basic physical characteristics:

- *Temperature.* The temperature of blood is roughly 38°C (100.4°F), slightly higher than normal body temperature.
- *Viscosity.* Blood is five times as viscous as water, because interactions between dissolved proteins, formed elements, and the surrounding water molecules make plasma relatively sticky, cohesive, and resistant to flow.
- *pH.* The pH of blood averages 7.4 and ranges from 7.35 to 7.45; it is therefore slightly alkaline. ∞ *p. 36*

PLASMA

Plasma contributes approximately 55 percent of the volume of whole blood, and water accounts for 92 percent of the plasma volume (Figure 12-1b•). Together, plasma and interstitial fluid account for most of the volume of extracellular fluid (ECF) in the body.

Differences Between Plasma and Interstitial Fluid

In many respects, the composition of the plasma resembles that of interstitial fluid (IF). ∞ *p. 93* In contrast to cytoplasm, for example, both plasma and IF have roughly the same concentrations of the major plasma ions (electrolytes). The chief differences between plasma and interstitial fluid involve the concentrations of dissolved proteins and respiratory gases (oxygen and carbon dioxide). The protein concentrations differ because plasma contains circulating plasma proteins that cannot cross the walls of blood vessels and thus cannot enter the interstitial fluids. The differences in the levels of respiratory gases will be discussed in Chapter 16.

Plasma Proteins

Plasma contains considerable quantities of dissolved proteins. As Figure 12-1b• indicates, there is about 7 g of protein in each 100 ml of plasma; this amount is almost five times the concentration in interstitial fluid. The large size and globular shapes of most blood proteins prevent them from crossing capillary walls, so they remain trapped within the circulatory system. The three primary classes of plasma proteins are: *albumins* (al-BŪ-minz), *globulins* (GLOB-ū-linz), and *fibrinogen* (fī-BRIN-ō-jen).

Albumins constitute roughly 60 percent of the plasma proteins. As the most abundant proteins, they are major contributors to the osmotic pressure of the plasma. **Globulins**, accounting for 35 percent of the protein

population, include immunoglobulins and transport proteins. **Immunoglobulins** (i-mū-nō-GLOB-ū-linz), also called **antibodies**, attack foreign proteins and pathogens. **Transport proteins** bind small ions, hormones, or compounds that might otherwise be filtered out of the blood at the kidneys. One example is thyroid-binding globulin, which binds and transports thyroid hormones.

Both albumins and globulins can become attached to lipids, such as triglycerides, fatty acids, or cholesterol. These lipids are not themselves water-soluble, but the protein-lipid combination readily dissolves in plasma. In this way, the cardiovascular system transports insoluble lipids to peripheral tissues. Globulins involved in lipid transport are called *lipoproteins* (lī-pō-PRŌ-tēnz).

The third type of protein, **fibrinogen**, functions in the clotting reaction. Under certain conditions, fibrinogen molecules interact and combine to form large, insoluble strands of **fibrin** (FĪ-brin), the basic framework of a blood clot. If steps are not taken to prevent clotting in a plasma sample, fibrinogen will convert to fibrin. The fluid left after the clotting proteins are removed is known as **serum**. *Prothrombin* is a much less abundant plasma protein that is also essential to the clotting reaction. Clotting will be discussed in a later section.

Immunoglobulins (antibodies) are produced by plasma cells of the immune system. The bulk of plasma proteins, however—more than 90 percent of them, including all of the albumin, fibrinogen, and prothrombin, and most of the globulins—are synthesized and released by the liver. Because the liver is the primary source of plasma proteins, liver disorders can alter the composition and functional properties of the blood. For example, some forms of liver disease can lead to uncontrolled bleeding, caused by inadequate synthesis of fibrinogen, prothrombin, and other plasma proteins involved in the clotting response.

FORMED ELEMENTS

The most abundant formed elements are red blood cells and white blood cells. In addition, blood contains noncellular formed elements—platelets, small packets of cytoplasm that function in the clotting response (Figure 12-1c•).

The Production of Formed Elements

Formed elements are produced through the process of **hemopoiesis** (hēm-ō-poy-Ē-sis), or *hematopoiesis*. Blood cells appear in the bloodstream during the third week of embryonic development. These cells divide repeatedly, increasing in number. The vessels of the yolk sac, an embryonic membrane, are the primary sites of blood formation for the first 8 weeks of development. As other organ systems appear, some of the embryonic blood cells move out of the bloodstream and into the liver, spleen, thymus, and bone marrow. These embryonic cells differentiate into **stem cells** whose divisions produce blood cells. The liver and spleen are the primary sites of hemopoiesis from the second to fifth month of development. As the skeleton enlarges, the bone marrow becomes increasingly important, and it is the primary site after the fifth developmental month. In adults, it is the only site of red blood cell production and the primary site of white blood cell formation.

Stem cells called **hemocytoblasts** produce all of the blood cells, but the process occurs in a series of steps. We will consider the results of hemocytoblast divisions later in this chapter when we discuss the formation of each type of formed element.

Red Blood Cells

Red blood cells (RBCs), or **erythrocytes** (e-RITH-rō-sītz; *erythros*, red), contain the pigment *hemoglobin*, which binds and transports oxygen and carbon dioxide. Red blood cells are the most abundant blood cells, accounting for 99.9 percent of the formed elements.

The number of erythrocytes in the blood of a normal individual staggers the imagination. A standard blood test checks the number per microliter (µl) of whole blood. One microliter, or cubic millimeter (mm^3), of whole blood from a man contains roughly 5.4 million erythrocytes; a microliter of blood from a woman contains about 4.8 million. Erythrocytes thus account for roughly one-third of all cells in the human body.

The **hematocrit** (hē-MA-tō-krit) is the percentage of whole blood occupied by cellular elements. In adult men, it averages 46 (range: 40–54); in adult women, 42 (range: 37–47). The difference in hematocrit between males and females reflects the fact that androgens stimulate red blood cell production, whereas estrogens have an inhibitory effect. Because whole blood contains roughly 1000 red blood cells for each white blood cell, the hematocrit closely approximates the volume of erythrocytes. For this reason, hematocrit values are often reported as the *volume of packed red cells (VPRC)* or simply the *packed cell volume (PCV)*.

Many factors can alter the hematocrit. For example, dehydration increases the hematocrit by reducing plasma volume, and internal bleeding or problems with RBC formation can decrease it through the loss of red blood cells. As a result, the hematocrit alone does not provide specific diagnostic information. However, a change in hematocrit is an indication that other, more specific tests are needed. (Some of those tests will be considered later in the chapter.)

The Structure of RBCs

Erythrocytes are specialized to transport oxygen and carbon dioxide within the bloodstream. As Figure 12-2● shows, each red blood cell has a thin central region and a thick outer margin. This unusual shape gives it a relatively large surface area that facilitates diffusion between its cytoplasm and the surrounding plasma and allows RBCs to squeeze through narrow capillaries.

Red blood cells lack several organelles found in most other cells. During their formation, RBCs lose their mitochondria, ribosomes, and nucleus. Without a nucleus or ribosomes, our RBCs can neither undergo cell division nor synthesize proteins. Without mitochondria, they can obtain energy only through anaerobic metabolism, relying on glucose obtained from the surrounding plasma. This characteristic makes RBCs relatively inefficient in terms of energy, but it ensures that absorbed oxygen will be carried to peripheral tissues, not "stolen" by mitochondria in the cell.

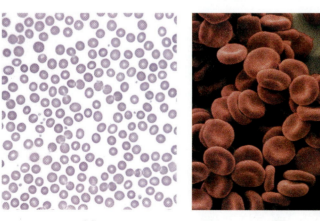
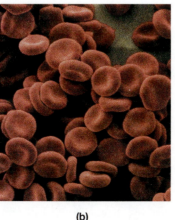
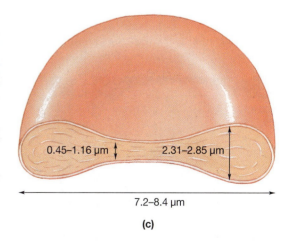

| (a) | (b) | (c) |

●**FIGURE 12-2**   **The Anatomy of Red Blood Cells**
(a) When viewed in a standard blood smear, red blood cells appear as two-dimensional objects because they are flattened against the surface of the slide. (LM × 320) **(b)** A scanning electron micrograph of red blood cells reveals their three-dimensional structure. (SEM × 1195) **(c)** A sectional view of a mature red blood cell, showing average dimensions.

Dimensions shown in (c): 0.45–1.16 µm, 2.31–2.85 µm, 7.2–8.4 µm

Hemoglobin Structure and Function

A mature red blood cell consists of a cell membrane surrounding a compact mass of transport proteins. The cytoplasm contains water (66 percent) and proteins (about 33 percent). Molecules of **hemoglobin** (HĒ-mō-glō-bin) **(Hb)** account for over 95 percent of the erythrocyte's proteins and give the cell its red color. Hemoglobin is responsible for the cell's ability to transport oxygen and carbon dioxide.

Four globular protein subunits combine to form a single molecule of hemoglobin. 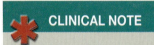 *p. 43* Each subunit contains a single molecule of an organic pigment called **heme**. Each heme molecule holds an iron ion in such a way that it can interact with an oxygen molecule. The iron-oxygen interaction is very weak, and the two can easily be separated without damage to either the hemoglobin or the oxygen molecule.

The amount of oxygen bound in each erythrocyte depends on the conditions in the surrounding plasma. When oxygen is abundant in the plasma, the hemoglobin molecules gain oxygen until all of the heme molecules are occupied. As plasma oxygen levels decline, plasma carbon dioxide levels are usually rising. Under these conditions, the hemoglobin molecules release their oxygen reserves and the globin portion of each hemoglobin molecule begins to bind carbon dioxide molecules in a process that is just as reversible as the binding of oxygen to heme.

As red blood cells circulate, they are exposed to varying combinations of oxygen and carbon dioxide concentrations. At the lungs, diffusion brings oxygen into the plasma and removes carbon dioxide. The hemoglobin molecules in red blood cells respond by absorbing oxygen and releasing carbon dioxide. In peripheral tissues, the situation is reversed, because active cells are consuming oxygen and producing carbon dioxide. As blood flows through these areas, oxygen diffuses out of the plasma and carbon dioxide diffuses in. Under these conditions, hemoglobin releases its stored oxygen and binds carbon dioxide.

Normal activity levels can be sustained only when tissue oxygen levels are kept within normal limits. The blood of a person who has a low hematocrit, or whose RBCs have a reduced hemoglobin content, has a reduced oxygen-carrying capacity. This condition is called **anemia**. Anemia causes a variety of symptoms, including premature muscle fatigue, weakness, and a general lack of energy.

RBC Life Span and Circulation

An erythrocyte is exposed to severe physical stresses. A single round-trip of the circulatory system usually takes

---

CLINICAL NOTE

SICKLE CELL DISEASE

Sickle cell disease is an inherited disorder caused by abnormal hemoglobin. Hemoglobin molecules consist of four hemoglobin chains. Most adults have *hemoglobin A,* which contains two alpha chains and two beta chains ($\alpha_2\beta_2$). In sickle cell disease, the beta chains are replaced with an abnormal hemoglobin chain called *hemoglobin S*. Sickle cell disease is passed from parent to child in an autosomal recessive pattern. That is, if a child receives hemoglobin S from one parent and a normal beta hemoglobin chain from the other parent, the child has *sickle cell trait* ($\alpha_2\beta S$). But, if the child receives an S chain from each parent, the child has *sickle cell disease* (α_2S_2).

Persons with sickle cell trait rarely have problems. However, persons with sickle cell disease have significant problems. When oxygenated, hemoglobin S functions normally. However, when deoxygenated, hemoglobin S polymerizes with the red blood cell (RBC) causing the classic sickle (crescent) shape. Sickled RBCs increase the viscosity of the blood, leading to sludging and obstruction of small blood vessels. Eventually, the cells become irreversibly sickled. Sickled RBCs are rapidly hemolyzed, resulting in an RBC life span of 10–20 days, compared with the normal RBC life span of 120 days.

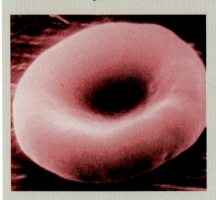

(a) **Normal RBC**

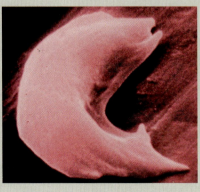

(b) **Sickled RBC**

•**FIGURE 12-3   Sickling in Red Blood Cells**
(a) When fully oxygenated, the cells of an individual with the sickling trait appear relatively normal. **(b)** At lower oxygen concentrations the RBCs change shape, becoming relatively rigid and sharply curved. (SEM × 67,500)

less than 30 seconds. In that time, a red blood cell is forced along vessels, where it bounces off the walls, collides with other red cells, and is squeezed through tiny capillaries. With all this mechanical battering and no repair mechanisms, a red blood cell has a relatively short life span, only about 120 days. The continuous elimination of RBCs usually goes unnoticed, because new erythrocytes enter the circulation at a comparable rate. About 1 percent of the circulating erythrocytes are replaced each day, and approximately 3 million new erythrocytes enter the circulation each second!

Hemoglobin Conservation and Recycling. As red blood cells age, they either rupture or are destroyed by phagocytic cells. If a damaged or aged erythrocyte ruptures, its hemoglobin breaks down into individual subunits small enough to pass through the filtration mechanism at the kidneys, where the subunits may be lost in the urine. When abnormally large numbers of erythrocytes break down in the circulation, the urine can turn reddish or brown. This condition, called **hemoglobinuria**, is usually prevented by specialized mechanisms that reclaim and recycle hemoglobin. Only about 10 percent of the RBCs survive long enough to rupture, or **hemolyze** (HĒ-mō-līz), within the bloodstream. Phagocytic cells of the liver, spleen, and bone marrow monitor the condition of circulating erythrocytes and usually recognize and engulf erythrocytes before they hemolyze. These phagocytes also remove hemoglobin and RBC fragments from the circulation. (Phagocytosis and phagocytic cells were introduced in Chapter 3; additional details are given in Chapter 15.) ∞ *p. 63*

Once a red blood cell has been engulfed and broken down by a phagocytic cell, the hemoglobin molecules begin to be recycled:

1. The globular proteins are disassembled into their component amino acids. These amino acids are either metabolized by the cell or released into the circulation for use by other cells.

2. Each heme molecule is stripped of its iron and converted to **biliverdin** (bil-ē-VER-din), a green substance. (Bad bruises often appear greenish because biliverdin forms in the blood-filled tissues.) Biliverdin is then converted to **bilirubin** (bil-ē-ROO-bin) and released into circulation. Liver cells absorb the bilirubin and excrete it in the bile. If the bile ducts are blocked (by gallstones, for example), bilirubin then diffuses into peripheral tissues, imparting a yellow coloration that is most apparent in the skin and eyes. This combination of yellow skin and eyes is called **jaundice** (JAWN-dis).

3. Iron extracted from the heme molecules may be stored in the phagocytic cell or released into the bloodstream, where it binds to **transferrin** (tranz-FER-in), a plasma protein. Red blood cells developing in the bone marrow absorb the amino acids and transferrins from the circulation and use them to synthesize new hemoglobin molecules. Excess transferrins are removed and stored by the liver and bone marrow, and the iron is stored in special protein-iron complexes.

In summary, most of the components of an individual erythrocyte are recycled following hemolysis or phagocytosis. The entire system is remarkably efficient; although roughly 26 mg of iron is incorporated into hemoglobin molecules each day, a dietary supply of 1–2 mg can keep pace with the incidental losses that occur at the kidney and the digestive tract.

Abnormalities in iron uptake, metabolism, or excretion can cause serious clinical problems. Women are especially dependent on a normal dietary supply of iron, because their iron reserves are smaller than those of men. The body of a normal man contains around 3.5 g of iron in the ionic form Fe^{2+}. Of that amount, 2.5 g is bound to the hemoglobin of circulating red blood cells, and the rest is stored in the liver and bone marrow. In women, the total body iron content averages 2.4 g, with roughly 1.9 g incorporated into red blood cells. Thus a woman's iron reserves consist of only 0.5 g, half that of a typical man. If dietary supplies of iron are inadequate, hemoglobin production slows down, and symptoms of iron deficiency anemia appear. Too much iron can also cause problems because of excessive buildup in the liver and cardiac muscle tissue. Excessive iron deposition has recently been linked to heart disease.

Red Blood Cell Formation

Red blood cell formation, or **erythropoiesis** (e-rith-rō-poy-Ē-sis), occurs in the bone marrow, or **myeloid tissue** (MĪ-e-loyd; *myelos*, marrow), of the adult. Red marrow, where active blood cell production occurs, is found in portions of the vertebrae, sternum, ribs, skull, scapulae, pelvis, and proximal limb bones. Other marrow areas contain a fatty tissue known as **yellow marrow**. Under extreme stimulation, such as a severe and sustained blood loss, areas of yellow marrow can convert to red marrow, increasing the rate of red blood cell formation.

Stages in RBC Maturation. During its maturation, a red blood cell passes through a series of stages (see Figure 12-7, p. 346). **Hematologists** (hē-ma-TOL-o-jists), specialists in blood formation and function, have given specific names to key stages. **Erythroblasts** are very immature red blood cells that are actively synthesizing hemoglobin. After roughly 4 days of differentiation and hemoglobin production, the erythroblast sheds its nucleus and becomes a **reticulocyte** (re-TIK-ū-lō-sīt). After 2 days in the bone marrow, reticulocytes enter the circulation. At this time they can still be detected in a blood smear with stains that specifically combine with RNA. Normally, reticulocytes account for about 0.8 percent of the circulating erythrocytes. After 24 hours in circulation, the reticulocytes complete their maturation and become indistinguishable from other mature RBCs.

The Regulation of Erythropoiesis. For erythropoiesis to proceed normally, the myeloid tissues must receive adequate supplies of amino acids, iron, vitamin B_{12}, and other vitamins (B_6 and folic acid) required for protein synthesis. It is stimulated directly by erythropoietin and indirectly by several hormones, including thyroxine, androgens, and growth hormone. As noted above, estrogens have an inhibitory effect on erythropoiesis.

Erythropoietin, also called **EPO** or *erythropoiesis-stimulating hormone*, appears in the plasma when peripheral tissues, especially the kidneys, are exposed to low oxygen concentrations, a condition called **hypoxia** (hī-POKS-ē-a; *hypo-*, below + *ox-*, presence of oxygen). For example, EPO is released during anemia and when blood flow to the kidneys declines (Figure 12-4•). Once in the circulation, EPO travels to areas of red marrow, where it stimulates stem cells and developing erythrocytes.

Erythropoietin has two major effects: (1) It stimulates increased rates of mitotic divisions in erythroblasts and in the progenitor cells that produce erythroblasts; and (2) it speeds up the maturation of red blood cells, primarily by accelerating the rate of hemoglobin synthesis. Under maximum EPO stimulation, the bone marrow can increase the rate of red blood cell formation tenfold, to around 30 million per second.

This reserve is important when recovering from a severe blood loss. If EPO is administered to a normal individual, however, the hematocrit may rise to 65 or more, placing an intolerable strain on the heart. Comparable strains can occur in the practice of blood doping, in which athletes reinfuse packed red blood cells removed and stored at an earlier date. The goal is to increase hematocrit and improve performance, but the result can be sudden death from heart failure.

RAPID BLOOD TESTS

In an emergency it is important to quickly determine baseline information about a patient's red blood cells (RBCs). The two most common rapid tests are the *hematocrit* and *hemoglobin* (H&H). The hematocrit determines the percentage of the blood occupied by RBCs. The hemoglobin test determines the concentration of hemoglobin in the RBC. Together, the H&H provides a quick evaluation of the quantity and quality of the patient's RBCs. Other tests routinely performed on RBCs are described in Table 12-1.

✓ What would be the effects of a decrease in the amount of plasma proteins?

✓ How would dehydration affect an individual's hematocrit?

✓ How would the level of bilirubin in the blood be affected by diseases that damage the liver?

✓ How would a decrease in the level of oxygen supplied to the kidneys affect the level of erythropoietin in the blood?

Blood Types

An individual's **blood type** is determined by the presence or absence of specific **surface antigens**, or *agglutinogens* (a-gloo-TIN-ō-jenz), in the erythrocyte cell membranes. The characteristics of RBC antigen molecules are genetically determined. At least 50 kinds of surface antigens exist on the surfaces of RBCs. Three of particular importance have been designated antigens **A**, **B**, and **Rh**.

All of the red blood cells of any individual have the same pattern of surface antigens. **Type A** blood has antigen A only, **Type B** has antigen B only, **Type AB**

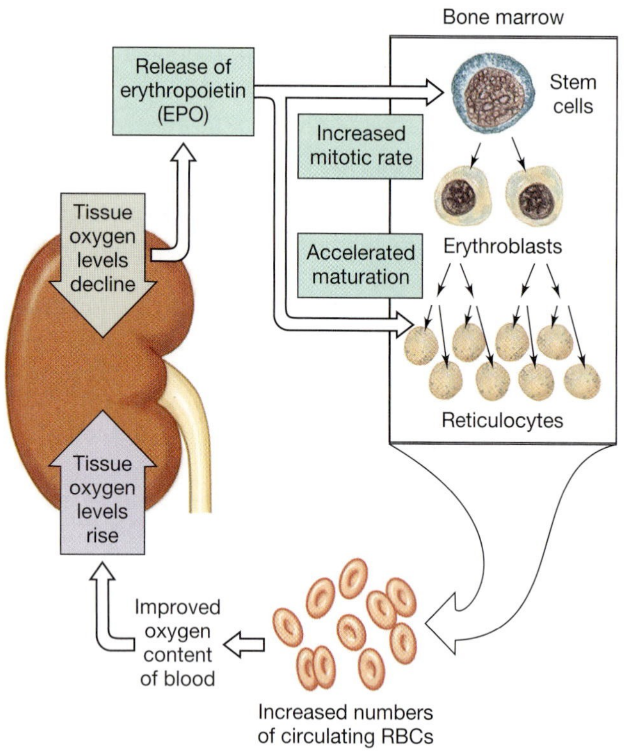

•FIGURE 12-4   The Control of Erythropoiesis
Tissues deprived of oxygen release EPO, which accelerates division of stem cells and the maturation of erythroblasts. More red blood cells then enter the circulation, improving the delivery of oxygen to peripheral tissues.

TABLE 12-1	RBC Tests and Related Terminology		
		Terms Associated with Abnormal Values	
Test	Determines	Elevated	Depressed
Hematocrit (Hct)	Percentage of formed elements in whole blood Normal = 37–54%	Polycythemia (may result from erythrocytosis or leukocytosis)	Anemia
Reticulocyte count (Retic.)	Circulating percentage of reticulocytes Normal = 0.8%	Reticulocytosis	
Hemoglobin concentration (Hb)	Concentration of hemoglobin in blood Normal = 12–18 g/dl		Anemia
RBC count	Number of RBCs per µl of whole blood Normal = 4.4–6.0 million/µl	Erythrocytosis	Anemia
Mean corpuscular volume (MCV)	Average volume of single RBC Normal = 82–101 µm³ (normocytic)	Macrocytic	Microcytic
Mean corpuscular hemoglobin concentration (MCHC)	Average amount of Hb in one RBC Normal = 27–34 pg/µl (normochromic)	Hyperchromic	Hypochromic

has both A and B, and **Type O** has neither A nor B. The average values for the U.S. population are Type O, 46 percent; Type A, 40 percent; Type B, 10 percent; and Type AB, 4 percent. Variations in these values result from racial and ethnic genetic differences (Table 12-2).

The presence or absence of the Rh antigen, sometimes called the Rh factor, is indicated by the terms Rh-positive (present) and Rh-negative (absent). Clinicians usually omit the term Rh and report the complete blood type as O-positive or O-negative, A-positive or A-negative, and so forth.

Antibodies and Cross-Reactions. Blood type is checked before an individual gives or receives blood. The surface antigens on a person's own red blood cells are ignored by that person's immune system. However, plasma contains antibodies, or *agglutinins* (a-GLOO-ti-ninz), which will attack "foreign" surface antigens (Figure 12-5a●). For example, the plasma of individuals with Type A blood contains circulating anti-B antibodies, which will attack Type B surface antigens. The plasma of Type B individuals contains anti-A antibodies, which will attack Type A surface antigens. The RBCs of an individual with Type O blood lack surface antigens A and B, so the plasma of such an individual contains both anti-A and anti-B. At the other extreme, Type AB individuals lack antibodies sensitive to either A or B surface antigens.

When an antibody meets its specific antigen, a **cross-reaction** occurs. Initially the RBCs clump together, a process called **agglutination** (a-gloo-ti-NĀ-shun); they may also hemolyze (Figure 12-5b●).

Clumps and fragments of RBCs under attack form drifting masses that can plug small vessels in the kidneys, lungs, heart, or brain, damaging or destroying tissues. Such reactions can be avoided by ensuring that the blood type of the donor and that of the recipient are **compatible**. A donor must be chosen whose blood cells will not undergo cross-reaction with the plasma of the recipient.

TABLE 12-2	Differences in Blood Group Distribution				
	Percentage with Each Blood Type				
Population	O	A	B	AB	Rh⁺
U.S. (AVERAGE)	46	40	10	4	85
Caucasian	45	40	11	4	85
African American	49	27	20	4	95
Chinese	42	27	25	6	100
Japanese	31	39	21	10	100
Korean	32	28	30	10	100
Filipino	44	22	29	6	100
Hawaiian	46	46	5	3	100
NATIVE NORTH AMERICAN	79	16	4	<1	100
NATIVE SOUTH AMERICAN	100	0	0	0	100
AUSTRALIAN ABORIGINE	44	56	0	0	100

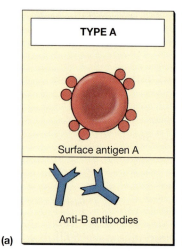
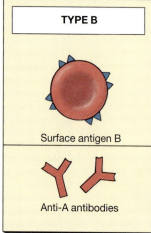
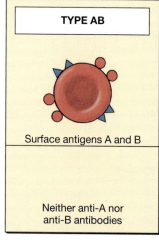
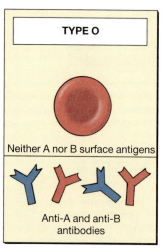

TYPE A	TYPE B	TYPE AB	TYPE O
Surface antigen A	Surface antigen B	Surface antigens A and B	Neither A nor B surface antigens
Anti-B antibodies	Anti-A antibodies	Neither anti-A nor anti-B antibodies	Anti-A and anti-B antibodies

(a)

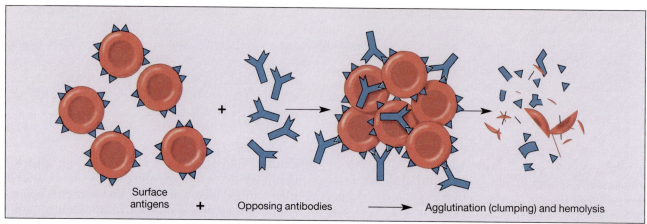

Surface antigens + Opposing antibodies → Agglutination (clumping) and hemolysis

(b)

● **FIGURE 12-5   Blood Typing and Cross-Reactions**
(a) Blood type depends on the presence of antigens on RBC surfaces. Blood plasma contains antibodies, which will react with foreign antigens. **(b)** A cross-reaction occurs when antibodies encounter their target antigens. The result is extensive clumping of the affected RBCs, followed by hemolysis.

✳ **CLINICAL NOTE** — **EMERGENCY TRANSFUSIONS**

Blood is a precious commodity and must be utilized so that it can provide the most benefit for the greatest number of people. A unit of whole blood consists of approximately 450 milliliters blood with about 65 grams of hemoglobin. In current medical practice, it is uncommon to administer whole blood. Instead, the blood is separated into its various elements, and those elements are administered as needed. Elements derived from whole blood include the red blood cells *(packed red blood cells)*, platelets, granulocytes, and plasma *(fresh frozen plasma)*. Patients receive only the blood elements that they need. A patient who has sustained hemorrhage, for instance, will receive packed RBCs and crystalloid fluids, while a patient with a platelet disorder will receive platelet transfusion.

In order to prevent a *hemolytic transfusion reaction,* blood must be tested for compatibility between the donor and the recipient. Blood products are tested for the major antigens (AB and Rh). In addition, they are tested for minor antigen compatibility. The analysis and selection of blood products for transfusion is a time-consuming process called *typing and cross matching.* In a critical emergency, there may not be time to wait for blood typing and cross matching.

In these situations, Type O-negative (O-) blood can be safely administered. Type O- blood does not contain the A, B, or Rh antigen. Thus, it will not induce a hemolytic reaction in a patient with a different blood type. Because of this, persons with type O- blood are referred to as *universal donors.*

Persons who have type AB blood are referred to as *universal recipients.* They have both the A and B antigens on their RBCs and thus lack circulating antibodies against both A and B. In an emergency, they can receive any type of blood, as they already have the antibodies.

In an emergency setting, if time permits, it is preferred to wait until the blood is fully typed and cross-matched. If there is not adequate time for this, the patient can be given *type specific blood.* Type-specific blood has been tested for the major (ABO and Rh) antigens. It has not been tested for the minor antigens. Finally, as described above, in critical situations, the patient may be given un-cross-matched type O- blood until typing and cross matching have been completed.

Platelets do not contain any minor blood antigens. Platelets should be of the same ABO and Rh type. They are rapidly destroyed by the body and must be frequently administered.

✳ TRANSFUSION REACTIONS

Blood and blood products must be compatible with the intended recipient. Modern blood-banking techniques have caused the incidence of transfusion reactions to markedly decline.

Transfusion reactions can be classified as immune and nonimmune. An immune transfusion reaction can result from incompatibility with the major antigens (AB and Rh) or the minor antigens. In this setting, antibodies are produced against the foreign blood type, resulting in RBC destruction *(hemolysis)*. Nonimmune reactions include circulatory overload and infection.

The signs and symptoms of a transfusion reaction include fever, chills, flushing, pain at the site of the transfusion, chest pain, shock, and kidney failure. If a transfusion reaction is suspected, the transfusion should be stopped immediately and the blood product saved for laboratory investigation. The patient should be well hydrated with intravenous fluids in order to maintain adequate urine output. In severe reactions, it may be necessary to administer a diuretic, such as furosemide (Lasix), to maintain brisk urinary output. Respirations, pulse, and blood pressure should be supported as required.

✓ Which blood types can be transfused into a person with Type AB blood?

✓ Why can't a person with Type A blood receive blood from a person with Type B blood?

White Blood Cells

White blood cells, also known as WBCs or **leukocytes** (LOO-kō-sīts; *leukos*, white), can easily be distinguished from RBCs because each has a nucleus and lacks hemoglobin. White blood cells help defend the body against invasion by pathogens and remove toxins, wastes, and abnormal or damaged cells. Traditionally, leukocytes have been divided into two groups on the basis of their appearance after staining: (1) *granulocytes* (with abundant stained granules) and (2) *agranulocytes* (with few if any stained granules). This categorization is convenient but somewhat misleading because the "granules" in granulocytes are actually secretory vesicles and lysosomes, and the "agranulocytes" contain lysosomes as well—they are just smaller and more difficult to see with the light microscope.

Typical leukocytes in the circulating blood are shown in Figure 12-6•. The three types of granulocytes are *neutrophils*, *eosinophils*, and *basophils*; the two kinds of agranulocytes are *monocytes* and *lymphocytes*. A microliter of blood typically contains 6000–9000 leukocytes. Circulating leukocytes, however, represent only a small fraction of the total population. Most of the WBCs in the body are located in peripheral tissues.

WBC Circulation and Movement

Unlike erythrocytes, leukocytes do not circulate for extended periods. The bloodstream provides rapid transportation to areas of invasion or injury, and in traversing

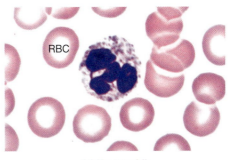

(a) Neutrophil

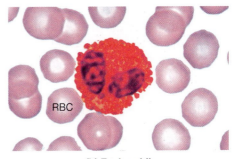

(b) Eosinophil

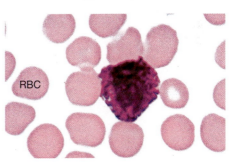

(c) Basophil

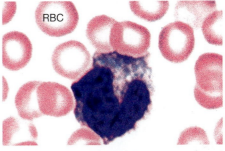

(d) Monocyte

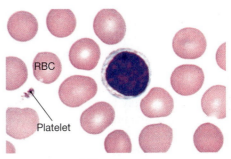

(e) Lymphocyte

•**FIGURE 12-6   White Blood Cells**
(LMs × 1500)

the miles of capillaries, leukocytes are sensitive to the chemical signs of damage to surrounding tissues. When problems are detected, these cells leave the circulation and enter the abnormal area.

Circulating leukocytes have four characteristics:

1. They are capable of *amoeboid movement*, which occurs when the cytoplasm of a WBC flows into slender cellular processes that are extended in front of the cell. This mobility allows WBCs to move along the walls of blood vessels and, when outside the bloodstream, through surrounding tissues.

2. They can migrate out of the bloodstream by squeezing between adjacent endothelial cells in the capillary wall. This process is known as **diapedesis** (dī-a-pe-DĒ-sis).

3. They are attracted to specific chemical stimuli. This characteristic, called **positive chemotaxis** (kē-mō-TAK-sis), guides them to invading pathogens, damaged tissues, and active WBCs.

4. Some of the circulating WBCs, specifically neutrophils, eosinophils, and monocytes, are capable of *phagocytosis.* ∞ *p. 63* These cells can engulf pathogens, cell debris, or other materials in or out of the bloodstream. Neutrophils and eosinophils are sometimes called microphages to distinguish them from the larger phagocytes found in the blood and peripheral tissues, the monocytes and macrophages.

General Functions

Neutrophils, eosinophils, basophils, and monocytes contribute to the body's *nonspecific defenses* of the immune system. These defenses respond to a variety of stimuli, but always in the same way—they do not discriminate between one type of threat and another. Lymphocytes, in contrast, are the cells responsible for *specific immunity*: the body's ability to attack invading pathogens or foreign proteins *on a specific, individual basis.* The interactions between WBCs and the relationships between specific and nonspecific defenses will be discussed in Chapter 15.

Neutrophils

Fifty to 70 percent of the circulating white blood cells are **neutrophils** (NOO-trō-filz). This name was selected because their granules are chemically neutral and thus difficult to stain with either acidic or basic dyes. A mature neutrophil (Figure 12-6a•) has a very dense, contorted nucleus that may be condensed into a series of lobes resembling beads on a chain.

Neutrophils are usually the first of the WBCs to arrive at an injury site. They are very active phagocytes, specializing in attacking and digesting bacteria. Most neutrophils have a short life span (about 12 hours). After engulfing one to two dozen bacteria, a neutrophil dies,

but its breakdown releases chemicals that attract other neutrophils to the site.

Eosinophils

Eosinophils (ē-ō-SIN-ō-filz) were so named because their granules stain darkly with the red dye eosin (Figure 12-6b•). They usually represent 2–4 percent of circulating WBCs and are similar in size to neutrophils. Their deep red granules and a two-lobed nucleus makes them easy to identify. Although they are phagocytes, eosinophils generally ignore bacteria and cellular debris. They are attracted instead to foreign compounds that have reacted with circulating antibodies. Their numbers increase dramatically during an allergic reaction or a parasitic infection.

Basophils

Basophils (BĀ-sō-filz) have numerous granules that stain darkly with basic dyes and that are a deep purple to blue in a standard blood smear (Figure 12-6c•). These cells are somewhat smaller than the other granulocytes and are relatively rare, accounting for less than 1 percent of the leukocyte population. Basophils migrate to sites of injury and cross the capillary endothelium to accumulate within the damaged tissues, where they discharge their granules into the interstitial fluids. The granules contain the chemicals *heparin*, which prevents blood clotting, and *histamine*. The release of histamine by basophils enhances the local inflammation initiated by the *mast cells* of damaged connective tissues. ∞ *p. 90* Other chemicals released by stimulated basophils attract eosinophils and other basophils to the area.

Monocytes

Monocytes (MON-ō-sīts) are nearly twice the size of a typical erythrocyte (Figure 12-6d•). The nucleus is large and commonly oval or shaped like a kidney bean. Monocytes normally account for 2–8 percent of circulating leukocytes. Outside the bloodstream in peripheral tissues they are called *free macrophages*, to distinguish them from the immobile *fixed macrophages* in many connective tissues. ∞ *p. 90* They are enthusiastic phagocytes that when active, release chemicals that attract and stimulate neutrophils, additional monocytes, and other phagocytes. Monocytes also secrete substances that lure fibroblasts to the region. The fibroblasts then begin producing scar tissue, which walls off the injured area.

Lymphocytes

Typical **lymphocytes** (LIM-fō-sīts) are roughly the same size as red blood cells and contain a relatively large nucleus surrounded by a thin halo of cytoplasm (Figure 12-6e•). Although lymphocytes account for 20–30 percent of the leukocyte population of the blood, this is only a minute segment of the entire lymphocyte population. Lymphocytes are the primary cells of the **lymphatic system**, a network of special vessels and organs distinct from those of the circulatory system.

The circulating blood contains three classes of lymphocytes, although they cannot be distinguished with a light microscope:

1. *T cells.* Lymphocytes called **T cells** attack foreign cells directly and stimulate or inhibit the activities of other lymphocytes.
2. *B cells.* Lymphocytes called **B cells** differentiate into plasma cells, tissue cells that secrete antibodies that can attack alien cells or proteins in distant parts of the body.
3. *Natural killer (NK) cells.* Lymphocytes called **natural killer (NK) cells** are responsible for immune surveil-

lance, the destruction of the body's own abnormal tissue cells.

The Differential Count and Changes in WBC Profiles

A variety of disorders, including pathogenic infection, inflammation, and allergic reactions, cause characteristic changes in the circulating populations of WBCs. A **differential count** of the WBC population, obtained by examining a stained blood smear, indicates the number of each type of cell encountered in a sample of 100 WBCs.

The normal range for each cell type is indicated in Table 12-3. **Leukopenia** (loo-kō-PĒ-nē-ah; *penia*, poverty) indicates inadequate numbers of WBCs. **Leukocytosis** (loo-kō-sī-TŌ-sis) refers to excessive numbers of WBCs. Leukocytosis with WBC counts of 100,000/µl or more usually indicates the presence of some form of

TABLE 12-3	A Review of the Formed Elements of the Blood		
Cell	*Abundance (Average per µl)*	*Functions*	*Remarks*
RED BLOOD CELLS	5.2 million (range: 4.4–6.0 million)	Transport oxygen from lungs to tissues and carbon dioxide from tissues to lungs	Remain in circulation; 120-day life expectancy; amino acids and iron recycled; produced in bone marrow
WHITE BLOOD CELLS	7000 (range: 6000–9000)		
Neutrophils	4150 (range: 1800–7300) Differential count: 50–70%	Phagocytic: Engulf pathogens or debris in tissues, release cytotoxic enzymes and chemicals	Move into tissues after several hours; survive minutes to days, depending on tissue activity; produced in bone marrow
Eosinophils	165 (range: 0–700) Differential count: <2–4%	Attack antibody-labeled materials through release of cytotoxic enzymes, and/or phagocytosis	Move into tissues after several hours; survive minutes to days, depending on tissue activity; produced in bone marrow
Basophils	44 (range: 0–150) Differential count: <1%	Enter damaged tissues and release histamine and other chemicals that reduce inflammation	Survival time unknown; assist mast cells of tissues in producing inflammation; produced in bone marrow
Monocytes	456 (range: 200–950) Differential count: 2–8%	Enter tissues to engulf pathogens or debris	Move into tissues after 1–2 days; survive months or or longer; primarily produced in bone marrow
Lymphocytes	2185 (range: 1500–4000) Differential count: 20–30%	Cells of lymphatic system, providing defense against specific pathogens or toxins	Survive months to decades; circulate from blood to tissues and back; produced in bone marrow and lymphatic tissues
PLATELETS	350,000 (range: 150,000–500,000)	Hemostasis: Clump together and stick to vessel wall (platelet phase); initiate coagulation cascade	Remain in circulation or in vascular organs; survive 7–12 days; produced by megakaryocytes in bone marrow

1
2

leukemia (loo-KĒ-mē-ah), a cancer of blood-forming tissues. Not all leukemias are characterized by leukocytosis; other indications are the presence of abnormal or immature WBCs. Unless treated, however, all leukemias are fatal. With treatment, many forms can be arrested or even cured.

White Blood Cell Formation

Stem cells responsible for the production of white blood cells originate in the bone marrow. Neutrophils, eosinophils, and basophils complete their development in myeloid tissue; monocytes begin their differentiation in the bone marrow, enter the circulation, and complete their development when they become free macrophages in peripheral tissues. Each of these cell types goes through a characteristic series of maturational stages. Figure 12-7• summarizes the relationships between the various WBC populations and compares the formation of WBCs and RBCs.

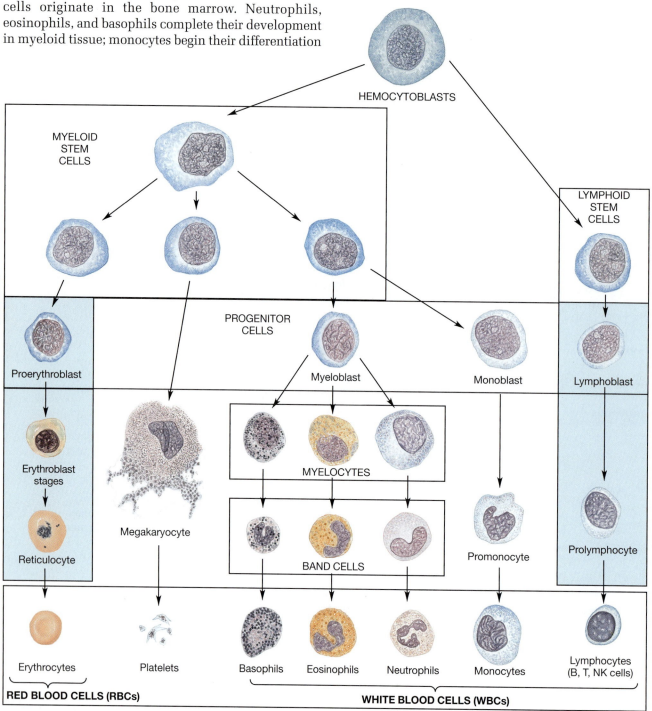

•FIGURE 12-7   The Origins and Differentiation of Blood Cells

Hemocytoblast divisions give rise to myeloid and lymphoid stem cells. Lymphoid stem cells produce the various classes of lymphocytes. Myeloid stem cells produce progenitor cells, which divide into various classes of blood cells.

Stem cells responsible for **lymphopoiesis**, the production of lymphocytes, also originate in the bone marrow. Many of these stem cells subsequently migrate to peripheral **lymphoid tissues**, including the thymus, spleen, and lymph nodes. As a result, lymphocytes are produced in these organs as well as in the bone marrow.

Factors that regulate lymphocyte maturation are not yet completely understood. Prior to maturity, the *thymosins* produced by the thymus gland promote the differentiation and maintenance of different T cell populations. ∞ *p. 318* The importance of the thymus gland in adulthood, especially in aging, is uncertain. In adults, the production of B and T lymphocytes is primarily regulated by exposure to antigens (foreign proteins, cells, or toxins). When foreign antigens appear, lymphocyte production escalates.

Several hormones, called *colony-stimulating factors (CSFs)*, are involved in the regulation of other white blood cell populations. Four CSFs have been identified, each targeting single stem cell lines or groups of stem cell lines.

Chemical communication between lymphocytes and other leukocytes assists in the coordination of the immune response. For example, active macrophages release chemicals that make lymphocytes more sensitive to antigens and accelerate the development of specific immunity. In turn, active lymphocytes release CSFs, reinforcing nonspecific defenses.

Platelets

Bone marrow contains enormous cells called **megakaryocytes** (meg-a-KĀR-ē-ō-sīts; *megas*, big + *karyon*, nucleus + *-cyte*, cell). These massive cells have large lobed or ring-shaped nuclei. As depicted in Figure 12-8•,

megakaryocytes continuously shed small membrane-enclosed packets of cytoplasm that enter the circulation. Now known as **platelets** (PLĀT-lets), they were once thought to be cells that had lost their nuclei, and histologists called them **thrombocytes** (THROM-bō-sīts; *thrombos*, clot). The term is still in use, although platelet is more suitable because these are cell fragments, not individual cells. Platelets initiate the clotting process and help close injured blood vessels. They are one participant in a vascular *clotting system*, detailed in the next section.

Platelets are continuously replaced. An individual platelet circulates for 10–12 days before being removed by phagocytes. Each microliter of circulating blood contains 150,000–500,000 platelets; 350,000/µl represents the average concentration. An abnormally low platelet count (80,000/µl or less) is known as *thrombocytopenia* (throm-bō-sī-tō-PĒ-nē-ah), and this condition usually results from excessive platelet destruction or inadequate platelet production. Symptoms include bleeding along the digestive tract, within the skin, and occasionally inside the CNS.

Platelet counts in *thrombocytosis* (throm-bō-sī-TŌ-sis) can exceed 1,000,000/µl. Thrombocytosis usually results from accelerated platelet formation in response to infection, inflammation, or cancer.

✓ Which type of white blood cell would you expect to find in the greatest numbers in an infected cut?

✓ Which cell type would you expect to find in elevated numbers in a person producing large amounts of circulating antibodies to combat a virus?

✓ A sample of bone marrow has fewer than normal numbers of megakaryocytes. What body process would you expect to be impaired as a result?

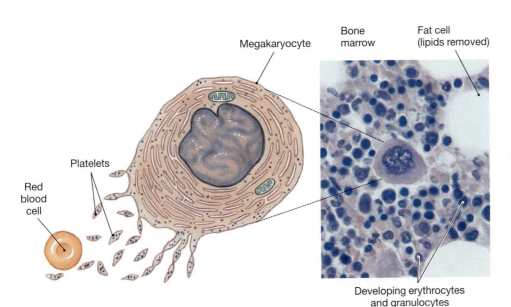

Megakaryocyte

Bone marrow

Fat cell (lipids removed)

Platelets

Red blood cell

Developing erythrocytes and granulocytes

•**FIGURE 12-8**
Megakaryocytes and Platelet Formation
In bone marrow sections, megakaryocytes stand out because of their relatively enormous size and the unusual shape of their large nuclei. These cells continuously shed chunks of cytoplasm that enter the circulation as platelets. (LM × 673)

HEMOSTASIS

The process of **hemostasis** (*haima*, blood + *stasis*, halt) prevents the loss of blood through the walls of damaged vessels. In restricting blood loss, this process also establishes a framework for tissue repairs. The major steps in hemostasis are the vascular, platelet, and coagulation phases, discussed next, followed by clot retraction and removal:

Step 1: *The vascular phase.* Cutting the wall of a blood vessel triggers a contraction in the smooth muscle fibers in the vessel wall that decreases the vessel's diameter. The contraction produces a local *vascular spasm*, which can slow or even stop the loss of blood through the wall of a small vessel. This period of local vascular spasm, called the **vascular phase** of hemostasis, lasts about 30 minutes. During the vascular phase, the membranes of endothelial cells at the injury site become "sticky," and in small capillaries endothelial cells may stick together and block the opening completely.

Step 2: *The platelet phase.* In larger vessels, platelets begin to attach to exposed endothelial surfaces. This attachment marks the start of the **platelet phase** of hemostasis. As more platelets arrive, they form a mass that may plug the break in the vascular lining.

Step 3: *The coagulation phase.* The vascular and platelet phases begin within a few seconds after the injury. The **coagulation** (kō-ag-ū-LĀ-shun) phase does not start until 15 seconds to several minutes later. Blood clotting, or **coagulation**, involves a complex sequence of steps leading to the conversion of circulating fibrinogen into the insoluble protein fibrin. As the fibrin network grows, blood cells and additional platelets are trapped within the fibrous tangle, forming a **blood clot** that effectively seals off the damaged portion of the vessel (Figure 12-9•).

The Clotting Process

Normal coagulation cannot occur unless the plasma contains the necessary **clotting factors**, which include calcium ions and 11 different plasma proteins. These proteins are converted to active enzymes that direct essential reactions in the clotting response. Most of the circulating clotting proteins are synthesized by the liver.

During the coagulation phase, the clotting proteins interact in sequence such that one protein is converted into an enzyme that activates a second protein and so on, in a chain reaction, or *cascade*. Figure 12-10• provides an overview of the cascades involved in the *extrinsic*, *intrinsic*, and *common pathways*.

The Extrinsic, Intrinsic, and Common Pathways

When a blood vessel is damaged, both the extrinsic and intrinsic pathways respond. Clotting usually begins in 15 seconds and is initiated by the shorter and faster extrinsic pathway. The slower, intrinsic path-

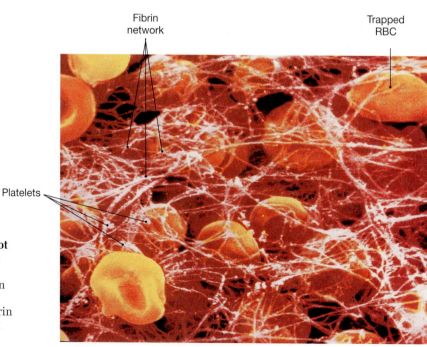

Fibrin network

Trapped RBC

Platelets

•**FIGURE 12-9   The Structure of a Blood Clot**
A scanning electron micrograph showing the fibrin network that forms the framework of a clot. (SEM × 4120) Red blood cells trapped in those fibers add to the mass of the blood clot and color it red. Platelets that stick to the fibrin strands gradually contract, shrinking the clot and tightly packing the RBCs.

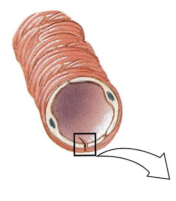

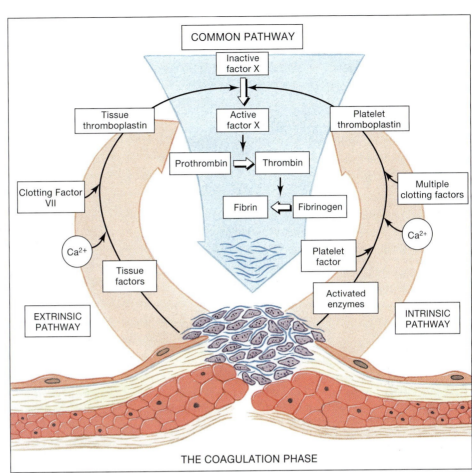

COMMON PATHWAY

Inactive
factor X

Tissue
thromboplastin

Active
factor X

Platelet
thromboplastin

Prothrombin → Thrombin

Clotting Factor
VII

Multiple
clotting factors

Fibrin ← Fibrinogen

Ca^{2+}

Ca^{2+}

Tissue
factors

Platelet
factor

EXTRINSIC
PATHWAY

Activated
enzymes

INTRINSIC
PATHWAY

THE COAGULATION PHASE

•FIGURE 12-10   The
Coagulation Phase of Hemostasis

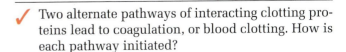

way reinforces the initial clot, making it larger and more effective.

The **extrinsic pathway** begins with the release of a lipoprotein called **tissue factor** by damaged endothelial cells or peripheral tissues. The greater the damage, the more tissue factor is released and the faster clotting occurs. Tissue factor then combines with calcium ions and one of the clotting proteins (Factor VII) to form an enzyme called **tissue thromboplastin**.

The **intrinsic pathway** begins with the activation of a clotting protein exposed to collagen fibers at the injury site. This pathway proceeds with the assistance of a platelet factor released by aggregating platelets. After a series of linked reactions involving various clotting proteins, the enzyme **platelet thromboplastin** is formed.

The **common pathway** begins after thromboplastin from either the extrinsic or the intrinsic pathway appears in the plasma. The first step involves the activation of a clotting protein (*Factor X*) responsible for the conversion of the clotting protein **prothrombin** into the enzyme **thrombin** (THROM-bin). Thrombin then completes the coagulation process by converting fibrinogen to fibrin.

Clot Retraction and Removal

Once the fibrin network has appeared, platelets and red blood cells stick to the fibrin strands. The platelets then contract and pull the torn edges of the wound closer together as the entire clot begins to undergo **clot retraction**. This process reduces the size of the damaged area, making it easier for the fibroblasts, smooth muscle cells, and endothelial cells in the area to carry out the necessary repairs.

As the repairs proceed, the clot gradually dissolves. This process, called **fibrinolysis** (fī-brin-OL-i-sis), begins with the activation of the plasma protein **plasminogen** (plaz-MIN-ō-jen), by **tissue plasminogen activator**, or **t-PA**, released by damaged tissues. The activation of plasminogen produces the enzyme **plasmin** (PLAZ-min), which begins digesting the fibrin strands and eroding the foundation of the clot.

✓   Two alternate pathways of interacting clotting proteins lead to coagulation, or blood clotting. How is each pathway initiated?

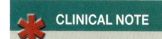

CLINICAL NOTE   **HEPARIN AND THROMBOLYTIC THERAPY**

The localized formation of a blood clot *(thrombosis)* is a normal part of the body's repair and healing response. A *physiological thrombus* serves to limit hemorrhage resulting from microscopic or macroscopic vascular injury. Physiological thrombosis is counterbalanced by physiological anticoagulation and physiological thrombolysis. In the normal setting, a physiological thrombus is confined to the immediate area of injury and does not obstruct blood flow to critical areas. Certain pathological conditions can lead to thrombus formation. In addition, under pathological conditions, a thrombus can expand into otherwise normal blood vessels, obstructing blood flow to critical tissues. An abnormal thrombus can occur anywhere in the body but is particularly problematic when it causes acute coronary syndrome, deep vein thrombosis, pulmonary embolism, acute nonhemorrhagic stroke, or blockage of peripheral arteries.

A thrombus in a coronary artery interrupts blood supply to a portion of the myocardium, resulting in acute coronary syndrome. Likewise, the formation of a thrombus within the vessels of the brain can cause a stroke. The time from blockage of the vessel until irreversible tissue injury occurs is short. In the setting of acute myocardial infarction, treatment must be provided in 6 hours or less in order to be most effective. When thrombolytics are administered to treat nonhemorrhagic strokes, they generally must be administered within 3 hours.

Therapy for abnormal thrombosis uses drugs that can be divided into three categories. The first is *thrombolytics,* agents that break down the offending thrombus *(thrombolysis).* Another is *anticoagulants,* agents that help prevent thrombus formation. Finally, *antiplatelet* drugs, which inhibit platelet aggregation, are helpful in preventing clot formation. All three categories play essential roles in emergency medicine.

- *Thrombolytic therapy.* Thrombolytic agents are able to dissolve preformed arterial and venous thrombi and restore blood flow to the affected tissues. They are derived from bacteria (streptokinase) or from recombinant DNA technology (tissue plasminogen activator, tPA). The effects of thrombolytic therapy are body-wide. Because of this, complications, most notably bleeding, can occur. Patients must be carefully screened before receiving thrombolytic therapy to assure that the possible benefits exceed the risks.

- *Anticoagulation therapy.* Anticoagulants are drugs that inhibit clot formation. They do not affect a clot that has already formed. These drugs are administered to patients at increased risk of clot formation or following removal of a clot. Heparin and warfarin (Coumadin) are the most frequently used. Heparin must be administered by injection, while warfarin must be administered orally. Recently, newer forms of heparin have been created that are much easier to administer and do not require frequent blood testing. These agents, called low-molecular-weight heparins (LMWH), include enoxaparin (Fragmin), dalteparin (Lovenox), and ardeparin (Fraxiparine). These drugs can be administered once or twice daily, allowing selected patients to be treated in the outpatient setting.

- *Antiplatelet therapy.* In addition to anticoagulants and thrombolytics, several other agents are beneficial in preventing thrombosis. Aspirin, a mainstay of medical therapy, inhibits platelet function and aggregation; it is inexpensive and highly effective. A new class of antiplatelet agents is the adenosine diphosphate (ADP) inhibitors. These agents are potent inhibitors of platelet aggregation through a mechanism that differs from aspirin. Drugs in this class include: abciximab (Reopro), epifabitide (Integrillin), and tirofibin (Aggrastat). These agents are being used with increasing frequency in the treatment of acute coronary syndrome.

Other thrombotic disorders, including deep venous thrombosis, pulmonary embolism, and peripheral arterial occlusion, are benefiting from these new therapies. With the development of safer and easier to administer medications, the use of thrombolytics and anticoagulants in prehospital care is increasing.

*C*hapter Review

KEY TERMS

blood, *p. 334*
cardiovascular system, *p. 334*
coagulation, *p. 348*
embolus, *p. 350*
erythrocyte, *p. 337*

fibrin, *p. 336*
fibrinolysis, *p. 349*
hematocrit, *p. 337*
hemoglobin, *p. 338*
hemopoiesis, *p. 336*

hemostasis, *p. 348*
leukocyte, *p. 343*
plasma, *p. 334*
platelets, *p. 334*

SUMMARY OUTLINE

INTRODUCTION   *p. 334*

1. The **cardiovascular system** provides a mechanism for the rapid transport of nutrients, waste products, and cells within the body.

THE FUNCTIONS OF BLOOD *p. 334*

1. **Blood** is a specialized connective tissue. Its functions include (1) transporting dissolved gases, nutrients, hormones, and metabolic wastes; (2) regulating the pH and electrolyte composition of the interstitial fluids; (3) restricting fluid losses through damaged vessels; (4) defending against pathogens and toxins; and (5) stabilizing body temperature through the absorption and redistribution of heat.

THE COMPOSITION OF BLOOD   *p. 334*

Blood Collection and Analysis   *p. 334*

1. Blood contains **plasma**, **red blood cells (RBCs)**, **white blood cells (WBCs)**, and **platelets**. The plasma and formed elements constitute whole blood, which can be **fractionated** for analytical or clinical purposes. *(Figure 12-1a)*

PLASMA   *p. 336*

1. Plasma accounts for about 55 percent of the volume of blood; roughly 92 percent of plasma is water. *(Figure 12-1b)*

Differences Between Plasma and Interstitial Fluid *p. 336*

2. Compared with interstitial fluid, plasma has a higher dissolved oxygen concentration and more dissolved proteins. The three classes of plasma proteins are *albumins*, *globulins*, and *fibrinogen*.

Plasma Proteins   *p. 336*

3. **Albumins** constitute about 60 percent of plasma proteins. **Globulins** constitute roughly 35 percent of plasma proteins; they include **immunoglobulins (antibodies)**, which attack foreign proteins and pathogens, and **transport proteins**, which bind ions, hormones, and other compounds. In the clotting reaction, **fibrinogen** molecules are converted to **fibrin**. Removing fibrinogen from plasma leaves a fluid called **serum**.

FORMED ELEMENTS   *p. 336*

The Production of Formed Elements   *p. 336*

1. **Hemopoiesis** is the process of blood cell formation. **Stem cells** called **hemocytoblasts** divide to form all of the blood cells.

Red Blood Cells   *p. 337*

2. **Erythrocytes (RBCs)** account for slightly less than half of the blood volume and 99.9 percent of the formed elements. The **hematocrit** is a value that indicates the percentage of whole blood occupied by cellular elements. *(Figure 12-1c)*

3. RBCs transport oxygen and carbon dioxide within the bloodstream. They are highly specialized cells with a large surface-to-volume ratio. Because RBCs lack mitochondria, ribosomes, and nuclei, these cells are unable to perform normal maintenance operations. As a result, they usually degenerate after about 120 days in the circulation. *(Figure 12-2)*

4. Molecules of **hemoglobin (Hb)** account for over 95 percent of RBC proteins. Hemoglobin is a globular protein formed from four subunits. Each subunit contains a single molecule of **heme** and can reversibly bind an oxygen molecule. Damaged or dead RBCs are recycled by phagocytes.

5. **Erythropoiesis**, the formation of erythrocytes, occurs mainly in the **myeloid tissue** (bone marrow) in adults. RBC formation increases under stimulation by **erythropoietin**, or **EPO** (erythropoiesis-stimulating hormone), which occurs when peripheral tissues are exposed to low oxygen concentrations. Stages in RBC development include **erythroblasts** and **reticulocytes**. *(Figures 12-4, 12-7)*

6. **Blood type** is determined by the presence or absence of specific **surface antigens** (*agglutinogens*) in the RBC cell membranes: antigens **A**, **B**, and **Rh**. Antibodies (agglutinins) in plasma will react with RBCs bearing different surface antigens. Anti-Rh antibodies are synthesized only after an Rh-negative individual becomes sensitized to the Rh surface antigen. *(Figure 12-5; Table 12-2)*

White Blood Cells   *p. 343*

7. White blood cells (**leukocytes**) defend the body against pathogens and remove toxins, wastes, and abnormal or damaged cells.

8. Leukocytes show **diapedesis** (the ability to move through vessel walls) and **positive chemotaxis** (attraction to specific chemicals).

9. *Granulocytes* (granular leukocytes) are often subdivided into *neutrophils*, *eosinophils*, and *basophils*. Fifty to 70 percent of circulating WBCs are **neutrophils**, which are highly mobile phagocytes. The much less common **eosinophils** are phagocytes attracted to foreign compounds that have reacted with circulating antibodies. The relatively rare **basophils** migrate to damaged tissues and release *histamines*, aiding the inflammation response. *(Figure 12-6)*

10. *Agranulocytes* (agranular leukocytes) are subdivided into *monocytes* and *lymphocytes*. **Monocytes** migrating into peripheral tissues become free macrophages. **Lymphocytes**, the primary cells of the **lymphatic system**, include **T cells** (which attack foreign cells directly), **B cells** (which produce antibodies), and **NK cells** (which destroy abnormal tissue cells). *(Figure 12-6)*

11. Granulocytes and monocytes are produced by stem cells in the bone marrow. Stem cells responsible for **lymphopoiesis** (production of lymphocytes) also originate in the bone marrow, but many migrate to peripheral lymphoid tissues. *(Figure 12-7)*

12. Factors that regulate lymphocyte maturation are not completely understood. *Colony-stimulating factors (CSFs)* are hormones involved in regulating other WBC populations.

Platelets *p. 347*

13. Megakaryocytes in the bone marrow release packets of cytoplasm (platelets) into the circulating blood. Platelets are essential to the clotting process. *(Figure 12-8)*

HEMOSTASIS *p. 348*

1. Hemostasis prevents the loss of blood through the walls of damaged vessels.

2. The initial step of hemostasis, the **vascular phase**, is a period of local contraction of vessel walls resulting from a vascular spasm at the injury site. The **platelet phase** follows as platelets stick to damaged surfaces.

The Clotting Process *p. 348*

3. The **coagulation phase** occurs as factors released by endothelial cells or peripheral tissues (**extrinsic pathway**) and platelets (**intrinsic pathway**) interact with **clotting factors** to form a **blood clot**. *(Figures 12-9, 12-10)*

Clot Retraction and Removal *p. 349*

4. During **clot retraction**, platelets contract and pull the torn edges closer together. During **fibrinolysis**, the clot gradually dissolves through the action of **plasmin**, the activated form of circulating **plasminogen**.

REVIEW QUESTIONS

LEVEL 1   Reviewing Facts and Terms

Match each item in column A with the most closely related item in column B. Use letters for answers in the spaces provided.

Column A

___ 1. interstitial fluid
___ 2. hemopoiesis
___ 3. stem cells
___ 4. hypoxia
___ 5. surface antigens
___ 6. antibodies
___ 7. diapedesis
___ 8. leukopenia
___ 9. agranulocyte
___ 10. leukocytosis
___ 11. granulocyte
___ 12. thrombocytopenia

Column B

a. hemocytoblasts
b. abundant WBCs
c. agglutinogens
d. neutrophil
e. WBC migration
f. extracellular fluid
g. monocyte
h. few WBCs
i. low platelet count
j. agglutinins
k. blood cell formation
l. low oxygen concentration

13. The formed elements of the blood include:
(a) plasma, fibrin, serum
(b) albumins, globulins, fibrinogen
(c) WBCs, RBCs, platelets
(d) a, b, and c are correct

14. Blood temperature is approximately _____, and the blood pH averages _____.
(a) 98.6°F, 7.0
(b) 104°F, 7.8
(c) 100.4°F, 7.4
(d) 96.8°F, 7.0

15. Plasma contributes approximately _____ percent of the volume of whole blood, and water accounts for _____ percent of the plasma volume.
(a) 55, 92   (b) 25, 55
(c) 92, 55   (d) 35, 72

16. When the clotting proteins are removed from plasma, _____ remains.
(a) fibrinogen   (b) fibrin
(c) serum   (d) heme

17. In an adult, the only site of red blood cell production, and the primary site of white blood cell formation, is the:
(a) liver   (b) spleen
(c) thymus   (d) red bone marrow

18. The most numerous WBCs found in a differential count of a "normal" individual are:
(a) neutrophils
(b) basophils
(c) lymphocytes
(d) monocytes

19. Stem cells responsible for the process of lymphopoiesis are located in the:
(a) thymus and spleen
(b) lymph nodes
(c) red bone marrow
(d) a, b, and c are correct

20. The first step in the process of hemostasis is:
(a) coagulation
(b) the platelet phase
(c) fibrinolysis
(d) vascular spasm

21. The complex sequence of steps leading to the conversion of fibrinogen to fibrin is called:
(a) fibrinolysis
(b) coagulation
(c) retraction
(d) the platelet phase

22. What five major functions are performed by the blood?

23. What three primary classes of plasma proteins are found in the blood? What is the major function of each?

24. What type of antibodies does the plasma contain for each of the following blood types?
    (a) Type A   (b) Type B
    (c) Type AB   (d) Type O

25. What three processes facilitate the movement of WBCs to areas of invasion or injury?

26. What contribution from the intrinsic and extrinsic pathways is necessary for the common pathway to begin?

27. Distinguish between an embolus and a thrombus.

LEVEL 2   Reviewing Concepts

28. Dehydration would cause:
    (a) an increase in the hematocrit
    (b) a decrease in the hematocrit
    (c) no effect in the hematocrit
    (d) an increase in plasma volume

29. Erythropoietin directly stimulates RBC formation by:
    (a) increasing rates of mitotic divisions in erythroblasts
    (b) speeding up the maturation of red blood cells
    (c) accelerating the rate of hemoglobin synthesis
    (d) a, b, and c are correct

30. A person with Type A blood has:
    (a) Anti-A in the plasma
    (b) Type B antigens in the plasma
    (c) Type A antigens on the red blood cells
    (d) Anti-B on the red blood cells

31. Hemolytic disease of the newborn can result if:
    (a) the mother is Rh-positive and the father is Rh-negative
    (b) both the father and the mother are Rh-negative
    (c) both the father and the mother are Rh-positive
    (d) an Rh-negative woman carries an Rh-positive fetus

32. How do red blood cells differ from typical cells found in the body?

LEVEL 3   Critical Thinking and Clinical Applications

33. Which of the formed elements would you expect to increase after you have donated a pint of blood?

34. Why do many individuals with advanced kidney disease become anemic?

ANSWERS TO CONCEPT CHECK QUESTIONS

Page 340
1. A decrease in the amount of plasma proteins in the blood could cause (1) a decrease in plasma osmotic pressure, (2) a decreased ability to fight infection, and (3) a decrease in the transport and binding of some ions, hormones, and other molecules.   **2.** The hematocrit measures the amount of formed elements (mostly red blood cells) as a percentage of the total blood. The loss of water during dehydration would decrease the plasma volume, resulting in an increased hematocrit. **3.** Diseases that damage the liver, such as hepatitis and cirrhosis, would impair the liver's ability to excrete bilirubin. As a result, bilirubin would accumulate in the blood, producing jaundice.   **4.** A decreased oxygen supply (and therefore a decreased blood flow) to the kidneys would trigger the release of erythropoietin. The elevated erythropoietin would lead to an increase in erythropoiesis (red blood cell formation).

Page 343
1. A person with Type AB blood can accept Type A, Type B, Type AB, or Type O blood.   **2.** If a person with Type A blood received a transfusion of Type B blood, the transfused RBCs would clump or agglutinate, because the anti-B antibodies in the blood of the Type A preson would attack the B antigens on the surfaces of Type B RBCs.

The agglutination would potentially block blood flow to various organs and tissues.

Page 347
1. In an infected cut, you would expect to find a large number of neutrophils. Neutrophils are phagocytic white blood cells that are usually the first to arrive at the site of an injury and that are specialized to attack infectious bacteria.   **2.** The type of white blood cell that produces circulating antibodies is the B lymphocyte, and these would be found in increased numbers.   **3.** Megakaryocytes are the precursors of platelets, which play an important role in hemostasis and the clotting process. A decreased number of megakaryocytes would result in fewer platelets, which in turn would interfere with the ability to clot properly.

Page 349
1. The faster, extrinsic pathway is initiated by damaged endothelial cells or damaged tissues when they release a lipoprotein called tissue factor. The slower, intrinsic pathway is initiated by the activation of a clotting protein exposed to damaged collagen fibers and by the release of platelet factor by aggregating platelets.

OVERVIEW

The circulating fluid of the body is blood. Whole blood is a living tissue that circulates through the body carrying nourishments, electrolytes, hormones, vitamins, antibodies, heat, and oxygen to the body's tissues. Whole blood contains red blood cells, white blood cells, and platelets that are suspended in a protein-containing liquid called plasma. Blood is a tissue that can be given to another individual when needed through a procedure referred to as a transfusion. It is a precious commodity that must be utilized so that it benefits the most people.

Physicians who specialize in diseases of the blood are called *hematologists.* Hematologists complete a residency in internal medicine and then serve a fellowship in hematology. Blood banking and laboratory analysis of blood is the domain of the *pathologist.* The pathologist specializes in laboratory medicine. Pathology residency programs generally last from three to four years.

BLOOD BANKING AND TRANSFUSION

Each year in the United States, approximately 13.9 million units of whole blood are donated and are transfused into approxi-

mately 4.5 million patients (Figure A12-1●). Typically, each donated unit of blood, referred to as whole blood, is separated, or *fractionated,* into multiple components, and each component is generally transfused into different individuals according to their specific needs. The components of whole blood include red blood cells, plasma, platelets, white blood cells, and plasma derivatives.

Red Blood Cells

Red blood cells (RBCs) are the most recognizable component of whole blood. The RBCs, also called *erythrocytes,* contain hemoglobin, which transports oxygen. With an average life of approximately 120 days, RBCs are continuously being produced and broken down by the body and are ultimately removed by the spleen. RBC transfusions, often called packed cells, are used in the treatment of acute blood loss and anemia.

Plasma

The plasma is the liquid portion of the blood in which the red cells, white cells, and platelets are suspended. It is a protein-salt solution that is 90 percent water. Plasma contains *albumin,* which is the principle protein in the blood. In addition, it contains *fibrino-*

●**FIGURE A12-1   Modern Blood Banking**
Modern blood banking techniques have made transfusion a safe procedure. Liquid blood can remain in storage for up to 42 days before it must be used or discarded.

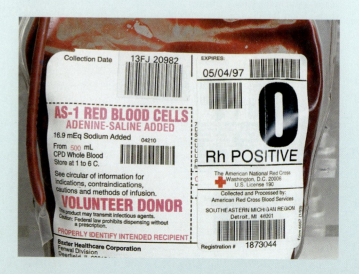

gen and other proteins that are part of the clotting system, and *globulins,* which include the antibodies that aid in fighting infection. Plasma is administered to patients with bleeding disorders

Cryoprecipitated AHF is the part of the plasma that contains certain clotting factors, including Factor VIII, fibrinogen, von Willebrand factor, and Factor XIII. Cryoprecipitated AHF is removed from plasma by freezing and then slowly thawing the plasma. Used only when specific factor concentrates are unavailable, it helps to control bleeding in individuals with hemophilia and von Willebrand's disease.

Platelets

Platelets, also called *thrombocytes,* are small blood components that aid in the clotting process by adhering to the lining of blood vessels. Platelets are manufactured in the bone marrow and remain viable in the circulation for an average of 9 to 10 days before being removed by the spleen. Units of platelets for transfusion are prepared by using a centrifuge to separate the platelets from plasma. Platelets can also be obtained through *apheresis,* a procedure in which blood is drawn from a patient, the platelets are removed, and the other blood components are returned to the patient. Platelets are used to treat thrombocytopenia or conditions involving an abnormality in platelet function.

White Blood Cells

White blood cells (WBCs), also called *leukocytes,* are responsible for protecting the body from invasion by foreign substances such as bacteria, viruses, fungi, and parasites. The majority of WBCs are produced in the bone marrow. There are several types of WBCs, which have been previously detailed in the text. WBCs must be used within 24 hours after collection. They are most frequently used for infections that are unresponsive to antibiotic therapy. However, the effectiveness of WBC transfusions is still not clear.

Plasma Derivatives

Plasma derivatives are concentrates of specific plasma proteins prepared from pools of many donors through a process known as *fractionation.* They are usually heat-treated or washed with a solvent-detergent that kills certain viruses including HIV and hepatitis B and C. Plasma derivatives include:

- Factor VIII concentrate
- Factor IX concentrate
- Anti-inhibitor coagulation complex (AICC)
- Albumin
- Immune globulins (including Rh immune globulin)
- Antithrombin III concentrate
- Alpha 1-proteinase inhibitor complex

Blood transfusions may be either allogenic or autologous. In *allogenic* blood transfusions, blood is transfused to someone other than the donor. In autologous transfusions, the blood donor and transfusion recipient are the same individual. The most common autologous donation is the preoperative donation of blood for transfusion back to the donor during elective surgery. Blood can be stored in its liquid form for up to 42 days. Preoperative autologous donation is not allowed within 72 hours of surgery due to the time necessary to recover from donation.

BLOOD TRANSFUSION REACTIONS

Human red blood cell membranes contain hundreds of different antigenic structures. Great care is taken to assure that blood products match the intended recipient before transfusion is undertaken. All blood products are tested to determine the ABO blood type and for the presence of the Rh antigen, as well as for several minor antigens. Blood that has been tested and deemed suitable for transfusion to a patient is said to be cross-matched. This means that the blood product in question has the lowest possible likelihood of causing a transfusion reaction.

Blood transfusion reactions can develop quite rapidly and are sometimes fatal. Transfusion reactions are usually classified as immune or nonimmune. Immune reactions are antibody-mediated reactions directed against a blood component. Nonimmune reactions include such complications as circulatory overload or transmission of an infectious agent.

A common type of blood transfusion reaction is the hemolytic reaction, in which red blood cell antibodies lyse (rupture) red cells within the circulatory system. This allows the contents of the cell to spill into the circulatory system. Hemoglobin can collect in the urine, adversely affecting renal function. Patients with hemolytic reactions often complain of flushing, pain at the infusion site, chest or back pain, restlessness, anxiety, nausea, or diarrhea. Fever and chills are common findings. Shock and renal failure also can occur. Treatment of a hemolytic transfusion reaction should begin with termination and removal of the product being transfused, which should be returned to the laboratory to determine the cause of the reaction. Fluids should be administered to maintain adequate renal output. On occasion, it may be necessary to administer a diuretic such as furosemide (Lasix) or an osmotic diuretic such as mannitol (Osmotrol) in order to maintain renal function and prevent fluid overload. Intravenous antihistamines and corticosteroids are sometimes required. Analgesics and anti-inflammatory agents may be required for the treatment of pain as well as fever and chills.

Nonimmune transfusion reactions are managed by treating the underlying problem. Circulatory overload is treated with fluid restriction and diuretics as needed. Infections are treated based on the type of infection present.

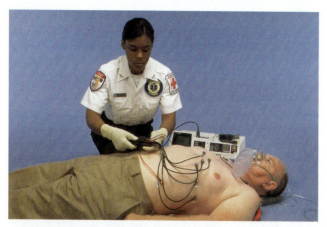

• **FIGURE A12-2   Battery-Powered ECG Monitor/Defibrillator**
The development of the battery-powered 12-lead ECG monitor/defibrillator now makes it possible to administer thrombolytic agents in the prehospital setting.

THROMBOLYTIC THERAPY: THE ERA OF REPERFUSION

Thrombolytic agents, also called *fibrinolytic agents,* are drugs that dissolve arterial and venous blood clots and restore blood flow to anoxic tissues. Thrombolytic therapy has become an essential component of emergency care in the twenty-first century (Figure A12-2•). Several life-threatening conditions result from the formation of blood clots in the vascular system. These can be localized clots (*thrombi*) or clots that move through the circulatory system (*emboli*). Conditions resulting from blood clot formation include acute coronary syndrome, acute ischemic stroke, pulmonary embolus, deep venous thrombosis, and peripheral arterial occlusion.

Acute Coronary Syndrome

Acute coronary syndrome results from the formation of a clot in one of the coronary arteries. The coronary arteries provide blood supply to the heart, and blockage of one of these vessels can cause death of myocardial tissue (acute myocardial infarction). The larger the affected vessel, the more severe is the resultant tissue damage. To be effective, thrombolytic therapy should be started within 6 hours after the onset of symptoms. Because of this, it is important to determine, if possible, when the patient's symptoms began. In rural areas and in areas subject to delays in getting patients to a hospital with invasive cardiology capabilities, paramedics in the field may have to initiate thrombolytic therapy.

Acute Ischemic Stroke

An acute ischemic stroke is the presence of a blood clot in the brain circulation interrupting blood flow to the part of the brain supplied by the affected artery. For many years, there was no effective therapy for strokes. Now, in selected patients, administration of a thrombolytic agent can dissolve the offending clot, restoring blood flow to the brain. The results can be striking. The best outcome occurs when thrombolytic therapy is started within 3 hours of the onset of symptoms.

Pulmonary Embolus

An acute pulmonary embolus is the presence of a blood clot in the pulmonary circulation. The clot develops in another part of the body, usually the large veins of the leg and pelvis, and travels through the circulatory system until it lodges in the lungs. This interrupts blood flow to the affected lung tissue, reduces pulmonary venous return, and can markedly decrease oxygenation of the blood and inhibit the removal of metabolic waste products. Thrombolytic therapy is usually limited to patients with massive emboli who have experienced symptoms for 48 hours or less and who show evidence of hemodynamic compromise.

Deep Venous Thrombosis

Deep venous thrombosis is the formation of a clot within one of the larger veins, usually in the lower extremity. These patients are at risk of the clot breaking loose and traveling to the lungs or brain, where it can be fatal. Thrombolytic therapy is limited to large clots that pose an immediate threat to the patient's life.

Peripheral Arterial Occlusion

The formation of a blood clot in a peripheral artery can adversely affect the tissues supplied by that artery. Thrombolytic agents can be administered directly into the affected artery or systemically.

Like clot formation, clot dissolution is an important body function. The process of clot dissolution is referred to as *fibrinolysis.* It begins with activation of the plasma protein *plasminogen* by *tissue plasminogen activator (tPA).* Damaged tissues release tPA. The activation of plasminogen produces the enzyme *plasmin,* which begins to digest the fibrin strands thus eroding the clot foundation. Thrombolytic agents cause the conversion of plasminogen to plasmin. *Alteplase (recombinant tPA, Activase)* is human tPA derived through recombinant DNA technology. Because it is chemically identical to natural tPA, the risks of an allergic reaction to the drug are minimized. Older thrombolytic agents were derived from beta-hemolytic streptococcal bacteria. The most common drug of this group is *streptokinase (Streptase).* It promotes thrombolysis by activating the conversion of plasminogen to plasmin. Plasmin in turn degrades fibrin, fibrinogen, and other procoagulant proteins. Because streptokinase is derived from bacteria, the risk of developing a serious allergic reaction is much higher. *Anistreplase (Eminase)* is a newer product that is derived from streptococcal bacteria. It appears to have less antigenicity than streptokinase and is much easier to administer.

Thrombolytic medications are very potent. In addition to dissolving the clot, they cause significant blood thinning that places the patient at increased risk of hemorrhage (Figure A12-3●). In fact, hemorrhage is the most common significant risk factor. Serious hemorrhage should be treated with transfusion of red blood cells to replace blood loss. Plasma and platelet administration may be indicated based upon laboratory evaluation of the patient's clotting system.

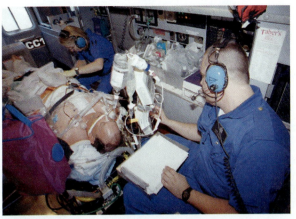

● **FIGURE A12-3   Monitoring for Hemorrhage**
It is essential that emergency personnel constantly monitor patients who have recently received a thrombolytic agent for signs and symptoms of hemorrhage.

SUMMARY

Blood is a precious body tissue with numerous biological functions. The science of blood banking allows us to take blood from one individual and administer it, or portions of it, to another patient. This is often life saving, especially in cases of trauma and complicated surgery.

The twenty-first century has been called the Era of Reperfusion because of treatment options now available that help limit or prevent tissue injury in acute coronary syndrome and in acute ischemic stroke. Treatment begins in the ambulance, before the patient is delivered to the hospital. Patients who have received successful reperfusion treatment often leave the hospital within days instead of weeks. In addition, patient screening occurs in the field to assure that patients are delivered to a hospital that has the facilities and physicians to provide whatever definitive care is needed.

A12

13

The Heart

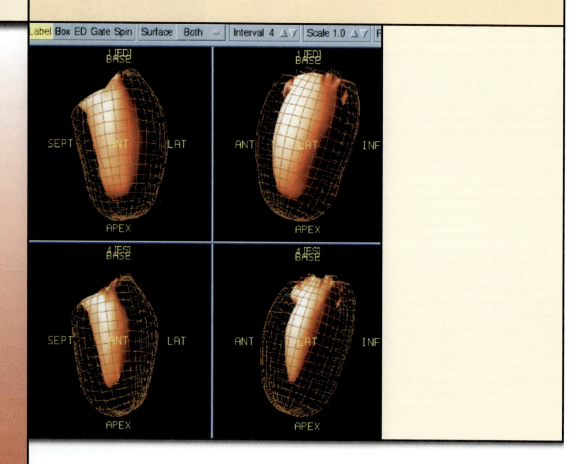

A stress Cardiolite scan is a noninvasive nuclear medicine test that can help determine the status of blood flow to the heart muscle. It also provides information about the heart's pumping ability through examination of ventricular-wall motion. The radioactive tracer sestamibi is injected during exercise. It is metabolized by the myocardium in a fashion similar to that of potassium. Following injection, a nuclear camera takes various images of the heart, which are entered into a computer for examination by the treating physician. The Cardiolite scan provides significant information about the condition of the heart without the need for surgery or cardiac catheterization.

Chapter Outline and Objectives

Vocabulary Development

anastomosis, outlet; *anastomoses*
*arter-, artery; *arteriosclerosis*
atrion, hall; *atrium*
auris, ear; *auricle*
bi-, two; *bicuspid*
bradys, slow; *bradycardia*
cuspis, point; *bicuspid valve*
diastole, expansion; *diastole*
-gram, record; *electrocardiogram*
luna, moon; *semilunar valve*
mitre, a bishop's hat; *mitral valve*
*myo-, muscle; *myocardial*
papilla, nipple-shaped elevation; *papillary muscles*
*-sclero, hard; *arteriosclerosis*
semi-, half; *semilunar valve*
septum, wall; *interatrial septum*
systole, a drawing together; *systole*
tachys, swift; *tachycardia*
tri-, three; *tricuspid valve*
ventricle, little belly; *ventricle*

Every living cell relies on the surrounding interstitial fluid for oxygen, nutrients, and waste disposal. Conditions in the interstitial fluid are kept stable through continuous exchange between the peripheral tissues and circulating blood. If the blood remains stationary, its oxygen and nutrient supplies are quickly exhausted, its capacity to absorb wastes is soon saturated, and neither hormones nor white blood cells can reach their intended targets. All cardiovascular functions ultimately depend on the heart. This muscular organ beats approximately 100,000 times each day, pumping roughly 8000 liters of blood—enough to fill forty 55-gallon drums, or 8800 quart-sized milk cartons.

We shall begin this chapter by examining the structural features that enable the heart to perform so reliably, even under widely varying physical demands. We will then consider the mechanisms that regulate the activities of the heart to meet the body's ever-changing needs.

THE HEART AND THE CIRCULATORY SYSTEM

Blood flows through a network of blood vessels that extend between the heart and peripheral tissues. Blood vessels are subdivided into a **pulmonary circuit**, which carries blood to and from exchange surfaces of the lungs, and a **systemic circuit**, which transports blood to and from the rest of the body. Each circuit begins and ends at the heart. **Arteries**, or *efferent* vessels, carry blood away from the heart; **veins**, or *afferent* vessels, return blood to the heart. **Capillaries** are small, thin-walled vessels between the smallest arteries and veins.

As Figure 13-1• shows, blood travels through these circuits in sequence. For example, blood returning to the heart in the systemic veins must complete the pulmonary circuit before reentering the systemic arteries. The heart contains four muscular chambers, two associated with each circuit. The **right atrium** (Ā-trē-um; hall; plural, *atria*) receives blood from the systemic (body) circuit, and the **right ventricle** (VEN-tri-kl; "little belly") discharges blood into the pulmonary (lungs) circuit. The **left atrium** collects blood from the pulmonary circuit, and the **left ventricle** ejects it into the systemic circuit. When the heart beats, the two ventricles contract at the same time and eject equal volumes of blood.

THE ANATOMY AND ORGANIZATION OF THE HEART

Despite its impressive workload, the heart is a small organ, roughly the size of a clenched fist. Located near the center of the thoracic cavity, it is enclosed by the connective tissues of the mediastinum, a tissue mass that divides the thoracic cavity into two pleural cavities and also contains the thymus, esophagus, and trachea.

The heart lies near the anterior chest wall, directly behind the sternum (Figure 13-2a•). It is surrounded by the **pericardial** (per-i-KAR-dē-al) **cavity**, one of the three ventral body cavities introduced in Chapter 1. ∞ *p. 21* This cavity is lined by a serous membrane called the **pericardium**. ∞ *p. 96* To visualize the relationship between

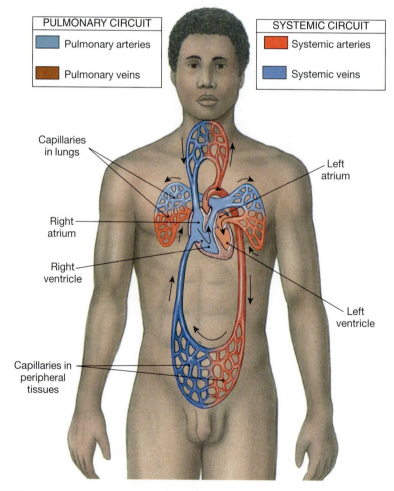

PULMONARY CIRCUIT		SYSTEMIC CIRCUIT	
■	Pulmonary arteries	■	Systemic arteries
■	Pulmonary veins	■	Systemic veins

Capillaries in lungs

Left atrium

Right atrium

Right ventricle

Left ventricle

Capillaries in peripheral tissues

•**FIGURE 13-1   An Overview of the Cardiovascular System**
Blood flows through separate pulmonary and systemic circuits, driven by the pumping of the heart. Each circuit begins and ends at the heart and contains arteries, capillaries, and veins.

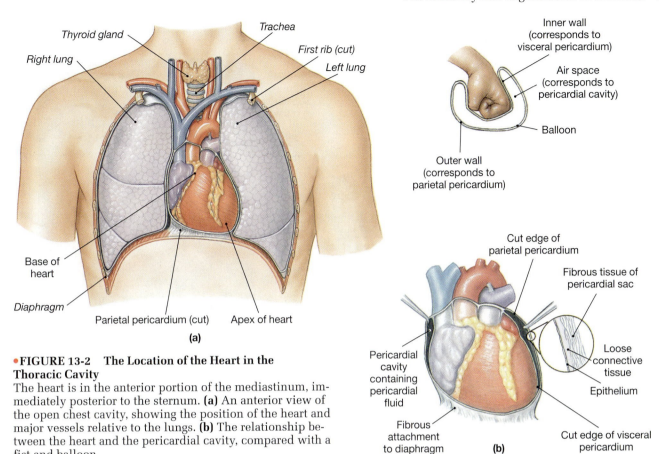

•FIGURE 13-2   The Location of the Heart in the Thoracic Cavity
The heart is in the anterior portion of the mediastinum, immediately posterior to the sternum. **(a)** An anterior view of the open chest cavity, showing the position of the heart and major vessels relative to the lungs. **(b)** The relationship between the heart and the pericardial cavity, compared with a fist and balloon.

the heart and the pericardial cavity, imagine pushing your fist toward the center of a large balloon (Figure 13-2b•). The balloon represents the pericardium, and your fist represents the heart. Your wrist, where the balloon folds back on itself, corresponds to the **base** of the heart. The space inside the balloon is the pericardial cavity.

The pericardium can be subdivided into the visceral pericardium and the parietal pericardium. The **visceral pericardium**, or **epicardium**, covers the outer surface of the heart, and the **parietal pericardium** lines the inner surface of the *pericardial sac*, which surrounds the heart (Figure 13-2b•). The pericardial sac is reinforced by a dense network of collagen fibers that stabilizes the positions of the pericardium, heart, and associated vessels in the mediastinum. The slender gap between the opposing parietal and visceral surfaces is the pericardial cavity. This space normally contains a small quantity of *pericardial fluid*, which acts as a lubricant, reducing friction as the heart beats.

The Surface Anatomy of the Heart

The heart's four chambers are easily identified in a surface view (Figure 13-3a•). Several external features distinguish the atria from the ventricles. The atria have relatively thin muscular walls and are highly distensible. When an atrium is not filled with blood, its outer

portion deflates into a lumpy, wrinkled flap called an **auricle** (AW-ri-kl; *auris*, ear). A deep groove, the **coronary sulcus**, marks the border between the atria and the ventricles. Another depression, the **interventricular sulcus**, marks the boundary between the left and right ventricles (Figure 13-3a,b•). The connective tissue of the epicardium at the coronary and interventricular sulci usually contains substantial amounts of fat, as well as the major arteries and veins that supply blood to cardiac muscle tissue.

The great veins and arteries of the circulatory system are connected to the superior end of the heart at the base. The inferior, pointed tip of the heart is the **apex** (Ā-peks) (Figure 13-2a•). A typical heart measures approximately 12.5 cm (5 in.) from the attached base to the apex.

The heart sits at an angle to the longitudinal axis of the body. It is also rotated slightly toward the left, so the anterior surface primarily consists of the right atrium and right ventricle (Figure 13-3a•). The wall of the left ventricle forms much of the posterior surface between the base and the apex of the heart (Figure 13-3b•).

Internal Anatomy and Organization

Figure 13-4• (p. 359) illustrates the four internal chambers of the heart. The two atria are separated by the **interatrial septum** (*septum*, wall), and the two ventricles

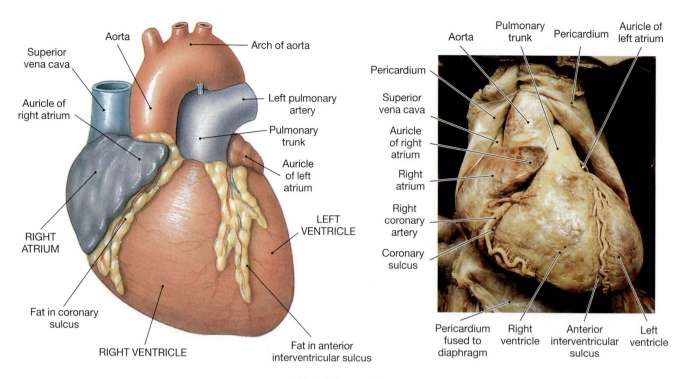

Aorta

Arch of aorta

Superior vena cava

Auricle of right atrium

Left pulmonary artery

Pulmonary trunk

Auricle of left atrium

LEFT VENTRICLE

RIGHT ATRIUM

Fat in coronary sulcus

RIGHT VENTRICLE

Fat in anterior interventricular sulcus

(a) Anterior surface

Pulmonary trunk

Aorta

Pericardium

Auricle of left atrium

Pericardium

Superior vena cava

Auricle of right atrium

Right atrium

Right coronary artery

Coronary sulcus

Pericardium fused to diaphragm

Right ventricle

Anterior interventricular sulcus

Left ventricle

•**FIGURE 13-3   The Surface Anatomy of the Heart**
(a) An anterior view of the heart, showing major anatomical features. **(b)** The posterior surface of the heart. (Coronary arteries are shown in red, cardiac veins in blue.)

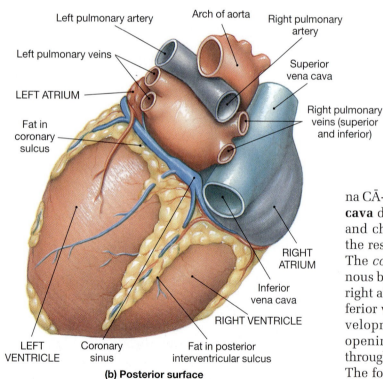

Left pulmonary artery

Arch of aorta

Right pulmonary artery

Left pulmonary veins

LEFT ATRIUM

Superior vena cava

Fat in coronary sulcus

Right pulmonary veins (superior and inferior)

RIGHT ATRIUM

Inferior vena cava

RIGHT VENTRICLE

LEFT VENTRICLE

Coronary sinus

Fat in posterior interventricular sulcus

(b) Posterior surface

are divided by the **interventricular septum**. Each atrium communicates with the ventricle on the same side through an **atrioventricular (AV) valve**, flaps of tissue arranged so as to ensure a one-way flow of blood from the atria into the ventricles.

The right atrium receives blood from the systemic circuit via two large veins, the superior vena cava (VĒ-

na CĀ-va) and the inferior vena cava. The **superior vena cava** delivers blood from the head, neck, upper limbs, and chest. The **inferior vena cava** carries blood from the rest of the trunk, the viscera, and the lower limbs. The *coronary*, or *cardiac*, *veins* of the heart return venous blood to the **coronary sinus**, which opens into the right atrium slightly below the connection with the inferior vena cava. From the fifth week of embryonic development until birth, the foramen ovale, an oval opening, permits blood flow between the two atria through the interatrial septum (see Figure 14-22, p. 403). The foramen ovale shunts blood away from the developing lungs. At birth, the foramen ovale closes, and after 48 hours it is permanently sealed. A small depression, the *fossa ovalis*, persists at this site in the adult heart (Figure 13-4•). Occasionally, the foramen ovale remains open and the circulation to the lungs does not increase at birth. The tissues of the newborn infant soon become starved for oxygen, and the cyanosis that develops makes the infant appear blue. ∞ *p. 111* Such infants are called "blue babies."

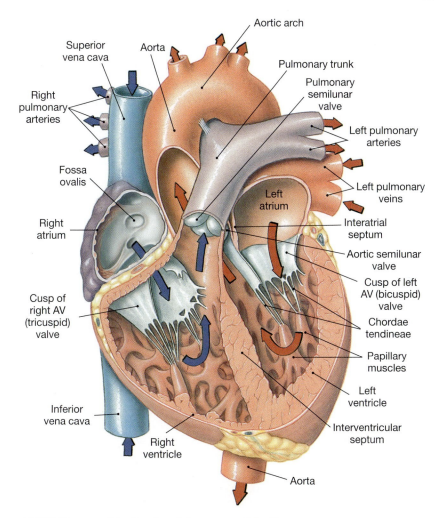

Superior
vena cava

Aortic arch

Aorta

Pulmonary trunk

Pulmonary
semilunar
valve

Right
pulmonary
arteries

Left pulmonary
arteries

Fossa
ovalis

Left pulmonary
veins

Left
atrium

Interatrial
septum

Right
atrium

Aortic semilunar
valve

Cusp of left
AV (bicuspid)
valve

Cusp of
right AV
(tricuspid)
valve

Chordae
tendineae

Papillary
muscles

Left
ventricle

Inferior
vena cava

Interventricular
septum

Right
ventricle

Aorta

•FIGURE 13-4   The Sectional Anatomy of the Heart
A diagrammatic frontal section through the heart, showing the major landmarks and the path of blood flow through the atria and ventricles.

Blood travels from the right atrium into the right ventricle through a broad opening bounded by three flaps of fibrous tissue. These flaps, or **cusps**, are part of the **right atrioventricular (AV) valve**, also known as the **tricuspid** (trī-KUS-pid; *tri-*, three + *cuspis*, point) **valve**. Each cusp is braced by the **chordae tendineae** (KŌR-dē TEN-di-nē-ē; "tendinous cords"). These tendinous cords are connected to **papillary** (PAP-i-ler-ē) **muscles** on the inner surface of the right ventricle. By tensing the chordae tendineae, these muscles limit the movement of the cusps and ensure proper valve function (Figure 13-4•).

Blood leaving the right ventricle flows into the **pulmonary trunk**, the start of the pulmonary circuit. The **pulmonary semilunar** (*semi-*, half + *luna*, moon; a crescent, or half-moon, shape) **valve** guards the entrance to this efferent trunk. Within the pulmonary trunk, blood flows into the **left** and **right pulmonary arteries**. These vessels branch repeatedly in the lungs, supplying the capillaries where gas exchange occurs. From these respiratory capillaries, oxygenated blood

collects into the **left** and **right pulmonary veins**, which deliver it to the left atrium.

Like the right atrium, the left atrium has an external auricle and a valve, the **left atrioventricular (AV) valve**, or **bicuspid** (bī-KUS-pid) **valve**. As the name bicuspid implies, the left AV valve contains a pair of cusps rather than a trio. Clinicians often use the term **mitral** (MĪ-tral; *mitre*, a bishop's hat) when referring to this valve.

The internal organization of the left ventricle resembles that of the right ventricle. A pair of papillary muscles braces the chordae tendineae that insert on the bicuspid valve. Blood leaving the left ventricle passes through the **aortic semilunar valve** and into the **aorta**, the start of the systemic circuit.

Structural Differences Between the Left and Right Ventricles

The function of an atrium is to collect blood returning to the heart and deliver that blood to the attached ventricle. The demands on the right and left atria are very similar, and the two chambers look almost identical. But the demands on the right and left ventricles are very different, and there are anatomical differences between the two.

The lungs are close to the heart, and the pulmonary arteries and veins are relatively short and wide. Thus the right ventricle normally does not need to push very hard to propel blood through the pulmonary circuit. The wall of the right ventricle is relatively thin, and in sectional view it resembles a pouch attached to the massive wall of the left ventricle. When the right ventricle contracts, it acts like a bellows pump, squeezing the blood against the left ventricle. This mechanism moves blood very efficiently with minimal effort, but it develops relatively low pressures.

A comparable pumping arrangement would not be suitable for the left ventricle, because pushing blood around the systemic circuit takes six to seven times more force than pushing blood around the pulmonary circuit. The left ventricle has an extremely thick muscular wall, and it is round in cross section. When this ventricle contracts, two things happen: (1) The distance between the base and apex decreases, and (2) the diameter of the ventricular chamber decreases. (If you imagine the effects of simultaneously squeezing and rolling up the end of a toothpaste tube, you will get the idea.) As the powerful left ventricle contracts, it also

1
3

bulges into the right ventricular cavity; reducing the volume of the left ventricle helps force blood out of the right ventricle. An individual whose right ventricular musculature has been severely damaged may survive because the contraction of the left ventricle helps push blood through the pulmonary circuit.

The Heart Valves

Details of the structure and function of the heart valves are shown in Figure 13-5●.

The Atrioventricular Valves.   The atrioventricular valves prevent the backflow of blood from the ven-

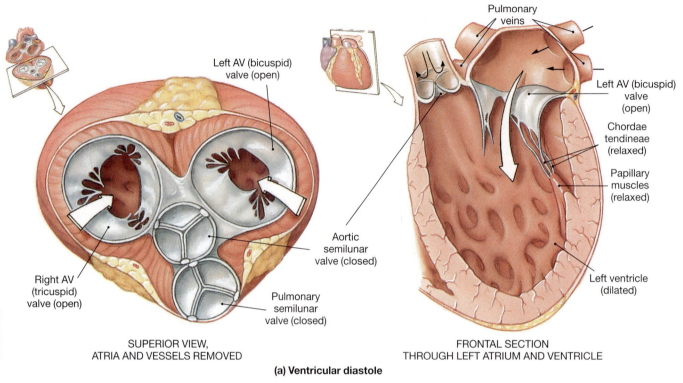

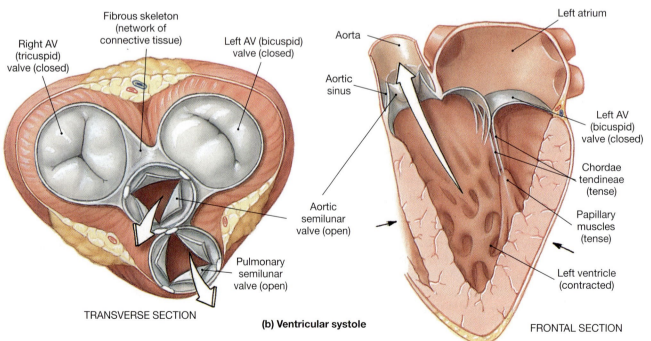

●**FIGURE 13-5   The Valves of the Heart**
(a) The valve position during ventricular relaxation (diastole), when the AV valves are open and the semilunar valves are closed. The chordae tendineae are slack, and the papillary muscles are relaxed. **(b)** The cardiac valves during ventricular contraction (systole), when the AV valves are closed and the semilunar valves are open. In the frontal section, notice that the chordae tendineae and papillary muscles prevent backflow through the left AV valve.

tricles into the atria. The chordae tendineae and papillary muscles play an important role in the normal function of the AV valves. When a ventricle is filling with blood (a phase called *diastole*), the papillary muscles are relaxed and the AV valve offers no resistance to the flow of blood from atrium to ventricle (Figure 13-5a•). When the ventricle begins to contract, blood moving back toward the atrium swings the cusps together, closing the valve (Figure 13-5b•). During ventricular contraction (a phase called *systole*), tension in the papillary muscles and chordae tendineae keeps the cusps from swinging into the atrium. This action prevents the backflow, or **regurgitation**, of blood into the atrium each time the ventricle contracts. A small amount of regurgitation often occurs, even in normal individuals. The swirling action creates a soft but distinctive sound called a *heart murmur*.

✳ CHAGAS' DISEASE

In many parts of Central and South America, heart disease is the number one cause of death. But, unlike the United States and Canada, the type of heart disease seen in those areas is called *Chagas' disease* and is due to infection by the parasite *Trypanosoma cruzi.* Thought to infect over 16 million persons, it is spread through the bite of an insect known as the "kissing bug." The initial signs and symptoms are mild. However, ten to twenty years later, the patient develops an enlarged heart and dysrhythmias and eventually dies from heart failure.

The Semilunar Valves. The pulmonary and aortic semilunar valves prevent the backflow of blood from the pulmonary trunk and aorta into the right and left ventricles. The semilunar valves do not require muscular braces, because the arterial walls do not contract; the relative positions of the cusps are stable. When these valves close, the cusps swing together. They don't swing back into the ventricles, because in the closed position, the three symmetrical cusps in each valve push against one another, preventing further movement (Figure 13-5a•).

✳ VALVULAR HEART DISEASE

Prior to the latter half of the twentieth century, valvular heart disease was the most common type of heart disease encountered. Many valvular heart problems began following rheumatic fever. Rheumatic fever can cause the body's immune system to mistakenly manufacture antibodies against the leaflets of the valves, causing vegetative growths. These growths prevent the valves from properly closing, which results in leaking that reduces pumping efficiency and eventually leads to congestive heart failure. Since the introduction of antibiotics, the incidence of rheumatic fever has dropped markedly.

The Heart Wall

The wall of the heart contains three distinct layers: the epicardium (visceral pericardium), the myocardium, and the endocardium (Figure 13-6a•). The **epicardium**, which covers the outer surface of the heart, is a serous membrane that consists of an exposed epithelium and an underlying layer of loose connective tissue. The **myocardium**, or muscular wall of the heart, contains cardiac muscle tissue and associated connective tissues, blood vessels, and nerves. The cardiac muscle tissue of the myocardium forms concentric layers that wrap around the atria and spiral into the walls of the ventricles. This arrangement results in squeezing and twisting contractions that increase the pumping efficiency of the heart (Figure 13-6b•). The inner surfaces, including the valves, are covered by the **endocardium** (en-dō-KAR-dē-um), a simple squamous epithelium continuous with the epithelial lining of the attached blood vessels.

Cardiac Muscle Cells

Typical cardiac muscle cells, or *cardiocytes*, are shown in Figure 13-6c,d•. These cells are relatively small and contain a single centrally located nucleus. Like skeletal muscle fibers, each cardiac muscle cell contains myofibrils, and contraction involves the shortening of individual sarcomeres. Since cardiac muscle cells are almost totally dependent on aerobic metabolism to obtain the energy needed to continue contracting, they have many mitochondria and abundant reserves of myoglobin (to store oxygen). Energy reserves are maintained in the form of glycogen and lipids.

Each cardiac muscle cell is in contact with several others at specialized sites known as **intercalated** (in-TER-ka-lā-ted) **discs**. ∞ *p. 99* Tight junctions, desmosomes, and gap junctions at these sites give the cells mechanical stability and a means of communication through the movement of ions and small molecules. ∞ *p. 83* As a result, action potentials travel from cell to cell without delay. In addition, myofibrils anchored to the discs of adjacent cells are locked together, increasing the efficiency of the cells as they "pull together." Because the cardiac muscle cells are mechanically, chemically, and electrically connected in this way, the entire tissue resembles a single, enormous muscle cell and has been called a *functional syncytium* (sin-SISH-ē-um; a fused mass of cells).

The Fibrous Skeleton

The connective tissues of the heart include large numbers of collagen and elastic fibers that wrap around each cardiac muscle cell and also tie together adjacent cells. These fibers are in turn interwoven with more extensive sheets of fibrous tissue that separate concentric layers of cardiac muscle cells and encircle each of the heart

13

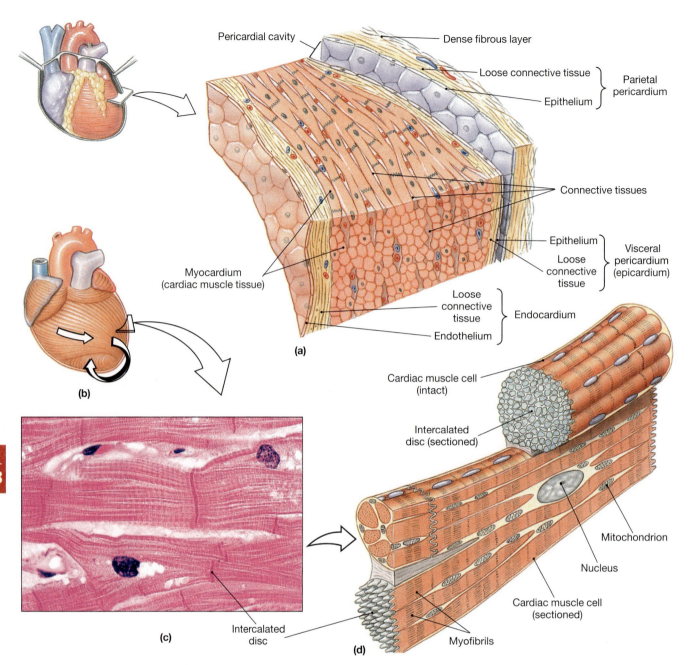

Pericardial cavity

Dense fibrous layer

Loose connective tissue

Epithelium

Parietal pericardium

Connective tissues

Epithelium

Loose connective tissue

Visceral pericardium (epicardium)

Myocardium (cardiac muscle tissue)

Loose connective tissue

Endocardium

Endothelium

(a)

(b)

Cardiac muscle cell (intact)

Intercalated disc (sectioned)

Mitochondrion

Nucleus

Cardiac muscle cell (sectioned)

Intercalated disc

Myofibrils

(c)

(d)

●FIGURE 13-6   The Heart Wall
(a) A diagrammatic section through the heart wall, showing the relative positions of the epicardium, myocardium, and endocardium. **(b)** Cardiac muscle tissue forms concentric layers that wrap around the atria and spiral within the walls of the ventricles. **(c,d)** Sectional and diagrammatic views of cardiac muscle tissue. Cardiac muscle cells are smaller than skeletal muscle fibers and have a single, central nucleus, branching interconnections between cells, and intercalated discs. (LM $\times$ 575)

valves. This internal connective tissue network is called the **fibrous skeleton** of the heart (see Figure 13-5●). The fibrous skeleton supports and stabilizes muscle cells and valves, and its elasticity limits overexpansion and helps the heart return to normal shape after contractions. It also physically isolates the atrial muscle tissue from the ventricular muscle tissue. This isolation is important to normal cardiac function because it means that the timing of ventricular contraction relative to atrial contraction can be precisely controlled.

The Blood Supply to the Heart

The heart works continuously, and cardiac muscle cells require reliable supplies of oxygen and nutrients. The **coronary circulation** supplies blood to the muscles of the heart. During maximum exertion, the oxygen demand rises considerably, and the blood flow to the heart can increase to nine times that of resting levels.

As Figure 13-7● illustrates, the coronary circulation involves an extensive network of vessels. The left and

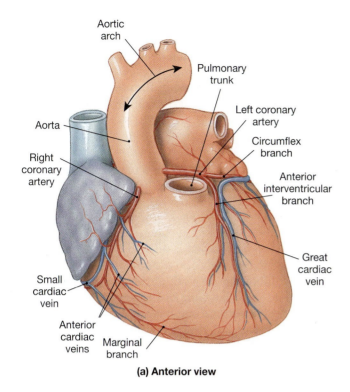

(a) Anterior view

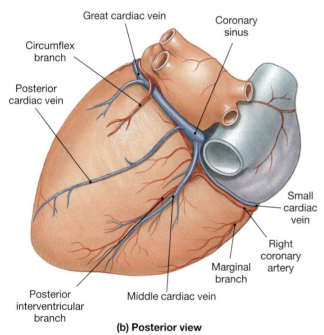

(b) Posterior view

●**FIGURE 13-7   The Coronary Circulation**
Coronary vessels supplying the **(a)** anterior and **(b)** posterior surfaces of the heart.

right **coronary arteries** originate at the base of the aorta (Figure 13-7a●). Blood pressure there is the highest anywhere in the systemic circuit, and this pressure ensures a continuous flow of blood to meet the demands of active cardiac muscle. Each coronary artery gives rise to two branches (the *marginal* and *posterior interventricular [descending]* branches from the right, and the *circumflex* and *anterior interventricular [descending]*

branches from the left). Small tributaries from these branches of the left and right coronary arteries form interconnections called **anastomoses** (a-nas-to-MŌ-sēz; *anastomosis*, outlet). Because the arteries are interconnected in this way, the blood supply to the cardiac muscle remains relatively constant, regardless of pressure fluctuations in the left and right coronary arteries. The **great** and **middle cardiac veins** carry blood away from the coronary capillaries. They drain into the **coronary sinus**, a large, thin-walled vein in the posterior portion of the coronary sulcus. The coronary sinus opens into the right atrium near the base of the inferior vena cava.

In a **myocardial** (mī-ō-KAR-dē-al) **infarction (MI)**, or *heart attack*, the coronary circulation becomes blocked and the cardiac muscle cells die from a lack of oxygen. The affected tissue then degenerates, creating a nonfunctional area known as an *infarct*. Heart attacks most often result from severe *coronary artery disease*, a condition characterized by the buildup of fatty deposits in the walls of the coronary arteries.

✓ Damage to the semilunar valves on the right side of the heart would interfere with blood flow to which vessel?

✓ What prevents the AV valves from opening back into the atria?

✓ Why are the left atrium and ventricle more muscular than the right atrium and ventricle?

1
3

THE HEARTBEAT

The heart's remarkably steady performance is a direct result of the unusual structural characteristics of its cardiac muscle tissue. Each time the heart beats, the contractions of individual cardiac muscle cells are coordinated and harnessed to ensure that blood flows in the right direction at the proper time. Two types of cardiac muscle cells are involved in a normal heartbeat. (1) *Contractile cells* produce the powerful contractions that propel blood, and (2) specialized muscle cells of the *conducting system* control and coordinate the activities of the contractile cells.

Contractile Cells

Contractile cells, which account for about 99 percent of all muscle cells in the heart, form the bulk of the heart's muscle tissue. The first step in triggering the contraction in a contractile cell, as in a skeletal muscle fiber, is the appearance of an action potential in the sarcolemma. ∞ *p. 172* In the 10 msec (millisecond) action potential of a skeletal muscle, a rapid depolarization is immediately followed by a rapid repolarization. In the sarcolemma of a cardiac muscle cell, the complete de-polarization-repolarization process lasts 250–300 msec, some 25–30 times longer than the duration of an action potential in a skeletal muscle sarcolemma. Until the membrane repolarizes, it cannot respond to further stimulation, and the refractory period of a cardiac muscle cell membrane is relatively long. Thus, a normal cardiac muscle cell is limited to a maximum rate of about 200 contractions per minute.

In skeletal muscle fibers, the refractory period ends before the muscle fiber develops peak tension and relaxes. As a result, twitches can build on one another until tension reaches a sustained peak; this state is called *tetanus*. ∞ *p. 177* In cardiac muscle cells, the refractory period continues until relaxation is under way. A summation of twitches is therefore not possible, and tetanic contractions cannot occur in a normal cardiac muscle cell, regardless of the frequency and intensity of stimulation. This feature is absolutely vital, since a heart in tetany could not pump blood.

The Conducting System

In contrast to skeletal muscle, cardiac muscle tissue contracts on its own in the absence of neural or hormonal stimulation. This property, called *automaticity*, or *autorhythmicity*, also characterizes some types of smooth muscle tissue discussed in Chapter 7.

In the normal pattern of blood flow, each contraction follows a precise sequence. The atria contract first, followed by the ventricles. Cardiac contractions are coordinated by two types of specialized cardiac muscle cells that do not contract: (1) **nodal cells**, which are responsible for establishing the rate of cardiac contraction, and (2) **conducting cells,** which distribute the contractile stimulus to the general myocardium.

Nodal Cells

Nodal cells are unusual because their cell membranes depolarize spontaneously and generate action potentials at regular intervals. Nodal cells are electrically coupled to one another, to conducting cells, and to normal cardiac muscle cells. As a result, when an action potential appears in a nodal cell, it sweeps through the conducting system, reaching all of the cardiac muscle tissue and causing a contraction. In this way, nodal cells determine the heart rate.

Not all nodal cells depolarize at the same rate, and the normal rate of contraction is established by **pacemaker cells**, the nodal cells that reach threshold first. These pacemaker cells are located in the **sinoatrial** (sī-nō-Ā-trē-al) **node (SA node)**, or *cardiac pacemaker*, a tissue mass embedded in the posterior wall of the right atrium near the entrance of the superior vena cava

(Figure 13-8a●). Pacemaker cells depolarize rapidly and spontaneously, generating 70–80 action potentials per minute. This results in a heart rate of 70–80 beats per minute (bpm). Artificial pacemakers generate 70–80 electrical impulses per minute, and each stimulation triggers the contraction of the ventricles.

Conducting Cells

The stimulus for a contraction is usually generated at the SA node, but it must be distributed so that (1) the atria contract together, before the ventricles, and (2) the ventricles contract together, in a wave that begins at the apex and spreads toward the base. When the ventricles contract in this way, blood is pushed toward the base of the heart, into the aorta and pulmonary trunk.

The conducting network of the heart is illustrated in Figure 13-8a●. The cells of the SA node are electrically connected to those of the larger **atrioventricular** (ā-trē-ō-ven-TRIK-ū-lar) **node (AV node)** by conducting cells in the atrial walls. Although the AV nodal cells also depolarize spontaneously, they generate only 40–60 action potentials per minute. Under normal circumstances, before an AV cell depolarizes to threshold spontaneously, it is stimulated by an action potential generated by the SA node. However, if the AV node does not receive this action potential, it will then become the pacemaker of the heart and establish a heart rate of 40–60 beats per minute.

The AV node is located in the floor of the right atrium near the opening of the coronary sinus. From there the action potentials travel to the **AV bundle**, also known as the *bundle of His* (hiss). This bundle of conducting cells travels along the interventricular septum before dividing into **left** and **right bundle branches**, which radiate across the inner surfaces of the left and right ventricles. At this point, specialized **Purkinje** (pur-KIN-jē) **fibers** (*Purkinje cells*) convey the impulses to the contractile cells of the ventricular myocardium.

Pacemaker cells in the SA node usually generate 60–100 action potentials per minute. It takes an action potential roughly 50 msec to travel from the SA node to the AV node over the conducting pathways (Figure 13-8b●). Along the way, the conducting cells pass the contractile stimulus to cardiac muscle cells of the right and left atria. The action potential then spreads across the atrial surfaces through cell-to-cell contact. The stimulus affects only the atria, because the fibrous skeleton electrically isolates the atria from the ventricles everywhere except at the AV bundle.

At the AV node, the impulse slows down, and another 100 msec passes before it reaches the AV bundle. This delay is important because the atria must be contracting and blood movement must be occurring before the ventricles are stimulated. Once the impulse enters the AV bundle, it flashes down the septum, along the bundle branches, and into the ventricular myocardium

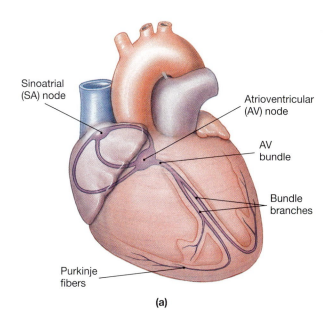

Sinoatrial (SA) node

Atrioventricular (AV) node

AV bundle

Bundle branches

Purkinje fibers

(a)

●**FIGURE 13-8   The Conducting System of the Heart**
(a) The stimulus for contraction is generated by pacemaker cells at the SA node. From there, impulses follow three different paths through the atrial walls to reach the AV node. After a brief delay, the impulses are conducted to the AV bundle (bundle of His) and then on to the left and right bundle branches, the Purkinje fibers, and the ventricular myocardial cells. **(b)** The movement of the contractile stimulus through the heart.

along the Purkinje fibers. Within another 75 msec, the stimulus to begin a contraction has reached all of the ventricular muscle cells.

A number of clinical problems result from abnormal pacemaker function. The normal heart rate averages 70–80 bpm. **Bradycardia** (brād-ē-KAR-dē-a; *bradys*, slow) refers to a slower than normal heart rate (less than 60 bpm). **Tachycardia** (tak-ē-KAR-dē-a; *tachys*, swift) indicates a faster than normal heart rate (100 bpm or more).

✓ Cardiac muscle does not undergo tetanus as skeletal muscle does. How does this characteristic affect the functioning of the heart?

✓ If the cells of the SA node were not functioning, how would the heart rate be affected?

✓ Why is it important for the impulses from the atria to be delayed at the AV node before passing into the ventricles?

The Electrocardiogram

The electrical events occurring in the heart are powerful enough that they can be detected by electrodes on the body surface. An **electrocardiogram** (ē-lek-trō-KAR-dē-ō-gram), also called an **ECG** or **EKG**, is a recording of

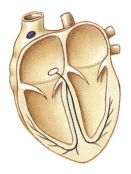
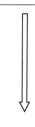

STEP 1:
SA node activity and atrial activation begin.

Time = 0

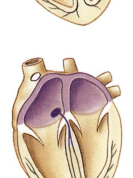

STEP 2:
Stimulus reaches the AV node.

Elapsed time = 50 msec

STEP 3:
There is a 100 msec delay at the AV node. Atrial contraction begins.

Elapsed time = 150 msec

1
3

STEP 4:
The impulse travels along the interventricular septum, within the AV bundle and the bundle branches, to the Purkinje fibers.

Elapsed time = 175 msec

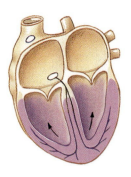

STEP 5:
The impulse is distributed by Purkinje fibers and relayed throughout the ventricular myocardium. Atrial contraction is completed, and ventricular contraction begins.

Elapsed time = 225 msec

(b)

these electrical activities. Each time the heart beats, a wave of depolarization radiates through the atria, reaches the AV node, travels down the interventricular septum to the apex, turns, and spreads through the ventricular myocardium toward the base.

The appearance of the ECG tracing varies with the placement of the monitoring electrodes. Figure 13-9• shows the important features of an electrocardiogram as analyzed with the leads in one of the standard configurations:

- The small **P wave** accompanies the depolarization of the atria. The atria begin contracting around 100 msec after the start of the P wave.

- The **QRS complex** appears as the ventricles depolarize. This electrical signal is relatively strong because the mass of the ventricular muscle is much larger than that of the atria. The ventricles begin contracting shortly after the peak of the R wave.

- The smaller **T wave** indicates ventricular repolarization. Atrial repolarization occurs while the ventricles are depolarizing, so the electrical events are masked by the QRS complex.

By comparing the information obtained from electrodes placed at different locations on the body surface, you can check the performance of specific nodal, conducting, and contractile components. For example,

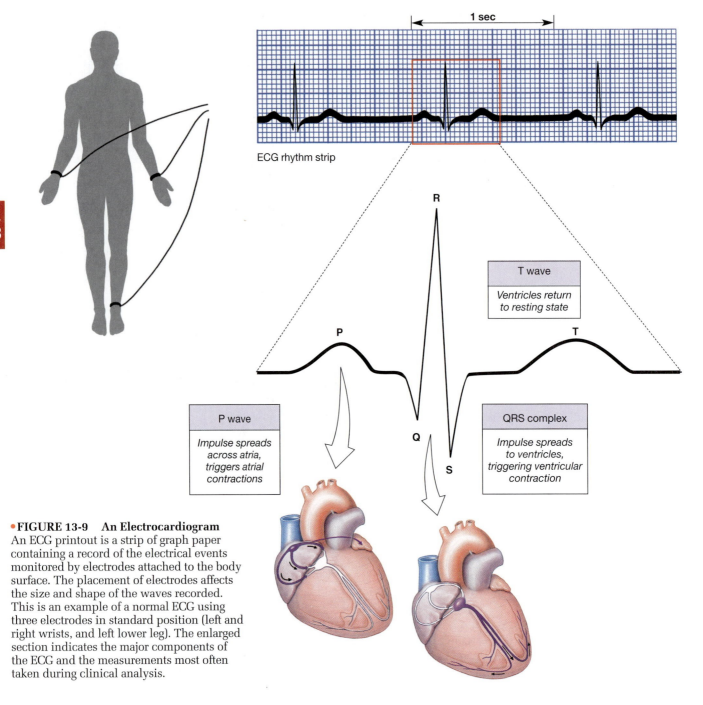

•**FIGURE 13-9   An Electrocardiogram**
An ECG printout is a strip of graph paper containing a record of the electrical events monitored by electrodes attached to the body surface. The placement of electrodes affects the size and shape of the waves recorded. This is an example of a normal ECG using three electrodes in standard position (left and right wrists, and left lower leg). The enlarged section indicates the major components of the ECG and the measurements most often taken during clinical analysis.

ECG rhythm strip

1 sec

R

T wave

Ventricles return to resting state

P

T

P wave

Impulse spreads across atria, triggers atrial contractions

Q

S

QRS complex

Impulse spreads to ventricles, triggering ventricular contraction

1
3

when a portion of the heart has been damaged, the affected muscle cells will no longer conduct action potentials, so an ECG will reveal an abnormal pattern of impulse conduction. Physicians thus rely on ECGs to detect structural or functional problems in the heart. Analyzing an ECG involves measuring the size of the voltage changes and determining the durations and temporal relationships of the various components. Attention usually focuses on the amount of depolarization occurring during the P wave and the QRS complex. For example, a smaller than normal electrical signal can mean that the mass of the heart muscle has decreased, and excessively strong depolarizations can mean that the heart muscle has become enlarged.

Electrocardiogram analysis is useful in detecting and diagnosing **cardiac arrhythmias** (ā-RITH-mē-az), abnormal patterns of cardiac activity. Momentary arrhythmias are not inherently dangerous, and about 5 percent of the normal population experiences a few abnormal heartbeats each day. Clinical problems appear when the arrhythmias reduce the heart's pumping efficiency. Serious arrhythmias can indicate damage to the myocardium, injuries to the pacemaker or conduction pathways, exposure to drugs, or variations in the electrolyte composition of the extracellular fluids.

The Cardiac Cycle

The coordinated contractions of cardiac muscle tissue underlie the approximately 100,000 beats per day of the heart. The period between the start of one heartbeat and the beginning of the next is a single **cardiac cycle** (Figure 13-10●). The cardiac cycle therefore includes both a period of contraction and one of relaxation. For any one chamber in the heart, the cardiac cycle can be divided into two phases. During contraction, or **systole** (SIS-to-lē), the chamber pushes blood into an adjacent chamber or into an arterial trunk. Systole is followed by the second phase, one of relaxation, or **diastole** (dī-AS-to-lē), when the chamber fills with blood and prepares for the start of the next cardiac cycle.

Fluids tend to move from an area of higher pressure to one of lower pressure. During the cardiac cycle, the pressure within each chamber rises during systole and falls during diastole. An increase in pressure in one chamber will cause the blood to flow to another chamber or vessel where the pressure is lower. The atrioventricular and semilunar valves ensure that blood flows in one direction only during the cardiac cycle.

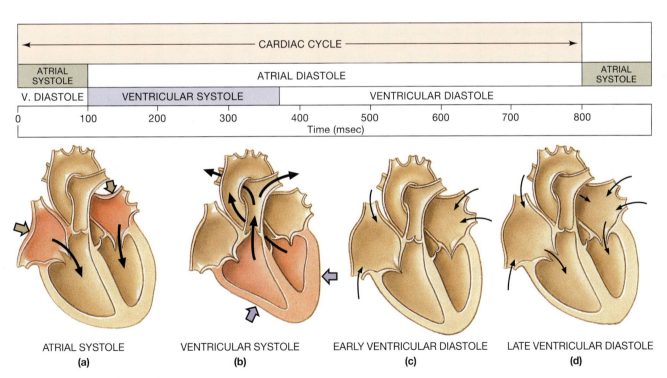

●**FIGURE 13-10 The Cardiac Cycle**
The atria and ventricles go through repeated cycles of systole and diastole. The timing of systole and diastole differs between the atria and ventricles. A cardiac cycle consists of one period of systole and diastole; here we consider a cardiac cycle as determined by the state of the atria. **(a)** Atrial systole: The atria contract, and the ventricles become filled with blood just before ventricular systole starts. **(b)** Ventricular systole: Blood is ejected into the aorta and pulmonary trunk. **(c)** Ventricular diastole: Once the AV valves open, passive filling of the ventricles occurs through the period of atrial systole in the next cardiac cycle. **(d)** The condition of the heart at the end of a cardiac cycle, with both the atria and ventricles in diastole.

The correct pressure relationships depend on the careful timing of contractions. The elaborate pacemaking and conduction systems normally provide the required spacing between atrial systole and ventricular systole. If the atria and ventricles were to contract at the same moment, blood could not leave the atria, because the AV valves would be closed. In the normal heart, atrial systole and atrial diastole are slightly out of phase with ventricular systole and diastole. Figure 13-10• shows the duration and timing of systole and diastole for a heart rate of 75 bpm.

The cardiac cycle begins with atrial systole. At the start of atrial systole, the ventricles are filled to around 70 percent of capacity; atrial systole essentially tops them off by providing the additional 30 percent. As atrial systole ends, ventricular systole begins. As pressures in the ventricles rise above those in the atria, the AV valves swing shut. But blood cannot begin moving into the arterial trunks until ventricular pressures exceed the arterial pressures. At this point, the blood pushes open the semilunar valves and flows into the aorta and pulmonary trunk. This blood flow continues for the duration of ventricular systole.

When ventricular diastole begins, ventricular pressures decline rapidly. As they fall below the pressures of the arterial trunks, the semilunar valves close. Ventricular pressures continue to drop; as they fall below atrial pressures, the AV valves open and blood flows from the atria into the ventricles. Both atria and ventricles are now in diastole; blood now flows from the major veins through the relaxed atria and into the ventricles. By the time atrial systole marks the start of another cardiac cycle, the ventricles are roughly 70 percent filled. The relatively minor contribution atrial systole makes to ventricular volume explains why individuals can survive quite normally when their atria have been so severely damaged that they can no longer function. In contrast, damage to one or both ventricles can leave the heart unable to maintain adequate cardiac output. A condition of *heart failure* then exists.

Heart Sounds

When you listen to a heart with a stethoscope, you hear the familiar "lubb-dupp" that accompanies each heartbeat. These sounds accompany the action of the heart valves. The first heart sound ("lubb") is produced as the AV valves close and the semilunars open. It marks the start of ventricular systole and lasts a little longer than the second sound. The second heart sound, "dupp," occurs at the beginning of ventricular diastole, when the semilunar valves close.

Third and *fourth heart sounds* may be audible as well, but they are usually very faint and are seldom detectable in healthy adults. These sounds are associated with atrial contraction and blood flowing into the ventricles rather than with valve action.

✓ Is the heart always pumping blood when pressure in the left ventricle is rising? Explain.

✓ What causes the "lubb-dupp" sounds of the heart that are heard with a stethoscope?

HEART DYNAMICS

Heart dynamics refers to the movements and forces generated during cardiac contractions. Each time the heart beats, the two ventricles eject equal amounts of blood. The amount ejected by a ventricle during a single beat is the **stroke volume (SV)**. The stroke volume can vary from beat to beat. Hence, physicians are often more interested in the **cardiac output (CO)**, or the amount of blood pumped by each ventricle in 1 minute.

Cardiac output can be calculated by multiplying the average stroke volume by the heart rate (HR):

$$\begin{array}{ccccc} \text{CO} & = & \text{SV} & \times & \text{HR} \\ \text{cardiac} & & \text{stroke} & & \text{heart} \\ \text{output} & & \text{volume} & & \text{rate} \\ \text{(ml/min)} & & \text{(ml)} & & \text{(bpm)} \end{array}$$

For example, if the average stroke volume is 80 ml and the heart rate is 70 beats per minute (bpm), the cardiac output will be:

$$\begin{aligned} \text{CO} &= 80 \text{ ml} \times 70/\text{min} \\ &= 5600 \text{ ml/min (5.6 liters per minute)} \end{aligned}$$

This value represents a cardiac output equivalent to the total volume of blood of an average adult every minute. Cardiac output is highly variable, however. A normal heart can increase both its rate of contraction and its stroke volume. When both the heart rate and stroke volume increase together, the cardiac output can increase by 600 to 700 percent, or up to 30 liters per minute.

Factors Controlling Cardiac Output

Cardiac output is precisely regulated so that peripheral tissues receive an adequate circulatory supply under a variety of conditions. The major factors that regulate cardiac output often affect both heart rate and stroke volume simultaneously. These primary factors include *blood volume reflexes*, *autonomic innervation*, and *hormones*. Secondary factors include the concentration of ions in the extracellular fluid and body temperature.

Blood Volume Reflexes

Cardiac muscle contraction is an active process, but relaxation is entirely passive. The force necessary to return cardiac muscle to its precontracted length is provided by the blood pouring into the heart, aided by the elasticity of the fibrous skeleton. As a result, there is a direct relationship between the amount of blood entering the heart and the amount of blood ejected during the next contraction.

Two heart reflexes respond to changes in blood volume. One of these occurs in the right atrium and affects heart rate. The other is a ventricular reflex that affects stroke volume.

The **atrial reflex** (*Bainbridge reflex*) involves adjustments in heart rate that are triggered by an increase in the **venous return**, the flow of venous blood to the heart. When the walls of the right atrium are stretched, the cells of the SA node depolarize faster, so the heart rate increases. This effect is due to (1) the response of the nodal cells to stretching and (2) an increase in sympathetic activity in response to the stimulation of stretch receptors in the atrial walls.

The amount of blood pumped out of a ventricle each beat depends on the venous return and the filling time. **Filling time** is the duration of ventricular diastole, the period during which blood can flow into the ventricles. Filling time depends primarily on the heart rate: The faster the heart rate, the shorter the available filling time. Venous return changes in response to alterations in cardiac output, peripheral circulation, and other factors that affect the rate of blood flow through the venae cavae.

Over the range of normal activities, the greater the volume of blood entering the ventricles, the more powerful the contraction. The greater the degree of stretching in the walls of the heart, the more force developed when a contraction occurs. In a resting individual, the venous return is relatively low, the walls are not stretched significantly, and the ventricles develop little power. If the venous return suddenly increases, more blood flows into the heart, the myocardium stretches farther, and the ventricles produce greater force on contraction. This general rule of "more in = more out" is often called the **Frank-Starling law of the heart**, in honor of the physiologists who first demonstrated the relationship.

Autonomic Innervation

The basic heart rate is established by the pacemaker cells of the SA node, but this rate can be modified by the autonomic nervous system (ANS). As shown in Figure 13-11•, both the sympathetic and parasympathetic divisions of the ANS innervate the heart. Postganglionic sympathetic fibers extend from neurons located in the cervical and upper thoracic ganglia. The vagus nerve (cranial nerve N X) carries parasympathetic preganglionic fibers to small ganglia near the heart. Both ANS divisions innervate the SA and AV nodes as well as the atrial and ventricular cardiac muscle cells.

Autonomic Effects on Heart Rate.   Autonomic effects on heart rate primarily reflect the responses of the SA node to acetylcholine (ACh) and to norepinephrine (NE). Acetylcholine released by parasympathetic motor neurons results in a lowering of the heart rate. Norepinephrine released by sympathetic neurons increases the heart rate. A more sustained rise in heart rate follows the release of epinephrine (E) and norepinephrine by the adrenal medullae during sympathetic activation.

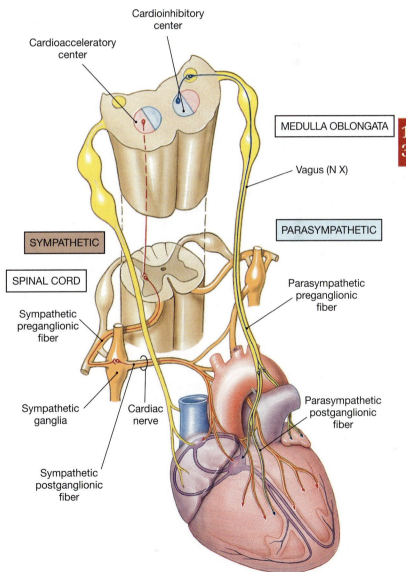

• **FIGURE 13-11**   **Autonomic Innervation of the Heart**

Autonomic Effects on Stroke Volume.   Through the release of NE, E, and ACh, the ANS also affects stroke volume by altering the force of myocardial contractions:

- **The Effects of NE and E**. The sympathetic release of NE at synapses in the myocardium and the release of NE and E by the adrenal medullae stimulate cardiac muscle cell metabolism and increase the force and degree of contraction. The result is an increase in stroke volume.

- **The Effects of ACh**. The primary effect of parasympathetic ACh release is inhibition, resulting in a decrease in the force of cardiac contractions. Because parasympathetic innervation of the ventricles is relatively limited, the atria show the greatest reduction in contractile force.

Both autonomic divisions are normally active at a steady background level, releasing ACh and NE both at the nodes and into the myocardium. Thus, cutting the vagus nerves increases the heart rate, and sympathetic blocking agents slow the heart rate. Through dual innervation and adjustments in autonomic tone, the ANS can make very delicate adjustments in cardiovascular function.

The Coordination of Autonomic Activity.   The cardiac centers of the medulla oblongata contain the autonomic headquarters for cardiac control. ∞ *p. 243* The stimulation of the **cardioacceleratory center** activates the necessary sympathetic motor neurons; the nearby **cardioinhibitory center** governs the activities of the parasympathetic motor neurons (Figure 13-11•). Information concerning the status of the cardiovascular system arrives at the cardiac centers over sensory fibers from the vagus nerve and from the sympathetic nerves of the cardiac plexus.

The cardiac centers respond to changes in blood pressure and in the arterial concentrations of dissolved oxygen and carbon dioxide. These properties are monitored by baroreceptors and chemoreceptors innervated by the glossopharyngeal (N IX) and vagus nerves. A decline in blood pressure or oxygen concentrations or an increase in carbon dioxide levels usually indicates that the oxygen demands of peripheral tissues have increased. The cardiac centers then call for an increase in the cardiac output, and the heart works harder.

In addition to making automatic adjustments in response to sensory information, the cardiac centers can be influenced by higher centers, especially centers in the hypothalamus. As a result, changes in emotional state (such as rage, fear, or arousal) have an immediate effect on heart rate.

EMERGENCY CARDIAC CARE

Emergency cardiac care (ECC) is a comprehensive system designed to deal with sudden, often life-threatening events that affect the cardiovascular, cerebrovascular, and respiratory systems. ECC specifically includes:

1. Recognition of the early warning signs of a heart attack and stroke, efforts to prevent complications, reassurance of the victim, activation of the EMS system, and prompt availability of monitoring equipment.
2. Provision of immediate basic life support (BLS) and cardiopulmonary resuscitation (CPR) at the scene when needed.
3. Provision of advanced cardiac life support (ACLS) at the scene as quickly as possible to defibrillate if necessary and to stabilize the victim prior to transport.
4. Transfer of the stabilized victim to a hospital where definitive cardiac care can be provided.

The key link in the ECC system is the layperson who recognizes the medical emergency, summons EMS, and provides initial CPR and other BLS measures.

Advanced prehospital care and paramedic practice were first developed to treat life-threatening cardiac emergencies. Now, in addition to ECC, paramedics treat all types of medical and traumatic emergencies providing effective on scene stabilization.

✓ What effect would stimulating the acetylcholine receptors of the heart have on cardiac output?

✓ What effect would an increased venous return have on the stroke volume?

✓ How would increased sympathetic stimulation of the heart affect stroke volume?

Chapter Review

KEY TERMS

atrioventricular valve, *p. 358*	electrocardiogram (ECG, EKG), *p. 365*	pericardium, *p. 356*
atrium, *p. 356*	endocardium, *p. 361*	Purkinje fibers, *p. 364*
cardiac cycle, *p. 367*	epicardium, *p. 361*	sinoatrial node, *p. 364*
cardiac output, *p. 368*	intercalated disc, *p. 361*	systole, *p. 367*
diastole, *p. 367*	myocardium, *p. 361*	ventricle, *p. 356*

SUMMARY OUTLINE

THE HEART AND THE CIRCULATORY SYSTEM p. 356

1. The circulatory system can be subdivided into the **pulmonary circuit** (which carries blood to and from the lungs) and the **systemic circuit** (which transports blood to and from the rest of the body). **Arteries** carry blood away from the heart; **veins** return blood to the heart. **Capillaries** are tiny vessels between the smallest arteries and smallest veins. *(Figure 13-1)*

2. The heart has four chambers: the **right atrium**, **right ventricle**, **left atrium**, and **left ventricle**.

THE ANATOMY AND ORGANIZATION OF THE HEART p. 356

1. The heart is surrounded by the **pericardial cavity** (lined by the **pericardium**). The **visceral pericardium (epicardium)** covers the heart's outer surface, and the **parietal pericardium** lines the inner surface of the *pericardial sac*, which surrounds the heart. *(Figure 13-2)*

The Surface Anatomy of the Heart p. 357

2. The **coronary sulcus**, a deep groove, marks the boundary between the atria and ventricles. *(Figure 13-3)*

Internal Anatomy and Organization p. 357

3. The atria are separated by the **interatrial septum**, and the ventricles are divided by the **interventricular septum**. The right atrium receives blood from the systemic circuit via two large veins, the **superior vena cava** and **inferior vena cava**. *(Figure 13-4)*

4. Blood flows from the right atrium into the right ventricle via the **right atrioventricular (AV) valve (tricuspid valve)**. This opening is bounded by three **cusps** of fibrous tissue braced by the tendinous **chordae tendineae**, which are connected to **papillary muscles**.

5. Blood leaving the right ventricle enters the **pulmonary trunk** after passing through the **pulmonary semilunar valve**. The pulmonary trunk divides to form the **left** and **right pulmonary arteries**. The **left** and **right pulmonary veins** return blood to the left atrium. Blood leaving the left atrium flows into the left ventricle via the **left atrioventricular (AV) valve (bicuspid valve** or **mitral valve)**. Blood leaving the left ventricle passes through the **aortic semilunar valve** and into the systemic circuit via the **aorta**. *(Figure 13-5)*

6. Anatomical differences between the ventricles reflect the functional demands on them. The wall of the right ventricle is relatively thin, while the left ventricle has a massive muscular wall.

7. Valves normally permit blood flow in only one direction, preventing the **regurgitation** (backflow) of blood.

The Heart Wall p. 361

8. The bulk of the heart consists of the muscular **myocardium**. The **endocardium** lines the inner surfaces of the heart. The **fibrous skeleton** supports the heart's contractile cells and valves. *(Figures 13-5, 13-6a)*

9. **Cardiac muscle cells** are interconnected by **intercalated discs**, which convey the force of contraction from cell to cell and conduct action potentials. *(Figure 13-6b–d)*

The Blood Supply to the Heart p. 362

10. The **coronary circulation** meets the high oxygen and nutrient demands of cardiac muscle cells. The coronary arteries originate at the base of the aorta. Arterial **anastomoses**, interconnections between arteries, ensure a constant blood supply. The **great** and **middle cardiac veins** carry blood from the coronary capillaries to the **coronary sinus**. *(Figure 13-7)*

THE HEARTBEAT p. 363

1. Two general classes of cardiac cells are involved in the normal heartbeat: *contractile cells* and cells of the conducting system.

Contractile Cells p. 363

2. Cardiac muscle cells have a long refractory period, so rapid stimulation produces isolated contractions rather than tetanic contractions.

The Conducting System p. 364

3. The conducting system includes **nodal cells** and **conducting cells**. The conducting system initiates and distributes electrical impulses in the heart. Nodal cells establish the rate of cardiac contraction; **pacemaker cells** are nodal cells that reach threshold first. Conducting cells distribute the contractile stimulus to the general myocardium.

4. Unlike skeletal muscle, cardiac muscle contracts without neural or hormonal stimulation. Pacemaker cells in the **sinoatrial (SA) node** *(cardiac pacemaker)* normally establish the rate of contraction. From the SA node, the stimulus travels to the **atrioventricular (AV) node** and then to the AV bundle, which divides into **bundle branches**. From there **Purkinje fibers** convey the impulses to the ventricular myocardium. *(Figure 13-8)*

The Electrocardiogram p. 365

5. A recording of electrical activities in the heart is an **electrocardiogram (ECG** or **EKG)**. Important landmarks of an ECG include the **P wave** (atrial depolarization), **QRS complex** (ventricular depolarization), and **T wave** (ventricular repolarization). *(Figure 13-9)*

The Cardiac Cycle p. 367

6. The **cardiac cycle** consists of **systole** (contraction) followed by **diastole** (relaxation). Both ventricles contract at the same time, and they eject equal volumes of blood. *(Figure 13-10)*

7. The closing of the heart valves and the rushing of blood through the heart cause characteristic heart sounds.

HEART DYNAMICS p. 368

1. *Heart dynamics* refers to the movements and forces generated during contractions. The amount of blood ejected by a ventricle during a single beat is the **stroke volume (SV)**; the amount of blood pumped each minute is the **cardiac output (CO)**.

Factors Controlling Cardiac Output p. 368

2. The major factors that affect cardiac output are blood volume reflexes, autonomic innervation, and hormones.

3. Blood volume reflexes are stimulated by changes in **venous return**, the amount of blood entering the heart. The

atrial reflex accelerates the heart rate when the walls of the right atrium are stretched. Ventricular contractions become more powerful and increase stroke volume when the ventricular walls are stretched (the **Frank-Starling law of the heart**).

4. The basic heart rate is established by the pacemaker cells, but it can be modified by the ANS. *(Figure 13-11)*

5. Acetylcholine (ACh) released by parasympathetic motor neurons lowers the heart rate and stroke volume. Norepinephrine (NE) released by sympathetic neurons increases the heart rate and stroke volume.

6. Epinephrine (E) and norepinephrine, hormones released by the adrenal medullae during sympathetic activation, increase both heart rate and stroke volume.

7. The **cardioacceleratory center** in the medulla oblongata activates sympathetic neurons; the **cardioinhibitory center** governs the activities of the parasympathetic neurons. The cardiac centers receive inputs from higher centers and from receptors monitoring blood pressure and the levels of dissolved gases.

REVIEW QUESTIONS

LEVEL 1   Reviewing Facts and Terms

Match each item in column A with the most closely related item in column B. Use letters for answers in the spaces provided.

Column A

___ 1. epicardium
___ 2. right AV valve
___ 3. left AV valve
___ 4. anastomoses
___ 5. myocardial infarction
___ 6. SA node
___ 7. systole
___ 8. diastole
___ 9. cardiac output
___ 10. HR slower than usual
___ 11. HR faster than normal
___ 12. atrial reflex

Column B

a. heart attack
b. cardiac pacemaker
c. tachycardia
d. SV × HR
e. tricuspid valve
f. bradycardia
g. mitral valve
h. interconnections between arteries
i. visceral pericardium
j. increased venous return
k. contractions of heart chambers
l. relaxation of heart chambers

13. The blood supply to the muscles of the heart is provided by the:
    (a) systemic circulation
    (b) pulmonary circulation
    (c) coronary circulation
    (d) coronary portal system

14. The autonomic centers for cardiac function are located in the:
    (a) myocardial tissue of the heart
    (b) cardiac centers of the medulla oblongata
    (c) cerebral cortex
    (d) a, b, and c are correct

15. The simple squamous epithelium covering the valves of the heart constitutes the:
    (a) epicardium
    (b) endocardium
    (c) myocardium
    (d) fibrous skeleton

16. The structure that permits blood flow from the right atrium to the left atrium while the lungs are developing is the:
    (a) foramen ovale
    (b) interatrial septum
    (c) coronary sinus
    (d) fossa ovalis

17. Blood leaves the left ventricle by passing through the:
    (a) aortic semilunar valve
    (b) pulmonary semilunar valve
    (c) mitral valve
    (d) tricuspid valve

18. The QRS complex of the ECG appears as the:
    (a) atria depolarize
    (b) ventricles depolarize
    (c) ventricles repolarize
    (d) atria repolarize

19. During diastole in the cardiac cycle, the chambers of the heart:
    (a) relax and fill with blood
    (b) contract and push blood into an adjacent chamber
    (c) experience a sharp increase in pressure
    (d) reach a pressure of approximately 120 mm Hg

20. What role do the chordae tendineae and papillary muscles have in the normal function of the AV valves?

21. What are the principal valves found in the heart, and what is the function of each?

22. Trace the normal pathway of an electrical impulse through the conducting system of the heart.

23. (a) What is the cardiac cycle? (b) What phases and events are necessary to complete the cardiac cycle?

LEVEL 2   Reviewing Concepts

24. Tetanic muscle contractions cannot occur in a normal cardiac muscle cell because:
    (a) cardiac muscle tissue contracts on its own
    (b) there is no neural or hormonal stimulation
    (c) the refractory period lasts until the muscle cell relaxes
    (d) the refractory period ends before the muscle cell reaches peak tension

25. The amount of blood forced out of the heart depends on:
    (a) the degree of stretching at the end of ventricular diastole
    (b) the contractility of the ventricle
    (c) the amount of pressure required to eject blood
    (d) a, b, and c are correct

26. The cardiac output cannot increase indefinitely because:
    (a) available filling time becomes shorter as the heart rate increases
    (b) cardiovascular centers adjust the heart rate
    (c) the rate of spontaneous depolarization decreases
    (d) the ion concentrations of pacemaker cell membranes decrease

27. Describe the association of the four muscular chambers of the heart with the pulmonary and systemic circuits.

28. What are the source and significance of the heart sounds?

29. (a) What effect does sympathetic stimulation have on the heart? (b) What effect does parasympathetic stimulation have on the heart?

LEVEL 3   Critical Thinking and Clinical Applications

30. A patient's ECG tracing shows a consistent pattern of two P waves followed by a normal QRS complex and T wave. What is the cause of this abnormal wave pattern?

31. Karen is taking the medication verapamil, a drug that blocks the calcium channels in cardiac muscle cells. What effect would you expect this medication to have on Karen's stroke volume?

ANSWERS TO CONCEPT CHECK QUESTIONS

Page 363

1. The semilunar valves on the right side of the heart guard the opening to the pulmonary artery. Damage to these valves would interfere with the blood flow through this vessel.   **2.** When the ventricles begin to contract, they force the AV valves to close, which in turn pulls on the chordae tendineae, which then pull on the papillary muscles. The papillary muscles respond by contracting, counteracting the force that is pushing the valves upward.   **3.** The wall of the left ventricle is more muscular than that of the right ventricle because the left ventricle must generate enough force to propel blood throughout all of the body's systems except the lungs. The right ventricle must generate only enough force to propel the blood a few centimeters to the lungs. Since the left ventricle is so muscular, more force is required to push blood into the chamber against the normal tension of the muscle; in turn, the left atrium must be more muscular than the right atrium.

Page 365

1. Unlike the situation in skeletal muscle fibers, tetanus is not possible. The longer refractory period in cardiac muscle cells results in a relatively long relaxation period, during which the heart's chambers can refill with blood. A heart in tetany could not fill with blood.   **2.** If these cells were not functioning, the heart would still continue to beat but at a slower rate.   **3.** If the impulses from the atria were not delayed at the AV node, they would be conducted through the ventricles so quickly by the bundle branches and Purkinje fibers that the ventricles would begin contracting immediately before the atria had finished contracting. As a result, the ventricles would not be as full

of blood as they could be and the pumping of the heart would not be as efficient, especially during activity.

Page 368

1. When pressure in the left ventricle is rising, the heart is contracting but no blood is leaving the heart. During this initial phase of contraction, both the AV valves and the semilunar valves are closed. The increase in pressure is the result of increased tension as the muscle contracts. When the pressure in the ventricle exceeds the pressure in the aorta, the aortic semilunar valves are forced open and the blood is rapidly ejected from the ventricle.   **2.** The first sound is produced by the simultaneous closing of the AV valves and the opening of the semilunar valves. The second sound is produced when the semilunar valves close.

Page 370

1. Stimulating the acetylcholine receptors of the heart would cause the heart to slow down. Since the cardiac output is the product of stroke volume times the heart rate, if the heart rate decreases, so will the cardiac output (assuming no change in the stroke volume).   **2.** The venous return fills the heart with blood, stretching the heart muscle. According to the Frank-Starling law, the more the heart muscle is stretched, the more forcefully it will contract (to a point). The more forceful the contraction, the more blood the heart will eject with each beat (stroke volume). Therefore, increased venous return will increase the stroke volume if all other factors are constant.   **3.** Increased sympathetic stimulation of the heart would result in an increased heart rate and an increased force of contraction.

Emergency Care Applications

OVERVIEW

Cardiovascular disease is the number-one cause of death in the United States and Canada. Advanced prehospital care was initially developed to treat cardiovascular emergencies. Although EMS has evolved to treat virtually any type of emergency, there is still an emphasis on cardiac care. Survival of cardiac arrest is enhanced if basic life support is provided within 4 minutes and advanced life support in 8 minutes. Many treatment modalities available in the twenty-first century provide the heart disease patient with the best possible chance of survival. These include automated external defibrillators (AEDs), thrombolytic therapy, and prehospital 12-lead ECG monitoring. Patients with heart disease are now promptly identified and routed to a medical facility with the capabilities of treating the suspected problem. Physicians who specialize in the treatment of heart disease are *cardiologists.* They must first complete a residency in internal medicine and then a fellowship in cardiology. Some cardiologists will classify themselves as *invasive cardiologists* or *noninvasive cardiologists* based on the nature of their practice. Invasive cardiologists perform cardiac catheterization and various interventions. Some cardiologists specialize in electrophysiology, which emphasizes evaluating and treating problems with the heart's conductive system including placement of pacemakers and implantable cardioverters/defibrillators.

CORONARY ARTERY DISEASE

The initial biological process in the progression of coronary artery disease is the development of microscopic *atherosclerosis.* Atherosclerosis is a form of *arteriosclerosis* where soft deposits of intra-arterial fat and fibrin cause thickening and hardening of the arterial wall. The initial occurence in this process is an endothelial injury, followed by a series of pathological events leading to the development of a fatty streak on the lining of the vessel. These lesions can be found in the walls of most people's arteries, even young children's. They are reversible with treatment that lowers *low-density lipoprotein (LDL)* levels. Once formed, however, fatty streaks produce toxic oxygen radicals and cause inflammatory changes that result in progressive damage to the arterial wall.

The next stage of *atherogenesis* is the incorporation of fibrous tissue and damaged smooth muscle cells into the area forming a *fibrous plaque* or *fibroadenoma.* This causes further endothelial dysfunction, necrosis of underlying vessel tissue, and narrowing of the vessel lumen. As the plaque continues to develop, it can ulcerate or rupture because of the mechanical shear forces and continued necrosis of the vessel wall. Platelets aggregate and adhere to the vessel surface, at the same time activating the coagulation cascade. In severe cases, a thrombus (blood clot) can form completely obstructing the vessel lumen and resulting in tissue ischemia and infarction.

The rate of progression of atherosclerosis can be significantly influenced by specific conditions and behaviors referred to as *risk factors* including age, gender, tobacco use, diabetes, obesity, hypertension, and many others. Atherosclerosis is a disease spectrum with various events occurring along the continuum. Cardiac arrest and myocardial infarction (heart attack) are, in the vast majority of cases, end points in a decades-long evolution of atherosclerotic arterial disease (Figure A13-1●). The rate of progression of atherosclerosis is the primary determinant of the age at which myocardial infarction or sudden death occurs. Control or elimination of risk factors can usually be achieved by establishing positive health attitudes and behaviors, especially in the young. Significant modifications in risk factors can occur by exercise, cessation of smoking, dietary modifications, control of hypertension, and use of medications to reduce lipid levels, blood pressure, and platelet aggregation. Atherosclerotic heart disease is a disease that must be identified and controlled in order to assure long-term health.

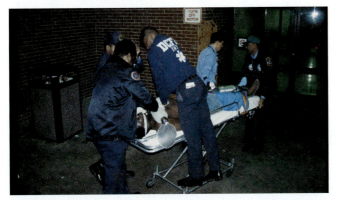

• **FIGURE A13-1   Cardiac Arrest**
Acute myocardial infarction and cardiac arrest are often the end points in the evolution of atherosclerotic arterial disease over a number of decades.

ACUTE CORONARY SYNDROME

Our knowledge and treatment of acute myocardial infarction (AMI) has evolved dramatically over the past decade. We now recognize that AMI and unstable angina are part of a spectrum of clinical disease referred to as *acute coronary syndrome.* Most patients with acute coronary syndrome have some level of underlying atherosclerotic coronary artery disease. Often, an atheromatous plaque will rupture and block the artery, or a thrombus (blood clot) will form blocking blood flow through the affected vessel. The degree and duration of the occlusion determine the type of infarction. The severity of the infarction can be reduced if collateral blood vessels supply some blood to the tissues distal to the obstruction.

Initially following coronary artery occlusion, the myocardial tissue supplied by the affected artery will become ischemic (Figures A13-2, A13-3, and A13-4•). If blood flow is restored in time, myocardial ischemia will resolve without permanent muscle injury; however, if myocardial ischemia continues, then actual tissue injury will begin. Tissue injury may or may not be reversed with the restoration of blood flow. Finally, if blood flow is interrupted long enough, then irreversible tissue damage (myocardial infarction) will occur (Figure A13-5•).

The signs and symptoms of acute coronary syndrome are due to coronary artery occlusion and related muscle injury and death. They include chest pain, difficulty breathing, sweating (diaphoresis), nausea, vomiting, and dizziness.

Half of all patients who die of AMI do so early, usually before reaching a hospital. Most of these patients develop *dysrhythmias,* irregularities in their heart's electrical activity, some of which can be immediately fatal. Common dysrhythmias associated with myocardial ischemia and sudden death are *ventricular fibrillation* or *ventricular tachycardia.* In ventricular fibrillation, no organized electrical activity occurs, and the myocardial muscle mass simply quivers, or fibrillates (Figure A13-6•). Thus, no

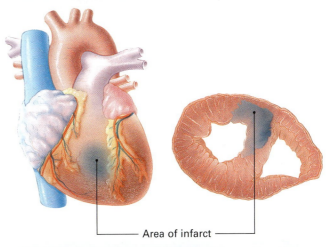

— Area of infarct —

• **FIGURE A13-2   Myocardial Infarction**
Blockage of a coronary artery results in injury and death to the myocardial tissue supplied by that artery.

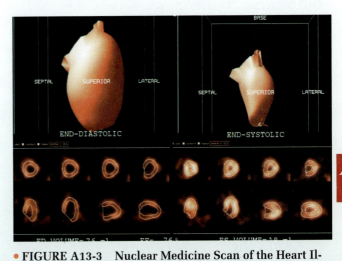

• **FIGURE A13-3   Nuclear Medicine Scan of the Heart Illustrating Good Ventricular Function**
Nuclear medicine technology allows detailed examination of cardiac perfusion and function.

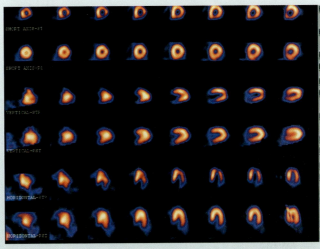

• **FIGURE A13-4   Myocardial Blood Flow Can Be Difficult to Visualize**
Nuclear medicine scanning of the heart, as indicated here, can show the heart in multiple projections and can readily identify areas that are poorly perfused.

A1
3

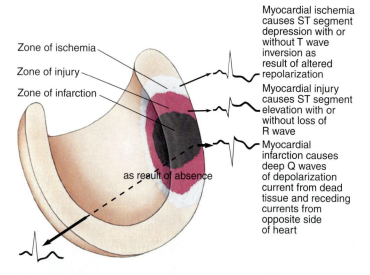

Zone of ischemia

Zone of injury

Zone of infarction

as result of absence

Myocardial ischemia causes ST segment depression with or without T wave inversion as result of altered repolarization

Myocardial injury causes ST segment elevation with or without loss of R wave

Myocardial infarction causes deep Q waves of depolarization current from dead tissue and receding currents from opposite side of heart

• FIGURE A13-5   Evolving Myocardial Infarction
The center of the lesion is the zone of infarction where tissue death has actually occurred. Adjacent to that is the zone of injury where some recovery is possible. At the periphery of the lesion is the zone of ischemia where actual tissue injury has not yet occurred.

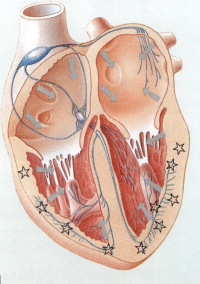

myocardial contraction takes place. Ventricular fibrillation can be effectively treated by defibrillation, the rapid application of an electrical countershock (Figure A13-7•). Defibrillation stops the irregular electrical activity of the heart allowing the normal pacemaker of the heart to resume control. Defibrillator technology has evolved significantly. Now, portable defibrillators are completely automated and readily available. Persons learning CPR and basic life support are now trained in the use of an automated defibrillator.

REPERFUSION

One of the most significant advances in emergency medicine over the last decade has been the development of reperfusion therapy, the process of restoring blood flow through an occluded artery. This can be achieved with medications, surgery, or both. Initially limited to acute myocardial infarction, reperfusion therapy is being used now in the treatment of selected stroke patients and patients with large blood clots in the lungs (pulmonary emboli).

The 12-lead electrocardiogram (ECG) is a major tool in diagnosing acute coronary syndrome. It is also used to stratify, or triage, patients into one of three groups for treatment:

1. ST-segment elevation or new left bundle branch block (LBBB)
2. ST-segment depression ($\geq$ 1 millimeter) or T wave inversion
3. Nondiagnostic or normal ECG

Patients who have signs and symptoms consistent with acute coronary syndrome and have demonstrable high-risk ECG changes (ST segment elevation or new left bundle branch block) should be considered candidates for thrombolytic therapy. Patients who meet the screening criteria and whose symptoms have been present for six hours or less should receive thrombolytic therapy. The thrombolytic agent varies depending upon local recommendations.

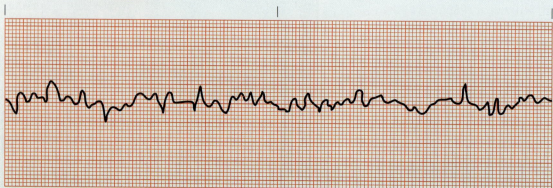

• FIGURE A13-6   Physiology of Ventricular Fibrillation and ECG
Ventricular fibrillation is a lethal dysrhythmia where cells throughout the heart fire in an uncoordinated fashion resulting in loss of the heart's pumping action.

Regardless of the agent, the patient should be monitored for the development of adverse effects such as intracranial hemorrhage. In addition to thrombolytic agents, patients usually will receive aspirin, heparin (blood thinner), beta blockers, and nitroglycerin. The treatment is based upon the assessment of the patient's overall condition.

Patients who have signs and symptoms consistent with acute coronary syndrome and demonstrable moderate-risk ECG changes (ST segment depression or T wave inversion) should be considered as strongly suspicious for myocardial ischemia. These patients should be treated with heparin, aspirin, beta blockers, and nitroglycerin. Some patients in this category might benefit from glycoprotein IIb/IIIa inhibitors. These agents provide benefits beyond those of aspirin and heparin. A commonly used drug from this classification is abciximab (ReoPro). Aggrastat and Integrilin are also commonly used in the non-catheterization setting.

Finally, patients who have signs and symptoms consistent with acute coronary syndrome but do not have demonstrable ECG changes or have a normal ECG should receive aspirin and other therapy as appropriate. The concept of risk-stratification in acute coronary syndrome is designed to assure that patients receive the best possible therapy as quickly as possible.

REVASCULARIZATION

Following thrombolytic therapy, or when thrombolytic therapy is not indicated or is ineffective, patients should be referred for coronary angiography and possible interventional therapy. In many cases, emergent cardiac catheterization is superior to thrombolytic therapy. It allows visualization of the coronary artery anatomy including the degree and magnitude of vessel blockage.

While in the cardiac catheterization lab for coronary angiography, patients with atherosclerotic lesions and occlusions suitable for angioplasty can be treated. The process, called *percutaneous transluminal coronary angioplasty (PTCA),* involves introducing a small catheter into the affected artery. An uninflated balloon catheter is placed at the site of the lesion, or lesions, and then inflated. This compresses the atheromatous plaque increasing the size of the vessel lumen. This procedure may need to be repeated several times until the artery remains open. If the vessel will not remain adequately open following balloon angioplasty, a metal stent can be placed at the site of the lesion. The metal stent is compressed for placement. Once placed, the stent is released and expands to hold back the plaque thus restoring patency to the blood vessel. Other technologies, such as intraluminal lasers and rotary files that break down inflammatory and atheromatous plaques, are used occasionally.

Some patients have severe and diffuse atherosclerotic coronary artery disease. Their coronary angiograms reveal multiple regions of obstruction making angioplasty impossible. These patients are evaluated for *coronary artery bypass grafting (CABG).* CABG is a major procedure that requires that the sternum be split, the heart stopped (cardioplegia), and the patient placed on a bypass pump for the duration of the surgery. The medial aspect of the leg is opened and a part of the saphenous vein harvested for the bypass grafts. The grafts are prepared and sewn into the aorta, just above the aortic valve. The distal end is then attached to the diseased coronary artery distal to the blockage. Some patients require multiple grafts. It is not uncommon to perform 4 or 5 grafts in one operation. In younger patients, arteries in the chest, such as the internal mammary artery, are used to provide blood to one of the new grafts. New technologies are making the surgical procedure less invasive thus shortening the patient's hospitalization and recovery period. In "keyhole surgery" a small camera and the necessary surgical instruments are introduced through several small incisions in the chest. This operation is referred to as "off pump" surgery as the entire procedure is performed while the heart remains beating. This significantly lessens the patient's pain and decreases the hospital stay because the patient has several small incisions instead of two large ones.

DEFIBRILLATION

Defibrillation is used to treat life-threatening dysrhythmias such as ventricular fibrillation and nonperfusing ventricular tachycardia. Defibrillation is the delivery of sufficient electrical energy to the heart to depolarize the myocardial muscle mass while at the same time causing minimal electrical injury to the heart. This allows a pacemaker cell within the heart to resume its rhythmic firing thus restoring a normal electrical pattern. A shock will not terminate the dysrhythmia if the energy or current is too low. Functional and structural damage to the heart can occur if the energy or current are too high.

When first developed, defibrillators were extremely large units that operated on standard electrical current. These older units used alternating current (AC) and were limited to hospitals. In the 1970s, portable defibrillators that could be used in the prehospital setting were developed. These units utilized direct current (DC) but were extremely heavy and bulky, often weighing 40 pounds or more (Figure A13-8●). Battery technology was limited and the unit required recharging immediately after use. Now, defibrillators are available that are approximately the size of a notebook. Many are completely automated allowing their use by nonmedical personnel (Figure A13-9●).

Technology has also allowed the development of a defibrillator unit that can be permanently implanted in patients deemed at risk for life-threatening dysrhythmias. These devices, referred to as *implantable cardioverter-defibrillators (ICDs),* have become the treatment of choice for sudden cardiac death. They have reduced mortality from 30 to 45

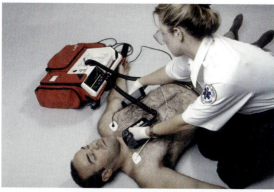

● **FIGURE A13-7   EMS-Provided Defibrillation**
Defibrillation can be life saving in the treatment of sudden death and acute coronary syndrome when complicated by ventricular fibrillation or nonperfusing ventricular tachycardia.

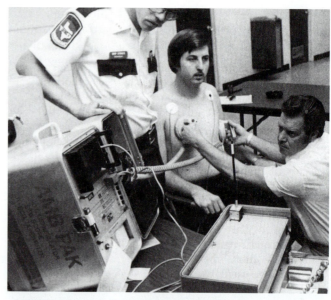

● **FIGURE A13-8   Early Portable Defibrillator**
Defibrillator and EMS technology has evolved significantly. This 1975 photo shows a portable defibrillator/monitor that weighed nearly 40 pounds. The large device at the bottom of the screen is a Motorola Apcor radio modified to operate as a mobile telephone.

percent per year to less than 2 percent per year. The ICD consists of a pulse generator, a lead system with both sensing and shocking electrodes, integrated circuitry to analyze the cardiac rhythm and trigger defibrillation, and a power supply. The life span of these units is approximately 8 years depending upon the frequency of discharge.

Today, there are three general types of external defibrillators: automated external defibrillators (AEDs), semi-automated external defibrillators (SAEDs), and manual defibrillators. Automated units simply require application of the electrodes and turning on the device. Semi-automated units require that the operator press a button to deliver the electrical shock as directed by the device. These extremely automated units are designed for use by first responders and nonmedical personnel. Most airlines now carry automated external defibrillators on flights longer than 3 hours. Soon, all large commercial passenger aircraft will carry these devices. The manual units are designed for use by trained medical personnel. They usually have several other features including continuous cardiac monitoring, synchronized cardioversion, hard-copy recording, and external cardiac pacing. Newer units allow recording and monitoring of a 12-lead ECG. They also contain a diagnostic module that provides a computerized interpretation of the ECG tracing.

The ability to defibrillate a fibrillating heart depends primarily on the electrical current delivered to the myocardium. All modern defibrillators use direct current (DC) and store the energy in a capacitor that discharges when triggered by the operator. Factors that impede the flow of energy to the myocardium include resistance to current flow by the chest wall (transthroracic impedance) and internal loss of energy within the defibrillator. The current delivered to the myocardium is a function of the energy delivered by the defibrillator, the electrical impedance within the device and chest, and the duration of current flow:

Energy = current × impedance × duration
(Joules = amperes × ohms × seconds)

An increase in either current or duration will increase the energy. An increase in transthoracic impedance (resistance to current flow) will reduce the delivered current.

Modern defibrillators deliver energy, or current, in waveforms. The energy levels vary with the type of device and type of waveform it uses. Modern defibrillators use two types of waveforms: monophasic and biphasic (Figure A13-10●). For years the standard DC waveform was monophasic, delivering current in one direction only. Biphasic waveforms, in contrast, deliver current that flows in a positive direction for a specific duration and then flows in a negative direction for the remaining millisecond of the electrical discharge. A biphasic waveform has been demonstrated to be superior in patients who have implantable cardioverter-defibrillators. However, research has not determined whether a biphasic waveform provides any advantage in external defibrillators. The recommended energy settings for defibrillation with a monophasic-type machine start at 200 Joules, then increase to 300 Joules with the second shock, and increase again to 360 Joules with the third and subsequent shocks. The optimum energy for biphasic-type machines has not been clearly identified.

Many of the manual defibrillator/monitors can provide synchronized cardioversion. This technology, monitors the patient's ECG, electronically marks the QRS complex, and triggers the shock at precisely the proper time in the cardiac cycle to depolarize the heart. Because the shock targets the vulnerable period, the amount of energy needed to depolarize the myocardium is markedly less.

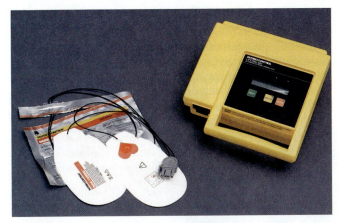

• **FIGURE A13-9   Modern Defibrillator**
Defibrillators are now compact and completely automated as illustrated by the device shown here.

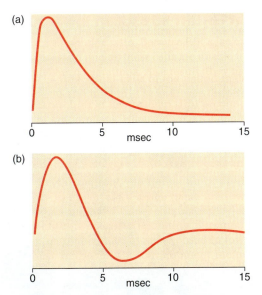

• **FIGURE A13-10   Examples of Defibrillator Waveforms**
The top waveform is monophasic, the lower waveform is biphasic. With a biphasic waveform, current travels in a positive direction for the first part of the energy delivery and then in a negative direction for the remainder.

BLUNT MYOCARDIAL INJURY

Blunt trauma to the myocardium can result in injuries ranging from contusions to concussion. In a myocardial contusion, blunt trauma to the anterior chest transmits energy to the underlying heart. The most common cause of blunt myocardial injury is high-speed motor vehicle collisions, often with crushing of the steering wheel. This can result in focal myocardial edema, interstitial hemorrhage, and occasionally subendocardial hemorrhage. The portions of the heart most frequently affected are the anterior right ventricular wall, the anterior interventricular septum, and anterior/apical aspect of the left ventricle.

A myocardial contusion usually causes chest pain similar to that seen in angina pectoris. There is often tachycardia associated with rhythm and conduction disturbances. Severe injuries can cause a reduction in cardiac output. Myocardial contusions can cause abnormalities in the ECG such as ST segment elevation in the leads over the injured myocardium. In some cases, an elevation of cardiac enzymes is often seen. Most patients who sustain a myocardial contusion have complete recovery within 3–6 weeks.

Commotio Cordis

A *myocardial concussion,* often called *commotio cordis,* is a blow to the myocardium where no obvious gross or microscopic injury can be found. However, the patient can develop a life-threatening dysrhythmia, such as ventricular fibrillation, and die. Myocardial concussion usually results from a direct force to the chest, often a seemingly minor blow during sporting activities. The

sports most frequently associated with *commotio cordis* are karate, hockey, softball, and baseball. Young male athletes aged 5–18 years are particularly at risk for this catastrophe. Death is usually instantaneous. In animal models, *commotio cordis* has been reproduced. The patient develops ventricular fibrillation immediately upon impact. The chest impact must fall within the vulnerable period of the cardiac cycle (during repolarization just before peaking of the T wave) to induce ventricular fibrillation. Successful resuscitation has been documented with prompt defibrillation, cardiopulmonary resuscitation, or application of a precordial thump. *Commotio cordis* is an extremely rare cause of death. The personal, physiological, and cardiovascular benefits of athletics far outweigh the risks. When possible, protective pads and similar devices should be used in those felt to be at increased risk.

SUMMARY

Heart disease is a major cause of death and disability. Fortunately, medications and technology have been developed that allow early intervention and treatment before permanent heart damage has occurred. Prehospital advanced life support was initially developed to provide emergency care to heart attack victims. Emergency cardiac care still remains a major priority of modern EMS.

14 Blood Vessels and Circulation

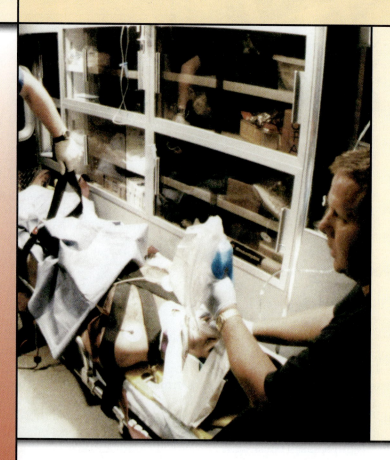

Intravenous access is an essential emergency medical procedure. Usually, intravenous access can be achieved by placing a plastic catheter into a peripheral vein. In cases where a peripheral venous access site cannot be obtained, placing a catheter into one of the three major central veins (subclavian, internal jugular, and femoral) may be necessary. Venous access allows a reliable route for the administration of essential intravenous fluids and medications.

Chapter Outline and Objectives

Vocabulary Development

alveolus, sac; *alveoli*
baro-, pressure; *baroreceptors*
capillaris, hairlike; *capillary*
manometer, device for measuring pressure; *sphygmomanometer*
porta, gate; *portal vein*
pulmo-, lung; *pulmonary*
pulsus, stroke; *pulse*
saphenes, prominent; *saphenous vein*
skleros, hard; *arteriosclerosis*
sphygmos, pulse; *sphygmomanometer*
*vaso-, vessel; *vasoconstriction; vascular*

The last two chapters examined the composition of blood and the structure and function of the heart, whose pumping action keeps blood in motion. We will now consider the vessels that carry blood to peripheral tissues and the nature of the exchange that occurs between the blood and interstitial fluids of the body.

Blood leaves the heart in the pulmonary and aortic trunks, each with a diameter of around 2.5 cm (1 in.). These vessels branch repeatedly, forming the major arteries that distribute blood to body organs. Within these organs further branching occurs, creating several hundred million tiny arteries that provide blood to more than 10 billion **capillaries** barely the diameter of a single red blood cell. These capillaries form extensive, branching networks with a combined length of 25,000 miles. If all of the capillaries in the body were placed end to end, they would circle the globe.

The vital functions of the cardiovascular system depend entirely on events at the capillary level: *All chemical and gaseous exchange between the blood and interstitial fluid takes place across capillary walls.* Tissue cells rely on capillary diffusion to obtain nutrients and oxygen and to remove metabolic wastes, such as carbon dioxide and urea.

This chapter examines the structural organization of the arteries, veins, and capillaries. We will then consider their functions and basic principles of cardiovascular regulation. The final section of the chapter examines the distribution of major blood vessels of the body.

THE ANATOMY OF BLOOD VESSELS

Blood flows to and from the lungs and other body organs through tubelike arteries and veins, with the heart providing the necessary propulsion. The large-diameter **arteries** that carry blood away from the heart branch repeatedly and gradually decrease in size until they become **arterioles** (ar-TĒ-rē-ōlz), the smallest vessels of the arterial system. From the arterioles, blood enters the capillary networks that service local tissues.

Blood flowing out of the capillary complex first enters the **venules** (VEN-ūlz), the smallest vessels of the venous system. These slender vessels subsequently merge with their neighbors to form small **veins**. Blood then passes through medium-sized and large veins before reaching the venae cavae (in the systemic circuit) or the pulmonary veins (in the pulmonary circuit) (see Figure 13-1•, p. 356).

The Structure of Vessel Walls

The walls of arteries and veins contain three distinct layers (Figure 14-1•):

1. The **tunica interna** (in-TER-na), or *tunica intima*, is the innermost layer of a blood vessel. It includes the endothelial lining of the vessel and an underlying layer of connective tissue dominated by elastic fibers.

2. The **tunica media**, the middle layer, contains smooth muscle tissue in a framework of collagen and elastic

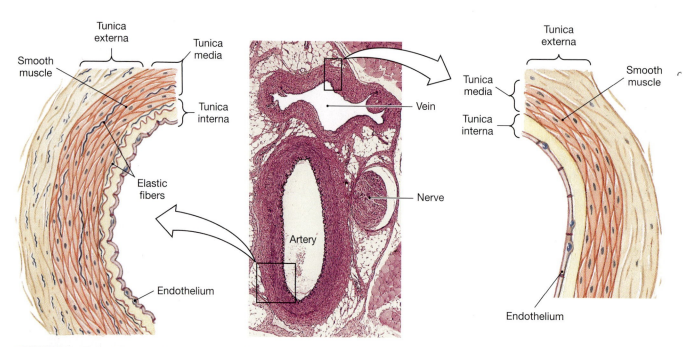

•**FIGURE 14-1   A Comparison of a Typical Artery and a Typical Vein** (LM × 74)

fibers. When these smooth muscles contract, the vessel decreases in diameter, and when they relax, the diameter increases.

3. The outer **tunica externa** (eks-TER-na), or *tunica adventitia* (ad-ven-TISH-ē-a), forms a sheath of connective tissue around the vessel. Its collagen fibers may intertwine with those of adjacent tissues, stabilizing and anchoring the blood vessel.

The multiple layers in their walls give arteries and veins considerable strength, and the muscular and elastic components permit controlled alterations in diameter as blood pressure or blood volume changes. Because the blood is under pressure, a weakness in the wall can lead to the rupture of the vessel, like a blowout in an old tire.

Arteries and veins often lie side by side in a narrow band of connective tissue, as in Figure 14-1•. The figure clearly shows the greater wall thickness characteristic of arteries. The thicker tunica media of an artery contains more smooth muscle and elastic fibers than does that of a vein. These contractile and elastic components resist the pressure generated by the heart as it forces blood into the arterial network.

Arteries

In traveling from the heart to the capillaries, blood passes through elastic arteries, muscular arteries, and arterioles. **Elastic arteries** are large, extremely resilient vessels with diameters of up to 2.5 cm (1 in.). Some examples are the pulmonary and aortic trunks and their major arterial branches. Their relatively thin walls contain a tunica media dominated by elastic fibers rather than smooth muscle cells. As a result, elastic arteries are able to absorb the pressure shock generated in systole, when the ventricles contract and blood leaves the heart. During ventricular systole, blood pressure rises quickly as additional blood is pushed into the systemic circuit. Over this period, the elastic arteries are stretched, and their diameter increases. During ventricular diastole, arterial blood pressure declines, and the elastic fibers recoil to their original dimensions. The net result is that arterial expansion cushions the rise in pressure during ventricular systole, and arterial recoil slows the decline in pressure during ventricular diastole. If the arteries were solid pipes rather than elastic tubes, pressures would rise much higher during systole and would fall much lower during diastole.

Muscular arteries, also known as *medium-sized arteries* or *distribution arteries*, distribute blood to peripheral organs. A typical muscular artery has a diameter of approximately 0.4 cm (0.15 in.). The carotid artery of the neck is one example. The thick tunica media in a muscular artery contains more smooth muscle and fewer elastic fibers than does an elastic artery.

Arterioles, with an average diameter of about 30 μm, are much smaller than muscular arteries. The tunica media of an arteriole of this size consists of one to three layers of smooth muscle fibers. These muscle layers enable muscular arteries and arterioles to change their diameter, thereby altering the blood pressure and the rate of flow through the dependent tissues.

Capillaries

Capillaries are the only blood vessels whose walls permit exchange between the blood and the surrounding interstitial fluid. Because the walls are relatively thin, the diffusion distances are small and exchange can occur quickly. In addition, blood flows through capillaries relatively slowly, allowing sufficient time for the diffusion or active transport of materials across the capillary walls.

A typical capillary consists of a single layer of endothelial cells inside a delicate basement membrane. The average diameter of a capillary is a mere 8 μm, very close to that of a single red blood cell. In most regions, the endothelium forms a complete lining, and most substances enter or leave the capillary by diffusing through gaps between adjacent endothelial cells. In some areas (notably, the choroid plexus of the brain, the hypothalamus, and filtration sites at the kidneys), small pores in the endothelial cells permit the passage of relatively large molecules, including proteins.

14

Capillary Beds

Capillaries function as part of an interconnected network called a **capillary bed**, simplified in Figure 14-2a•. On reaching its target area, a single arteriole usually gives rise to dozens of capillaries, which will in turn collect into several venules, the smallest vessels of the venous system. The entrance to each capillary is guarded by a **precapillary sphincter**, a band of smooth muscle. Contraction of the smooth muscle fibers narrows the diameter of the capillary entrance and reduces the flow of blood. The relaxation of the sphincter dilates the opening, allowing blood to enter the capillary more rapidly.

Although blood usually flows from the arterioles to the venules at a constant rate, the blood flow within a single capillary can be quite variable. Each precapillary sphincter goes through cycles of activity, alternately contracting and relaxing perhaps a dozen times each minute. As a result of this cyclical change, called **vasomotion** (*vaso-*, vessel), the blood flow within any one capillary occurs in a series of pulses rather than as a steady and constant stream. The net effect is that blood may reach the venules by one route now and by a quite different route later. This process is regulated at the tissue level, as smooth muscle fibers respond to local changes in the composition of the interstitial fluid. This regulation at the tissue level is called *autoregulation*.

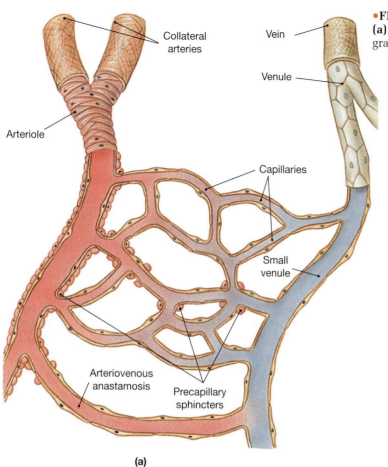

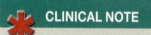

(a)

● **FIGURE 14-2   The Organization of a Capillary Bed**
(a) Basic features of a typical capillary bed. **(b)** A micrograph of a capillary network.

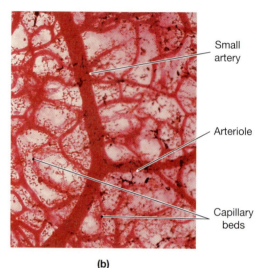

(b)

ARTERIOSCLEROSIS

Arteriosclerosis is a chronic disease of the arterial system. Complications of this disease account for half of all deaths in the United States. Arteriosclerosis is characterized by thickening and hardening of the vessel walls. In arteriosclerosis, the innermost lining of the artery *(tunica intima)* undergoes a series of changes that reduce the vessel's ability to change the diameter of the lumen. Smooth muscle cells and collagen fibers migrate into the tunica intima causing it to stiffen and thicken. This process gradually narrows the arterial lumen.

Atherosclerosis is a form of arteriosclerosis where the thickening and hardening of the arterial walls are caused by soft deposits of intra-arterial fat and fibrin. These deposits, called *atheromatous plaques,* harden over time. Atherosclerosis is the leading contributor to coronary artery and cerebrovascular disease.

The formation of atherosclerosis results from a process called *atherogenesis.* Initially, there is an injury to the *endothelium.* The endothelial cells then stop making normal substances such as *nitric oxide* and *prostaglandin* that prevent thrombosis and provide vasodilation. Growth factors are released that cause the smooth muscle in the wall of the affected vessel to proliferate. *Macrophages,* the body's scavenger cells, then start adhering to the damaged endothelial surface due to the production of adhesion molecules *(athero-elam).* Fats in the form of *low-density lipoproteins (LDL)* are oxidized by the macrophages. This recruits more macrophages, which fill with oxidized LDL and become *foam cells* that form a lesion called a *fatty streak.* Fatty streaks are found on the walls of most people's arteries, even young children's. They are reversible if the levels of LDL are decreased.

The fatty streaks will incorporate fibrous tissue and damaged smooth muscle cells into the area overlying the foam cells causing the *atheromatous plaques.* Ultimately, this causes further endothelial dysfunction, necrosis of underlying vessel tissue, and narrowing of the lumen of the vessel as the plaque sticks out from the vessel wall. As the plaque continues to develop, it can ulcerate or rupture due to mechanical shear forces and continued necrosis of the vessel wall. Platelets will aggregate and adhere to the surface of the ruptured plaque, activating the coagulation cascade, and a *thrombus* forms over the lesion. This thrombus, called a *complicated lesion,* may completely obstruct the lumen of the vessel. Depending on its location, the blockage may compromise blood flow to essential organs such as the heart and brain.

Under certain conditions, the blood will completely bypass the capillary bed through an **arteriovenous anastomosis** (a-nas-tō-MŌ-sis; "outlet"; plural, *anastomoses*), a vessel that connects an arteriole to a venule (Figure 14-2a●). An anastomosis may also interconnect two arterioles; such a vessel is called an **arterial anastomosis**. An arterial anastomosis provides a second blood supply for capillary beds. This anastomosis thus acts like an insurance policy: If one artery is compressed or blocked, the other can continue to deliver blood to the capillary bed, and the dependent tissues will not be damaged. Arterial anastomoses occur in the brain and in the coronary circulation. ∞ *p. 363*

Veins

Veins collect blood from all tissues and organs and return it to the heart. Veins are classified on the basis of their internal diameters. The smallest, the venules, resemble expanded capillaries, and venules with diameters smaller than 50 μm lack a tunica media altogether. **Medium-sized veins** range from 2 to 9 mm in diameter. In these veins, the tunica media contains several smooth muscle layers, and the relatively thick tunica externa has longitudinal bundles of elastic and collagen fibers. **Large veins** include the two venae cavae and their tributaries in the abdominopelvic and thoracic cavities. In these vessels, the thin tunica media is surrounded by a thick tunica externa composed of elastic and collagenous fibers.

Veins have relatively thin walls because they do not have to withstand much pressure. In venules and medium-sized veins, the pressure is so low that it cannot oppose the force of gravity. In the limbs, medium-sized veins contain **valves** that act like the valves in the heart, preventing the backflow of blood (Figure 14-3●). As long as the valves function normally, any movement that distorts or compresses a vein will push blood toward the heart. If the walls of the veins near the valves weaken or become stretched and distorted, the valves may not work properly. Blood then pools in the veins, and the vessels become distended. The effects range from mild discomfort and a cosmetic problem, as in superficial *varicose veins* in the thighs and legs, to painful distortion of adjacent tissues, as in *hemorrhoids*.

✓ Several small, thin-walled vessels have very little smooth muscle tissue in the tunica media. Which type of vessels are these?

✓ How would the relaxation of precapillary sphincters affect the blood flow through a tissue?

✓ Why are valves found in veins but not in arteries?

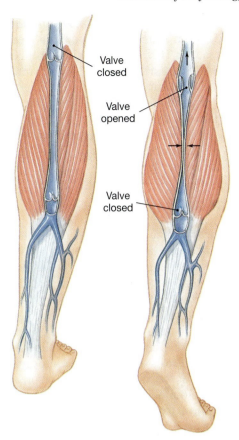

●**FIGURE 14-3   The Function of Valves in the Venous System**
Valves in the walls of medium-sized veins prevent the backflow of blood. Venous compression caused by the contraction of adjacent skeletal muscles helps maintain venous blood flow.

CIRCULATORY PHYSIOLOGY

The components of the cardiovascular system (the blood, heart, and blood vessels) are functionally integrated to maintain an adequate blood flow through peripheral tissues and organs. Under normal circumstances, blood flow is equal to cardiac output. When cardiac output goes up, so does capillary blood flow; when cardiac output declines, blood flow is reduced. Two factors—*pressure* and *resistance*—affect the flow rates of blood through the capillaries.

Pressure

Liquids, including blood, will flow from an area of higher pressure toward an area of relatively lower pressure. The flow rate is directly proportional to the pressure difference: The greater the difference in pressure, the faster the flow. In the systemic circuit, the overall pressure difference is measured between the base of the aorta (as blood leaves the left ventricle) and the entrance to the right atrium (as it returns). This pressure difference, called the *circulatory pressure*, averages around 100 mm Hg (mm Hg = millimeters of mercury, a standardized unit of pressure). This relatively high circulatory pressure is needed primarily to force blood through the arterioles and into the capillaries.

Circulatory pressure is often divided into three components: (1) *arterial pressure*, (2) *capillary pressure*, and (3) *venous pressure*. The term **blood pressure** will be used when referring to arterial pressure rather than to the total circulatory pressure.

Resistance

A *resistance* is a force that opposes movement. For circulation to occur, the circulatory pressure must be greater than the *total peripheral resistance*, the resistance of the entire circulatory system. Because the resistance of the venous system is very low, attention focuses on the **peripheral resistance**, the resistance of the arterial system.

Neural and hormonal control mechanisms regulate blood pressure, keeping it relatively stable. Adjustments in the peripheral resistance of vessels supplying specific organs allow the rate of blood flow to be precisely controlled. For example, Chapter 7 discussed the increase in blood flow to skeletal muscles during exercise. That increase occurs because there is a drop in the peripheral resistance of the arteries supplying active muscles.

Sources of peripheral resistance include *vascular resistance*, *viscosity*, and *turbulence*. Only vascular resistance can be adjusted by the nervous or endocrine system to regulate blood flow. Viscosity and turbulence, which affect peripheral resistance, are normally constant.

Vascular Resistance

Vascular resistance, the resistance of the blood vessels, is the largest component of peripheral resistance. *The most important factor in vascular resistance is friction between the blood and the vessel walls.* The amount of friction depends on the length of the vessel and its diameter. Vessel length is constant, so vascular resistance is controlled by changing the diameter of blood vessels by contracting or relaxing smooth muscle in the vessel walls.

Large arteries such as the *aorta*, *brachiocephalic artery*, or *carotid artery* contribute little to the peripheral resistance. Most of the resistance occurs in the arterioles and capillaries. As noted earlier in this chapter, arterioles are extremely muscular; an arteriole 30 μm in diameter is wrapped in a 20 μm thick layer of smooth muscle. Local, neural, and hormonal stimuli that stimulate or inhibit the arteriolar smooth muscle tissue can adjust the diameters of these vessels, and a small change in diameter can produce a very large change in resistance.

Viscosity

Viscosity is resistance to flow. It is caused by interactions among molecules and suspended materials in a liquid. Liquids of low viscosity, such as water, flow even at low pressures, whereas thick, syrupy liquids such as molasses flow only under relatively high pressures. Whole blood has a viscosity about five times that of water, due to the presence of plasma proteins and suspended blood cells. Under normal conditions, the viscosity of the blood remains stable. But disorders that affect the hematocrit or the plasma protein content can change blood viscosity and increase or decrease peripheral resistance. For example, in **anemia**, the hematocrit is reduced due to inadequate production of hemoglobin, RBCs, or both. As a result, both the oxygen-carrying capacity of the blood and blood viscosity are reduced. A reduction in blood viscosity can also result from protein deficiency diseases, in which the liver cannot synthesize normal amounts of plasma proteins.

Turbulence

Blood flow through a vessel is usually smooth, with the slowest flow near the walls and the fastest flow at the center of the vessel. High flow rates, irregular surfaces caused by injury or disease processes, or sudden changes in vessel diameter upset this smooth flow, creating eddies and swirls. This phenomenon, called *turbulence*, increases resistance and thereby slows the rate of flow.

Turbulence normally occurs when blood flows between the heart's chambers and from the heart into the aortic and pulmonary trunks. In addition to increasing resistance, this turbulence generates the *third* and *fourth heart sounds* often heard through a stethoscope. Turbulent blood flow across damaged or misaligned heart valves produces the sound of *heart murmurs*. ∞ *p. 361*

Circulatory Pressure

Blood pressure varies from one vessel to another within the systemic circuit. Systemic pressures are highest in the aorta, peaking at around 120 mm Hg, and lowest at the venae cavae, averaging about 2 mm Hg.

Arterial Blood Pressure

The graph in Figure 14-4• shows that blood pressure in large and small arteries rises and falls, rising during ventricular systole and falling during ventricular diastole. **Systolic pressure** is the peak blood pressure measured during ventricular systole, and **diastolic pressure** is the minimum blood pressure at the end of ventricular diastole. The difference between the systolic and diastolic pressures is the **pulse pressure** (*pulsus*, stroke).

Pulse pressure lessens as the distance from the heart increases. As already discussed, the average pressure declines as a result of friction between the blood and the vessel walls. The pulse pressure fades because arteries are elastic tubes rather than solid pipes. Much like a puff of air expands a partially inflated balloon, the elasticity of the arteries allows them to expand with blood during

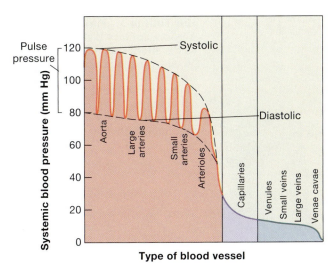

• **FIGURE 14-4   Pressures in the Circulatory System**
Notice the general reduction of circulatory pressures within the systemic circuit and the elimination of the pulse pressure in the arterioles, capillaries, and veins.

systole. When diastole begins and blood pressures fall, the arteries recoil to their original dimensions. Because the aortic semilunar valve prevents the return of blood to the heart, the arterial recoil adds an extra push to the flow of blood. The magnitude of this phenomenon, called **elastic rebound**, is greatest near the heart and drops in succeeding arterial sections. By the time blood reaches a precapillary sphincter, there are no pressure oscillations and the blood pressure remains steady at about 35 mm Hg. Along the length of a typical capillary, blood pressure gradually falls from about 35 mm Hg to roughly 18 mm Hg, the pressure at the start of the venous system.

Capillary Pressures and Capillary Dynamics

The blood pressure within a capillary, or **capillary pressure**, pushes against the capillary walls, just as it does in the arteries. But unlike other portions of the circulatory system, capillary walls are quite permeable to small ions, nutrients, organic wastes, dissolved gases, and water.

Capillary Exchange.   Since Chapter 3 described the forces that move water and solutes across membranes, only a brief overview is provided here. ∞ *p. 59* Solute molecules tend to diffuse across the capillary lining, driven by their individual concentration gradients. Water-soluble materials, including ions and small organic molecules such as glucose, amino acids, or urea, diffuse through small spaces between adjacent endothelial cells. Larger water-soluble molecules, such as plasma proteins, cannot normally leave the bloodstream. Lipid-soluble materials, including steroids, fatty acids, and dissolved gases, diffuse across the endothelial lining, passing through the membrane lipids.

Water molecules will move when driven by either hydrostatic pressure or osmotic pressure. ∞ *p. 60* Hy-

drostatic pressure is a physical force that pushes water molecules from an area of high pressure to an area of lower pressure. At a capillary, the hydrostatic pressure, or *capillary blood pressure* (*BP*), is greatest at the arteriolar end and least where it empties into a venule. The tendency for water and solutes to move out of the blood is therefore greatest at the start of a capillary, where the capillary pressure is highest, and declines along the length of the capillary as capillary pressure falls.

Osmosis, in contrast, is the movement of water across a semipermeable membrane separating two solutions of different solute concentrations. Water will move into the solution with the higher solute concentration, and the force of this water movement is called osmotic pressure. Because blood contains more dissolved proteins than does the interstitial fluid ∞ *p. 336*, water tends to move from the interstitial fluid into the blood. Thus, capillary blood pressure tends to push water out of the capillary, while *capillary osmotic pressure* (*COP*) tends to pull it back in (Figure 14-5•).

✳ CAPILLARY PHYSIOLOGY

The exchange of fluid through the capillary membranes is an important physiological process. Normally, capillaries are able to maintain normal fluid volume distribution between the plasma and the interstitial fluid. Normal capillary pressure at the arterial end of the capillaries is 15–25 mm Hg greater than at the venous end. Because of this difference, fluid "filters" out of the capillaries at the arterial end and is reabsorbed back into the capillaries at the venous end. This results in a small amount of fluid "flowing" through the tissues from the arterial ends of the capillaries to the venous ends.

Forces at the arterial end of the capillary move fluid outward. These include the *capillary blood pressure* and the *interstitial fluid colloid osmotic pressure*. At the same time, *plasma colloid osmotic pressure* tends to move fluid inward. At the arterial end, the outward pressures, called the *net filtration pressure,* exceed the inward pressures, resulting in loss of fluid from the capillaries to the interstitial space.

At the venous end of the capillary, *plasma colloid osmotic pressure* tends to move fluid inward. Likewise, *capillary blood pressure* and *interstitial fluid colloid osmotic pressure* tend to move fluids outward. Here, the inward pressure, called the *reabsorption pressure,* exceeds the outward pressure, causing fluid to move into the capillaries.

In hemorrhage or dehydration, the loss in blood volume causes a drop in blood pressure. Also, as water is lost from the plasma, the blood becomes more concentrated. This results in increased plasma colloid osmotic pressure that pulls fluid from the interstitial space into the intravascular space. The loss of fluid in the interstitial spaces causes a decrease in *skin turgor,* a characteristic finding of dehydration.

An increase in circulating fluid volume increases the capillary blood pressure at the arterial end. Plasma colloids are diluted by the excess fluid, decreasing the plasma colloid osmotic pressure. This causes the accumulation of fluid in the interstitial spaces, commonly called *edema.*

1
4

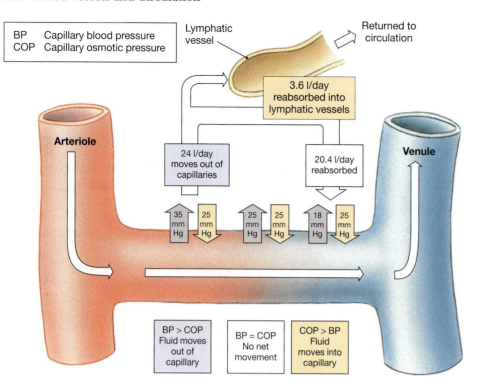

| BP | Capillary blood pressure |
| COP | Capillary osmotic pressure |

•FIGURE 14-5   Forces Acting Across Capillary Walls
At the arterial end of the capillary, blood hydrostatic pressure (BP) is stronger than capillary osmotic pressure (COP), and fluid moves out of the capillary. Near the venule, BP is lower than COP, and fluid moves into the capillary.

Lymphatic vessel

Returned to circulation

3.6 l/day reabsorbed into lymphatic vessels

Arteriole

24 l/day moves out of capillaries

20.4 l/day reabsorbed

Venule

| 35 mm Hg | 25 mm Hg | 25 mm Hg | 25 mm Hg | 18 mm Hg | 25 mm Hg |

BP > COP
Fluid moves out of capillary

BP = COP
No net movement

COP > BP
Fluid moves into capillary

Normally, hydrostatic and osmotic forces are not in balance along the length of a capillary, and the arterioles deliver more fluid to the capillaries than the venules carry away (Figure 14-5•). The water and dissolved materials that leave the plasma flow through the tissues and eventually enter a network of **lymphatic vessels**, which drain into the venous system. (This topic will be discussed further in Chapter 15.)

Venous Pressure

Although blood pressure at the start of the venous system is only about one-tenth that at the start of the arterial system, the blood must still travel through a vascular network as complex as the arterial system before returning to the heart. However, venous pressures are low, and the veins offer little resistance. As a result, once blood enters the venous system, pressure declines very slowly.

As blood travels through the venous system toward the heart, the veins become larger, resistance drops further, and the flow rate increases. Pressures at the entrance to the right atrium fluctuate, but they average around 2 mm Hg. This means that the driving force pushing blood through the venous system is a mere 16 mm Hg (18 mm Hg in the venules −2 mm Hg in the venae cavae = 16 mm Hg) as compared to the 85 mm Hg pressure acting along the arterial system (120 mm Hg at the aorta −35 mm Hg at the capillaries).

When you are lying down, a 16 mm Hg pressure gradient is sufficient to maintain venous flow. But when you are standing, the venous blood from the body below the heart must overcome gravity as it ascends within the inferior vena cava. Two factors help overcome gravity and propel venous blood toward the heart:

1. **Muscular compression**. The contractions of skeletal muscles near a vein compress it, helping push blood toward the heart. The valves in medium-sized veins ensure that blood flow occurs in one direction only (see Figure 14-3•, p. 379).

2. The **respiratory pump**. As you inhale, decreased pressure in the thoracic cavity draws air into the lungs. This drop in pressure also pulls blood into the venae cavae and atria, increasing venous return. On exhalation, the increased pressure that forces air out of the lungs compresses the venae cavae, pushing blood into the right atrium.

During exercise, both factors cooperate to elevate venous return and push cardiac output to maximal levels. However, when an individual stands at attention, with knees locked and leg muscles immobile, these mechanisms are impaired and the reduction in venous return leads to a fall in cardiac output. The blood supply to the brain is in turn reduced, sometimes enough to cause *fainting*, a temporary loss of consciousness. The person then collapses; in the horizontal position, both venous return and cardiac output return to normal.

✓ In a normal individual, where would you expect the blood pressure to be greater, in the aorta or in the inferior vena cava? Explain.

✓ While standing in the hot sun, Sally begins to feel light-headed and faints. Explain.

CLINICAL NOTE

VITAL SIGNS

Vital signs are outward indicators of what is going on inside the body. They include blood pressure (BP), heart rate, respiratory rate, and temperature. These measurements provide a great deal of information about a patient's condition and should be measured frequently.

The *pulse rate* is a measure of the number of times the heart beats per minute. The pulse is best measured where an artery lies close to the body's surface and crosses over a bone. Common locations for pulse determination are illustrated in Figure 14-6a. To measure the pulse rate, locate a suitable site and palpate the pulse. Then, count the number of pulse waves that occur in one minute. Alternatively, you can count the number of pulse waves in 30 seconds and multiply by two. In order to ensure accuracy, it is not recommended that intervals less than 30 seconds be measured.

The *respiratory rate* is a measure of the number of times a person breathes in one minute. To measure the respiratory rate, have the patient assume a comfortable position. While the patient is at rest, count the number of respirations that occur in one minute. People will alter their respiratory pattern if they feel it is being watched, so it is best to distract the patient. Skilled personnel will often take a patient's wrist and measure the pulse. Then, while still holding the wrist, they will count the respiratory rate while the patient thinks that the pulse is being measured.

The *blood pressure* is a function of the amount of blood being pumped by the heart (cardiac output) and the peripheral vascular resistance. To determine the blood pressure, a *blood pressure cuff (sphygmomanometer)* is placed on the arm 3–4 centimeters above the elbow (Figure 14-6b). A stethoscope is placed over the brachial artery. The blood pressure cuff is inflated to approximately 30 mm Hg above the point where it occludes the brachial artery and stops the flow of blood. Then, the pressure in the cuff is slowly released. When the pressure in the cuff falls below systolic pressure, blood flow resumes in the artery and produces *Korotkoff sounds.* As the pressure falls, the vessel remains open longer and the sounds in the artery change. When the cuff pressure falls below the diastolic pressure, blood flow becomes continuous and the Korotkoff sounds disappear completely.

The *temperature* is not often measured in EMS. However, electronic thermometers have made this a simple procedure. The temperature is measured in the mouth (under the tongue), rectally, or through the ear (tympanic membrane). Normal body temperature is 37° C (98.6° F).

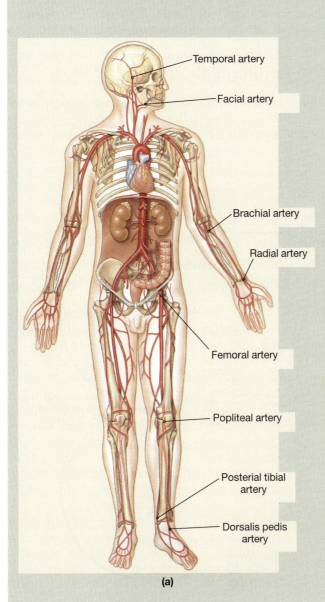

Temporal artery

Facial artery

Brachial artery

Radial artery

Femoral artery

Popliteal artery

Posterial tibial artery

Dorsalis pedis artery

(a)

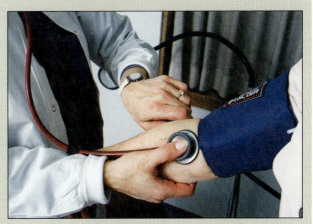

(b)

● **FIGURE 14-6 Checking the Pulse and Blood Pressure**
(a) Pressure points used to check the presence and strength of the pulse. **(b)** The use of a sphygmomanometer to check arterial blood pressure.

CARDIOVASCULAR REGULATION

Homeostatic mechanisms regulate cardiovascular activity to ensure that tissue blood flow, also called *tissue perfusion*, meets the demand for oxygen and nutrients. The three variable factors that influence tissue blood flow are cardiac output, peripheral resistance, and blood pressure. Cardiac output was discussed in Chapter 13, and peripheral resistance and blood pressure were considered earlier in this chapter (p. 380).

Most cells are relatively close to capillaries (within 135 µm). When a group of cells becomes active, the circulation to that region must increase to deliver the necessary oxygen and nutrients and to carry away the waste products and carbon dioxide that they generate. The goal of cardiovascular regulation is to ensure that these blood flow changes occur (1) at an appropriate time, (2) in the right area, and (3) without drastically altering blood pressure and blood flow to vital organs.

Factors involved in the regulation of cardiovascular function include (Figure 14-7●):

• *Local factors.* Local factors change the pattern of blood flow within capillary beds in response to chemical changes in the interstitial fluids. For example, at any moment some of the precapillary sphincters are open and others are closed. As long as the proportion remains constant, the total blood flow through the tissues will remain constant. This is an example of *autoregulation* at the tissue level.

• *Neural mechanisms.* Neural control mechanisms respond to changes in arterial pressure or blood gas levels at specific sites. When those changes occur, the autonomic nervous system adjusts cardiac output and peripheral resistance to maintain adequate blood flow.

• *Endocrine factors.* The endocrine system releases hormones that enhance short-term adjustments and direct long-term changes in cardiovascular performance.

Short-term responses adjust cardiac output and peripheral resistance to stabilize blood pressure and tissue blood flow. Long-term adjustments involve alterations in blood volume that affect cardiac output and the transport of oxygen and carbon dioxide to and from active tissues.

The Autoregulation of Blood Flow

Under normal resting conditions, cardiac output remains stable, and peripheral resistance in individual tissues is adjusted to control local blood flow. When

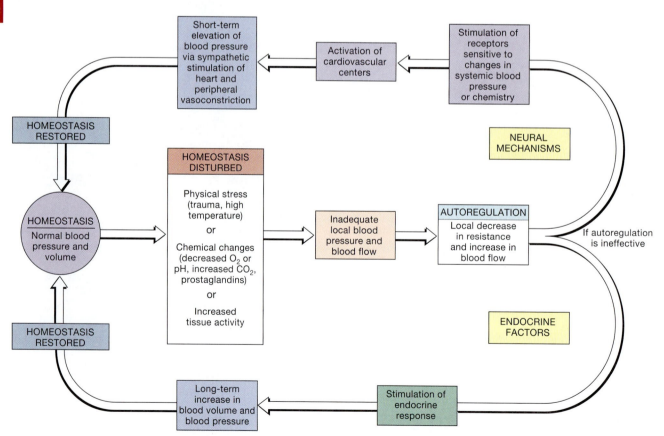

●FIGURE 14-7   **Local, Neural, and Endocrine Adjustments that Maintain Blood Pressure and Blood Flow**

a precapillary sphincter constricts, blood flow decreases; when it relaxes, blood flow increases. Precapillary sphincters can respond automatically to alterations in the local environment. For example, when oxygen is abundant, the smooth muscles contract and slow down the flow of blood. Oxygen levels decline in active tissues as the cells absorb O_2 for use in aerobic respiration. As tissue oxygen supplies dwindle, carbon dioxide levels rise, and the pH falls. This combination causes the smooth muscle cells in the precapillary sphincter to relax and blood flow to increase. The appearance of specific chemicals in the interstitial fluids can produce the same effect. For example, in the inflammation response, vasodilation occurs at an injury site because histamine, bacterial toxins, and prostaglandins cause the relaxation of the precapillary sphincters.

Factors that promote the dilation of precapillary sphincters are called *vasodilators*, and those that stimulate the constriction of precapillary sphincters are called *vasoconstrictors*. Together, such factors control blood flow in a single capillary bed. When present in high concentrations, these factors also affect arterioles, increasing or decreasing blood flow to all of the capillary beds in a given region. Such an event will often trigger a neural response, because significant changes in blood flow to one region of the body will have an immediate effect on circulation to other regions.

The Neural Control of Blood Pressure and Blood Flow

The nervous system is responsible for adjusting cardiac output and peripheral resistance to maintain adequate blood flow to vital tissues and organs. The *cardiac centers* and *vasomotor centers* of the medulla oblongata are the cardiovascular centers responsible for these regulatory activities. As noted in Chapter 13, the cardiac centers include a *cardioacceleratory center*, which increases cardiac output through sympathetic innervation, and a *cardioinhibitory center*, which reduces cardiac output through parasympathetic innervation. ∞ *p. 370*

The vasomotor center of the medulla oblongata primarily controls the diameters of the arterioles. Inhibition of the vasomotor center leads to **vasodilation**, a dilation of arterioles that reduces peripheral resistance. The stimulation of the vasomotor center causes **vasoconstriction** (the constriction of peripheral arterioles) and, with very strong stimulation, **venoconstriction** (the constriction of peripheral veins), both of which increase peripheral resistance.

The cardiovascular centers detect changes in tissue demand by monitoring arterial blood, especially blood pressure, pH, and dissolved gas concentrations. The *baroreceptor reflexes* respond to changes in blood pressure, and the *chemoreceptor reflexes* respond to changes in chemical composition.

Baroreceptor Reflexes

Baroreceptor reflexes (*baro-*, pressure) are autonomic reflexes that adjust cardiac output and peripheral resistance to maintain normal arterial pressures. When blood pressure climbs, the increased neural output from the baroreceptors travels to the medulla oblongata, where it inhibits the cardioacceleratory center, stimulates the cardioinhibitory center, and inhibits the vasomotor center (Figure 14-8•).

Under the command of the cardioinhibitory center, the vagus nerves release ACh, which reduces the rate and strength of the cardiac contractions, lowering cardiac output. The inhibition of the vasomotor center leads to the dilation of peripheral arterioles throughout the body. This combination of reduced cardiac output and decreased peripheral resistance then reduces the blood pressure.

This pattern is reversed if blood pressure becomes abnormally low. In that case, a corresponding reduction in baroreceptor output stimulates the cardioacceleratory center, inhibits the cardioinhibitory center, and stimulates the vasomotor center. The cardioacceleratory center stimulates sympathetic neurons innervating the SA node, AV node, and general myocardium. This stimulation increases heart rate and stroke volume, leading to an immediate increase in cardiac output. Vasomotor activity, also carried by sympathetic motor neurons, produces a rapid vasoconstriction, increasing peripheral resistance. These adjustments, increased cardiac output and increased peripheral resistance, work together to elevate blood pressure.

Baroreceptors monitor the degree of stretch in the walls of distensible organs. The three major baroreceptor populations respond to alterations in blood pressure at key locations in the cardiovascular system:

1. *Aortic baroreceptors* are located within the **aortic sinuses**, pockets in the walls of the aorta adjacent to the heart (Figure 13-5•, p. 360).
2. *Carotid sinus baroreceptors* are located in the walls of the **carotid sinuses**, expanded chambers near the bases of the internal carotid arteries of the neck (Figure 14-15a•, p. 395). Because pressure changes at this location affect the blood flow to the brain, the carotid sinus reflex is both extremely sensitive and quite important.
3. *Atrial baroreceptors*, in the wall of the right atrium, monitor the blood pressure there and at the venae cavae, the end of the systemic circuit. The responses produced by the atrial reflex differ from those of the aortic and carotid reflexes. Under normal circumstances, the heart pumps blood into the aorta at the same rate that it is arriving at the right atrium. When blood pressure rises in the atrium, it means

14

•**FIGURE 14-8   The Carotid and Aortic Sinus Baroreceptor Reflexes**

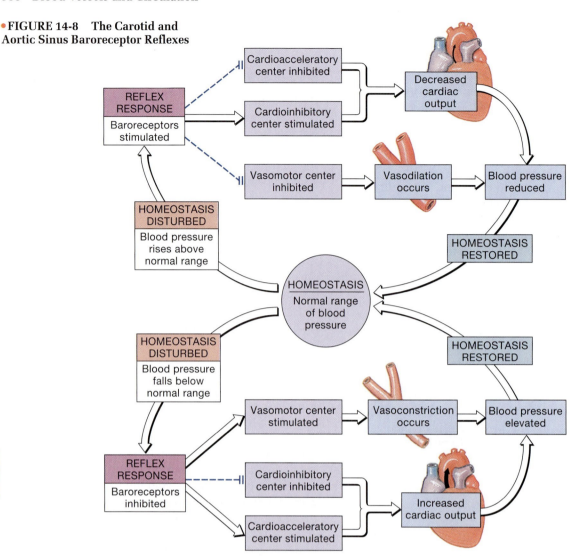

that a circulatory traffic jam exists, with blood arriving at the heart faster than it is being pumped out. The atrial baroreceptors solve the problem by stimulating the cardioacceleratory center, increasing cardiac output until the backlog of venous blood is removed and atrial pressure returns to normal.

Chemoreceptor Reflexes

The **chemoreceptor reflexes** respond to changes in the carbon dioxide levels, oxygen levels, or pH in the blood and cerebrospinal fluid (Figure 14-9•). The chemoreceptors involved are sensory neurons found in the carotid bodies, located in the neck near the carotid sinus, and the aortic bodies, situated near the arch of the aorta. These receptors monitor the composition of the arterial blood. Additional chemoreceptors on the medulla oblongata monitor the composition of the cerebrospinal fluid (CSF).

The activation of chemoreceptors occurs through a drop in pH or in plasma O_2, or a rise in CO_2 levels. Any of these changes leads to a stimulation of the cardioacceleratory and vasomotor centers. This ele-

vates arterial pressure and increases blood flow through peripheral tissues. Chemoreceptor output also affects the respiratory centers in the medulla oblongata. As a result, a rise in blood flow and blood pressure is associated with an elevated respiratory rate. The coordination of cardiovascular and respiratory activity is vital, because accelerating tissue blood flow is useful only if the circulating blood contains adequate oxygen. In addition, a rise in the respiratory rate accelerates venous return through the action of the respiratory pump. ∞ *p. 382*

The Influence of the ANS and Higher Brain Centers

The cardiac and vasomotor centers can also be influenced by the activities of other areas of the brain. Stimulation by sympathetic neurons of the ANS, assisted by the release of epinephrine and norepinephrine by the adrenal medullae, acts on these centers to increase cardiac output and cause vasoconstriction. In contrast, parasympathetic stimulation affects the cardioinhibitory center, reducing cardiac output. It does not directly af-

• **FIGURE 14-9**   **The Chemoreceptor Reflexes**

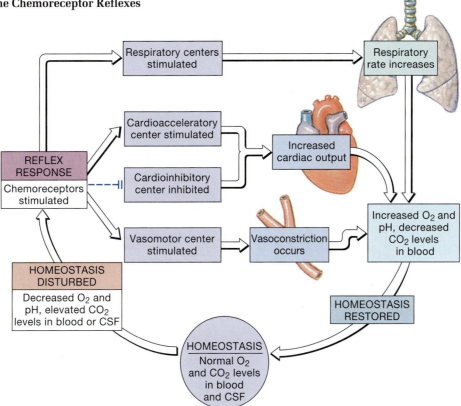

fect the vasomotor center, but vasodilation occurs as sympathetic activity declines.

The activities of higher brain centers can also affect blood pressure. Our thought processes or emotional states can produce significant changes in blood pressure by influencing cardiac output. For example, strong emotions of anxiety, fear, or rage are accompanied by an elevation in blood pressure, caused by cardiac stimulation and vasoconstriction.

Hormones and Cardiovascular Regulation

The endocrine system provides both short-term and long-term regulation of cardiovascular performance. Epinephrine (E) and norepinephrine (NE) from the adrenal medullae stimulate cardiac output and peripheral vasoconstriction. Other regulatory hormones include antidiuretic hormone (ADH), angiotensin II, erythropoietin (EPO), and atrial natriuretic peptide (ANP), introduced in Chapter 11. ∞ *pp. 313, 320* Although ADH and angiotensin II affect blood pressure, all four hormones affect primarily the long-term regulation of blood volume, as diagrammed in Figure 14-10•.

Angiotensin II

Angiotensin II appears in the blood following the release of renin by specialized kidney cells stimulat-

ed by a fall in blood pressure. Renin starts a chain reaction that ultimately converts an inactive protein, *angiotensinogen*, to the hormone angiotensin II. Angiotensin II causes an extremely powerful vasoconstriction that elevates blood pressure almost at once. It also stimulates the secretion of ADH by the pituitary and aldosterone by the adrenal cortex, and the two complement one another. The ADH stimulates water conservation at the kidneys, and the aldosterone stimulates the reabsorption of sodium ions and water from the urine. In addition, angiotensin II stimulates thirst, and the presence of ADH and aldosterone ensures that the additional water consumed will be retained, elevating the plasma volume.

Antidiuretic Hormone

In addition to its water-conserving effect on the kidneys, ADH also responds to an increase in the osmotic concentration of the plasma. The immediate result is a peripheral vasoconstriction that elevates blood pressure.

Erythropoietin

Erythropoietin is released by the kidneys if the blood pressure declines or if the oxygen content of the blood becomes abnormally low. This hormone stimulates red blood cell production, elevating the blood volume and improving the oxygen-carrying capacity of the blood.

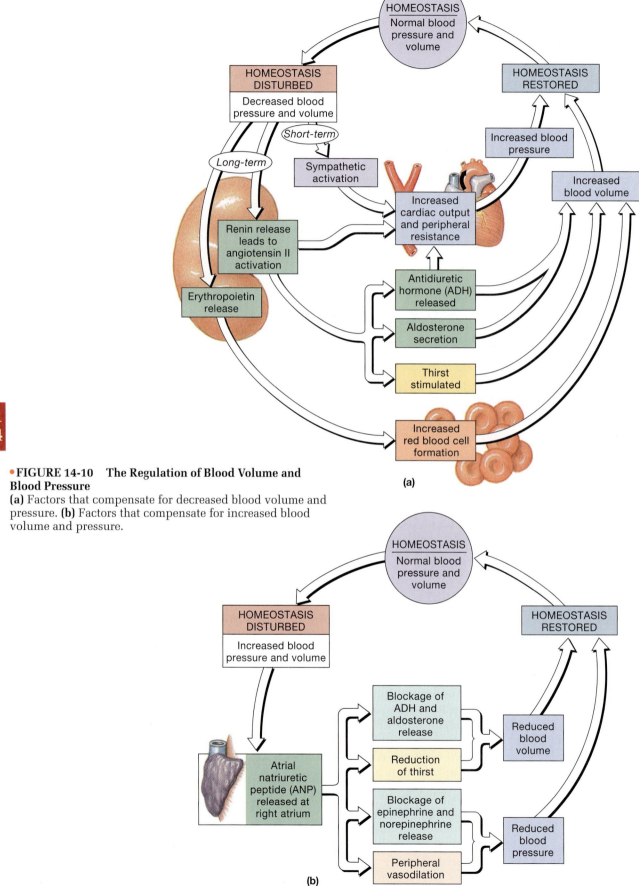

•FIGURE 14-10   **The Regulation of Blood Volume and Blood Pressure**
(a) Factors that compensate for decreased blood volume and pressure. (b) Factors that compensate for increased blood volume and pressure.

Atrial Natriuretic Peptide

In contrast to the three hormones just described, ANP release is stimulated by *increased* blood pressure (Figure 14-10b•). This hormone is produced by specialized cardiac muscle cells in the atrial walls when they are stretched by excessive venous return. The ANP reduces blood volume and blood pressure by (1) promoting the loss of sodium ions and water at the kidneys, (2) increasing water losses at the kidneys by blocking the release of ADH and aldosterone, (3) reducing thirst, (4) blocking the release of E and NE, and (5) stimulating peripheral vasodilation. As blood volume and blood pressure decline, the stress on the atrial walls is removed and ANP production ceases.

PATTERNS OF CARDIOVASCULAR RESPONSE

In our day-to-day lives, the cardiovascular system operates as an integrated complex of quite diverse components. Two common stresses, exercise and blood loss, illustrate the adaptability of this system and its ability to maintain homeostasis. We will also consider the physiological mechanisms involved in shock and heart failure, two important cardiovascular disorders.

Exercise and the Cardiovascular System

At rest, the cardiac output averages around 5.6 liters per minute. During exercise, both cardiac output and the pattern of blood distribution change markedly. As exercise begins, a number of interrelated changes occur:

- *Extensive vasodilation occurs* as the rate of skeletal muscle oxygen consumption increases. Peripheral resistance drops, blood flow through the capillaries increases, and blood enters the venous system at an accelerated rate.
- *The venous return increases* as skeletal muscle contractions squeeze blood along the peripheral veins and an increased breathing rate pulls blood into the venae cavae (the respiratory pump).
- *Cardiac output rises* as a result of the increased venous return. This increase occurs in direct response to ventricular stretching (the Frank-Starling law) and in a reflexive response to atrial stretching (the atrial reflex). ∞ *p. 369* The increased cardiac output keeps pace with the elevated demand, and arterial pressures are maintained despite the drop in peripheral resistance.

This regulation by venous feedback gradually increases cardiac output to about double resting levels.

Over this range, typical of light exercise, the pattern of blood distribution remains relatively unchanged.

At higher levels of exertion, other physiological adjustments occur as the sympathetic nervous system stimulates the cardiac and vasomotor centers. Cardiac output increases, arterial blood pressure increases, and blood flow is severely restricted to "nonessential" organs, such as those of the digestive system, in order to increase the blood flow to active skeletal muscles. When you exercise at maximal levels, your blood essentially races among your skeletal muscles, lungs, and heart. Only the blood supply to the brain is unaffected.

✱ HYPERTENSION

A consistent elevation of the blood pressure is called *hypertension*. Approximately 50 million Americans have hypertension. The diagnosis is made when the average of two or more diastolic blood pressure measurements taken on two different occasions is 90 mm Hg or higher or when the average of two or more systolic blood pressure measurements taken on two different occasions is 140 mm Hg or higher.

The blood pressure is a function of cardiac output and peripheral vascular resistance. An increase in cardiac output, peripheral vascular resistance, or both will increase the blood pressure. A specific cause of hypertension has not been determined. However, both genetic and environmental factors appear responsible for its development.

Chronic hypertension damages the walls of systemic blood vessels. Prolonged vasoconstriction and high pressures within these vessels, particularly the arteries and arterioles, causes the vessels to thicken and strengthen to withstand the stress.

Treatment of hypertension depends on the severity. Exercise, dietary changes, weight control, and medications can keep blood pressure under control and reduce the long-term complications.

Cardiovascular Response to Hemorrhaging

In Chapter 12 we considered the local circulatory reaction to a break in the wall of a blood vessel. ∞ *p. 348* When the clotting response fails to prevent a significant blood loss and arterial blood pressure falls, the entire cardiovascular system begins making adjustments. The immediate goal is to maintain adequate blood pressure and peripheral blood flow. The long-term goal is to restore normal blood volume. Short-term and long-term responses are diagrammed in Figure 14-10a•.

The Elevation of Blood Pressure

Short-term responses appear almost as soon as blood pressures start to decline, when the carotid and aortic reflexes increase cardiac output and cause peripheral vasoconstriction. When you donate blood at a blood bank, the amount collected is usually 500 ml, roughly 10 percent of your total blood volume. Such a loss initially causes a drop in cardiac output, but the vasomotor center quickly improves venous return and restores cardiac output to normal levels by a combination of vasoconstriction and mobilization of the **venous reserve** (large reservoirs of slowly moving venous blood in the liver, bone marrow, and skin). This venous compensation can restore normal arterial pressures and peripheral blood flow after losses that amount to 15–20 percent of the total blood volume. With a more substantial blood loss, cardiac output is maintained by increasing the heart rate, often to 180–200 bpm. Sympathetic activation assists by constricting the muscular arteries and arterioles and elevating blood pressure.

Sympathetic activation also causes the secretion of E and NE by the adrenal medullae. At the same time, ADH is released by the posterior pituitary gland, and at the kidneys the fall in blood pressure causes the release of renin, initiating the activation of angiotensin II. The E and NE increase cardiac output, and in combination with ADH and angiotensin II, they cause a powerful vasoconstriction that elevates blood pressure and improves peripheral blood flow.

The Restoration of Blood Volume

After a serious hemorrhage, several days may pass before the blood volume returns to normal. When the short-term responses are unable to maintain normal cardiac output and blood pressure, the decline in capillary blood pressure promotes the reabsorption of fluid from the interstitial spaces. Over this period, ADH and aldosterone promote fluid retention and reabsorption at the kidneys, preventing further reductions in blood volume. Thirst increases, and additional water is absorbed across the digestive tract. This intake of fluid elevates plasma volume and ultimately replaces the interstitial fluids "borrowed" at the capillaries. Erythropoietin targets the bone marrow, stimulating the maturation of red blood cells, which increase the blood volume and improve oxygen delivery to peripheral tissues.

✓ How would applying a small pressure to the carotid artery affect your heart rate?

✓ Why does blood pressure increase during exercise?

✓ What effect would the vasoconstriction of the renal artery have on blood pressure and blood volume?

THE BLOOD VESSELS

As discussed in Chapter 13, the circulatory system is divided into the **pulmonary circuit** and the **systemic circuit**. 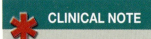 *p. 356* The pulmonary circuit is composed of arteries and veins that transport blood between the heart and the lungs. This circuit begins at the right ventricle and ends at the left atrium. From the left ventricle, the arteries of the systemic circuit transport oxygenated blood and nutrients to all organs and tissues, ultimately returning deoxygenated blood to the right atrium.

Arteries and veins on the left and right sides of the body are usually identical—except near the heart, where large vessels connect to the atria or ventricles. For example, the distribution of the *left* and *right sub-*

CLINICAL NOTE　　　　　　　　　　**SHOCK**

Shock (hypoperfusion) is a state of inadequate tissue perfusion and is often the end product of many disease and injury processes. During shock, body tissues are deprived of oxygen and essential nutrients. At the same time, carbon dioxide and other waste products accumulate. Regardless of the cause, shock results from one of three physiological problems. These include an inadequate pump (*cardiogenic shock*), inadequate fluid (*hypovolemic shock*), or an inadequate container (*neurogenic shock*). All of these can result in a fall in blood pressure and, ultimately, inadequate tissue perfusion.

Cardiogenic shock occurs when the heart fails as an effective pump. This is a complication of heart attack or congestive heart failure. *Hypovolemic shock* results from the loss of blood or plasma from the intravascular space. It is seen following severe hemorrhage, burns, crush injuries, and severe nausea and vomiting. *Neurogenic shock* occurs when autonomic control of peripheral blood vessels is lost, resulting in marked dilation and a marked decrease in peripheral vascular resistance. This can be seen following a spinal cord injury where nerve fibers are severed. It can also be seen in severe allergic reactions (*anaphylactic shock*) where histamine and other chemical mediators cause marked peripheral vascular dilation and loss of plasma from the capillaries. Thus, anaphylactic shock involves problems with both fluid loss and peripheral vascular dilation. Another form of neurogenic shock, *septic shock*, occurs following a severe bacterial infection, whereby bacteria release potent *endotoxins* that cause marked peripheral vasodilation resulting in shock.

The signs and symptoms of shock, which can often be subtle, include altered mental status; pale, cool, clammy skin; nausea and vomiting; increased pulse rate; increased respiratory rate; and a fall in blood pressure. A fall in blood pressure is considered a late sign. Shock is best treated when it is promptly identified and emergency interventions are provided before the blood pressure falls.

clavian, axillary, brachial, and *radial arteries* parallels the *left* and *right subclavian, axillary, brachial,* and *radial veins.* In addition, vessels often change names as they pass specific anatomical boundaries. For example, the *external iliac artery* becomes the *femoral artery* as it leaves the trunk and enters the thigh. Lastly, both arteries and veins often make anastomotic, or direct, connections. These connections reduce the impact of a temporary or permanent blockage (*occlusion*) of a single vessel. For example, the *radial* and *ulnar arteries* form an anastomosis from which the *digital arteries* originate.

The Pulmonary Circulation

Blood entering the right atrium has just returned from a trip to peripheral capillary beds, where oxygen was released and carbon dioxide absorbed. After traveling through the right atrium and ventricle, blood enters the **pulmonary trunk** (*pulmo-*, lung), the start of the pulmonary circuit. In this circuit, oxygen stores will be replenished, carbon dioxide excreted, and the "renewed"

blood returned to the heart for distribution in the systemic circuit.

Figure 14-11• details the anatomy of the pulmonary circuit. The arteries of the pulmonary circuit differ from those of the systemic circuit in that they carry deoxygenated blood. (For this reason, color-coded diagrams usually show the pulmonary arteries in blue, the same color as systemic veins.) As the pulmonary trunk curves over the superior border of the heart, that vessel gives rise to the **left** and **right pulmonary arteries**. These large arteries enter the lungs before branching repeatedly, giving rise to smaller and smaller arteries. The smallest branches, the pulmonary arterioles, provide blood to capillary networks that surround small air pockets, or **alveoli** (al-VĒ-ōl-ī; *alveolus*, sac). The walls of alveoli are thin enough for gas exchange to occur between the capillary blood and inspired air, a process detailed in Chapter 16. As it leaves the alveolar capillaries, oxygenated blood enters venules, which in turn unite to form larger vessels carrying blood to the **pulmonary veins**. These four veins, two from each lung, empty into the left atrium, completing the pulmonary circuit.

•**FIGURE 14-11   The Pulmonary Circuit**

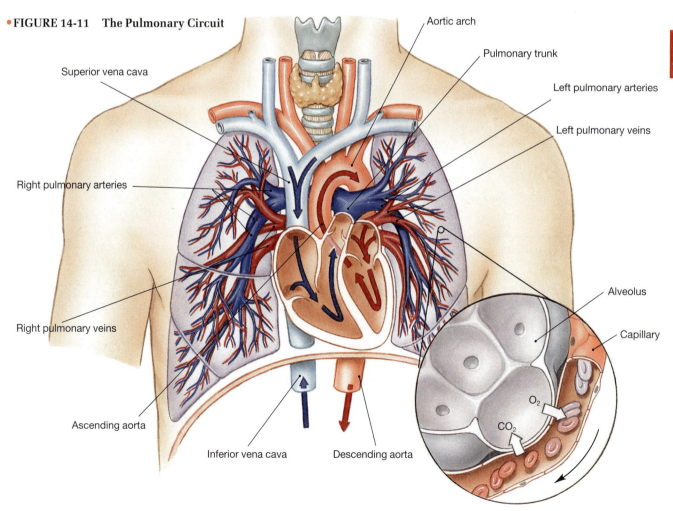

Superior vena cava

Right pulmonary arteries

Right pulmonary veins

Ascending aorta

Inferior vena cava

Descending aorta

Aortic arch

Pulmonary trunk

Left pulmonary arteries

Left pulmonary veins

Alveolus

Capillary

O_2

CO_2

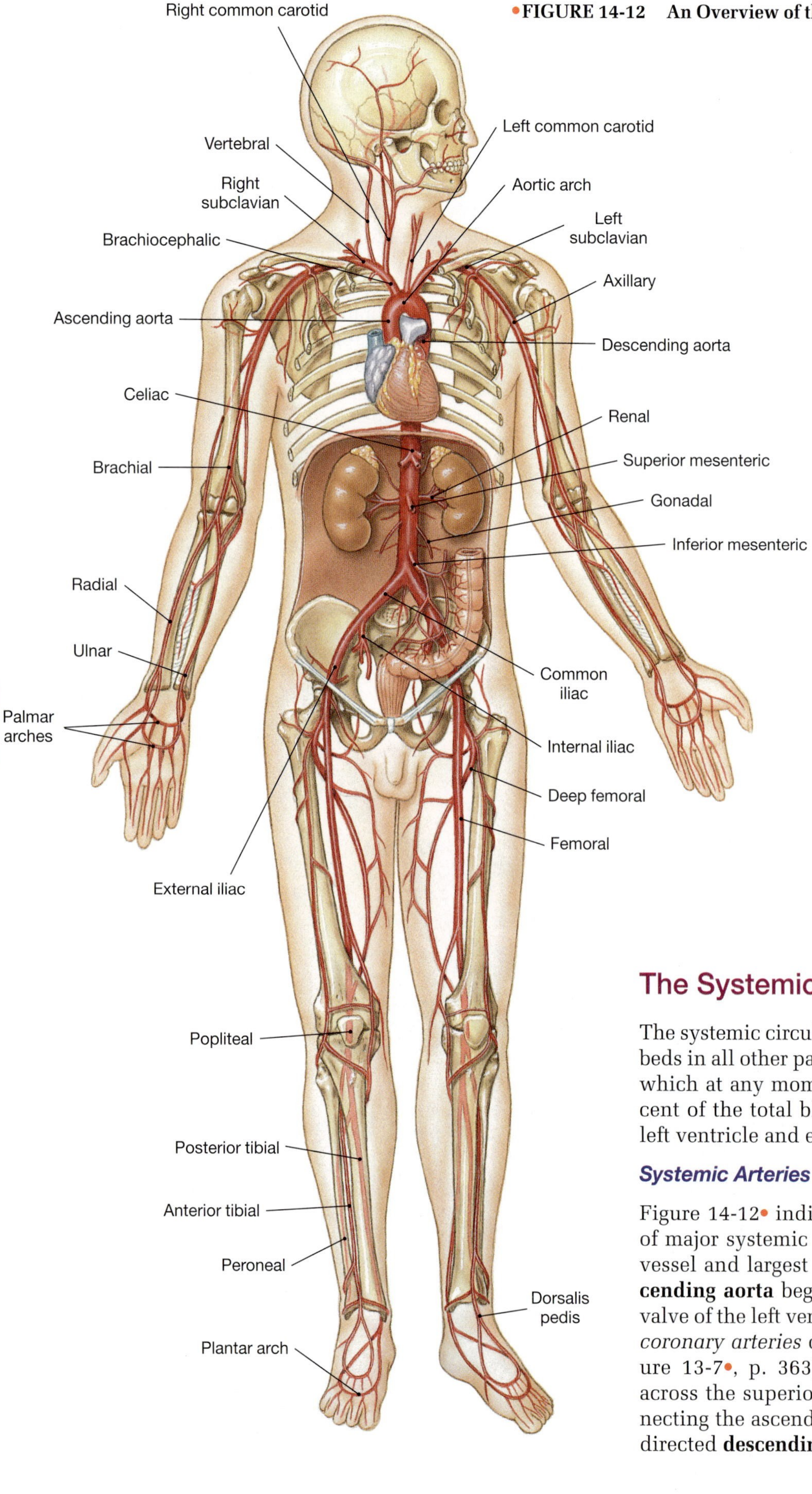

•FIGURE 14-12   An Overview of the Arterial System

Labels on figure (clockwise):
- Right common carotid
- Vertebral
- Right subclavian
- Brachiocephalic
- Ascending aorta
- Celiac
- Brachial
- Radial
- Ulnar
- Palmar arches
- External iliac
- Popliteal
- Posterior tibial
- Anterior tibial
- Peroneal
- Plantar arch
- Dorsalis pedis
- Left common carotid
- Aortic arch
- Left subclavian
- Axillary
- Descending aorta
- Renal
- Superior mesenteric
- Gonadal
- Inferior mesenteric
- Common iliac
- Internal iliac
- Deep femoral
- Femoral

The Systemic Circulation

The systemic circulation supplies the capillary beds in all other parts of the body. This circuit, which at any moment contains about 84 percent of the total blood volume, begins at the left ventricle and ends at the right atrium.

Systemic Arteries

Figure 14-12• indicates the relative locations of major systemic arteries. The first systemic vessel and largest artery is the aorta. The **ascending aorta** begins at the aortic semilunar valve of the left ventricle, and the *left* and *right coronary arteries* originate near its base (Figure 13-7•, p. 363). The **aortic arch** curves across the superior surface of the heart, connecting the ascending aorta with the caudally directed **descending aorta**.

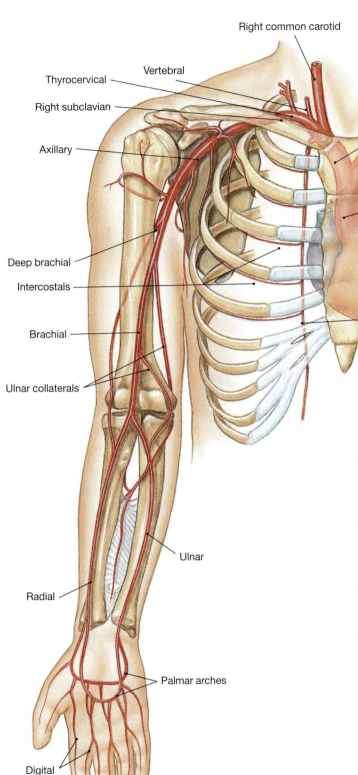

Right common carotid

Thyrocervical
Vertebral

Right subclavian

Axillary

Deep brachial

Intercostals

Brachial

Ulnar collaterals

Radial

Ulnar

Palmar arches

Digital arteries

Left common carotid

Brachiocephalic

Left subclavian

Aortic arch

Ascending aorta

Descending aorta

Heart

Internal thoracic

Descending aorta

•FIGURE 14-13   Arteries of the Chest and Upper Limb

Arteries of the Aortic Arch.   Three elastic arteries originate along the aortic arch (Figure 14-13•). These arteries, the **brachiocephalic** (brāk-ē-ō-se-FAL-ik), the **left common carotid**, and the **left subclavian** (sub-CLĀ-vē-an), deliver blood to the head, neck, shoulders, and upper limbs. The brachiocephalic artery ascends for a short distance before branching to form the **right common carotid artery** and the **right subclavian artery**. Thus, as the figure makes clear, there is only one brachiocephalic artery, and the left common carotid and left subclavian arteries arise separately from the aortic arch. In terms of their peripheral distribution, however, the vessels on the left side are mirror images of those on the right side. Because the following descriptions focus on major branches found on both sides of the body, the terms *right* and *left* will not be used. Figures 14-12• and 14-13• illustrate the major branches of these arteries, and additional details are included in the flow chart in Figure 14-14•.

The Subclavian Arteries.   The subclavian arteries supply blood to the upper limbs, chest wall, shoulders, back, and central nervous system. Before a subclavian artery leaves the thoracic cavity (Figure 14-13•), it gives rise to an *internal thoracic artery*, which supplies the pericardium and anterior wall of the chest, and a **vertebral artery**, which provides blood to the brain and spinal cord.

After passing the first rib, the subclavian gets a new name, the axillary artery (Figure 14-13•). The **axillary artery** crosses the axilla (armpit) to enter the arm, where

1
4

its name changes again, becoming the **brachial artery**. The brachial artery provides blood to the arm before branching to create the **radial artery** and **ulnar artery** of the forearm. These arteries are connected by anastomoses at the palm, and the *digital arteries* originate from these arterial connections.

The Carotid Artery and the Blood Supply to the Brain.

Figure 14-15a● follows the arterial supply to the brain. The common carotids ascend deep in the tissues of the neck. A carotid artery can usually be located by pressing gently along either side of the trachea until a strong pulse is felt. Each common carotid artery divides into an **external carotid** and an **internal carotid artery** at an expanded chamber, the **carotid sinus**. (This sinus, which contains baroreceptors involved in cardiovascular regulation, was introduced in Chapter 10.) ∞ *p. 274* The external carotids supply blood to the pharynx, esophogus, larynx, and face. The internal carotids enter the skull to deliver blood to the brain.

The brain is extremely sensitive to changes in its circulatory supply. An interruption of circulation for several seconds will produce unconsciousness, and after 4 minutes there may be permanent neural damage. Such circulatory crises are rare, because blood reaches the

brain through the vertebral arteries and by way of the internal carotids. The vertebral arteries ascend within the transverse foramina of the cervical vertebrae, penetrating the skull at the foramen magnum. Inside the cranium, they fuse to form a large **basilar artery**, which continues along the ventral surface of the brain. This artery gives rise to the vessels in Figure 14-15b●.

Normally, the internal carotids supply the arteries of the anterior half of the cerebrum, and the rest of the brain receives blood from the vertebral arteries. But this circulatory pattern can easily change, because the internal carotids and the basilar artery are interconnected in the **cerebral arterial circle**, or *circle of Willis*, a ring-shaped anastomosis that encircles the infundibulum (stalk) of the pituitary gland. Thus the brain can receive blood from either the carotids or the vertebrals, and the chances for a serious interruption of circulation are reduced. However, a plaque, blood clot, or rupture in one of the smaller arteries supplying the brain will injure or kill the dependent tissues. Symptoms of a *stroke*, or *cerebrovascular accident (CVA)*, then appear.

The Descending Aorta.

The descending aorta is divided—in name only—into a superior **thoracic aorta** and an inferior **abdominal aorta**, with the diaphragm

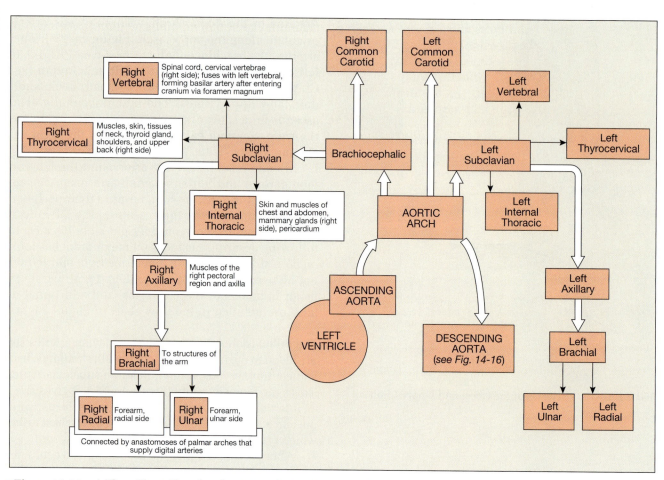

● **Figure 14-14**   **A Flow Chart Showing the Arterial Distribution to the Head, Chest, and Upper Limbs**

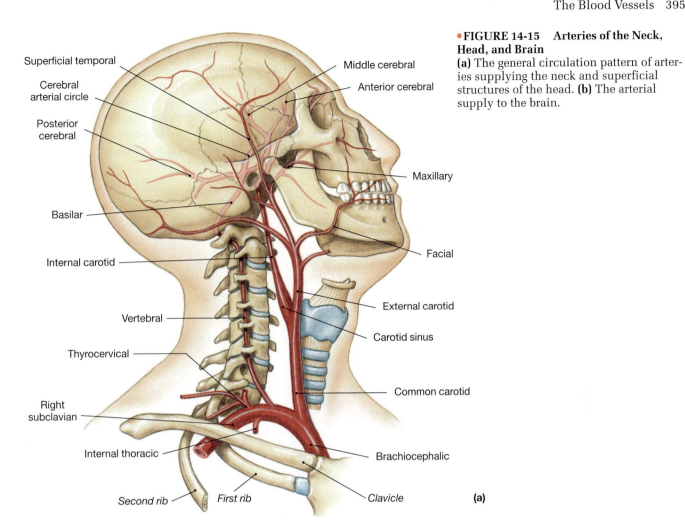

Superficial temporal

Cerebral arterial circle

Posterior cerebral

Basilar

Internal carotid

Vertebral

Thyrocervical

Right subclavian

Internal thoracic

Second rib

First rib

Middle cerebral

Anterior cerebral

Maxillary

Facial

External carotid

Carotid sinus

Common carotid

Brachiocephalic

Clavicle

(a)

•FIGURE 14-15   Arteries of the Neck, Head, and Brain
(a) The general circulation pattern of arteries supplying the neck and superficial structures of the head. (b) The arterial supply to the brain.

1
4

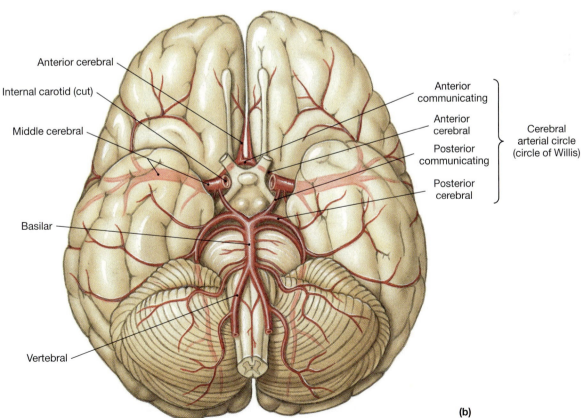

Anterior cerebral

Internal carotid (cut)

Middle cerebral

Basilar

Vertebral

Anterior communicating

Anterior cerebral

Posterior communicating

Posterior cerebral

Cerebral arterial circle (circle of Willis)

(b)

marking the boundary between the two regions (Figure 14-16•). The thoracic aorta travels within the mediastinum, providing blood to the intercostal arteries, which carry blood to the spinal cord and the body wall. The thoracic aorta also gives rise to small arteries that end in capillary beds in the esophagus, pericardium, and other mediastinal structures. Near the diaphragm, the **phrenic** (FREN-ik) **arteries** deliver blood to the

muscular diaphragm that separates the thoracic and abdominopelvic cavities. The branches of the thoracic aorta are detailed in Figure 14-16•.

The abdominal aorta delivers blood to elastic arteries that distribute blood to visceral organs of the digestive system and to the kidneys and adrenal glands. The **celiac** (SĒ-lē-ak) **artery**, **superior mesenteric** (mez-en-TER-ik) **artery**, and **inferior mesenteric artery** arise

• **FIGURE 14-16**
Major Arteries of the Trunk

(a) A diagrammatic view.

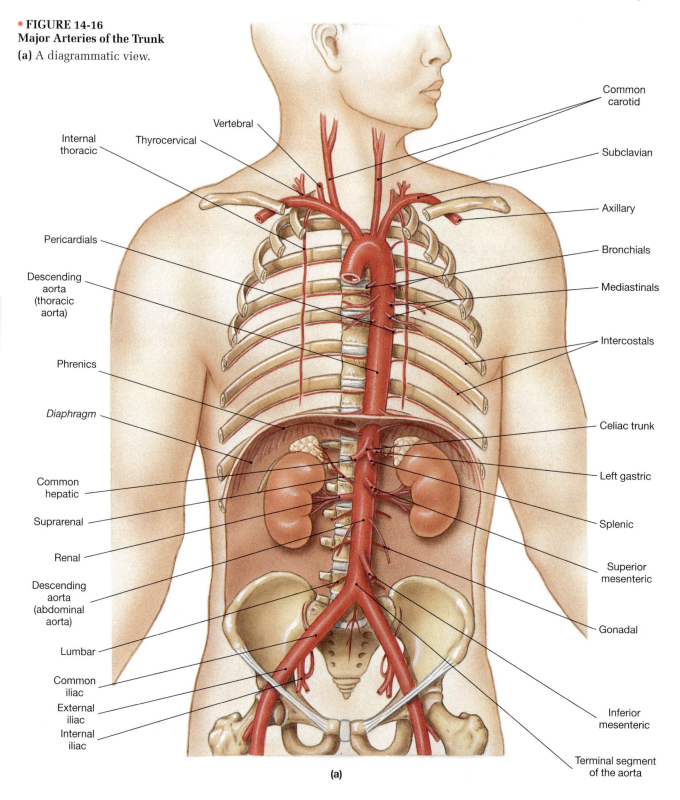

(a)

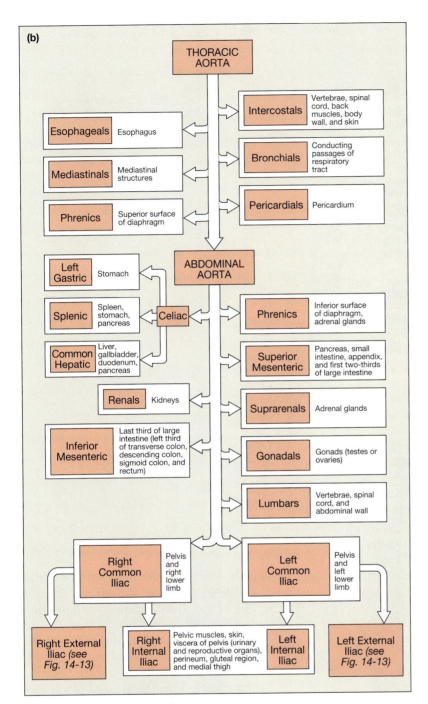

(b)

THORACIC AORTA

Intercostals	Vertebrae, spinal cord, back muscles, body wall, and skin
Bronchials	Conducting passages of respiratory tract
Pericardials	Pericardium

Esophageals	Esophagus
Mediastinals	Mediastinal structures
Phrenics	Superior surface of diaphragm

ABDOMINAL AORTA

Left Gastric	Stomach
Splenic	Spleen, stomach, pancreas
Common Hepatic	Liver, gallbladder, duodenum, pancreas

Celiac

Renals	Kidneys
Inferior Mesenteric	Last third of large intestine (left third of transverse colon, descending colon, sigmoid colon, and rectum)

Phrenics	Inferior surface of diaphragm, adrenal glands
Superior Mesenteric	Pancreas, small intestine, appendix, and first two-thirds of large intestine
Suprarenals	Adrenal glands
Gonadals	Gonads (testes or ovaries)
Lumbars	Vertebrae, spinal cord, and abdominal wall

Right Common Iliac	Pelvis and right lower limb
Left Common Iliac	Pelvis and left lower limb

Right External Iliac (see Fig. 14-13)	
Right Internal Iliac	Pelvic muscles, skin, viscera of pelvis (urinary and reproductive organs), perineum, gluteal region, and medial thigh
Left Internal Iliac	
Left External Iliac (see Fig. 14-13)	

•**FIGURE 14-16 (continued)**
(b) A flow chart.

Paired **gonadal** (gō-NAD-al) **arteries** originate between the superior and inferior mesenteric arteries. In males they are called *testicular arteries*; in females, *ovarian arteries.*

The **suprarenal arteries** and **renal arteries** arise along the lateral surface of the abdominal aorta and travel behind the peritoneal lining to reach the adrenal glands and kidneys. Small **lumbar arteries** begin on the posterior surface of the aorta and supply the spinal cord and the abdominal wall.

Near the level of vertebra L_4, the abdominal aorta divides to form a pair of muscular arteries. These **common iliac** (IL-ē-ak) **arteries** carry blood to the pelvis and lower limbs (see Figure 14-12•). As it travels along the inner surface of the ilium, each common iliac divides to form an **internal iliac artery**, which supplies smaller arteries of the pelvis, and an **external iliac artery**, which enters the lower limb.

Once in the thigh, the external iliac artery branches, forming the **femoral artery** and the **deep femoral artery**. When it reaches the back of the knee, the femoral artery becomes the **popliteal artery**, which almost immediately branches to form the **anterior tibial**, **posterior tibial**, and **peroneal arteries**. These arteries are connected by two anastomoses, one on the top of the foot (the *dorsalis pedis*) and one on the bottom (the *plantar arch*).

Systemic Veins

Figure 14-17• illustrates the major vessels of the venous system. Complementary arteries and veins often run side by side, and in many cases they have comparable names. For example, the axillary arteries run alongside the axillary veins. In addition, arteries and veins often travel in the company of peripheral nerves that have the same names and innervate the same structures.

on the anterior surface of the abdominal aorta and branch in the connective tissues of the mesenteries. These three vessels provide blood to all of the digestive organs in the abdominopelvic cavity. The celiac divides into three branches that deliver blood to the liver, gallbladder, stomach, and spleen. The superior mesenteric artery supplies the pancreas, small intestine, and most of the large intestine. The inferior mesenteric delivers blood to the last portion of the large intestine and rectum.

One significant difference between the arterial and venous systems concerns the distribution of major veins in the neck and limbs. Arteries in these areas are not found at the body surface; instead, they are deep beneath the skin, protected by bones and surrounding soft tissues. In contrast, there are usually two sets of peripheral veins, one superficial and the other deep. The superficial veins are so close to the surface that they can be seen quite easily. This location makes them easy targets for obtaining blood samples; most blood

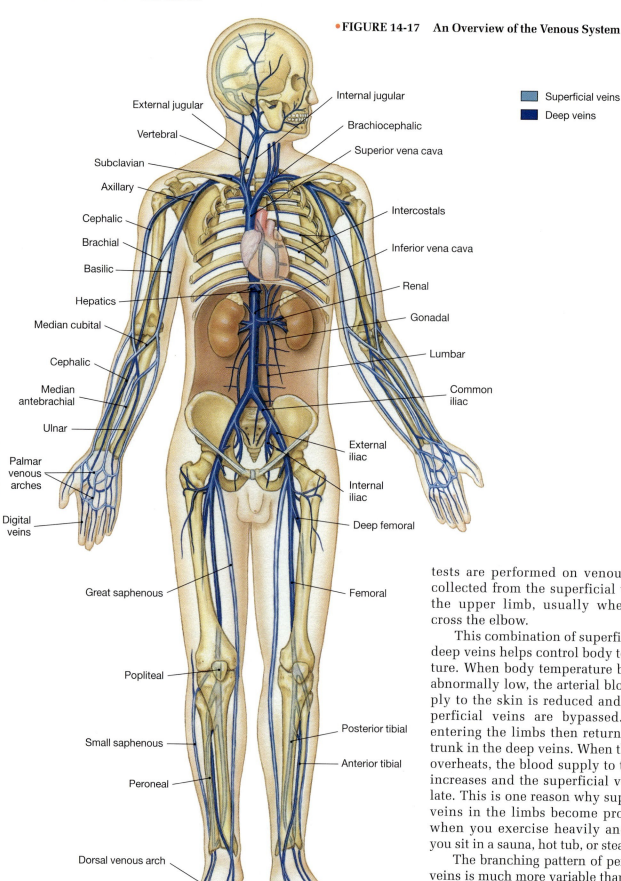

•FIGURE 14-17   **An Overview of the Venous System**

Superficial veins
Deep veins

External jugular

Internal jugular

Vertebral

Brachiocephalic

Subclavian

Superior vena cava

Axillary

Cephalic

Intercostals

Brachial

Inferior vena cava

Basilic

Hepatics

Renal

Median cubital

Gonadal

Cephalic

Lumbar

Median antebrachial

Common iliac

Ulnar

External iliac

Palmar venous arches

Internal iliac

Digital veins

Deep femoral

Great saphenous

Femoral

Popliteal

Posterior tibial

Small saphenous

Anterior tibial

Peroneal

Dorsal venous arch

Plantar venous arch

tests are performed on venous blood collected from the superficial veins of the upper limb, usually where they cross the elbow.

This combination of superficial and deep veins helps control body temperature. When body temperature becomes abnormally low, the arterial blood supply to the skin is reduced and the superficial veins are bypassed. Blood entering the limbs then returns to the trunk in the deep veins. When the body overheats, the blood supply to the skin increases and the superficial veins dilate. This is one reason why superficial veins in the limbs become prominent when you exercise heavily and when you sit in a sauna, hot tub, or steam bath.

The branching pattern of peripheral veins is much more variable than that of arteries. Arterial pathways are usually direct because developing arteries grow toward active tissues. By the time blood

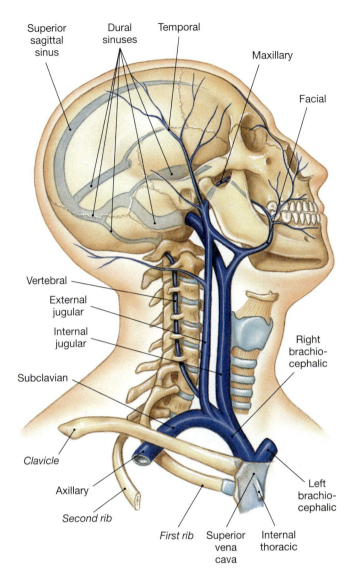

Superior sagittal sinus

Dural sinuses

Temporal

Maxillary

Facial

Vertebral

External jugular

Internal jugular

Subclavian

Clavicle

Axillary

Second rib

First rib

Superior vena cava

Internal thoracic

Right brachio-cephalic

Left brachio-cephalic

•FIGURE 14-18   Major Veins of the Head and Neck
Veins draining superficial and deep portions of the head and neck.

reaches the venous system, pressures are low and routing variations make little functional difference.

The Superior Vena Cava.

The **superior vena cava (SVC)** receives blood from the head and neck (Figure 14-18•), and the chest, shoulders, and upper limbs (Figure 14-19•).

Venous Return from the Head and Neck.

Small veins in the neural tissue of the brain empty into a network of thin-walled channels, the **dural sinuses**. The largest and most important sinus, the **superior sagittal sinus**, is located within the fold of dura mater lying between the cerebral hemispheres. Most of the blood leaving the brain passes through one of the dural sinuses and enters one of the **internal jugular veins**, which penetrate the jugular foramen and descend in the deep tissues of the neck. The more superficial **external jugular veins** collect blood from the overlying structures of the head and neck. These veins travel just beneath the skin, and a *jugular venous pulse (JVP)* can sometimes be detected at the base of the neck. **Vertebral veins** drain the cervical spinal cord and the posterior surface of the skull, descending within the transverse foramina of the cervical vertebrae along with the vertebral arteries.

Venous Return from the Limbs and Chest.

The major veins of the upper body are indicated in Figure 14-19•, and information concerning the venous tributaries of the superior vena cava can be found in Figure 14-20a• (p. 401). A venous network in the palms collects blood from the digital veins. These vessels drain into the **cephalic vein** and the **basilic vein**. The deeper veins of the forearm consist of a **radial vein** and an **ulnar vein**. After crossing the elbow, these veins fuse to form the **brachial vein**. As the brachial vein continues toward the trunk, it joins the basilic vein before entering the axilla as the **axillary vein**. The cephalic vein drains into the axillary vein at the shoulder.

The axillary vein then continues into the trunk; at the level of the first rib it becomes the **subclavian vein**. After traveling a short distance inside the thoracic cavity, the subclavian meets and merges with the external and internal jugular veins of that side. This fusion creates the large **brachiocephalic vein**, also known as the *innominate vein*. Near the heart, the two brachiocephalic veins (one from each side of the body) combine to create the superior vena cava. The SVC receives blood from the thoracic body wall via the **azygos (AZ-i-gos) vein** before arriving at the right atrium.

The Inferior Vena Cava.

The **inferior vena cava (IVC)** collects most of the venous blood from organs below the diaphragm. (A small amount reaches the superior vena cava via the azygos vein.) A flow chart of the tributaries of the IVC is shown in Figure 14-20b•, and the veins of the abdomen are illustrated in Figure 14-19•. Refer to Figure 14-17• for the veins of the lower limbs.

Blood leaving the capillaries in the sole of each foot collects into a network of **plantar veins**. The plantar network provides blood to the **anterior tibial vein**, the **posterior tibial vein**, and the **peroneal vein**, the deep veins of the leg. A *dorsal venous arch* drains blood from capillaries on the superior surface of the foot. This arch is drained by two superficial veins, the **great saphenous vein** (sa-FĒ-nus; *saphenes*, prominent) and the **small saphenous vein**. (Surgeons use segments of the great saphenous vein, the largest superficial vein, as a bypass vessel during *coronary bypass surgery*.) The plantar arch and the dorsal arch interconnect extensively, so the path of blood flow can easily shift from superficial to deep veins.

Behind the knee, the small saphenous, tibial, and peroneal veins unite to form the **popliteal vein**. When the popliteal vein reaches the femur, it becomes the

14

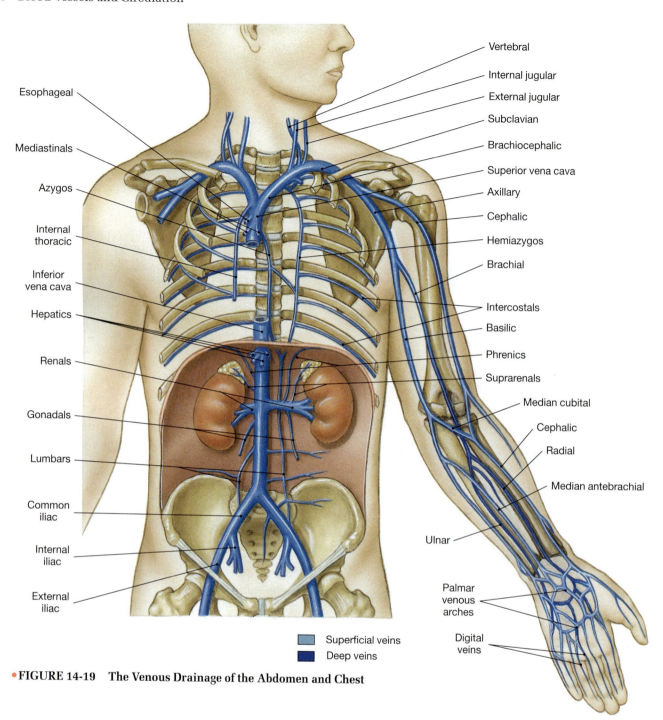

Esophageal

Mediastinals

Azygos

Internal
thoracic

Inferior
vena cava

Hepatics

Renals

Gonadals

Lumbars

Common
iliac

Internal
iliac

External
iliac

Vertebral

Internal jugular

External jugular

Subclavian

Brachiocephalic

Superior vena cava

Axillary

Cephalic

Hemiazygos

Brachial

Intercostals

Basilic

Phrenics

Suprarenals

Median cubital

Cephalic

Radial

Median antebrachial

Ulnar

Palmar
venous
arches

Digital
veins

　Superficial veins
　Deep veins

•FIGURE 14-19　The Venous Drainage of the Abdomen and Chest

femoral vein. Immediately before penetrating the abdominal wall, the femoral, great saphenous, and **deep femoral** veins unite. The large vein that results penetrates the body wall as the **external iliac vein**. As it travels across the inner surface of the ilium, the external iliac fuses with the **internal iliac vein**, which drains the pelvic organs. The resulting common iliac vein then meets its counterpart from the opposite side to form the IVC.

Like the aorta, the IVC lies posterior to the abdominopelvic cavity. As it ascends to the heart, it collects blood from several lumbar veins. In addition, the IVC receives blood from the *gonadal, renal, suprarenal,*

phrenic, and *hepatic veins* before reaching the right atrium (Figure 14-19•).

The Hepatic Portal System.　You may have noticed that the list of veins did not include any names that refer to digestive organs other than the liver. Instead of traveling directly to the inferior vena cava, blood leaving the capillaries supplied by the celiac, superior, and inferior mesenteric arteries flows to the liver via the **hepatic portal system** (*porta,* a gate). Blood in this system is quite different from that in other systemic veins, because the hepatic portal vessels contain substances ab-

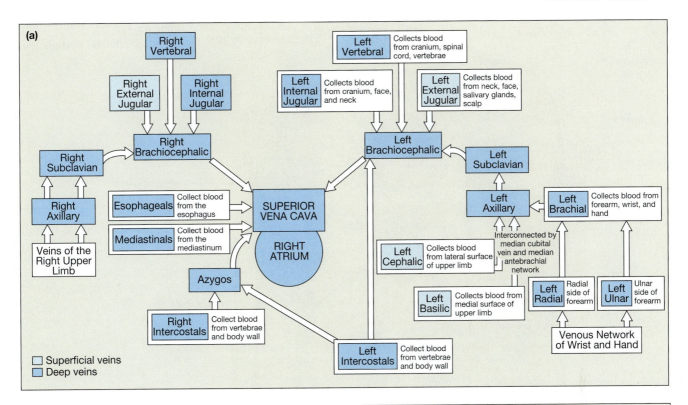

•FIGURE 14-20   **A Flow Chart of the Circulation to the Superior and Inferior Venae Cavae** (a) The tributaries of the SVC. (b) The tributaries of the IVC.

sorbed by the digestive tract. For example, levels of blood glucose, amino acids, fatty acids, and vitamins in the hepatic portal vein often exceed those found anywhere else in the circulatory system.

A portal system carries blood from one capillary bed to another and, in the process, prevents its contents from mixing with the entire bloodstream. The liver regulates the concentrations of nutrients, such as glucose or amino acids, in the circulating blood. When digestion is under way, the digestive tract absorbs high concentrations of nutrients, along with various wastes and an occasional toxin. The hepatic portal system delivers these compounds directly to the liver, where liver cells absorb them for storage, metabolic conversion, or excretion. After passing through the liver capillaries, blood collects into the hepatic veins, which empty into the inferior vena cava. Because blood goes to the liver first, the composition of the blood in the general circulation remains relatively stable, regardless of the digestive activities under way.

Blood delivered to the liver by the hepatic portal system often contains high concentrations of absorbed nutrients, but it is venous blood that contains relatively little oxygen. The liver cells obtain oxygen from arterial blood from the hepatic artery, a branch of the celiac trunk. Liver cells are thus exposed to a mixture of portal blood and arterial blood.

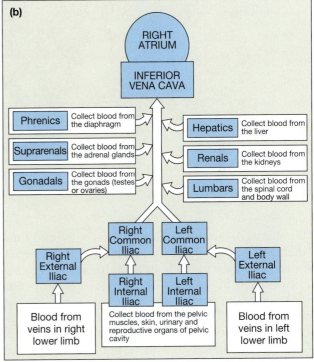

Figure 14-21• shows the anatomy of the hepatic portal system. The system begins in the capillaries of the digestive organs. Blood from capillaries along the lower portion of the large intestine enters the **inferior mesenteric vein**. As it nears the liver, veins from the spleen, the lateral border of the stomach, and the pancreas fuse with the inferior mesenteric, forming the **splenic vein**. The **superior mesenteric vein** also drains the lateral border

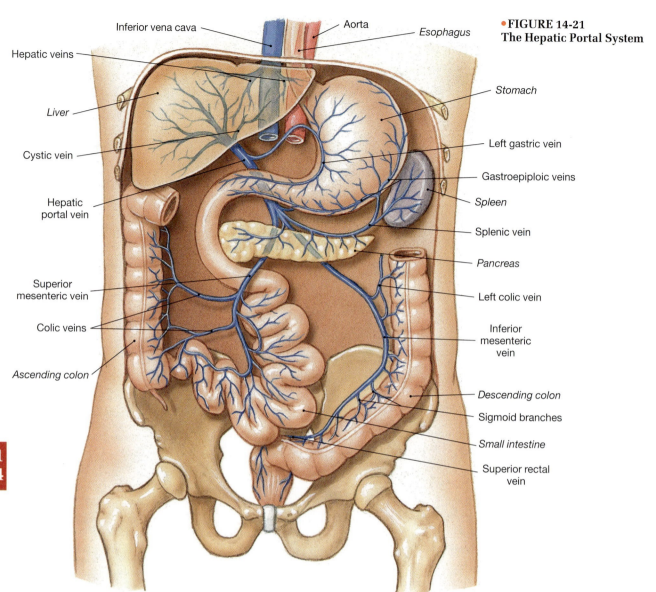

● **FIGURE 14-21**
The Hepatic Portal System

Inferior vena cava

Aorta

Esophagus

Hepatic veins

Liver

Cystic vein

Hepatic portal vein

Superior mesenteric vein

Colic veins

Ascending colon

Stomach

Left gastric vein

Gastroepiploic veins

Spleen

Splenic vein

Pancreas

Left colic vein

Inferior mesenteric vein

Descending colon

Sigmoid branches

Small intestine

Superior rectal vein

of the stomach, through an anastomosis with one of the branches of the splenic vein. In addition, the superior mesenteric collects blood from the entire small intestine and two-thirds of the large intestine. The system ends with the **hepatic portal vein**, which empties into the liver capillaries. The hepatic portal vein forms through the fusion of the superior mesenteric and splenic veins. Of the two, the superior mesenteric normally contributes the greater volume of blood and most of the nutrients.

✓ The blockage of which branch of the aortic arch would interfere with the blood flow to the left arm?

✓ Why would the compression of one of the common carotid arteries cause a person to lose consciousness?

✓ Grace is in an automobile accident and ruptures her celiac artery. Which organs would be affected most directly by this injury?

Fetal Circulation

The fetal and adult circulatory systems are significantly different, reflecting different sources of respiratory and nutritional support. The embryonic lungs are collapsed and nonfunctional, and the digestive tract has nothing to digest. All of the embryonic nutritional and respiratory needs are provided by diffusion across the *placenta*, a structure within the uterine wall where the maternal and fetal circulatory systems are in close contact.

Placental Blood Supply

Fetal circulation is diagrammed in Figure 14-22●. Blood flow to the placenta is provided by a pair of **umbilical arteries**, which arise from the internal iliac arteries and enter the umbilical cord. Blood returns from the placenta in the **umbilical vein**, bringing oxygen and nutrients to

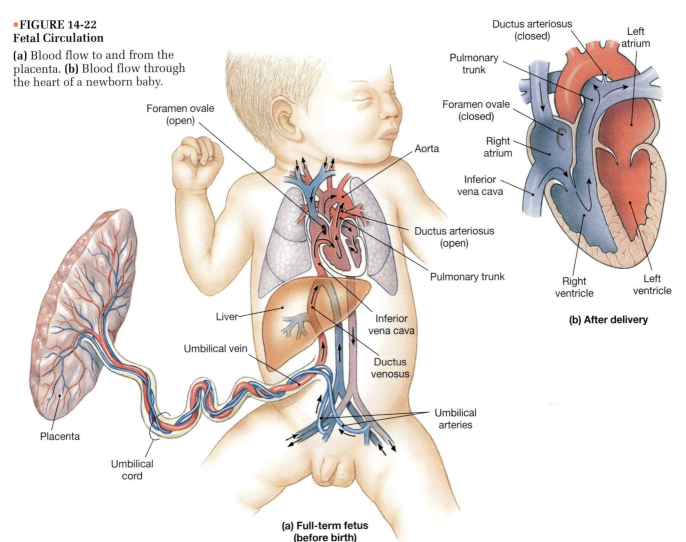

●**FIGURE 14-22**
Fetal Circulation

(a) Blood flow to and from the placenta. **(b)** Blood flow through the heart of a newborn baby.

Foramen ovale (open)

Aorta

Ductus arteriosus (open)

Pulmonary trunk

Liver

Inferior vena cava

Umbilical vein

Ductus venosus

Umbilical arteries

Placenta

Umbilical cord

(a) Full-term fetus (before birth)

Ductus arteriosus (closed)

Left atrium

Pulmonary trunk

Foramen ovale (closed)

Right atrium

Inferior vena cava

Right ventricle

Left ventricle

(b) After delivery

the developing fetus. The umbilical vein delivers blood to capillaries within the developing liver and to the inferior vena cava by the **ductus venosus**. When the placental connection is broken at birth, blood flow ceases along the umbilical vessels, and they soon degenerate.

Circulation in the Heart and Great Vessels

One of the most interesting aspects of circulatory development reflects the differences between the life of an embryo or fetus and that of an infant. Throughout embryonic and fetal life, the lungs are collapsed; yet after delivery, the newborn infant must be able to extract oxygen from inspired air rather than across the placenta.

Although the interatrial and interventricular septa of the heart develop early in fetal life, the interatrial partition remains functionally incomplete up to the time of birth. The interatrial opening, or **foramen ovale**, is associated with an elongate flap that acts as a valve. Blood can flow freely from the right atrium to the left atrium, but any backflow will close the valve and isolate the two chambers. Thus blood can enter the heart

at the right atrium and bypass the pulmonary circuit. A second short-circuit exists between the pulmonary and aortic trunks. This connection, the **ductus arteriosus**, consists of a short, muscular vessel.

With the lungs collapsed, the capillaries are compressed and little blood flows through the lungs. During diastole, blood enters the right atrium and flows into the right ventricle, but it also passes into the left atrium via the foramen ovale. About 25 percent of the blood arriving at the right atrium bypasses the pulmonary circuit in this way. In addition, over 90 percent of the blood leaving the right ventricle passes through the ductus arteriosus and enters the systemic circuit rather than continuing to the lungs.

Circulatory Changes at Birth

At birth, dramatic changes occur in circulatory patterns. When the infant takes its first breath, the lungs expand, and so do the pulmonary vessels. Within a few seconds, the smooth muscles in the ductus arteriosus contract, isolating the pulmonary and aortic trunks, and blood begins flowing through the pulmonary circuit. As pressures rise in the left atrium, the valvular flap closes the foramen ovale and completes the circulatory remodeling (Figure 14-22b•). In adults, the interatrial septum bears a shallow depression, the *fossa ovalis*, that marks the site of the foramen ovale (see Figure 13-4•, p. 359). The remnants of the ductus arteriosus persist as a fibrous cord, the **ligamentum arteriosum**.

If the proper circulatory changes do not occur at birth or shortly thereafter, problems will eventually develop because the blood flow to the lungs will not be sufficient to provide adequate amounts of oxygen. Treatment may involve surgical closure of the foramen ovale, the ductus arteriosus, or both. Other forms of congenital heart defects result from abnormal cardiac development or inappropriate connections between the heart and major arteries and veins.

AGING AND THE CARDIOVASCULAR SYSTEM

The capabilities of the cardiovascular system gradually decline with age. Major changes affect all parts of the cardiovascular system: blood, heart, and vessels.

In the blood, age-related changes may include (1) decreased hematocrit; (2) the constriction or blockage of peripheral veins by the formation of a *thrombus* (stationary blood clot), which can become detached, pass through the heart, and become wedged in a small artery, most often in the lungs, causing a *pulmonary embolism*; (3) the pooling of blood in the veins of the legs because valves are not working effectively.

In the heart, age-related changes include (1) a reduction in the maximum cardiac output; (2) changes in the activities of the nodal and conducting cells; (3) a reduction in the elasticity of the fibrous skeleton; (4) a progressive atherosclerosis, which can restrict coronary circulation; and (5) the replacement of damaged cardiac muscle cells by scar tissue.

In blood vessels, age-related changes are often related to arteriosclerosis, a thickening and toughening of the arterial wall. For example, (1) the inelastic walls of arteries become less tolerant of sudden pressure increases, which can lead to a localized dilation, or *aneurysm*, whose subsequent rupture may cause a stroke, infarct, or massive blood loss, depending on the vessel involved; (2) calcium salts can be deposited on weakened vascular walls, increasing the risk of a stroke or infarct; (3) thrombi can form at atherosclerotic plaques.

INTEGRATION WITH OTHER SYSTEMS

The cardiovascular system is both anatomically and functionally linked to all other systems, as vessel distribution makes clear. Figure 14-23• summarizes the physiological relationships between the cardiovascular system and other organ systems. The most extensive communication occurs between the cardiovascular system and the lymphatic system. Not only are the two systems physically interconnected, but cell populations of the lymphatic system use the cardiovascular system as a highway to move from one part of the body to another. Chapter 15 examines the lymphatic system in detail.

Chapter Review

KEY TERMS

anastomosis, *p. 379*	peripheral resistance, *p. 380*	vasoconstriction, *p. 385*
arteriole, *p. 376*	pulmonary circuit, *p. 390*	vasodilation, *p. 385*
artery, *p. 376*	pulse pressure, *p. 380*	vein, *p. 376*
blood pressure, *p. 380*	respiratory pump, *p. 382*	venule, *p. 376*
capillary, *p. 376*	systemic circuit, *p. 390*	
hepatic portal system, *p. 400*	valve, *p. 379*	

SUMMARY OUTLINE

INTRODUCTION *p. 376*

1. Blood flows through a network of arteries, veins, and capillaries. The vital functions of the cardiovascular system depend on events at the capillary level: All chemical and gaseous exchange between the blood and interstitial fluid takes place across **capillary** walls.

THE ANATOMY OF BLOOD VESSELS *p. 376*

1. Arteries and veins form an internal distribution system, propelled by the heart. **Arteries** branch repeatedly, decreasing in size until they become **arterioles**; from the arterioles, blood enters the capillary networks. Blood flowing from the capillaries enters small **venules** before entering larger **veins**.

INTEGUMENTARY SYSTEM

Stimulation of mast cells produces localized changes in blood flow and capillary permeability

Delivers immune system cells to injury sites; clotting response seals breaks in skin surface; carries away toxins from sites of infection; provides heat

THE CARDIOVASCULAR SYSTEM

FOR ALL SYSTEMS

Delivers oxygen, hormones, nutrients, and WBCs; removes carbon dioxide and metabolic wastes; transfers heat

SKELETAL SYSTEM

Provides calcium needed for normal cardiac muscle contraction; protects blood cells developing in bone marrow

Provides Ca^{2+} and PO_4^{3-} for bone deposition; delivers EPO to bone marrow, parathyroid hormone and calcitonin to osteoblasts and osteoclasts

MUSCULAR SYSTEM

Skeletal muscle contractions assist in moving blood through veins; protects superficial blood vessels, especially in neck and limbs

Delivers oxygen and nutrients, removes carbon dioxide, lactic acid, and heat during skeletal muscle activity

NERVOUS SYSTEM

Controls patterns of circulation in peripheral tissues; modifies heart rate and regulates blood pressure; releases ADH

Endothelial cells maintain blood–brain barrier, help generate CSF

ENDOCRINE SYSTEM

Erythropoietin regulates production of RBCs; several hormones elevate blood pressure; epinephrine stimulates cardiac muscle, elevating heart rate and contractile force

Distributes hormones throughout the body; heart secretes ANP

LYMPHATIC SYSTEM

Defends against pathogens or toxins in blood; fights infections of cardiovascular organs; returns tissue fluid to circulation

Distributes WBCs; carries antibodies that attack pathogens; clotting response assists in restricting spread of pathogens; granulocytes and lymphocytes produced in bone marrow

RESPIRATORY SYSTEM

Provides oxygen to cardiovascular organs and removes carbon dioxide

RBCs transport oxygen and carbon dioxide between lungs and peripheral tissues

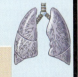

DIGESTIVE SYSTEM

Provides nutrients to cardiovascular organs; absorbs water and ions essential to maintenance of normal blood volume

Distributes digestive tract hormones; carries nutrients, water, and ions away from sites of absorption; delivers nutrients and toxins to liver

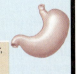

URINARY SYSTEM

Releases renin to elevate blood pressure and erythropoietin to accelerate red blood cell production

Delivers blood to capillaries, where filtration occurs; accepts fluids and solutes reabsorbed during urine production

Maintenance of healthy vessels and a slowing of development of atherosclerosis with age by estrogens

Distributes reproductive hormones; provides nutrients, oxygen, and waste removal for developing fetus; local blood pressure changes responsible for physical changes during sexual arousal

REPRODUCTIVE SYSTEM

• **FIGURE 14-23** **Functional Relationships Between the Cardiovascular System and Other Systems**

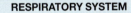
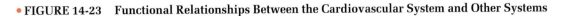
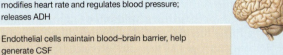
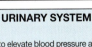
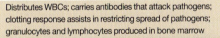
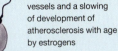

The Structure of Vessel Walls   *p. 376*

2. The walls of arteries and veins contain three layers: the **tunica interna**, **tunica media**, and outermost **tunica externa**. *(Figure 14-1)*

Arteries   *p. 377*

3. In general, the walls of arteries are thicker than the walls of veins. The arterial system includes the large **elastic arteries**, medium-sized **muscular arteries**, and smaller arterioles. As we proceed toward the capillaries, the number of vessels increases, but the diameter of the individual vessels decreases and the walls become thinner.

Capillaries   *p. 377*

4. Capillaries are the only blood vessels whose walls permit exchange between blood and interstitial fluid.

5. Capillaries form interconnected networks called **capillary beds**. A **precapillary sphincter** (a band of smooth muscle) adjusts blood flow into each capillary. Blood flow in a capillary changes as **vasomotion** occurs. *(Figure 14-2)*

Veins   *p. 379*

6. Venules collect blood from capillaries and merge into **medium-sized veins** and then **large veins**. The arterial system is a high-pressure system; pressure in veins is much lower. **Valves** in these vessels prevent backflow of blood. *(Figure 14-3)*

CIRCULATORY PHYSIOLOGY   *p. 379*
Pressure   *p. 379*

1. Flow is proportional to the difference in pressure; blood will flow from an area of higher pressure to one of relatively lower pressure.

Resistance   *p. 380*

2. For circulation to occur, the *circulatory pressure* must be greater than the *total peripheral resistance* (the resistance of the entire circulatory system). For blood to flow into peripheral capillaries, **blood pressure** (arterial pressure) must be greater than the **peripheral resistance** (the resistance of the arterial system). Neural and hormonal control mechanisms regulate blood pressure.

3. The most important determinant of peripheral resistance is the diameter of arterioles.

Circulatory Pressure   *p. 380*

4. The high arterial pressures overcome peripheral resistance and maintain blood flow through peripheral tissues. **Capillary pressures** are normally low; small changes in capillary pressure determine the rate of fluid movement into or out of the bloodstream. Venous pressure, normally low, determines venous return and affects cardiac output and peripheral blood flow.

5. Arterial pressure rises in ventricular systole and falls in ventricular diastole. The difference between the **systolic** and **diastolic pressures** is **pulse pressure**. *(Figures 14-4, 14-6)*

6. At the capillaries, solute molecules diffuse across the capillary lining, and water-soluble materials diffuse through small spaces between endothelial cells. Water will move when driven by either hydrostatic or osmotic pressure. The direction of water movement is determined by the balance between these two opposing pressures. *(Figure 14-5)*

7. Valves, **muscular compression**, and the **respiratory pump** help the relatively low venous pressures propel blood toward the heart. *(Figure 14-3)*

CARDIOVASCULAR REGULATION   *p. 384*

1. Homeostatic mechanisms ensure that tissue blood flow (*tissue perfusion*) delivers adequate oxygen and nutrients.

2. Blood flow varies directly with cardiac output, peripheral resistance, and blood pressure.

3. Local, autonomic, and endocrine factors influence the coordinated regulation of cardiovascular function. Local factors change the pattern of blood flow within capillary beds in response to chemical changes in interstitial fluids. Central nervous system mechanisms respond to changes in arterial pressure or blood gas levels. Hormones can assist in short-term adjustments (changes in cardiac output and peripheral resistance) and long-term adjustments (changes in blood volume that affect cardiac output and gas transport). *(Figure 14-7)*

The Autoregulation of Blood Flow   *p. 384*

4. Peripheral resistance is adjusted at the tissues by local factors that result in the dilation or constriction of precapillary sphincters.

The Neural Control of Blood Pressure and Blood Flow   *p. 385*

5. **Baroreceptor reflexes** are autonomic reflexes that adjust cardiac output and peripheral resistance to maintain normal arterial pressures. Baroreceptor populations include the **aortic** and **carotid sinuses** and *atrial baroreceptors*. *(Figure 14-8)*

6. **Chemoreceptor reflexes** respond to changes in the oxygen or carbon dioxide levels in the blood and cerebrospinal fluid. Sympathetic activation leads to stimulation of the *cardioacceleratory* and *vasomotor centers*; parasympathetic activation stimulates the *cardioinhibitory center*. *(Figure 14-9)*

Hormones and Cardiovascular Regulation   *p. 387*

7. The endocrine system provides short-term regulation of cardiac output and peripheral resistance with epinephrine and norepinephrine from the adrenal medullae. Hormones involved in long-term regulation of blood pressure and volume are antidiuretic hormone (ADH), angiotensin II, erythropoietin (EPO), and atrial natriuretic peptide (ANP). *(Figure 14-10)*

8. ADH and angiotensin II also promote peripheral vasoconstriction in addition to their other functions. ADH and aldosterone promote water and electrolyte retention and stimulate thirst. EPO stimulates red blood cell production. ANP encourages sodium loss, fluid loss, reduces blood pressure, inhibits thirst, and lowers peripheral resistance.

PATTERNS OF CARDIOVASCULAR RESPONSE   *p. 389*
Exercise and the Cardiovascular System   *p. 389*

1. During exercise, blood flow to skeletal muscles increases at the expense of circulation to nonessential organs, and cardiac output rises. Cardiovascular performance improves with training. Athletes have larger stroke volumes, slower resting heart rates, and greater cardiac reserves than do nonathletes.

Cardiovascular Response to Hemorrhaging   *p. 389*

2. Blood loss causes an increase in cardiac output, mobilization of venous reserves, peripheral vasoconstriction, and the liberation of hormones that promote fluid retention and the manufacture of red blood cells.

THE BLOOD VESSELS *p. 390*

1. The peripheral distributions of arteries and veins are usually identical on both sides of the body except near the heart.

The Pulmonary Circulation *p. 391*

2. The **pulmonary circuit** includes the **pulmonary trunk**, the **left** and **right pulmonary arteries**, and the **pulmonary veins**, which empty into the left atrium. *(Figure 14-11)*

The Systemic Circulation *p. 392*

3. In the **systemic circuit**, the **ascending aorta** gives rise to the coronary circulation. The **aortic arch** communicates with the **descending aorta**. *(Figures 14-12 to 14-16)*

4. Arteries in the neck and limbs are deep beneath the skin; in contrast, there are usually two sets of peripheral veins, one superficial and one deep. This dual-venous drainage is important for controlling body temperature.

5. The **superior vena cava (SVC)** receives blood from the head, neck, chest, shoulders, and arms. *(Figures 14-17 to 14-20)*

6. The **inferior vena cava (IVC)** collects most of the venous blood from organs below the diaphragm. *(Figure 14-20)*

7. The **hepatic portal system** directs blood from the other digestive organs to the liver before the blood returns to the heart. *(Figure 14-21)*

Fetal Circulation *p. 402*

8. The *placenta* receives blood from the two **umbilical arteries**. Blood returns to the fetus via the **umbilical vein**, which delivers blood to the **ductus venosus** in the liver. *(Figure 14-22a)*

9. Prior to delivery, blood bypasses the pulmonary circuit by flowing (1) from the right atrium into the left atrium through the **foramen ovale**, and (2) from the pulmonary trunk into the aortic arch via the **ductus arteriosus**. *(Figure 14-22b)*

AGING AND THE CARDIOVASCULAR SYSTEM *p. 404*

1. Age-related changes in the blood can include (1) decreased hematocrit, (2) the constriction or blockage of peripheral veins by a *thrombus* (stationary blood clot), (3) the pooling of blood in the veins of the legs because the valves are not working effectively.

2. Age-related changes in the heart include (1) a reduction in the maximum cardiac output, (2) changes in the activities of the nodal and conducting cells, (3) a reduction in the elasticity of the fibrous skeleton, (4) a progressive **atherosclerosis** that can restrict coronary circulation, and (5) the replacement of damaged cardiac muscle cells by scar tissue.

3. Age-related changes in blood vessels, often related to **arteriosclerosis**, include (1) a reduced tolerance of inelastic walls of arteries to sudden pressure increases, which can lead to an aneurysm; (2) the deposition of calcium salts on weakened vascular walls, increasing the risk of a stroke or infarct; (3) the formation of thrombi at atherosclerotic plaques.

INTEGRATION WITH OTHER SYSTEMS *p. 404*

1. The cardiovascular system delivers oxygen, nutrients, and hormones to all the body systems. *(Figure 14-23)*

REVIEW QUESTIONS

LEVEL 1 Reviewing Facts and Terms

Match each item in column A with the most closely related item in column B. Use letters for answers in the spaces provided.

Column A

___ 1. diastolic pressure

___ 2. arterioles

___ 3. hepatic vein

___ 4. renal vein

___ 5. aorta

___ 6. precapillary sphincter

___ 7. medulla oblongata

___ 8. internal iliac artery

___ 9. external iliac artery

___ 10. baroreceptors

___ 11. systolic pressure

___ 12. saphenous vein

Column B

a. drains the liver

b. largest superficial vein in body

c. carotid sinus

d. minimum blood pressure

e. blood supply to leg

f. blood supply to pelvis

g. peak blood pressure

h. vasomotion

i. largest artery in body

j. drains the kidney

k. vasomotor center

l. smallest arterial vessels

13. Blood vessels that carry blood away from the heart are called:
(a) veins
(b) arterioles
(c) venules
(d) arteries

14. The layer of the arteriole wall that provides the properties of contractility and elasticity is the:
(a) tunica adventitia
(b) tunica media
(c) tunica interna
(d) tunica externa

15. The two-way exchange of substances between blood and body cells occurs only through:
    (a) arterioles   (b) capillaries
    (c) venules   (d) a, b, and c are correct

16. The blood vessels that collect blood from all tissues and organs and return it to the heart are the:
    (a) veins   (b) arteries
    (c) capillaries   (d) arterioles

17. Blood is compartmentalized within the veins because of the presence of:
    (a) venous reservoirs   (b) muscular walls
    (c) clots   (d) valves

18. The most important factor in vascular resistance is:
    (a) the viscosity of the blood
    (b) friction between the blood and the vessel walls
    (c) turbulence due to irregular surfaces of blood vessels
    (d) the length of the blood vessels

19. In a blood pressure reading of 120/80, the 120 represents _____ and the 80 represents _____.
    (a) diastolic pressure; systolic pressure
    (b) pulse pressure; mean arterial pressure
    (c) systolic pressure; diastolic pressure
    (d) mean arterial pressure; pulse pressure

20. Hydrostatic pressure forces water _____ a solution; osmotic pressure forces water _____ a solution.
    (a) into, out of
    (b) out of, into
    (c) out of, out of
    (d) a, b, and c are incorrect

21. The two factors that assist the relatively low venous pressures in propelling blood toward the heart are:
    (a) ventricular systole and valve closure
    (b) gravity and vasomotion
    (c) muscular compression and the respiratory pump
    (d) atrial and ventricular contractions

22. The arteries of the pulmonary circuit differ from those of the systemic circuit in that they carry:
    (a) oxygen and nutrients
    (b) deoxygenated blood
    (c) oxygenated blood
    (d) oxygen, carbon dioxide, and nutrients

23. The two arteries formed by the division of the brachiocephalic artery are the:
    (a) aorta and internal carotid
    (b) axillary and brachial
    (c) external and internal carotid
    (d) common carotid and subclavian

24. The unpaired arteries supplying blood to the visceral organs include the:
    (a) suprarenal, renal, lumbar
    (b) iliac, gonadal, femoral
    (c) celiac, superior and inferior mesenterics
    (d) a, b, and c are correct

25. The artery generally used to feel the pulse at the wrist is the:
    (a) ulnar
    (b) radial
    (c) peroneal
    (d) dorsalis

26. The vein that drains the dural sinuses of the brain is the:
    (a) cephalic
    (b) great saphenous
    (c) internal jugular
    (d) superior vena cava

27. The vein that collects most of the venous blood from below the diaphragm is the:
    (a) superior vena cava
    (b) great saphenous
    (c) inferior vena cava
    (d) azygos

28. (a) What are the primary forces that cause fluid to move out of a capillary and into the interstitial fluid at its arterial end? (b) What are the primary forces that cause fluid to move into a capillary from the interstitial fluid at its venous end?

29. What two effects occur when the baroreceptor response to elevated blood pressure is triggered?

30. What factors affect the activity of chemoreceptors in the carotid and aortic bodies?

31. What circulatory changes occur at birth?

32. What age-related changes take place in the blood, heart, and blood vessels?

LEVEL 2   Reviewing Concepts

33. When dehydration occurs:
    (a) water reabsorption at the kidneys accelerates
    (b) fluids are reabsorbed from the interstitial fluid
    (c) blood osmotic pressure increases
    (d) a, b, and c are correct

34. Increased CO_2 levels in tissues would promote:
    (a) the constriction of precapillary sphincters
    (b) an increase in the pH of the blood
    (c) the dilation of precapillary sphincters
    (d) a decrease of blood flow to tissues

35. Elevated levels of the hormones ADH and angiotensin II will produce:
    (a) increased peripheral vasodilation
    (b) increased peripheral vasoconstriction
    (c) increased peripheral blood flow
    (d) increased venous return

36. Relate the anatomical differences between arteries and veins to their functions.

37. Why do capillaries permit the diffusion of materials whereas arteries and veins do not?

38. Why is blood flow to the brain relatively continuous and constant?

39. An accident victim displays the following symptoms: hypotension; pale, cool, moist skin; confusion and disorientation. Identify her condition and explain why these symptoms occur. If you took her pulse, what would you find?

LEVEL 3   Critical Thinking and Clinical Applications _____

40. Bob is sitting outside on a warm day and is sweating profusely. His friend Mary wants to practice taking blood pressures, and he agrees to play patient. Mary finds that Bob's blood pressure is elevated, even though he is resting and has lost fluid from sweating. (She reasons that fluid loss should lower blood volume and thus blood pressure.) Mary asks you why Bob's blood pressure is high instead of low. What should you tell her?

41. People with allergies frequently take antihistamines and decongestants to relieve their symptoms. The medication's box warns that the medication should not be taken by individuals being treated for high blood pressure. Why?

42. Gina awakens suddenly to the sound of her alarm clock. Realizing she is late for class, she jumps to her feet, feels light-headed, and falls back on her bed. What probably caused this to happen? Why doesn't this always happen?

ANSWERS TO CONCEPT CHECK QUESTIONS

Page 379

1. The blood vessels are veins. Arteries and arterioles have a relatively large amount of smooth muscle tissue in a thick, well-developed tunica media.   **2.** The relaxation of precapillary sphincters would increase the blood flow to a tissue.   **3.** Blood pressure in the arterial system pushes blood into the capillaries. Blood pressure on the venous side is very low, and other forces help keep the blood moving. Valves prevent the blood from flowing backward whenever the venous pressure drops.

Page 382

1. In a normal individual, the pressure should be greater in the aorta and least in the venae cavae. Blood, like other fluids, moves along a pressure gradient from high pressure to low pressure. If the pressure were higher in the inferior vena cava, the blood would flow backward.   **2.** When a person stands for periods of time, blood tends to pool in the lower extremities. The venous return to the heart decreases, and in turn the cardiac output decreases, sending less blood to the brain, causing light-headedness and fainting. A hot day adds to the effect, because body water is lost through sweating.

Page 390

1. Pressure at this site would decrease blood pressure at the carotid sinus, where the carotid baroreceptors are located. This decrease causes a decreased frequency of action potentials along the glossopharyngeal nerve (IX) to the medulla, and more sympathetic impulses will be sent to the heart. The net result will be an increase in the heart rate. **2.** During exercise, (1) blood flow to muscles increases, (2) cardiac output increases, and (3) resistance in visceral tissues increases.   **3.** The vasoconstriction of the renal artery would decrease both blood flow and blood pressure at the kidney. In response, the kidney would increase the amount of renin that it releases, which in turn would lead to an increase in the level of angiotensin II. The angiotensin II will bring about increased blood pressure and increased blood volume.

Page 402

1. The blockage of the left subclavian artery would interfere with blood flow to the left arm, because that artery is the branch of the aortic arch that sends blood to the left arm.   **2.** The common carotid arteries carry blood to the head. A compression of one these arteries would decrease blood flow to the brain and lead to the loss of consciousness or even death.   **3.** Organs served by the celiac artery include the stomach, spleen, liver, and pancreas; these organs would be affected most directly.

1
4

OVERVIEW

The vascular system is responsible for transporting important substances throughout the body. It consists of the arterial system, which delivers blood to the peripheral tissues, and the venous system, which returns the blood to the heart and lungs. Several disease processes arise from the vascular system including aneurysms, deep venous thrombosis, pulmonary emboli, arterial occlusions, and others. Some conditions, such as a ruptured aneurysm, are rapidly fatal. Others, such as varicose veins, rarely cause significant problems. Physicians who specialize in the treatment of blood vessel injuries and illnesses are *vascular surgeons*. These physicians complete a general surgical residency and then fellowship training that concentrates on surgery of the vascular system.

ANEURYSM

An *aneurysm* is a bulging in the weakened wall of a blood vessel. Aneurysms are at risk for rupture, and rupture of aneurysms in the brain, aorta, or heart can be rapidly fatal. The several types of aneurysms include:

- Atherosclerotic
- Dissecting
- Infectious
- Congenital
- Traumatic

Most aneurysms result from atherosclerosis and involve the aorta because the blood pressure there is higher than at any other vessel in the body (Figures A14-1● and A14-2●). An aneurysm usually occurs grad-

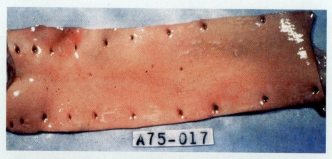

● **FIGURE A14-1**
Postmortem specimen of large artery, opened to reveal only minimal atherosclerotic changes.

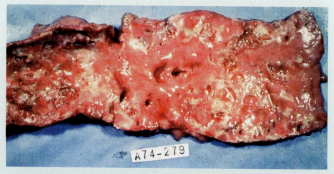

● **FIGURE A14-2**
Marked atherosclerosis in a medium-sized artery causing turbulent blood flow and marked blood flow restriction.

ually. Eventually, blood surges into the aortic wall through a tear in the aortic *tunica intima.* Infectious aneurysms are most commonly associated with syphilis and are rare in the United States. Congenital aneurysms can occur with several disease states, such as Marfan's syndrome, a hereditary disease that affects the connective tissue. Aortic aneurysm occurs in people with Marfan's syndrome because it involves the connective tissue within the vessel wall. Those affected may experience sudden death, usually from spontaneous rupture of the aorta, often at a fairly young age. Aortic aneurysms can occur in the chest or in the abdomen. Thoracic aortic aneurysms usually involve the arch of the aorta. They cause symptoms by eroding into nearby structures. Rupture of a thoracic aortic aneurysm is usually a catastrophic event.

Abdominal Aortic Aneurysm

Abdominal aortic aneurysm usually results from atherosclerosis and occurs most frequently in the aorta, below the renal arteries and above the bifurcation of the common iliac arteries (Figure A14-3●). It is ten times more common in men than in women and most prevalent between ages 60 and 70. Many abdominal aortic aneurysms are detected by physical exam or by diagnostic imaging (X-rays, ultrasound). Nondissecting aneurysms less than 5 centimeters in diameter are usually monitored. Larger aneurysms, or those that are rapidly expanding, require surgical repair.

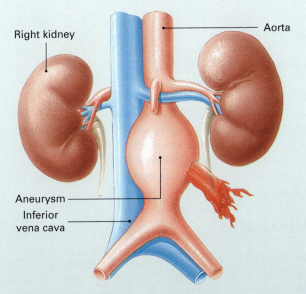

Right kidney

Aorta

Aneurysm

Inferior vena cava

● **FIGURE A14-3   Abdominal Aortic Aneurysm**
Most abdominal aortic aneurysms occur below the branches of the renal arteries and extend down to the bifurcation of the iliac arteries. Rupture can cause rapid exsanguination that will be rapidly fatal without emergent surgical repair.

The signs and symptoms of an abdominal aneurysm include:

- Abdominal pain
- Back and flank pain
- Hypotension
- Urge to defecate, caused by the retroperitoneal leakage of blood

Rupture or leaking of an aortic aneurysm is a surgical emergency. Patients suspected of having this condition should be promptly taken to surgery for repair and grafting. Massive transfusion of blood in these cases is common.

Dissecting Aneurysm

Some aneurysms will begin to dissect within the wall of the blood vessel. Most dissecting aortic aneurysms result from degenerative changes in the smooth muscle and elastic tissue of the aortic tunica media that can result in hematoma and, subsequently, aneurysm. The original tear often is due to *cystic medial necrosis,* a degenerative disease of connective tissue commonly associated with hypertension and to a certain extent, aging. Predisposing factors include hypertension, which is present in 75–85 percent of cases. It occurs more frequently in patients older than 40–50, although it can occur in younger individuals, especially pregnant women. A tendency for this disease also runs in families.

Of dissecting aortic aneurysms, 67 percent involve the ascending aorta. Once dissection has started, it can extend to all of the abdominal aorta as well as its branches, including the coronary arteries, aortic valve, subclavian arteries, and carotid arteries. The aneurysm can rupture at any time, usually into the pericardial or pleural cavity, often causing death.

ACUTE PULMONARY EMBOLISM

Acute pulmonary embolism (PE) occurs when a blood clot or other particle lodges in a pulmonary artery and blocks blood flow through that vessel. Pulmonary emboli may be composed of air, fat, amniotic fluid, or blood clots. Factors that predispose a patient to blood clots include prolonged immobilization, thrombophlebitis (inflammation and clots in a vein), use of certain medications, and atrial fibrillation. Long periods of travel in airplanes and automobiles increase an individual's chances of developing a PE.

When a PE blocks the blood flow through a pulmonary vessel, the right heart must pump against increased resistance, which in turn increases pulmonary capillary pressure (Figure A14-4●). The area of the lung supplied by the occluded vessel then stops functioning, and gas exchange decreases. The larger the volume of the lung affected, the more significant will be the problems with gas exchange.

• FIGURE A14-4

Massive acute pulmonary embolism can cause a sudden increase in pulmonary vascular resistance resulting in right heart failure. This initially causes tachycardia and distended neck veins. If it continues, it can cause accumulation of fluid in the liver (hepatomegaly), spleen (splenomegaly), and in the peritoneal cavity (ascites). Eventually, edema of the extremities develops.

RIGHT HEART FAILURE

Signs
- Tachycardia

- Neck veins engorging and pulsating

- Edema of body and lower extremities

- Engorged liver and spleen

- Abdominal distention (ascites)

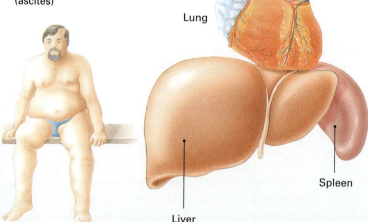

Lung

Spleen

Liver

The signs and symptoms of pulmonary embolism depend upon the size of the obstruction. The patient suffering acute pulmonary embolism may report a sudden onset of severe and unexplained dyspnea that may or may not be associated with chest pain. The signs and symptoms of an acute pulmonary embolism can be subtle and easily overlooked. The diagnosis can be made using several imaging techniques. A frequently used test is the ventilation/perfusion scan (V/Q scan), for which the patient inhales radioactive material and also has radioactive material injected into his or her venous system. Two sets of images of the patient's lungs are obtained, one showing pulmonary ventilation through the respiratory tree and the other showing pulmonary perfusion in the pulmonary circulatory system. Areas of the lung that are ventilated but not perfused indicate a PE. The gold standard for the diagnosis of PE is a pulmonary arteriogram that will show any blockage in the pulmonary circulation. Pulmonary angiograms are higher risk procedures than V/Q scans and require specialized facilities.

The treatment of a PE varies depending upon its size. With small to moderate emboli, the patient will usually receive a blood thinner and be closely monitored in the hospital. Large emboli, as evidenced by marked hypoxia and low blood pressure, may require thrombolytic therapy. In most severe cases, the affected pulmonary artery is catheterized and a thrombolytic agent injected directly into the affected vessel.

ACUTE ARTERIAL OCCLUSION

An acute arterial occlusion is the sudden occlusion of arterial blood flow due to trauma, thrombosis, tumor, embolus, or idiopathic means. Emboli are probably the most common cause of acute arterial occlusion. They can arise from within a chamber of the heart (mural emboli), as from a thrombus in the left ventricle, from an atrial thrombus secondary to atrial fibrillation, or from a thrombus caused by abdominal aortic atherosclerosis. Arterial occlusions most commonly involve vessels in the abdomen or lower extremities.

Acute arterial occlusions are usually treated by an embolectomy, the surgical removal of the clot. In this procedure, a balloon catheter or similar device is inserted in the artery distal to the obstruction. The balloon is inflated, the catheter withdrawn, and the embolus removed from the vessel lumen.

VASCULITIS

Vasculitis is an inflammation of a blood vessel. Most vasculitis stems from a variety of rheumatic diseases and syndromes. The inflammatory process is usually segmental, and inflammation within the tunica media of a muscular artery tends to destroy the internal elastic lamina. Necrosis and hypertrophy (enlarging) of the vessel occur, and the vessel wall has a high likelihood of breaching, leaking fibrin and red blood cells into the surrounding tissue. This potentially can lead to partial or total vascular occlusion and subsequent necrosis.

Raynaud's phenomenon is a type of vasculitis that is characterized by episodic ischemia of the fingers or toes as evidenced by digital blanching, cyanosis, and pain. Cold weather or emotional upset have been identified as triggers. Treatment of Raynaud's involves reassurance and having the patient dress warmly and wear gloves. In severe cases, medications that dilate the blood vessels (calcium-channel blockers) are used.

OTHER PERIPHERAL VASCULAR CONDITIONS

Many peripheral vascular conditions are not considered life threatening but may require prehospital care. They include peripheral arterial atherosclerotic disease, intermittent claudication, deep venous thrombosis, and varicose veins.

Peripheral arterial atherosclerotic disease is a progressive degenerative disease of the medium-sized and large arteries. It affects the aorta and its branches, the brachial and femoral peripheral arteries, and the cerebral arteries. For reasons unknown it does not affect the coronary arteries. It is a gradual, progressive disease, often associated with diabetes mellitus. In extreme cases, significant arterial insufficiency may lead to ulcers and gangrene. Occlusion of the peripheral arteries causes chronic and acute ischemia.

In the chronic setting, intermittent claudication (diminished blood flow in exercising muscle) produces pain with exertion. It occurs most commonly with the calf, but can affect any leg muscle. Rest initially relieves this pain. Most patients with intermittent claudication report being able to walk a given distance before leg pain develops. After they rest and the pain resolves, they can resume walking, but as the disease progresses, the pain begins to occur even at rest. The extremity usually appears normal, but pulses will be reduced or absent. As the ischemia worsens, the extremity becomes painful, cold, and numb, and ulceration, gangrene, and necrosis may be present. There usually is no edema. In the acute setting of intermittent claudication, arterial occlusion from an embolus, aneurysm, or thrombosis occurs. The patient experiences a sudden onset of pain, coldness, numbness, and pallor. Pulses are absent distal to the occlusion. Acute occlusion may cause severe ischemia with motor and sensory deficits. Edema is not present.

Deep venous thrombosis is a blood clot in a vein. It most commonly occurs in the larger veins of the thigh and calf, although the subclavian vein is sometimes involved. Predisposing factors include a recent history of trauma, inactivity, pregnancy, or varicose veins. The patient frequently complains of gradually increasing pain and calf tenderness. Often the leg and foot are swollen because of occluded venous drainage. Leg elevation may alleviate the signs and symptoms. In some cases, the patient may be asymptomatic. Gentle palpation of the calf and thigh may reveal tenderness and, on occasion, cordlike clotted veins. Dorsiflexion of the foot may cause *Homan's sign,* discomfort behind the knee. This is associated with deep venous thrombosis. The skin may be warm and red. Deep venous thrombosis has traditionally been treated with a blood thinner (heparin) and hospitalization with the affected leg elevated. Heparin must be administered by continuous intravenous infusion, and the patient's coagulation profile must be checked frequently to assure proper dosing. In many cases, patients are hospitalized at complete bed rest for 7 to 10 days. With the development of low-molecular-weight heparin (Lovenox), which can be administered by periodic subcutaneous injections, patients with deep venous thrombosis can be treated as outpatients. Patients are instructed to self-administer the drug at home and keep the affected extremity elevated.

Varicose veins are dilated superficial veins, usually in the lower extremities. Predisposing factors include pregnancy, obesity, and genetics. Signs and symptoms include the visible distention of the leg veins, lower leg swelling and discomfort (especially at the end of the day), and skin color and texture changes in the legs and ankles. If the condition is chronic, venous stasis ulcers can develop. Although venous stasis ulcers can rupture, direct pressure usually can control the bleeding, which occasionally is significant. Venous stasis ulcers are usually slow healing and require proper care to prevent additional complications. Treatment of varicose veins primarily involves use of support stockings. Laser therapy and injection of the veins with a sclerosing agent will help improve the legs' cosmetic appearance.

VASCULAR TRAUMA

Injury to the vascular system can interrupt blood flow to the part of the body supplied by the artery. Also, some fractures and dislocations can impinge upon nearby arteries, obstructing blood flow; the blood flow often returns when the affected extremity is returned to its anatomical position. Any vascular structure is subject to injury. Laceration of a moderate-sized artery or vein can cause life-threatening hemorrhage. If the vessel is cut cleanly, however, as with a knife, the muscles in the wall of the vessel contract, which constricts the vessel lumen and retracts the end of the severed vessel into the nearby soft-tissue. As the muscle is drawn back from the wound, it thickens and further restricts the vessel lumen, thus restricting blood flow. This, in turn, reduces the rate of blood loss and assists the body's clotting mechanisms. Clean lacerations and amputations therefore do not bleed profusely, but if the vessel is not cleanly lacerated, muscle contraction may actually open the wound, increasing blood flow and loss (Figure A14-5●).

A14

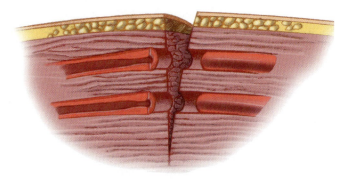

a. A clean lateral cut permits the vessel
to retract and thicken its wall.

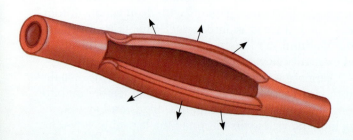

b. A longitudinal cut to the vessel
causes the wound to open.

FIGURE A14-5   Arterial Lacerations
(a) Clean, transverse lacerations of arteries cause spasm and contraction of the vessel slowing bleeding. **(b)** In longitudinal lacerations, the muscle fibers can actually hold the wound open, worsening blood loss.

Traumatic Aneurysm or Rupture of the Aorta

Aortic aneurysm and rupture are extremely life-threatening injuries resulting from either blunt or penetrating trauma. The aorta is most commonly injured by blunt trauma and carries an overall mortality of 85 to 95 percent. It is responsible for 15 percent of all thoracic trauma deaths. Aneurysm and rupture are usually associated with high-speed automobile crashes (most commonly lateral impact) and, in some cases, with high falls. Unlike myocardial rupture, a significant proportion of these victims, possibly as high as 20 percent, will survive the initial insult and aneurysm. Some 30 percent of those initial survivors will die in 6 hours if not treated, increasing to about 50 percent at 24 hours, and to just under 70 percent by the end of the first week. It is this subset of patients who survive the initial impact and are alive at the scene whom you can most benefit by recognizing their potential injury and then rapidly extricating, packaging, and transporting them to a trauma center.

The aorta is a large, high-pressure vessel that provides outflow from the left ventricle for distribution to the body. It is relatively fixed at three points as it passes through the thoracic cavity: the aortic annulus, where the aorta joins the heart; the aortic isthmus, where it is joined by the ligamentum arteriosum; and the diaphragm, where it exits the chest. Because of this, the aorta experiences shear forces secondary to severe deceleration of the chest. Traumatic dissecting aneurysm occurs most commonly to the descending aorta and, infrequently, to the ascending aorta. With severe deceleration, shear forces separate the layers of the artery, specifically the interior surface (the *tunica intima*) from the muscle layer (the *tunica media*). This allows blood to enter the area between the layers, and because the blood is under great pressure, it begins to dissect the aortic lining like a bulging inner tube (Figure A14-6•). The aorta is likely to rupture if it is not surgically repaired.

The patient with aortic rupture will be severely hypotensive, quickly lose all vital signs, and die unless taken immediately to surgery. Dissecting aortic aneurysm progresses more slowly, though the aneurysm may rupture at any moment. The patient will probably have a history of a high fall or severe auto impact and deceleration. Lateral impact is an especially high risk factor for aortic aneurysm. The patient may complain of severe tearing chest pain that may radiate to the back. The patient may have a pulse deficit between the left and right upper extremities and/or reduced pulse strength in the lower extremities. Blood pressure may be high (hypertension) due to stretching of sympathetic nerve fibers in the aorta near the ligamentum arteriosum, or the pressure may be low due to leakage and hypovolemia. Turbulence as the blood exits the heart and passes the disrupted blood vessel wall may create a harsh systolic murmur.

Other Vascular Injuries

Other thoracic vascular structures that can sustain injury during chest trauma are the pulmonary arteries and vena cava. Their injury, and the resulting hemorrhage, may cause significant hemothorax, possibly leading to hypotension and respiratory insufficiency. The blood may also flow into the mediastinum and compress the great vessels, esophagus, and heart. Penetrating trauma is the primary cause of injury to the pulmonary arteries and vena cava. The patient with pulmonary artery or vena cava injuries will likely have a penetrating wound to the central chest, or elsewhere with a likelihood of central chest involvement. These injuries initially present with the signs and symptoms of hypovolemia and shock and then present with the signs and symptoms of hemothorax or hemomediastinum as those conditions develop.

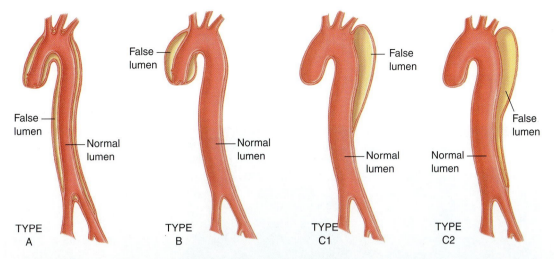

● FIGURE A14-6 Different Types of Thoracic Aortic Dissection
(A) The dissecting aneurysm begins near the aortic valve in the ascending aorta and extends throughout the aorta down to the external iliac arteries. **(B)** Dissecting aneurysm limited to the ascending aorta (as seen with Marfan's syndrome). **(C1)** Dissecting thoracic aneurysm that originates distal to the left subclavian artery. The localized nature of this lesion makes it readily accessible for surgical excision. **(C2)** Dissecting aneurysm arising distal to the left subclavian artery but extending into the abdominal aorta. Only partial excision is possible.

SUMMARY

The blood vessels are an important component of the cardiovascular system. Emergencies involving the blood vessels can require prompt care. Rupture of aortic or cerebrovascular aneurysms can be fatal. Ideally, these lesions will be identified before they rupture, so that they can be repaired. You may encounter several vascular conditions, and it is important to carefully assess the vascular system as a part of your focused patient examination.

A14

15 The Lymphatic System and Immunity

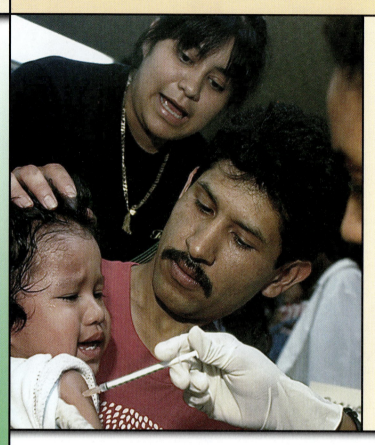

Virtually no other medical development in the last 100 years has done so much to alleviate human suffering and save lives as vaccination. Vaccinations protect patients from diseases that were, in many instances, fatal. Smallpox, a viral disease, was once one of humankind's greatest scourges. However, because of an effective vaccination program, smallpox was officially wiped off the face of the earth on May 8, 1980. The last patient to succumb to smallpox was a medical photographer at the University of Birmingham who accidentally contracted the disease during a laboratory accident. Current plans call for the destruction of all remaining smallpox cultures stored at the CDC in Atlanta and the Institute for Viral Preparations in Moscow.

Chapter Outline and Objectives

1 *Identify the major components of the lymphatic system, and explain their functions.*
2 *Discuss the importance of lymphocytes, and describe where they are found in the body.*

3 *List the body's nonspecific defenses, and explain how each one functions.*

4 *Define specific resistance, and identify the forms and properties of immunity.*
5 *Distinguish between cell-mediated immunity and antibody-mediated (humoral) immunity.*
6 *Discuss the different types of T cells and the role played by each in the immune response.*
7 *Describe the structure of antibody molecules, and explain how they function.*
8 *Describe the primary and secondary immune responses to antigen exposure.*

9 *Relate allergic reactions and autoimmune disorders to immune mechanisms.*
10 *Describe the changes in the immune system that occur with aging.*

11 *Discuss the structural and functional interactions among the lymphatic system and other body systems.*

Vocabulary Development

anamnesis, a memory; *anamnestic response*
*-phylaxis, a guard; *anaphylaxsis*
apo-, away; *apoptosis*
chemo-, chemistry; *chemotaxis*
dia-, through; *diapedesis*
-gen, to produce; *pyrogen*
humor, a liquid; *humoral immunity*
immunis, safe; *immune*
inflammare, to set on fire; *inflammation*
lympha, water; *lymph*
nodulus, little knot; *nodule*
pathos, disease; *pathogen*
pedesis, a leaping; *diapedesis*
ptosis, a falling; *apoptosis*
pyr, fire; *pyrogen*
taxis, arrangement; *chemotaxis*

The world is not always kind to the human body. Accidental bumps, cuts, and scrapes, chemical and thermal burns, extreme cold, and ultraviolet radiation are just a few of the hazards in the physical environment. Making matters worse, an assortment of viruses, bacteria, fungi, and parasites thrive in the environment. Many of these organisms are perfectly capable of not only surviving but thriving inside our bodies—and potentially causing us great harm. These microorganisms, called **pathogens** (*pathos*, disease + *-gen*, to produce), are responsible for many human diseases. Each has a different mode of life and attacks the body in a characteristic way. For example, viruses spend most of their time hiding within cells, many bacteria multiply in the interstitial fluids, and the largest parasites burrow through internal organs.

Many different organs and systems work together in an effort to keep us alive and healthy. In this ongoing struggle, the **lymphatic system** plays a central role.

Lymphocytes, the dominant cells of the lymphatic system, were introduced in Chapter 12. ∞ *p. 344* These cells are vital to our ability to resist or overcome infection and disease. They respond to the presence of (1) invading pathogens, such as bacteria or viruses; (2) abnormal body cells, such as virus-infected cells or cancer cells; and (3) foreign proteins, such as the toxins released by some bacteria. Lymphocytes attempt to eliminate these threats or render them harmless by a combination of physical and chemical attack.

Lymphocytes respond to specific threats, such as a bacterial invasion of a tissue, by organizing a defense against that specific, or particular, type of bacterium. Such a *specific defense* of the body is known as an **immune response**. **Immunity** is the ability to resist infection and disease through the activation of specific defenses.

This chapter begins by examining the organization of the lymphatic system. We will then consider how the lymphatic system interacts with cells and tissues of other systems to defend the body against infection and disease.

ORGANIZATION OF THE LYMPHATIC SYSTEM

One of the least familiar organ systems, the lymphatic system includes the following three components:

1. *Vessels.* A network of **lymphatic vessels** begins in peripheral tissues and ends at connections to the venous system.
2. *Fluid.* A fluid called **lymph** flows through the lymphatic vessels. Lymph resembles plasma but contains a much lower concentration of suspended proteins.
3. *Lymphoid organs.* **Lymphoid organs** are connected to the lymphatic vessels and contain large numbers of lymphocytes. Examples are the lymph nodes, the spleen, and the thymus.

Figure 15-1• provides an overview of the lymphatic system.

Functions of the Lymphatic System

The primary functions of the lymphatic system are:

- *The production, maintenance, and distribution of lymphocytes.* Lymphocytes are produced and stored within lymphoid organs, such as the spleen, thymus, and bone marrow.
- *The return of fluid and solutes from peripheral tissues to the blood.* The return of tissue fluids through

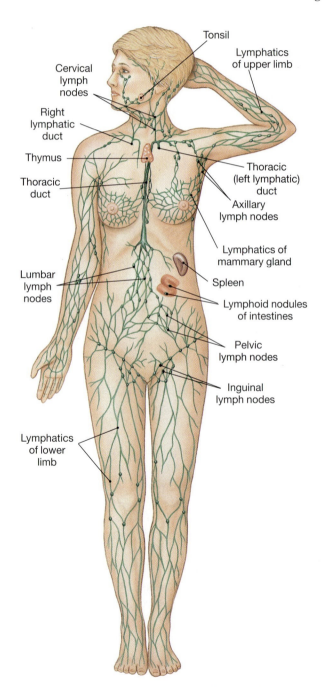

Tonsil

Lymphatics of upper limb

Cervical lymph nodes

Right lymphatic duct

Thymus

Thoracic duct

Thoracic (left lymphatic) duct

Axillary lymph nodes

Lymphatics of mammary gland

Lumbar lymph nodes

Spleen

Lymphoid nodules of intestines

Pelvic lymph nodes

Inguinal lymph nodes

Lymphatics of lower limb

•**FIGURE 15-1** **The Components of the Lymphatic System**

the lymphatic system maintains normal blood volume and eliminates local variations in the composition of the interstitial fluid. The volume of flow is considerable—roughly 3.6 liters per day—and a break in a major lymphatic vessel can cause a rapid and potentially fatal decline in blood volume.

- *The distribution of hormones, nutrients, and waste products from their tissues of origin to the general circulation.* Substances unable to enter the bloodstream directly may do so by way of the lymphatic vessels. For example, lipids absorbed by the digestive tract often fail to enter the circulation at the capillary level. However, they still reach the bloodstream by passage along lymphatic vessels (a process explored further in Chapter 17).

Lymphatic Vessels

Lymphatic vessels, often called *lymphatics*, carry lymph from the peripheral tissues to the venous system in all parts of the body except the central nervous system. The smallest vessels begin as blind pockets and are called **lymphatic capillaries** (Figure 15-2a●). The arrangement of endothelial cells in a lymphatic capillary permits fluid to flow into a lymphatic but prevents backflow into the intercellular spaces.

From the lymphatic capillaries, lymph flows into larger lymphatic vessels that lead toward the trunk. The walls of these lymphatics contain layers comparable to those of veins, and like veins, the larger lymphatics contain valves (Figure 15-2b●). The valves in lymphatic vessels are closer together than are those of veins. Pressures within the lymphatic system are extremely low, and the valves are essential to maintaining normal lymph flow.

The lymphatic vessels ultimately empty into two large collecting ducts (Figure 15-3●). The **thoracic duct** collects lymph from the lower abdomen, pelvis, and lower limbs and from the left half of the head, neck, and chest. It empties its collected lymph into the venous system near the junction between the left internal jugular vein and the left subclavian vein. The smaller **right lymphatic duct**, which ends at the comparable location on the right side, delivers lymph from the right side of the body above the diaphragm. The blockage of lymphatic drainage in a region can cause peripheral swelling due to the accumulation of interstitial fluid. This condition is called *lymphedema.*

Lymphocytes

Lymphocytes were introduced in Chapter 12 because they account for roughly 25 percent of the circulating white blood cell population. ∞ *p. 344* But circulating lymphocytes are only a small fraction of the total lymphocyte population. The body contains around 10^{12}

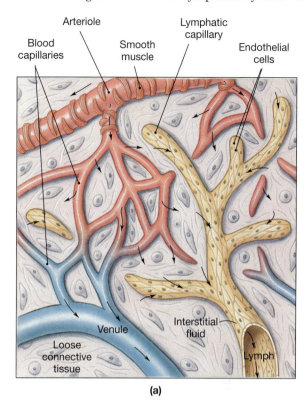

(a)

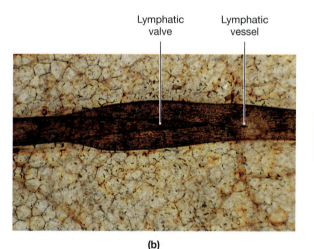

(b)

●**FIGURE 15-2   Lymphatic Capillaries**
(a) A three-dimensional view of the association of blood capillaries, tissue, interstitial fluid, and lymphatic capillaries. Arrows show the directions of interstitial fluid and lymph movement. **(b)** A valve within a small lymphatic vessel. (LM × 43)

lymphocytes, with a combined weight of over a kilogram. At any given moment, most of the lymphocytes are found within lymphoid organs or other tissues. The bloodstream provides a rapid transport system for lymphocytes moving from one tissue to another.

Types of Lymphocytes

The blood contains three classes of lymphocytes in the blood: *T cells* (thymus-dependent), *B cells* (bone

15

●FIGURE 15-3   **The Lymphatic Ducts and the Venous System**
The thoracic duct carries lymph originating in tissues inferior to the diaphragm and from the left side of the upper body. The right lymphatic duct drains the right half of the body superior to the diaphragm and empties into the right subclavian vein.

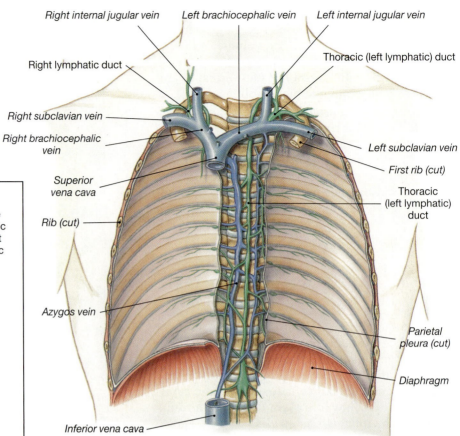

Right internal jugular vein
Left brachiocephalic vein
Left internal jugular vein
Right lymphatic duct
Thoracic (left lymphatic) duct
Right subclavian vein
Right brachiocephalic vein
Left subclavian vein
First rib (cut)
Superior vena cava
Thoracic (left lymphatic) duct
Rib (cut)
Azygos vein
Parietal pleura (cut)
Diaphragm
Inferior vena cava

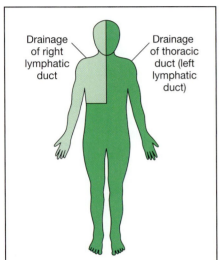

Drainage of right lymphatic duct
Drainage of thoracic duct (left lymphatic duct)

marrow–derived), and *NK cells* (*natural killers*). Each lymphocyte class has distinctive functions.

T Cells.   Approximately 80 percent of circulating lymphocytes are **T cells.** *Cytotoxic T cells* directly attack foreign cells or body cells infected by viruses. These lymphocytes are the primary cells that provide *cell-mediated immunity*, or *cellular immunity. Helper T cells* stimulate the activities of both T cells and B cells, and *suppressor T cells* inhibit both T cells and B cells. Helper and suppressor T cells are also called **regulatory T cells.**

B Cells.   **B cells** constitute 10–15 percent of circulating lymphocytes. B cells can differentiate into **plasma cells,** cells responsible for the production and secretion of **antibodies.** Antibodies are globular proteins that are often called **immunoglobulins.** ∞ *p. 336* Antibodies react with specific chemical targets called **antigens.** Antigens are usually pathogens, parts or products of pathogens, or other foreign compounds. When an antigen-antibody complex forms, it starts a chain of events leading to the destruction of the target compound or organism. Because the blood is the primary distribution route for antibodies, B cells are said to be responsible for *antibody-mediated immunity*, or *humoral* ("liquid") *immunity.*

NK Cells.   The remaining 5–10 percent of circulating lymphocytes are **natural killer (NK) cells.** These lymphocytes will attack foreign cells, normal cells infected with viruses, and cancer cells that appear in normal tissues. Their continual monitoring of peripheral tissues, a process known as *immunological surveillance*, is discussed in more detail later in the chapter.

The Origin and Circulation of Lymphocytes

Lymphocytes in the blood, bone marrow, spleen, thymus, and peripheral lymphoid tissues are visitors, not residents. Lymphocytes move throughout the body; they wander through a tissue and then enter a blood vessel or lymphatic for transport to another site. In general, lymphocytes have relatively long life spans. Roughly 80 percent survive for four years, and some last 20 years or more. Throughout life, normal lymphocyte populations are maintained through the divisions of stem cells in the bone marrow and lymphoid tissues.

Lymphocyte production, or **lymphopoiesis** (lim-fō-poy-Ē-sis), involves the bone marrow and thymus (Figure 15-4●). As they develop, each B cell and T cell gains the ability to respond to the presence of a specific antigen, and NK cells gain the ability to recognize abnormal cells. *Hemocytoblasts* in the bone marrow produce lymphoid stem cells with two distinct fates. One group

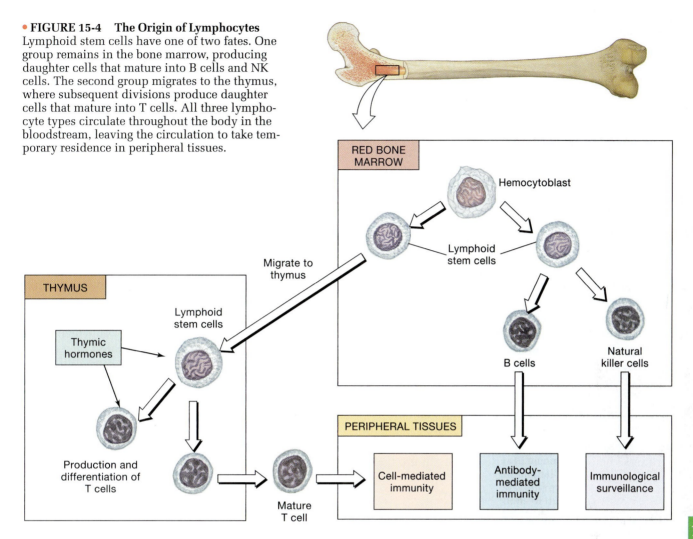

• **FIGURE 15-4   The Origin of Lymphocytes**
Lymphoid stem cells have one of two fates. One group remains in the bone marrow, producing daughter cells that mature into B cells and NK cells. The second group migrates to the thymus, where subsequent divisions produce daughter cells that mature into T cells. All three lymphocyte types circulate throughout the body in the bloodstream, leaving the circulation to take temporary residence in peripheral tissues.

1
5

remains in the bone marrow and generates functional NK cells and B cells that enter the circulation and travel throughout the body. The second group of lymphoid stem cells migrates to the thymus. Under the influence of hormones collectively known as the *thymosins*, these cells divide repeatedly, producing large numbers of T cells that reenter the circulation.

As these lymphocyte populations migrate through peripheral tissues, they retain the ability to divide and produce daughter cells of the same type. For example, a dividing B cell produces other B cells, not T cells or NK cells. As we shall see, the ability to increase the number of lymphocytes of a specific type is important to the success of the immune response.

Lymphoid Nodules

Lymphoid tissues are made up of loose connective tissue and lymphocytes. **Lymphoid nodules** are masses of lymphoid tissue that are not surrounded by a fibrous capsule. As a result, their size can increase or decrease, depending on the number of lymphocytes present at

any given moment. In large lymphoid nodules, there is often a pale central region, called a *germinal center*, where lymphocytes are actively dividing.

Lymphoid nodules are found beneath the epithelia lining various organs of the respiratory, digestive, and urinary systems. All of these systems are open to the external environment and therefore provide a route of entry into the body for potentially harmful organisms and toxins.

Because our food usually contains foreign proteins and often contains bacteria, lymphoid nodules associated with the digestive tract play a particularly important role in the defense of the body. The **tonsils**, large lymphoid nodules in the walls of the pharynx, guard the entrance to the digestive and respiratory tracts. Five tonsils are usually present: a single *pharyngeal tonsil*, or *adenoids*; a pair of *palatine tonsils*; and a pair of *lingual tonsils*. Lymphoid nodules also lie in clusters beneath the epithelial lining of the intestines, and lymphoid tissues dominate the walls of the *appendix*, a blind pouch located near the junction of the small and large intestines.

The lymphocytes in a lymphoid nodule are not always able to destroy bacterial or viral invaders, and if pathogens become established in a lymphoid nodule, an infection develops. Two examples are probably familiar to you: *tonsillitis*, an infection of one of the tonsils (usually the pharyngeal tonsil), and *appendicitis*, an infection of lymphoid nodules in the appendix.

Lymphoid Organs

Lymphoid organs have a stable internal structure and are separated from surrounding tissues by a fibrous capsule. Important lymphoid organs include the *lymph nodes*, the *thymus*, and the *spleen*.

Lymph Nodes

Lymph nodes are small, oval lymphoid organs covered by a fibrous capsule and ranging in diameter from 1–25 mm (up to 1 in.) (Figure 15-5●). One set of lymphatics delivers lymph to a lymph node, and another carries the lymph onward, toward the venous system. The lymph node functions like a kitchen water filter: It filters and purifies the lymph before it reaches the venous system. As lymph flows through a lymph node, at least 99 percent of the antigens present in the arriving lymph will be removed. As the antigens are detected and removed, T cells and B cells are stimulated, and an immune response is initiated. Lymph nodes are located in regions where they can detect and eliminate harmful "intruders" before they reach vital organs of the body (see Figure 15-1●, p. 412).

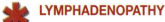

LYMPHADENOPATHY

An enlargement of the lymph nodes is called *lymphadenopathy*. Localized enlargement of lymph nodes, such as in the neck, is usually due to infection. However, generalized lymph node enlargement may indicate a systemic process such as a malignancy or a viral illness. Several disorders cause marked lymphadenopathy. *Infectious mononucleosis,* for example, causes enlargement and tenderness of lymph nodes throughout the body. *Strep throat,* a bacterial infection, typically causes swelling and tenderness of the lymph nodes in the neck. Painless, widespread lymphadenopathy is suggestive of a malignant process such as HIV, cancer of the lymphatic system (*lymphoma*), or cancer of the blood (*leukemia*).

The Thymus

The **thymus**, the site of T cell maturation, lies behind the sternum (Figure 15-6●). The thymus reaches its greatest size (relative to body size) in the first year or two after birth and its maximum absolute size during puberty, when it weighs between 30 and 40 g (1.06 to 1.41 oz.). Thereafter, the thymus gradually decreases in size.

The thymus has two lobes, each divided into *lobules* by fibrous partitions, or *septae* (*septum,* a wall). Each lobule consists of a densely packed outer *cortex* and a paler central *medulla.* Lymphocytes in the cortex are dividing, and as the T cells mature, they migrate into the medulla, eventually entering one of the blood vessels in that region. Other cells within the lobules produce the thymic hormones collectively known as *thymosins.*

The Spleen

The adult **spleen** contains the largest collection of lymphatic tissue in the body. It is around 12 cm (5 in.) long and can weigh about 160 g (5.6 oz.). As indicated in Figure 15-7a●, it sits wedged between the stomach, the left kidney, and the muscular diaphragm. The spleen normally has a deep red color because of the blood it contains. The cellular components constitute the **pulp** of the spleen. Areas of *red pulp* contain large quantities of blood, whereas areas of *white pulp* resemble lymphoid nodules. As blood flows through the spleen, macrophages identify and engulf any damaged or infected cells. The presence of lymphocytes nearby ensures that any microorganisms or other abnormal antigens will stimulate an immune response.

15

●**FIGURE 15-5   The Structure of a Lymph Node**
The arrows indicate the direction of lymph flow

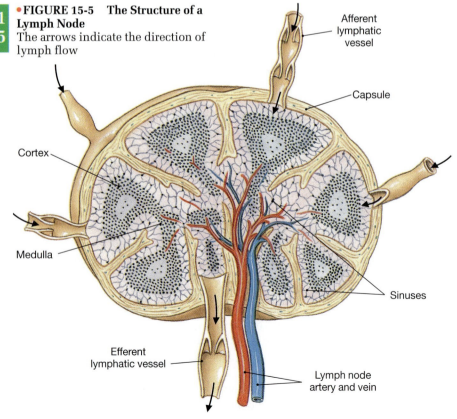

Afferent lymphatic vessel

Capsule

Cortex

Medulla

Sinuses

Efferent lymphatic vessel

Lymph node artery and vein

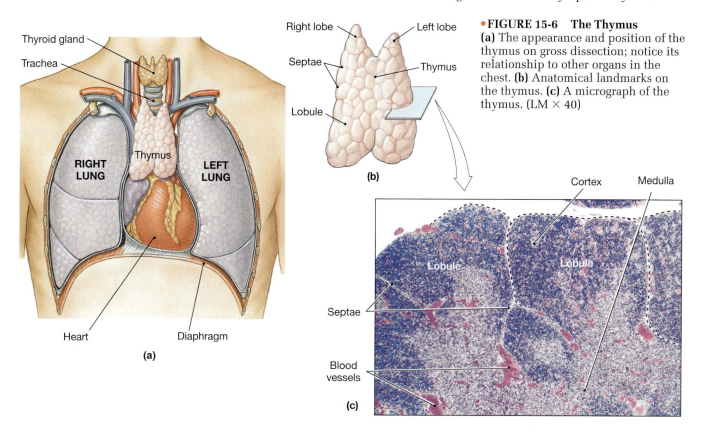

•FIGURE 15-6   The Thymus
(a) The appearance and position of the thymus on gross dissection; notice its relationship to other organs in the chest. (b) Anatomical landmarks on the thymus. (c) A micrograph of the thymus. (LM × 40)

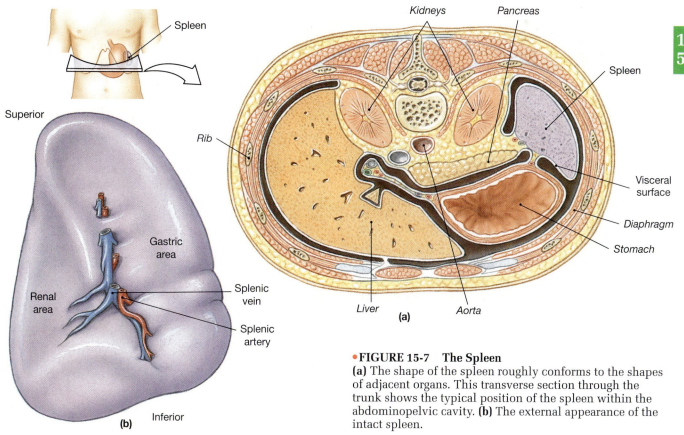

•FIGURE 15-7   The Spleen
(a) The shape of the spleen roughly conforms to the shapes of adjacent organs. This transverse section through the trunk shows the typical position of the spleen within the abdominopelvic cavity. (b) The external appearance of the intact spleen.

1
5

The spleen performs similar functions for the blood that the lymph nodes perform for lymph: (1) removing abnormal blood cells and components, and (2) initiating immune responses by B cells and T cells in response to antigens in the circulating blood. In addition, the spleen stores iron from recycled red blood cells.

✳ SPLENIC INJURY

The *spleen* is the most frequently injured organ in blunt abdominal trauma. It is a highly vascular organ, and its rupture can cause life-threatening intra-abdominal hemorrhage. In addition, splenic injury is often associated with other intra-abdominal injuries. In the past, treatment of splenic injury has primarily been *splenectomy*. However, the trend in recent years has been to try to avoid splenectomy by carefully observing the patient and obtaining serial *computed tomography (CT)* scans.

The spleen plays an important role in combating disease. Its loss places the patient at increased risk of infection. All patients who have undergone splenectomy should receive vaccine prophylaxis against the bacteria that commonly causes pneumonia *(pneumococcus)*.

✓ How would blockage of the thoracic duct affect the circulation of lymph?

✓ If the thymus gland failed to produce thymosin, which population of lymphocytes would be affected?

✓ Why do the lymph nodes enlarge during some infections?

Body Defenses and the Lymphatic System

The human body relies on two general mechanisms for its defense:

1. **Nonspecific defenses**, which do not discriminate between one threat and another. These defenses, which are present at birth, include *physical barriers, phagocytic cells, immunological surveillance, interferons, complement, inflammation,* and *fever*. They provide the body with a defensive capability known as **nonspecific resistance**.

2. **Specific defenses**, which provide protection against threats on an individual basis. For example, a specific defense may protect against infection by one type of bacterium but ignore other bacteria and viruses. Specific defenses are dependent upon the activities of lymphocytes. Together, they produce a state of protection known as **specific resistance**, or immunity.

Nonspecific and specific resistance do not function in complete isolation from each other; both are necessary to provide adequate resistance to infection and disease.

NONSPECIFIC DEFENSES

Nonspecific defenses are defenses that deny entrance to, or limit the spread of, microorganisms or other environmental agents to the body (Figure 15-8•).

Physical Barriers

To cause infection or disease, a foreign (antigenic) compound or pathogen must enter the body tissues, which requires crossing an epithelium. The epithelial covering of the skin, described in Chapter 5, has multiple layers, a keratin coating, and a network of desmosomes that lock adjacent cells together. ∞ *p. 109* These create a very effective barrier that protects underlying tissues.

The exterior surface of the body has several layers of defense. The hairs found in most areas provide some protection against mechanical abrasion (especially on the scalp), and they often prevent hazardous materials or insects from contacting the skin's surface. The epidermal surface also receives the secretions of sebaceous glands and sweat glands. These secretions flush the surface, washing away microorganisms and chemical agents. The secretions also contain bactericidal chemicals, destructive enzymes (*lysozymes*), and antibodies.

The epithelia lining the digestive, respiratory, urinary, and reproductive tracts are more delicate, but they are equally well defended. Mucus bathes most surfaces of the digestive tract, and the stomach contains a powerful acid that can destroy many potential pathogens. Mucus moves across the lining of the respiratory tract, urine flushes the urinary passageways, and glandular secretions do the same for the reproductive tract. Special enzymes, antibodies, and an acidic pH add to the effectiveness of these secretions.

Phagocytes

Phagocytes in peripheral tissues remove cellular debris and respond to invasion by foreign compounds or pathogenic organisms. These cells represent the "first line" of cellular defense, often attacking and removing the microorganisms before lymphocytes become aware of the incident. Two general classes of phagocytic cells are found in the human body: *microphages* and *macrophages*.

Microphages are the neutrophils and eosinophils normally found in the circulating blood. These phagocytic cells leave the bloodstream and enter peripheral tissues subjected to injury or infection. As noted in Chapter 12, neutrophils are abundant, mobile, and quick to phagocytize cellular debris or invading bacteria. ∞ *p. 344* The less abundant eosinophils target foreign compounds or pathogens that have been coated with antibodies.

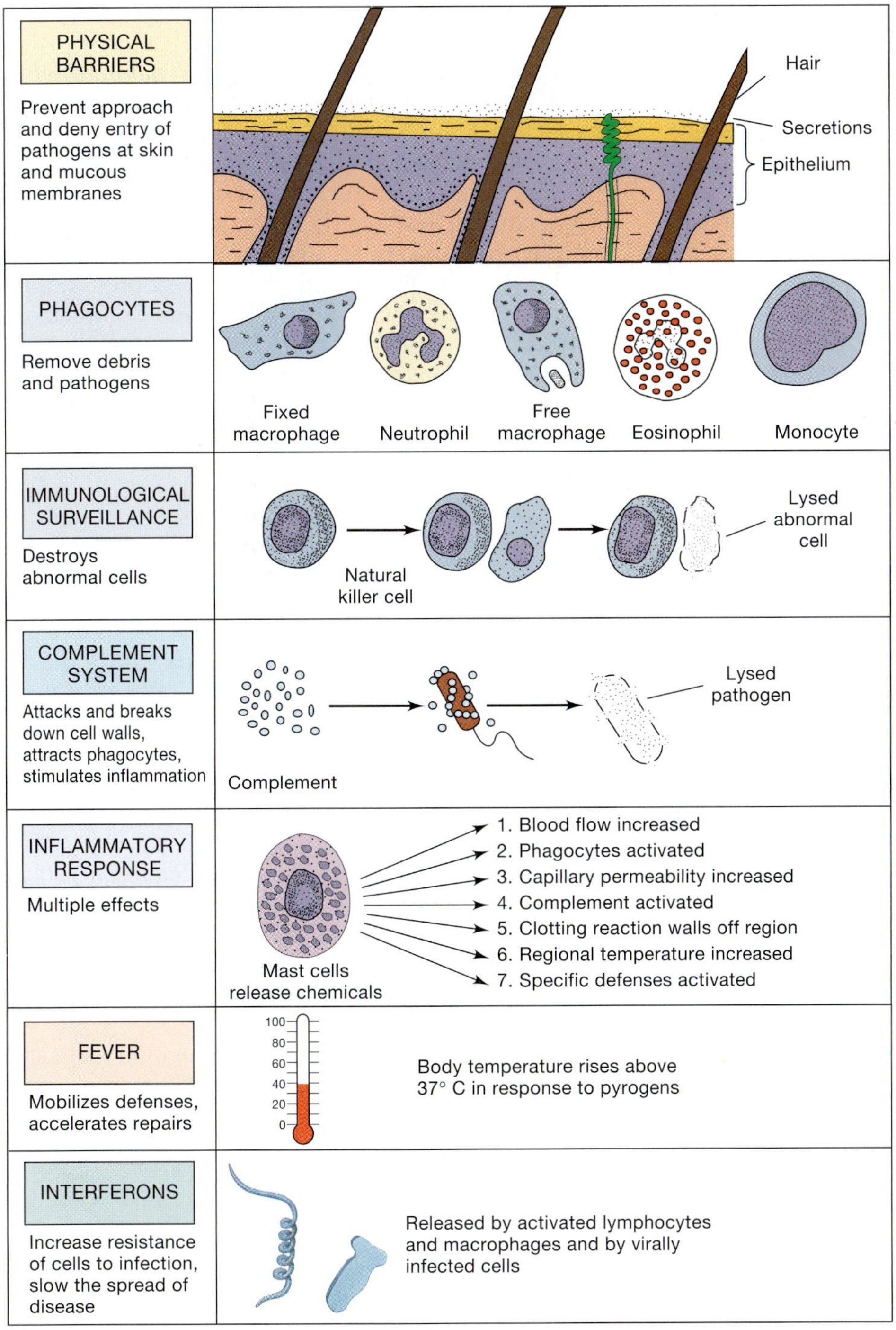

•FIGURE 15-8
Nonspecific Defenses

PHYSICAL BARRIERS — Prevent approach and deny entry of pathogens at skin and mucous membranes	Hair / Secretions / Epithelium
PHAGOCYTES — Remove debris and pathogens	Fixed macrophage / Neutrophil / Free macrophage / Eosinophil / Monocyte
IMMUNOLOGICAL SURVEILLANCE — Destroys abnormal cells	Natural killer cell → Lysed abnormal cell
COMPLEMENT SYSTEM — Attacks and breaks down cell walls, attracts phagocytes, stimulates inflammation	Complement → Lysed pathogen
INFLAMMATORY RESPONSE — Multiple effects	Mast cells release chemicals → 1. Blood flow increased / 2. Phagocytes activated / 3. Capillary permeability increased / 4. Complement activated / 5. Clotting reaction walls off region / 6. Regional temperature increased / 7. Specific defenses activated
FEVER — Mobilizes defenses, accelerates repairs	Body temperature rises above 37° C in response to pyrogens
INTERFERONS — Increase resistance of cells to infection, slow the spread of disease	Released by activated lymphocytes and macrophages and by virally infected cells

The body also contains several different types of **macrophages**—large, actively phagocytic cells derived from the monocytes of the blood. Almost every tissue in the body shelters resident or visiting macrophages. In some organs, the macrophages have special names. For example, in the CNS they are called *microglia*. The relatively diffuse collection of phagocytic cells throughout the body is called the **monocyte-macrophage system.**

All phagocytic cells function in much the same way, although the items selected for phagocytosis may differ from one cell type to another. Mobile macrophages and microphages also share a number of other functional characteristics in addition to phagocytosis. They can all move through capillary walls by squeezing between adjacent endothelial cells, a process known as *diapedesis* (*dia*, through + *pedesis*, a leaping). They may also be attracted to or repelled by chemicals in the surrounding fluids, a phenomenon called **chemotaxis** (*chemo-*, chemistry + *taxis*, arrangement). They are particularly sensitive to chemicals released by other body cells or by pathogens.

15

Immunological Surveillance

Our immune defenses generally ignore normal cells in the body's tissues, but abnormal cells are attacked and destroyed. The constant monitoring of normal tissues is called **immunological surveillance**, and it primarily involves the lymphocytes known as NK (natural killer) cells. These cells are sensitive to the presence of antigens that are characteristic of abnormal cell membranes. When they encounter these antigens on a cancer cell or a cell infected with viruses, NK cells secrete proteins that kill the abnormal cell by destroying its cell membrane.

Killing the abnormal cells can slow the spread of a viral infection and may eliminate cancer cells before they spread to other tissues. Unfortunately, some cancer cells avoid detection, a process called *immunological escape*. Once immunological escape has occurred, cancer cells can multiply and spread without interference by NK cells.

Interferons

Interferons (in-ter-FER-onz) are small proteins released by activated lymphocytes, macrophages, and tissue cells infected with viruses. Cells exposed to these molecules respond by producing proteins that interfere with viral replication. In addition, interferons stimulate the activities of macrophages and NK cells. Interferons are examples of **cytokines** (SĪ-tō-kīnz), chemical messengers released by tissue cells to coordinate local activities. In effect, cytokines are the hormones of the immune system; they are released to alter the activities of cells and tissues throughout the body. Their role in the regulation of specific defenses will be discussed later in the chapter.

Complement

The plasma contains 11 special *complement proteins*, which form the **complement system**. The name refers to the fact that this system "complements," or supplements, the action of antibodies. These proteins interact with one another in chain reactions comparable to those of the clotting system. The reaction is begun when a complement binds to an antibody molecule or to bacterial cell walls. The bound complement protein then interacts with other complement proteins. Complement activation is known to (1) attract phagocytes, (2) enhance phagocytosis, (3) destroy cell membranes, and (4) promote inflammation.

Inflammation

Inflammation, a localized tissue response to injury introduced in Chapter 4, produces local sensations of swelling, redness, heat, and pain. ∞ *p. 100* Inflammation can be produced by any stimulus that kills cells or damages loose connective tissue. *Mast cells* within the affected tissue play a pivotal role in this process. ∞ *p. 90* When stimulated by mechanical stress or chemical changes in the local environment, mast cells release chemicals, including *histamine* and *heparin*, into the interstitial fluid. These chemicals initiate the process of inflammation. Inflammation initiates the replacement or repair of damaged tissue—a process called *regeneration*.

Figure 15-9• summarizes the events that occur during inflammation of the skin. Comparable events will occur in almost any tissue subjected to physical damage or to infection. The purposes of inflammation are:

- To perform a temporary repair at the injury site and prevent the access of additional pathogens.

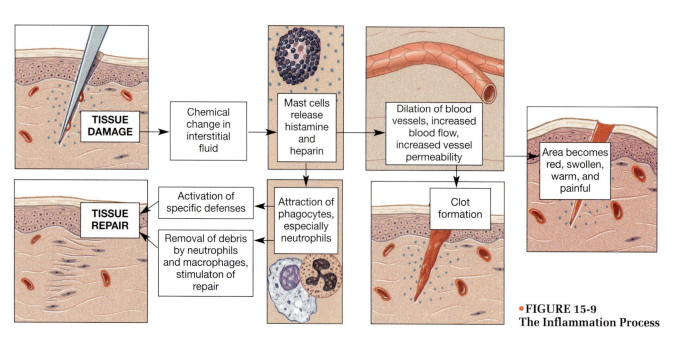

•**FIGURE 15-9**
The Inflammation Process

- To slow the spread of pathogens from the injury site.
- To mobilize a wide range of defenses that can overcome the pathogens and facilitate permanent tissue repair.

Fever

A **fever** is the maintenance of a body temperature greater than 37.2°C (99°F). The hypothalamus, which contains nuclei that regulate body temperature, acts as the body's thermostat. ∞ *p. 14* Circulating proteins called **pyrogens** (PĪ-rō-jenz; *pyr*, fire + *-gen*, to produce) can reset the thermostat in the hypothalamus and cause a rise in body temperature. Pathogens, bacterial toxins, and antigen-antibody complexes may act as pyrogens or stimulate the release of pyrogens by macrophages.

Within limits, a fever may be beneficial. High body temperatures can accelerate the activities of the immune system. However, high fevers (over 40°C, or 104°F) can damage many physiological systems. For example, a high fever can cause CNS problems, such as nausea, disorientation, hallucinations, or convulsions.

✓ What types of cells would be affected by a decrease in the monocyte-forming cells in the bone marrow?

✓ A rise in the level of interferon in the body would suggest what kind of infection?

✓ What effects do pyrogens have in the body?

SPECIFIC DEFENSES: THE IMMUNE RESPONSE

The body's specific defenses that produce specific resistance, or immunity, are provided by the coordinated activities of T cells and B cells, which respond to the presence of *specific* antigens. T cells provide a defense against abnormal cells and pathogens that are inside living cells; this process is called **cell-mediated immunity**, or *cellular immunity*. B cells provide a defense against antigens and pathogenic organisms that are in body fluids. This process is called **antibody-mediated immunity**, or *humoral immunity*.

Forms of Immunity

Immunity can be either innate or acquired (Figure 15-10•). **Innate immunity** is genetically determined; it is present at birth and has no relation to previous exposure to the antigen involved. For example, people are not subject to the same diseases as goldfish.

Acquired immunity can be either active or passive. **Active immunity** appears following exposure to an antigen, as a consequence of the immune response. The immune system has the *capability* of defending against an enormous number of antigens. However, the appropriate defenses are mobilized only after an individual's lymphocytes encounter a particular antigen. Active

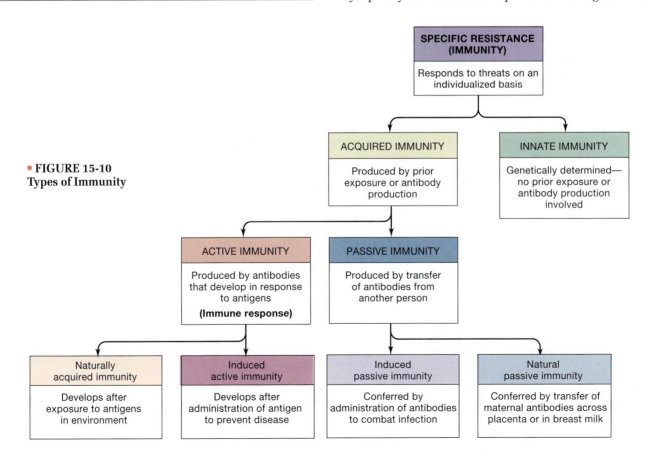

• **FIGURE 15-10**
Types of Immunity

immunity may develop as a result of natural exposure to an antigen in the environment (naturally acquired immunity) or from deliberate exposure to an antigen (induced active immunity).

Naturally acquired immunity normally begins to develop after birth, and it is continually enhanced as the individual encounters "new" pathogens or other antigens. You might compare this process to vocabulary development—a child begins with a few basic common words and learns new ones as needed. The purpose of *induced active immunity*, also known as *artificially acquired immunity*, is to stimulate antibody production under controlled conditions so that the individual will be able to overcome any natural exposure to the same type of pathogen at some time in the future. This is the basic principle behind immunization to prevent disease.

Passive immunity is the result of the transfer of antibodies from another individual. *Natural passive immunity* results when antibodies produced by the mother cross the placental barrier to provide protection against embryonic or fetal infections. In *induced passive immunity*, antibodies are administered to fight infection or prevent disease.

Properties of Immunity

Four general properties of immunity are recognized:

1. *Specificity*. A specific defense is activated by an antigen, and the response targets only that particular antigen in a process known as *antigen recognition*. **Specificity** occurs because the cell membrane of each T cell and B cell has receptors that will bind only one specific antigen, ignoring all other types of antigens. Either lymphocyte will destroy or inactivate that specific antigen without affecting other antigens or normal tissues.

2. *Versatility*. In the course of a normal lifetime, an individual encounters tens of thousands of antigens. The immune system cannot anticipate which antigens it will encounter, so it must be ready to confront *any* antigen at *any* time. It does this by producing millions of different lymphocyte populations, each with different antigen receptors. In this way, the immune system can produce appropriate and specific responses to each antigen when exposure does occur.

3. *Memory*. The immune system "remembers" antigens that it encounters. During the initial response to an antigen, lymphocytes sensitive to its presence undergo repeated cell divisions. Two kinds of cells are produced: some that attack the invader and others that remain inactive unless they are exposed to the same antigen at a later date. These latter cells are

memory cells, which enable the immune system to "remember" previously encountered antigens and launch a faster, stronger counterattack if one of them ever appears again.

4. *Tolerance*. **Tolerance** is said to exist when the immune system does not respond to a particular antigen. During their differentiation in the bone marrow (B cells) and thymus (T cells), cells that react to antigens normally present in the body are destroyed. As a result, B and T cells will ignore normal, or **self**, antigens and attack foreign, or **nonself**, antigens.

An Overview of the Immune Response

The purpose of the **immune response** is to destroy or inactivate pathogens, abnormal cells, and foreign molecules such as toxins. The process begins with the appearance of an antigen. Lymphocytes sensitive to a particular antigen have receptors in their membranes that can bind that particular antigen, a process known as **antigen recognition**. As Figure 15-11● shows, the precise nature of the resulting immune response varies depending on whether the activated lymphocyte is a T cell or a B cell.

T Cells and Cell-Mediated Immunity

Before an immune response can begin, T cells must be activated by exposure to an antigen. However, this activation seldom happens by direct lymphocyte-antigen interaction, and foreign compounds or pathogens entering a tissue often fail to stimulate an immediate response.

T cells recognize antigens when they are bound to receptors on the membranes of other cells. The receptors involved are called *major histocompatibility complex (MHC) proteins*. MHC proteins are found on the surfaces of all of our cells. To trigger an immune response, foreign cells (including bacteria) and foreign proteins must first be engulfed by macrophages. The macrophages break down the foreign antigens, creating antigenic fragments that are displayed on their cell surfaces, bound to MHC proteins. T cells that contact this macrophage membrane become activated, initiating an immune response. In the case of viruses, T cells can be activated by contact with an infected cell. An infected cell displays viral antigens on its surface, also bound to MHC proteins. The activation of T cells by these antigens can rally a defense against the viral infection.

On activation, T cells divide and differentiate into cells with specific functions in the immune response. The major cell types are *cytotoxic T cells*, *memory T cells*, *suppressor T cells*, and *helper T cells*.

● **FIGURE 15-11**
An Overview of the Immune Response

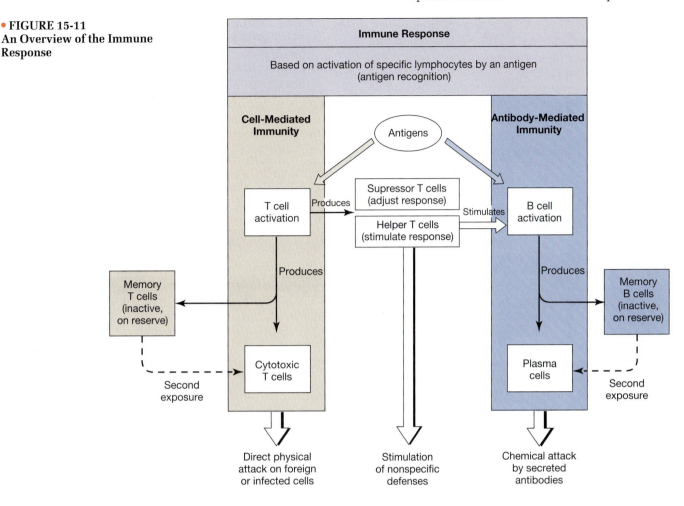

Immune Response

Based on activation of specific lymphocytes by an antigen (antigen recognition)

Cell-Mediated Immunity

Antibody-Mediated Immunity

Antigens

T cell activation

Produces

Supressor T cells (adjust response)

Helper T cells (stimulate response)

Stimulates

B cell activation

Produces

Memory T cells (inactive, on reserve)

Produces

Cytotoxic T cells

Second exposure

Produces

Memory B cells (inactive, on reserve)

Plasma cells

Second exposure

Direct physical attack on foreign or infected cells

Stimulation of nonspecific defenses

Chemical attack by secreted antibodies

Cytotoxic T Cells

Cytotoxic T cells are responsible for cell-mediated immunity. These cells, also called *killer T cells*, track down and attack the bacteria, fungi, protozoa, or foreign tissues that contain the target antigen. For example, cytotoxic T cells are responsible for the rejection of skin grafts or organ transplants from other individuals.

A cytotoxic T cell may accomplish its destruction in several ways (Figure 15-12●):

• By rupturing the antigenic cell membrane through the release of a destructive protein called *perforin*.
• By killing the target cell by secreting a poisonous *lymphotoxin* (lim-fō-TOK-sin).
• By activating genes within the target cell that tell it to die. The process of genetically programmed cell death is called *apoptosis* (ap-op-TŌ-sis; *apo-*, away + *ptosis*, a falling).

Memory T Cells

During the cell divisions that follow T cell activation, some of the cells develop into cytotoxic T cells and others develop into **memory T cells**. Memory T cells re-

main "in reserve." If the same antigen appears a second time, these cells will immediately differentiate into cytotoxic T cells, producing a more rapid and effective cellular response.

Suppressor T Cells

Activated **suppressor T cells** depress the responses of other T cells and B cells by secreting *suppression factors*. This suppression does not occur immediately, because suppressor T cells take much longer to become activated than other types of T cells. As a result, suppressor T cells act *after* the initial immune response. In effect, these cells "put on the brakes" and limit the degree of immune system activation from a single stimulus.

Helper T Cells

On activation, some T cells undergo a series of divisions that produce **helper T cells**. Helper T cells release a variety of cytokines that (1) coordinate specific and nonspecific defenses and (2) stimulate cell-mediated immunity and antibody-mediated immunity. The mechanism involved will be discussed in the next section.

15

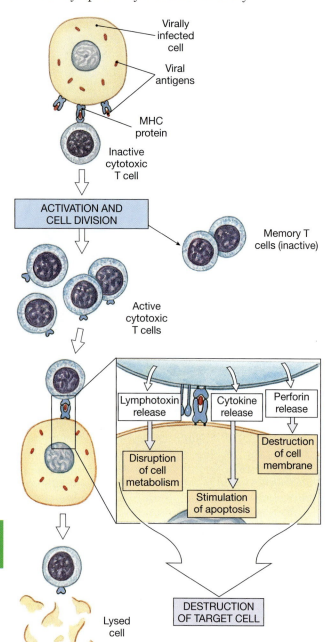

•FIGURE 15-12   The Activation of Cytotoxic T Cells
For activation, an inactive cytotoxic T cell must encounter an appropriate antigen bound to MHC proteins. Once activated, the T cell undergoes divisions that produce memory T cells and active cytotoxic T cells. When one of these active cells encounters a membrane displaying the target antigen, the cytotoxic T cell will use one of several methods to destroy the cell.

B Cells and Antibody-Mediated Immunity

B cells are responsible for launching a chemical attack on antigens by producing appropriate antibodies. B cell activation proceeds in a series of steps diagrammed in Figure 15-13•.

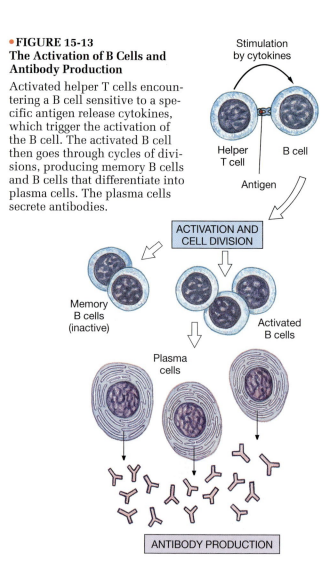

•FIGURE 15-13
The Activation of B Cells and Antibody Production
Activated helper T cells encountering a B cell sensitive to a specific antigen release cytokines, which trigger the activation of the B cell. The activated B cell then goes through cycles of divisions, producing memory B cells and B cells that differentiate into plasma cells. The plasma cells secrete antibodies.

B Cell Activation

B cells are activated primarily by the activities of helper T cells. Activated helper T cells bind to inactive B cells and and secrete cytokines that (1) promote B cell activation, (2) stimulate B cell division, (3) accelerate plasma cell production, and (4) enhance antibody production.

As Figure 15-13• shows, the activated B cell divides several times, producing daughter cells that differentiate into plasma cells and **memory B cells**. Plasma cells begin synthesizing and secreting large numbers of antibodies that have the same target as the antibodies on the surface of the sensitized B cell. Memory B cells perform the same role for antibody-mediated immunity that memory T cells perform for cellular-mediated immunity. They will remain in reserve to deal with subsequent exposure to the same antigens. At that time, they will respond and differentiate into antibody-secreting plasma cells.

Antibody Structure

Figure 15-14• shows different representations of a single antibody molecule. The molecule consists of two parallel

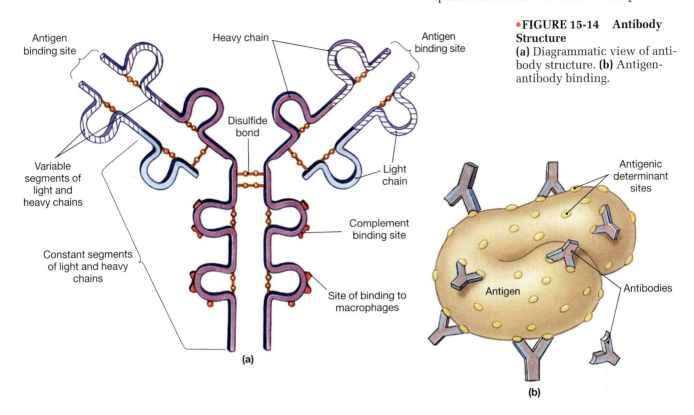

●FIGURE 15-14   **Antibody
Structure**
(a) Diagrammatic view of antibody structure. **(b)** Antigen-
antibody binding.

pairs of polypeptide chains: one pair of long *heavy chains*
and one pair of shorter *light chains*. Each chain contains
constant and *variable segments*. The constant segments of
the heavy chains resemble those of every other antibody
molecule of that particular class. (The various classes of
antibodies are described in the following section.) The
specificity of the antibody molecule depends on the structure of the variable segments of the light and heavy chains.
The free tips of the two variable segments contain the
antigen binding sites of the antibody molecule. Small differences in the amino acid sequence of the variable segments affect the precise shape of the antigen binding sites.
The different shapes of these sites account for the differences in specificity between the antibodies produced by
different B cells. It has been estimated that the 10 trillion
or so B cells of a normal adult can produce an estimated
100 million different antibodies.

When an antibody molecule binds to its proper antigen, an **antigen-antibody complex** is formed. The specificity of that binding depends on the three-dimensional
"fit" between the variable segments of the antibody molecule and the corresponding sites of the antigen.

Antigens come in a variety of sizes, ranging from a
single polypeptide to an entire bacterium. Antibodies do
not target the antigen as a whole, but instead focus on
certain portions of its exposed surface called *antigenic
determinant sites*. To be a *complete antigen*, a molecule
must have at least two antigenic determinant sites, one
for each arm of the antibody molecule. Most environmental antigens have multiple antigenic determinant
sites; entire microorganisms may have thousands.

Classes of Antibodies

Body fluids contain five classes of antibodies, or
immunoglobulins (Ig): *IgG, IgM, IgA, IgE,* and *IgD*
(Table 15-1). The most important is **immunoglobulin
G,** or **IgG,** the largest class of antibodies. Several types
of IgG collectively account for 80 percent of all immunoglobulins. The IgG antibodies are responsible for
resistance to many viruses, bacteria, and bacterial toxins. Circulating *IgM* antibodies are responsible for the
cross-reactions between incompatible blood types, described in Chapter 12. ⊷ *p. 341*

Antibody Function

The function of antibodies is to destroy antigens. The
formation of an antigen-antibody complex may cause
their elimination in several ways:

1. *Neutralization.* Antibodies can bind to toxins or
   viruses, making them incapable of attaching to a cell.
   This mechanism is called **neutralization**.
2. *Agglutination and precipitation.* When large numbers
   of antibodies bind to antigens, they can create large
   complexes. Antigenic cells may clump together; this
   process is called **agglutination**. The clumping of red
   blood cells that occurs when incompatible blood types
   are mixed is an example of agglutination. ⊷ *p. 341*
   Smaller antigens may form insoluble masses that settle
   out of body fluids. This process is called **precipitation**.
3. *Activation of complement.* Upon binding to an
   antigen, portions of the antibody molecule change

TABLE 15-1   **Classes of Antibodies**

Class	Function	Remarks
IgG	Responsible for defense against many viruses, bacteria, and bacterial toxins	Largest class of antibodies, with several subtypes
IgM	Anti-A, anti-B, anti-D forms responsible for cross-reactions between incompatible blood types; other forms attack bacteria insensitive to IgG	First antibody type secreted following arrival of antigen; levels decline as IgG production accelerates
IgA	Attack pathogens before they enter the body tissues	Found in glandular secretions (tears, mucus, and saliva)
IgE	Accelerate inflammation on exposure to antigen	Bound to surfaces of mast cells and basophils; important in allergic response
IgD	Bind antigens to B cells	May play a role in B cell activation

---

CLINICAL NOTE   INFECTIOUS DISEASES AND EMS

Infectious diseases are caused by infestation of the body with biological organisms such as bacteria, viruses, fungi, protozoa, and helminthes (worms). They pose a real and significant risk for emergency personnel. Although most infectious diseases are not life threatening, some types of infection, such as human immunodeficiency virus (HIV), hepatitis B (HBV), hepatitis C (HCV), and tuberculosis, are particularly dangerous and may cause death or permanent disability. Early recognition and management of these patients may make a difference in how the patient is treated and may also ensure that care providers take necessary precautions to prevent the spread of the disease to others.

Human immunodeficiency virus (HIV) is the causative agent of *acquired immunodeficiency syndrome (AIDS)*. HIV is an example of a *retrovirus*. In retroviruses, the genetic information is carried as RNA instead of DNA. The virus enters the target cell, specifically lymphocytes, and starts using enzyme systems within the host cell to manufacture DNA from the viral RNA strands. Cells infected with HIV are ultimately killed. The gradual destruction of *helper T cells* impairs the immune response. *Suppressor T cells* are relatively unaffected by the virus, and over time, the excess of suppressing factors "turns off" the normal immune response. Circulating antibody levels fall, cellular immunity is reduced, and the body is left without protection against many diseases.

With immune function so reduced, normally harmless biological agents can cause infections, many potentially lethal. Examples of opportunistic infections include infection with the fungus *Candida albicans*, infection with the protozoan *Pneumocystis carinii*, infection with *herpes virus* and *cytomegalovirus*, and development of cancerous lesions from *Kaposi's sarcoma*.

Infection with HIV occurs through intimate contact with the body fluids of an infected individual. Most AIDS patients become infected through sexual contact with an HIV-infected person. Another common cause is sharing needles with a patient who carries the virus for AIDS.

Hepatitis is an inflammation of the liver. The most common cause of inflammation is infection, although several agents, both biological and chemical, can cause hepatitis. It is the viral agents that cause hepatitis that pose risks to EMS personnel and health care workers.

Hepatitis A (HAV) is a common type of hepatitis. Formerly called *infectious hepatitis*, it is commonly seen in periodic outbreaks. HAV is transmitted by the fecal-oral route, with most infections picked up by handling or eating contaminated food products, often leafy vegetables. HAV infection is less severe than HBV and does not result in a chronic infection or carrier state. A vaccine for HAV is now available.

Hepatitis B (HBV), also known as *serum hepatitis*, is transmitted as a blood borne pathogen and can stay active in bodily fluids outside the body for days. Because HBV is more common and transmission following exposure is more efficient, emergency personnel are at a much greater risk of contacting HBV infections than HIV. Hepatitis B results in a severe form of hepatitis and can leave some patients with a chronic infection, which in turn can cause cirrhosis of the liver and liver cancer. Some patients infected with HBV will become carriers of the disease. In fact, it is estimated that well over 310 million persons worldwide are HBV carriers. An effective vaccine is available for HBV and should be administered to all health care workers.

Hepatitis C (HCV), formerly called *non-A, non-B hepatitis*, is becoming more of a problem for emergency personnel. HAC is spread through blood borne transmission and can cause chronic and debilitating liver damage. HCV was most often transmitted through blood transfusions. Now, however, blood tests are available to detect HCV, and this risk factor is markedly reduced. There is currently no vaccine available and there is no effective post-exposure prophylaxis.

Hepatitis D (HDV), also called *delta hepatitis*, is relatively uncommon. HDV must be activated by HBV and occurs only as a superinfection of HBV.

Hepatitis E (HEV) is typically seen only in Central America and sub-Saharan Africa. It is waterborne and responsible for epidemics in these areas.

There has been a resurgence of *tuberculosis* in the last decade or so. Tuberculosis is spread by airborne respiratory droplets but may also be contracted through contact with mucous membranes and broken skin. The risk of transmitting tuberculosis is not high but remains noteworthy for emergency personnel.

Because of the significant risk of infectious diseases, emergency personnel must follow all recommended guidelines to prevent disease transmission. Use of personal protective equipment (PPE) is a must.

1
5

shape, exposing areas that bind complement proteins. The bound complement molecules then activate the complement system, destroying the antigen.

4. *Attraction of phagocytes.* Antigens covered with antibodies attract eosinophils, neutrophils, and macrophages, which can phagocytize pathogens and destroy foreign or abnormal cell membranes.

5. *Enhancement of phagocytosis.* A coating of antibodies and complement proteins increases the effectiveness of phagocytosis.

6. *Stimulation of inflammation.* Antibodies may promote inflammation by stimulating basophils and mast cells. This can help mobilize nonspecific defenses and slow the spread of the infection to other tissues.

Primary and Secondary Responses to Antigen Exposure

The initial response to antigen exposure is called the **primary response**. When an antigen appears a second time, it triggers a more extensive and prolonged **secondary response**. The secondary response reflects the presence of large numbers of memory cells that are already "primed" for the arrival of the antigen.

Because the antigen must activate the appropriate B cells and the B cells must then respond by differentiating into plasma cells, the primary response does not appear immediately (Figure 15-15•). Instead, there is a gradual, sustained rise in the concentration of circulating antibodies, and the antibody activity, or *antibody titer*, in the blood does not peak until several weeks after the initial exposure. Thereafter the antibody concentration declines, assuming that the person is no longer exposed to the antigen.

Memory B cells do not differentiate into plasma cells unless they are exposed to the same antigen a second time. If and when that exposure occurs, these cells respond immediately, dividing and differentiating into plasma cells that secrete antibodies in massive quantities. This represents the secondary response, or *anamnestic response* (an-am-NES-tik; *anamnesis*, a memory), to antigen exposure.

The secondary response produces an immediate rise in IgG concentrations to levels many times higher than those of the primary response. This response is so much faster and stronger than the primary response because the numerous memory cells can produce massive quantities of antibodies in a short time. The secondary response appears even if the second exposure occurs years after the first, for memory cells are long-lived, potentially surviving for 20 years or more.

The relatively slow primary response is much less effective at disease prevention than the more rapid and intense secondary response. Immunization is effective because it stimulates the production of memory B cells under controlled conditions; it is the secondary response that prevents disease.

Hormones of the Immune System

The specific and nonspecific defenses of the body are coordinated by physical interaction and by the release of chemical messengers. An example of physical interaction is the displaying of antigens by activated macrophages or helper T cells. Examples of chemical messengers are the release of cytokines by many cell types. Cytokines of the immune response are sometimes classified according to their sources: *lymphokines*, secreted by lymphocytes, and *monokines*, released by active macrophages and other antigen-presenting cells. The general term cytokine is preferable, however, since lymphocytes, macrophages, and cells involved with nonspecific defenses and tissue repair may secrete the same chemical messenger.

Table 15-2 contains examples of some of the cytokines identified to date. **Interleukins (Il)** are probably the most diverse and important chemical messengers in the immune system. These proteins have widespread effects that include increasing T cell and B cell sensitivities and enhancing nonspecific defenses, such as inflammation or fever. Massive production of interleukins can cause problems at least as severe as those of the primary infection. For example, in *Lyme disease*, the release of Il-1 by activated macrophages produces symptoms of fever, pain, skin rash, and arthritis that affect the entire body in response to a localized bacterial infection.

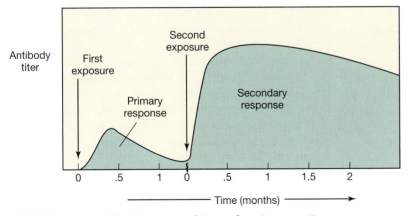

•**FIGURE 15-15** **The Primary and Secondary Immune Responses** The primary response takes several weeks to develop peak antibody titers, and antibody concentrations do not remain elevated. The secondary response is characterized by a very rapid increase in antibody titer, to levels much higher than those of the primary response. Antibody activity remains elevated for an extended period following the second exposure to the antigen.

TABLE 15-2   **Examples of Chemical Mediators (Cytokines) of the Immune Response**

Compound	Functions
INTERLEUKINS	
Il-1	Stimulates T cells, promotes inflammation, causes fever
Il-2, -12	Stimulate T cells and NK cells
Il-3	Stimulates production of blood cells
Il-4, -5, -6, -7, -10, -11	Promote differentiation and growth of B cells, and stimulate plasma cell formation and antibody production
INTERFERONS	Activate other cells to prevent viral entry and replication, stimulate NK cells and macrophages
TUMOR NECROSIS FACTORS (TNFs)	Kill tumor cells, stimulate activities of T cells and eosinophils, inhibit parasites and viruses
PHAGOCYTIC REGULATORS	
Monocyte-chemotactic factor (MCF)	Attracts monocytes, activates them to macrophages
Macrophage-inhibitory factor (MIF)	Prevents macrophage migration from the area
COLONY-STIMULATING FACTORS (CSFs)	
M-CSF	Stimulates activity in the monocyte-macrophage line
GM-CSF	Stimulates production of both microphages and monocytes

Interferons make the synthesizing cell and its neighbors resistant to viral infection, thereby slowing the spread of the virus. These compounds may have other beneficial effects in addition to their antiviral activity.

Tumor necrosis factors (TNFs) slow tumor growth and kill sensitive tumor cells. In addition to their effects on tumor cells, tumor necrosis factors (1) stimulate the production of neutrophils, eosinophils, and basophils; (2) promote eosinophil activity; (3) cause fever; and (4) increase T cell sensitivity to interleukins.

Phagocytic regulators include several cytokines that coordinate the specific and nonspecific defenses by adjusting the activities of phagocytic cells. These cytokines include factors that attract free macrophages and microphages to the area and prevent their premature departure.

Colony-stimulating factors (CSFs) are produced by a wide variety of cells including active T cells, cells of the monocyte-macrophage group, and fibroblasts. CSFs stimulate the production of blood cells in the bone marrow and lymphocytes in lymphoid tissues and organs.

✓ A decrease in the number of cytotoxic T cells would affect what type of immunity?

✓ How would a lack of helper T cells affect the humoral immune response?

✓ A sample of lymph contains an elevated number of plasma cells. On the basis of this observation, would you expect the amount of antibodies in the blood to be increasing or decreasing? Why?

PATTERNS OF IMMUNE RESPONSE

We have discussed the basic chemical and cellular interactions that follow the appearance of a foreign antigen. Figure 15-16• presents a broader, integrated view of the immune response and its relationship to nonspecific defenses.

Immune Disorders

Because the immune response is so complex, there are many opportunities for things to go wrong. A great variety of clinical conditions can result from disorders of immune function. General classes of such disorders include *immunodeficiency diseases*, *autoimmune disorders*, and *allergies.* Immunodeficiency diseases and autoimmune disorders are relatively rare conditions—clear evidence of the effectiveness of the immune system's control mechanisms. Allergies make up a far more common, and usually far less dangerous, class of immune disorders. In an **immunodeficiency disease**, either the immune system fails to develop normally or the immune response is blocked in some way. AIDS, an important example of an immunodeficiency disease, was considered on p. 426. We will consider autoimmune disorders and allergies next.

Autoimmune Disorders

Autoimmune disorders develop when the immune response mistakenly targets normal body cells and tissues. The immune system usually recognizes and

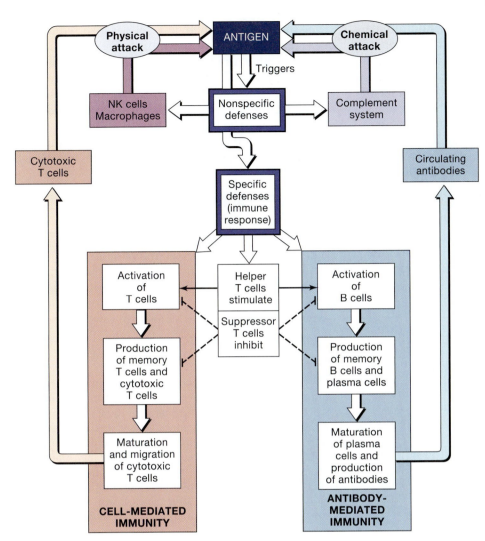

•FIGURE 15-16
An Integrated Summary of the
Immune Response

ignores the antigens normally found in the body. The recognition system can malfunction, however, and when it does, the activated B cells begin to manufacture antibodies against other cells and tissues. The resulting symptoms depend on the identity of the antigen attacked by these misguided antibodies, called *autoantibodies*. For example, *rheumatoid arthritis* occurs when autoantibodies attack joint surfaces.

Many autoimmune disorders appear to be cases of mistaken identity. For example, proteins associated with the measles, influenza, and other viruses contain amino acid sequences that are similar to those of myelin proteins. As a result, antibodies that target these viruses may also attack myelin sheaths, producing the neurological complications sometimes associated with a vaccination or viral infection.

Similarly, unusual types of MHC proteins have been linked to at least 50 clinical conditions. These disorders include psoriasis, rheumatoid arthritis, myasthenia gravis, multiple sclerosis, narcolepsy, Type 1 diabetes, Graves' disease, Addison's disease, pernicious anemia, systemic lupus erythematosus, and chronic hepatitis.

Allergies

Allergies are inappropriate or excessive immune responses to antigens. The sudden increase in cellular activity or antibody titers can have a number of unpleasant side effects. For example, neutrophils or cytotoxic T cells may destroy normal cells while attacking the antigen, or the antigen-antibody complex may trigger a massive inflammatory response. Antigens that trigger allergic reactions are often called **allergens**.

Four types of allergies are recognized: *immediate hypersensitivity (Type I), cytotoxic reactions (Type II), immune complex disorders (Type III),* and *delayed hypersensitivity (Type IV).* Immediate hypersensitivity is probably the most common type, and it includes "hay fever" and environmental allergies that may affect 15 percent of the U.S. population. The cross-reactions that occur following the transfusion of an incompatible blood type is an example of Type II hypersensitivity. ∞ p. 341

Immediate hypersensitivity begins when B cells and helper T cells are first exposed and *sensitized* to an allergen. Sensitization leads to the production of large quantities of IgE antibodies. The tendency to produce IgE antibodies in response to an allergen may be genetically determined. The first exposure to an allergen does not produce allergic symptoms. However, the IgE antibodies that are produced at this time become attached to the cell membranes of basophils and mast cells throughout the body. When exposed to the same allergen later, these cells are stimulated to release histamine, heparin, several cytokines, prostaglandins, and other chemicals into the surrounding tissues. The result is a sudden inflammation of the affected tissues.

The severity of the allergic reaction depends on the person's sensitivity and the location involved. If the allergen exposure occurs at the body surface, the response is usually restricted to that area. If the allergen enters the bloodstream, the response may be more dramatic and occasionally lethal.

✳ ANAPHYLAXIS

The most severe type of allergic reaction is an *anaphylactic reaction.* Anaphylactic reactions often develop when a specific allergen is injected directly into the circulation (such as occurs following a bee sting or penicillin injection). When the allergen enters the circulation, it is widely distributed through the blood, where it interacts with both basophils and mast cells. Once activated, these cells begin dumping *histamine* and other substances associated with anaphylaxis into the blood, including the *slow-reacting substance of anaphylaxis (SRS-A).* Together, these cause widespread peripheral vasodilation and increased capillary permeability. The patient develops characteristic skin lesions (urticaria) and significant bronchoconstriction. Hypotension, airway obstruction, and respiratory failure may ensue. Death can rapidly follow if appropriate emergency measures are not provided.

Age and the Immune Response

With advancing age, the immune system becomes less effective at combating disease. T cells become less responsive to antigens, so fewer cytotoxic T cells respond to an infection. This effect may, at least in part, be associated with the gradual decrease in size (*involution*) of the thymus and with reduced thymosin production. Because the number of helper T cells is also reduced, B cells are less responsive, and antibody levels do not rise as quickly after antigen exposure. The net result is an increased susceptibility to viral and bacterial infection. For this reason, vaccinations for acute viral diseases, such as the flu (influenza), are strongly recommended for elderly people. The increased incidence of cancer in the elderly reflects the fact that immune surveillance declines, and tumor cells are not eliminated as effectively.

INTEGRATION WITH OTHER SYSTEMS

Figure 15-17● summarizes the interactions between the lymphatic system and other physiological systems. The relationships between the cells and tissues involved with the immune response and the nervous and endocrine systems are now the focus of intense research.

✳ RABIES

Few diseases today invoke fear like *rabies.* Rabies is an oftentimes fatal disease contracted through the saliva of infected carnivores and bats. In the United States, rabies is present in all 48 contiguous states. Fortunately, through pet vaccination programs, the incidence of human rabies in the United States is quite low. Once rabies disease occurs, there is no successful treatment. However, survival is excellent if an immunization program is started promptly after the exposure and before the disease begins. Treatment includes administration of *human rabies immunoglobulin (HRIG),* which provides immediate *passive immunity.* Concurrently, *active immunity* is provided by the administration of *human diploid cell vaccine (HDCV).* Passive immunity lasts for 21 days while active immunity begins on day 3 and lasts for at least 2 years.

✓ Would the primary response or the secondary response be more affected by a lack of memory B cells for a particular antigen?

✓ Which kind of immunity protects a growing fetus, and how does that immunity develop?

*C*hapter Review

KEY TERMS

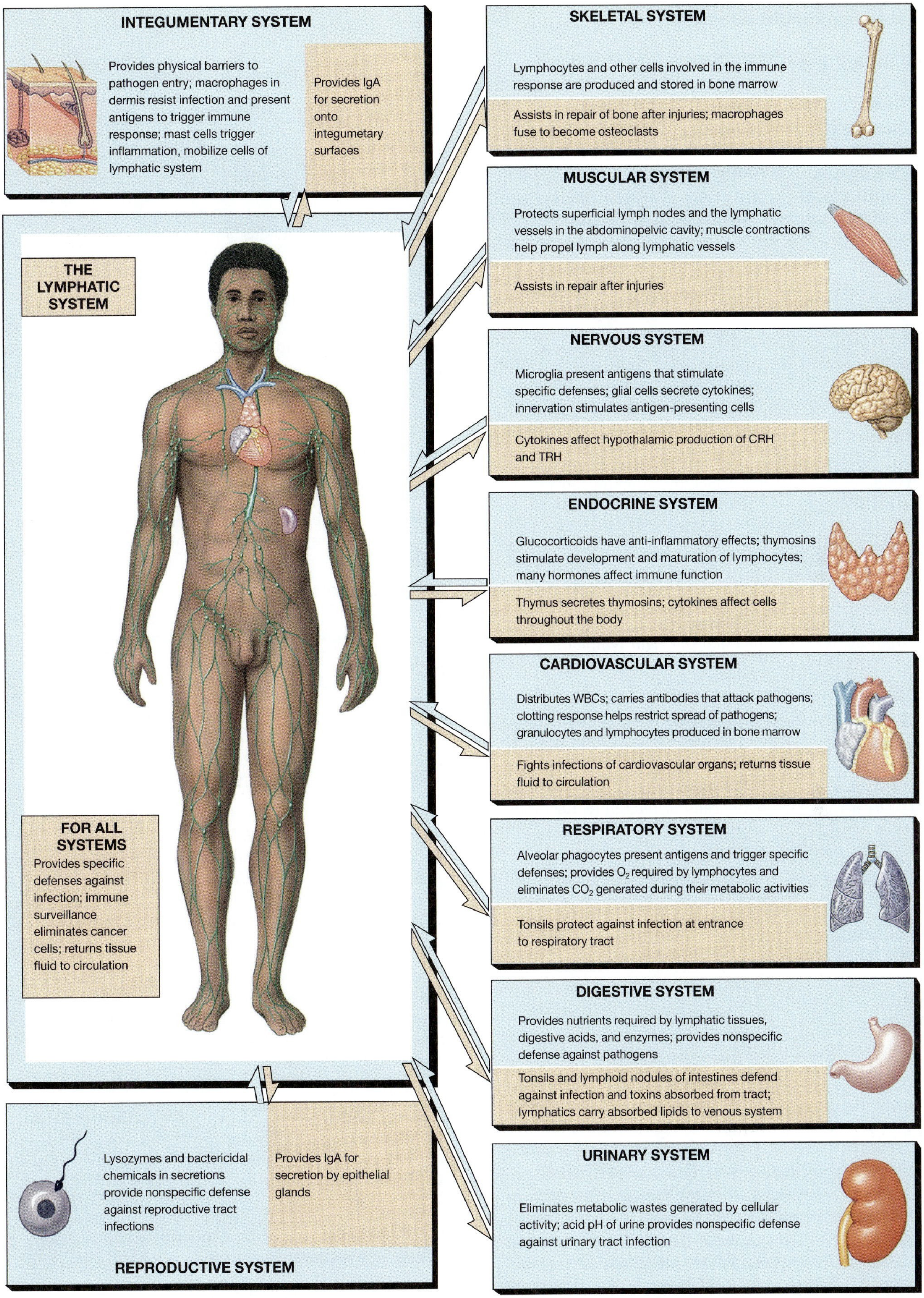

INTEGUMENTARY SYSTEM

Provides physical barriers to pathogen entry; macrophages in dermis resist infection and present antigens to trigger immune response; mast cells trigger inflammation, mobilize cells of lymphatic system

Provides IgA for secretion onto integumetary surfaces

THE LYMPHATIC SYSTEM

FOR ALL SYSTEMS

Provides specific defenses against infection; immune surveillance eliminates cancer cells; returns tissue fluid to circulation

Lysozymes and bactericidal chemicals in secretions provide nonspecific defense against reproductive tract infections

Provides IgA for secretion by epithelial glands

REPRODUCTIVE SYSTEM

SKELETAL SYSTEM

Lymphocytes and other cells involved in the immune response are produced and stored in bone marrow

Assists in repair of bone after injuries; macrophages fuse to become osteoclasts

MUSCULAR SYSTEM

Protects superficial lymph nodes and the lymphatic vessels in the abdominopelvic cavity; muscle contractions help propel lymph along lymphatic vessels

Assists in repair after injuries

NERVOUS SYSTEM

Microglia present antigens that stimulate specific defenses; glial cells secrete cytokines; innervation stimulates antigen-presenting cells

Cytokines affect hypothalamic production of CRH and TRH

ENDOCRINE SYSTEM

Glucocorticoids have anti-inflammatory effects; thymosins stimulate development and maturation of lymphocytes; many hormones affect immune function

Thymus secretes thymosins; cytokines affect cells throughout the body

CARDIOVASCULAR SYSTEM

Distributes WBCs; carries antibodies that attack pathogens; clotting response helps restrict spread of pathogens; granulocytes and lymphocytes produced in bone marrow

Fights infections of cardiovascular organs; returns tissue fluid to circulation

RESPIRATORY SYSTEM

Alveolar phagocytes present antigens and trigger specific defenses; provides O_2 required by lymphocytes and eliminates CO_2 generated during their metabolic activities

Tonsils protect against infection at entrance to respiratory tract

DIGESTIVE SYSTEM

Provides nutrients required by lymphatic tissues, digestive acids, and enzymes; provides nonspecific defense against pathogens

Tonsils and lymphoid nodules of intestines defend against infection and toxins absorbed from tract; lymphatics carry absorbed lipids to venous system

URINARY SYSTEM

Eliminates metabolic wastes generated by cellular activity; acid pH of urine provides nonspecific defense against urinary tract infection

15

•FIGURE 15-17   Functional Relationships Between the Lymphatic System and Other Systems

SUMMARY OUTLINE

INTRODUCTION *p. 412*

1. The cells, tissues, and organs of the **lymphatic system** play a central role in the body's defenses against a variety of **pathogens**, or disease-causing organisms.

2. **Lymphocytes**, the primary cells of the lymphatic system, provide an **immune response** to specific threats to the body. **Immunity** is the ability to resist infection and disease through the activation of specific defenses.

ORGANIZATION OF THE LYMPHATIC SYSTEM *p. 412*

1. The lymphatic system includes a network of **lymphatic vessels** that carry **lymph** (a fluid similar to plasma but with a lower concentration of proteins). A series of **lymphoid organs** are connected to the lymphatic vessels. *(Figure 15-1)*

Functions of the Lymphatic System *p. 412*

2. The lymphatic system produces, maintains, and distributes lymphocytes (cells that attack invading organisms, abnormal cells, and foreign proteins). The system also helps maintain blood volume and eliminate local variations in the composition of the interstitial fluid.

Lymphatic Vessels *p. 413*

3. Lymph flows along a network of *lymphatics* that originate in the **lymphatic capillaries**. The lymphatic vessels empty into the **thoracic duct** and the **right lymphatic duct**. *(Figures 15-1 to 15-3)*

Lymphocytes *p. 413*

4. The three classes of lymphocytes are **T cells** (*thymus-dependent*), **B cells** (*bone marrow-derived*), and **natural killer (NK) cells**.

5. *Cytotoxic T cells* attack foreign cells or body cells infected by viruses; they provide *cellular immunity*. **Regulatory T cells** (*helper* and *suppressor T cells*) regulate and coordinate the immune response.

6. B cells can differentiate into **plasma cells**, which produce and secrete antibodies that react with specific chemical targets, or **antigens**. Antibodies in body fluids are also called **immunoglobulins**. B cells are responsible for *antibody-mediated immunity*, or *humoral immunity*.

7. NK cells attack foreign cells, normal cells infected with viruses, and cancer cells. They provide a monitoring service called *immunological surveillance*.

8. Lymphocytes continuously migrate in and out of the blood through the lymphoid tissues and organs. *Lymphopoiesis* (lymphocyte production) involves the bone marrow, thymus, and peripheral lymphoid tissues. *(Figure 15-4)*

Lymphoid Nodules *p. 415*

9. A **lymphoid nodule** consists of loose connective tissue containing densely packed lymphocytes.

Lymphoid Organs *p. 416*

10. Important lymphoid organs include the *lymph nodes*, the *thymus*, and the *spleen*. Lymphoid tissues and organs are distributed in areas especially vulnerable to injury or invasion.

11. **Lymph nodes** are encapsulated masses of lymphoid tissue containing lymphocytes. Lymph nodes monitor the lymph before it drains into the venous system, removing antigens and initiating appropriate immune responses. *(Figure 15-5)*

12. The **thymus** lies behind the sternum. T cells become mature in the thymus. *(Figure 15-6)*

13. The adult **spleen** contains the largest mass of lymphoid tissue in the body. The cellular components form the **pulp** of the spleen. *Red pulp* contains large numbers of red blood cells, and areas of *white pulp* resemble lymphoid nodules. The spleen removes antigens and damaged blood cells from the circulation, initiates appropriate immune responses, and stores iron obtained from recycled red blood cells. *(Figure 15-7)*

Body Defenses and the Lymphatic System *p. 418*

14. The lymphatic system is a major component of the body's defenses. These fall into two categories: (1) **nonspecific defenses**, which do not discriminate between one threat and another; and (2) **specific defenses**, which protect against threats on an individual basis.

NONSPECIFIC DEFENSES *p. 418*

1. Nonspecific defenses prevent the approach, deny the entrance, or limit the spread of living or nonliving hazards. *(Figure 15-8)*

Physical Barriers *p. 418*

2. Physical barriers include hair, epithelia, and various secretions of the integumentary and digestive systems.

Phagocytes *p. 418*

3. Two types of cells are **phagocytes**: **microphages** (neutrophils and eosinophils) and **macrophages** (cells of the *monocyte-macrophage system*).

4. Phagocytes move between cells through *diapedesis*, and they show *chemotaxis* (sensitivity and orientation to chemical stimuli).

Immunological Surveillance *p. 420*

5. **Immunological surveillance** involves constant monitoring of normal tissues by NK cells sensitive to abnormal antigens on the surfaces of otherwise normal cells. Cancer cells with tumor-specific antigens on their surfaces are killed.

Interferons *p. 420*

6. **Interferons**, small proteins released by cells infected with viruses, trigger the production of antiviral proteins that interfere with viral replication inside the cell. Interferons are *cytokines*, chemical messengers released by tissue cells to coordinate local activities.

Complement *p. 420*

7. Eleven *complement proteins* make up the **complement system**. They interact with each other in chain reactions to destroy target cell membranes, stimulate inflammation, attract phagocytes, and enhance phagocytosis.

Inflammation *p. 420*

8. **Inflammation** represents a coordinated nonspecific response to tissue injury. *(Figure 15-9)*

Fever *p. 421*

9. A **fever** (body temperature greater than 37.2°C or 99°F) can inhibit pathogens and accelerate metabolic processes.

SPECIFIC DEFENSES: THE IMMUNE RESPONSE
p. 421

1. Specific defenses are provided by T cells and B cells. T cells provide **cell-mediated immunity**; B cells provide **antibody-mediated immunity**.

Forms of Immunity *p. 421*

2. Specific immunity may involve **innate immunity** (genetically determined and present at birth) or **acquired immunity**. The two types of acquired immunity are **active immunity** (which appears following exposure to an antigen) and **passive immunity** (produced by the transfer of antibodies from another person). *(Figure 15-10)*

Properties of Immunity *p. 422*

3. Lymphocytes provide specific immunity, which has four general characteristics: specificity, versatility, memory, and tolerance. **Specificity** occurs because only specific antigens can bind to T cell and B cell membranes. The immune system is versatile in that it can respond to any of the tens of thousands of antigens it encounters. **Memory cells** enable the immune system to "remember" previous target antigens. **Tolerance** refers to the ability of the immune system to ignore some antigens, such as those of body cells.

An Overview of the Immune Response *p. 422*

4. The goal of the **immune response** is to destroy or inactivate pathogens, abnormal cells, and foreign molecules. It is based on the activation of lymphocytes by specific antigens through the process of **antigen recognition**. *(Figure 15-11)*

T Cells and Cell-Mediated Immunity *p. 422*

5. Foreign antigens must usually be processed by macrophages and incorporated into their cell membranes bound to *MHC proteins* before they can activate T cells. T cells can also be activated by viral antigens displayed on the surfaces of virus-infected cells.

6. Activated T cells may differentiate into *cytotoxic T cells, memory T cells, suppressor T cells,* or *helper T cells.*

7. Cell-mediated immunity results from the activation of **cytotoxic**, or *killer*, **T cells**. Activated **memory T cells** remain on reserve to guard against future such attacks. *(Figure 15-12)*

8. **Suppressor T cells** depress the responses of other T and B cells. *(Figure 15-16)*

9. **Helper T cells** secrete cytokines that help coordinate specific and nonspecific defenses and regulate cellular and humoral immunity. *(Figure 15-13)*

B Cells and Antibody-Mediated Immunity *p. 424*

10. B cells, responsible for antibody-mediated immunity, normally become activated by helper T cells sensitive to the same antigen.

11. An activated B cell divides and produces plasma cells and **memory B cells**. Antibodies are produced by the plasma cells. *(Figure 15-13)*

12. An antibody molecule consists of two parallel pairs of polypeptide chains containing *fixed segments* and *variable segments.* *(Figure 15-14)*

13. When an antibody molecule binds to an antigen, they form an **antigen-antibody complex**. Antibodies focus on specific *antigenic determinant sites*.

14. Five classes of antibodies exist in body fluids: (1) **immunoglobulin G (IgG)**, responsible for resistance against many viruses, bacteria, and bacterial toxins; (2) *IgM*, the first antibody type secreted after an antigen arrives; (3) *IgA*, found in glandular secretions; (4) *IgE*, which releases chemicals that accelerate local inflammation; and (5) *IgD*, found on the surfaces of B cells. *(Table 15-1)*

15. Antibodies can destroy antigens through **neutralization**, **precipitation** and **agglutination**, the activation of complement, the attraction of phagocytes, the enhancement of phagocytosis, and the stimulation of inflammation.

16. The antibodies produced by plasma cells on first exposure to an antigen are the agents of the **primary response**. The maximum antibody titer appears during the **secondary** *(anamnestic)* **response**, which follows subsequent exposure to the same antigen. *(Figure 15-15)*

Hormones of the Immune System *p. 427*

17. **Interleukins (Il)** increase T cell sensitivity to antigens exposed on macrophage membranes; stimulate B cell activity, plasma cell formation, and antibody production; and enhance nonspecific defenses.

18. Interferons slow the spread of a virus by making the cell that synthesized them, and that cell's neighbors, resistant to viral infections.

19. **Tumor necrosis factors (TNFs)** slow tumor growth and kill tumor cells.

20. Several **phagocytic regulators** adjust the activities of phagocytic cells to coordinate specific and nonspecific defenses. *(Table 15-2)*

PATTERNS OF IMMUNE RESPONSE *p. 428*

1. Foreign antigens may undergo physical or chemical attack by specific and nonspecific defenses. *(Figure 15-16)*

Immune Disorders *p. 428*

2. In an **immunodeficiency disease**, either the immune system does not develop normally or the immune response is somehow blocked.

3. **Autoimmune disorders** develop when the immune response mistakenly targets normal body cells and tissues.

4. **Allergies** are inappropriate or excessive immune responses to **allergens** (antigens that trigger allergic reactions). The four types of allergies are *immediate hypersensitivity (Type I), cytotoxic reactions (Type II), immune complex disorders (Type III),* and *delayed hypersensitivity (Type IV).*

Age and the Immune Response *p. 430*

5. With aging, the immune system becomes less effective at combating disease.

INTEGRATION WITH OTHER SYSTEMS *p. 430*

1. The lymphatic system has extensive interactions with the nervous and endocrine systems.

REVIEW QUESTIONS

LEVEL 1   Reviewing Facts and Terms

Match each item in column A with the most closely related item in column B. Use letters for answers in the spaces provided.

Column A

___ 1. humoral immunity

___ 2. lymphoma

___ 3. complement

___ 4. microphages

___ 5. macrophages

___ 6. microglia

___ 7. interferon

___ 8. pyrogens

___ 9. innate immunity

___10. active immunity

___11. passive immunity

___12. apoptosis

Column B

a. induce fever

b. system of circulating proteins

c. CNS macrophages

d. monocytes

e. genetically programmed cell death

f. transfers of antibodies

g. neutrophils, eosinophils

h. secretion of antibodies

i. present at birth

j. cytokine

k. lymphatic system cancer

l. exposure to antigen

13. Lymph from the lower abdomen, pelvis, and lower limbs is received by the:
    (a) right lymphatic duct   (b) inguinal duct
    (c) thoracic duct   (d) aorta

14. Lymphocytes responsible for providing cell-mediated immunity are called:
    (a) macrophages
    (b) B cells
    (c) plasma cells
    (d) cytotoxic T cells

15. B cells are responsible for:
    (a) cellular immunity
    (b) immunological surveillance
    (c) antibody-mediated immunity
    (d) a, b, and c are correct

16. Lymphoid stem cells that can form all types of lymphocytes occur in the:
    (a) bloodstream   (b) thymus
    (c) bone marrow   (d) spleen

17. Lymphatics are found in all portions of the body except the:
    (a) lower limbs
    (b) central nervous system
    (c) head and neck region
    (d) hands and feet

18. The largest collection of lymphoid tissue in the body is contained in the:
    (a) adult spleen   (b) adult thymus
    (c) bone marrow   (d) tonsils

19. Red blood cells that are damaged or defective are removed from the circulation by the:
    (a) thymus   (b) lymph nodes
    (c) spleen   (d) tonsils

20. Phagocytes move through capillary walls by squeezing between adjacent endothelial cells, a process known as:
    (a) diapedesis
    (b) chemotaxis
    (c) adhesion
    (d) perforation

21. Perforins are destructive proteins associated with the activity of:
    (a) T cells
    (b) B cells
    (c) macrophages
    (d) plasma cells

22. Complement activation:
    (a) stimulates inflammation
    (b) attracts phagocytes
    (c) enhances phagocytosis
    (d) a, b, and c are correct

23. Inflammation:
    (a) aids in temporary repair at an injury site
    (b) slows the spread of pathogens
    (c) facilitates permanent repair
    (d) a, b, and c are correct

24. Memory B cells:
    (a) respond to a threat on first exposure
    (b) secrete large numbers of antibodies into the interstitial fluid
    (c) deal with subsequent injuries or infections that involve the same antigens
    (d) contain binding sites that can activate the complement system

25. Which two large collecting vessels are responsible for returning lymph to the veins of the circulatory system? What areas of the body does each serve?

26. Give a function for each of the following:
    (a) cytotoxic T cells
    (b) helper T cells
    (c) suppressor (regulatory) T cells
    (d) plasma cells
    (e) NK cells
    (f) interferons
    (g) T cells
    (h) B cells
    (i) interleukins

27. What seven defenses, present at birth, provide the body with the defensive capability known as nonspecific resistance?

15

LEVEL 2   Reviewing Concepts

28. Compared with nonspecific defenses, *specific* defenses:
    (a) do not discriminate between one threat and another
    (b) are always present at birth
    (c) provide protection against threats on an individual basis
    (d) deny entrance of pathogens to the body

29. T cells and B cells can be activated only by:
    (a) pathogenic microorganisms
    (b) interleukins, interferons, and colony-stimulating factors
    (c) cells infected with viruses, bacterial cells, or cancer cells
    (d) exposure to a specific antigen at a specific site on a cell membrane

30. List and explain the four general properties of immunity.
31. How does the formation of an antibody-antigen complex cause elimination of an antigen?
32. What effects follow activation of the complement system?

LEVEL 3   Critical Thinking and Clinical Applications

33. An investigator at a crime scene discovers some body fluid on the victim's clothing. The investigator carefully takes a sample and sends it to the crime lab for analysis. On the basis of analysis of immunoglobulins, could the crime lab determine whether the sample was blood plasma or semen? Explain.

34. Ted finds out that he has been exposed to the measles. He is concerned that he might have contracted the disease. His physician takes a blood sample and sends it to a lab for antibody titers. The results show an elevated level of IgM antibodies to rubella (measles) virus but very few IgG antibodies to the virus. Did Ted contract the disease?

ANSWERS TO CONCEPT CHECK QUESTIONS

Page 418
1. The thoracic duct drains lymph from the area beneath the diaphragm and the left side of the head and thorax. Most of the lymph enters the venous blood by way of this duct. A blockage of this duct would not only impair circulation of lymph through most of the body, but also it would promote the accumulation of fluid in the extremities (lymphedema).   **2.** The thymosins from the thymus play a role in the differentiation of stem lymphocytes into T lymphocytes. A lack of these hormones would result in an absence of T lymphocytes.   **3.** During an infection, the lymphocytes and phagocytes in the lymph nodes in the affected region undergo cell division to deal with the infectious agent better. This increase in the number of cells in the nodes causes the nodes to become enlarged or swollen.

Page 421
1. A decrease in the number of monocyte-forming cells in the bone marrow would result in a decreased number of macrophages in the body, since all of the different macrophages are derived from monocytes. The macrophages would include the microglia of the CNS, the Kuppfer's cells of the liver, and alveolar macrophages.   **2.** A rise in interferon levels would indicate a viral infection. Interferon is released from cells that are infected with viruses. It does not help the infected cell but "interferes" with the virus's ability to infect other cells.   **3.** Pyrogens stimulate the temperature control area within the hypothalamus. The result is an increase in body temperature, or fever.

Page 428
1. Cytotoxic T cells function in cell-mediated immunity. A decrease in the number of cytotoxic T cells would interfere with the ability to kill foreign cells and tissues as well as cells infected by viruses.   **2.** Helper T cells promote B cell division, the maturation of plasma cells, and the production of antibody by plasma cells. Without helper T cells, the humoral immune response would be much slower and less efficient.   **3.** Since plasma cells produce and secrete antibodies, we would expect to see increased levels of circulating antibodies in the blood if the number of plasma cells were increased.

Page 430
1. The secondary response would be affected by the lack of memory B cells for a specific antigen. The ability to produce a secondary response depends on the presence of memory B cells and T cells that are formed during the primary response to an antigen. These cells are not involved in the primary response but are held in reserve against future contact with the same antigen.   **2.** The developing fetus is protected primarily by passive immunity, the product of IgG antibodies that cross the placenta from the mother's circulation. In addition, the fetus may show some degree of active cellular immunity by the third month of development.

1
5

Emergency Care Applications

OVERVIEW

The immune system is the principle body system involved in fighting disease. Much of immune system function occurs in the lymphatic system, which consists of the lymphatic vessels, the lymph, and the lymph organs. Its primary functions are the production, maintenance, and distribution of lymphocytes (white blood cells); the return of fluid and solutes from the peripheral tissues to the blood; and the distribution of hormones, nutrients, and waste products from their tissues of origin to the general circulation. Immunity is one of the body's major defense mechanisms. It is provided by the coordinated activities of T cells and B cells, which respond to the presence of specific antigens. T cells provide cellular immunity, while B cells provide humoral immunity.

Physicians who specialize in the immune system disorders are referred to as *allergists* or *allergists/immunologists.* They usually train in general internal medicine or pediatrics and take additional training in allergy and immunology. An *immunologist* is a scientist (Ph.D., M.D., or D.O.) who specializes in the study of the immune system. A closely related medical discipline is infectious disease. Because infectious disease processes almost always involve the body's immune system, *infectious disease* specialists often treat immune system disorders. Like an allergist/immunologist, an infectious disease specialist first trains in general internal medicine or pediatrics and then serves a fellowship in infectious disease.

IMMUNITY

The ability of the body's defenses to combat infection with specific responses is called *immunity.* The immune response is a complex cascade of events that occurs following activation by an invading substance, or *pathogen.* Its goal is the destruction or inactivation of pathogens, abnormal cells, or foreign molecules such as toxins. The body can accomplish this through two mechanisms, cellular immunity and humoral immunity. Cellular immunity involves a direct attack on the foreign substance by specialized cells of the immune system. These cells physically engulf and deactivate or destroy the offending agent. Humoral immunity, on the other hand, is much more complicated. Humoral immunity is basically a chemical attack on the invading substance. The principal chemical agents of this attack are antibodies, also called immunoglobulins (Igs). Antibodies are a unique class of chemicals that are manufactured by specialized cells of the immune system called B cells. There are five different classes of antibodies: IgA, IgD, IgE, IgG, and IgM.

The humoral immune response begins with exposure of the body to an antigen. An antigen is any substance capable of inducing an immune response. Most antigens are proteins. Following exposure to an antigen, antibodies are released from cells of the immune system and attach themselves to the invading substance to facilitate its removal from the body by other cells of the immune system.

The immune system responds differently to a particular antigen depending upon if the body has or has not been exposed previously to that antigen. The initial response to an antigen is called the *primary response.* Following exposure to a new antigen, both the cellular and humoral components of the immune system require several days to respond. Generalized antibodies (IgG and IgM) are first released to help fight the antigen.

At the same time, other components of the immune system begin to develop antibodies specific for the antigen. These cells also develop a memory of the particular antigen. If the body is exposed to the same antigen again, the immune system responds much faster. This is called the *secondary response.* As a part of the secondary response, antibodies specific for the offending antigen are released. Antigen-specific antibodies are much more effective in facilitating removal of the offending antigen than are the generalized antibodies released during the primary response.

Immunity may be either natural or acquired. *Natural immunity,* also called *innate immunity,* is genetically predetermined. It is present at birth and has no relation to previous exposure to a particular antigen. All humans are born with some innate immunity. *Acquired immunity* develops over time and results from exposure to an antigen. The immune system's production of antibodies specific for the antigens to which the body is exposed protects the organism, as subsequent exposure to the same antigen will result in a vigorous immune response. Naturally acquired immunity normally begins to develop after birth and is continually enhanced by exposure to new pathogens and antigens throughout life. For example, a child contracts chicken pox (varicella) at age 18 months. Following the infection, the child's immune system creates antibodies specific for the varicella virus. Repeated exposure to the varicella virus usually will not result in another infection. In fact, it is not unusual for a patient exposed to varicella to develop lifelong immunity to the infection.

Induced active immunity, also called *artificially acquired immunity,* is designed to provide protection from exposure to an antigen at some time in the future. This is achieved through vaccination and provides relative protection against serious infectious agents. In vaccination, an antigen is injected into the body so as to generate an immune response. This results in the development of antibodies specific for the antigen and provides protection against future infection. Most vaccines contain antigenic proteins from a particular virus or bacterium. Later, when the individual is actually exposed to the pathogen, the immune response will be vigorous and will often be enough to prevent the infection from developing.

An example of a commonly used vaccine is the DPT (diphtheria/pertussis/tetanus) vaccine. This vaccine contains antigenic proteins from the bacteria that cause diphtheria, whooping cough, and tetanus. It is administered at several intervals during the first five years of life and provides protection against infection from these bacteria. Some vaccinations will impart lifelong immunity, while others must be periodically followed with a "booster dose" to assure continued protection.

Acquired immunity can be either active or passive. *Active immunity* occurs following exposure to an antigen and results in the production of antibodies specific for the antigen. Most vaccinations result in the development of active immunity. However, it takes some time for a patient to develop specific antibodies. In certain cases, it is necessary to administer antibodies to provide protection until the active immunity can take effect. *Passive immunity* results from the introduction of antibodies. There are two types of passive immunity. *Natural passive immunity* occurs when antibodies cross the placental barrier from the mother to the infant to provide protection against embryonic or fetal infections. *Induced passive immunity* is the administration of antibodies to an individual to help fight infection or prevent diseases.

An example of the clinical use of both active and passive immunity is the regimen used for the prevention of tetanus. Most people from developed countries have received some form of tetanus vaccination during their life. These people typically have some antibodies to tetanus and often need nothing more than a tetanus booster. However, some people have never received any sort of tetanus vaccination. When they seek treatment for a tetanus-prone wound, they must receive prophylaxis for tetanus in addition to care for their wound. This is best achieved by providing both passive and active immunity. To provide immediate protection, the patient is administered antibodies specific for tetanus (tetanus immune globulin [TIG], Hypertet). Then, the patient is also administered a tetanus vaccination (Td or Dt). The tetanus immune globulin (TIG) provides passive immunity until the body's immune system can respond to the vaccination and develop antibodies specific for tetanus. This should be followed by periodic tetanus boosters until the patient's immunization program is complete.

IMMUNIZATION

Immunization is the manipulation of the immune system by administering antigens under controlled conditions or by providing antibodies that can combat an existing infection. Active immunization is the process of inducing the immune system to produce specific antibodies through the administration of a *vaccine.* A vaccine is a preparation of antigens derived from a specific pathogen (*Table A15-1*). The vaccine can be given orally or by injection. Most vaccines contain the pathogenic organism. They may contain either the entire organism or just the antigenic proteins found on the organism. Some vaccines may contain the living organism, while others achieve satisfactory results with a dead organism. If a living organism is used, it is usually weakened, or *attenuated,* to lessen the chances of inducing a real infection. Despite attenuation, some vaccines may contain enough of the pathogenic organism to cause mild signs or symptoms. Regardless, the risks of developing a serious illness are quite low compared to those of contracting the disease because of lack of vaccination.

Inactivated, or "killed," vaccines consist of bacterial cell walls or viral protein coats. These vaccines cannot cause the development of even mild disease symptoms. However, they do not induce as strong an immune response as live or attenuated vaccines. Some attenuated vaccines do not induce long-lasting immunity but require periodic booster injections to keep antibody titers at a protective level.

The administration of a vaccine induces the immune system to produce antibodies specific for the antigen or antigens contained within the vaccine. This is a form of active immunity, and protective antibody levels may take several weeks to develop. Immediate protection can, in some cases, be provided by the administration of antibodies. This process, called *passive immunization,* is effective only for certain infections. Antibody preparations may be general or may be specific for a particular disease.

A15

TABLE A15-1 **Common Immunizations**

Immunization Target	Type of Immunity Provided	Vaccine Type	Remarks
VIRUSES			
Poliovirus	Active	Live, attenuated	Oral
	Active	Killed	Boosters every 2–3 years
Rubella	Active	Live, attenuated	
	Passive	Human antibodies (pooled)	
Mumps	Active	Live, attenuated	
Measles (rubeola)	Active	Live, attenuated	May need second booster
Varicella	Active	Live, attenuated	
Hepatitis A	Passive	Human antibodies (pooled)	
Hepatitus B	Active	Killed	May need periodic boosters
	Passive	Human antibodies (pooled)	
Smallpox	Active	Live, related virus	Boosters every 3–5 years (no longer required as disease appears to have been eliminated)
Yellow fever	Active	Live, attenuated	Boosters every 10 years
Herpes zoster	Passive	Human antibodies (pooled)	
Rabies	Passive	Human antibodies (pooled)	
	Passive	Horse antibodies	
	Active	Killed	Boosters required
BACTERIA			
Typhoid	Active	Killed	Boosters every 2, 3, or 5 years, depending on vaccine type
Tuberculosis	Active	Live, Attenuated	
Plague	Active	Killed	Boosters every 1–2 years
Tetanus	Active	Toxins only	Boosters every 5–10 years
	Passive	Human antibodies (pooled)	
Diptheria	Active	Toxins only	Boosters every 10 years
	Passive	Horse antibodies	
Streptococcal pneumonia	Active	Bacteria and cell wall components	
Botulism	Passive	Horse antibodies	
Rickettsia: Typhus	Active	Killed	Boosters yearly
Hemophilus influenza H (HIB)	Active	Killed	May need periodic boosters
OTHER TOXINS			
Snake bite	Passive	Horse antibodies	
Spider bite	Passive	Horse antibodies	
Venomous fish spine	Passive	Horse antibodies	

The development of specific antibodies is limited primarily to life-threatening diseases such as tetanus, rabies, diphtheria, and hepatitis that cannot be treated by other methods. Usually, specific passive immunizations are very expensive. General passive immunization involves the injection of various antibodies obtained from the blood donor pool. Referred to as *gamma globulin,* these agents can provide limited protection until the immune system responds to an administered vaccine.

More and more vaccines are being developed. It is important that emergency personnel be vaccinated against diseases for which they are deemed to be at increased risk. The most important of these is hepatitis B. The hepatitis B vaccine is effective and should be started as soon as possible. It is usually administered in three doses over six-months. Hepatitis B vaccine is now a part of most infant immunization programs.

Influenza vaccines are important in the prevention of that disease. However, they must be administered on a yearly basis. Because the influenza viruses often have different antigenic proteins on their surfaces, epidemiologists must try to predict which influenza viruses are going to be a problem in the coming year. They then prepare an influenza vaccine that contains antigenic portions of the predicted influenza viruses. The epidemiologists' predictions are usually accurate, but in some years, inaccurate predictions have resulted in outbreaks of particular strains of influenza.

ALLERGIES

An *allergic reaction* is an exaggerated response by the immune system to a foreign substance. Allergic reactions can range from mild skin rashes to severe, life-threatening reactions that involve virtually every body system. The most severe type of allergic reaction is called *anaphylaxis*. Anaphylaxis is a life-threatening emergency that requires prompt recognition and treatment.

The immune system is the principal body system involved in allergic reactions, although other body systems are affected also. These include the cardiovascular system, the respiratory system, the gastrointestinal system, and the nervous system, among others.

An individual's initial exposure, referred to as *sensitization,* results in an immune response. Subsequent exposure induces a much stronger secondary response. Some individuals can become hypersensitive (overly sensitive) to a particular antigen. *Hypersensitivity* is an unexpected and exaggerated reaction to a particular antigen. In many instances, hypersensitivity is used synonymously with the term *allergy.* There are two types of hypersensitivity reactions, delayed and immediate.

Delayed Hypersensitivity

Delayed hypersensitivity results from cellular immunity and therefore does not involve antibodies. It usually occurs in the hours and days following exposure and is the sort of allergy that occurs in normal people. Delayed hypersensitivity most commonly results in a skin rash and is often due to exposure to certain drugs and chemicals. The rash associated with poison ivy is an example of delayed hypersensitivity (Figure A15-1•).

Immediate Hypersensitivity

When people use the term *allergy* they usually are referring to immediate hypersensitivity reactions. Examples of immediate hypersensitivity reactions include hay fever,

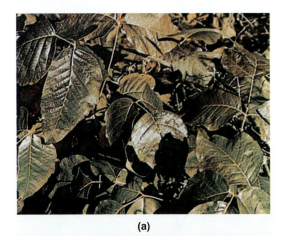
(a)

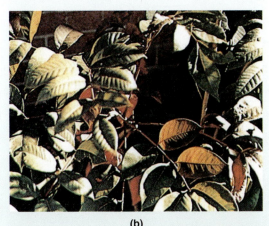
(b)

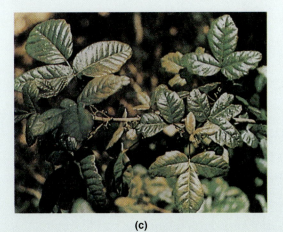
(c)

• **FIGURE A15-1   Poisonous Plants**
Plants of the genus *Toxicodendron* contain the antigenic resin urushiol, which causes a cell-mediated reaction and rash. They are: **(a)** poison ivy, **(b)** poison sumac, and **(c)** poison oak.

drug allergies, food allergies, eczema, and asthma. Some individuals have an allergic tendency. This allergic tendency is usually genetic, meaning it is passed from parent to child and is characterized by the presence of large quantities of IgE antibodies. Any antigen that causes

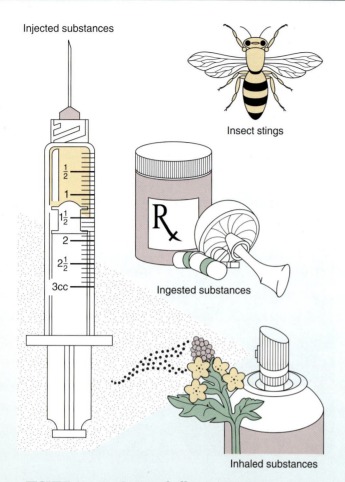

Injected substances

Insect stings

R

Ingested substances

Inhaled substances

• **FIGURE A15-2   Causes of Allergic Reactions**

release of the IgE antibodies is referred to as an allergen. Common allergens include:

- Drugs
- Foods and food additives
- Animals
- Insects (*Hymenoptera* stings) and insect parts
- Fungi and molds
- Radiology contrast materials

Allergens can enter the body through various routes, including oral ingestion, inhalation, topical absorption, injection, and envenomation (Figure A15-2•). The vast majority of anaphylactic reactions result from injection or envenomation.

Parenteral penicillin injections are the most common cause of fatal anaphylactic reactions. Insect stings are the second most frequent cause of fatal anaphylactic reactions. The most frequent offending insects are those in the order *Hymenoptera*. There are three families in this order: fire ants (*Formicoidea*); wasps, yellow jackets, and hornets (*Vespidae*); and honey bees (*Apoidea*). Although these families' venoms all have similar components, each is unique. Honeybees often will leave their stinger embedded in the victim following a sting.

Following the body's exposure to a particular allergen, large quantities of IgE antibodies are released. These antibodies attach to the membranes of basophils and mast cells—specialized cells of the immune system containing chemicals that assist in the immune response. When the allergen binds to IgE attached to the basophils and mast cells, those cells release histamine, heparin, and other substances into the surrounding tissues. Histamine and other substances are stored in granules found within the basophils and mast cells. (Because of this, basophils and mast cells are often called granulocytes.) The process of releasing these substances from the cells, termed *degranulation,* results in what people call an allergic reaction, which can range from very mild to very severe.

The principal chemical mediator of an allergic reaction is *histamine,* a potent substance that activates specialized histamine receptors present throughout the body. This causes bronchoconstriction, increased intestinal motility, vasodilation, and increased vascular permeability. Increased vascular permeability causes fluid from the circulatory system to leak into the surrounding tissues. Thus, a common manifestation of severe allergic reactions and anaphylaxis is *angioneurotic edema,* a marked edema of the skin that usually involves the head, neck, face, and upper airway (Figure A15-3•).

There are two classes of histamine receptors. H_1 receptors, when stimulated, cause bronchoconstriction and contraction of the intestines. H_2 receptors cause peripheral vasodilation and secretion of gastric acids. The goal of histamine release is to minimize the body's exposure to the antigen. Bronchoconstriction decreases the antigen's possibility of entering through the respiratory tract, while increased gastric acid production helps destroy an ingested antigen. Increased intestinal motility serves to move the antigen quickly though the gastrointestinal system with minimal absorption of the antigen into the body. Vasodilation and capillary permeability help remove the allergen from the circulation, where it has the potential to do the most harm.

Anaphylaxis

The most severe type of allergic reaction is *anaphylaxis.* Anaphylaxis usually occurs when a specific allergen is injected directly into the circulation. Thus, anaphylaxis is more common following injections of drugs and diagnostic agents and following bee stings (*Table A15-2*). When the allergen enters the circulation, it is rapidly distributed throughout the body. It interacts with both basophils and mast cells, resulting in the massive dumping of histamine and other substances associated with anaphylaxis. The principal body systems affected by anaphylaxis are the cardiovascular system, the respiratory system, the gastrointestinal system, and the skin. Histamine causes widespread peripheral vasodilation as well as increased permeability of the capillaries. In turn, increased capillary permeability results in marked loss of

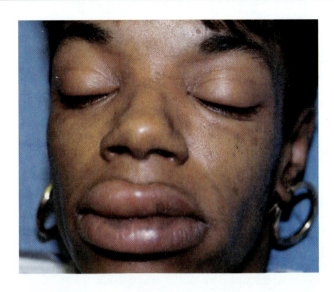

● FIGURE A15-3   Example of Angioneurotic Edema
Swelling of the face and lips can be severe.

TABLE A15-2	Agents That May Cause Anaphylaxis

Antibiotics and other drugs
Foreign proteins (e.g., horse serum, Streptokinase)
Foods (nuts, eggs, shrimp)
Allergen extracts (allergy shots)
Hymenoptera stings (bees, wasps)
Hormones (insulin)
Blood products
Aspirin
Nonsteroidal anti-inflammatory drugs (NSAIDs)
Preservatives (sulfiting agents)
X-ray contrast media
Dextran

plasma from the circulation. People sustaining anaphylaxis can die from circulatory shock.

Also released from the basophils and mast cells is a substance called *slow-reacting substance of anaphylaxis (SRS-A)*. This substance causes spasm of the bronchial smooth muscle, resulting in an asthma-like attack and occasionally asphyxia. SRS-A potentiates the effects of histamine, especially on the respiratory system.

The signs and symptoms of anaphylaxis typically begin within 30–60 seconds following exposure to the offending allergen. In a small percentage of patients, their onset may be delayed more than an hour. The signs and symptoms of anaphylaxis can vary significantly. The severity of the reaction is often proportional to the speed of onset: reactions that develop very quickly tend to be much more severe. Patients suffering an anaphylactic reaction often have a sense of impending doom. In addition to angioneurotic edema involving the face and neck, laryngeal edema is a frequent complication and can threaten the airway. Initially, laryngeal edema will cause hoarseness, and as the edema worsens, the patient may develop stridor. Finally, this may culminate in complete airway obstruction from either massive laryngeal edema, laryngospasm, or-pharyngeal edema, or any combination of these.

The respiratory system is significantly involved in anaphylactic reactions. Initially, the patient will become tachypneic. Later, as lower airway edema and bronchospasm develop, respirations will become labored as evidenced by retractions, accessory muscle usage, and prolonged expiration. Wheezing commonly results from bronchospasm and edema of the smaller airways and may be so pronounced that it can be heard without the aid of a stethoscope. Ultimately, anaphylaxis can result in markedly diminished lung sounds, which reflect decreased air movement and hypoventilation.

The skin is typically involved early in severe allergic reactions and anaphylaxis. Generally, a fine red rash will appear diffusely on the body. As histamine is released, fluid will diffuse from leaky capillaries, resulting in *urticaria*. Urticaria, also called hives, is a wheal and flare reaction characterized by red raised bumps that may appear and disappear across the body (Figure A15-4●). As

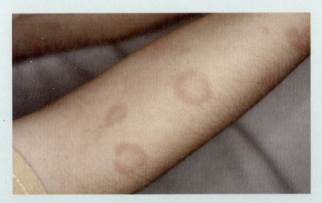

● FIGURE A15-4   Urticaria (Hives) on the Arm

cardiovascular collapse and dyspnea progress, the patient will become diaphoretic. This may, if untreated, progress to cyanosis and pallor.

Histamine's affect on the gastrointestinal system is pronounced. Initially, the patient may note a rumbling sensation in the abdomen as gastrointestinal motility increases. Later, nausea, vomiting, cramping, and diarrhea develop as the body tries to rid itself of the offending allergen.

Emergency treatment of anaphylaxis includes monitoring the patient with all available devices, including the cardiac monitor, the pulse oximeter, and if the patient is intubated, an end-tidal carbon dioxide detector. As anaphylaxis progresses, the end-tidal carbon dioxide level may climb due to the development of both respiratory and metabolic acidosis, which results in increased carbon dioxide elimination. High concentrations of oxygen should be administered and intravenous fluids should be initiated. Emergency medications used in the treatment of anaphylaxis include oxygen, epinephrine, antihistamines, corticosteroids, and vasopressors. Occasionally, inhaled beta agonists, such as albuterol, may be required. Of these, epinephrine remains the primary treatment.

A severe allergic or anaphylactic reaction is a harrowing experience for the patient. Many of the patients you treat will be suffering from forms of allergic reaction less severe than anaphylaxis. An allergic reaction, as contrasted with an anaphylactic reaction, will have a more gradual onset with milder signs and symptoms, and the patient will have a normal mental status. Common manifestations of mild (nonanaphylactic) allergic reactions include itching, rash, and urticaria. Patients with simple itching and nonurticarial rashes may be treated with antihistamines alone. In addition to antihistamines, epinephrine is often necessary for the treatment of urticaria.

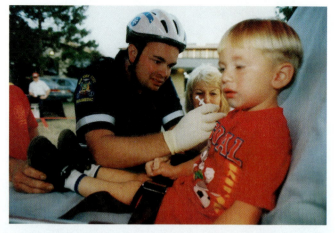

●FIGURE A15-5
Epinephrine remains the primary treatment for all significant allergic reactions, including anaphylaxis.

Lesser allergic reactions that are not accompanied by hypotension or airway problems can be adequately treated with epinephrine 1:1,000 administered subcutaneously (Figure A15-5●).

SUMMARY

The majority of the body's immune functions occur within the lymphatic system, an important body system that is closely associated with the circulatory system. The immune response can be categorized as cellular or humoral. Cellular immunity involves specialized cells that directly attack and remove offending agents, while humoral immunity involves a complex system of antibodies, chemicals that help mark and remove antigenic substances. Emergency personnel should be familiar with the anatomy and physiology of the lymphatic system and the associated immune response.

A15

16

The Respiratory System

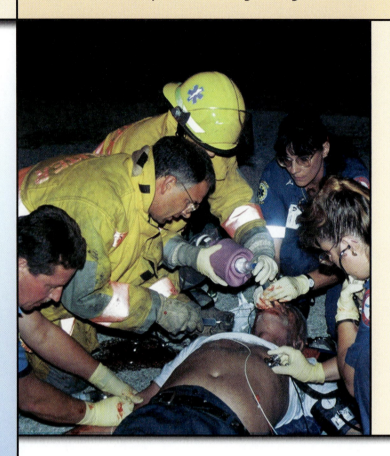

Your initial task in any medical emergency is to evaluate the status of the patient's airway. However, you can learn little about the status of the airway if the patient is not breathing. The respiratory system is a major body system that is closely interfaced with the circulatory system. A change in the respiratory system is often one of the earliest indicators of deterioration in a patient's condition. Such change should prompt immediate and detailed reevaluation.

Chapter Outline and Objectives

Vocabulary Development

alveolus, a hollow cavity; *alveolus, alveolar duct*
ateles, imperfect; *atelectasis*
*bronchus, windpipe, airway; *bronchitis*
cricoid, ring-shaped; *cricoid cartilage*
ektasis, expansion; *atelectasis*
-ia, condition; *pneumonia*
kentesis, puncture; *thoracentesis*
oris, mouth; *oropharynx*
*pneuma, air; *pneumothorax*
pneumon, lung; *pneumonia*
stoma, mouth; *tracheostomy*
thorac-, chest; *thoracentesis*
thyroid, shield-shaped; *thyroid cartilage*

Living cells need energy for maintenance, growth, defense, and replication. Our cells obtain that energy through aerobic respiration, a process that requires oxygen and produces carbon dioxide. ∞ *p. 69* Therefore, the cells in the body must have a way to obtain oxygen and eliminate carbon dioxide. Our respiratory exchange surfaces are inside the lungs, where diffusion occurs between the air and the blood. The exchange surfaces are relatively delicate—they must be very thin to encourage rapid diffusion. The cardiovascular system provides the link between the interstitial fluids of the body and the exchange surfaces of the lungs. The circulating blood carries oxygen from the lungs to peripheral tissues; it also accepts and transports the carbon dioxide generated by those tissues, delivering it to the lungs.

We begin our discussion of the respiratory system by following air as it travels from the exterior to the alveoli of the lungs. We will then consider the mechanics of breathing, or *pulmonary ventilation* (the physical movement of air into and out of the lungs), and the physiology of respiration, which includes the processes of breathing and gas transport and exchange between the air, blood, and tissues.

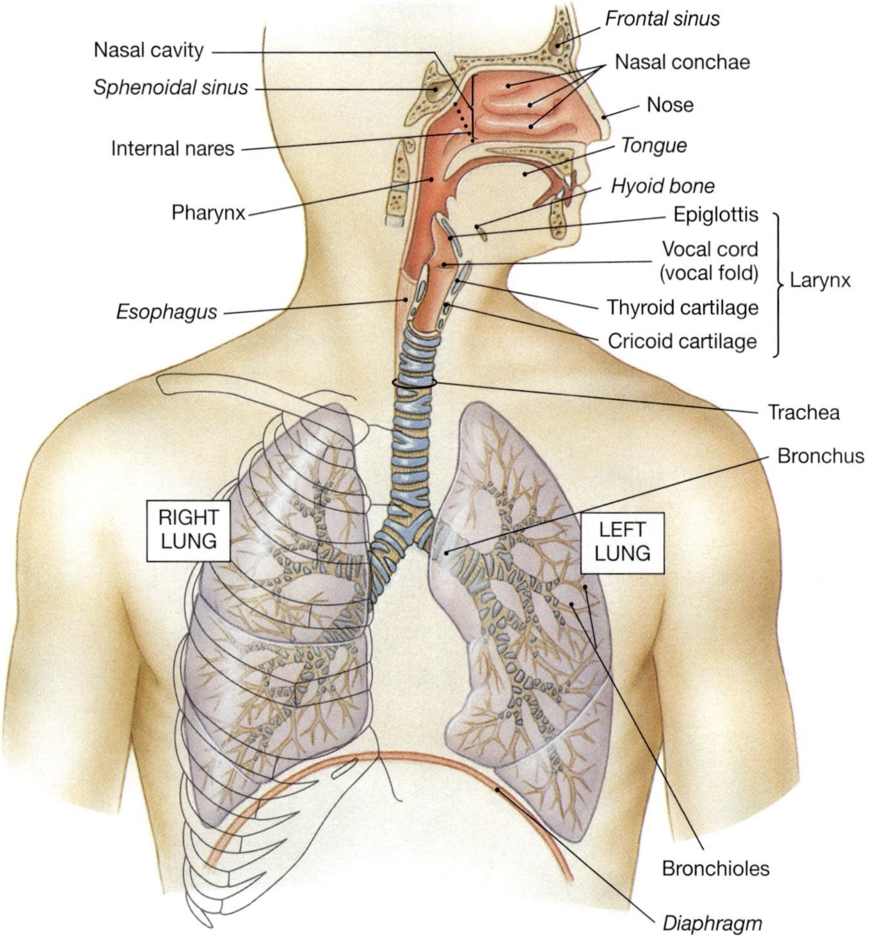

THE FUNCTIONS OF THE RESPIRATORY SYSTEM

The **respiratory system** performs the following range of functions: It (1) moves air to and from the gas-exchange surfaces where diffusion occurs between air and circulating blood, (2) provides nonspecific defenses against pathogenic invasion, (3) permits vocal communication, and (4) helps control the pH of body fluids.

THE ORGANIZATION OF THE RESPIRATORY SYSTEM

The respiratory system consists of the nose, nasal cavity, and sinuses; the pharynx (throat); the larynx (voice box); the trachea (windpipe); and the bronchi and bronchioles (conducting passageways) and alveoli (exchange surfaces) of the lungs (Figure 16-1•).

The Respiratory Tract

Your **respiratory tract** consists of the airways that carry air to and from the exchange surfaces of your lungs. The respiratory tract can be divided into a *conducting portion* and a *respiratory portion*. The conducting portion begins at the entrance to the nasal cavity and continues through the pharynx, larynx, trachea, bronchi, and the larger bronchioles. The respiratory portion includes the smallest and most delicate bronchioles and the alveoli, which are the site of gas exchange.

In addition to delivering air to the lungs, the conducting passageways filter, warm, and humidify the air, thereby protecting the alveoli from debris, pathogens, and environmental extremes. By the time the air reaches the alveoli, most foreign particles and pathogens have been removed, and the humidity and temperature are within acceptable limits.

The Nose

Air normally enters the respiratory system via the paired **external nares** (NĀ-rēz, or nostrils, which communicate with the **nasal cavity**. The **vestibule** (VES-ti-būl) is the anterior portion of the nasal cavity enclosed by the flexible tissues of the nose.

Nasal cavity
Sphenoidal sinus
Internal nares
Pharynx
Esophagus

Frontal sinus
Nasal conchae
Nose
Tongue
Hyoid bone
Epiglottis
Vocal cord (vocal fold)
Thyroid cartilage
Cricoid cartilage
Larynx
Trachea
Bronchus

RIGHT LUNG
LEFT LUNG

Bronchioles
Diaphragm

•FIGURE 16-1   **The Components of the Respiratory System**

1
6

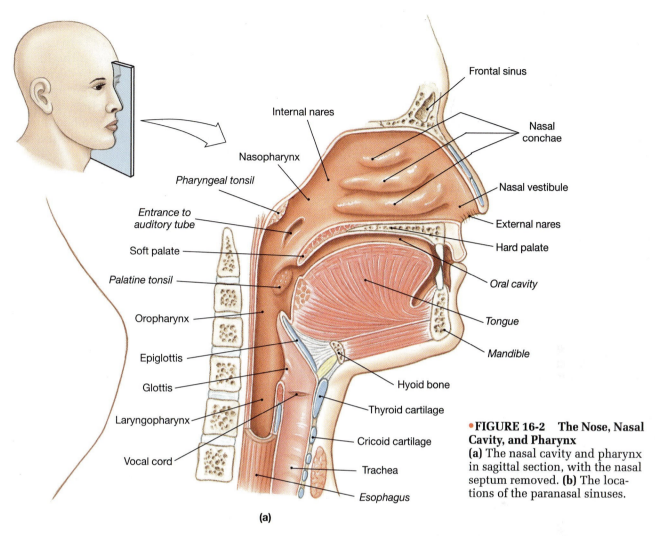

●**FIGURE 16-2   The Nose, Nasal Cavity, and Pharynx**
(a) The nasal cavity and pharynx in sagittal section, with the nasal septum removed. **(b)** The locations of the paranasal sinuses.

Here coarse hairs guard the nasal cavity from large airborne particles such as sand, dust, and insects.

The maxillary, nasal, frontal, ethmoid, and sphenoid bones form the lateral and superior walls of the nasal cavity. The nasal septum divides the nasal cavity into left and right sides. The bony posterior septum includes portions of the vomer and the ethmoid bone. A bony **hard palate**, formed by the palatine and maxillary bones, separates the oral and nasal cavities. A fleshy **soft palate** extends behind the hard palate, marking the boundary line between the superior **nasopharynx** (nā-zō-FĀR-inks) and the rest of the pharynx. The nasal cavity opens into the nasopharynx at the **internal nares**.

Superior, middle, and *inferior nasal conchae* project toward the nasal septum from the lateral walls of the nasal cavity (Figure 16-2a●). To pass from the vestibule to the internal nares, air tends to flow between adjacent conchae. As the air eddies and swirls, like water flowing over rapids, small airborne particles come in contact with the mucus that coats the lining of the nasal cavity. In addition to promoting filtration, the turbulent flow allows extra time for warming and humidifying the incoming air.

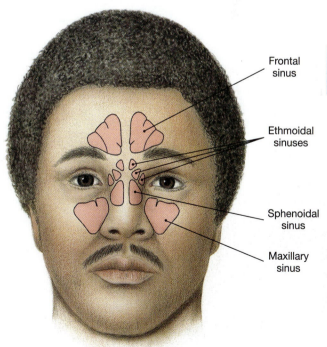

1
6

(b)

The nasal cavity and much of the rest of the respiratory tract are lined by a protective, mucous membrane. ∞ *p. 96* This membrane is made up of the *respiratory epithelium*, a ciliated epithelium containing many *goblet cells*, and an underlying loose connective tissue layer (*the lamina propria*) containing mucous glands (Figure 16-3•). The goblet cells and mucous glands produce mucus that bathes the exposed surfaces of the nasal cavity and lower respiratory tract. Cilia sweep that mucus and any trapped debris or microorganisms toward the pharynx, where they can be swallowed and exposed to the acids and enzymes of the stomach. The respiratory surfaces of the nasal cavity are also flushed by mucus produced in the *paranasal sinuses* (the *frontal, sphenoid, ethmoid,* and *maxillary sinuses*), and by tears flowing through the nasolacrimal duct (Figure 16-2b•). Exposure to noxious vapors, large quantities of dust and debris, allergens, or pathogens usually causes a rapid increase in the rate of mucus production, and a "runny nose" develops.

The Pharynx

The **pharynx**, or *throat*, is a chamber shared by the digestive and respiratory systems that extends between the internal nares and the entrances to the larynx and esophagus. Its three subdivisions are shown in Figure 16-2a•. The nasopharynx is connected to the nasal cavity by the internal nares and extends to the posterior edge of the soft palate. The nasopharynx, lined by a typical respiratory epithelium, contains the entrances to the *auditory tubes* and the *pharyngeal tonsil*. The **oropharynx** extends between the soft palate and the base of the tongue at the level of the hyoid bone. The palatine tonsils lie in the lateral walls of the oropharynx. The narrow **laryngopharynx** (lā-rin-gō-FĀR-inks) includes that portion of the pharynx between the hyoid bone and entrance to the esophagus. Materials entering the digestive tract pass through both the oropharynx and laryngopharynx. These regions are lined by a stratified squamous epithelium that can resist mechanical abrasion, chemical attack, and pathogenic invasion.

✳ RESPIRATORY SYNCTIAL VIRUS (RSV) INFECTIONS

Bronchiolitis, an infection of the smaller airways, is a common disease in children less than 2 years of age. Most cases of bronchiolitis are caused by the *respiratory syncytial virus (RSV).* It often occurs in epidemics during the midwinter and primarily affects children between the ages of 2 and 6 months. Typically, the child with an RSV infection will develop a runny nose, low-grade fever, and decreased appetite. Then, there will be an increase in the respiratory rate and depth and in the work of breathing. As the disease progresses, there is often a fall in the oxygen level, wheezing, and trapping of air within the lungs, causing hyperexpansion of the chest. Treatment includes intensive monitoring, supplemental oxygen, bronchodilators, and occasionally, ventilatory support. Usually, children develop lifelong immunity following infection.

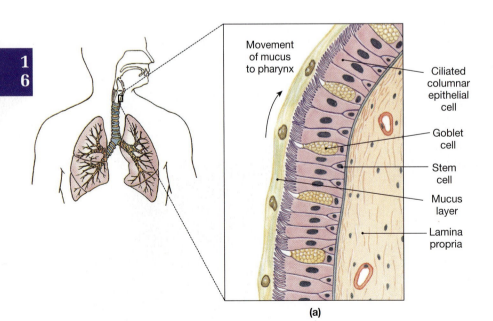

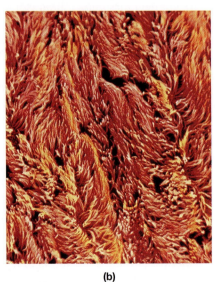

(b)

• **FIGURE 16-3   The Respiratory Epithelium**
(a) A sketch showing the sectional appearance of the respiratory epithelium and its role in mucus transport. **(b)** A surface view of the epithelium. The cilia of the epithelial cells form a dense layer that resembles a shag carpet. The movement of these cilia propels mucus across the epithelial surface. (SEM × 1614)

The Larynx

Incoming air leaves the pharynx by passing through the **glottis** (GLOT-is), a narrow opening surrounded and protected by the **larynx** (LAR-inks), or *voice box*. The larynx contains nine cartilages that are stabilized by ligaments, skeletal muscles, or both (Figure 16-4•). There are three large cartilages: the *epiglottis*, *thyroid cartilage*, and *cricoid cartilage*.

The elastic **epiglottis** (ep-i-GLOT-is) projects above the glottis. During swallowing, the larynx is elevated and the epiglottis folds back over the glottis, preventing the entry of liquids or solid food into the respiratory passageways. The curving **thyroid** (*thyroid*; shield-shaped) **cartilage** forms much of the anterior and later-al surfaces of the larynx. A prominent ridge on the anterior surface of this cartilage forms the "Adam's apple." The thyroid sits atop the **cricoid** (KRĪ-koyd; ring-shaped) **cartilage**, which provides posterior support to the larynx. The thyroid and cricoid cartilages protect the glottis and the entrance to the trachea, and their broad surfaces provide sites for the attachment of important laryngeal muscles and ligaments.

The larynx also contains three pairs of smaller cartilages. The *arytenoid*, *corniculate*, and *cuneiform cartilages* are supported by the cricoid. Two pairs of ligaments, enclosed by folds of epithelium, extend across the larynx between the thyroid cartilage and these cartilages, considerably reducing the size of the glottis. The upper pair, known as the **false vocal cords**,

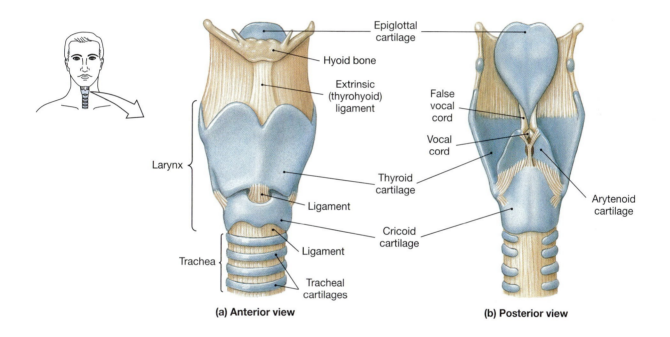

(a) Anterior view

(b) Posterior view

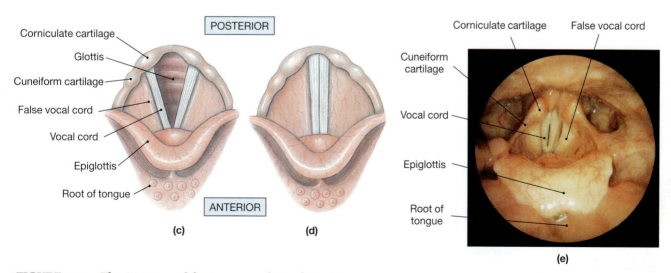

(c)   **(d)**   **(e)**

•**FIGURE 16-4   The Anatomy of the Larynx and Vocal Cords**
(a) An anterior view of the larynx. **(b)** A posterior view of the larynx. **(c)** A superior view of the larynx with the glottis open and **(d)** with the glottis closed. **(e)** A fiber-optic view of the larynx with the glottis closed.

are relatively inelastic. They help prevent foreign objects from entering the glottis, and they protect a more delicate pair of folds. These lower folds, the **true vocal cords**, contain elastic ligaments that extend between the thyroid cartilage and the arytenoids. Small muscles that insert on these cartilages change their position and alter the tension in these ligaments.

The Vocal Cords and Sound Production

The vocal cords vibrate when air passes through the glottis. These vibrations generate sound waves. As on a guitar or violin, short, thin strings vibrate rapidly, producing a high-pitched sound; large, long strings vibrate more slowly, producing a low-pitched tone. Because both boys and girls have slender, short vocal cords, their voices tend to be high-pitched. At puberty, the larynx of males enlarges more than that of females. The true vocal cords of adult males are thicker and longer and produce lower tones than those of adult females.

The pitch of the voice is regulated by the amount of tension in the vocal cords, which is controlled by skeletal muscles that change the position of the arytenoid cartilages. The volume depends on the force of the air movement. Further amplification and resonance occur in the pharynx, the oral cavity, the nasal cavity, and the paranasal sinuses. The final production of distinct words further depends on voluntary movements of the tongue, lips, and cheeks.

The Trachea

The **trachea** (TRĀ-kē-a), or *windpipe*, is a tough, flexible tube with a diameter of about 2.5 cm (1 in.) and a length of approximately 11 cm (4.25 in.) (Figure 16-5●). It extends between the level of the sixth cervical vertebra, where it attaches to the cricoid cartilage of the larynx, and the level of the fifth thoracic vertebra, where it branches to form a pair of primary bronchi.

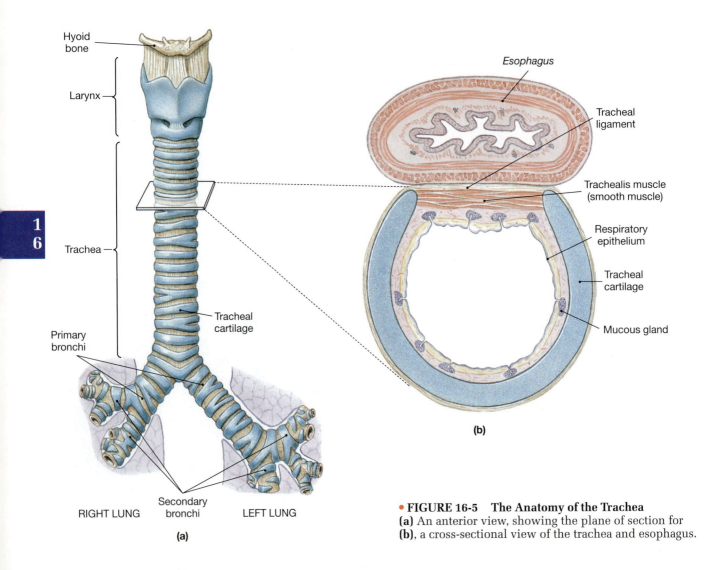

● **FIGURE 16-5   The Anatomy of the Trachea**
(a) An anterior view, showing the plane of section for **(b)**, a cross-sectional view of the trachea and esophagus.

The walls of the trachea are supported by about 20 **tracheal cartilages**. These C-shaped cartilages stiffen the tracheal walls and protect the airway. They also prevent its collapse or overexpansion as pressures change in the respiratory system. The open portions of the C-shaped tracheal cartilages face posteriorly, toward the esophagus. Because the cartilages do not continue around the trachea, the posterior tracheal wall can easily distort, allowing large masses of food to pass along the esophagus. The diameter of the trachea is adjusted by the contractions of muscles under autonomic control. Sympathetic stimulation increases the diameter of the trachea and makes it easier to move large volumes of air along the respiratory passageways.

✳ BRONCHIAL ANGLES

The division of the trachea into the right and left primary bronchi occurs at the *carina*. The *right primary bronchus* angulates less acutely from the trachea than does the *left primary bronchus*. Because of this, foreign objects that inadvertently enter the respiratory tract usually enter the right primary bronchus and the right lung. The aspirated foreign body can act as a one-way valve allowing air to enter the lung but not exit. This results in overexpansion of the lung and can eventually lead to a pneumothorax.

In an emergency, it is common for rescue personnel to place a breathing tube into the trachea (endotracheal intubation). Accidentally inserting the tube too far can cause the tip of the tube to enter the right primary bronchus. This results in only the right lung being effectively ventilated and can lead to hypoxia. Endobronchial intubation results in the absence of breath sounds over the left chest, decreased compliance, and possibly hypoxia. The situation can be remedied by simply withdrawing the tube until bilateral breath sounds return. It is important to frequently reassess tube placement to assure that dislodgement or endobronchial intubation does not occur.

The Bronchi

The trachea branches within the mediastinum, giving rise to the **right** and **left primary bronchi** (BRONG-kī) (Figure 16-5•). The histological organization of the primary bronchi resembles that of the trachea, complete with cartilaginous C-shaped rings. The primary bronchi and their branches form the **bronchial tree**. As it enters the lung, each primary bronchus gives rise to **secondary bronchi**, which enter the lobes of that lung. The secondary bronchi divide to form 9–10 **tertiary bronchi** in each lung. Each tertiary bronchus branches repeatedly.

The cartilages of the secondary bronchi are quite massive, but farther along the branches of the bronchial tree they become smaller and smaller. When the diameter of the passageway has narrowed to around 1 mm, cartilages disappear completely. This narrow passage is a **bronchiole**.

The Bronchioles

Bronchioles are to the respiratory system what arterioles are to the circulatory system. Varying the diameter of the bronchioles controls the amount of resistance to airflow and the distribution of air in the lungs. Sympathetic activation leads to a relaxation of smooth muscles in the walls of bronchioles, causing a dilation of the respiratory passageways. Constriction of these smooth muscles can almost completely block the passageways. For example, acute bronchiolar constriction can occur during an asthma attack or an allergic reaction, due to inflammation of the bronchioles.

After further branching, we reach the level of the *terminal bronchioles*, with diameters of 0.3–0.5 mm. Each terminal bronchiole supplies air to a lobule of the lung. A **lobule** is a segment of lung tissue that is bounded by connective tissue partitions and supplied by a single bronchiole, accompanied by branches of the pulmonary arteries and pulmonary veins. Within a lobule, a terminal bronchiole divides to form several respiratory bronchioles. These passages, the finest branches of the bronchial tree, deliver air to the respiratory surfaces of the lungs.

The Alveolar Ducts and Alveoli

Figure 16-6a• shows the basic structure of a lobule. Respiratory bronchioles open into expansive chambers called **alveolar ducts**. These passageways end at **alveolar sacs**, common chambers connected to individual **alveoli**—the exchange surfaces of the lungs. Each lung contains approximately 150 million alveoli, and their abundance gives the lung an open, spongy appearance (Figure 16-6b•).

To meet our metabolic requirements, the alveolar exchange surfaces of the lungs must be very large, equal to around 140 square meters—roughly the size of a tennis court. The alveolar epithelium primarily consists of an unusually thin and delicate simple squamous epithelium (Figure 16-6c•). Roaming **alveolar macrophages** (*dust cells*) patrol the epithelium, phagocytizing dust or debris that has reached the alveolar surfaces. **Surfactant** (sur-FAK-tant) **cells** produce surfactant, an oily secretion that forms a superficial coating over the alveolar epithelium. Surfactant is important because it reduces surface tension within the alveolus. Surface tension results from the attraction between water molecules at an air-water boundary. The alveolar walls are so delicate that without surfactant, the surface tension would be strong enough to collapse them. If surfactant levels are inadequate, as a result of injury or genetic abnormalities, each inhalation must be forceful enough to pop open the alveoli. An individual with this condition, called **respiratory distress syndrome**, is soon exhausted by the effort required to keep inflating and deflating the lungs.

16

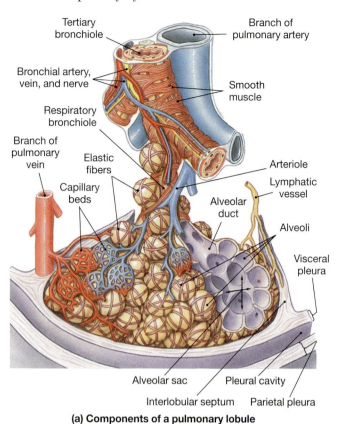

Tertiary bronchiole

Branch of pulmonary artery

Bronchial artery, vein, and nerve

Smooth muscle

Respiratory bronchiole

Branch of pulmonary vein

Elastic fibers

Capillary beds

Arteriole

Lymphatic vessel

Alveolar duct

Alveoli

Visceral pleura

Alveolar sac

Interlobular septum

Pleural cavity

Parietal pleura

(a) Components of a pulmonary lobule

● **FIGURE 16-6   Alveolar Organization**
(a) The basic structure of a lobule. A network of capillaries surrounds each alveolus. **(b)** An SEM of the lung. **(c)** A diagrammatic view of alveolar structure. **(d)** The respiratory membrane.

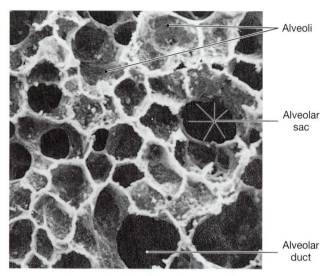

Alveoli

Alveolar sac

Alveolar duct

(b) Alveolar ducts and alveoli (SEM × 270)

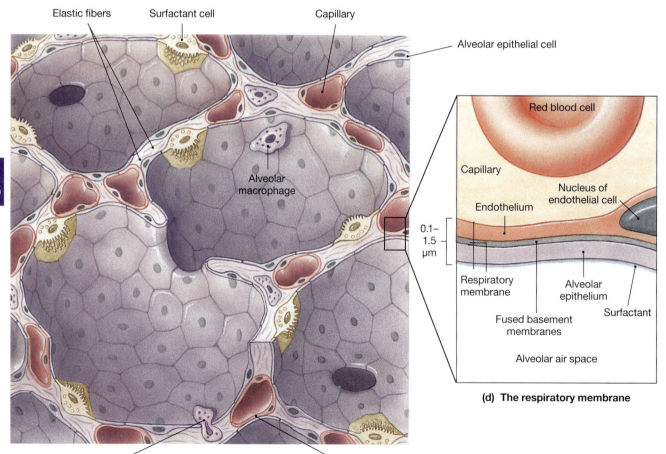

Elastic fibers   Surfactant cell   Capillary

Alveolar epithelial cell

Alveolar macrophage

Red blood cell

Capillary

Nucleus of endothelial cell

Endothelium

0.1–1.5 μm

Respiratory membrane

Alveolar epithelium

Fused basement membranes

Surfactant

Alveolar air space

(d) The respiratory membrane

Alveolar macrophage

Endothelial cell of capillary

(c) Alveolar structure

1
6

The Respiratory Membrane

Gas exchange occurs across the **respiratory membrane** of the alveoli. The respiratory membrane (Figure 16-6d●) consists of three components:

1. The squamous epithelial cells lining the alveolus.
2. The endothelial cells lining an adjacent capillary.
3. The fused basement membranes that lie between the alveolar and endothelial cells.

At the respiratory membrane, the total distance separating the alveolar air and the blood can be as little as 0.1 μm. Diffusion across the respiratory membrane proceeds very rapidly, because (1) the distance is small, and (2) both oxygen and carbon dioxide are lipid-soluble. The membranes of the epithelial and endothelial cells thus do not pose a barrier to the movement of oxygen and carbon dioxide between the blood and alveolar air spaces.

Circulation to the Respiratory Membrane

The respiratory exchange surfaces receive blood from arteries of the *pulmonary circuit.* ∞ *pp. 390, 391* The pulmonary arteries enter the lungs and branch, following the bronchi to the lobules. Each lobule receives an arteriole and a venule, and a network of capillaries surrounds each alveolus directly beneath the epithelium. After passing through the pulmonary venules, venous blood enters the pulmonary veins, which deliver it to the left atrium.

Blood pressure in the pulmonary circuit is usually relatively low, with systemic pressures of 30 mm Hg or less. With pressures that low, pulmonary vessels can easily become blocked by small blood clots, fat masses, or air bubbles in the pulmonary arteries. Because the lungs receive the entire cardiac output, any drifting masses in the blood are likely to cause problems almost at once. The blockage of a branch of a pulmonary artery will stop blood flow to a group of lobules or alveoli. This condition is called a **pulmonary embolism**.

✳ PULMONARY EMBOLISM

Pulmonary embolism (PE) is a common and potentially deadly disorder that can be extremely difficult to diagnose. It usually arises from the large veins of the leg or pelvis. A blood clot in the leg, referred to as *deep venous thrombosis (DVT),* usually develops over a period of minutes to hours. Prolonged immobilization, such as occurs during hospitalization or a long plane or car ride, has been identified as a risk factor for the development of DVT. Ultimately, the clot breaks loose, travels through the circulatory system, and enters the pulmonary circulation. When it reaches the part of the blood vessel that is smaller than itself, the clot lodges there. Blood flow to the lung is restricted and oxygenation is impaired. Large clots can obstruct a significant portion of the lung and may be rapidly fatal.

The Lungs

The left and right **lungs** (Figure 16-7●) occupy the left and right pleural cavities. ∞ *p. 21* Each lung has distinct **lobes** separated by deep fissures. The right lung has three lobes (*superior, middle,* and *inferior*), and the left lung has two (*superior* and *inferior*). The bluntly rounded

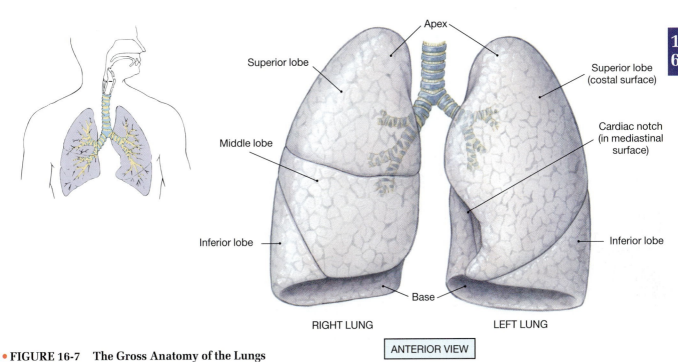

Superior lobe

Apex

Superior lobe (costal surface)

Middle lobe

Cardiac notch (in mediastinal surface)

Inferior lobe

Inferior lobe

Base

RIGHT LUNG

LEFT LUNG

ANTERIOR VIEW

● **FIGURE 16-7   The Gross Anatomy of the Lungs**

apex of each lung extends into the base of the neck above the first rib, and the concave *base* rests on the superior surface of the diaphragm, the muscular sheet that separates the thoracic and abdominopelvic cavities. The curving *costal surface* follows the inner contours of the rib cage. The *mediastinal surface* has a more irregular shape. The mediastinal surface of the left lung bears the *cardiac notch*, an indentation that conforms to the shape of the pericardium, and both lungs bear grooves that mark the passage of vessels traveling to and from the heart.

Because most of the actual volume of each lung consists of air-filled passageways and alveoli, the lung has a light and spongy consistency. An abundance of elastic fibers gives the lungs the ability to tolerate large changes in volume.

The Pleural Cavities

The thoracic cavity has the shape of a broad cone. Its walls are the rib cage, and its floor is the muscular diaphragm. The mediastinum divides the thoracic cavity into two pleural cavities (Figure 16-8•). Each lung occupies a single pleural cavity, lined by a serous membrane, or **pleura** (PLOO-ra). The *parietal pleura* covers the inner surface of the body wall and extends over the diaphragm and mediastinum. The *visceral pleura* covers the outer surfaces of the lungs, extending into the fissures between the lobes.

The pleural cavity represents a potential space rather than an open chamber, because the parietal and visceral layers are usually in close contact. A thin layer of fluid covering these surfaces provides lubrication that reduces friction and irritation of the pleura. Pleural fluid is sometimes obtained for diagnostic purposes by means of a long needle inserted between the ribs. This procedure is called *thoracentesis* (thor-a-sen-TĒ-sis; *thorac-*, chest + *kentesis*, puncture). The fluid is examined for the presence of bacteria, blood cells, and other abnormal components.

Respiratory Changes at Birth

Several important differences exist between the respiratory systems of a fetus and a newborn infant. Before delivery, the pulmonary vessels are collapsed, so pulmonary arterial resistance is high. The rib cage is compressed, and the lungs and conducting passageways contain only small amounts of fluid and no air. At birth, the newborn infant takes a truly heroic first breath through powerful contractions of the diaphragm and external intercostal muscles. The inspired air enters the passageways with enough force to push the contained fluids out of the way and to inflate the entire bronchial tree and most of the alveolar complexes. The same drop in pressure that pulls air into the lungs pulls blood into the pulmonary circulation.

The exhalation that follows fails to empty the lungs completely, because the rib cage does not return to its former, fully compressed state. Cartilages and connective tissues keep the conducting passageways open, and the surfactant covering the alveolar surfaces prevents their collapse. Subsequent breaths complete the inflation of the alveoli. These physical changes are sometimes used by pathologists to determine whether a newborn infant died before or shortly after delivery. Before the first breath, the lungs are completely filled with fluid, and they will sink if placed in water. After the first breath, even the collapsed lungs contain enough air to keep them afloat.

✓ When the tension in the vocal cords increases, what happens to the pitch of the voice?

✓ Why are the cartilages that reinforce the trachea C-shaped instead of complete circles?

✓ What would happen to the alveoli if surfactant were not produced?

16

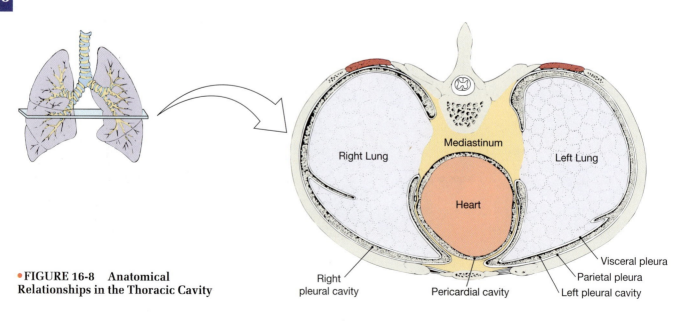

•**FIGURE 16-8   Anatomical Relationships in the Thoracic Cavity**

Right Lung

Mediastinum

Left Lung

Heart

Right pleural cavity

Pericardial cavity

Visceral pleura

Parietal pleura

Left pleural cavity

RESPIRATORY PHYSIOLOGY

The process of respiration involves four integrated steps:

Step 1: *Pulmonary ventilation*, or breathing, which refers to the physical movement of air into and out of the lungs.

Step 2: *Gas diffusion across the respiratory membrane*, which separates the alveolar air from the blood within the alveolar capillaries.

Step 3: *The storage and transport of oxygen and carbon dioxide.* In this step, the blood stores and carries the respiratory gases between the alveolar capillaries and the capillary beds in other tissues.

Step 4: *The exchange of oxygen and carbon dioxide between the blood and the interstitial fluids.* In this step, the blood delivers oxygen to body tissues and receives carbon dioxide for transport to the lungs.

Abnormalities affecting any single step will ultimately affect the gas concentrations of the interstitial fluids. If the oxygen content declines, the affected tissues will suffer from **hypoxia** (hī-POKS-ē-a), which places severe limits on the metabolic activities of peripheral tissues. If the supply of oxygen gets cut off completely, **anoxia** (a-NOKS-ē-a) results, and cells die very quickly. For example, much of the damage caused by strokes and heart attacks is the result of localized anoxia.

✳ PNEUMONIA

Pneumonia is an infection of the lungs and a common medical problem. The elderly and patients with chronic disease, such as acquired immune deficiency syndrome (AIDS), are at increased risk. In fact, pneumonia is one of the leading causes of death in both groups. Bacteria and viruses are the most common causes of pneumonia. Viral pneumonia is more common in children and tends to be diffuse and less severe. Bacterial pneumonia is seen more often in adults and is usually isolated to one part of the lungs. In pneumonia, fluid and inflammatory cells collect in the infected alveoli, often causing alveolar collapse. When this occurs, the ventilatory capacity of the affected lung is lost and oxygen exchange is impaired. Severe disease can result in profound ventilatory impairment, hypoxia, and even death.

Pulmonary Ventilation

Pulmonary ventilation is the physical movement of air into and out of the respiratory tract. A single breath, or *respiratory cycle*, consists of an inhalation, or *inspiration*, and an exhalation, or *expiration*. Breathing functions to maintain adequate **alveolar ventilation**, the movement of air into and out of the alveoli.

✳ MECHANICAL VENTILATION

When respirations are inadequate or oxygen exchange is impaired, it is often necessary to provide *mechanical ventilation* for a patient. Mechanical ventilators are designed to deliver a predetermined volume of air to the patient or to shut down when a predetermined airway pressure has been reached. With *volume-cycled ventilators,* inspiration is terminated and expiration begins when a preset tidal volume has been reached. With *pressure-cycled ventilators,* inspiration is terminated and expiration begins when a preset pressure limit is reached. However, changes in a patient's chest wall and lung *compliance* can adversely affect airway pressures. Because of this, volume-cycled ventilators have become the standard for mechanical ventilation in adults because they deliver a relatively constant tidal volume despite changes in compliance.

Pressure and Airflow to the Lungs

As we know from television weather reports, air will flow from an area of higher pressure to an area of lower pressure. The greater the *pressure gradient*, the difference between the high and low pressures, the faster the air will move. This relationship applies both to the movement of atmospheric winds and to the movement of air into and out of the lungs (pulmonary ventilation). Pressure gradients between the atmosphere and the lungs occur when the volume of the lungs changes. Because gases can be compressed, the pressure of a gas in a closed container (such as a lung) can be altered by increasing or decreasing its volume. When the lungs expand, pressure inside the airways falls and air moves into the respiratory tract. When the lungs contract, pressure increases and air moves out of the respiratory tract.

The volume of the lungs depends on the volume of the pleural cavities. The parietal and pleural membranes are separated by only a thin film of pleural fluid, and although the two membranes can slide across each other, they are held together by that fluid film. You encounter the same principle when you set a wet glass on a smooth surface. You can slide the glass quite easily, but when you try to lift it, you encounter considerable resistance from this fluid bond. A comparable fluid bond exists between the parietal pleura and the visceral pleura covering the lungs. As a result, the surface of each lung sticks to the inner wall of the chest and the superior surface of the diaphragm. Movements of the chest wall or the diaphragm thus have a direct effect on the volume of the lungs. The basic principle is shown in Figure 16-9a●.

At the start of a breath, pressures inside and outside the lungs are identical and there is no movement of air (Figure 16-9b●). When the thoracic cavity enlarges, the pressure inside the lungs decreases. Air now enters the respiratory passageways because the pressure inside the lungs (P_i) is lower than atmospheric pressure (pressure outside, or P_o) (Figure 16-9c●). During quiet breathing, the enlargement of the thoracic cavity involves the contractions of the diaphragm, aided by the *external intercostal muscles*:

16

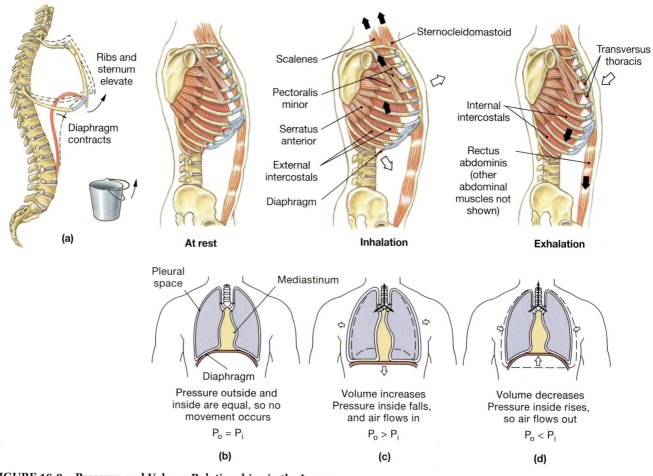

• FIGURE 16-9   Pressure and Volume Relationships in the Lungs
(a) Raising the curved handle of the bucket increases the amount of space between it and the bucket. Similarly, the volume of the thoracic cavity is increased when the ribs are elevated or the diaphragm is depressed when it contracts. **(b)** An anterior view at rest, with no air movement. **(c)** Inhalation: Elevation of the rib cage and depression of the diaphragm increase the size of the thoracic cavity. Pressure decreases, and air flows into the lungs. **(d)** Exhalation: When the rib cage returns to its original position or the diaphragm relaxes, the volume of the thoracic cavity decreases. Pressure rises, and air moves out of the lungs. Accessory muscles may assist such movements of the rib cage to increase the depth and rate of respiration.

- *The diaphragm forms the floor of the thoracic cavity.* The abdominal viscera normally push upward on its inferior surface. As a result, the relaxed diaphragm has the shape of a dome and projects upward into the thoracic cavity, compressing the lungs. When the diaphragm contracts, it flattens and increases the volume of the thoracic cavity, expanding the lungs. The contraction of the diaphragm is controlled by the *phrenic nerves*, branches of the *cervical plexus.* ∞ *p. 256*

- *The external intercostals elevate the rib cage.* Because of the way the ribs and the vertebrae articulate, this movement increases the volume of the thoracic cavity. Contraction of the external intercostals is controlled by *intercostal nerves*, branches of the thoracic spinal nerves. ∞ *p. 255* When you breathe heavily, accessory muscles, such as the sternocleidomastoid, can help the external intercostals elevate the ribs.

Downward movement of the rib cage and upward movement of the diaphragm reverse the process and reduce the size of the lungs. Pressure inside the lungs now exceeds atmospheric pressure, and air moves out of the lungs (Figure 16-9d•). During quiet breathing, the expansion of the lungs stretches their elastic fibers. In addition, the elevation of the rib cage stretches opposing skeletal muscles and the elastic fibers in the body wall. When the inspiratory muscles relax, these elastic components recoil, returning the diaphragm and rib cage to their original positions. When you breathe heavily, contractions of the internal intercostal muscles and the abdominal muscles may assist in exhalation.

The **compliance** of the lungs is an indication of their expandability. The lower the compliance, the greater the force required to fill and empty the lungs. When you are at rest, the muscular activity involved in pulmonary ventilation usually accounts for less than 5 percent of your resting energy demand. If compliance is reduced, the energy demand increases dramatically and you can become exhausted simply trying to continue breathing. For example, if the alveoli collapse due to inadequate surfactant production, compliance is reduced and breathing becomes very difficult. Breathing can also become difficult if movement of the rib cage is restricted by arthritis or by other skeletal disorders.

An injury to the chest wall that penetrates the parietal pleura or damages the alveoli and the visceral pleura can allow air into the pleural cavity. This **pneumothorax** (noo-mō-THŌ-raks; *pneuma*, air) breaks the fluid bond between the pleurae and allows the elastic fibers to contract. The result is a collapsed lung, or *atelectasis* (at-e-LEK-ta-sis; *ateles*, imperfect + *ektasis*, expansion). Treatment involves removing as much of the air as possible before sealing the opening. This procedure restores the fluid bond and reinflates the lung. Lung volume can also be reduced by the accumulation of blood in the pleural cavity. This condition is called a **hemothorax**.

Modes of Breathing

Respiratory movements are classified as forced breathing or quiet breathing by the pattern of muscle activity in the course of a single respiratory cycle. In *forced* breathing, both inhalation and exhalation are active. In *quiet breathing*, inhalation involves muscular contractions, but exhalation is passive. Inhalation results from the contraction of the diaphragm and the external intercostals. Diaphragm contraction accounts for around 75 percent of the air movement in normal quiet breathing. That percentage can change, however. For example, pregnant women increasingly rely on movements of the rib cage as expansion of the uterus forces abdominal organs against the diaphragm.

Respiratory Volumes and Rates

As noted earlier, a respiratory cycle is a single cycle of inhalation and exhalation. The **tidal volume** is the amount of air moved into or out of the lungs during a single respiratory cycle. Only a small proportion of the air in the lungs is exchanged during a single quiet respiratory cycle; the tidal volume can be increased by more vigorous inhalation and more complete exhalation. The total volume of the lungs can be divided into *volumes* and *capacities* graphically shown in Figure 16-10•:

- *Expiratory reserve volume.* During a normal quiet respiratory cycle, the tidal volume averages about 500 ml. The amount of air that could be voluntarily

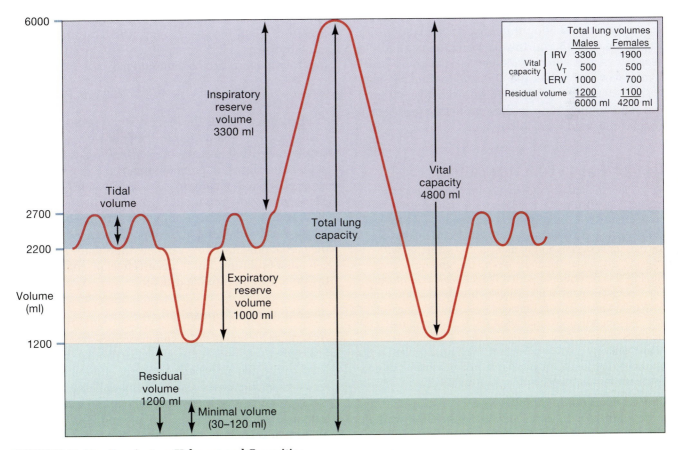

•**FIGURE 16-10   Respiratory Volumes and Capacities**
The graph diagrams the relationships between the respiratory volumes and capacities of an average male. The table compares the values for males and females.

expelled at the end of a tidal cycle is about 1000 ml. This volume is the **expiratory reserve volume (ERV)**.

- *Inspiratory reserve volume.* The **inspiratory reserve volume (IRV)** is the amount of air that can be taken in over and above the tidal volume. Because the lungs of males are larger than those of females, the IRV of males averages 3300 ml versus 1900 ml in females.

- *Vital capacity.* The sum of the inspiratory reserve volume, the expiratory reserve volume, and the tidal volume is the **vital capacity**—the maximum amount of air that can be moved into and out of the respiratory system in a single respiratory cycle.

- *Residual volume.* Roughly 1200 ml of air remains in the respiratory passageways and alveoli, even after the expiratory reserve volume has been exhausted. Most of this **residual volume** exists because the lungs are held against the thoracic wall, preventing their elastic fibers from contracting further.

- *Minimal volume.* When the chest cavity is opened, as in a pneumothorax, the lungs collapse and the amount of air in the respiratory system is reduced to the **minimal volume**. Some air remains in the lungs, even at minimal volume, because the surfactant coating the alveolar surfaces prevents their collapse.

Not all of the inspired air reaches the alveolar exchange surfaces within the lungs. A typical tidal inspiration pulls around 500 ml of air into the respiratory system. The first 350 ml travels along the conducting passageways and enters the alveolar spaces. The last 150 ml never gets farther than the conducting passageways and does not participate in gas exchange with the blood. The volume of air in the conducting passages is known as the dead space of the lungs.

PULMONARY FUNCTION TESTING

The efficiency of pulmonary function, especially in obstructive lung disease, can be rapidly determined through *pulse oximetry* and *peak expiratory flow rate (PEFR)* testing. A pulse oximeter is an electronic device that measures the amount of hemoglobin saturated with oxygen. This device is small, easy to use, and quite accurate. PEFR is determined with a *Wright peak expiratory flow meter*. The patient takes a deep breath and blows into the Wright meter. This is repeated twice and the highest reading is recorded. Normal adult PEFR varies from 400 to 600 liters/minute. Any reading less than 400 indicates some degree of airflow obstruction. Peak flow testing should be repeated throughout care in order to determine the degree of improvement.

✓ Mark breaks a rib, and it punctures the chest wall on his left side. What will happen to his left lung?

✓ In pneumonia, fluid accumulates in the alveoli of the lungs. How would vital capacity be affected?

Gas Exchange at the Respiratory Membrane

In pulmonary ventilation, the alveoli are supplied with oxygen and the accumulated carbon dioxide is removed. The actual process of gas exchange occurs between the blood and alveolar air across the respiratory membrane. This process depends on (1) the *partial pressures* of the gases involved and (2) the diffusion of molecules from a gas into a liquid. (You may wish to review diffusion in Chapter 3 before proceeding.) ∞ *p. 58*

Mixed Gases and Partial Pressures

The air we breathe is not a single gas but a mixture of gases. Nitrogen molecules (N_2) are the most abundant, accounting for about 78.6 percent of the atmospheric gas molecules. Oxygen molecules (O_2), the second most abundant, constitute roughly 20.8 percent of the atmospheric gas population. Most of the remaining 0.5 percent consists of water molecules, with carbon dioxide (CO_2) contributing a mere 0.04 percent to the total number of gas molecules in the atmosphere.

Atmospheric pressure at sea level is approximately 760 mm Hg. Each of the gases contributes to the total pressure in proportion to its relative abundance. The pressure contributed by a single gas is the **partial pressure** of that gas, abbreviated as P. The sum of the partial pressures of all the gases equals the total pressure exerted by the gas mixture. In the case of the atmosphere, this relationship can be summarized as:

$$P_{N_2} + P_{O_2} + P_{H_2O} + P_{CO_2} = 760 \text{ mm Hg}$$

Because we know the individual percentages, we can easily calculate the partial pressure of each gas. For example, the partial pressure of oxygen, P_{O_2}, is 20.8 percent of 760 mm Hg, or roughly 159 mm Hg. The partial pressures of other atmospheric gases are given in Table 16-1. These values are important because the partial pressure of an individual gas determines its rate of diffusion between the alveolar air and the bloodstream. For instance, the partial pressure of oxygen determines how much oxygen enters solution, but it has no effect on the rate of nitrogen or carbon dioxide diffusion.

Alveolar versus Atmospheric Air

As soon as air enters the respiratory tract, its characteristics begin to change. For example, in passing through the nasal cavity, the air becomes warmer and the amount of water vapor increases. On reaching the alveoli, the incoming air mixes with air that remained in the alveoli after the previous respiratory cycle. The resulting alveolar gas mixture thus contains more carbon dioxide and less oxygen than does atmospheric air. As noted earlier, the last 150 ml of inspired air never gets farther than the conducting passageways and remains in the dead space of the

TABLE 16-1	Partial Pressures (mm Hg) and Normal Gas Concentrations in Air			
Source of Sample	Nitrogen (N₂)	Oxygen (O₂)	Water Vapor (H₂O)	Carbon Dioxide (CO₂)
Inspired air (dry)	597 (78.6 percent)	159 (20.8 percent)	3.7 (0.5 percent)	0.3 (0.04 percent)
Alveolar air (saturated)	573 (75.4 percent)	100 (13.2 percent)	47 (6.2 percent)	40 (5.2 percent)
Expired air (saturated)	569 (74.8 percent)	116 (15.3 percent)	47 (6.2 percent)	28 (3.7 percent)

lungs. During expiration, the departing alveolar air mixes with air in the dead space to produce yet another mixture that differs from both atmospheric and alveolar samples. The differences in composition between atmospheric (inspired) and alveolar air can be seen in Table 16-1.

TENSION PNEUMOTHORAX

Injuries to the chest can sometimes allow air into the pleural space. Known as a *pneumothorax,* the amount of air in the pleural space can increase, compressing the lung on the affected side and, ultimately, displacing the heart and great vessels. Increasing pressure within the chest can impair filling of the heart, resulting in shock and even death. This emergency, known as a *tension pneumothorax,* requires prompt decompression of the chest to relieve the pressure. This is accomplished by placing a needle in the chest on the affected side. The entrapped air leaves the chest through the needle, and the affected lung reexpands. Following emergency decompression, emergency personnel usually place a tube into the pleural space in order to maintain lung expansion.

Partial Pressures within the Circulatory System

Figure 16-11• details the partial pressures of oxygen and carbon dioxide in the alveolar air and capillaries and in the arteries and veins of the pulmonary and systemic circuits. The blood delivered by the pulmonary arteries has a higher P_{CO_2} and a lower P_{O_2} than does alveolar air. Diffusion between the alveolar air and the pulmonary capillaries thus elevates the P_{O_2} of the blood while lowering its P_{CO_2}. By the time it enters the pulmonary venules, the blood has reached equilibrium with the alveolar air, so it departs the alveoli with a P_{O_2} of about 100 mm Hg and a P_{CO_2} of roughly 40 mm Hg.

Normal interstitial fluid has a P_{O_2} of 40 mm Hg and a P_{CO_2} of 45 mm Hg. As a result, oxygen diffuses out of the capillaries and carbon dioxide diffuses in until the capillary partial pressures are the same as those in the adjacent tissues. At a normal tissue P_{O_2}, the blood entering the venous system still contains around 75 percent of its total oxygen content. The remaining oxygen represents a reserve that can be called on when tissue activity increases or when the oxygen supply is temporarily reduced (such as when you hold your breath). When the blood returns to the alveolar capillaries, it will replace the oxygen released in the tissues at the same time that the excess CO₂ is lost.

ARTERIAL BLOOD GAS MEASUREMENTS

The partial pressure of the respiratory gases can be determined with an *arterial blood gas (ABG)* measurement. For this, a sample of arterial blood is obtained from the radial, brachial, or femoral artery. The sample is immediately placed into a blood-gas machine and measured. Most blood-gas machines will provide readings of the partial pressure of oxygen (pO_2), the partial pressure of carbon dioxide (pCO_2), the pH, the bicarbonate level (HCO_{32}), and the hemoglobin (Hg). These parameters provide a great deal of information about the efficiency of ventilation and oxygenation and will readily detect acid-base abnormalities. ABGs are an essential tool in the treatment of most severe respiratory disease processes.

Gas Pickup and Delivery

Oxygen and carbon dioxide have limited solubilities in blood plasma. This limitation poses certain functional problems because peripheral tissues need more oxygen and generate more carbon dioxide than the plasma can absorb and transport. The extra oxygen and carbon dioxide diffuse into the red blood cells, where the gas molecules are either tied up (in the case of oxygen) or used to manufacture soluble compounds (in the case of carbon dioxide). The important thing about these reactions is that they are temporary and completely reversible. When plasma oxygen or carbon dioxide concentrations are high, the excess molecules are removed by the red blood cells; when the plasma concentrations are falling, the red blood cells release their stored reserves.

Oxygen Transport

Only around 1.5 percent of the oxygen content of arterial blood consists of oxygen molecules in solution. All the rest is bound to hemoglobin (Hb) molecules, specifically to the iron atoms in the center of heme units. ∞ *p. 338* This reversible reaction can be summarized as follows:

$$Hb + O_2 \longleftrightarrow HbO_2$$

The amount of oxygen retained by hemoglobin depends primarily on the P_{O_2} in its surroundings. As a result, the lower the oxygen content of a tissue, the more oxygen released by hemoglobin molecules as they circulate through the region. At a normal tissue P_{O_2} of 40 mm Hg,

16

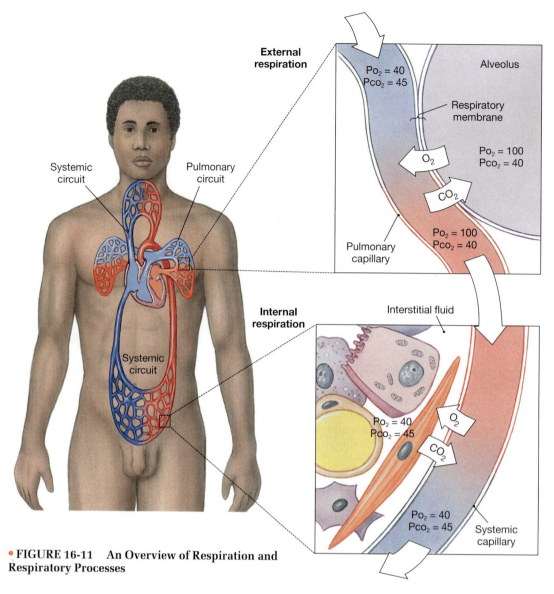

External respiration

Alveolus

$Po_2 = 40$
$Pco_2 = 45$

Respiratory membrane

$Po_2 = 100$
$Pco_2 = 40$

O_2

CO_2

$Po_2 = 100$
$Pco_2 = 40$

Pulmonary capillary

Systemic circuit

Pulmonary circuit

Systemic circuit

Internal respiration

Interstitial fluid

$Po_2 = 40$
$Pco_2 = 45$

O_2

CO_2

$Po_2 = 40$
$Pco_2 = 45$

Systemic capillary

● **FIGURE 16-11   An Overview of Respiration and Respiratory Processes**

16

hemoglobin releases roughly 25 percent of its stored oxygen. Active tissues consume oxygen at an accelerated rate. When the P_{O_2} declines, it automatically increases the amount of oxygen released by hemoglobin molecules passing through local capillaries.

In addition to the effect of P_{O_2}, the amount of oxygen released by hemoglobin is influenced by pH and temperature. Active tissues generate acids that lower the pH of the interstitial fluids. When the pH declines, the hemoglobin molecules release their bound oxygen molecules more readily. Hemoglobin also releases more oxygen when the temperature rises.

All three of these factors (P_{O_2}, pH, and temperature) are important during periods of maximal exertion. When a skeletal muscle works hard, its temperature rises and the local pH and P_{O_2} decline. The combination makes the hemoglobin entering the area release much more oxygen. Without this automatic adjustment, tissue P_{O_2} would fall to very low levels almost immediately and the exertion would come to a premature halt.

✳ CARBON MONOXIDE POISONING

Carbon monoxide (CO) is an odorless, tasteless gas that is often the byproduct of incomplete combustion. Because of its chemical structure, CO has more than 200 times the affinity of oxygen to bind with hemoglobin in the red blood cells. The binding of CO to hemoglobin causes hypoxia as the oxygen-carrying capacity of the blood is markedly decreased.

Causes of carbon monoxide poisoning include improperly ventilated heating systems, enclosed structure fires, and automobile exhaust fumes. Signs and symptoms of CO poisoning depend on the severity. Initially, the signs are mild and nonspecific. They include headache, nausea, vomiting, altered mental status, and rapid breathing. With severe poisonings, coma and death can ensue.

Treatment includes maximizing oxygen delivery to assure that all available hemoglobin is oxygenated. Some experts advocate placing the patient into a hyperbaric chamber. Increasing the environmental pressure to several atmospheres can drive oxygen to unbound hemoglobin. Often, however, the patient must wait on new red blood cell production for complete recovery.

Carbon Dioxide Transport

Carbon dioxide is generated by aerobic metabolism in peripheral tissues. After entering the bloodstream, a CO_2 molecule may be (1) dissolved in the plasma, (2) bound to the hemoglobin of red blood cells, or (3) converted to a molecule of carbonic acid (H_2CO_3) (Figure 16-12a●). These reactions are completely reversible.

Plasma Transport. Roughly 7 percent of the carbon dioxide absorbed by peripheral capillaries is transported in the form of dissolved gas molecules. The rest diffuses into the red blood cells.

Hemoglobin Binding. Once in the red blood cells, some of the carbon dioxide molecules are bound to the protein "globin" portions of hemoglobin molecules, forming **carbaminohemoglobin** (kar-ba-mē-nō-hē-mō-GLŌ-bin). Normally, about 23 percent of the carbon dioxide entering the blood in peripheral tissues is transported as carbaminohemoglobin. On arriving at the pulmonary capillaries, the plasma P_{CO_2} declines, and then the bound carbon dioxide is released.

Carbonic Acid Formation. The rest of the carbon dioxide molecules, roughly 70 percent of the total, are converted to carbonic acid through the activity of the enzyme carbonic anhydrase. The carbonic acid mole-

cules do not remain intact, however; almost immediately, each of these molecules breaks down into a hydrogen ion and a bicarbonate ion. The entire sequence can be summarized as follows:

$$\overset{\text{carbonic}}{\underset{}{\text{anhydrase}}}$$
$$CO_2 + H_2O \longleftrightarrow H_2CO_3 \longleftrightarrow H^+ + HCO_3^-$$

The reactions occur very rapidly and are completely reversible. Because most of the carbonic acid formed immediately dissociates into bicarbonate and hydrogen ions, we can ignore the intermediary step and summarize the reaction as follows:

$$\overset{\text{carbonic}}{\underset{}{\text{anhydrase}}}$$
$$CO_2 + H_2O \longleftrightarrow H^+ + HCO_3^-$$

In peripheral capillaries, this reaction proceeds vigorously, tying up large numbers of carbon dioxide molecules. The reaction is driven from left to right because carbon dioxide continues to arrive, diffusing out of the interstitial fluids, and the hydrogen ions and bicarbonate ions are continuously being removed. Most of the hydrogen ions get tied up by hemoglobin molecules. Bicarbonate ions diffuse into the surrounding plasma, where they associate with sodium ions to form sodium bicarbonate ($NaHCO_3$).

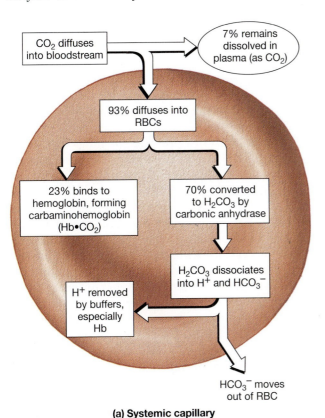

(a) Systemic capillary

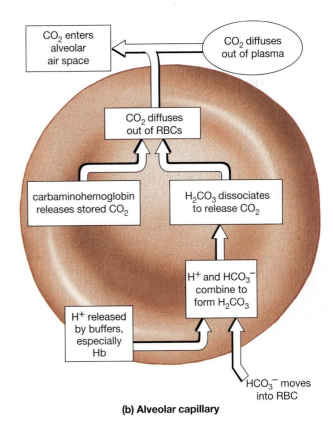

(b) Alveolar capillary

●**FIGURE 16-12   Carbon Dioxide Transport in the Blood**
(a) Carbon dioxide uptake in peripheral capillaries. **(b)** Carbon dioxide release at alveolar capillaries.

When venous blood reaches the alveoli, carbon dioxide diffuses out of the plasma and the P_{CO_2} declines. Because all of the carbon dioxide transport mechanisms are reversible, as carbon dioxide diffuses out of the red blood cells, the reactions shown in Figure 16-12b• proceed in the opposite direction. Hydrogen ions leave the hemoglobin molecules, and bicarbonate ions diffuse into the cytoplasm of the red blood cells, to be converted to water and CO_2.

✓ Why does it take more energy to breathe on a hot, humid day than on a cool, dry day?

✓ During exercise, hemoglobin releases more oxygen to the active skeletal muscles than it does when the muscles are at rest. Why?

✓ How would an obstruction of the airways affect the body's pH?

THE CONTROL OF RESPIRATION

Cells continuously absorb oxygen from the interstitial fluids and generate carbon dioxide. Under normal conditions, cellular rates of absorption and generation are matched by capillary rates of delivery and removal, and these rates are identical to those of oxygen absorption and carbon dioxide excretion at the lungs. If these rates become seriously unbalanced, the activities of the cardiovascular and respiratory systems must be adjusted.

The Respiratory Centers of the Brain

The **respiratory centers** integrating large-scale responses include three pairs of loosely organized nuclei in the reticular formation of the pons and medulla. These nuclei regulate the activities of the respiratory muscles and control the respiratory rate and the depth of breathing. The **respiratory rate** is the number of breaths per minute. This rate in normal adults at rest ranges from 12 to 18 breaths per minute. Children breathe more rapidly, about 18 to 20 breaths per minute.

The **respiratory rhythmicity center** of the medulla oblongata sets the pace for respiration. It can be subdivided into a *dorsal respiratory group* (*DRG*), which contains an *inspiratory center*, and a *ventral respiratory group* (*VRG*), which contains an *expiratory center*. Other areas of the brain—notably, the respiratory centers of the pons—can adjust the output of the rhythmicity center. For example, these centers may adjust the respiratory rate and the depth of respiration in response to sensory stimuli, emotional states, or speech patterns.

The Activities of the Respiratory Rhythmicity Center

The inspiratory center functions in every respiratory cycle, whether quiet or forced. During quiet respiration, the neurons of the inspiratory center gradually increase stimulation of the inspiratory muscles for two seconds, and then the inspiratory center becomes silent for the next three seconds. During that period of inactivity, the respiratory muscles relax, and passive exhalation occurs. The inspiratory center will maintain this basic rhythm even in the absence of sensory or regulatory stimuli. The expiratory center remains inactive during quiet respiration and functions only during forced breathing, when it activates the accessory muscles involved in inhalation and exhalation. The relationships between the inspiratory and expiratory centers during quiet and forced ventilation are diagrammed in Figure 16-13•.

The performance of these respiratory centers can be affected by any factor that alters the metabolic or chemical activities of neural tissues. For example, elevated body temperatures or CNS stimulants, such as amphetamines or caffeine, increase the respiratory rate. Decreased body temperature or CNS depressants, such as barbiturates or opiates, reduce the respiratory rate. Respiratory activities are also strongly influenced by reflexes that are triggered by mechanical or chemical stimuli.

The Reflex Control of Respiration

Normal breathing occurs automatically, without conscious control. Two types of reflexes are involved in respiration: *mechanoreceptor reflexes* and *chemoreceptor reflexes*.

Mechanoreceptor Reflexes

Mechanoreceptor reflexes respond to changes in the volume of the lungs or to changes in arterial blood pressure. Chapter 10 described several populations of baroreceptors involved in respiratory function. ∞ *p. 274*

The **inflation reflex** prevents the lungs from overexpanding during forced breathing. The receptors involved are stretch receptors that are stimulated when the lungs expand. Sensory fibers leaving these receptors reach the inspiratory and expiratory centers through the vagus nerve. As the volume of the lungs increases, the inspiratory center is gradually inhibited and the expiratory center is stimulated. Thus inspiration stops as the lungs near maximum volume, and active expiration then begins. In contrast, the **deflation reflex** inhibits the expiratory center and stimulates the inspiratory center when the lungs are collapsing. The smaller the volume of the lungs, the greater the inhibition.

Although neither the inflation nor the deflation reflex is involved in normal quiet breathing, both are important in regulating the forced ventilations that accompany strenuous exercise. Together, the inflation and deflation reflexes are known as the *Hering-Breuer reflexes*, after the physiologists who described them in 1865.

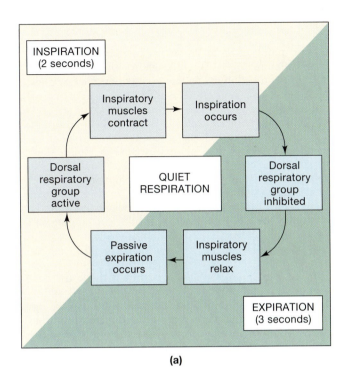

(a)

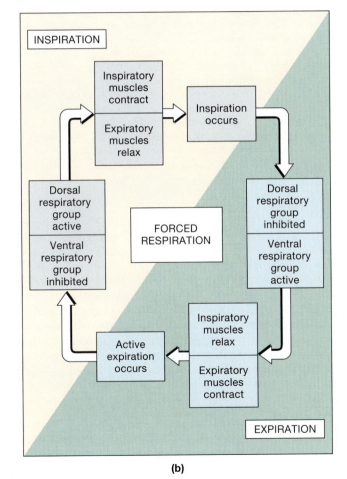

(b)

• **FIGURE 16-13   Basic Regulatory Patterns**
(a) Quiet respiration. **(b)** Forced respiration.

The effects of the carotid and aortic baroreceptors on systemic blood pressure were described in Chapter 14. ∞ *p. 385* The output from these baroreceptors affects the respiratory centers as well as the cardiac and vasomotor centers. When blood pressure falls, the respiratory rate increases; when blood pressure rises, the respiratory rate declines. This adjustment results from the stimulation or inhibition of the inspiratory and expiratory centers by sensory fibers in the glossopharyngeal (IX) and vagus (X) nerves.

Chemoreceptor Reflexes

Chemoreceptor reflexes respond to changes in the blood and cerebrospinal fluid. Centers in the carotid bodies (adjacent to the carotid sinus) and the aortic bodies (near the aortic arch) are sensitive to the pH, P_{CO_2}, and P_{O_2} in arterial blood; receptors in the medulla oblongata respond to the pH and P_{CO_2} in the cerebrospinal fluid. Under normal conditions, the P_{O_2} has very little effect on the respiratory centers, and it is carbon dioxide that sets the respiratory pace.

✳ HYPOXIC DRIVE

Respiratory drive is controlled primarily by the amount of carbon dioxide in the blood (PCO_2). An increase in the PCO_2 stimulates respirations, while a fall in PCO_2 inhibits respirations. In chronic obstructive pulmonary diseases, such as *emphysema* or *chronic bronchitis,* the level of carbon dioxide in the blood gradually rises (*hypercapnia*). As the disease progresses, the chemoreceptors become accustomed to chronic hypercapnia. When this occurs, the body begins to rely on oxygen levels (PO_2), instead of PCO_2 levels, to regulate respirations. This change, referred to as *hypoxic drive,* occurs only in advanced and severe disease. Administration of supplemental oxygen, a routine part of emergency care, can significantly increase PO_2 levels and can inhibit respirations. In severe cases, administration of high levels of supplemental oxygen can cause respiratory arrest.

Respiratory Drive and P_{CO_2}.   Under normal conditions, carbon dioxide levels have a much more powerful effect on respiratory activity than does oxygen because arterial P_{O_2} does not usually decline enough to activate the oxygen receptors. But when arterial P_{O_2} does fall, the two receptor populations cooperate. Carbon dioxide is generated during oxygen consumption, so when oxygen concentrations are falling rapidly, carbon dioxide levels are usually increasing.

Chemoreceptor reflexes are extremely powerful respiratory stimulators, and they cannot be consciously suppressed. For example, you can hold your breath before you dive into a swimming pool to avoid the inhalation of water. But you cannot hold your breath "till you turn blue." Once the P_{CO_2} rises to critical levels, you will be forced to take a breath. People may take deep, full breaths to extend their breath-holding times. Most

1
6

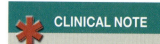

CLINICAL NOTE   **ASTHMA**

Asthma is a common respiratory illness. Although deaths from other respiratory diseases are steadily declining, deaths from asthma have increased significantly during the last decade. Most of the increased asthma deaths have occurred in patients who are 45 years of age or older. In addition, the death rate for black asthmatics is more than twice as high as for their white counterparts. Asthma is a common reason people summon EMS and a common reason for emergency department visits.

Asthma is a chronic inflammatory disorder of the airways. In susceptible individuals, this inflammation causes symptoms usually associated with widespread but variable airflow obstruction. In addition to airflow obstruction, the airways become hyperresponsive. The airflow obstruction and hyperresponsiveness often are reversible with treatment.

Asthma may be induced by one of many different factors. These factors, commonly referred to as *triggers,* vary from one individual to another. Within minutes of exposure to the offending trigger, a two-phase reaction occurs. The first phase of the reaction is characterized by the release of chemical mediators such as *histamine.* These mediators cause contraction of the bronchial smooth muscle and leakage of fluid from the peribronchial capillaries. This results in both bronchoconstriction and bronchial edema. These two factors can significantly decrease expiratory air flow, causing the typical "asthma attack."

Often, the attack will resolve spontaneously in 1–2 hours or may be aborted by the use of inhaled bronchodilator medication. However, within 6–8 hours after exposure to the trigger, a second reaction occurs. This late phase is characterized by inflammation of the bronchioles as cells of the immune system invade the mucosa of the respiratory tract. This leads to additional edema and swelling of the bronchioles and a further decrease in expiratory airflow.

The second-phase reaction will not typically respond to inhaled beta-agonist drugs such as albuterol. Instead, anti-inflammatory medications, such as corticosteroids, are often required. It is important to point out that the severe inflammatory changes seen in an acute asthma attack do not develop over a few hours or even a few days. The inflammation will often begin several days or several weeks before the onset of the asthma attack.

The patient with asthma usually presents with dyspnea, wheezing, and cough. Wheezing results from turbulent airflow through the inflamed and narrowed bronchioles. Many asthmatics will have a persistent cough. This is due primarily to hyperresponsiveness of the airway. It is important to point out that some asthmatics do not wheeze. Instead, they may present with a frequent and persistent cough. As asthma's severity increases, the patient may exhibit air trapping and hyperinflation of the chest. In addition, the patient may begin using the accessory muscles of respiration to aid breathing. Measurement of the peak expiratory flow rate (PEFR) provides a good indication of the degree of airway obstruction. Patients should be familiar with their normal PEFRs and be able to detect deterioration before it becomes life threatening.

The treatment of asthma is typically divided into chronic therapy and acute therapy. Chronic therapy consists of medications that keep the disease under control. These include inhaled corticosteroid medications and long-acting bronchodilators that are taken on a regular schedule. However, when there is an exacerbation of asthma, it must be treated rapidly to prevent life-threatening deterioration. Initially, acute therapy consists of high concentrations of oxygen and inhaled bronchodilators. These are usually beta-agonists and are chemically similar to epinephrine. Beta-agonist therapy can be repeated as needed or, in severe cases, administered continuously. In addition, potent corticosteroids are administered intravenously or by mouth to prevent and minimize inflammation. If an asthma attack cannot be aborted, there is a risk of the patient's becoming fatigued and developing respiratory failure. In this case, emergency personnel may have to provide mechanical ventilation.

16

believe this helps by providing "extra" oxygen. But the real reason is they are driving down levels of carbon dioxide. If the P_{CO_2} is reduced enough, breath-holding ability may increase to the point that an individual becomes unconscious from oxygen starvation in the brain without ever feeling the urge to breathe.

Control by Higher Centers

Higher centers influence respiration through their effects on the respiratory centers of the pons and by the direct control of respiratory muscles. For example, the contractions of respiratory muscles can be voluntarily suppressed or exaggerated; this control is necessary during talking or singing. The depth and pace of respiration also change following the activation of centers involved with rage, eating, or sexual arousal. These changes, directed by the limbic system, occur at an involuntary level. Figure 16-14• summarizes factors involved in the regulation of respiration.

SIDS

Sudden infant death syndrome (SIDS) is the sudden death of an infant under one year of age that remains unexplained after a thorough case investigation including a complete autopsy, an examination of the death scene, and a review of the clinical history. In the United States, SIDS is the leading cause of death among infants between 1 month and 1 year of age. SIDS deaths occur quickly, with no signs of suffering, and are often associated with sleep. SIDS deaths occur more frequently in the fall and winter, and most take place in children between 2 and 4 months of age. Boys are affected more often than girls.

SIDS occurs in all types of families and is largely indifferent to race or socioeconomic status. The mother's health and behavior during her pregnancy and the baby's health before birth seem to influence the occurrence of SIDS. Maternal risk factors include cigarette smoking during pregnancy, age less than 20 years, poor prenatal care, low weight gain, anemia, and use of illegal drugs. SIDS is extremely tragic and extremely difficult for the family.

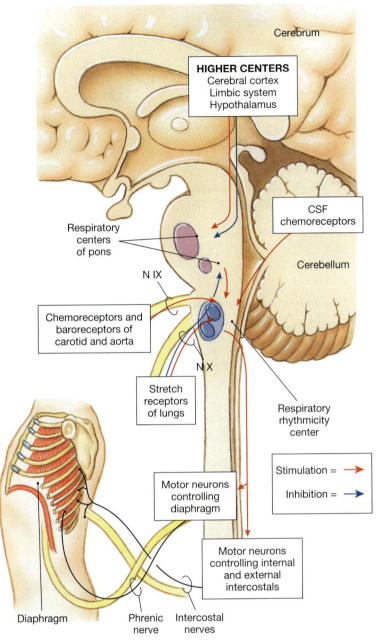

Cerebrum

HIGHER CENTERS
Cerebral cortex
Limbic system
Hypothalamus

CSF chemoreceptors

Respiratory centers of pons

Cerebellum

N IX

Chemoreceptors and baroreceptors of carotid and aorta

N X

Stretch receptors of lungs

Respiratory rhythmicity center

Stimulation = →
Inhibition = →

Motor neurons controlling diaphragm

Motor neurons controlling internal and external intercostals

Diaphragm

Phrenic nerve

Intercostal nerves

•FIGURE 16-14   **The Control of Respiration**

AGING AND THE RESPIRATORY SYSTEM

The efficiency of the respiratory system is reduced in elderly individuals as a result of the interaction of many factors. Three examples are noteworthy:

1. With increasing age, an individual's elastic tissue deteriorates throughout the body, lowering the resilience of the lungs and the vital capacity.

2. Movements of the chest cage are restricted by arthritic changes in the rib articulations and by decreased flexibility at the costal cartilages. With the changes noted in (1), the stiffening and reduction in chest movement limit pulmonary ventilation. This restriction contributes to the reduction in exercise performance and capabilities with increasing age.

3. Some emphysema is normally found in individuals age 50–70, but the extent varies widely with the lifetime exposure to cigarette smoke and other respiratory irritants. Comparative studies of nonsmokers and those who have smoked for varying lengths of time clearly show the negative effect of smoking on respiratory performance.

✓ Are peripheral chemoreceptors as sensitive to carbon dioxide levels as to oxygen levels?

✓ Strenuous exercise would stimulate which set of respiratory reflexes?

✓ Johnny tells his mother he will hold his breath until he turns blue and dies. Should she worry?

INTEGRATION WITH OTHER SYSTEMS

1 6

The respiratory system has extensive anatomical connections to the cardiovascular system. It is functionally linked to all other systems, as Figure 16-15• shows.

Chapter Review

KEY TERMS

alveolus/alveoli, *p. 443*
bronchial tree, *p. 443*
bronchiole, *p. 443*
bronchus/bronchi, *p. 443*
larynx, *p. 441*

lungs, *p. 445*
nasal cavity, *p. 438*
partial pressure, *p. 450*
pharynx, *p. 440*
respiratory membrane, *p. 445*

respiratory rhythmicity center, *p. 454*
respiratory system, *p. 438*
surfactant, *p. 443*
trachea, *p. 442*
vital capacity, *p. 450*

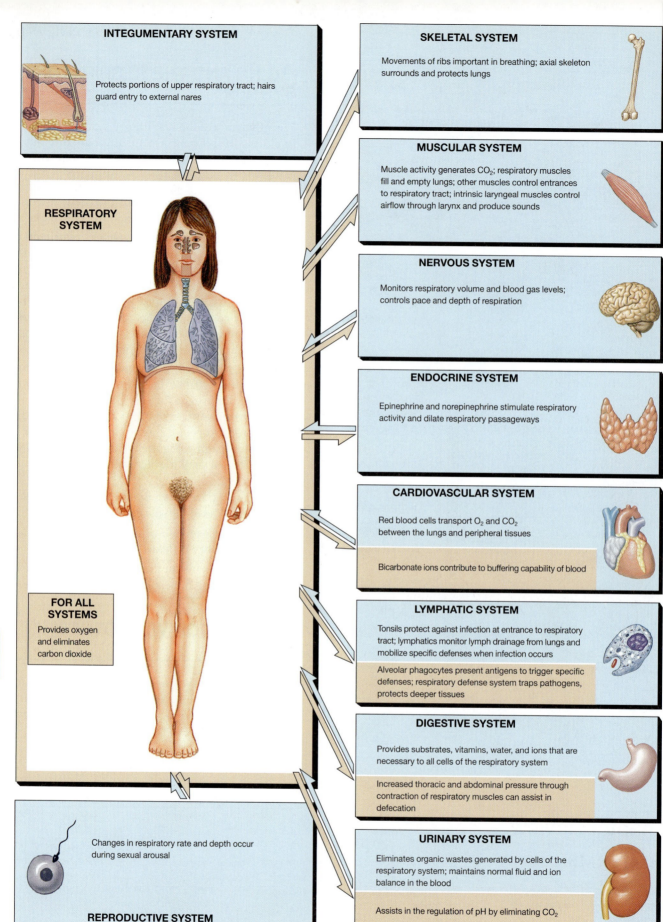

INTEGUMENTARY SYSTEM

Protects portions of upper respiratory tract; hairs guard entry to external nares

RESPIRATORY SYSTEM

FOR ALL SYSTEMS

Provides oxygen and eliminates carbon dioxide

SKELETAL SYSTEM

Movements of ribs important in breathing; axial skeleton surrounds and protects lungs

MUSCULAR SYSTEM

Muscle activity generates CO_2; respiratory muscles fill and empty lungs; other muscles control entrances to respiratory tract; intrinsic laryngeal muscles control airflow through larynx and produce sounds

NERVOUS SYSTEM

Monitors respiratory volume and blood gas levels; controls pace and depth of respiration

ENDOCRINE SYSTEM

Epinephrine and norepinephrine stimulate respiratory activity and dilate respiratory passageways

CARDIOVASCULAR SYSTEM

Red blood cells transport O_2 and CO_2 between the lungs and peripheral tissues

Bicarbonate ions contribute to buffering capability of blood

LYMPHATIC SYSTEM

Tonsils protect against infection at entrance to respiratory tract; lymphatics monitor lymph drainage from lungs and mobilize specific defenses when infection occurs

Alveolar phagocytes present antigens to trigger specific defenses; respiratory defense system traps pathogens, protects deeper tissues

DIGESTIVE SYSTEM

Provides substrates, vitamins, water, and ions that are necessary to all cells of the respiratory system

Increased thoracic and abdominal pressure through contraction of respiratory muscles can assist in defecation

URINARY SYSTEM

Eliminates organic wastes generated by cells of the respiratory system; maintains normal fluid and ion balance in the blood

Assists in the regulation of pH by eliminating CO_2

Changes in respiratory rate and depth occur during sexual arousal

REPRODUCTIVE SYSTEM

•**FIGURE 16-15** Functional Relationships Between the Respiratory System and Other Systems

1 6

SUMMARY OUTLINE

INTRODUCTION   *p. 438*

1. To continue functioning, body cells must obtain oxygen and eliminate carbon dioxide.

THE FUNCTIONS OF THE RESPIRATORY SYSTEM   *p. 438*

1. The functions of the **respiratory system** include: (1) moving air to and from exchange surfaces where diffusion can occur between air and circulating blood; (2) defending the respiratory system and other tissues from pathogens; (3) permitting vocal communication; and (4) helping control body fluid pH.

THE ORGANIZATION OF THE RESPIRATORY SYSTEM   *p. 438*

1. The respiratory system includes the nose, nasal cavity, and sinuses as well as the pharynx, larynx, trachea, and conducting passageways leading to the surfaces of the lungs. *(Figure 16-1)*

The Respiratory Tract   *p. 438*

2. The **respiratory tract** consists of the conducting passageways that carry air to and from the alveoli.

The Nose   *p. 438*

3. Air normally enters the respiratory system via the **external nares**, which open into the **nasal cavity**. The **vestibule** (entrance) is guarded by hairs that screen out large particles. *(Figure 16-2)*

4. The **hard palate** separates the oral and nasal cavities. The **soft palate** separates the superior nasopharynx from the rest of the pharynx. The **internal nares** connects the nasal cavity and nasopharynx. *(Figure 16-2)*

5. Much of the respiratory epithelium is ciliated and produces mucus that traps incoming particles. *(Figure 16-3)*

The Pharynx   *p. 440*

6. The **pharynx** (throat) is a chamber shared by the digestive and respiratory systems.

The Larynx   *p. 441*

7. Inhaled air passes through the **glottis** en route to the lungs; the **larynx** surrounds and protects the glottis. The **epiglottis** projects into the pharynx. *(Figure 16-4a,b)*

8. Air passing through the glottis vibrates the **true vocal cords** and produces sound. *(Figure 16-4c–d)*

The Trachea   *p. 442*

9. The wall of the **trachea** ("windpipe") contains C-shaped tracheal cartilages, which protect the airway. The posterior tracheal wall can distort to permit large masses of food to pass. *(Figure 16-5)*

The Bronchi   *p. 443*

10. The trachea branches within the mediastinum to form the **right** and **left primary bronchi**. *(Figure 16-5)*

11. The primary bronchi, **secondary bronchi**, and their branches form the *bronchial tree*. As the **tertiary bronchi** branch within the lung, the amount of cartilage in their walls decreases and the amount of smooth muscle increases. *(Figures 16-5, 16-6)*

The Bronchioles   *p. 443*

12. Each terminal **bronchiole** delivers air to a single pulmonary **lobule**. Within the lobule, the terminal bronchiole branches into respiratory bronchioles. *(Figure 16-6a)*

The Alveolar Ducts and Alveoli   *p. 443*

13. The respiratory bronchioles open into **alveolar ducts**, which end at **alveolar sacs**. Many alveoli are interconnected at each alveolar sac. *(Figure 16-6a,b)*

The Respiratory Membrane   *p. 445*

14. The **respiratory membrane** consists of (1) a simple squamous alveolar epithelium, (2) a capillary endothelium, and (3) their fused basement membranes. **Surfactant cells** scattered among the alveolar epithelial cells produce an oily secretion that keeps the alveoli from collapsing. **Alveolar macrophages** patrol the epithelium and engulf foreign particles. *(Figure 16-6c,d)*

The Lungs   *p. 445*

15. The **lungs** are made up of five **lobes**. The right lung has three and the left lung has two. *(Figure 16-7)*

The Pleural Cavities   *p. 446*

16. Each lung occupies a single pleural cavity lined by a **pleura** (serous membrane). *(Figure 16-8)*

Respiratory Changes at Birth   *p. 446*

17. Before delivery, the fetal lungs are fluid-filled and collapsed. After the first breath, the alveoli normally remain inflated for the life of the individual.

RESPIRATORY PHYSIOLOGY   *p. 446*

1. Respiratory physiology focuses on a series of integrated processes: *pulmonary ventilation*, or breathing (movement of air into and out of the lungs); gas diffusion between the alveoli and circulating blood; and gas storage, transport, and exchange between the blood and interstitial fluids. If oxygen content declines, the affected tissues will suffer from **hypoxia**; if the oxygen supply is completely shut off, **anoxia** and tissue death result.

Pulmonary Ventilation   *p. 447*

2. A single breath, or **respiratory cycle**, consists of an inhalation (*inspiration*) and an exhalation (*expiration*).

3. The relationship between the pressure inside the respiratory tract and atmospheric pressure determines the direction of airflow. *(Figure 16-9)*

4. The diaphragm and the external intercostal muscles are involved in *quiet breathing*, in which exhalation is passive. Accessory muscles become active during the active inspiratory and expiratory movements of *forced breathing*, in which exhalation is active. *(Figure 16-9)*

5. The **vital capacity** includes the **tidal volume** plus the **expiratory reserve volume** and the **inspiratory reserve volume**. The air left in the lungs at the end of maximum expiration is the **residual volume**. *(Figure 16-10)*

Gas Exchange at the Respiratory Membrane   *p. 450*

6. **Alveolar ventilation** is the amount of air reaching the alveoli each minute. Alveolar air and atmospheric air differ in their composition. *(Figure 16-11; Table 16-1)*

16

Gas Pickup and Delivery *p. 451*

7. Blood entering peripheral capillaries delivers oxygen and absorbs carbon dioxide. The transport of oxygen and carbon dioxide in the blood involves reactions that are completely reversible.

8. Over the range of oxygen pressures normally present in the body, a small change in plasma P_{O_2} will mean a large change in the amount of oxygen bound or released.

9. Aerobic metabolism in peripheral tissues generates carbon dioxide. Roughly 7 percent of the CO_2 transported in the blood is dissolved in the plasma; another 23 percent is bound as **carbaminohemoglobin**; the rest is converted to carbonic acid, which dissociates into a hydrogen ion and a bicarbonate ion. *(Figure 16-12)*

THE CONTROL OF RESPIRATION *p. 454*

1. Large-scale changes in oxygen demand require the integration of cardiovascular and respiratory responses.

The Respiratory Centers of the Brain *p. 454*

2. The **respiratory centers** include three pairs of nuclei in the reticular formation of the pons and medulla oblongata. These nuclei regulate the respiratory muscles and control the respiratory rate and the depth of breathing. The **respiratory rhythmicity center** sets the basic pace for respiration. *(Figure 16-13)*

The Reflex Control of Respiration *p. 454*

3. The **inflation reflex** prevents overexpansion of the lungs during forced breathing; the **deflation reflex** stimulates inspiration when the lungs are collapsing. Chemoreceptor reflexes respond to changes in the pH, P_{O_2} and P_{CO_2} of the blood and cerebrospinal fluid.

Control by Higher Centers *p. 456*

4. Conscious and unconscious thought processes can affect respiration by affecting the respiratory centers or the motor neurons controlling respiratory muscles. *(Figure 16-14)*

AGING AND THE RESPIRATORY SYSTEM *p. 457*

1. The respiratory system is generally less efficient in the elderly because: (1) elastic tissue deteriorates, lowering the vital capacity of the lungs; (2) movements of the chest cage are restricted by arthritic changes and decreased flexibility of costal cartilages; and (3) some degree of emphysema is normal in the elderly.

INTEGRATION WITH OTHER SYSTEMS *p. 457*

1. The respiratory system has extensive anatomical connections to the cardiovascular system. *(Figure 16-15)*

REVIEW QUESTIONS

LEVEL 1   Reviewing Facts and Terms

Match each item in column A with the most closely related item in column B. Use letters for answers in the spaces provided.

Column A

___ 1. nasopharynx
___ 2. laryngopharynx
___ 3. thyroid cartilage
___ 4. surfactant cells
___ 5. dust cells
___ 6. parietal pleura
___ 7. visceral pleura
___ 8. hypoxia
___ 9. anoxia
___10. collapsed lung
___11. inhalation
___12. exhalation

Column B

a. no O_2 supply to tissues
b. alveolar macrophages
c. produce oily secretion
d. covers inner surface of thoracic wall
e. low O_2 content in tissue fluids
f. inferior portion of pharynx
g. inspiration
h. superior portion of pharynx
i. Adam's apple
j. covers outer surface of lungs
k. expiration
l. atelectasis

13. The structure that prevents the entry of liquids or solid food into the respiratory passageways during swallowing is the:
    (a) glottis
    (b) arytenoid cartilage
    (c) epiglottis
    (d) thyroid cartilage

14. The amount of air moved into or out of the lungs during a single respiratory cycle is the:
    (a) respiratory minute volume
    (b) tidal volume
    (c) residual volume
    (d) inspiratory capacity

1
6

LEVEL 2   Reviewing Concepts

15. When the diaphragm contracts, it tenses and moves inferiorly, causing:
    (a) an increase in the volume of the thoracic cavity
    (b) a decrease in the volume of the thoracic cavity
    (c) decreased pressure on the contents of the abdominopelvic cavity
    (d) increased pressure in the thoracic cavity

16. Gas exchange at the respiratory membrane is efficient because:
    (a) the differences in partial pressure are substantial
    (b) the gases are lipid-soluble
    (c) the total surface area is large
    (d) a, b, and c are correct

17. What is the functional significance of the decrease in the amount of cartilage and increase in the amount of smooth muscle in the lower respiratory passageways?

18. Why is breathing through the nasal cavity more desirable than breathing through the mouth?

19. How would you justify the statement "The bronchioles are to the respiratory system what the arterioles are to the cardiovascular system"?

20. How are surfactant cells involved with keeping the alveoli from collapsing?

LEVEL 3   Critical Thinking and Clinical Applications

21. A decrease in blood pressure will trigger a baroreceptor reflex that leads to increased ventilation. What is the possible advantage of this reflex?

22. You spend the night at a friend's house during the winter. Your friend's home is quite old, and the hot-air furnace lacks a humidifier. When you wake up in the morning, you have a fair amount of nasal congestion and decide you might be coming down with a cold. After you take a steamy shower and drink some juice for breakfast, the nasal congestion disappears. Explain.

ANSWERS TO CONCEPT CHECK QUESTIONS

Page 446
1. Increased tension in the vocal cords will cause a higher pitch in the voice. 2. The tracheal cartilages are C-shaped to allow room for esophageal expansion when large portions of food or liquid are swallowed. 3. Without surfactant, surface tension in the thin layer of water that moistens their surfaces would cause the alveoli to collapse.

Page 450
1. Since the rib penetrates the chest wall, atmospheric air will enter the thoracic cavity. This condition is called a pneumothorax. Pressure within the pleural cavity is normally lower than atmospheric pressure. When air enters the pleural cavity, the natural elasticity of the lung may cause it to collapse. The resulting condition is called atelectasis, or a collapsed lung. 2. Since the fluid produced in pneumonia takes up space that would normally be occupied by air, the vital capacity would decrease.

Page 454
1. On a hot, humid day, the air contains more water vapor, which means that the partial pressure of oxygen in the air is less than on a cool, dry day. Since gases expand when heated, on a hot day the same volume of gas would contain fewer molecules. Thus, an individual must breathe deeper or faster (or both) to gain the same amount of oxygen as on a cool, dry day. 2. As skeletal muscles become more active, they generate more heat and more acid waste products and so lower the pH of surrounding fluid. The combination of lower pH and higher temperature causes the hemoglobin to release more oxygen than it would under conditions of lower temperature and higher pH. 3. An obstruction of the airways would interfere with the body's ability to gain oxygen and eliminate carbon dioxide. Since most carbon dioxide is carried in the blood as bicarbonate ion that is formed from the dissociation of carbonic acid, an inability to eliminate carbon dioxide would result in an excess of hydrogen ions, thus lowering the body's pH.

Page 457
1. Chemoreceptors are more sensitive to carbon dioxide levels than to oxygen levels. When carbon dioxide dissolves, it produces hydrogen ions, which lower pH and alter cell or tissue activity. 2. Strenuous exercise would stimulate the inflation and deflation reflexes, also known as the Hering-Breuer reflexes. In the inflation reflex, the stimulation of stretch receptors in the lungs results in an inhibition of the inspiratory center and a stimulation of the expiratory center. In contrast, collapse of the lungs initiates the deflation reflex. This reflex results in an inhibition of the expiratory center and a stimulation of the inspiratory center. 3. Johnny's mother shouldn't worry. When Johnny holds his breath, the level of carbon dioxide in his blood will increase. This will lead to increased stimulation of the inspiratory center, forcing Johnny to breathe again.

16

OVERVIEW

The respiratory system is a major body system responsible for supplying oxygen to the blood, at the same time removing carbon dioxide and other waste products. It includes the airway and associated structures, and the lungs. It is closely related to the cardiovascular system. A considerable portion of emergency care is devoted to the assessment and management of respiratory system problems. Emergencies involving the respiratory system can arise from either medical problems or trauma. Because the respiratory system affects so many other body systems, correction of respiratory system problems is a high-priority component of emergency care.

Physicians who specialize in the care of respiratory system problems are called *pulmonologists.* They are initially trained in internal medicine or pediatrics and then take fellowship training in pulmonary medicine. Surgeons who specialize in lower respiratory tract problems are *thoracic surgeons.* They are initially trained in general surgery and then take fellowship training in noncardiac thoracic surgery. *Otorhinolaryngologists,* commonly referred to as ear, nose, and throat (ENT) specialists, limit their practice to the medical and surgical care of the upper airway and adjoining structures including the sinuses, the ears, and the larynx. They must complete a five- to six-year residency following medical school.

RESPIRATORY SYSTEM PROBLEMS

A multitude of problems can arise from the respiratory system. Many of these can develop over weeks or months, while others develop over hours. The following discussion details the more common types of respiratory system problems seen in the emergency setting.

Obstructive Lung Disease

Obstructive lung disease is widespread in our society. The most common obstructive lung diseases encountered in prehospital care are asthma, emphysema, and chronic bronchitis (the last two are often discussed together as chronic obstructive pulmonary disease, or COPD). Asthma afflicts 4–5 percent of the U.S. population, and COPD is found in 25 percent of all adults. Chronic bronchitis alone affects one in five adult males. Patients with COPD have a 50 percent mortality within 10 years of the diagnosis.

Although asthma may have a genetic predisposition, COPD is known to be caused directly by cigarette smoking and environmental toxins. Other factors have been shown to precipitate symptoms in patients who already have obstructive airway disease. Intrinsic factors include stress, upper respiratory infections, and exercise. Extrinsic factors include tobacco smoke, drugs, occupational hazards (chemical fumes, dust, etc.), and allergens such as foods, animal dander, dusts, and molds.

Abnormal ventilation is a common feature of all obstructive lung diseases. This abnormal ventilation is a result of obstruction that occurs primarily in the bronchioles, where several changes occur. One of these changes is bronchospasm (sustained smooth muscle contraction), which may be reversed by beta-adrenergic receptor stimulation. Agents such as terbutaline, albuterol, and epinephrine are used to accomplish this. Increased mucus production by goblet cells that line the respiratory tree also contribute to obstruction. This effect may be worsened by the fact that in many patients the cilia are destroyed, resulting in poor clearance of excess mucus. Finally, inflammation of the bronchial passages results in the accumulation of fluid and inflammatory cells. Depending on the underlying cause, some elements of bronchial obstruction are reversible, whereas others are not.

During inspiration, the bronchioles will naturally dilate, allowing air to be drawn into the alveoli. As the patient begins to exhale, the bronchioles constrict. When this natural constriction occurs—in addition to the underlying bronchospasm, increased mucus production, and inflammation in patients with obstructive airway disease—the result is significant air trapping distal to the obstruction. This is one of the hallmarks of obstructive lung disease.

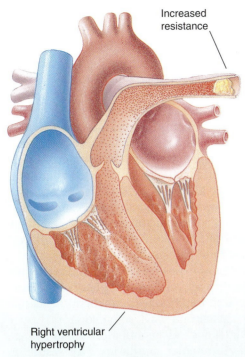

Increased
resistance

Right ventricular
hypertrophy

• **FIGURE A16-1   Pulmonary Hypertension**
Increased pulmonary vascular resistance causes an increase
in cardiac work. Over time, the right ventricle will enlarge
(hypertrophy) in order to pump against the increased
pressure. In the later stages, it can cause a type of heart
failure referred to as cor pulmonale.

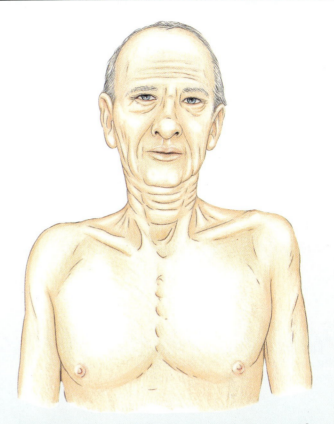

• **FIGURE A16-2   Typical Appearance of a Patient with
Chronic Emphysema**
Note hypertrophy of the accessory muscles of respiration,
most notably the strap muscles of the neck. These patients are
usually thin as most of their caloric intake goes to respiration.

Emphysema

Emphysema results from destruction of the alveolar walls
distal to the terminal bronchioles. It is more common in
men than in women. The major factor contributing to
emphysema in our society is cigarette smoking. Significant exposure to environmental toxins is another contributing factor.

Continued exposure to noxious substances, such as
cigarette smoke, results in the gradual destruction of the
walls of the alveoli. This process decreases the alveolar
membrane surface area, thus lessening the area available
for gas exchange. The progressive loss of the respiratory
membrane results in an increased ratio of air to lung tissue. The result is diffusion defects. Additionally, the
number of pulmonary capillaries in the lung is decreased,
thus increasing resistance to pulmonary blood flow. This
condition ultimately causes pulmonary hypertension,
which in turn may lead to right-heart failure, cor pulmonale, and death (Figure A16-1•).

Emphysema also causes weakening of the walls of
the small bronchioles. When the walls of the alveoli and
small bronchioles are destroyed, the lungs lose their capacity to recoil and air becomes trapped in the lungs.
Thus, residual volume increases while vital capacity remains relatively normal. The destroyed lung tissue (called

blebs) results in alveolar collapse. To counteract this effect,
patients tend to breathe through pursed lips. This creates
continued positive pressure similar to PEEP (positive end-
expiratory pressure) and prevents alveolar collapse.

As the disease progresses, the PaO_2 further decreases, which may lead to increased red blood cell production and polycythemia (an excess of red blood cells
resulting in an abnormally high hematocrit). The $PaCO_2$
also increases and becomes chronically elevated, forcing
the body to depend upon hypoxic drive to control respirations. Finally, remember that emphysema is characterized by irreversible airway obstruction.

Patients with emphysema are more susceptible to acute
respiratory infections, such as pneumonia, and to cardiac
dysrhythmias. Chronic emphysema patients ultimately become dependent on bronchodilators, corticosteroids, and
in the final stages, supplemental oxygen (Figure A16-2•).

Chronic Bronchitis

Chronic bronchitis results from an increase in the number of the goblet (mucus-secreting) cells in the respiratory
tree (Figure A16-3•). It is characterized by the production
of a large quantity of sputum. This often occurs after prolonged exposure to cigarette smoke.

A16

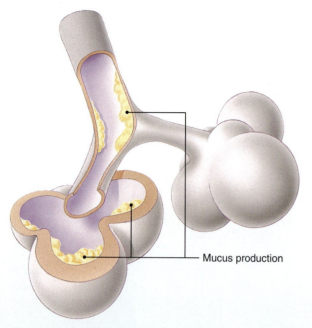

Mucus production

● **FIGURE A16-3 Chronic Bronchitis**
Increased mucus production by goblet cells within the airways results in air trapping and carbon dioxide retention.

Unlike emphysema, in chronic bronchitis the alveoli are not severely affected and diffusion remains normal. Gas exchange is decreased because alveolar ventilation is lowered, which ultimately results in hypoxia and hypercarbia. Hypoxia may increase red blood cell production, which in turn leads to polycythemia (as occurs in emphysema). Increased $PaCO_2$ levels may lead to irritability, somnolence, decreased intellectual abilities, headaches, and personality changes. Physiologically, an increased $PaCO_2$ causes pulmonary vasoconstriction, resulting in pulmonary hypertension and, eventually, cor pulmonale. Unlike emphysema, the vital capacity is decreased, while the residual volume is normal or decreased.

Asthma

Asthma is a common respiratory illness that affects many persons. Although deaths from other respiratory diseases are steadily declining, deaths from asthma have significantly increased during the last decade. Most of the increased asthma deaths have occurred in patients who are 45 years of age or older. In addition, the death rate for black asthmatics has been twice as high as for their white counterparts. Approximately 50 percent of patients who die from asthma do so before reaching the hospital. Thus, EMS personnel are frequently called upon to treat patients suffering an asthma attack. Prompt recognition followed by appropriate treatment can significantly improve the patient's condition and enhance his chance of survival.

Asthma is a chronic inflammatory disorder of the airways. In susceptible individuals, this inflammation causes symptoms usually associated with widespread but variable airflow obstruction. In addition to airflow obstruction, the airway becomes hyperresponsive. The airflow obstruction and hyperresponsiveness are often reversible with treatment. These conditions may also reverse spontaneously.

Asthma may be induced by one of many different factors. These factors, commonly referred to as triggers or inducers, vary from one individual to the next. In allergic individuals, environmental allergens are a major cause of inflammation. These may occur both indoors and outdoors. In addition to allergens, asthma may be triggered by cold air, exercise, foods, irritants, stress, and certain medications. Often, no specific trigger can be identified. Extrinsic triggers tend predominantly to affect children, whereas intrinsic factors trigger asthma in adults.

Within minutes of exposure to the offending trigger, a two-phase reaction occurs. The first phase of the reaction is characterized by the release of chemical mediators such as histamine. These mediators cause contraction of the bronchial smooth muscle and leakage of fluid from peribronchial capillaries. This results in both bronchoconstriction and bronchial edema. These two factors can significantly decrease expiratory air flow causing the typical asthma attack.

Often, the asthma attack will resolve spontaneously in 1–2 hours or may be aborted by the use of inhaled bronchodilator medications such as albuterol. However, within 6–8 hours after exposure to the trigger, a second reaction occurs. This late phase is characterized by inflammation of the bronchioles as cells of the immune system (eosinophils, neutrophils, and lymphocytes) invade the mucosa of the respiratory tract. This leads to additional edema and swelling of the bronchioles and a further decrease in expiratory airflow.

The second phase reaction will not typically respond to inhaled beta-agonist drugs such as metaproterenol or albuterol. Instead, anti-inflammatory agents such as corticosteroids are often required. It is important to point out that the severe inflammatory changes seen in an acute asthma attack do not develop over a few hours or even a few days. The inflammation will often begin several days or several weeks before the onset of the actual asthma attack. Many asthmatic patients will wait before summoning EMS. The longer the time interval from the onset of the asthma attack until treatment, the less likely it will be that bronchodilator medications will work. Often, after a prolonged asthma attack, the patient may become fatigued. A fatigued patient can quickly develop respiratory failure and subsequently require intubation and mechanical ventilation. Always be prepared to provide airway and respiratory support for the asthmatic.

Status Asthmaticus

Status asthmaticus is a severe, prolonged asthma attack that cannot be broken by repeated doses of bronchodilators. It is a serious medical emergency that requires prompt recognition, treatment, and transport. The patient suffering status asthmaticus frequently will have a greatly distended chest from continued air trapping. Breath sounds, and often wheezing, may be absent. The patient is usually exhausted, severely acidotic, and dehydrated. The management of status asthmaticus is basically the same as for asthma. Recognize that respiratory arrest is imminent and be prepared for endotracheal intubation. The patient should be transported immediately with aggressive treatment continued en route.

Upper Respiratory Infection (URI)

Among the most common infections for which patients seek medical attention are those involving the upper airway and respiratory tract. Although these conditions are rarely life threatening, upper respiratory infections can make many existing pulmonary diseases worse or lead to direct pulmonary infection. The best defense against the spread of upper respiratory infection is to practice common hygiene such as good hand washing and covering the mouth during coughing and sneezing. Attention to such details is important when caring for patients with underlying pulmonary disease or those who are immunosuppressed (HIV infection, cancer) because URIs are more severe in these populations. Due to the prevalence of such infections, complete protection is impossible.

Remember that the upper airway begins at the nose and mouth, passes through the pharynx, and ends at the larynx. Other related structures are the paranasal sinuses and the eustachian tubes that connect the pharynx and the middle ear. In addition, several collections of lymphoid tissue found in the pharynx (palatine, pharyngeal, and lingual tonsils) produce antibodies and provide immune protection.

Viruses cause the vast majority of upper respiratory infections (URIs). A variety of bacteria may also produce infection of the upper respiratory tract. The most significant is *group A streptococcus*, which is the causative organism in "strep throat" and accounts for up to 30 percent of URIs. These bacteria are also implicated in sinusitis and middle-ear infections. Up to 50 percent of patients who have pharyngitis (inflammation of the pharynx) are not found to have a viral or bacterial cause. Fortunately, most URIs are self-limiting illnesses that resolve after several days of symptoms.

The major symptoms of URI are dependent upon the portion of the upper respiratory tract that is predominantly affected. Patients with URIs will often have accompanying symptoms such as fever, chills, myalgias (muscle pains), and fatigue. Most upper respiratory infections are treated symptomatically. Acetaminophen or ibuprofen is prescribed for fever, headache, and myalgias. Encourage patients to drink plenty of fluids. Saltwater gargles may be used for throat discomfort. Decongestants and antihistamines may be used to reduce mucus secretion. Encourage patients being treated with antibiotics for bacterial causes of URI to continue these agents.

Pneumonia

Pneumonia is an infection of the lungs and a common medical problem, especially in the aged and those infected with the human immunodeficiency virus (HIV). In fact, pneumonia is one of the leading causes of death in both groups of patients and is the fifth leading overall cause of death in the U.S.

Patients with HIV infection and those on immune suppressive therapy (cancer patients) are at high risk of developing pneumonia. In addition, the very young and very old are at higher risk of acquiring pneumonia because of ineffective protective mechanisms. Other risk factors include a history of alcoholism, cigarette smoking, and exposure to cold temperatures.

Pneumonia is a collection of related respiratory diseases caused when a variety of infectious agents invade the lungs. It is crucial to remember the importance of adequate mucus production and the action of respiratory tract cilia in protecting the body against bacterial invasion. When considering which patients are at risk, the unifying concept is that there is a defect in mucus production, ciliary action, or both.

Bacterial and viral pneumonias occur the most frequently, although fungal and other forms of pneumonia do exist. More unusual forms of pneumonia are seen in those patients who are currently or recently have been hospitalized, where they are exposed to a more unusual variety of microorganisms. This is referred to as hospital-acquired pneumonia. (Cases that develop in the out-of-hospital setting are described as community-acquired pneumonia.) The infection begins in one part of the lung and often spreads to nearby alveoli. The infection may ultimately involve the entire lung. As the disease progresses, fluid and inflammatory cells collect in the alveoli, and alveolar collapse may occur. Pneumonia is primarily a ventilation disorder. Occasionally, the infection will extend beyond the lungs into the bloodstream and to more distant sites in the body. This systemic spread may lead to septic shock.

A patient with pneumonia will generally appear ill. He may report a recent history of fever and chills, commonly described as "bed shaking." There is usually a generalized weakness and malaise. The patient will tend to complain of a deep, productive cough and may expel yellow to brown sputum, often streaked with blood. Many cases involve associated pleuritic chest pain; therefore, pneumonia should be considered in any patient who presents complaining of chest pain, especially if accompanied by fever and/or chills. In pneumonia involving the lower lobes of the lungs, a patient may complain of nothing more than upper abdominal pain.

In the forms of pneumonia involving viral, fungal, and rare bacterial causes, the typical symptoms described above are not seen. Instead, these patients may report a nonproductive cough with less prominent lung findings. Systemic symptoms such as headache, malaise, fatigue, muscle aches, sore throat, and abdominal complaints including nausea, vomiting, and diarrhea are more prominent. Fever and chills are not as impressive as in bacterial pneumonia.

Lung Cancer

Lung cancer (neoplasm) is the leading cause of cancer-related death in the U.S. in both men and women. Most patients with lung cancer are between the ages of 55 and 65 years. The mortality rate for patients with lung cancer is high after only one year with the disease.

There are currently four major types of lung cancer based on the predominant cell type. Twenty percent of cases involve only the lung tissue. Another 35 percent involve spread to the lymphatic system, and 45 percent have distant metastases (cancer cells spreading to other tissues). In those cases involving lung tissue invasion, the primary problem is disruption of diffusion. In some larger cancers, there may also be alterations in ventilation by obstruction of the conducting bronchioles.

Cigarette smoking has long been known to be a risk factor for development of lung cancer. Environmental exposure to asbestos, hydrocarbons, radiation, and fumes from metal production have also been identified as risk factors. Finally, home exposure to radon has been implicated in the development of lung cancer. Preventive strategies include educating teenagers about the dangers of cigarette smoking and encouraging current smokers to quit. Implementing environmental safety standards that reduce the risk of exposure to such substances as asbestos will also reduce the risk of lung cancer. Finally, cancer screening of populations at risk is encouraged.

Although cancers that start elsewhere in the body can spread to the lungs, the vast majority of lung cancers are caused by carcinogens (cancer-producing substances) from cigarette smoking. A small portion of lung cancers are caused by inhalation of occupational agents such as asbestos and arsenic. These substances irritate and adversely affect the various tissues of the lung, ultimately leading to the development of abnormal (cancerous) cells.

There are four major types of lung cancers depending upon the type of lung tissue involved. The most common type, *adenocarcinoma,* arises from glandular-type (i.e., mucus-producing) cells found in the lungs and bronchioles. The next most frequently encountered type of lung cancer, *small cell carcinoma* (also called *oat cell carcinoma*), arises from bronchial tissues. The third type is *epidermoid carcinoma,* and the fourth is *large cell carcinoma.* Like small cell carcinoma, epidermoid and large cell carcinomas typically arise from the bronchial tissues. Lung cancers generally have a bad prognosis, with most patients dying within a year of the diagnosis.

Patients with lung cancer will present with a variety of complaints, depending on whether they are related to direct lung involvement, invasion of local structures, or metastatic spread. Patients with localized disease will present with cough, dyspnea, hoarseness, vague chest pain,

Cigarette smoking and the abuse of tobacco products are significant risk factors for the development of respiratory and cardiovascular illnesses. Always question the patient about cigarette and tobacco usage. Patients will generally underreport tobacco usage. A better picture of tobacco usage might be obtained from the patient's spouse or another family member.

A patient's cigarette smoking history is generally reported in pack/years. If possible, determine the number of cigarette packs (20 cigarettes/pack) smoked per day and the number of years the patient has smoked. Multiply the number of packs smoked per day by the number of years. For example, a man who has smoked two packs per day for 15 years would have a 30 pack/year smoking history. Medical problems related to smoking, such as emphysema, chronic bronchitis, and lung cancer, usually begin after a patient surpasses a 20-pack/year history, although this can vary significantly. This is an important part of the history and should be determined if the patient's condition allows it. Patients should also be questioned about the use of smokeless tobacco. Although smokeless tobacco has less impact on the respiratory system than smoke products, it still increases the patient's risk for developing cancers of the mouth and throat.

and hemoptysis (coughing up blood). Fever, chills, and pleuritic chest pain are seen in patients who develop pneumonia. Symptoms related to local invasion include pain on swallowing (dysphagia), weakness or numbness in the arm, and shoulder pain. Metastatic symptoms are related to the area of spread and include headache, seizures, bone pain, abdominal pain, nausea, and malaise.

Physical findings are nonspecific. Patients with advanced disease have profound weight loss and cachexia (general physical wasting and malnutrition). Crackles (rales), rhonchi, wheezes, and diminished breath sounds may be heard in the affected lung. If the superior vena cava is occluded, venous distention in the arms and neck (superior vena cava syndrome) may be present. The rapid progression of lung cancer can be striking.

RESPIRATORY SYSTEM INTERVENTIONS

Several emergency interventions are used in the care of respiratory system emergencies. Oftentimes it is necessary to actually take over a patient's breathing until the underlying problem is corrected. This is done with mechanical ventilation, which uses a device to generate a volume of air that can be administered to a patient. Initially, this is done with a bag-valve mask unit, a common emergency device that can provide adequate respirations. However, if it is necessary to provide respirations over a prolonged period, a mechanical ventilator is used.

Mechanical Ventilation

Patients who require prolonged ventilation are usually placed on a mechanical ventilator. The mechanical ventilator is a device that provides ventilatory support for patients in respiratory failure.

Mechanical ventilators can be classified as: *pressure-cycled, volume-cycled,* or *time-cycled.* In pressure-cycled ventilators, the inspiratory phase is terminated when a preset pressure limit is reached. This type of ventilator works well if the patient's airway compliance remains constant. The airway compliance is the respiratory system's resistance to airflow. The greater the airway resistance, the lower the compliance. Conversely, the less the airway resistance, the greater will be the airway compliance. In the emergency setting, a patient's airway compliance can change. An increase in airway resistance, or a decrease in airway compliance, can cause a decrease in tidal volume (V_T). In severe cases, this may lead to hypoventilation. Because of this, most pressure-cycled ventilators have been replaced with volume-cycled ventilators. Pressure-cycled ventilators nonetheless have several distinct advantages. First, they are more compact and can be powered by compressed gas without the need for electrical power. This makes them suitable for ambulance and helicopter usage.

With volume-cycled ventilators, inspiration is terminated when a preset tidal volume is reached. The gas is usually delivered from compressible bellows. Most volume-cycled respirators are powered by an external electrical source.

With time-cycled ventilators, inspiration is terminated and expiration begins after a preset time has expired. Time-cycled ventilators are like volume-cycled ventilators in that they deliver a fairly constant tidal volume despite changes in the patient's airway compliance. They can also function as pressure-cycled ventilators when the secondary pressure limits are adjusted. Time-cycled ventilators are becoming increasingly popular.

Ventilator Settings

Important ventilator parameters can be controlled on most mechanical ventilators. These include: respiratory rate, tidal volume, inspired oxygen concentration, positive-end expiratory pressure, and ventilation mode. The *respiratory rate* is the number of ventilatory cycles per minute. The *tidal volume (V_T)* is the amount of air delivered during each ventilatory cycle. The tidal volume usually is set initially at 10–15 milliliters per kilogram of body weight. The inspired oxygen concentration, or *FiO_2,* can also be set. This is usually expressed in percentages or in decimals (i.e., FiO_2 of 0.5 = 50% inspired oxygen concentration or FiO_2 of 1.0 = 100% inspired oxygen concentration). The *positive-end expiratory pressure (PEEP)* is the pressure within the airway at the end of expiration. PEEP is usually expressed in centimeters of water (cm/H_2O) and can be adjusted to meet the patient's

needs. Normal PEEP ranges from 0 cm/H_2O to 2 cm/H_2O. Increasing the PEEP improves oxygenation by keeping alveoli open during expiration. It also helps to reexpand any collapsed alveoli, which in turn will help to decrease shunting and improve the PaO_2.

Finally, the ventilatory mode can be set on most ventilators. There are several ventilator modes including:

- *Controlled mechanical ventilation (CMV).* Usually used in situations where the patient is apneic. In CMV mode, the patient is ventilated at the rate set by the operator. The patient cannot breathe between machine breaths.
- *Assist control mode ventilation (ACMV).* With ACMV, the operator sets the minimum rate at which the patient is to be ventilated. If the patient makes no respiratory effort, then only the prescribed number of breaths will be delivered. If the patient tries to breathe, the machine will deliver an extra breath with the same tidal volume as has been set. The amount of negative inspiratory pressure necessary to trigger a ventilation can be adjusted by the operator.
- *Intermittent mandatory ventilation (IMV).* With IMV, as with ACMV, the patient may breathe at a rate faster than set on the ventilator. However, the machine offers no assistance to the patient-generated ventilation, and the patient receives only the tidal volume that is self-generated. This allows medical personnel to determine the rate and depth of the patient's native respiratory efforts.
- *Synchronized intermittent mandatory ventilation (SIMV).* A problem with IMV is that the ventilator sometimes delivers a ventilation just as the patient has completed a spontaneous inspiration. Because of this, SIMV was developed. With SIMV, the mode is the same as IMV except that the ventilator times the machine breaths to fall in a pause between the patient's spontaneous respiratory cycle or to coincide with the initiation of a spontaneous breath.
- *Pressure support ventilation (PSV).* PSV mode was the basic mode used by intermittent positive-pressure breathing machines. When the patient initiates a breath, the machine delivers a constant inspiratory pressure until inspiratory flow drops below 25 percent of the peak level. Thus, the patient determines the rate, and tidal volume is dependent on patient airway compliance. PSV is usually used when weaning a patient from the ventilator.

Prehospital Mechanical Ventilation

Several mechanical ventilators have been developed for use in prehospital care. Most of these are pressure-cycled and powered by compressed oxygen. With most units, the respiratory rate and V_T can be adjusted. With some units, the inspiratory-to-expiratory ratio can be adjusted for use with pediatric patients. Prehospital mechanical ventilators, also called *automatic transport* ventilators, are common

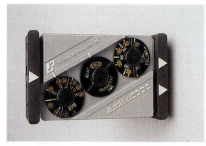

• **FIGURE A16-4   Prehospital Mechanical Ventilator**
Newer technologies have allowed the development of small, portable ventilators that can be used in out-of-hospital settings. These units allow the selection of respiratory rate, tidal volume, and inspiratory time.

on EMS units that provide interhospital transport, particularly critical care interhospital transport (Figure A16-4•). It is important not to become overly reliant on mechanical ventilators. Bag-valve mask (BVM) units should be immediately available in case of respiratory failure.

Complications of Mechanical Ventilation

Mechanical ventilation is safe and effective; however, several complications can develop, especially with prolonged mechanical ventilation and use of positive-end expiratory pressure (PEEP). A relatively common complication of ventilator therapy is barotrauma. Pneumothorax is the most common form of barotrauma. Typically, the pneumothorax is simple, but failure to recognize and treat a ventilator-induced pneumothorax can potentially lead to a tension pneumothorax and cardiovascular collapse. A less common manifestation of barotrauma is pneumoperitoneum. This is often mistaken as a ruptured abdominal viscus and can result in unnecessary surgery. Other complications of mechanical ventilation include diminished cardiac output, pneumonia, and oxygen toxicity.

Positive End-Expiratory Pressure (PEEP)

Positive-end expiratory pressure (PEEP), or continuous positive airway pressure (CPAP), can be used to reclaim lost lung volumes and to increase oxygenation. PEEP or CPAP should be considered in cases where decreased pulmonary compliance prevents adequate tidal volumes or when hypoxemia exists despite delivery of 100% oxygen.

PEEP and CPAP are usually measured in centimeters of water (cm/H_2O). Initially, a PEEP of 2.5–5.0 cm/H_2O should be tried. This can be slowly increased to 10–15 cm/H_2O. A PEEP of greater than 12–15 cm/H_2O will usually affect cardiac output. PEEP pressures greater than 20 cm/H_2O affect ventricular filling to the point where the benefits of PEEP are not being outweighed by the risks. High levels of PEEP result in increased intrathoracic pressure, which decreases venous return to the heart. This reduces ventricular filling and,

ultimately, cardiac output. Thus, PEEP should be used with caution in any patient with a head injury, as increased intrathoracic pressure will impair venous return from the brain, effectively increasing intracranial pressure.

Devices are available that allow delivery of CPAP through a tightly fitted facemask. These were initially developed for treatment of obstructive sleep apnea. However, it has been found that use of CPAP can enhance oxygenation and, in many cases, prevent the need for endotracheal intubation. As CPAP devices have become more compact, they are used with increasing frequency in prehospital care.

Chest Decompression

In certain thoracic emergencies, decompression of the chest by emergency personnel can be life saving. The most frequently encountered condition that requires pleural decompression is *tension pneumothorax*. With tension pneumothorax, a leak or tear develops in one of the lungs. Air begins to leak into the pleural space, and because it has no way to exit the chest, it begins to accumulate. Eventually, it will start to compress the affected lung leading to decreased ventilation and decreased perfusion. If allowed to progress untreated, the expanding mass of air will start to displace the mediastinum away from the injured side. This can decrease ventricular filling, which in turn decreases cardiac output. To prevent continued deterioration, emergency personnel must equalize the pressure in the chest with that of the environment. This will allow removal of the pressurized air mass, reexpansion of the lung, and movement of the mediastinum back to its normal position.

The simplest way to decompress the chest is to place a needle through the chest wall into the pleural space. This procedure is safest at the fifth intercostal space in a midaxillary line or at the second intercostal space in a midclavicular line. Remember that the intercostal neurovascular bundle runs immediately beneath and slightly behind each rib. Accidental puncture of the intercostal artery or vein can cause significant bleeding, and puncture or laceration of the intercostal nerve can cause pain or a loss in sensation to the dermatome it supplies. Because of this, it is important to palpate the rib and insert the needle along the superior border of the rib. The same warning is especially important when placing a thoracostomy tube (chest tube). The incision and tube insertion should be guided across the superior surface of the rib (Figure A16-5•).

Remember, too, that the pleural pain fibers are located in the parietal pleura and not the visceral pleura. The patient will experience the most pain as the needle exits the chest wall. When placing larger tubes, such as chest tubes, it is important to inject an adequate amount of local anesthetic into the parietal pleura to assure that the patient is as comfortable as possible.

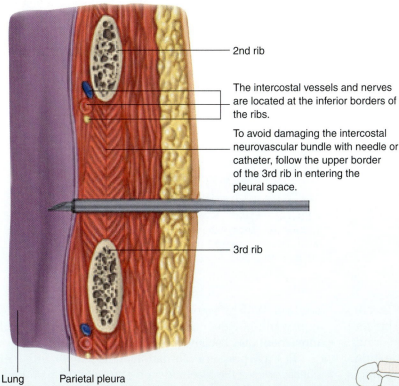

2nd rib

The intercostal vessels and nerves are located at the inferior borders of the ribs.

To avoid damaging the intercostal neurovascular bundle with needle or catheter, follow the upper border of the 3rd rib in entering the pleural space.

3rd rib

Lung   Parietal pleura

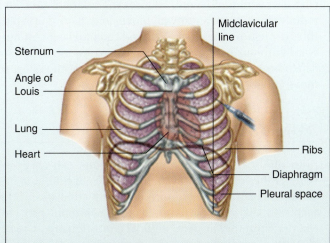

Sternum

Angle of Louis

Lung

Heart

Midclavicular line

Ribs

Diaphragm

Pleural space

● **FIGURE A16-5   Proper Needle Placement for Decompression of the Chest**
The needle should be inserted along the upper border of the rib to avoid puncturing the intercostal neurovascular bundle.

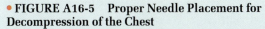

● **FIGURE A16-6   Flail Segment**
Note the free-floating segment of the chest wall resulting from the fracture of multiple ribs in multiple places.

Flail Chest

Flail chest is a segment of the chest that becomes free to move with the pressure changes of respiration. This occurs when three or more adjacent ribs fracture in two or more places (Figure A16-6●). It is one of the most serious chest wall injuries as it is often associated with severe underlying pulmonary injury (contusion) and it reduces the volume of respiration and increases the effort associated with it. This underlying injury adds to mortality

in serious thoracic trauma (between 20 and 40 percent), as do age, head injury, shock, and other associated injuries. The most common mechanisms of injury causing flail chest are blunt traumas from falls, motor vehicle crashes, industrial accidents, and assaults.

The flail segment created by this injury is no longer a controlled component of the chest wall and bellows system. Increasing intrathoracic pressure associated with expiration moves the flail segment outward while the rest of the chest moves inward, pushing air under the

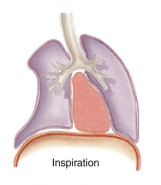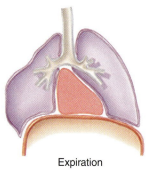

Inspiration   Expiration

● **FIGURE A16-7**   **Flail Chest**
In flail chest, the flail segment will move paradoxically to the remainder of the chest. Large flail segments can significantly reduce ventilation leading to hypoxia.

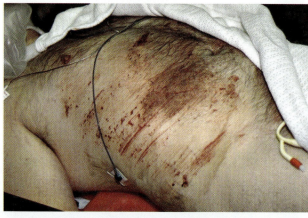

● **FIGURE A16-8**   **Signs of Internal Injury**
In most instances, chest trauma affects more than the chest wall. Always suspect problems with underlying structures such as the heart, lungs, or great vessels.

moving segment that would normally be exhaled. This reduces the change in chest volume caused by the breathing effort as well as the volume of air expired and draws the mediastinum toward the injury. During inspiration, the intrathoracic pressure falls as the respiratory muscles move the chest wall outward and the diaphragm drops caudally (tail-ward). The reduced pressure draws the flail segment inward. The lung beneath it moves away from the inward-moving segment, reducing the volume of air moving into the thorax and displacing the mediastinum away from the injury. In summary, the injury produces a segment of the chest wall that moves in opposition to the chest's normal respiratory effort (paradoxical movement); it reduces the volume of air moved with each breath; and it displaces the mediastinum toward and then away from the injury site with each breath (Figure A16-7●). In flail chest, the patient takes more energy to move less air and the respiratory volume is further reduced as the rib fracture pain produces a natural splinting of the chest.

It takes tremendous energy to create these six fracture sites (three or more ribs fractured in two or more places), and accordingly, flail chest is often associated with serious internal injury (Figure A16-8●). In addition, the movement of the flail segment, which is opposite to the rest of the chest wall, damages surrounding tissue. With each breath, the bone fracture sites move against one another causing further muscle damage, soft tissue damage, and pain. Small flail segments may go undetected as the associated intercostal muscle spasm naturally splints the

segment. With time however, these muscles suffer further injury and fatigue, and the flail segment's paradoxical movement may become more and more apparent.

Positive pressure ventilation of the patient with flail chest reverses the mechanism that causes the paradoxical chest wall movement, restores the tidal volume, and reduces the pain of chest wall movement. It accomplishes this by pushing the chest wall and the flail segment outward with positive pressure. Passive expiration then may cause both the flail segment and the rest of the chest to move inward again together.

SUMMARY

Both medical and traumatic conditions can arise involving the respiratory system. Because of this, it is important to perform a comprehensive evaluation of the respiratory system as part of your assessment process. Many respiratory system medical conditions require little more than oxygen and supportive care. Others, however, require aggressive care, sometimes involving use of a mechanical ventilator. Thoracic trauma can range from simple contusions to collapse of the lung. Respiratory system and thoracic trauma often requires emergent care in order to prevent significant disability or even death. Because of the importance of the respiratory system, it is essential that emergency personnel have a detailed understanding of the anatomy, physiology, and pathophysiology of this major body system.

The Digestive System

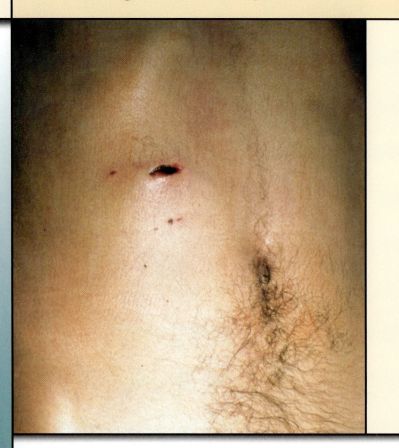

When you encounter patients with abdominal trauma, you must evaluate them based upon the severity of their presentation. When examining the victim of penetrating trauma, such as a stab wound to the right upper abdominal quadrant, you must be able to mentally visualize the possible injuries that occurred internally. For example, with a wound such as shown here, you should assume a high index of suspicion for injury to the liver, hepatic flexure of the colon, diaphragm, lung, small intestine, gall bladder, and possibly the kidney. Of these, a laceration to the liver can pose the greatest risk to the patient's life because of massive bleeding into the peritoneum. Wounds that penetrate the peritoneum typically require surgical exploration.

Chapter Outline and Objectives

Vocabulary Development

chymos, juice; *chyme*

deciduus, falling off; *deciduous*

enteron, intestine; *myenteric plexus*

frenulum, small bridle; *lingual frenulum*

*gastr, stomach; *gastric juice; gastrointestinal*

*hepati-, liver; *hepatocyte;* hepatitis

hiatus, gap or opening; *esophageal hiatus*

lacteus, milky; *lacteal*

nutrients, nourishing; *nutrient*

odonto-, tooth; *periodontal ligament*

omentum, fat skin; *greater omentum*

pyle, gate; *pyloric sphincter*

rugae, wrinkles; *rugae*

sigmoides, Greek letter S; *sigmoid colon*

stalsis, constriction; *peristalsis*

vermis, worm; *vermiform appendix*

villus, shaggy hair; *intestinal villus*

Few people give any serious thought to the digestive system unless it malfunctions. Yet we spend hours of conscious effort filling and emptying it. References to this system are part of our everyday language. We "have a gut feeling," "want to chew on" something, or find someone's opinions "hard to swallow." When something does go wrong with the digestive system, even something minor, most people seek relief immediately. For this reason, every hour of television programming contains advertisements that promote toothpaste and mouthwash, diet supplements, antacids, and laxatives.

Chapter 16 discussed the respiratory system, which delivers the oxygen needed to "burn" metabolic fuels. The digestive system provides the fuel and performs many other chemical exchanges. It consists of a muscular tube—the **digestive tract**—and **accessory organs**, including the salivary glands, gallbladder, liver, and pancreas.

Digestive functions involve six related processes:

1. **Ingestion** occurs when foods enter the digestive tract through the mouth.

2. **Mechanical processing** is the physical manipulation of solid foods, first by the tongue and the teeth and then by swirling and mixing motions of the digestive tract.

3. **Digestion** refers to the chemical breakdown of food into small organic fragments that can be absorbed by the digestive epithelium.

4. **Secretion** aids digestion through the release of water, acids, enzymes, and buffers by the digestive tract and accessory organs.

5. **Absorption** is the movement of small organic molecules, electrolytes, vitamins, and water across the digestive epithelium and into the interstitial fluid of the digestive tract.

6. **Excretion** is the removal of waste products from the body. Within the digestive tract, these waste products are compacted and discharged through the process of *defecation* (def-e-KĀ-shun).

The lining of the digestive tract also plays a defensive role by protecting surrounding tissues against the corrosive effects of digestive acids and enzymes and against pathogens that are either swallowed with food or residing inside the digestive tract. The digestive epithelium and its secretions provide a nonspecific defense against these bacteria, and bacteria reaching the underlying tissues are attacked by macrophages and other cells of the immune system.

AN OVERVIEW OF THE DIGESTIVE TRACT

The major components of the digestive tract are shown in Figure 17-1•. This tract begins with the oral cavity and continues through the pharynx, esophagus, stomach, small intestine, and large intestine before ending at the rectum and anus. Although these subdivisions of the digestive tract have overlapping functions, each region has certain areas of specialization and shows distinctive histological features that reflect those specializations.

Histological Organization

The digestive tract has four major layers (Figure 17-2•): the *mucosa*, the *submucosa*, the *muscularis externa*, and the *serosa*.

The Mucosa

The **mucosa**, or inner lining of the digestive tract, is an example of a *mucous membrane*. It consists of an epithelial surface moistened by glandular secretions and an underlying layer of loose connective tissue, the *lamina propria*. Along most of the length of the digestive tract, the mucosa is thrown into folds that increase the surface area available for absorption and permit expansion after a large meal. In the small intestine, the mucosa forms fingerlike projections, called *villi* (*villus*, shaggy hair), that further increase the area for absorption.

Most of the digestive tract is lined by a simple columnar epithelium, often containing various types of secretory cells. Ducts opening onto the epithelial surfaces carry the secretions of glands located in the lamina propria, in the surrounding submucosa, or within accessory glandular organs. In most regions of the digestive tract, the outer portion of the mucosa contains a narrow band of smooth muscle and elastic fibers. Contractions of this layer, the *muscularis* (mus-kū-LAR-is) *mucosae*, move the mucosal folds and villi.

The Submucosa

The **submucosa** is a second layer of loose connective tissue that surrounds the muscularis mucosae. It contains large blood vessels and lymphatics as well as a network of nerve fibers, sensory neurons, and parasympathetic motor neurons. This neural tissue, the *submucosal plexus*, helps control and coordinate the contractions of smooth muscle layers and also helps regulate the secretion of digestive glands.

The Muscularis Externa

The **muscularis externa** is a collection of smooth muscle cells arranged in an inner circular layer and an outer longitudinal layer. Contractions of these layers in various combinations agitate the contents and propel materials along the digestive tract. These are autonomic reflex movements controlled primarily by a network of nerves, the *myenteric plexus* (*mys*, muscle + *enteron*, intestine), sandwiched between the inner and outer smooth muscle layers. Parasympathetic stimulation increases muscular tone and activity, and sympathetic stimulation promotes muscular inhibition and relaxation.

17

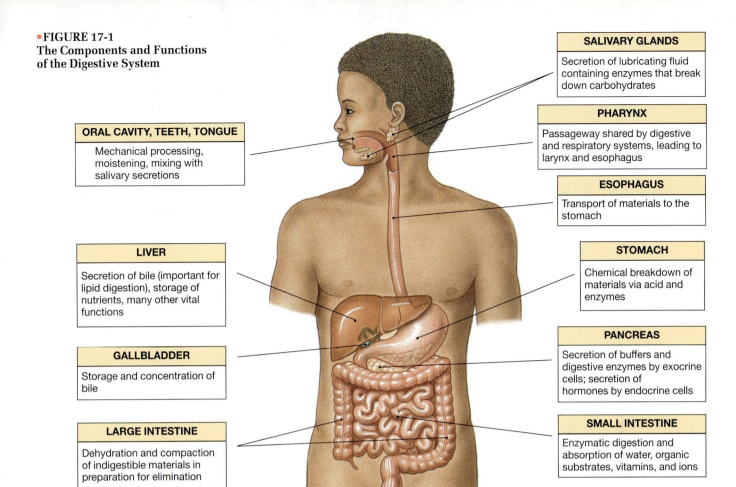

● FIGURE 17-1
The Components and Functions of the Digestive System

ORAL CAVITY, TEETH, TONGUE
Mechanical processing, moistening, mixing with salivary secretions

LIVER
Secretion of bile (important for lipid digestion), storage of nutrients, many other vital functions

GALLBLADDER
Storage and concentration of bile

LARGE INTESTINE
Dehydration and compaction of indigestible materials in preparation for elimination

SALIVARY GLANDS
Secretion of lubricating fluid containing enzymes that break down carbohydrates

PHARYNX
Passageway shared by digestive and respiratory systems, leading to larynx and esophagus

ESOPHAGUS
Transport of materials to the stomach

STOMACH
Chemical breakdown of materials via acid and enzymes

PANCREAS
Secretion of buffers and digestive enzymes by exocrine cells; secretion of hormones by endocrine cells

SMALL INTESTINE
Enzymatic digestion and absorption of water, organic substrates, vitamins, and ions

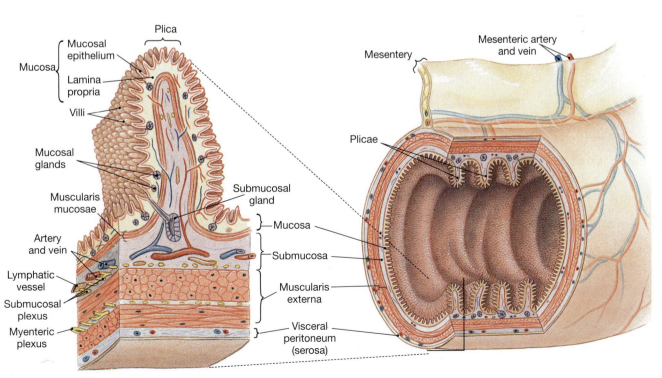

Plica

Mucosal epithelium

Mucosa

Lamina propria

Villi

Mucosal glands

Muscularis mucosae

Artery and vein

Lymphatic vessel

Submucosal plexus

Myenteric plexus

Submucosal gland

Mucosa

Submucosa

Muscularis externa

Visceral peritoneum (serosa)

Mesentery

Mesenteric artery and vein

Plicae

Mucosa

Submucosa

Muscularis externa

Visceral peritoneum (serosa)

1
7

● FIGURE 17-2   **Layers and Structures of the Digestive Tract**
A representative portion of the digestive tract—the small intestine.

The Serosa

The **serosa**, a serous membrane, covers the muscularis externa along most portions of the digestive tract inside the peritoneal cavity. This *visceral peritoneum* is continuous with the *parietal peritoneum* that lines the inner surfaces of the body wall. ∞ *p. 96* In some areas, the parietal and visceral peritoneum are connected by double sheets of serous membrane called **mesenteries** (MEZ-en-ter-ēz). The loose connective tissue sandwiched between the epithelia provides an access route for the passage of the blood vessels, nerves, and lymphatics servicing the digestive tract.

There is no serosa covering the muscularis externa of the oral cavity, pharynx, esophagus, and rectum. Instead, the muscularis externa is surrounded by a dense network of collagen fibers that firmly attaches these regions of the digestive tract to adjacent structures. This fibrous wrapping is called an *adventitia* (ad-ven-TISH-a).

✳ RETROPERITONEAL ORGANS

The organs of the *abdominal cavity* are partially or completely enclosed by the *peritoneum.* However, certain organs lie between the peritoneal lining and the muscular posterior wall of the abdominal cavity. These organs behind the peritoneum, said to be *retroperitoneal,* include the kidneys, ureters, adrenal glands, pancreas, descending colon, and the majority of the duodenum.

The Movement of Digestive Materials

Smooth muscle tissue is found within almost every organ, forming sheets, bundles, or sheaths around other tissues. *Pacesetter cells* in the smooth muscle of the digestive tract trigger waves of contraction, resulting in rhythmic cycles of activity. The coordinated contractions of the smooth muscle in the walls of the digestive tract play a vital role in moving materials along the tract, through *peristalsis* (*peri-*, around + *stalsis*, constriction), and in mechanical processing, through *segmentation*.

Peristalsis and Segmentation

The muscularis externa propels materials from one part of the digestive tract to another by means of **peristalsis** (per-i-STAL-sis), waves of muscular contractions that move along the length of the digestive tract (Figure 17-3a•). During a peristaltic movement, the circular muscles first contract behind the digestive contents. Then longitudinal muscles contract, shortening adjacent segments. A wave of contraction in the circular muscles then forces the materials in the desired direction.

Regions of the small intestine also undergo **segmentation**, movements that churn and fragment digestive materials (Figure 17-3b•). Over time, this action

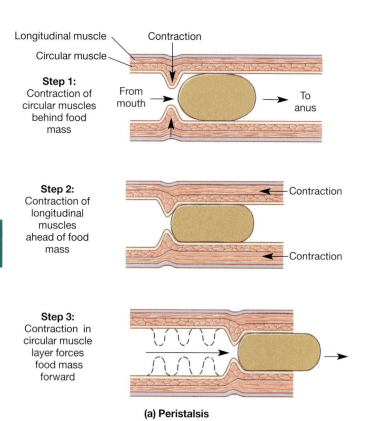

Step 1:
Contraction of circular muscles behind food mass

Step 2:
Contraction of longitudinal muscles ahead of food mass

Step 3:
Contraction in circular muscle layer forces food mass forward

(a) Peristalsis

•**FIGURE 17-3   Peristalsis and Segmentation**
(a) Peristalsis propels materials along the length of the digestive tract. (b) Segmentation promotes mixing but does not produce net movement in any direction.

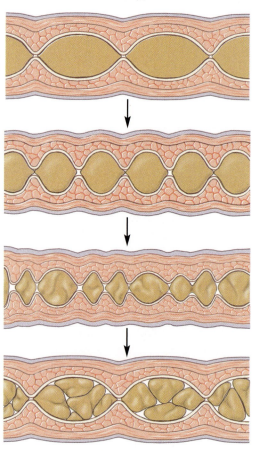

(b) Segmentation

results in a thorough mixing of the contents with intestinal secretions. Because they do not follow a set pattern, segmentation movements do not propel materials in a particular direction.

THE ORAL CAVITY

The mouth opens into the **oral cavity**, the part of the digestive tract that receives food. The oral cavity (1) analyzes material before swallowing; (2) mechanically processes material through the actions of the teeth, tongue, and surfaces of the palate; (3) lubricates material by mixing it with mucus and salivary secretions; and (4) begins the digestion of carbohydrates with the help of salivary enzymes.

Figure 17-4• shows the boundaries of the oral cavity, also known as the **buccal** (BUK-al) **cavity**. The **cheeks** form the lateral walls of this chamber; anteriorly they are continuous with the lips, or **labia** (LĀ-bē-a; singular, *labium*). The **vestibule**, a subdivision of the oral cavity, includes the space between the cheeks or lips and the teeth. A pink ridge, the gums, or **gingivae** (JIN-ji-vē; singular, *gingiva*), surrounds the bases of the teeth. The gums cover the tooth-bearing surfaces of the upper and lower jaws.

The **hard palate** and **soft palate** provide a roof for the oral cavity, while the tongue dominates its floor. The free anterior portion of the tongue is connected to the underlying epithelium by a thin fold of mucous membrane, the **lingual frenulum** (FREN-ū-lum; *frenulum*, a small bridle). The dividing line between the oral cavity and pharynx extends between the base of the tongue and the dangling *uvula*.

The Tongue

The muscular **tongue** manipulates materials inside the mouth and may occasionally be used to bring food into the oral cavity. The primary functions of the tongue are (1) mechanical processing by compression, abrasion, and distortion; (2) manipulation to assist in chewing and to prepare the material for swallowing; and (3) sensory analysis by touch, temperature, and taste receptors. Most of the tongue lies within the oral cavity, but the base of the tongue extends into the pharynx. A pair of prominent lateral swellings at the base of the tongue marks the location of the *lingual tonsils*, lymphoid nodules that help resist infections. ∞ *p. 415*

Salivary Glands

Figure 17-5• shows the locations and relative sizes of the three pairs of salivary glands (compare to Figure 17-4•). On each side, the large **parotid salivary gland** lies below the zygomatic arch under the skin of the face. ∞ *p. 136* The **parotid duct** empties into the vestibule at the level of the second upper molar. The **sublingual salivary glands** are located beneath the mucous membrane of the floor of the mouth, and numerous sublingual ducts open along either side of the lingual frenulum. The **submandibular salivary glands** are in the floor of the mouth along the inner surfaces of the mandible; their ducts open into the mouth behind the teeth on either side of the lingual frenulum.

These salivary glands produce 1.0–1.5 liters of saliva each day, with a composition of 99.4 percent water, plus an assortment of ions, buffers, waste products,

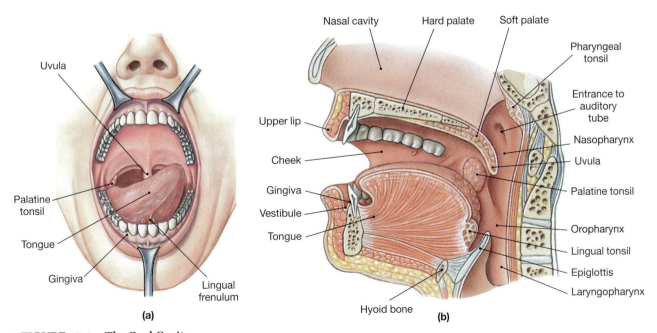

•**FIGURE 17-4   The Oral Cavity**
(a) An anterior view of the oral cavity, as seen through the open mouth. **(b)** A sagittal section of the oral cavity.

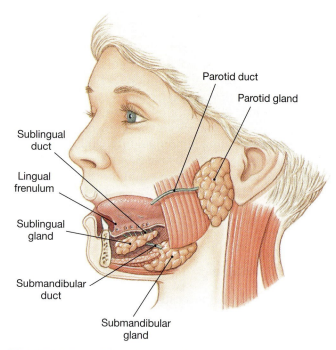

Parotid duct

Parotid gland

Sublingual
duct

Lingual
frenulum

Sublingual
gland

Submandibular
duct

Submandibular
gland

● **FIGURE 17-5   The Salivary Glands**
A lateral view, showing the relative positions of the salivary glands and ducts on the left side of the head.

metabolites, and enzymes. At mealtimes, large quantities of saliva lubricate the mouth and dissolve chemicals that stimulate the taste buds. Coating the food with slippery mucus reduces friction and makes swallowing possible. A continuous background level of secretion flushes the oral surfaces, and salivary immunoglobulins (IgA) and lysozymes help control populations of oral bacteria. When salivary secretions are reduced or eliminated, such as by radiation exposure, emotional distress, or other factors, the bacterial population in the oral cavity explodes. This condition soon leads to recurring infections and the progressive erosion of the teeth and gums.

✳ SALIVARY GLAND DISORDERS

Salivary gland disorders usually cause pain and swelling of the affected gland. Infections of the salivary glands (*siloadenitis*) are the most common disorders and can be either viral or bacterial. Mumps is the most common viral infection and primarily occurs in children. Bacterial infections are seen most frequently in dehydrated or debilitated patients and often result from slowing of the flow of saliva. Stones (*salivary calculi*) can develop in the salivary glands and can block the flow of saliva through the duct, resulting in gland enlargement. Treatment includes the use of substances such as hard lemon-drop candy to increase salivary flow.

Salivary Secretions

Each of the salivary glands produces a slightly different kind of saliva. The parotid glands produce a secretion rich in **salivary amylase**, an enzyme that breaks down complex carbohydrates, such as starches or glycogen, into smaller molecules that can be absorbed by the digestive tract. Saliva originating in the submandibular and sublingual salivary glands contains fewer enzymes but more buffers and mucus. During eating, all three salivary glands increase their rates of secretion, and salivary production may reach 7 ml per minute, with about half of that volume provided by the parotid glands. The pH also rises, shifting from slightly acidic (pH 6.7) to slightly basic (pH 7.5). These secretory activities are controlled by the autonomic nervous system.

Teeth

Movements of the tongue are important in passing food across the surfaces of the **teeth**. The opposing surfaces of the teeth perform chewing, or **mastication** (mas-ti-KĀ-shun), of food. Mastication breaks down tough connective tissues and plant fibers and helps saturate the materials with salivary lubricants and enzymes.

Figure 17-6a● shows the parts of a tooth. The **neck** of the tooth marks the boundary between the **root** and the **crown**. The crown is covered by a layer of **enamel**, which contains a crystalline form of calcium phosphate, the hardest biologically manufactured substance. Adequate amounts of calcium, phosphates, and vitamin D_3 during childhood are essential if the enamel coating is to be complete and resistant to decay. Fluoride treatment or fluoridation of the water over the same period also helps, probably by increasing the density and hardness of the enamel layer.

The bulk of each tooth consists of **dentin** (DEN-tin), a mineralized matrix similar to that of bone. Dentin differs from bone in that it does not contain living cells. Instead, cytoplasmic processes extend into the dentin from cells within the central **pulp cavity**. The pulp cavity receives blood vessels and nerves via a narrow **root canal** at the base, or **root**, of the tooth. The root sits within a bony socket, or *alveolus* (a hollow cavity). Collagen fibers of the **periodontal ligament** (*peri-*, around + *odonto-*, tooth) extend from the dentin of the root to the surrounding bone. A layer of **cementum** (se-MEN-tum) covers the dentin of the root, providing protection and firmly anchoring the periodontal ligament. Cementum also resembles bone, but it is softer, and remodeling does not occur following its deposition. Where the tooth penetrates the gum surface, epithelial cells form tight attachments to the tooth and prevent bacterial access to the easily eroded cementum of the root.

Adult teeth are shown in Figure 17-6c●. Each of the four types of teeth has a specific function: (1) **Incisors** (in-SĪ-zerz), blade-shaped teeth found at the front of the mouth, are useful for clipping or cutting, as when nipping off the tip of a carrot. (2) **Cuspids** (KUS-pidz),

1
7

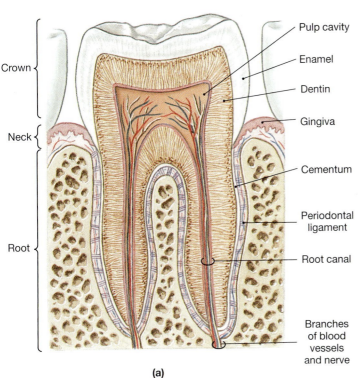

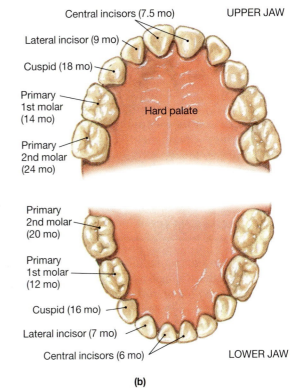

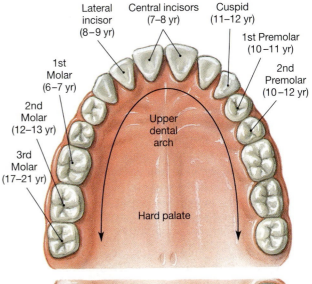

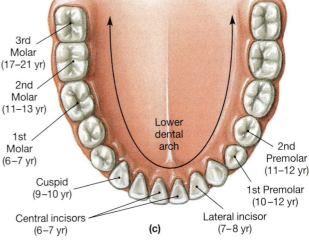

●FIGURE 17-6   Teeth: Structural Components and Dental Succession
(a) A diagrammatic section through a typical adult tooth.
(b) The primary teeth of a child. (c) The normal orientation of adult teeth, with the age at eruption given in years.

or *canines*, are conical with a sharp ridgeline and a pointed tip. They are used for tearing or slashing. A tough piece of celery might be weakened by the clipping action of the incisors, but then moved to one side to take advantage of the shearing action provided by the cuspids. (3) **Bicuspids** (bī-KUS-pidz), or *premolars*, and (4) **molars** have flattened crowns with prominent ridges. They are used for crushing, mashing, and grinding. A tough piece of meat will usually be shifted to the premolars and molars.

Dental Succession

During development, two sets of teeth begin to form. The first to appear are the **deciduous teeth** (de-SID-ū-us; *deciduus*, falling off), also known as *primary teeth*, *milk teeth*, or *baby teeth*. There are usually 20 deciduous teeth (Figure 17-6b●). These teeth will later be replaced by the adult **secondary dentition**, or *permanent dentition* (Figure 17-6c●). Three additional teeth appear on each side of the upper and lower jaws as the person ages, extending the length of the tooth rows posteriorly and bringing the permanent tooth count to 32. The last teeth to appear are the *third molars*, or *wisdom teeth*.

17

THE PHARYNX

The **pharynx** serves as a common passageway for solid food, liquids, and air. The three major subdivisions of the pharynx were discussed in Chapter 16. ∞ *p. 440* Food normally passes through the oropharynx and laryngopharynx on its way to the esophagus. The pharyngeal muscles cooperate with muscles of the oral cavity and esophagus to initiate the process of swallowing. The muscular contractions during swallowing force the food mass along the esophagus and into the stomach.

THE ESOPHAGUS

The **esophagus** is a muscular tube that begins at the pharynx and ends at the stomach (see Figure 17-1•). It is about 25 cm (1 ft) long with a diameter of about 2 cm (0.75 in.). The esophagus lies posterior to the trachea in the neck, passes through the mediastinum in the thoracic cavity, and enters the peritoneal cavity through an opening in the diaphragm, the *esophageal hiatus* (hī-Ā-tus; a gap or opening), before emptying into the stomach.

The esophagus is lined with a stratified squamous epithelium that resists abrasion, hot or cold temperatures, and chemical attack. The secretions of mucous glands lubricate this surface and prevent materials from sticking to the sides of the esophagus during swallowing.

Swallowing

Swallowing, or **deglutition**, involves both voluntary actions and involuntary reflexes that transport food from the pharynx to the stomach (Figure 17-7•). Before swallowing can occur, the food must have the proper texture and consistency. Once the material has been shredded or torn by the teeth, moistened with salivary secretions, and approved by the taste receptors, the tongue begins compacting the debris into a small mass, or **bolus**.

Swallowing occurs in three phases. In the **oral phase**, swallowing begins with the compression of the bolus against the hard palate. The tongue then retracts, forcing the bolus into the pharynx and helping to elevate the soft palate, thus preventing the bolus from entering the nasopharynx (Figure 17-7a,b•). The oral phase is the only phase of swallowing that can be consciously controlled.

The **pharyngeal phase** begins when the bolus comes in contact with the posterior pharyngeal wall (Figure 17-7c,d•). The larynx elevates, and the epiglottis folds to direct the bolus past the closed glottis. In less than a second the contraction of pharyngeal muscles forces the bolus through the entrance to the esophagus, which is guarded by the *upper esophageal sphincter*.

The **esophageal phase** begins as the bolus enters the esophagus. During this phase, the bolus is pushed toward the stomach by a peristaltic wave. The approach of the bolus triggers the opening of the *lower esophageal sphincter*, and the bolus enters the stomach (Figure 17-7e–h•).

For a typical bolus, the entire trip takes about 9 seconds to complete. Fluids may make the journey in a few seconds, arriving ahead of the peristaltic contractions; a relatively dry or bulky bolus travels much more slowly, and repeated peristaltic waves may be required to drive it into the stomach. A completely dry bolus cannot be swallowed at all, for friction with the walls of the esophagus will make peristalsis ineffective.

ORAL PHASE

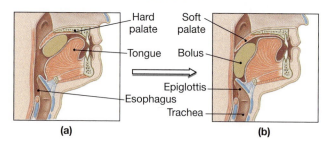

(a)   (b)

PHARYNGEAL PHASE

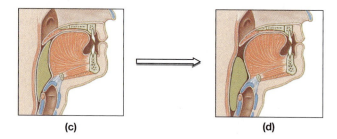

(c)   (d)

ESOPHAGEAL PHASE

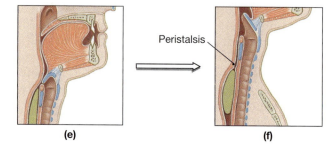

(e)   (f)

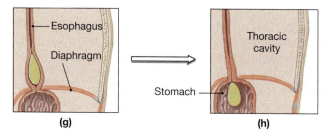

(g)   (h)

•**FIGURE 17-7   The Swallowing Process**
This sequence, based on a series of X-rays, shows the stages of swallowing and the movement of materials from the mouth to the stomach. (See also Figure 16-4•.)

✳ SWALLOWED FOREIGN BODIES

Swallowed foreign bodies are a common reason people seek emergency care. Approximately 80 percent of ingested foreign bodies occur in children. Dentures in adults account for the second most frequent type of swallowed foreign body. The presence of dentures impairs the ability to determine how well food is chewed.

Most swallowed foreign bodies pass spontaneously. However, 10–20 percent require some medical intervention. Once an object has passed the pylorus and enters the stomach, it usually passes without further incident. Objects that lodge in the esophagus, however, usually require intervention.

A barium swallow and esophageal X-ray can aid in the diagnosis of an esophageal foreign body. Alternatively, direct examination with a fiber-optic endoscope will confirm the diagnosis.

The type of foreign body present dictates treatment. Food impactions often pass following administration of medications that relax smooth muscle and decrease lower esophageal sphincter pressures. These include glucagon, nifedipine, and nitroglycerin. Sharp objects may require surgical removal. Swallowed batteries are a true emergency, as the alkaline substance in the battery rapidly burns the esophageal mucosa, and thus may result in perforation.

✓ Would peristalsis or segmentation be more efficient in propelling intestinal contents from one place to another?

✓ What effect would a drug that blocks parasympathetic stimulation of the digestive tract have on peristalsis?

✓ What is occurring when the soft palate and larynx elevate and the glottis closes?

✓ What prevents the backflow of materials from the stomach into the esophagus?

THE STOMACH

The **stomach**, located within the left upper quadrant of the abdominopelvic cavity, receives the food from the esophagus. The stomach has four primary functions: (1) the temporary storage of ingested food, (2) the mechanical breakdown of resistant materials, (3) the beginning of digestion by breaking chemical bonds through the action of acids and enzymes, and (4) the production of *intrinsic factor*, a compound necessary for the absorption of vitamin B_{12}. The agitation of ingested materials with the gastric juices secreted by the glands of the stomach produces a viscous, soupy mixture called **chyme** (kīm).

Figure 17-8a● shows the four regions of the stomach, a muscular organ with the shape of an expanded J. The esophagus connects to the stomach at the **cardia** (KAR-dē-a). The bulge of the stomach superior to the cardia is the **fundus** (FUN-dus) of the stomach, and the large area between the fundus and the curve of the J is the **body**. The curve of the J, the **pylorus** (pī-LOR-us; *pyle*, gate +

ouros, guard), connects the stomach with the small intestine. A muscular **pyloric sphincter** regulates the flow of chyme between the stomach and small intestine.

The dimensions of the stomach are extremely variable. When empty, the stomach resembles a muscular tube with a narrow and constricted lumen. When full, it can expand to contain 1–1.5 liters. This degree of expansion is possible because the stomach wall contains thick layers of smooth muscle, and the mucosa of the relaxed stomach contains a number of prominent ridges and folds, called **rugae** (ROO-gē; wrinkles). As the stomach expands, the smooth muscle stretches and the rugae gradually disappear.

Unlike the two-layered muscularis externa of other portions of the digestive tract, that of the stomach contains a longitudinal layer, a circular layer, and an inner oblique layer. This extra layer adds strength and assists in the mixing and churning activities essential to forming chyme.

The visceral peritoneum covering the outer surface of the stomach is continuous with a pair of mesenteries. The **greater omentum** (ō-MEN-tum; *omentum*, a fatty skin) extends below the greater curvature and forms an enormous pouch that hangs over and protects the abdominal viscera (Figure 17-8b●). The much smaller **lesser omentum** extends from the lesser curvature to the liver.

The Gastric Wall

The stomach is lined by an epithelium dominated by mucous cells. The secreted mucus helps protect the stomach lining from the acids, enzymes, and abrasive materials it contains. Shallow depressions, called **gastric pits**, open onto the gastric surface (Figure 17-8c●). Each gastric pit communicates with **gastric glands** that extend deep into the underlying lamina propria (Figure 17-8d●). These glands are dominated by two types of secretory cells: *parietal cells* and *chief cells*. Together these cells secrete about 1500 ml of **gastric juice** each day.

Parietal Cells

Parietal cells secrete intrinsic factor and hydrochloric acid (HCl). **Intrinsic factor** facilitates the absorption of vitamin B_{12} across the intestinal lining. Hydrochloric acid lowers the pH of the gastric juice, kills microorganisms, breaks down cell walls and connective tissues in food, and activates the enzymatic secretions of the chief cells.

Chief Cells

Chief cells secrete **pepsinogen** (pep-SIN-ō-jen), an inactive form of the enzyme **pepsin**. The hydrochloric acid released by the parietal cells converts pepsinogen to pepsin. Pepsin is an example of a proteolytic, or

17

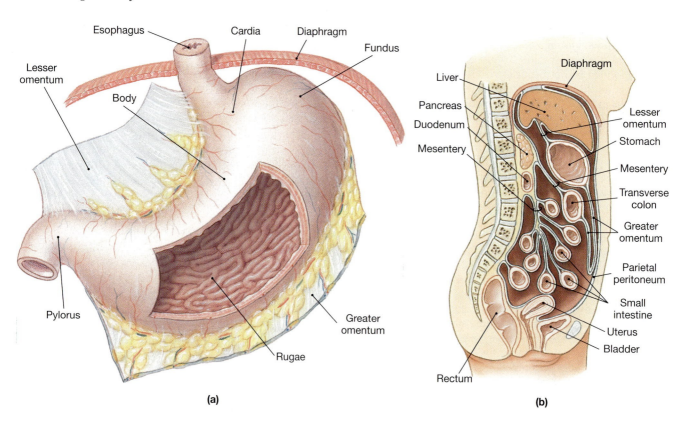

(a)

(b)

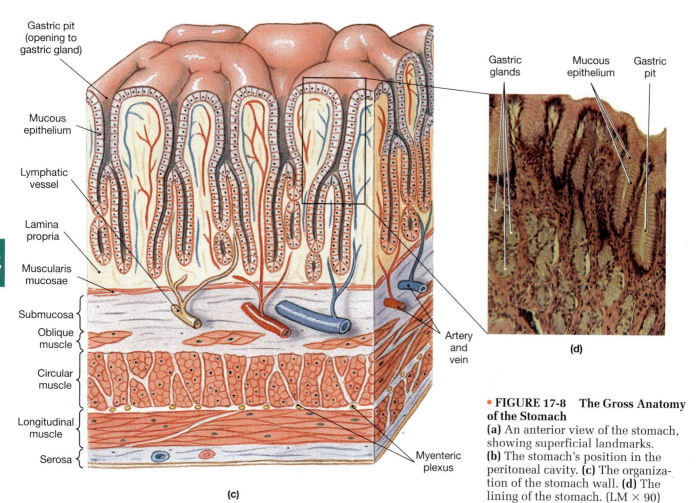

(c)

(d)

17

• **FIGURE 17-8   The Gross Anatomy of the Stomach**
(a) An anterior view of the stomach, showing superficial landmarks.
(b) The stomach's position in the peritoneal cavity. **(c)** The organization of the stomach wall. **(d)** The lining of the stomach. (LM × 90)

protein-splitting, enzyme that breaks down proteins. The stomachs of newborn infants also produce additional enzymes important for the digestion of milk, *rennin* and *gastric lipase*. Rennin coagulates milk proteins, and gastric lipase initiates the digestion of milk fats.

✳ PEPTIC ULCER DISEASE

Ulceration of the stomach or duodenum due to gastric acids or enzymes is called *peptic ulcer disease*. Normally, the stomach and duodenum are protected from the effects of gastric acids and enzymes by the mucosal lining. However, an increase in gastric acids and enzymes or damage to the protective mucosa can cause erosion of the lining of the stomach or duodenum.

Risk factors for the development of peptic ulcers include the ingestion of alcohol, strongly acidic or alkaline chemicals, and anti-inflammatory drugs. Physical and emotional stress and cigarette smoking can cause increased acid secretion. Recently, infection with the bacteria *Helicobacter pylori* has been identified as a major cause of peptic ulcer development. In fact, over 80 percent of peptic ulcers may be due to bacterial infection.

Treatment of peptic ulcer disease is directed at the underlying cause. Bacterial infection is treated with a course of antibiotics. Increased acid secretion can be managed with the use of medications (H_2 blockers and proton-pump inhibitors) and by acid neutralizing agents (antacids).

The Regulation of Gastric Activity

The production of acid and enzymes by the stomach can be controlled by the central nervous system as well as by local hormonal mechanisms. Three stages can be identified, although considerable overlap exists between them (Figure 17-9•):

1. *Cephalic phase.* The sight, smell, taste, or thought of food initiates the **cephalic phase** of gastric secretion. This stage, which is directed by the CNS, prepares the stomach to receive food. Under the control of the vagus nerve, parasympathetic fibers innervate parietal cells, chief cells, and mucous cells of the stomach. In response to stimulation, the production of gastric juice accelerates, reaching rates of around 500 ml per hour. This phase usually lasts for a relatively brief period before the gastric phase commences.

2. *Gastric phase.* The **gastric phase** begins with the arrival of food in the stomach. The stimulation of stretch receptors in the stomach wall and of chemoreceptors in the mucosa triggers the release of the hormone **gastrin** into the circulatory system. Proteins, alcohol in small doses, and caffeine are potent stimulators of gastric secretion because they excite the mucosal chemoreceptors. Both parietal and chief cells respond to the presence of gastrin by accelerating their secretory activities. The effect on the parietal cells is the most pronounced, and the pH of the gastric contents drops sharply. This phase may

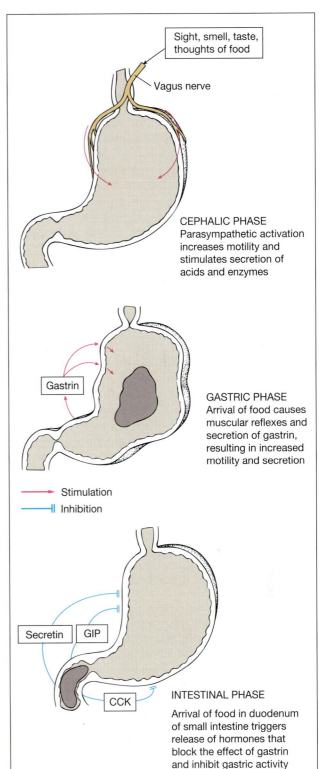

•**FIGURE 17-9   The Phases of Gastric Secretion**

continue for several hours while the ingested materials are processed by the acids and enzymes.

During this period, stomach contractions begin to swirl and churn the gastric contents, mixing the ingested materials with the gastric secretions to form chyme. As digestion proceeds, the contractions begin sweeping down the length of the stomach, and each time the pylorus contracts, a small quantity of chyme squirts through the pyloric sphincter.

3. *Intestinal phase.* The **intestinal phase** begins when chyme starts to enter the small intestine. The purpose of this phase is to control the rate of gastric emptying and ensure that the secretory, digestive, and absorptive functions of the small intestine can proceed efficiently. Most of the regulatory controls are inhibitory, providing a brake for gastric activities. Both endocrine and neural mechanisms are involved. Intestinal hormones, such as *secretin*, *cholecystokinin (CCK)*, and *gastric inhibitory peptide (GIP)*, are released when chyme enters the small intestine. These hormones reduce gastric activity and give the small intestine time to deal with the arriving acids.

Inhibitory reflexes that depress gastric activity are stimulated when the proximal portion of the small intestine becomes too full, too acidic, unduly irritated by the chyme, or filled with partially digested proteins, carbohydrates, or fats. For example, as the small intestine distends, inhibitory feedback slows the contractions in the stomach walls, inhibits the parasympathetic nervous system, and stimulates sympathetic innervation. The combination significantly reduces gastric activity.

✳ ABDOMINAL PAIN

Abdominal pain is one of the most frequent reasons people seek emergency care. The cause of abdominal pain can be difficult to determine. Inflammation, distension, or an interruption in blood supply to an organ causes a pain signal to be transmitted to the spinal cord and brain. Hollow organs, such as the stomach, gall bladder, small intestine, and large intestine, tend to cause diffuse, poorly localized pain. However, pain from solid organs, such as the liver, pancreas, and kidneys, tends to be more localized. Finally, problems in other parts of the body, such as pneumonia, can cause abdominal pain. This is called *referred pain* and can further complicate the diagnostic work-up. The patient with abdominal pain can be a challenge for emergency personnel. A systematic approach and a good knowledge of the pathophysiology of abdominal disorders will help identify the cause.

Digestion in the Stomach

The stomach performs preliminary digestion of proteins by pepsin and, for a variable period, permits the digestion of carbohydrates by salivary amylase. This enzyme remains active until the pH throughout the material in the stomach falls below 4.5, usually within 1–2 hours after a meal.

As the stomach contents become more fluid and the pH approaches 2.0, pepsin activity increases and protein disassembly begins. Protein digestion is not completed in the stomach, but there is usually enough time

for pepsin to break down complex proteins into smaller peptide and polypeptide chains before the chyme enters the small intestine.

Although digestion begins in the stomach, little if any nutrient absorption occurs there because (1) the epithelial cells are covered by a blanket of alkaline mucus and are not directly exposed to the chyme; (2) the epithelial cells lack the specialized transport mechanisms found in cells lining the small intestine; (3) the gastric lining is impermeable to water; and (4) digestion has not proceeded to completion by the time chyme leaves the stomach.

THE SMALL INTESTINE

The **small intestine** is about 6 meters (20 ft) long and has a diameter ranging from 4 cm at the stomach to about 2.5 cm at the junction with the large intestine. It has three subdivisions: the duodenum, the jejunum, and the ileum (Figure 17-10●):

1. The **duodenum** (doo-AH-de-num or doo-ō-DĒ-num) is the 25 cm (1 ft) closest to the stomach. This portion receives chyme from the stomach and exocrine secretions from the pancreas and liver.

2. A rather abrupt bend marks the boundary between the duodenum and the **jejunum** (je-JOO-num). The jejunum, which is supported by a sheet of mesentery, is about 2.5 meters (8 ft) long. The bulk of chem-

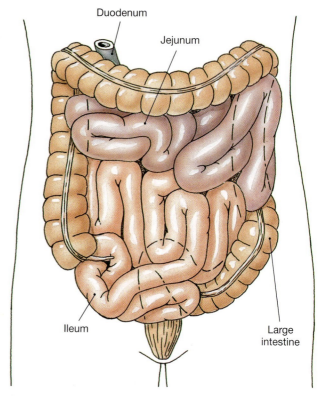

●**FIGURE 17-10   The Location and Parts of the Small Intestine**

ical digestion and nutrient absorption occurs in the jejunum. One rather drastic approach to weight control involves the surgical removal of a significant portion of the jejunum.

3. The jejunum leads to the third segment, the **ileum** (IL-ē-um). The ileum ends at a sphincter, the *ileocecal valve*, which controls the flow of materials from the ileum into the *cecum* of the large intestine.

The small intestine fits in the relatively small peritoneal cavity because it is well packed, and the position of each of the segments is stabilized by mesenteries attached to the dorsal body wall (Figure 17-8b•, p. 472).

The Intestinal Wall

The intestinal lining bears a series of transverse folds called **plicae** (PLĪ-sē), or *plicae circulares* (Figure 17-11a•). The lining of the intestine is composed of a series of fin-

gerlike projections, the **villi** (Figure 17-11b•). These villi are covered by a simple columnar epithelium carpeted with microvilli. If the small intestine were a simple tube with smooth walls, it would have a total absorptive area of around 3300 square centimeters, or roughly 3.6 square feet. Instead, the epithelium contains folds, each fold supports a forest of villi, and each villus is covered by epithelial cells blanketed in microvilli. This arrangement increases the total area for absorption to approximately 2 million square centimeters, or more than 2200 square feet!

Each villus contains a network of capillaries (Figure 17-11c•) that transports respiratory gases and carries

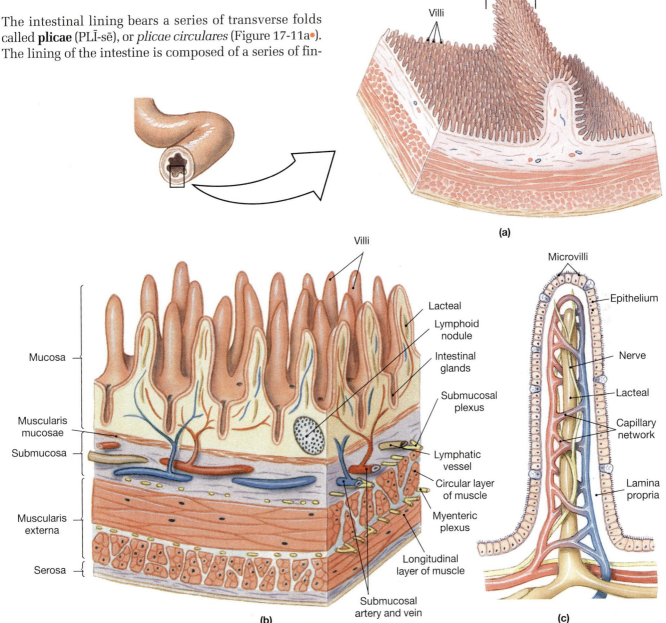

•**FIGURE 17-11   The Intestinal Wall**
(a) One plica and multiple villi. (b) The histological structure of the intestinal wall. (c) The internal structure of a single villus.

absorbed nutrients to the hepatic portal circulation. In addition to capillaries and nerve endings, each villus contains a terminal lymphatic called a **lacteal** (LAK-tē-al; *lacteus*, milky). This name refers to the pale, cloudy appearance of the lymph in these channels. Lacteals transport materials that are unable to cross the walls of local capillaries. For example, absorbed fatty acids are assembled into protein-lipid packages that are too large to diffuse into the bloodstream. These packets, called *chylomicrons* (*chylos*; juice), reach the circulation by passage through the lymphatic system.

At the bases of the villi are entrances to intestinal glands that secrete a watery *intestinal juice*. In the duodenum, large intestinal glands secrete an alkaline mucus that helps buffer the acids in chyme. Intestinal glands also contain endocrine cells responsible for the production of intestinal hormones considered in a later section.

Intestinal Movements

Once the chyme is within the small intestine, segmentation contractions mix it with mucous secretions and enzymes before absorption can occur. As absorption occurs, weak peristaltic contractions slowly move the remaining materials along the length of the small intestine. These contractions are local reflexes not under CNS control, and the effects are limited to within a few centimeters of the site of the original stimulus. More elaborate reflexes coordinate activities along the entire length of the small intestine. Two examples are the gastroenteric reflex and the gastroileal reflex.

Distension of the stomach initiates the *gastroenteric* (gas-trō-en-TER-ik) *reflex*, which immediately accelerates glandular secretion and peristaltic activity in all segments. The increased peristalsis distributes materials along the length of the small intestine and empties the duodenum.

The *gastroileal* (gas-trō-IL-ē-al) *reflex* is a response to circulating levels of the hormone gastrin. The entry of food into the stomach triggers the release of gastrin, which relaxes the ileocecal valve at the entrance to the large intestine. Because the valve is relaxed, the increased peristalsis pushes materials from the ileum into the large intestine. On average, it takes about 5 hours for ingested food to pass from the duodenum to the end of the ileum, so the first of the materials to enter the duodenum after breakfast may leave the small intestine at lunch.

Intestinal Secretions

Roughly 1.8 liters of watery **intestinal juice** enters the intestinal lumen each day. Intestinal juice moistens the intestinal contents, helps buffer acids, and dissolves both the digestive enzymes provided by the pancreas and the products of digestion. Much of this fluid arrives through osmosis, as water flows out of the mucosa, and the rest is provided by intestinal glands stimulated by the activation of touch and stretch receptors in the intestinal walls.

Hormonal and CNS controls are important in regulating the secretions of the digestive tract and accessory organs. Because the duodenum is the initial region of the intestine to receive chyme, it is the focus of these regulatory mechanisms. Here, the acid content of the chyme must be neutralized and the appropriate enzymes added. The submucosal glands protect the duodenal epithelium from gastric acids and enzymes. They increase their secretions in response to local reflexes and also to parasympathetic (vagal) stimulation. As a result of vagal activity, the duodenal glands begin secreting long before chyme reaches the pyloric sphincter. Sympathetic stimulation inhibits their activation, leaving the duodenal lining relatively unprepared for the arrival of the acid chyme. This is probably why duodenal ulcers can be caused by chronic stress or by other factors that promote sympathetic activation.

✴ VOMITING

Vomiting, also called *emesis*, is a forceful emptying of the stomach and intestinal contents through the mouth. There are several things that can stimulate the vomiting reflex. Locally, distention of the stomach or duodenum can cause vomiting. On a systemic level, vomiting can result from activation of the *chemoreceptor trigger zone* (*CTZ*) in the medulla of the brain by the neurotransmitter *serotonin*. Serotonin appears to be released from cells within the intestinal wall and from neurons in the brain stem which then stimulate the vomiting center.

Nausea and retching usually precede vomiting. Nausea is a subjective sensation that is seen with many medical conditions. Increased salivation and an increase in heart rate are often seen. Retching involves contraction of the abdominal muscles and movement of stomach contents into the esophagus, but not out into the mouth.

Vomiting usually follows retching. Peristalsis in the duodenum, stomach, and esophagus is reversed. Accompanied by contraction of the abdominal muscles, this results in forceful emptying of the stomach. Medications are available that help alleviate vomiting. Most appear to block serotonin receptors in the chemoreceptor trigger zone.

Intestinal Hormones

Duodenal endocrine cells produce hormones that coordinate the secretory activities of the stomach, duodenum, pancreas, and liver. These hormones were introduced in the discussion of gastric activity (see p. 473).

Secretin (sē-KRĒ-tin) is released when the pH falls in the duodenum. This occurs when acid chyme arrives from the stomach. The primary effect of secretin is to increase the secretion of water and buffers by the pancreas and liver.

Cholecystokinin (kō-lē-sis-tō-KĪ-nin), or **CCK**, is secreted when chyme arrives in the duodenum, especially when it contains lipids and partially digested proteins. This hormone also targets the pancreas and

TABLE 17-1 | **Important Gastrointestinal Hormones and Their Primary Effects**

Hormone	Stimulus	Origin	Target	Effects
Gastrin	Vagal stimulation or arrival of food in the stomach	Stomach	Stomach	Stimulates production of acids and enzymes, increases motility
	Arrival of chyme containing large quantities of undigested proteins	Duodenum	Stomach	Stimulates gastric secretion and motion
Secretin	Arrival of acid chyme in the duodenum	Duodenum	Pancreas	Stimulates production of alkaline buffers
			Stomach	Inhibits gastric secretion and motility
Cholecystokinin (CCK)	Arrival of acid chyme containing lipids and partially digested proteins	Duodenum	Pancreas	Stimulates production of pancreatic enzymes
			Gallbladder	Stimulates contraction of gallbladder
			Duodenum	Causes relaxation of sphincter at base of bile duct
			Stomach	Inhibits gastric secretion and motion
Gastric inhibitory peptide (GIP)	Arrival of chyme containing large quantities of glucose	Duodenum	Pancreas	Stimulates release of insulin by pancreatic islets

liver. In the pancreas, CCK accelerates the production and secretion of all types of digestive enzymes. At the liver, it causes the ejection of *bile* from the gallbladder into the duodenum. The presence of either secretin or CCK in high concentrations also reduces gastric motility and secretory rates.

Gastric inhibitory peptide, or **GIP**, is released when fats and glucose enter the small intestine. This peptide hormone inhibits gastric activity and causes the release of insulin from the pancreatic islets.

Functions of the major gastrointestinal hormones are summarized in Table 17-1, and their interactions are diagrammed in Figure 17-12●.

Digestion in the Small Intestine

In the stomach, food becomes saturated with gastric juices and exposed to the digestive effects of a strong acid and a proteolytic enzyme, pepsin. Most of the important digestive processes are completed in the small intestine, where the final products of digestion—simple sugars, fatty acids, and amino acids—are absorbed, along with most of the water content. Approximately 80 percent of

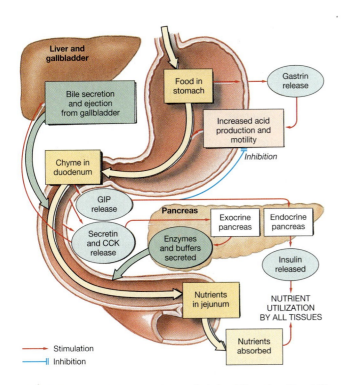

●**FIGURE 17-12** **The Activities of Major Digestive Tract Hormones**
The primary actions of gastrin, GIP, secretin, and CCK.

all absorption takes place in the small intestine, with the rest divided between the stomach and the large intestine. However, the small intestine produces only a few of the enzymes needed to break down the complex materials found in the diet. Most of the enzymes and buffers are contributed by the liver and pancreas, which are discussed in the next section.

✓ Which muscle regulates the flow of chyme from the stomach to the small intestine?

✓ When a person suffers from chronic ulcers in the stomach, treatment sometimes involves cutting the branches of the vagus nerve that serve the stomach. Why?

✓ How is the small intestine adapted for the absorption of nutrients?

✓ How would a meal that is high in fat affect the level of cholecystokinin in the blood?

THE PANCREAS

The **pancreas**, shown in Figure 17-13a•, lies behind the stomach, extending laterally from the duodenum toward the spleen. It is an elongate, pinkish-gray organ with a length of approximately 15 cm (6 in.) and a weight of around 80 g (3 oz.). The surface of the pancreas has a knobbly texture, and its tissue is soft and easily torn.

Histological Organization

The pancreas is primarily an exocrine organ, producing digestive enzymes and buffers. **Pancreatic islets**, which secrete insulin and glucagon, account for only around 1 percent of the cellular population of the pancreas. Exocrine cells and their associated ducts account for the rest. The numerous ducts that branch throughout the pancreas begin at saclike pouches called the **pancreatic acini** (AS-i-nī; singular *acinus*, grape) (Figure 17-13b•). Enzymes and buffers are secreted by the *acinar cells* of these pouches and by the cells that line the ducts. The smaller ducts converge to form larger ducts; these ultimately fuse to form the **pancreatic duct**, which carries these secretions to the duodenum. The pancreatic duct penetrates the duodenal wall with the *common bile duct* from the liver and gallbladder.

Pancreatic enzymes are broadly classified according to their intended targets. **Lipases** (LĪ-pā-sez) attack lipids, **carbohydrases** (kar-bō-HĪ-drā-sez) digest sugars and starches, and **proteases** (prō-tē-ā-sez) (proteolytic enzymes) break proteins apart.

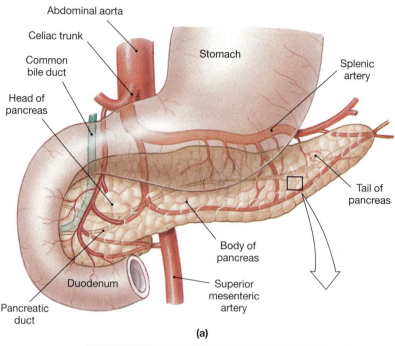

(a)

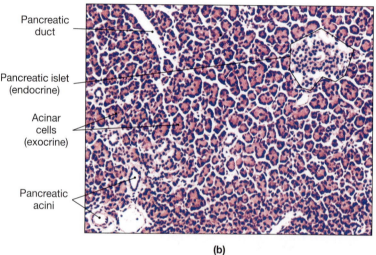

(b)

•**FIGURE 17-13   The Pancreas**
(a) Gross anatomy. The head of the pancreas is tucked into a curve of the duodenum that begins at the pylorus of the stomach. (b) The pancreatic duct and exocrine and endocrine tissues. (LM × 168)

✳ PANCREATITIS

Pancreatitis can be either acute or chronic and is often associated with alcoholism, obstruction of the biliary tract by gallstones (*cholelithiasis*), and a high level of circulating lipids (*hyperlipidemia*). *Acute pancreatitis* is a severe inflammation resulting from injury or disruption of the pancreatic ducts, or acini, that permits leakage of pancreatic enzymes into the pancreas. The enzymes become activated, causing *autodigestion* and acute pancreatitis.

The signs and symptoms of pancreatitis include severe epigastric or midabdominal pain, fever, hypovolemia and severe vomiting that is refractory to antiemetic medications. From 10 to 15 percent of patients with acute pancreatitis will go on to develop *chronic pancreatitis*.

The Control of Pancreatic Secretion

The pancreatic exocrine cells produce a watery **pancreatic juice** in response to hormonal instructions from the duodenum. When acid chyme arrives in the small intestine, secretin is released, triggering the pancreatic production of an alkaline fluid with a pH of 7.5 to 8.8. Among its other components, this secretion contains buffers, primarily *sodium bicarbonate*, that help bring the pH of the chyme under control. A different intestinal hormone, CCK, controls the production and secretion of pancreatic enzymes. The specific enzymes involved are **pancreatic amylase**, similar to salivary amylase, **pancreatic lipase**, **nucleases** that break down nucleic acids, and several proteolytic enzymes.

Proteolytic enzymes account for around 70 percent of the total pancreatic enzyme production. The most abundant proteases are **trypsin** (TRIP-sin), **chymotrypsin** (kī-mō-TRIP-sin), and **carboxypeptidase** (kar-bok-sē-PEP-ti-dās). Together they shatter complex proteins into a mixture of short peptide chains and amino acids. The enzymes are quite powerful, and the pancreatic cells protect themselves by secreting them as inactive *proenzymes*, which are activated by other enzymes within the intestinal tract.

THE LIVER

The **liver** is the largest visceral organ, weighing about 1.5 kg (3.3 lb) and accounting for roughly 2.5 percent of the total body weight. This large, firm, reddish-brown organ has three general categories of essential metabolic and synthetic functions: *metabolic regulation*, *hematological regulation*, and *bile production*.

Anatomy of the Liver

Figure 17-14• illustrates the anatomy of the liver. Although its overall shape conforms to its surroundings, the liver is divided into four lobes: The large **left** and **right lobes**, and the smaller **caudate** and **quadrate lobes**. A tough connective tissue fold, the *falciform ligament*, marks the division between the left and right lobes. Its thickened posterior margin is the *round ligament*, a fibrous band remnant of the fetal umbilical vein.

Lodged within a recess under the right lobe of the liver is the *gallbladder*, a muscular sac that stores and concentrates bile before it is excreted into the small intestine. The gallbladder and associated structures will be described in a later section.

Histological Organization

The basic functional unit of the liver is the **liver lobule** (Figure 17-15•). The liver contains about 100,000 lobules. Because their orientation usually varies, a single histological section seldom reveals all of their details.

Liver cells, called *hepatocytes* (he-PAT-ō-sīts), within a lobule are arranged into a series of irregular plates like the spokes of a wheel. *Sinusoids*, specialized and

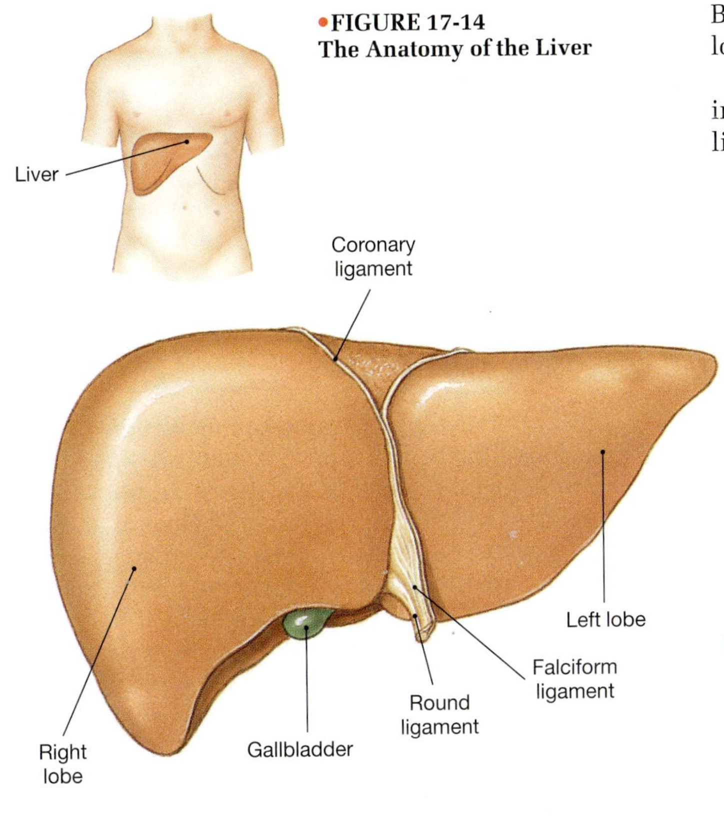

•**FIGURE 17-14**
The Anatomy of the Liver

(a) Anterior (parietal) surface

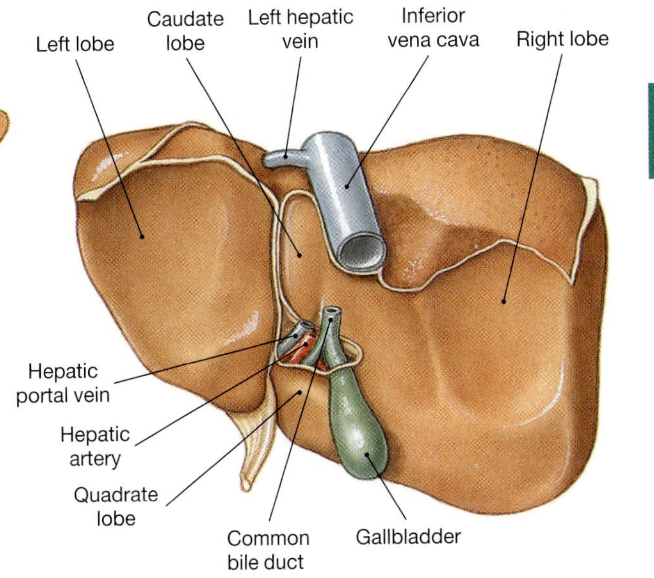

(b) Posterior (visceral) surface

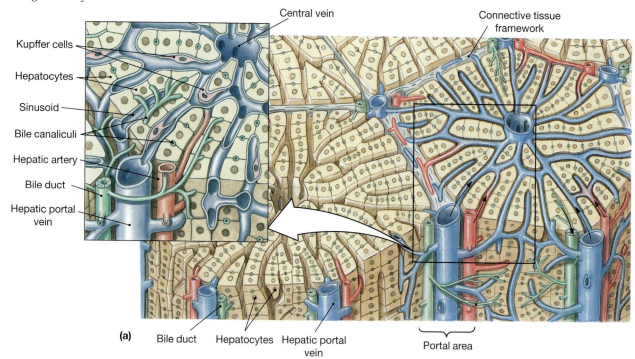

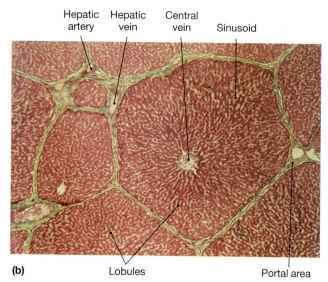

(a)   Bile duct   Hepatocytes   Hepatic portal vein   Portal area

•**FIGURE 17-15   Liver Histology**
(a) Lobular organization. **(b)** Typical liver lobules. (LM × 38)

(b)   Lobules   Portal area

highly permeable capillaries, form passageways between the adjacent plates that empty into the *central vein*. In addition to typical endothelial cells, the sinusoidal lining includes a large number of phagocytic *Kupffer* (KOOP-fer) *cells*. Part of the monocyte-macrophage system, these cells engulf pathogens, cell debris, and damaged blood cells.

Blood enters the sinusoids from branches of the hepatic portal vein and hepatic artery, and as blood flows past, the liver cells absorb and secrete materials into the bloodstream. Blood then leaves the sinusoids and enters the **central vein** of the lobule. The central veins of all of the lobules ultimately merge to form the *hepatic veins* that empty into the inferior vena cava. Liver diseases, such as the various forms of *hepatitis*, and conditions such as alcoholism can lead to degenerative changes in the liver tissue and constriction of the circulatory supply.

Bile is a secretory product released into a network of narrow channels called **bile canaliculi** between adjacent liver cells. These canaliculi carry bile away from the central vein, toward a network of ever-larger bile ducts within the liver until it eventually leaves the liver through the **common hepatic duct**. The bile in the common hepatic duct may either flow into the **common bile duct**, which empties into the duodenum, or enter the **cystic duct**, which leads to the gallbladder. Liver cells produce roughly 1 liter of bile each day, but a sphincter at the intestinal end of the common bile duct stays opens only during eating. When bile cannot flow along the common bile duct, however, it can enter the cystic duct for storage within the expandable gallbladder.

Liver Functions

Metabolic Regulation

The liver is vital to metabolic regulation. As noted in the discussion of the hepatic portal system, all blood leaving the absorptive areas of the digestive tract flows through the liver before reaching the general circulation. ∞ *p. 400* Thus liver cells can (1) extract absorbed nutrients or toxins from the blood before it reaches the rest of the body and (2) monitor and adjust the circulating levels of organic nutrients. Excesses are removed and stored, and deficiencies are corrected by mobilizing stored reserves or synthesizing the necessary compounds. For example, when blood glucose levels rise, the liver removes glucose and synthesizes glycogen. When blood glucose levels fall, the liver breaks down glycogen and releases glucose into the circulation. Cir-

**1
7**

culating toxins and metabolic wastes are also removed for later inactivation or excretion. Finally, fat-soluble vitamins (A, D, K, and E) are absorbed and stored.

Hematological Regulation

The liver is the largest blood reservoir in the body. In addition to the blood arriving over the hepatic portal vein, the liver receives about 25 percent of the cardiac output. As blood passes by, phagocytic cells in the liver remove aged or damaged red blood cells, debris, and pathogens from the circulation. Equally important, liver cells synthesize the plasma proteins that determine the osmotic concentration of the blood, transport nutrients, and establish the clotting and complement systems. ∞ *p. 336*

The Synthesis and Secretion of Bile

Bile is synthesized in the liver and excreted into the lumen of the duodenum. Bile consists mostly of water, ions, *bilirubin* (a pigment derived from hemoglobin), cholesterol, and an assortment of lipids collectively known as **bile salts**. The water and ions help dilute and buffer acids in chyme as it enters the small intestine. Bile salts are synthesized from cholesterol in the liver and are required for the normal digestion and absorption of fats.

Other Liver Functions

To date, more than 200 liver functions have been identified. (Table 17-2 contains a partial listing.) Therefore, any condition that severely damages the liver represents a serious threat to life. Although the liver has the ability to regenerate partially after injury, complete liver function is often not fully restored. The extensive blood supply complicates the treatment of severe injuries to the liver, because bleeding can be difficult to control and the texture of the liver makes normal suturing ineffective. Thus, liver transplants are becoming increasingly common since the development of immunosuppressive drugs, and there is now an 80 percent survival rate. Clinical trials are also under way to test an artificial liver known as *ELAD* (*extracorporeal liver assist device*), which may prove suitable for the long-term support of people with chronic liver disease.

The Gallbladder

The **gallbladder** is a muscular organ shaped like a pear (Figure 17-16•). It has two major functions: bile storage and bile modification. When filled to capacity, the gallbladder contains 40–70 ml of bile. As bile remains in the gallbladder, its composition gradually changes. Water is absorbed, and the bile salts and other components of bile become increasingly concentrated. If they become too concentrated, the bile salts may precipitate, forming *gallstones* that can cause a variety of clinical problems.

TABLE 17-2	Major Functions of the Liver

Digestive and Metabolic Functions

Synthesis and secretion of bile

Storage of glycogen and lipid reserves

Maintenance of normal blood glucose, amino acid, and fatty acid concentrations

Synthesis and interconversion of nutrient types (e.g., transamination of amino acids or conversion of carbohydrates to lipids)

Synthesis and release of cholesterol bound to transport proteins

Inactivation of toxins

Storage of iron reserves

Storage of fat-soluble vitamins

Other Major Functions

Synthesis of plasma proteins

Synthesis of clotting factors

Synthesis of the inactive hormone angiotensinogen

Phagocytosis of damaged red blood cells (by Kupffer cells)

Blood storage (major contributor to venous reserve)

Absorption and breakdown of circulating hormones (insulin, epinephrine) and immunoglobulins

Absorption and inactivation of lipid-soluble drugs

The Physiological Role of Bile

Most dietary lipids are not water-soluble. Mechanical processing along the digestive tract creates large drops containing various lipids that are much too massive to be attacked by digestive enzymes. Bile salts break the drops apart by **emulsification** (ē-mul-si-fi-KĀ-shun), which creates tiny emulsion droplets with a superficial coating of bile salts. The formation of tiny droplets increases the surface area available for enzymatic attack. In addition, the layer of bile salts facilitates interaction between the lipids and lipid-digesting enzymes from the pancreas. (We will return to the mechanism of lipid digestion later.)

The arrival of the intestinal hormone cholecystokinin, or CCK, in the circulating blood stimulates bile excretion. Cholecystokinin relaxes the biliary sphincter, and contractions of the walls of the gallbladder then push bile into the small intestine. CCK is released whenever chyme enters the intestine, but the amount secreted increases if the chyme contains large amounts of fat.

✓ A narrowing of the ileocecal valve would hamper movement of materials between what two organs?

✓ The digestion of which nutrient would be most impaired by damage to the exocrine pancreas?

✓ How would a decrease in the amount of bile salts in bile affect the digestion and absorption of fat?

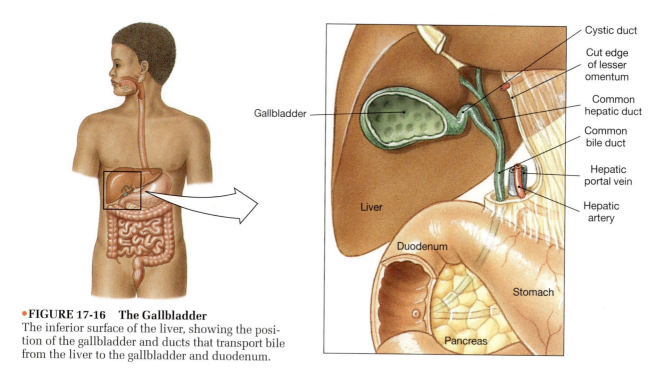

● **FIGURE 17-16   The Gallbladder**
The inferior surface of the liver, showing the position of the gallbladder and ducts that transport bile from the liver to the gallbladder and duodenum.

THE LARGE INTESTINE

The horseshoe-shaped **large intestine** begins at the end of the ileum and ends at the anus (Figure 17-17●). The large intestine lies below the stomach and liver and almost completely frames the small intestine. The main functions of the large intestine include (1) the reabsorption of water and compaction of feces, (2) the absorption of important vitamins liberated by bacterial action, and (3) the storing of fecal material prior to defecation.

The large intestine, often called the *large bowel*, has an average length of approximately 1.5 meters (5 ft) and a width of 7.5 cm (3 in.). It can be divided into three major regions: (1) the pouchlike *cecum*, the first portion; (2) the *colon*, the largest portion; and (3) the *rectum*, the last 15 cm (6 in.) of the large intestine and the end of the digestive tract.

The Cecum

Material arriving from the ileum first enters an expanded chamber, the **cecum** (SĒ-kum), where compaction begins. A muscular sphincter, the **ileocecal** (il-ē-ō-SĒ-kal) **valve**, guards the connection between the ileum and the cecum. The cecum usually has the shape of a rounded sac, and the slender **vermiform** (*vermis*, worm) **appendix** attaches to the cecum along its posteromedial surface. The appendix is generally about 9 cm (3.5 in.) long, but its size and shape are quite variable. The walls of the appendix are dominated by lymphoid nodules, and it functions primarily as an organ of the lymphatic system. Inflammation of the appendix produces the symptoms of *appendicitis*.

The Colon

The most striking external feature of the **colon** is the pouches, or **haustra** (singular, *haustrum*), that permit considerable distension and elongation (Figure 17-17●). Longitudinal bands of muscle, the **taeniae coli** (TĒ-nē-a KŌ-lī), are visible on the outer surface of the colon just beneath the serosa. Muscle tone within these bands produces the haustra.

The **ascending colon** begins at the ileocecal valve. It ascends along the right side of the peritoneal cavity until it reaches the inferior margin of the liver. It then turns horizontally, becoming the **transverse colon**. The transverse colon continues toward the left side, passing below the stomach and following the curve of the body wall. Near the spleen, it turns inferiorly to form the **descending colon**. The descending colon continues along the left side until it curves and recurves as the **sigmoid** (SIG-moyd; *sigmoides*, the Greek letter S) **colon**. The sigmoid colon empties into the rectum.

✳ DIVERTICULITIS

Diverticula are saclike outpouchings of mucosa through the muscle layers of the colon. The two most frequent complications of diverticular disease are diverticulitis and diverticulosis. In diverticulitis, a piece of fecal material obstructs the lumen of a diverticulum, causing infection. Signs and symptoms include abdominal pain (usually on the left side as the *descending colon* is most often affected), fever, nausea, and vomiting. Because diverticulitis develops in much the same manner as acute appendicitis, it is occasionally referred to as left-sided appendicitis. Diverticulitis usually responds well to a course of antibiotics.

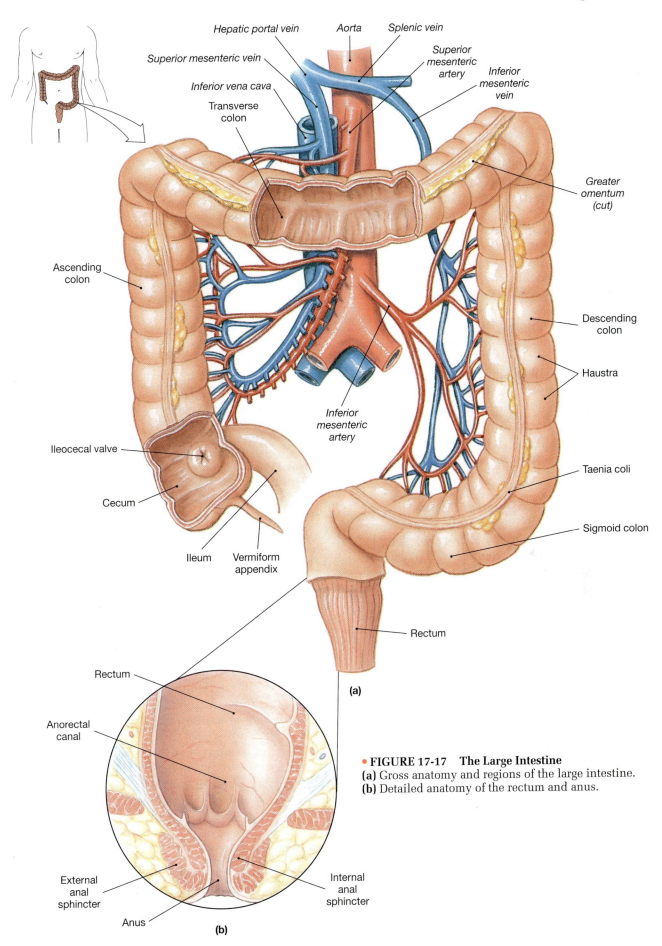

Hepatic portal vein

Aorta

Splenic vein

Superior mesenteric vein

Superior mesenteric artery

Inferior vena cava

Inferior mesenteric vein

Transverse colon

Greater omentum (cut)

Ascending colon

Descending colon

Haustra

Ileocecal valve

Inferior mesenteric artery

Cecum

Taenia coli

Sigmoid colon

Ileum

Vermiform appendix

Rectum

(a)

Rectum

Anorectal canal

External anal sphincter

Internal anal sphincter

Anus

(b)

• **FIGURE 17-17   The Large Intestine**
(a) Gross anatomy and regions of the large intestine.
(b) Detailed anatomy of the rectum and anus.

1
7

The Physiology of the Large Intestine

The major functions of the large intestine are absorption and preparation of the fecal material for elimination.

Absorption in the Large Intestine

The reabsorption of water is an important function of the large intestine. Although roughly 1500 ml of watery material arrives in the colon each day, some 1300 ml of water is recovered from it and only about 200 ml of feces is ejected. The remarkable efficiency of digestion can best be appreciated by considering the average composition of fecal wastes: 75 percent water, 5 percent bacteria, and the rest a mixture of indigestible materials, small quantities of inorganic matter, and the remains of epithelial cells.

In addition to reabsorbing water, the large intestine absorbs a variety of other substances:

Vitamins.   Bacteria within the colon generate three vitamins that supplement the dietary supply:

- Vitamin K, a fat-soluble vitamin needed by the liver to synthesize four clotting factors.
- Biotin, a water-soluble vitamin important in glucose metabolism.
- Vitamin B_5, a water-soluble vitamin required in the manufacture of steroid hormones and that of some neurotransmitters.

Deficiencies of biotin or vitamin B_5 are extremely rare after infancy because the intestinal bacteria produce enough to make up for any shortage in the diet. Vitamin K deficiencies, which interfere with blood clotting, may result from inadequate dietary fats, metabolic problems, or chronic diarrhea.

Bilirubin Products.   Chapter 12 discussed the breakdown of heme and its release as bilirubin in the bile. ∞ *p. 339* Inside the large intestine, bacteria convert the bilirubin into other products, some of which are absorbed and excreted in the urine. Others, on exposure to oxygen, are further modified into the pigments that give feces a brown color.

Bile Salts.   Most of the bile salts remaining in the material reaching the cecum will be reabsorbed and transported to the liver for secretion at a later date.

Toxins.   Bacterial action breaks down peptides remaining in the feces into various compounds. Some of these will be reabsorbed and processed by the liver into relatively nontoxic compounds and eventually will be excreted at the kidneys. Other bacterial activities are responsible for the odor of feces or result in the generation of hydrogen sulfide (H_2S), a gas that produces a "rotten egg" odor.

Indigestible carbohydrates are not altered by intestinal enzymes and arrive in the colon intact. These molecules provide a nutrient source for colonic bacteria, whose metabolic activities are responsible for the small quantities of intestinal gas, or *flatus*. Beans often trigger gas because they contain a high concentration of indigestible polysaccharides.

Movements of the Large Intestine

The gastroileal reflex moves material into the cecum at mealtimes. Movement from the cecum to the transverse colon is very slow, allowing hours for the reabsorption of water. Movement from the transverse colon through the rest of the large intestine results from *mass movements*, powerful peristaltic contractions, a few times a day. The normal stimulus is distension of the stomach and duodenum. The commands are relayed over the intestinal nerve plexuses. The contractions force fecal materials into the rectum and cause the urge to defecate.

✳ DIVERTICULOSIS

In *diverticulosis* (dī-ver-tik-ū-LŌ-sis), pockets (*diverticula*) form in the mucosa, usually in the sigmoid colon. These get forced outward, probably by the pressures generated during defecation. If the pockets push through weak points in the muscularis externa, they form semi-isolated chambers that are subject to recurrent infection and inflammation. The infections cause pain and occasional bleeding, a condition known as *diverticulitis* (dī-ver-tik-ū-LĪ-tis). Inflammation of other portions of the colon is called *colitis* (ko-LĪ-tis).

The Rectum

The **rectum** (REK-tum) forms the end of the digestive tract (see Figure 17-17b•). The last portion of the rectum, the **anorectal** (ā-nō-REK-tal) **canal**, contains small longitudinal folds joined by transverse folds that mark the boundary between the columnar epithelium of the rectum and a stratified squamous epithelium similar to that found in the oral cavity. Very close to the **anus**, the opening of the anorectal canal, the epidermis becomes keratinized and identical to that on the skin surface.

The circular muscle layer of the muscularis externa in this region forms the **internal anal sphincter**. The **external anal sphincter** guards the exit of the anorectal canal. This sphincter, which consists of skeletal muscle fibers, is under voluntary control.

Defecation

The rectum is usually empty until a powerful peristaltic contraction forces fecal materials out of the sigmoid colon. Distension of the rectal wall then triggers the **defecation reflex**, with two positive feedback loops:

1
7

1. Stretch receptors in the rectal walls order a series of peristaltic contractions in the colon and rectum, moving feces toward the anus.
2. The sacral parasympathetic system, also activated by the stretch receptors, stimulates peristalsis via motor commands distributed by the pelvic nerves.

The movement of feces through the anorectal canal requires relaxation of the internal anal sphincter, but when it relaxes, the external sphincter automatically clamps shut. Thus, the actual release of feces requires conscious effort to open the external sphincter voluntarily. If the commands do not arrive, the peristaltic contractions cease until additional rectal expansion triggers the defecation reflex a second time.

In addition to opening the external sphincter, consciously directed activities, such as tensing the abdominal muscles or making expiratory movements while closing the glottis (called the *Valsalva maneuver*), elevate intra-abdominal pressures and help to force fecal materials out of the rectum. Such pressures also force blood into the network of veins in the lamina propria and submucosa of the anorectal canal, causing them to stretch. Repeated incidents of straining to force defecation can cause the veins to be permanently distended, producing *hemorrhoids*.

✳ LIVER TRANSPLANT

Liver transplantation is the replacement of a native, diseased liver with a liver from a brain-dead donor (*allograft*). This operation allows a patient who otherwise would have died from liver failure to live a relatively full and normal life. The donor liver contains several tissue antigens that can induce an immune response in the recipient. Because of this, the donor and recipient must be checked for tissue antigen compatibility. A good match will decrease the likelihood of *organ rejection*. Patients receiving a liver transplant will be placed on *immunosuppressive drugs* and will remain on them for the rest of their lives.

Patients with *fulminate liver failure,* regardless of the cause, will die within hours or days if a suitable organ donor cannot be located. In an extreme situation, a liver from a lower animal (*xenograft*), most commonly a pig, can be used temporarily until a human donor becomes available.

On rare occasions, liver tissue may be harvested from a suitable living donor. Although the procedure is technically more complicated and places a second patient at risk, it is being used with increasing frequency when a suitable donor cannot be found. A lobe of the liver is taken from the donor and placed in the recipient. The liver is unique in that it will regenerate. Thus, in a living donor operation, the livers will grow to normal size in both the donor and the recipient within 6–8 weeks.

DIGESTION AND ABSORPTION

A typical meal contains a mixture of carbohydrates, proteins, lipids, water, electrolytes, and vitamins. The digestive system handles each of these components differently. Large organic molecules must be broken down through digestion before absorption can occur. Water, electrolytes, and vitamins can be absorbed without preliminary processing, but special transport mechanisms are often involved.

The Processing and Absorption of Nutrients

Food contains large organic molecules, many of them insoluble. The digestive system first breaks down the physical structure of the ingested material and then disassembles the component molecules into smaller fragments. This disassembly produces small organic molecules that can be absorbed. Once absorbed, they will be used by the body to generate ATP and to synthesize complex carbohydrates, proteins, and lipids. This section will focus on the mechanics of digestion and absorption; the fate of the compounds in the body will be considered in Chapter 18.

Foods are usually complex chains of simpler molecules. In a typical dietary carbohydrate, the basic molecules are simple sugars. In a protein, the building blocks are amino acids, and in lipids they are usually fatty acids. Digestive enzymes break the bonds between the component molecules in a process called *hydrolysis*. (The hydrolysis of carbohydrates, lipids, and proteins was detailed in Chapter 2.) ∞ *p. 39*

Digestive enzymes differ in their specific targets. Carbohydrases break the bonds between sugars, proteinases split the linkages between amino acids, and lipases separate the fatty acids from glycerides. Specific enzymes in each class may be even more selective, breaking bonds between specific molecular participants. For example, a carbohydrase might ignore all bonds except those connecting two glucose molecules. Table 17-3 reviews the major digestive enzymes and their functions.

Carbohydrate Digestion and Absorption

Carbohydrate digestion begins in the mouth through the action of salivary amylase. Amylase breaks down complex carbohydrates into smaller fragments, producing a mixture primarily composed of disaccharides (two sugars) and trisaccharides (three sugars). Salivary amylase continues to digest the starches and glycogen in the meal for an hour or two before stomach acids render it inactive. In the duodenum, the remaining complex carbohydrates are broken down through the action of pancreatic amylase.

17

TABLE 17-3	Digestive Enzymes and Their Functions				
Enzyme	Source	Optimal pH	Target	Products
Amylase	Salivary glands, pancreas	6.7–7.5	Bonds between carbohydrates	Disaccharides and trisaccharides
Pepsin	Chief cells of stomach	1.5–2.0	Bonds between amino acids in proteins	Short polypeptides
Trypsin, chymotrypsin, carboxypeptidase	Pancreas	7–8	Bonds between amino acids in proteins	Short peptide chains
Pancreatic lipase	Pancreas	7–8	Triglycerides	Fatty acids and monoglycerides
Nuclease	Pancreas	7–8	Nucleic acids	Nitrogenous bases and simple sugars

Epithelial Processing and Absorption.   Before they are absorbed, disaccharides and trisaccharides are fragmented into simple sugars by enzymes found on the surfaces of the intestinal microvilli. The intestinal epithelium then absorbs simple sugars through carrier-mediated transport mechanisms, such as facilitated diffusion. ∞ *p. 62* Simple sugars entering an intestinal cell diffuse through the cytoplasm and across the basement membrane to enter the interstitial fluid. They then enter the intestinal capillaries for delivery to the hepatic portal vein.

✳ LACTOSE INTOLERANCE

Have you ever wondered why there is no cheese in Chinese food? People of Asian and African descent develop a deficiency in the enzyme *lactase* during puberty. Because of this, they inadequately break down *lactose* (mild sugar). People with *lactose intolerance* who ingest a milk product develop abdominal cramps, bloating, distension, and diarrhea. Supplementing the diet with lactase tablets helps minimize symptoms.

Lipid Digestion and Absorption

Chapter 2 introduced the structure of triglycerides, the most abundant dietary lipids (see Figure 2-11•, p. 41). A triglyceride molecule consists of three fatty acids attached to a single molecule of glycerol. Triglycerides and other dietary fats are relatively unaffected by conditions in the stomach and enter the duodenum in the form of large lipid drops. As noted earlier in the chapter, bile salts emulsify these drops into tiny droplets that can be attacked by pancreatic lipase. This enzyme breaks the triglycerides apart, and the lipids released interact with bile salts to form small complexes called **micelles** (mī-SELZ) (Figure 17-18•). When a micelle contacts the intestinal epithelium, the enclosed lipids diffuse across the cell membrane and enter the cytoplasm. The intestinal cells use the arriving lipids to manufacture new triglycerides that are then coated with proteins. This step creates a soluble complex known as a **chylomicron** (kī-lō-MĪ-kron). The chylomicrons are secreted into the interstitial fluids, where they enter the intestinal lacteals through the large gaps between adjacent endothelial cells. From the lacteals they proceed along the lymphatics, through the thoracic duct, and finally enter the circulation at the left subclavian vein.

Protein Digestion and Absorption

Proteins have very complex structures, and their breakdown involves both mechanical and chemical processes. Mechanical processing in the oral cavity increases the surface area of food exposed to gastric juices following ingestion. Placing the bolus into a strongly acid environment kills most pathogenic microorganisms, breaks down cell walls, and provides the proper environment for the efforts of pepsin, the proteolytic enzyme secreted by chief cells of the stomach. Pepsin does not complete the process, but it does reduce the relatively huge proteins of the chyme into smaller polypeptide fragments.

After the acid bath has ended and the pH has risen in the duodenum, pancreatic enzymes come into play. Working together, each with its own specificities, trypsin, chymotrypsin, and carboxypeptidase complete the disassembly of the fragments into a mixture of short peptide chains and individual amino acids. Enzymes on the surfaces of the microvilli complete the process by breaking the peptide chains into their component amino acids, and the amino acids are absorbed through carrier-mediated transport. Carrier proteins at the inner surface of the cell then dump the absorbed amino acids into the interstitial fluid. Once within the interstitial fluids, most of the amino acids diffuse into intestinal capillaries.

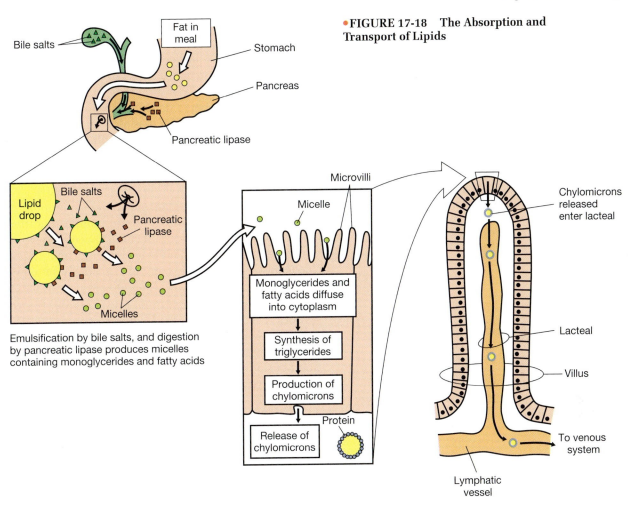

•FIGURE 17-18   **The Absorption and Transport of Lipids**

Emulsification by bile salts, and digestion by pancreatic lipase produces micelles containing monoglycerides and fatty acids

Water and Electrolyte Absorption

Each day, 2–2.5 liters of water enters the digestive tract in the form of food or drink. The salivary, gastric, intestinal, and accessory gland secretions provide another 6–7 liters. Out of that total, only about 150 ml is lost in the fecal wastes. This water conservation occurs passively, following osmotic gradients; water always tends to flow into the solution containing the higher concentration of solutes.

The epithelial cells are continually absorbing dissolved nutrients and ions, and these activities gradually lower the solute concentration of the intestinal contents. As the solute concentration decreases, water moves into the surrounding tissues, "following" the solutes and maintaining osmotic equilibrium. The absorption of sodium and chloride ions is the most important factor promoting water movement. Other ions absorbed in smaller quantities are calcium, potassium, magnesium, iodine, bicarbonate, and iron. Calcium absorption occurs under hormonal control, requiring the presence of parathyroid hormone and calcitriol. Regulatory mechanisms governing the absorption or excretion of the other ions are poorly understood.

The Absorption of Vitamins

Vitamins are organic compounds related to lipids and carbohydrates that are required in very small quantities. The nine **water-soluble vitamins** function primarily as participants in enzymatic reactions. All but one, vitamin B_{12}, are easily absorbed by the digestive epithelium. Vitamin B_{12} cannot be absorbed by the intestinal mucosa unless it has been bound to *intrinsic factor*, a protein secreted by the parietal cells of the stomach. ∞ *p. 471* The bacteria residing in the intestinal tract are an important source for several water-soluble vitamins.

The **fat-soluble vitamins** enter the duodenum in fat droplets, mixed with dietary lipids. The vitamins remain in association with those lipids when micelles form. The fat-soluble vitamins are then absorbed from the micelles along with the products of lipid digestion. One fat-soluble vitamin, vitamin K, is also produced by the action of resident bacteria and is absorbed in the colon. (This vitamin was introduced in Chapter 12 in the discussion of blood clotting.) ∞ *p. 350*

✳ EMERGENCY VITAMINS?

Vitamins are not generally thought of as emergency medications. However, two vitamins play an important role in emergency and critical care: vitamin B₁ and vitamin K.

Vitamin B₁, commonly referred to as *thiamine,* is important in many of the body's biochemical systems. It is a coenzyme for the first step of Kreb's cycle and plays an important role in several other metabolic processes. Thiamine deficiency is usually seen in chronic alcoholics and can result in altered mental status and other problems. Because of this, administration of thiamine is often a part of the emergency treatment of patients with altered mental status.

Vitamin K is necessary for blood coagulation. Deficiency can occur in chronic liver disease and causes bleeding. Vitamin K administration stimulates the coagulation system, causing blood clotting. In the United States, all hospital-born babies are prophylactically treated with intramuscular vitamin K.

AGING AND THE DIGESTIVE SYSTEM

Essentially normal digestion and absorption occur in elderly individuals. But many changes in the digestive system parallel age-related changes already described for other systems:

- *The rate of epithelial stem cell division declines.* The digestive epithelium becomes more susceptible to damage by abrasion, acids, or enzymes. Peptic ulcers therefore become more likely. In the mouth, esophagus, and anus, the stratified epithelium becomes thinner and more fragile.

- *Smooth muscle tone decreases.* General motility decreases, and peristaltic contractions are weaker. This change slows the rate of intestinal movement and promotes constipation. Sagging walls of haustra in the colon can produce symptoms of diverticulitis. Straining to eliminate compacted fecal materials can stress the less-resilient walls of blood vessels, causing hemorrhoids. Problems are not restricted to the lower digestive tract. For example, weakening of muscular sphincters can lead to esophageal reflux and frequent bouts of "heartburn."

- *The effects of cumulative damage become apparent.* One example is the gradual loss of teeth due to *dental caries* ("cavities") or *gingivitis* (inflammation of the gums). Cumulative damage can involve internal organs as well. Toxins such as alcohol and other injurious chemicals absorbed by the digestive tract are transported to the liver for processing. Liver cells are not immune to these compounds. Chronic exposure can lead to *cirrhosis* or other types of liver disease.

- *Cancer rates increase.* Cancers are most common in organs where stem cells divide to maintain epithelial cell populations. Rates of colon cancer and stomach cancer rise in the elderly; oral and pharyngeal cancers are particularly common in elderly smokers.

- *Changes in other systems have direct or indirect effects on the digestive system.* For example, the reduction in bone mass and calcium content in the skeleton is associated with erosion of the tooth sockets and eventual tooth loss. The decline in olfactory and gustatory sensitivity with age can lead to dietary changes that affect the entire body.

✓ What component of a meal would increase the number of chylomicrons in the lacteals?

✓ The absorption of which vitamin would be impaired by the removal of the stomach?

✓ Why is diarrhea potentially life-threatening but constipation is not?

INTEGRATION WITH OTHER SYSTEMS

The digestive system is functionally linked to all other systems, and it has extensive anatomical connections to the nervous, cardiovascular, endocrine, and lymphatic systems. Figure 17-19● summarizes the physiological relationships between the digestive system and other organ systems.

Chapter Review

KEY TERMS

bile, *p. 480*	**gastric glands,** *p. 471*	**pancreatic juice,** *p. 479*
chylomicrons, *p. 486*	**gallbladder,** *p. 481*	**peristalsis,** *p. 466*
chyme, *p. 471*	**lacteal,** *p. 476*	**stomach,** *p. 471*
digestion, *p. 464*	**liver,** *p. 479*	**teeth,** *p. 468*
defecation reflex, *p. 484*	**mesentery,** *p. 466*	**villus/villi,** *p. 475*
duodenum, *p. 474*	**mucosa,** *p. 464*	
esophagus, *p. 470*	**pancreas,** *p. 478*	

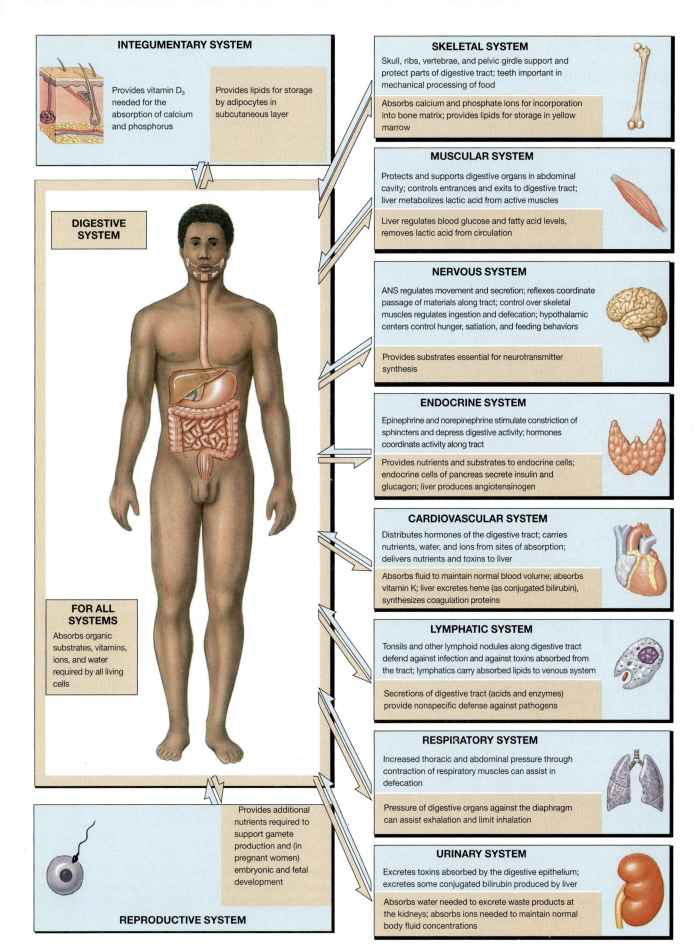

INTEGUMENTARY SYSTEM

Provides vitamin D₃ needed for the absorption of calcium and phosphorus

Provides lipids for storage by adipocytes in subcutaneous layer

DIGESTIVE SYSTEM

FOR ALL SYSTEMS

Absorbs organic substrates, vitamins, ions, and water required by all living cells

Provides additional nutrients required to support gamete production and (in pregnant women) embryonic and fetal development

REPRODUCTIVE SYSTEM

SKELETAL SYSTEM

Skull, ribs, vertebrae, and pelvic girdle support and protect parts of digestive tract; teeth important in mechanical processing of food

Absorbs calcium and phosphate ions for incorporation into bone matrix; provides lipids for storage in yellow marrow

MUSCULAR SYSTEM

Protects and supports digestive organs in abdominal cavity; controls entrances and exits to digestive tract; liver metabolizes lactic acid from active muscles

Liver regulates blood glucose and fatty acid levels, removes lactic acid from circulation

NERVOUS SYSTEM

ANS regulates movement and secretion; reflexes coordinate passage of materials along tract; control over skeletal muscles regulates ingestion and defecation; hypothalamic centers control hunger, satiation, and feeding behaviors

Provides substrates essential for neurotransmitter synthesis

ENDOCRINE SYSTEM

Epinephrine and norepinephrine stimulate constriction of sphincters and depress digestive activity; hormones coordinate activity along tract

Provides nutrients and substrates to endocrine cells; endocrine cells of pancreas secrete insulin and glucagon; liver produces angiotensinogen

CARDIOVASCULAR SYSTEM

Distributes hormones of the digestive tract; carries nutrients, water, and ions from sites of absorption; delivers nutrients and toxins to liver

Absorbs fluid to maintain normal blood volume; absorbs vitamin K; liver excretes heme (as conjugated bilirubin), synthesizes coagulation proteins

LYMPHATIC SYSTEM

Tonsils and other lymphoid nodules along digestive tract defend against infection and against toxins absorbed from the tract; lymphatics carry absorbed lipids to venous system

Secretions of digestive tract (acids and enzymes) provide nonspecific defense against pathogens

RESPIRATORY SYSTEM

Increased thoracic and abdominal pressure through contraction of respiratory muscles can assist in defecation

Pressure of digestive organs against the diaphragm can assist exhalation and limit inhalation

URINARY SYSTEM

Excretes toxins absorbed by the digestive epithelium; excretes some conjugated bilirubin produced by liver

Absorbs water needed to excrete waste products at the kidneys; absorbs ions needed to maintain normal body fluid concentrations

17

•**FIGURE 17-19** **Functional Relationships Between the Digestive System and Other Systems**

SUMMARY OUTLINE

INTRODUCTION *p. 464*

1. The digestive system consists of the muscular **digestive tract** and various **accessory organs**.

2. Digestive functions include **ingestion**, **mechanical processing**, **digestion**, **secretion**, **absorption**, **compaction**, and **excretion**.

AN OVERVIEW OF THE DIGESTIVE TRACT *p. 464*

1. The digestive tract includes the oral cavity, pharynx, esophagus, stomach, small intestine, large intestine, rectum, and anus. *(Figure 17-1)*

Histological Organization *p. 464*

2. The epithelium and underlying connective tissue, the *lamina propria*, form the **mucosa** (mucous membrane) of the digestive tract. Next, outward, are the **submucosa**, the **muscularis externa**, and the *adventitia*, a layer of loose connective tissue. In the peritoneal cavity, the muscularis externa is covered by the **serosa**, a serous membrane *(Figure 17-2)*

3. Double sheets of peritoneal membrane called **mesenteries** suspend the digestive tract.

The Movement of Digestive Materials *p. 466*

4. The neurons that innervate the smooth muscle of the muscularis externa are not under voluntary control.

5. The muscularis externa propels materials through the digestive tract by means of the contractions of **peristalsis**. **Segmentation** movements in areas of the small intestine churn digestive materials. *(Figure 17-3)*

THE ORAL CAVITY *p. 467*

1. The functions of the **oral cavity** are (1) analysis of potential foods; (2) mechanical processing using the teeth, tongue, and palatal surfaces; (3) lubrication by mixing with mucus and salivary secretions; and (4) digestion by salivary enzymes.

2. The oral cavity, or **buccal cavity**, is lined by oral mucosa. The **hard palate** and **soft palate** form its roof, and the tongue forms its floor. *(Figure 17-4)*

The Tongue *p. 467*

3. The primary functions of the **tongue** include (1) mechanical processing, (2) manipulation to assist in chewing and swallowing, and (3) sensory analysis.

Salivary Glands *p. 467*

4. The **parotid**, **sublingual**, and **submandibular salivary glands** discharge their secretions into the oral cavity. Saliva lubricates the mouth, dissolves chemicals, flushes the oral surfaces, and helps control bacteria. Salivation is usually controlled by the ANS. *(Figure 17-5)*

Teeth *p. 468*

5. **Mastication** (chewing) occurs through the contact of the opposing surfaces of the **teeth**. The **periodontal ligament** anchors the tooth in a bony socket. **Dentin** forms the basic structure of a tooth. The **crown** is coated with **enamel**, and the **root** is covered with **cementum**. *(Figure 17-6a)*

6. The 20 primary teeth, or **deciduous teeth**, are replaced by the 32 teeth of the **secondary dentition** during development. *(Figure 17-6b,c)*

THE PHARYNX *p. 470*

1. The **pharynx** serves as a common passageway for solid food, liquids, and air. Pharyngeal muscle contractions during swallowing propel the food mass along the esophagus and into the stomach.

THE ESOPHAGUS *p. 470*

1. The **esophagus** carries solids and liquids from the pharynx to the stomach through an opening in the diaphragm, the *esophageal hiatus*.

Swallowing *p. 470*

2. **Deglutition** (swallowing) can be divided into **oral**, **pharyngeal**, and **esophageal phases**. Swallowing begins with the compaction of a **bolus** and its movement into the pharynx, followed by the elevation of the larynx, reflection of the epiglottis, and closure of the glottis. After opening of the *upper esophageal sphincter*, peristalsis moves the bolus down the esophagus to the *lower esophageal sphincter*. *(Figure 17-7)*

THE STOMACH *p. 471*

1. The **stomach** has four major functions: (1) the temporary bulk storage of ingested matter, (2) the mechanical breakdown of resistant materials, (3) the disruption of chemical bonds using acids and enzymes, and (4) the production of *intrinsic factor*. **Chyme** forms in the stomach as gastric and salivary secretions are mixed with food.

2. The four regions of the stomach are the **cardia**, **fundus**, **body**, and **pylorus**. The **pyloric sphincter** guards the exit from the stomach. In a relaxed state the stomach lining contains numerous **rugae** (ridges and folds). *(Figure 17-8)*

The Gastric Wall *p. 471*

3. Within the **gastric glands**, **parietal cells** secrete **intrinsic factor** and hydrochloric acid. **Chief cells** secrete **pepsinogen**, which acids in the gastric lumen convert to the enzyme **pepsin**.

The Regulation of Gastric Activity *p. 473*

4. Gastric secretion includes: (1) the **cephalic phase**, which prepares the stomach to receive ingested materials; (2) the **gastric phase**, which begins with the arrival of food in the stomach; and (3) the **intestinal phase**, which controls the rate of gastric emptying. *(Figure 17-9)*

THE SMALL INTESTINE *p. 474*

1. The **small intestine** includes the **duodenum**, the **jejunum**, and the **ileum**. The *ileocecal valve*, a sphincter, marks the transition between the small and large intestines. *(Figure 17-10)*

The Intestinal Wall *p. 475*

2. The intestinal mucosa bears transverse folds called **plicae**, or *plicae circulares*, and small projections called intestinal **villi**. These increase the surface area for absorption. Each villus contains a terminal lymphatic called a **lacteal**. *(Figure 17-11)*

3. Some of the smooth muscle cells in the musularis externa of the small intestine contract periodically, without stim-

ulation, to produce brief, localized peristaltic contractions that slowly move materials along the tract. More extensive peristaltic activities along the entire length of the small intestine are coordinated by the *gastroenteric* and the *gastroileal reflexes.*

4. On average, it takes about 5 hours for materials to pass from the duodenum to the end of the ileum. Along the way, absorptive effectiveness is enhanced by segmentation movements, which stir and mix the intestinal contents.

Intestinal Secretions *p. 476*

5. Intestinal glands secrete **intestinal juice**, mucus, and hormones. Intestinal juice moistens the chyme, helps buffer acids, and dissolves digestive enzymes and the products of digestion.

6. Intestinal hormones include **secretin, cholecystokinin (CCK)**, and **gastric inhibitory peptide (GIP)**. *(Figure 17-12; Table 17-1)*

Digestion in the Small Intestine *p. 477*

7. Most of the important digestive and absorptive functions occur in the small intestine. Digestive enzymes and buffers are provided by the pancreas, liver, and gallbladder.

THE PANCREAS *p. 478*

1. The **pancreatic duct** penetrates the wall of the duodenum, where it delivers the secretions of the **pancreas**. *(Figure 17-13a)*

Histological Organization *p. 478*

2. Exocrine gland ducts branch repeatedly before ending in the **pancreatic acini** (blind pockets). *(Figure 17-13b)*

3. The pancreas has two functions: endocrine (secreting insulin and glucagon into the blood) and exocrine (secreting water, ions, and digestive enzymes into the small intestine). Pancreatic enzymes include **lipases, carbohydrases**, and **proteases**.

The Control of Pancreatic Secretion *p. 479*

4. The pancreatic exocrine cells produce a watery **pancreatic juice** in response to hormonal instructions from the duodenum. When chyme arrives in the small intestine, (1) secretin triggers the pancreatic production of a fluid containing buffers, primarily sodium bicarbonate, that help bring the pH of the chyme under control; and (2) CCK is released.

5. CCK stimulates the pancreas to produce and secrete **pancreatic amylase, pancreatic lipase, nucleases**, and several proteolytic enzymes—notably, **trypsin, chymotrypsin**, and **carboxypeptidase**.

THE LIVER *p. 479*

1. The **liver** is the largest and most versatile visceral organ in the body, with over 200 known functions. *(Figure 17-14)*

Anatomy of the Liver *p. 479*

2. The **liver lobule** is the organ's basic functional unit. Blood is supplied to the lobules by the hepatic artery and hepatic portal vein. Within the lobules, blood flows past *hepatocytes* through *sinusoids* to the **central vein**. **Bile canaliculi** carry bile away from the central vein and toward bile ducts. *(Figure 17-15)*

3. The bile ducts from each lobule unite to form the **common hepatic duct**, which meets the **cystic duct** to form the common bile duct, which empties into the duodenum.

Liver Functions *p. 480*

4. The liver performs metabolic and hematological regulation and produces **bile**. *(Table 17-2)*

The Gallbladder *p. 481*

5. The **gallbladder** stores and concentrates bile for release into the duodenum. During **emulsification**, bile salts break apart large drops of lipids and make them accessible to pancreatic lipases. *(Figure 17-16)*

THE LARGE INTESTINE *p. 482*

1. The main functions of the **large intestine** are to (1) reabsorb water and compact the feces, (2) absorb vitamins liberated by bacteria, and (3) store fecal material prior to defecation. *(Figure 17-17a)*

The Cecum *p. 482*

2. The **cecum** collects and stores material from the ileum and begins the process of compaction. The **vermiform appendix** is attached to the cecum.

The Colon *p. 482*

3. The **colon** has a larger diameter and a thinner wall than the small intestine. It bears **haustra** (pouches) and the **taeniae coli** (longitudinal bands of muscle).

The Physiology of the Large Intestine *p. 484*

4. The large intestine reabsorbs water and other substances, such as *vitamins, bilirubin products, bile salts*, and *toxins*. Bacteria residing in the large intestine are responsible for intestinal gas, or *flatus*.

5. Distension of the stomach and duodenum stimulates peristalsis, or *mass movements*, of feces from the colon into the rectum.

The Rectum *p. 484*

6. The **rectum** terminates in the **anorectal canal**, leading to the **anus**. *(Figure 17-17b)*

7. Muscular sphincters control the passage of fecal material to the anus. Distension of the rectal wall triggers the *defecation reflex*. Under normal circumstances, the release of feces cannot occur unless the **external anal sphincter** is voluntarily relaxed.

DIGESTION AND ABSORPTION *p. 485*

The Processing and Absorption of Nutrients *p. 485*

1. The digestive system breaks down the physical structure of the ingested material and then disassembles the component molecules into smaller fragments through *hydrolysis*. *(Table 17-3)*

2. Amylase breaks down complex carbohydrates into disaccharides and trisaccharides. These are broken down into monosaccharides by enzymes at the epithelial surface and are absorbed by the intestinal epithelium through facilitated diffusion and cotransport.

3. *Triglycerides* are emulsified into large lipid drops. The resulting fatty acids and other lipids interact with bile salts to form **micelles**, from which they diffuse across the

1
7

intestinal epithelium. The intestinal cells absorb fatty acids and synthesize new triglycerides. These are packaged in **chylomicrons**, which are released into the interstitial fluid and transported to the venous system by lymphatics. *(Figure 17-18)*

4. Protein digestion involves the gastric enzyme pepsin and the various pancreatic proteases. Peptidases liberate amino acids that are absorbed by the intestinal epithelium and released into the interstitial fluids.

Water and Electrolyte Absorption *p. 487*

5. About 2–2.5 liters of water is ingested each day, and digestive secretions provide 6–7 liters. Nearly all is reabsorbed by osmosis.

6. Various processes are responsible for the movement of cations (such as sodium and calcium) and anions (such as chloride and bicarbonate).

The Absorption of Vitamins *p. 487*

7. The nine **water-soluble vitamins** are important as cofactors in enzymatic reactions. **Fat-soluble vitamins** are enclosed within fat droplets and are absorbed with the products of lipid digestion.

AGING AND THE DIGESTIVE SYSTEM *p. 488*

1. Age-related changes include a thinner and more fragile epithelium due to a reduction in epithelial stem cell division and weaker peristaltic contractions as smooth muscle tone decreases.

INTEGRATION WITH OTHER SYSTEMS *p. 488*

1. The digestive system has extensive anatomical connections to the nervous, cardiovascular, endocrine, and lymphatic systems. *(Figure 17-19)*

REVIEW QUESTIONS

LEVEL 1   Reviewing Facts and Terms

Match each item in column A with the most closely related item in column B. Use letters for answers in the spaces provided.

Column A

___ 1. pyloric sphincter
___ 2. liver cells
___ 3. mucosa
___ 4. mesentery
___ 5. chief cells
___ 6. palate
___ 7. parietal cells
___ 8. parasympathetic stimulation
___ 9. sympathetic stimulation
___10. peristalsis
___11. bile salts
___12. salivary amylase

Column B

a. serous membrane sheet
b. moves materials along digestive tract
c. regulates flow of chyme
d. increases muscular activity of digestive tract
e. starch digestion
f. inhibits muscular activity of digestive tract
g. inner lining of digestive tract
h. roof of oral cavity
i. pepsinogen
j. hydrochloric acid
k. hepatocytes
l. emulsification of fats

13. The enzymatic breakdown of large molecules into their basic building blocks is called:
    (a) absorption
    (b) secretion
    (c) mechanical digestion
    (d) chemical digestion

14. The activities of the digestive system are regulated by:
    (a) hormonal mechanisms
    (b) local mechanisms
    (c) neural mechanisms
    (d) a, b, and c are correct

15. The layer of the peritoneum that lines the inner surfaces of the body wall is the:
    (a) visceral peritoneum
    (b) parietal peritoneum
    (c) greater omentum
    (d) lesser omentum

16. Protein digestion in the stomach results primarily from secretions released by:
    (a) hepatocytes   (b) parietal cells
    (c) chief cells   (d) goblet cells

17. The part of the gastrointestinal tract that plays the primary role in the digestion and absorption of nutrients is the:
    (a) large intestine   (b) small intestine
    (c) stomach   (d) cecum and colon

18. The duodenal hormone that stimulates the production and secretion of pancreatic enzymes is:
    (a) pepsinogen
    (b) gastrin
    (c) secretin
    (d) cholecystokinin

19. The essential metabolic and synthetic service(s) provided by the liver is (are):
    (a) metabolic regulation
    (b) hematological regulation
    (c) bile production
    (d) a, b, and c are correct

20. Bile release from the gallbladder into the duodenum occurs only under the stimulation of:
    (a) cholecystokinin   (b) secretin
    (c) gastrin   (d) pepsinogen

1
7

21. The major function(s) of the large intestine is (are):
    (a) reabsorption of water and compaction of feces
    (b) absorption of vitamins liberated by bacterial action
    (c) storage of fecal material prior to defecation
    (d) a, b, and c are correct
22. The part of the colon that empties into the rectum is the:
    (a) ascending colon   (b) descending colon
    (c) transverse colon   (d) sigmoid colon
23. What are the primary digestive functions?
24. What is the purpose of the transverse or longitudinal folds in the mucosa of the digestive tract?
25. Name and describe the layers of the digestive tract, proceeding from the innermost to the outermost layer.

26. What are the four primary functions of the oral (buccal) cavity?
27. What specific function does each of the four types of teeth perform in the oral cavity?
28. What three subdivisions of the small intestine are involved in the digestion and absorption of food?
29. What are the primary functions of the pancreas, liver, and gallbladder in the digestive process?
30. What are the three major functions of the large intestine?
31. What five age-related changes occur in the digestive system?

LEVEL 2   Reviewing Concepts

32. If the lingual frenulum is too restrictive, an individual:
    (a) has difficulty tasting food
    (b) cannot swallow properly
    (c) cannot control movements of the tongue
    (d) cannot eat or speak normally
33. The gastric phase of secretion is initiated by:
    (a) distension of the stomach
    (b) an increase in the pH of the gastric contents
    (c) the presence of undigested materials in the stomach
    (d) a, b, and c are correct

34. A drop in pH to 4.0 in the duodenum stimulates the secretion of:
    (a) secretin   (b) cholecystokinin
    (c) gastrin   (d) a, b, and c are correct
35. Differentiate between the action and outcome of peristalsis and segmentation.
36. How does the stomach promote and assist in the digestive process?
37. What changes in gastric function occur during the three phases of gastric secretion?

LEVEL 3   Critical Thinking and Clinical Applications

38. Some patients with gallstones develop pancreatitis. How could this occur?
39. Barb suffers from Crohn's disease, a regional inflammation of the intestine that is thought to have some genetic basis, although the actual cause is as yet unknown. When the disease flares up, she experiences abdominal pain, weight loss, and anemia. Which part(s) of the intestine is (are) probably involved, and what is the cause of her symptoms?

ANSWERS TO CONCEPT CHECK QUESTIONS

Page 471
1. Peristalsis would be more efficient in propelling intestinal contents. Segmentation is essentially a churning action that mixes intestinal contents with digestive fluids.   2. Parasympathetic stimulation increases muscle tone and motility in the digestive tract. A drug that blocks this activity would decrease the rate of peristalsis.   3. The process that is being described is swallowing.   4. The lower esophageal sphincter normally prevents the backflow of the stomach contents into the esophagus.

Page 478
1. The pyloric sphincter regulates the flow of chyme into the small intestine.   2. The vagus nerve contains parasympathetic motor fibers that can stimulate gastric secretions even if no food is in the stomach (cephalic phase of gastric digestion). Cutting the branches of the vagus that supply the stomach would prevent this type of secretion and would decrease the chance of ulcer formation.   3. The small intestine has several adaptations that increase surface area to increase its absorptive capacity. First, walls of the small intestine form folds called plicae. The tissue that covers the plicae forms villi, fingerlike projections. The cells that cover the villi have an exposed surface that in turn is covered by small fingerlike projections called microvilli. In addition, the small intestine has a very rich blood supply and lymphatic supply to transport the nutrients that are absorbed.   4. It would increase.

Page 481
1. A narrowing of the ileocecal valve would interfere with the flow of chyme from the small intestine to the large intestine.   2. Damage to the exocrine pancreas would most affect the digestion of fats (lipids) because that organ is the primary source of lipases.   3. A decrease in the amount of bile salts would decrease the effectiveness of fat digestion and absorption.

Page 488
1. Chylomicrons are formed from the fats that are digested in a meal. A meal that is high in fat would increase the number of chylomicrons in the lacteals.   2. The removal of the upper portion of the stomach would interfere with the absorption of vitamin B_{12}. This vitamin requires intrinsic factor, a molecule produced by the parietal cells in the stomach.   3. Diarrhea is potentially life-threatening because a person could lose fluid and electrolytes faster than these substances can be replaced. This would result in dehydration and possibly death. Although it can be quite uncomfortable, constipation does not interfere with any major body process. The few toxic waste products that are normally eliminated via the digestive system can move into the blood and be eliminated by the kidneys.

1
7

OVERVIEW

The digestive system, also referred to as the gastrointestinal (GI) system, is responsible for the ingestion, processing, and elimination of food. It also plays a defensive role by protecting surrounding tissues from the corrosive effects of digestive acids and enzymes and by protecting the body against pathogens ingested with food or residing in the GI tract. Several common emergency conditions involve the GI system, including appendicitis, gall bladder disease, diverticulitis, and many others.

Physicians who specialize in the treatment of digestive system problems are *gastroenterologists.* They normally complete a fellowship in gastroenterology following an internal medicine residency. Much of modern gastroenterology practice involves the use of fiberoptic endoscopes for examining and treating the gastrointestinal system. The esophagogastroduodenoscope (EGD) is used to examine the esophagus, stomach, and first part of the duodenum. Small pinch biopsies and some treatment procedures can be performed through this scope. The colonoscope is used to examine the entire colon. It is inserted through the rectum and can usually be guided all the way to the ileocecal valve. Pinch biopsies and snare removal of polyps are all possible through the colonoscope. Some surgeons choose to specialize in surgery of the colon and associated structures. They are referred to as *colon/rectal* surgeons. They complete a one- to two-year fellowship following a general surgery residency program.

APPENDICITIS

Appendicitis is an inflammation of the vermiform appendix, which is located at the junction of the small intestine and the large intestine (ileocecal junction). Appendicitis occurs in approximately 10 to 20 percent of the United States population. The maximum incidence occurs in the second and third decades of life and is relatively rare at the extremes of age.

The most common cause of acute appendicitis is obstruction of the lumen of the appendix, usually by fecal material (fecalith). The shape and location of the appendix makes it particularly vulnerable to obstruction by feces or other material, such as food particles or tumor. This inflames the lymphoid tissue and often leads to bacterial infection that subsequently ulcerates the mucosa. The inflammation causes the appendix's internal diameter to expand, which can block blood flow through the appendicular artery and cause thrombosis. With its blood supply cut off, the appendix becomes ischemic, and infarction, tissue necrosis, and gangrene follow. At this point, the walls of the appendix weaken to the point of rupture, spilling the appendiceal contents into the peritoneal cavity. Rupture of the appendix can lead to peritonitis and systemic infection.

The signs and symptoms of appendicitis can vary. Older patients and diabetics tend to have less classical symptoms. Initially, the patient with appendicitis will develop diffuse, colicky abdominal pain, usually associated with nausea and vomiting and low-grade fever. Often the pain is located in the periumbilical region. As the illness progresses, the pain localizes to the right lower quadrant. A common location of appendicitis pain is McBurney's point. McBurney's point is 1½ to 2 inches above the anterior iliac crest along a direct line from the anterior iliac crest to the umbilicus (Figure A17-1•). Once the appendix ruptures, the pain becomes diffuse due to the development of peritonitis. Occasionally, the appendix can be affixed to the posterior aspect of the large intestine (cecum). This condition, referred to as retrocecal appendicitis, often causes low-back pain or flank pain instead of pain over McBurney's point. Retrocecal appendicitis can be more difficult to diagnose.

The diagnosis of appendicitis can often be made based on the history and physical examination. Usually, the patient will have an elevated white blood cell count. In uncertain cases, ultrasound examination of the abdomen can aid in diagnosis. Normally, the appendix cannot be seen on ultrasound examination. If

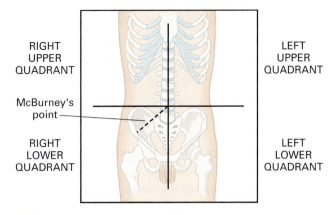

● **FIGURE A17-1** **McBurney's Point**
McBurney's point is located along approximately 1½ to 2 inches above the right anterior iliac crest along an imaginary line drawn between the right anterior iliac crest and the umbilicus.

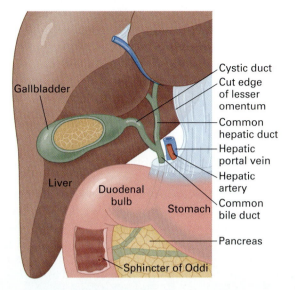

● **FIGURE A17-2** **Cholecystitis**
The gall bladder is located immediately under the liver in the right upper abdominal quadrant. Gallstones can enter the cystic duct or the common bile duct. The latter can result in partial or complete obstruction of the duct.

seen, then it is highly suggestive of acute appendicitis. Computed tomography (CT) of the abdomen is very helpful in confirming the diagnosis of acute appendicitis.

Treatment of appendicitis is surgical removal of the appendix (appendectomy). Today, most appendectomies can be performed using a laparoscope that markedly decreases pain and recovery time. Surgery for appendicitis should be prompt to prevent rupture of the appendix. If appendiceal rupture occurs, the patient often develops bacterial peritonitis. This usually requires a prolonged hospital stay and intravenous antibiotics.

BILIARY COLIC AND CHOLECYSTITIS

Cholecystitis is an inflammation of the gallbladder. Cholelithiasis (the formation of gallstones), which causes 90 percent of cholecystitis cases, occurs in approximately 15 percent of the adult population in the United States, with over one million new cases diagnosed annually. There are two types of gallstones, cholesterol-based and bilirubin-based. Cholesterol-based stones are far more common and are associated with a specific risk profile: obese, middle-aged women with more than one biological child.

Definitive treatment of acute cholecystitis includes antibiotic therapy, laparoscopic surgery, lithotripsy (ultrasound treatment to break up the stones), and surgery if the other, less invasive, therapies fail. With the advent of laparoscopic surgery, mortality has fallen to less then 1 percent, with an overall morbidity of approximately 6 percent.

Cholecystitis caused by gallstones can be chronic or acute (Figure A17-2●). The liver produces bile, the primary vehicle for removing cholesterol from the body. The bile travels down the common bile duct to empty into the small intestine at the sphincter of Oddi. The sphincter of Oddi opens when chyme exits the stomach through the cardiac sphincter. When the sphincter of Oddi closes, the flow of bile backs up into the gallbladder via the cystic duct. The bile remains in the gallbladder until the sphincter of Oddi opens again.

The bile can become supersaturated and calculi—stone-like masses based on bilirubin, cholesterol, or both—form. These calculi travel down the cystic duct, frequently lodging in the common bile duct. When they obstruct the flow of bile, gallbladder inflammation and irritation result. The bile salts subsequently attack the mucosal membrane lining the gallbladder, leaving the underlying epithelial tissue without protection. Prostaglandins are also released, further irritating the epithelial wall. As irritation continues, the inflammation grows; increasing intraluminal pressure and ultimately reducing blood flow to the epithelium.

Other causes of cholecystitis include acalculus cholecystitis (cholecystitis without associated stones) and chronic inflammation caused by bacterial infection. Acalculus cholecystitis usually results from burns, sepsis, diabetes, and multiple organ failure. Chronic cholecystitis resulting from a bacterial infection (*Escherichia coli* and enterococci) presents with an inflammatory process similar to cholelithiasis.

An inflamed gallbladder usually causes an acute attack of upper right quadrant abdominal pain. The inflammation can cause an irritation of the diaphragm with referred pain in the right shoulder. If the gallstones are lodged in the cystic duct, the pain may be colicky, due to expansion and contraction of the duct. Often the pain occurs after a meal that is high in fat content because of the secondary release of bile from the gallbladder. The right subcostal region may be tender because of abdominal muscle spasms. Patients may experience extreme pain as the epithelium in the gallbladder erodes away. Sympathetic stimulation because of the pain may cause pale, cool, clammy skin. If peritonitis occurs, the skin

A17

may be warm due to increased blood flow to the inflamed peritoneum. Nausea and vomiting are common, due to cystic duct spasm. Many patients will have tenderness under the right costal margin referred to as a positive Murphy's sign.

PANCREATITIS

Pancreatitis is an inflammation of the pancreas. There are four main categories of pancreatitis: metabolic, mechanical, vascular, and infectious. Metabolic causes, especially alcoholism, account for 80 per cent of all cases. Pancreatitis is common in the United States because of the high incidence of alcoholism. Mechanical obstruction caused by gallstones or elevated serum lipids account for another 9 percent of cases. Overall, mortality in acute pancreatitis is high, approaching 30 to 40 percent, mainly due to accompanying sepsis and shock.

As discussed in the text, the pancreas produces digestive enzymes that empty into the duodenum at the ampulla of Vater, near the junction with the stomach. The other function of the pancreas is endocrine. The islets of Langerhans secrete glucagon, insulin, and somatostatin directly into the circulatory system. Occasionally, gallstones leaving the common bile duct become lodged at the ampulla of Vater and obstruct the pancreatic duct. These obstructions back up pancreatic digestive enzymes into the pancreatic duct and the pancreas itself. The digestive enzymes then inflame the pancreas causing edema. This reduces blood flow, similar to the pathogenesis of acute appendicitis. In turn, the decreased blood flow causes ischemia and, finally, acinar destruction. This process is called acute pancreatitis because of the rapidity of onset.

Chronic pancreatitis results from acinar tissue destruction. This results from chronic alcohol intake, drug toxicity, ischemia, and infectious disease. Alcohol ingestion results in the formation and deposit of platelet plugs in the acinar tissue. The plugs disrupt the enzymes' flow from the pancreas. When digestive juices back up into the pancreas from the ampulla of Vater, the digestive enzymes become activated and begin to digest the pancreas itself. This autodigestion causes lesions and fatty tissue changes to appear in the pancreas. Chronic pancreatitis can result in destruction of a significant portion of the pancreas, affecting both endocrine and exocrine tissues. In these cases, patients may be required to take digestive enzyme supplements. If a significant portion of the endocrine tissue occurs, diabetes mellitus can occur requiring insulin replacement.

As tissue digestion continues, the lesion can erode and begin to hemorrhage (hemorrhagic pancreatitis). This causes severe abdominal pain, usually located in the epigastrium or the left upper quadrant. The pain often radiates straight through to the back and often requires high doses of narcotics to control. Morphine is contraindicated as it causes spasm of the sphincter of Oddi. The patient will appear acutely ill with diaphoresis, tachycardia, and possible hypotension if massive hemorrhage occurs. Intractable vomiting may be present and will require placement of a nasogastric tube. Cessation of alcohol intake must occur for recovery from pancreatitis.

UPPER GASTROINTESTINAL BLEEDING

Upper gastrointestinal bleeding can be defined as bleeding within the gastrointestinal tract proximal to the ligament of Treitz, which supports the duodenojejunal junction, the point where the first two sections of the small intestine (the duodenum and the jejunum) meet.

Upper gastrointestinal bleeds account for over 300,000 hospitalizations per year. The mortality rate has remained fairly steady at approximately 10 percent over the past years (Figure A17-3•). Many factors contribute to this high mortality. First, the number of patients who treat their symptoms with home remedies and over-the-counter medications is increasing rapidly. Many of these patients come under medical care only when their disease has caused significant damage, such as large-scale hemorrhage from an ulcerated lesion. Second, the overall age of the population is increasing. The infirmities of age and its greater likelihood of coexisting illnesses, such as hypertension, atherosclerosis, diabetes, and substance abuse (including abuse of medications), make this older population more vulnerable to the effects of upper gastrointestinal bleeds. The mortality rate is highest in those over 60 years of age. One prevention strategy for the field is to check for such coexisting problems, especially in elderly patients, and to treat accordingly. In particular, look at the history and physical for evidence of tobacco or alcohol use, or both.

The six major identifiable causes of upper GI hemorrhage, in descending order of frequency, are peptic ulcer

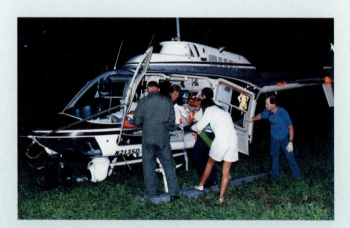

• **FIGURE A17-3   Gastrointestinal Emergency**
An acute gastrointestinal hemorrhage is as serious a medical emergency as external hemorrhage. The patient should be aggressively treated with IV fluids and promptly transported to a facility where transfusion and surgical capabilities are available.

disease, gastritis, variceal rupture, Mallory-Weiss syndrome (esophageal laceration, usually secondary to vomiting), esophagitis, and duodenitis. Peptic ulcer disease accounts for approximately 50 percent of upper GI bleeds, with gastritis accounting for an additional 25 percent. Overall, irritation or erosion of the gastric lining of the stomach causes more than 75 percent of upper GI bleeds. Most cases of upper GI bleeding are chronic irritations or inflammations that cause minimal discomfort and minor hemorrhage. Physicians can manage these conditions on an outpatient basis; however, if a peptic ulcer erodes through the gastric mucosa, if the esophagus is lacerated in Mallory-Weiss syndrome, or if varices (often secondary to alcoholic liver damage) rupture, an acute-onset, life-threatening, and difficult-to-control hemorrhage can result.

Upper GI bleeds may be obvious, or they may present quite subtly. Most often patients will complain of some type of abdominal discomfort ranging from a vague burning sensation to an upset stomach, gas pain, or tearing pain in the upper quadrants. Because blood severely irritates the GI system, most cases present with nausea and vomiting. If the bleeding is in the upper GI tract, the patient may experience hematemesis (bloody vomitus) or, if it passes through the lower GI tract, melena. The partially digested blood will turn the stool black and tarry. For melena to be recognizable, approximately 150 cc of blood must drain into the GI tract and remain there for from five to eight hours. Blood in emesis may be bright red (new, fresh blood) or look like coffee grounds (old, partially digested blood).

Upper GI bleeding may be light or it may be brisk and life threatening. Patients who suffer a rupture of an esophageal varix or a tear or disruption in the esophageal or gastric lining may vomit copious amounts of blood. These hemorrhages can cause the classic signs and symptoms of shock, including alteration in mental status, tachycardia, peripheral vasoconstriction, diaphoresis (sweating producing pale, cool, clammy skin), and hemodynamic instability. Besides shock, the vomitus itself can compromise the airway, resulting in impaired respirations, aspiration, and ultimately, respiratory arrest.

A frequently employed clinical indicator is the tilt test, which indicates if the patient has orthostatic hypotension (a 10-mm Hg change in blood pressure or a 20-bpm change in heart rate when the patient rises from supine to standing). Hypotension suggests a decreased circulating volume. The human body can compensate for a circulating volume deficit of approximately 15 percent before clinical indicators such as the tilt test show positive results. Thus, those patients whose systolic blood pressure drops 10 mm Hg or whose heart rate increases 20 bpm or more need aggressive fluid resuscitation.

PEPTIC ULCERS

Peptic ulcers are erosions caused by gastric acid (Figure A17-4●). They can occur anywhere in the gastrointestinal tract; terminology is based on the portion of the GI tract

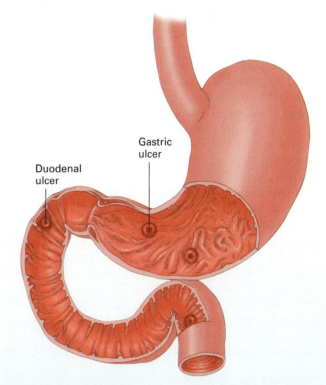

● **FIGURE A17-4   Types of Peptic Ulcers**
Peptic ulcers are erosions in the mucosa of the stomach or duodenum. They can erode completely through the wall of the organ resulting in perforation and life-threatening hemorrhage.

affected. Duodenal ulcers most frequently occur in the proximal portion of the duodenum; gastric ulcers occur exclusively in the stomach. Overall, peptic ulcers occur in males four times more frequently than in females, and duodenal ulcers occur from two to three times more frequently than do gastric ulcers. Current statistics place the number of peptic ulcers at 4–5 million, with approximately 500,000 new cases diagnosed yearly. Those patients who are more likely to have gastric ulcers are over 50 years old and work in jobs requiring physical activity. Their pain usually increases after eating or with a full stomach, and they usually have no pain at night. Duodenal ulcers are more common in patients from 25 to 50 years old who are executives or leaders under high stress. There is also some familial tendency toward duodenal ulcer, suggesting genetic predisposition. Patients with duodenal ulcers commonly have pain at night or whenever their stomach is empty.

Nonsteroidal anti-inflammatory medications (aspirin, Motrin, Advil, Naprosyn), acid-stimulating products (alcohol, nicotine), or *Helicobacter pylori* bacteria are the most common causes of peptic ulcers. To help break down food boluses, the stomach secretes hydrochloric acid. One of the enzymes that control this secretion is pepsinogen. The hydrochloric acid helps to convert pepsinogen into its active form, pepsin. Between them, the pepsin and the hydrochloric acid can make the digestive enzymes very irritating to the GI tract's mucosal lining. Ordinarily, mucous gland secretions protect the stomach's mucosal barrier from these irritants. But when nonsteroidal anti-inflammatory medications, acid stimulators, or *H. pylori* damage the barrier, the mucosa is exposed to the highly acidic fluid, and peptic ulcers result. Prostaglandin, an important locally acting hormone, decreases the stimulation for blood flow through the gastric mucosa, thus allowing its further destruction.

The recent discovery that *Helicobacter pylori* bacteria appear in over 80 percent of gastric and duodenal ulcers has enabled physicians to treat the disease by eliminating its cause with antacids and antibiotics rather than merely treating its symptoms.

A blocked pancreatic duct can also contribute to duodenal ulcers. As chyme passes through the pyloric sphincter from the stomach into the duodenum, the pancreas secretes an alkalotic solution laden with bicarbonate ions that neutralize the acidic hydrogen ions in the chyme. If the pancreatic duct is blocked, however, the acidic chyme can cause ulcerations throughout the intestine. One other cause of duodenal ulcers is Zollinger-Ellison syndrome, in which an acid-secreting tumor provokes the ulcerations.

Acute, severe pain is probably due to a rupture of the ulcer into the peritoneal cavity causing hemorrhage. Depending on the ulcer's location, the patient may have hematemesis or may have melena-colored stool. Bouts of nausea and vomiting due to the irritation of the mucosa are common. If the ulcer has eroded through a highly vascular area, massive hemorrhage can occur. Along with the signs of hemorrhage on visual inspection, these patients will appear very ill and have signs of hemodynamic instability, such as pale, cool, and clammy skin, tachycardia, decreased blood pressure, and possibly, altered mental status. Most patients will lie still to decrease the pain. They may have surgical scars from previous ulcer repair. Bowel sounds will usually be absent.

DIVERTICULITIS

Diverticulitis is a relatively common complication of diverticulosis. Diverticulosis is a condition characterized by the presence in the intestine of diverticula, small outpouchings of mucosal and submucosal tissue that push through the outermost layer of the intestine, the muscle. Colonic diverticula are far more common in developed countries such as the United States and increase markedly in prevalence with increased age. They are present in more than half of patients over 60 years of age. Diverticulitis is an inflammation of diverticula secondary to infection. Unlike diverticulosis, it is symptomatic; patients will complain of lower left-sided pain (because most diverticula are in the sigmoid colon); exam and testing will show fever and an increased white blood cell count.

The pathogenesis of an acquired diverticulum is twofold. First, stool passes sluggishly through the colon, a condition associated with the relatively low fiber diets

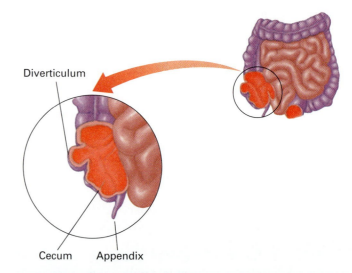

● **FIGURE A17-5   Diverticulum**
Diverticula, outpouchings of the wall of the colon, can become infected (diverticulitis) or bleed (diverticulosis).

common in developed countries. The colon responds with muscle spasms that increase bulk movement by raising the pressure on the contents inside the colon and pushing the fecal material forward. Second, the outermost layer of colon tissue is made up of fibrous bands of muscle wrapped around one another. Among them are muscles called the teniae coli. Nerves and blood vessels enter the colon through small openings within the teniae coli. These openings become weakened with age, and the increased pressure of muscle spasms can cause the inner layers of tissue, the mucosa and submucosa, to herniate through the openings, forming diverticula (Figure A17-5●).

These diverticula commonly trap small amounts of fecal material, including sunflower seeds, popcorn fragments, okra seeds, sesame seeds, and others. The entrapped feces may allow bacteria other then the normal flora to grow and cause an infection. The problem is compounded when the diverticula become inflamed, causing diverticulitis. Complications secondary to diverticulitis include possible hemorrhage or larger perforations of the colon wall through which the infected fecal contents can spill into the peritoneal cavity and cause peritonitis.

The most common presentation of diverticulitis is colicky pain associated with a low-grade fever, nausea and vomiting, and tenderness upon palpation. The pain is usually localized to the lower left side because the sigmoid colon is involved in 95 percent of reported cases. Thus diverticulitis is often called left-sided appendicitis. If the diverticula begin to bleed significantly, the usual signs and symptoms associated with severe lower GI bleeding may be present: cool, clammy skin, tachycardia, and diaphoresis. Bleeding diverticula can also result in bright red and bloody feces (hematochezia) because of their close proximity to the rectum. Patients may additionally complain of the perception that they cannot empty their rectums, even after defecation.

HEMORRHOIDS

The *rectum* is drained by the *internal* and *external hemorrhoidal veins*. Swelling of these veins is referred to as *hemorrhoids*. *Internal hemorrhoids* may be asymptomatic or may cause rectal pain, itching, or bright red bleeding (usually with defecation). *External hemorrhoids* tend to thrombose, especially after lifting, causing severe rectal pain and pressure. Internal hemorrhoids usually respond to rectal creams and analgesics. External hemorrhoids require drainage of the thrombosed hemorrhoid, which usually provides immediate relief.

PORTAL HYPERTENSION

The portal system is a specialized component of the circulatory system. Veins from the spleen, stomach, pancreas, gall bladder, and intestines do not drain directly into the inferior vena cava, as do the veins from other abdominal organs. Instead, they drain into the portal vein that delivers the blood to the liver. In the liver, blood from the portal circulation mixes with the arterial blood in the hepatic capillaries and is eventually drained from the liver by the hepatic veins. The hepatic veins drain into the inferior vena cava.

Blood in the hepatic portal system contains substances absorbed by the digestive tract. Blood entering the liver via the portal vein contains greater concentrations of glucose, amino acids, and fats than does blood leaving the liver via the hepatic vein. The liver regulates the concentration of nutrients, such as glucose or amino acids, in the circulating blood.

The pressure within the portal system is normally 3 mm Hg. An increase in portal pressure to at least 10 mm Hg is referred to as *portal hypertension*. Portal hypertension is caused by disorders that impede or obstruct blood flow through any part of the portal system or the vena cava. The obstruction can occur in the liver or in the hepatic veins that drain the liver. The most common cause of portal hypertension is obstruction caused by cirrhosis of the liver. *Cirrhosis* is an irreversible inflammatory disease that disrupts the structure and function of the liver. The most common cause of cirrhosis in the United States is chronic alcohol abuse (Figure A17-6●). Chronic infectious hepatitis also can cause cirrhosis resulting in portal hypertension.

Increased pressure within the portal system causes collateral blood vessels between the portal veins and the systemic veins to open. Blood pressure in the systemic veins is considerably lower than that in the portal system, which enables blood to bypass the obstructed portal vessels. The collateral veins develop in the esophagus, anterior abdominal wall, and rectum. High pressure and increased blood flow are transmitted through these veins from the portal to the systemic venous circulation. Blood that is shunted into the systemic circulation bypasses the liver where toxic metabolic waste products are usually re-

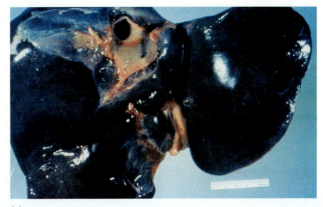

(a)

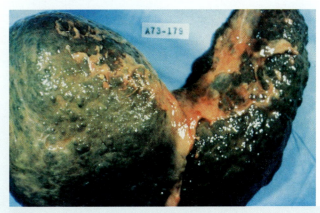

(b)

● FIGURE A17-6   Postmortem Specimens Comparing (a) Normal Liver and (b) Cirrhotic Liver
Note the cirrhotic liver is irregular and smaller than the normal specimen.

moved. This results in an accumulation of these waste products in the systemic circulation.

Long-term portal hypertension results in numerous problems that are quite difficult to treat. These include:

- *Varices*. Varices are tortuous, distended collateral veins that develop secondary to long-standing increased portal pressure. They are found in the lower esophagus, upper stomach, and rectum. They are prone to bleeding that can be difficult to control (Figure A17-7●).

- *Ascites*. Ascites is the accumulation of fluid in the space between the parietal and visceral peritoneum. It is caused by increased pressure in the mesenteric tributaries of the portal vein. Hydrostatic pressure within the veins forces water out of these vessels and into the peritoneal cavity.

- *Splenomegaly*. Splenomegaly, an enlargement of the spleen, results from increased pressure in the splenic vein, which is a branch of the portal vein.

- *Hepatic encephalopathy*. Hepatic encephalopathy is characterized by central nervous system disturbances

A17

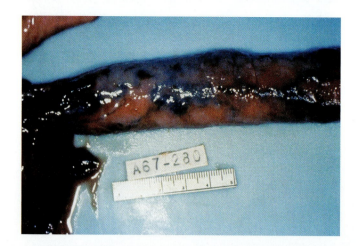

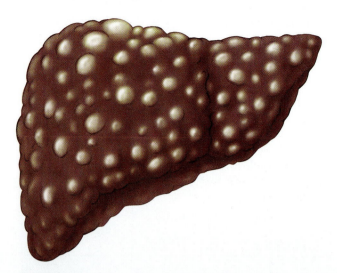

Hepatitis can lead to liver failure, and some types can lead to chronic infection causing cirrhosis and, in some cases, liver cancer.

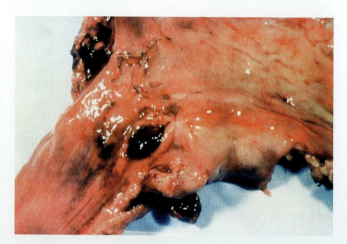

• **FIGURE A17-7   Esophageal Varices in a Patient with Portal Hypertension Secondary to Alcoholic Cirrhosis**

such as confusion, somnolence, and unconsciousness. Hepatic encephalopathy results from increased amounts of metabolic waste products in the blood, especially ammonia.

Portal hypertension develops over years. The most common clinical manifestation is vomiting of blood from bleeding esophageal varices. Slow, chronic variceal bleeding can cause anemia or melena. Rupture of esophageal varices is painless and can cause massive hemorrhage that is notoriously difficult to control and often fatal. Variceal bleeding can sometimes be controlled by injecting a sclerosing agent into the bleeding varix or banding of the bleeding varix with a fiberoptic esophagogastroduodenoscope (EGD). Placing a Sengstaken-Blakemore tube can sometimes control massive hemorrhages. This is a cylindrical balloon with a bulb at the end that is inserted into the distal esophagus and inflated. Inflation of the balloon and the bulb compresses the bleeding varices, slowing or stopping bleeding. Unfortunately, there are numerous, potentially lethal, complications associated with

the Sengstaken-Blakemore tube use. Because of this, it is rarely used except as a last resort.

The viable treatment options for portal hypertension are exceedingly limited. Surgical construction of a portacaval shunt (connection of the portal vein to the inferior vena cava) can reduce portal pressure. However, it can cause liver failure or encephalopathy due to reduced hepatic blood flow. In selected cases, liver transplantation can be curative if the disease is not too advanced. Overall, there is no effective, definitive treatment for portal hypertension.

HEPATITIS

Hepatitis is an inflammation of the liver and can result from both infectious and noninfectious causes. Medications, toxins, chemicals, and autoimmune disorders may cause *noninfectious hepatitis. Infectious hepatitis* can result from infection with viruses, bacteria, fungi, and parasites. The vast majority of infectious hepatitis cases are viral (Figure A17-8•).

Several viruses have been identified as causative agents for hepatitis. These include: hepatitis A virus (HAV), hepatitis B virus (HBV), hepatitis C virus (HCV), hepatitis D virus (HDV), hepatitis E virus (HEV), hepatitis F virus (HFV), and hepatitis G virus (HGV). HAV, HBV, and HCV cause more than 90 percent of cases of acute viral hepatitis in the United States. Emergency personnel are at particular risk for exposure to HBV and HCV because of the increased risk of exposure to body fluids. HAV, HBV, HCV, and HDV are the only hepatitis viruses endemic to the United States.

The hepatitis viruses impair liver function by attacking and destroying liver cells. Hepatitis may be either acute or chronic. All hepatitis viruses cause an acute infection. The severity of the infection can vary from asymptomatic to fulminant liver failure. Patients who contract hepatitis A and hepatitis E usually do not develop a chronic infection. However, patients who are infected with hepatitis B, hepatitis C, hepatitis D, and hepatitis G are at risk of developing chronic active hepatitis. Chronic active hepatitis is progressive, leading to deterioration in liver function and eventually cirrhosis. Many patients will develop hepatocellular cancer. Complications associated with chronic active hepatitis include portal hypertension, ascites, and eventually, hepatic encephalopathy (CNS dysfunction). As liver failure progresses, toxic metabolic waste products are not effectively cleared by the liver and start to accumulate in the blood. Among the more important of these waste products is ammonia. An increase in serum ammonia can cause hepatic encephalopathy resulting in disorientation, confusion, somnolence, and eventually unconsciousness. As hepatic encephalopathy worsens, the patient will develop asterixis, an involuntary "flapping" of the hands when the patient holds his hands up, flexed at the wrist (such as the motion for stopping traffic).

The signs and symptoms of infectious hepatitis depend on the type of hepatitis involved. Typically, patients will develop a low-grade fever, loss of appetite, and malaise. The skin, sclera, and mucous membranes may become jaundiced (icteric) due to the accumulation of bilirubin in the body. In more severe cases, the patient may develop significant nausea and vomiting that can lead to dehydration as evidenced by tachycardia, dry mucous membranes, and decreased skin turgor. The liver may be diffusely enlarged and tender to palpation.

There are several different types of infectious viral hepatitis depending on the virus involved. These include:

- *Hepatitis A.* Hepatitis A, often called infectious hepatitis, is the primary cause of viral hepatitis in the United States. It is transmitted via the fecal/oral route, often through food, water, milk, and shellfish contaminated by fecal wastes. The incubation period is typically 2 to 6 weeks. Hepatitis A often occurs in epidemics that can be attributed to a community source such as a restaurant. Hepatitis A is usually a mild self-limited disease. Infection with HAV confers life-long immunity, and chronic infection with HAV does not occur. A vaccine is available for those deemed to be at increased risk.
- *Hepatitis B.* Hepatitis B, also called serum hepatitis, is a major cause of hepatitis worldwide. Hepatitis B is transmitted via blood or other body products, often through mucous membranes. Saliva, serum, and semen have all been demonstrated to be infectious. In addition, HBV can be transmitted perinatally from an infected mother to her unborn child. The incubation period for hepatitis B is consider-

ably longer than for hepatitis A, ranging from 1 to 6 months. Hepatitis B is a serious infection and can develop into a chronic infection. Chronic hepatitis B can lead to cirrhosis of the liver and, eventually, hepatocellular cancer. An effective vaccine against hepatitis B is available and should be administered to emergency personnel.

- *Hepatitis C.* Hepatitis C, formerly referred to as non-A, non-B hepatitis, is a serious infection and the most common cause of chronic viral hepatitis in the United States. Emergency personnel are at increased risk of infection by hepatitis C due to exposure to infected blood or body fluids. The incubation period can range from 1 to 6 months. The signs and symptoms of hepatitis C are similar to those of hepatitis B. Approximately 80 percent of those infected with HCV will go on to develop chronic HCV infection. Chronic hepatitis C infection is the leading reason for liver transplantation in the United States. There is no effective vaccine against hepatitis C or post-exposure prophylaxis.
- *Hepatitis D.* Hepatitis D, also called delta hepatitis, is a unique type of hepatitis. It requires the presence of hepatitis B virus in order to replicate. Thus, hepatitis D is often considered to be a coinfection or superinfection of hepatitis B. The transmission of hepatitis D is similar to that for hepatitis B. Patients with both hepatitis B and hepatitis D tend to have a more severe course than those with hepatitis B alone. Hepatitis D tends to lead to chronic infection. A vaccine for hepatitis D is not yet available.
- *Hepatitis E.* Hepatitis E is similar to hepatitis A and is transmitted via the fecal-oral route. The incubation period for hepatitis E ranges from 2 to 9 weeks. Like hepatitis A, the disease is usually self-limited and chronic infection does not occur. Hepatitis E is the most common cause of hepatitis worldwide, but seldom seen in the United States. A vaccine against hepatitis E is not yet available.
- *Hepatitis F.* Hepatitis F is proposed as another hepatitis virus transmitted by the fecal-oral route. A small number of cases have been reported in France. Little else is known about the infection.
- *Hepatitis G.* Hepatitis G virus was identified in 1996 and is associated with both acute and chronic liver disease. The incidence is approximately 0.3 percent of all cases of acute viral hepatitis. Transmission of HGV is blood borne. Chronic infection is common, occurring in 90–100 percent of infected persons. Much remains to be learned about hepatitis G. A vaccine is not yet available.

HEPATIC ABSCESSES

The liver is the organ most commonly subject to the development of abscesses. Liver abscesses are uncommon, especially in industrialized countries. When they do occur, they most frequently result from parasitic infection. The amoeba *Entamoeba histolytica* is the most common etiological agent, especially in developing countries. Approximately half of all patients with amoebic liver abscess will be asymptomatic. The other half will have low-grade fever, nausea, vomiting, diarrhea, and abdominal pain. The abscesses appear like "anchovy paste" on gross examination. The diagnosis can usually be established by identifying the parasite through stool testing.

In the United States, hepatic abscesses are usually the result of a surgical procedure, especially one that involves the biliary tract and gallbladder. The principle treatment is drainage of the abscess. This may be accomplished through open surgical drainage or placement of a catheter into the abscess.

SUMMARY

Emergencies involving the digestive system are common. They can arise from the actual digestive tract or from accessory organs such as the vermiform appendix or gallbladder. Life-threatening hemorrhage also can occur from either the upper or lower parts of the gastrointestinal system. GI bleeding is often difficult to control and can require massive transfusion and surgery. Hepatitis is an inflammation and infection of the liver. Hepatitis B and C pose significant risk for emergency personnel. It is important always to follow body substance isolation procedures and, when possible, obtain vaccination for hepatitis.

A17
7

18 Nutrition and Metabolism

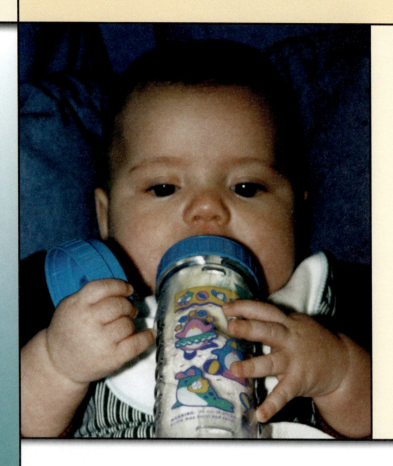

We must obtain our nutritional needs from outside sources. During infancy, milk provides the sole source of nutrition for the first few months of the child's life. As the child gets older, other foods are slowly added to the diet. Despite this, infant formula, which provides 20 calories per milliliter, remains the child's principal energy source through much of the first year of life.

Chapter Outline and Objectives

1 *Define metabolism, and explain why cells need to synthesize new organic structures.*
2 *Describe the basic steps in glycolysis, the TCA cycle, and the electron transport system.*
3 *Describe the pathways involved in lipid metabolism.*
4 *Discuss protein metabolism and the use of proteins as an energy source.*
5 *Discuss nucleic acid metabolism.*

6 *Explain what constitutes a balanced diet and why it is important.*
7 *Discuss the functions of vitamins, minerals, and other important nutrients.*

8 *Describe the significance of the caloric value of foods.*
9 *Define metabolic rate, and discuss the factors involved in determining an individual's metabolic rate.*
10 *Discuss the homeostatic mechanisms that maintain a constant body temperature*

11 *Describe the change in nutritional requirements with age.*

Vocabulary Development

anabole, a building up; *anabolism*
genesis, an origin; *thermogenesis*
glykus, sweet; *glycolysis*
katabole, a throwing down; *catabolism*
lipos, fat; *lipogenesis*
lysis, breakdown; *glycolysis*
neo-, new; *gluconeogenesis*
therme, heat; *thermogenesis*
vita, life; *vitamin*

Metabolism refers to all the chemical reactions of the body. ∞ *p. 34* Living cells are chemical factories that use chemical reactions to break down organic molecules and to obtain energy, usually in the form of ATP. To carry out these processes, cells in the human body must also obtain water, vitamins, ions, and oxygen. Oxygen is absorbed at the lungs, but all the other required substances, usually called **nutrients**, are obtained by absorption at the digestive tract. The cardiovascular system distributes oxygen and nutrients to cells throughout the body.

The energy released in a cell supports growth, cell division, contraction, secretion, and other special functions that vary from cell to cell. Each tissue type contains different populations of cells, and the energy and nutrient requirements of any two tissues (such as loose connective tissue and cardiac muscle) are quite different. Furthermore, when cells, tissues, and organs change their patterns or levels of activity, they change their nutrient requirements. Thus, our nutrient requirements vary from moment to moment (resting versus active), hour to hour (asleep versus awake), and year to year (child versus adult).

When organic nutrients, such as carbohydrates or lipids, are abundant, energy reserves are built up. Different tissues and organs are specialized to store excess nutrients; the storage of lipids in adipose tissue is one familiar example. These reserves can then be called on when the diet cannot provide the right quantity or quality of nutrients. The endocrine system, with the assistance of the nervous system, adjusts and coordinates the metabolic activities of the body's tissues and controls the storage and release of nutrient reserves.

The absorption of nutrients from food is called *nutrition*. The mechanisms involved in absorption through the lining of the digestive tract were detailed in Chapter 17. ∞ *p. 485–487* This chapter considers what happens to nutrients after they are inside the body.

CELLULAR METABOLISM

Figure 18-1• reviews the ways cells use organic nutrients absorbed from the extracellular fluid. Most of these nutrients are obtained from the food we eat. After food has been mechanically and chemically digested, simple sugars, amino acids, and lipids are absorbed by the digestive tract and distributed by the bloodstream. After diffusing into the interstitial fluid, these nutrients cross the cell membrane and join other nutrients already in the cytoplasm. All of the cell's metabolic operations rely on the resulting *nutrient pool.*

Catabolism breaks down organic molecules, releasing energy that can be used to synthesize ATP or other high-energy compounds. ∞ *p. 35* Catabolism proceeds in a series of steps. In general, preliminary processing occurs in the cytosol, where enzymes break down large organic molecules into smaller fragments. For example, carbohydrates are broken down into short carbon chains, triglycerides are split into fatty acids and glycerol, and proteins are broken down to individual amino acids.

Relatively little ATP is formed during these initial steps. However, the simple molecules produced can be absorbed and processed by mitochondria, and the mitochondrial steps release significant amounts of energy. As mitochondrial enzymes break the covalent bonds that hold these molecules together, they capture roughly 40 percent of the energy released. The captured energy is used to

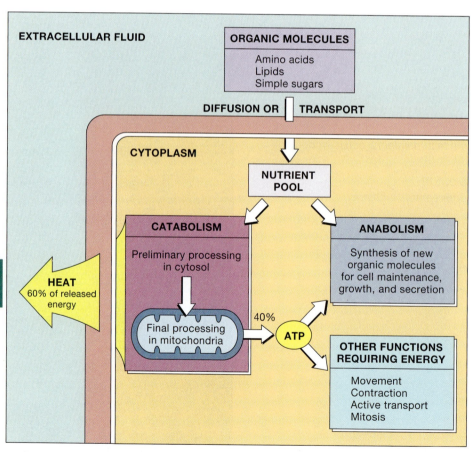

•**FIGURE 18-1   Cellular Metabolism**
The cell obtains organic molecules from the extracellular fluid and breaks them down to obtain ATP. Only about 40 percent of the energy released through catabolism is captured in ATP; the rest is radiated as heat. The ATP generated through catabolism provides energy for all vital cellular activities, including anabolism.

convert ADP to ATP, and the rest escapes as heat that warms the interior of the cell and the surrounding tissues.

Anabolism, the synthesis of new organic molecules, involves the formation of new chemical bonds. ∞ *p. 35* The ATP produced by mitochondria provides energy to support anabolism as well as other cell functions. Those additional functions, such as contraction, ciliary or cell movement, active transport, and cell division, vary from one cell to another. For example, muscle fibers need ATP to provide energy for contraction, whereas gland cells need ATP to synthesize and transport their secretions.

Cells synthesize new organic components for three basic reasons:

1. *To perform structural maintenance and repairs.* All cells must expend energy to perform ongoing maintenance and repairs, because most organic molecules and structures in the cell, including organelles, are temporary rather than permanent. The removal and replacement of these molecules and structures are part of the process of **metabolic turnover**.

2. *To support growth.* Cells preparing for division enlarge and synthesize extra proteins and organelles.

3. *To produce secretions.* Secretory cells must synthesize their products and deliver them to the interstitial fluid.

The nutrient pool is the source of organic molecules for both catabolism and anabolism. As you might expect, the cell tends to conserve the materials needed to build new compounds and breaks down the rest to provide ATP. The cell is continuously replacing membranes, organelles, enzymes, and structural proteins. These anabolic activities require more amino acids than lipids, and relatively few carbohydrates. Catabolic activities, however, tend to process these organic molecules in the reverse order. In general, *a cell with excess carbohydrates, lipids, and amino acids will break down carbohydrates first.* Lipids are broken down when carbohydrates are no longer available, and amino acids are seldom broken down.

The next few sections will examine some of the major catabolic and anabolic reactions that occur in our cells.

Carbohydrate Metabolism

Carbohydrates, most familiar to us as sugars and starches, are important sources of energy. Most cells generate ATP and other high-energy compounds by breaking down carbohydrates, especially glucose. The complete reaction sequence can be summarized as:

$$C_6H_{12}O_6 \; + \; 6 \, O_2 \; \rightarrow \; 6 \, CO_2 \; + \; 6 \, H_2O$$
$$\text{glucose} \qquad \text{oxygen} \qquad \text{carbon} \qquad \text{water}$$
$$\text{dioxide}$$

The breakdown occurs in a series of small steps, and several of the steps release sufficient energy to support the conversion of ADP to ATP. During the complete catabolism of glucose, a typical cell gains 36 ATP molecules.

Although most of the actual energy production occurs inside mitochondria, the preliminary steps take place in the cytosol. The steps involved were outlined in Chapter 7. ∞ *p. 180* This reaction sequence is called *glycolysis*. These steps are said to be *anaerobic* because oxygen is not needed. Glycolysis is therefore a form of **anaerobic metabolism**. The products of glycolysis can then be absorbed by mitochondria and used for energy production. Mitochondrial activity, which requires oxygen, is called **aerobic metabolism**, or *cellular respiration*.

Glycolysis

Glycolysis (glī-KOL-i-sis; *glykus*, sweet + *lysis*, breakdown) is the breakdown of glucose to *pyruvic acid*. This process occurs in the cytosol. In this process, a series of enzymatic steps breaks the six-carbon glucose molecule into two three-carbon molecules of pyruvic acid (CH_3-CO-COOH).

Glycolysis requires (1) glucose molecules, (2) appropriate cytoplasmic enzymes, (3) ATP and ADP, and (4) **NAD** (*n*icotinamide *a*denine *d*inucleotide), a coenzyme that removes hydrogen atoms. *Coenzymes* are organic molecules, usually derived from vitamins, that must be present for an enzymatic reaction to occur. If the cell lacks any of these four required participants, glycolysis cannot take place.

The basic steps of glycolysis are summarized in Figure 18-2•. This reaction sequence provides a net gain of two ATP molecules for each glucose molecule converted to two pyruvic acid molecules. A few highly specialized cells, such as red blood cells, lack mitochondria and derive all of their ATP by glycolysis. Skeletal muscle fibers rely on glycolysis for energy production during periods of active contraction, and most cells can survive brief periods of hypoxia (low oxygen levels) by using the ATP glycolysis provides. When oxygen is readily available, however, mitochondrial activity provides most of the ATP required by our cells.

Mitochondrial Energy Production

Glycolysis yields an immediate net gain of two ATP molecules for the cell, but a great deal of additional energy is still locked in the chemical bonds of pyruvic acid. The ability to capture that energy depends on the availability of oxygen. If oxygen supplies are adequate, mitochondria will absorb the pyruvic acid molecules and break them down completely. The hydrogen atoms are removed by coenzymes and will ultimately be the source of most of the energy gain for the cell. The carbon and oxygen atoms are removed and released as carbon dioxide.

Once inside the mitochondrion, a pyruvic acid molecule first loses one carbon atom in a complicated reaction involving the molecule *coenzyme A* (or *CoA*).

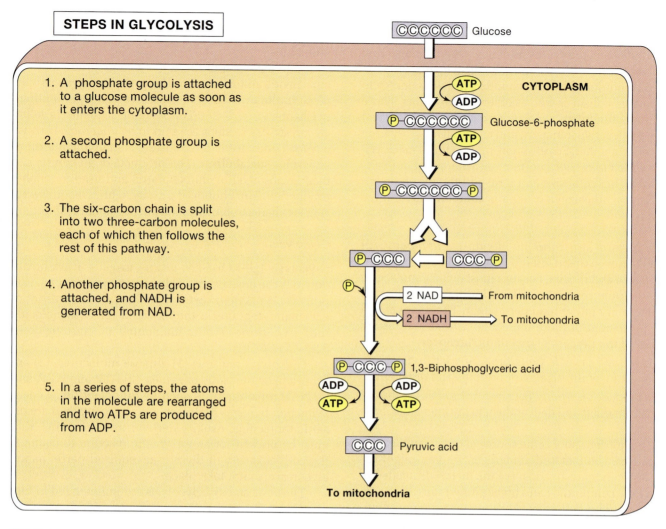

STEPS IN GLYCOLYSIS

1. A phosphate group is attached to a glucose molecule as soon as it enters the cytoplasm.

2. A second phosphate group is attached.

3. The six-carbon chain is split into two three-carbon molecules, each of which then follows the rest of this pathway.

4. Another phosphate group is attached, and NADH is generated from NAD.

5. In a series of steps, the atoms in the molecule are rearranged and two ATPs are produced from ADP.

Glucose

CYTOPLASM

Glucose-6-phosphate

2 NAD — From mitochondria
2 NADH — To mitochondria

1,3-Biphosphoglyceric acid

Pyruvic acid

To mitochondria

• **FIGURE 18-2   Glycolysis**
Glycolysis breaks down a six-carbon glucose molecule into two three-carbon molecules of pyruvic acid. This process involves a series of enzymatic steps. There is a net gain of two ATPs for each glucose molecule converted to pyruvic acid.

This reaction yields one molecule of carbon dioxide and one molecule of **acetyl-CoA** (as-Ē-til-KŌ-ā). Acetyl-CoA consists of a two-carbon *acetyl group* ($CH_3C=O$) bound to coenzyme A. Next, the acetyl group is transferred from CoA to a four-carbon molecule, producing *citric acid.*

The TCA Cycle.   The formation of citric acid is the first step in a sequence of enzymatic reactions called the **tricarboxylic** (trī-kar-bok-SIL-ik) **acid (TCA) cycle**, also known as the *citric acid cycle*. This cycle, which occurs inside mitochondria, removes hydrogen atoms from organic molecules and transfers them to coenzymes. The electrons in these hydrogen atoms contain energy that can be used by the mitochondria to generate ATP. An overview of the TCA cycle, sometimes known as the *Krebs cycle* in honor of Hans Krebs, the biochemist who described these reactions in 1937, is shown in Figure 18-3•.

At the start of the TCA cycle, the two-carbon acetyl group carried by CoA is attached to a four-carbon molecule to make the six-carbon citric acid molecule. Coenzyme A is then released intact to bind another acetyl group. A complete revolution of the TCA cycle removes the two added carbon atoms, regenerating the four-carbon chain. (This is why the reaction sequence is called a *cycle*.) The two removed carbon atoms generate two molecules of carbon dioxide (CO_2), a metabolic waste product. The hydrogen atoms of the acetyl group are removed by coenzymes.

The only immediate energy benefit of the TCA cycle is the formation of a single molecule of ATP. The real value of the TCA cycle can be seen by following the hydrogen atoms that are removed by coenzymes. The coenzymes (NAD and **FAD, flavine adenine dinucleotide**) deliver the hydrogen atoms to the *electron transport system.*

18

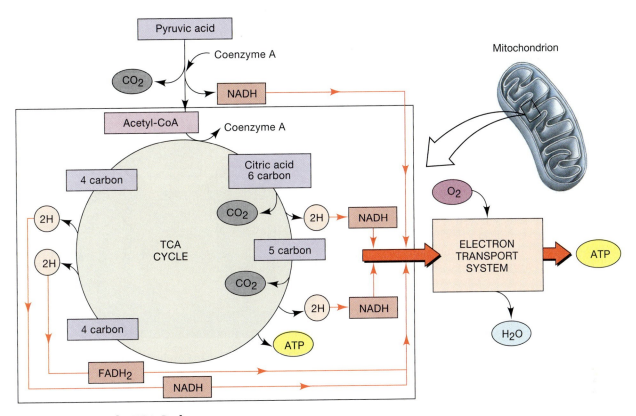

•**FIGURE 18-3   The TCA Cycle**
The TCA cycle completes the breakdown of organic molecules begun by glycolysis and other catabolic pathways.

The Electron Transport System.   The **electron transport system** (**ETS**), or *electron transport chain*, is embedded in the inner mitochondrial membrane. The ETS consists of a series of protein-pigment complexes called *cytochromes*. Coenzymes in the mitochondrial matrix deliver hydrogen atoms to the electron transport chain; the electrons are removed and passed from cytochrome to cytochrome, losing energy in a series of small steps. At several steps along the way, enough energy is released to attach a phosphate group to ADP, forming ATP. At the end of the electron transport system, an oxygen atom accepts the electrons, creating an oxygen ion (O^{2-}). This ion is very reactive, and it quickly combines with hydrogen ions (H^+) to form a molecule of water.

The electron transport system is the most important mechanism for the generation of ATP; in fact, it provides roughly 95 percent of the ATP needed to keep our cells alive. Halting or significantly reducing the rate of mitochondrial activity will usually kill a cell. If many cells are affected, the individual may die. For example, if the supply of oxygen is cut off, mitochondrial ATP production will cease because the ETS will be unable to get rid of its electrons. With the last reaction in the chain stopped, the entire ETS comes to

a halt, like cars at a washed-out bridge. The affected cells quickly die of energy starvation.

Energy Yield of Glycolysis and Cellular Respiration

For most cells, the series of chemical reactions that begin with glucose and end with carbon dioxide and water is the primary method of generating ATP. A cell gains ATP at several steps along the way:

- Through glycolysis in the cytoplasm, the cell gains two molecules of ATP for each glucose molecule broken down to pyruvic acid.
- Inside the mitochondria, the two pyruvic acid molecules derived from each glucose molecule are fully broken down in the TCA cycle. Two revolutions of the TCA cycle, each yielding a molecule of ATP, provide a net gain of two additional molecules of ATP.
- For each molecule of glucose broken down, activity at the electron transport chain in the mitochondrial membrane will provide 32 molecules of ATP.

Summing up, for each glucose molecule processed, a typical cell gains 36 molecules of ATP. *All but two of them are produced by the mitochondria.*

18

✳ CELLULAR HYPOXIA

Oxygen is essential for normal glucose metabolism. Glucose breakdown and energy production begins in the cytosol with *glycolysis.* Glycolysis, which does not require oxygen, produces two molecules of ATP as it converts the glucose molecule to *pyruvic acid.* If oxygen supplies are adequate, pyruvic acid enters the *mitochondria* and enters the *TCA cycle.* The TCA cycle breaks down the pyruvic acid to *carbon dioxide,* generating two additional molecules of ATP. The hydrogen ions removed through the TCA cycle then enter the *electron transport system (ETS).* There, the hydrogen ions eventually bind with *oxygen* forming *water.* However, through the ETS, 32 molecules of ATP are produced. When completely processed, one glucose molecule yields 36 molecules of ATP. A lack of oxygen, referred to as *hypoxia,* inhibits or stops the TCA cycle and electron transport resulting in the accumulation of pyruvic acid. Glycolysis continues unheeded. As pyruvic acid accumulates, it is converted to *lactic acid* and released into the extracellular fluid where it can cause dangerous shifts in body pH. If oxygen is restored, lactic acid is converted back to pyruvic acid and the normal processes resume.

Other Catabolic Pathways

Aerobic metabolism is relatively efficient and capable of generating large amounts of ATP. It is the cornerstone of normal cellular metabolism, but it has one obvious limitation—the cell must have adequate supplies of both oxygen and glucose. Cells can survive only briefly without oxygen. Low glucose concentrations have a much smaller effect on most cells, because cells can break down other nutrients to provide organic molecules for the TCA cycle, as shown in Figure 18-4•. Many cells can switch from one nutrient source to another as the need arises. For example, many cells can shift from glucose-based to lipid-based ATP production when necessary.

Cells break down proteins for energy only when lipids or carbohydrates are unavailable; this makes sense because the enzymes and organelles that the cell needs to survive are composed of proteins. Nucleic acids are present only in small amounts, and they are seldom catabolized for energy, even when the cell is dying of acute starvation. This restraint makes sense, too, as it is the DNA in the nucleus that determines all of the structural and functional characteristics of the cell. We will consider the catabolism of other compounds in later sections as we discuss the metabolism of lipids, proteins, and nucleic acids.

Gluconeogenesis

The synthesis of glucose from precursors other than glucose is called **gluconeogenesis** (gloo-kō-nē-ō-JEN-e-sis; *glykus,* sweet + *neo-,* new + *genesis,* an origin). Because some of the steps in glycolysis are not reversible, car-

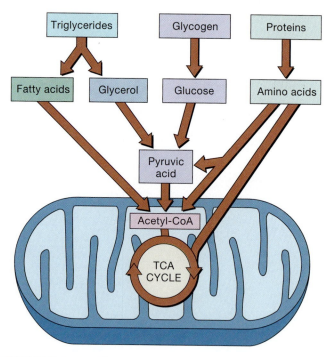

•**FIGURE 18-4   Alternate Catabolic Pathways**

bohydrate synthesis involves a different set of regulatory enzymes, and carbohydrate breakdown and synthesis are independently regulated. Pyruvic acid or other three-carbon molecules can be used as starting materials. As indicated in Figure 18-5•, this reaction sequence enables a cell to create glucose molecules from other carbohydrates, glycerol, or some amino acids. Acetyl-CoA cannot be used to make glucose, because the reaction that removes the carbon dioxide molecule (a *decarboxylation*) between pyruvic acid and acetyl-CoA

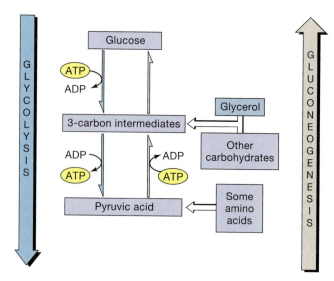

•**FIGURE 18-5   Carbohydrate Metabolism**
A flow chart of the major pathways of glycolysis and gluconeogenesis. Some amino acids, other carbohydrates, and glycerol can be converted to glucose. All these reactions occur in the cytosol.

cannot be reversed. Because their breakdown yields acetyl-CoA, neither fatty acids nor many amino acids can be converted to glucose.

Glucose molecules created by gluconeogenesis can be used to manufacture other simple sugars, complex carbohydrates, or nucleic acids. In the liver and in skeletal muscle, glucose molecules are stored as **glycogen**. Glycogen is an important energy reserve that can be broken down when the cell cannot obtain enough glucose from the interstitial fluid. Although glycogen molecules are large, glycogen reserves take up very little space because they form compact, insoluble granules.

Lipid Metabolism

Lipid molecules, like carbohydrates, contain carbon, hydrogen, and oxygen, but in different proportions. Because triglycerides are the most abundant lipid in the body, our discussion will focus on pathways for triglyceride breakdown and synthesis. ∞ p. 41

Lipid Catabolism

During lipid catabolism, or **lipolysis**, lipids are broken down into pieces that can be converted to pyruvic acid or channeled directly into the TCA cycle (Figure 18-4●). A triglyceride is first split into its component parts through hydrolysis. This step yields one molecule of glycerol and three fatty acid molecules. Glycerol enters the TCA cycle after cytoplasmic enzymes convert it to pyruvic acid. The catabolism of fatty acids, known as *beta-oxidation*, involves a different set of enzymes that break the fatty acids down into two-carbon fragments. The fragments enter the TCA cycle or combine to form *ketone bodies*, short carbon chains discussed in a later section. Beta-oxidation occurs inside mitochondria, so

the carbon chains can enter the TCA cycle immediately. The cell gains 144 ATP molecules from the breakdown of one 18-carbon fatty acid molecule—almost 1.5 times the energy obtained from the breakdown of three 6-carbon glucose molecules.

Lipids and Energy Production

Lipids are important as an energy reserve because they can provide large amounts of ATP. Being insoluble, they can be stored in compact droplets in the cytosol. This feature also makes it difficult for water-soluble enzymes to reach them; as a result, lipid reserves are harder to mobilize than carbohydrate reserves. In addition, most lipids are processed inside mitochondria, and mitochondrial activity is limited by the availability of oxygen. The net result is that lipids cannot provide large amounts of ATP in a short amount of time. However, cells with modest energy demands can shift to lipid-based energy production when glucose supplies are limited. Skeletal muscle fibers normally cycle between lipid metabolism and carbohydrate metabolism. When you are at rest, your energy demands are low, and your skeletal muscle fibers break down fatty acids. When you are active, your energy demands are both large and immediate, and your skeletal muscle fibers then metabolize glucose.

Lipid Synthesis

The synthesis of lipids is known as **lipogenesis** (li-pō-JEN-e-sis; *lipos*, fat). It usually begins with acetyl-CoA, but almost any organic molecule can be used because lipids, amino acids, and carbohydrates can easily be converted to acetyl-CoA (Figure 18-6●). Our cells cannot *build* every fatty acid they can break down. *Linoleic acid*, an 18-carbon, unsaturated fatty acid, cannot be

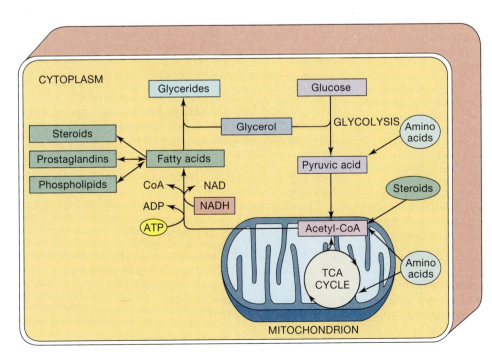

●**FIGURE 18-6   Lipid Synthesis**
Pathways of lipid synthesis begin with acetyl-CoA. Molecules of acetyl-CoA can be strung together in the cytosol, yielding fatty acids. Those fatty acids can be used to synthesize glycerides or other lipid molecules. Lipids can also be synthesized from amino acids or carbohydrates.

synthesized at all. Thus, a diet poor in linoleic acid slows growth and alters the appearance of the skin. *Arachidonic* and *linolenic acids* are other long-chain unsaturated fatty acids that the human body cannot synthesize. These three **essential fatty acids** must be included in the diet, because they are needed to synthesize prostaglandins and phospholipids for cell membranes. These unsaturated fatty acids are synthesized by plants; common sources are corn, peanut, safflower, and soy oils.

Lipid Transport and Distribution

Lipids circulate in the bloodstream as lipoproteins and free fatty acids. **Lipoproteins** are lipid-protein complexes that contain large insoluble glycerides, cholesterol, or both, with a superficial coating dominated by phospholipids and proteins. The proteins and phospholipids make the entire complex soluble, and the proteins help regulate lipid absorption by cells.

One group of lipoproteins, the *chylomicrons*, forms in the intestinal tract. ∞ *p. 486* Chylomicrons enter the venous circulation via lymphatic capillaries. The chylomicrons transport triglycerides, which are absorbed by skeletal muscle, cardiac muscle, adipose tissue, and the liver.

Two other major groups of lipoproteins are the **low-density lipoproteins (LDLs)** and **high-density lipoproteins (HDLs)**. These lipoproteins transport cholesterol between the liver and other tissues. The LDLs deliver cholesterol to peripheral tissues. Because this cholesterol may end up in arterial plaques, LDL cholesterol is often called "bad cholesterol." The HDL cholesterol transports excess cholesterol from peripheral tissues to the liver for storage or excretion in the bile. Because HDL cholesterol is returning cholesterol that will not cause circulatory problems, it is called "good cholesterol."

Free fatty acids (FFA) are lipids that can diffuse easily across cell membranes. Those circulating in the blood are usually bound to albumin, the most abundant plasma protein. Liver cells, cardiac muscle cells, skeletal muscle fibers, and many other body cells can metabolize free fatty acids. They are an important energy source during periods of starvation, when glucose supplies are limited.

Protein Metabolism

There are roughly 100,000 different proteins in the human body, with varied forms, functions, and structures. All contain some combination of the same 20+ amino acids. Under normal conditions, there is a continuous turnover of cellular proteins in the cytosol. Peptide bonds are broken, and the free amino acids are used to manufacture new proteins. If other energy sources are inadequate, mitochondria can break down amino acids in the TCA cycle to generate ATP. Not all amino

acids enter the TCA cycle at the same point, so the ATP outputs vary. However, the average yield is comparable to that of carbohydrate catabolism.

Amino Acid Catabolism

The first step in amino acid catabolism is the removal of the amino group, which requires a coenzyme derivative of **vitamin B_6** (*pyridoxine*). The amino group can be removed by transamination or deamination. *Transamination* (trans-am-i-NĀ-shun) attaches the amino group of an amino acid to another carbon chain, creating a "new" amino acid. Transaminations enable a cell to synthesize many of the amino acids needed for protein synthesis. Cells of the liver, skeletal muscles, heart, lung, kidney, and brain, which are particularly active in protein synthesis, perform many transaminations.

Several inherited metabolic disorders result from an inability to produce specific enzymes involved with amino acid metabolism. Individuals with **phenylketonuria** (fen-il-kē-tō-NOO-rē-a), or **PKU**, cannot convert the amino acid phenylalanine to the amino acid tyrosine, because of a defect in the enzyme *phenylalanine hydroxylase*. This reaction is an essential step in the synthesis of norepinephrine, epinephrine, and melanin. If PKU is not detected in infancy, central nervous system development is inhibited and severe brain damage results.

Deamination (dē-am-i-NĀ-shun) is the removal of an amino group in a reaction that generates an ammonia molecule (NH_3). Ammonia is highly toxic, even in low concentrations. The liver, the primary site of deamination, has the enzymes needed to deal with the problem of ammonia generation. Liver cells convert the ammonia to **urea**, a relatively harmless, water-soluble compound that is excreted in the urine. The fate of a carbon chain after deamination in the liver depends on its structure. The carbon chains of some amino acids can be converted to pyruvic acid and then used in gluconeogenesis. Other carbon chains are converted to acetyl-CoA and broken down or are converted to ketone bodies. **Ketone bodies** are organic acids that are also produced when lipid catabolism is under way. *Acetone* is an example of a ketone body generated by the body. It is a small molecule that can diffuse into the alveoli of the lungs, giving the breath a distinctive odor.

Ketone bodies are not metabolized by the liver, and they diffuse into the general circulation. The ketone bodies are used by other cells, which reconvert them into acetyl-CoA for breakdown in the TCA cycle and the production of ATP. The increased production of ketone bodies that occurs during protein and lipid catabolism by the liver results in high ketone body concentrations in body fluids, a condition called **ketosis** (kē-TŌ-sis).

COMPLICATIONS OF DIABETES MELLITUS

Diabetes mellitus is a disorder of glucose metabolism. The diabetic under treatment can develop complications that result from an inadequate amount of available glucose (*hypoglycemia*) or an excess amount of available glucose (*hyperglycemia*). Patients with Type 1 diabetes require *insulin.* An excess dose of insulin or inadequate food intake after a standard dose of insulin can cause life-threatening hypoglycemia. Likewise, a lack of insulin or increased food intake with a standard dose of insulin can cause hyperglycemia. Type 2 diabetics usually do not require insulin. Instead, they are able to manage their blood-sugar levels through diet, exercise, or use of an *oral hypoglycemic agent.* Although much less common, a Type 2 diabetic can develop hypoglycemia if an excess of oral hypoglycemic medication is taken or if food intake decreases significantly. Like the Type 1 diabetic, the Type 2 diabetic can develop hypoglycemia if food intake is increased or if the oral hypoglycemic agent being used does not adequately lower blood-glucose levels.

The extremes of blood sugar can affect many body systems. Prolonged poor control of blood-sugar levels markedly increases the patient's chances of developing many of the long-term complications associated with diabetes. The extremes of blood sugar require prompt treatment by emergency personnel.

- *Hypoglycemia.* The blood-glucose level at which hypoglycemia occurs varies from individual to individual. However, a blood-glucose level less than 50 mg/dl results in hypoglycemia in most diabetics. Hypoglycemia is a true medical emergency and the most life-threatening complication of diabetes mellitus. The central nervous system (CNS) relies almost exclusively on glucose as its sole source of energy. Thus, an inadequate blood-glucose level can cause CNS injury. The symptoms of hypoglycemia are due to CNS dysfunction. Prompt recognition of hypoglycemia and administration of glucose is essential if CNS injury is to be prevented.

- *Hyperglycemia.* An abnormal elevation in blood glucose is termed hyperglycemia. Unlike hypoglycemia, which can develop in minutes, hyperglycemia can take hours or even days to develop. In most patients, there is an inadequate level of the insulin necessary for glucose entry into the cells. When glucose entry is impaired, cellular starvation occurs. In addition to its effect on glu-

cose metabolism, insulin is also responsible for the manufacture and storage of *lipids* (fats) by the body. Inadequate insulin levels cause the breakdown of lipids into glucose, further increasing blood-glucose levels. As a byproduct of lipid breakdown, free-fatty acids are converted to *ketone bodies.* As ketone bodies accumulate, systemic acidosis occurs. The sequence of events results in *diabetic ketoacidosis (DKA).* In severe DKA, the pH can fall to 7.0 or lower.

—*Diabetic ketoacidosis.* Most Type 1 diabetics develop DKA if their blood-glucose levels are allowed to rise unchecked. The signs and symptoms of DKA are related to the various biochemical derangements described above. They include dehydration, hypotension, and reflex tachycardia. As the disease progresses, the patient will develop nausea, vomiting, and abdominal pain. Because of the acidosis, hyperventilation occurs as a compensatory mechanism. The hyperventilation is quite exaggerated and is referred to as *Kussmaul's respiration.* The sweet smell of ketones can sometimes be detected in the patient's breath. Eventually, the patient will develop altered mental status and, in time, unconsciousness. Treatment includes massive intravenous fluid replacement and the administration of insulin.

—*Non-ketotic hyperosmolar coma.* A certain subset of patients, most of whom have Type 2 diabetes, will not develop ketones as a complication of hyperglycemia. In these patients, there appears to be enough insulin present to prevent ketone formation. As their blood glucose levels rise, they can develop *non-ketotic hyperosmolar coma (NKHC).* In NKHC, the blood glucose level can rise to 1,000 mg/dl or more. As the glucose is spilled into the urine, the resultant *osmotic diuresis* causes severe dehydration. The *osmolarity* of the blood, a measure of concentration of molecules in the blood climbs significantly. NKHC most commonly occurs in middle-aged or elderly diabetics and is often associated with another disease process such as infection. It typically takes days for NKHC to occur, and the signs and symptoms are similar to those seen in DKA. Kussmaul's respirations are not seen. Treatment is similar to DKA. However, the mortality rate for NHKC is higher than for DKA.

18

Several factors make protein catabolism an impractical source of quick energy:

- Proteins are more difficult to break apart than are complex carbohydrates or lipids.
- One of the byproducts, ammonia, is a toxin that can damage cells.
- Proteins form the most important structural and functional components of any cell. Extensive protein catabolism therefore threatens homeostasis at the cellular and systems levels.

Amino Acids and Protein Synthesis

The basic mechanism of protein synthesis was detailed in Chapter 3 (Figures 3-17• and 3-18•). ∞ *pp. 71–73* The human body can synthesize roughly half of the different amino acids needed to build proteins. There are ten *essential amino acids.* Eight of them (*isoleucine, leucine, lysine, threonine, tryptophan, phenylalanine, valine,* and *methionine*) cannot be synthesized; the other two (*arginine* and *histidine*) can be synthesized, but in amounts that are insufficient for growing children. The other amino acids, which can be synthesized on demand, are called the *nonessential amino acids.*

Protein deficiency diseases develop when an individual does not consume adequate amounts of all essential amino acids. All amino acids must be available if protein synthesis is to occur. Every transfer RNA molecule must appear at the proper location bearing its individual amino acid; as soon as the amino acid called for by a particular codon is missing, the entire process comes to a halt. Regardless of the energy content of the diet, if the diet is deficient in essential amino acids, the individual will be malnourished to some degree. Examples of protein deficiency diseases include *marasmus* and *kwashiorkor.* Although over 100 million children worldwide have symptoms of these disorders, neither condition is common in the United States today.

✳ BERIBERI

A deficiency of *thiamine (vitamin B₁)* causes *beriberi.* In developing countries, beriberi is due to consumption of milled (polished) rice. In developed nations, thiamine deficiency is due to inadequate thiamine intake and absorption in chronic alcoholics.

Thiamine deficiency primarily affects the cardiovascular system (*wet beriberi*) and the nervous system (*dry beriberi*). Beriberi heart disease includes peripheral vasodilation, retention of sodium and water leading to edema, and biventricular myocardial failure. *Acute fulminate cardiovascular beriberi* can end in cardiovascular collapse. Improvement occurs with thiamine replacement.

Two primary nervous system diseases are due to thiamine deficiency. *Wernicke's encephalopathy (WE),* or *cerebral beriberi,* causes vomiting, dysfunction of the extraocular muscles, fever, ataxia, and mental deterioration. *Korsakoff's syndrome (KS),* also called *Korsakoff's psychosis (KP),* is a continuation of *WE* and includes retrograde amnesia and impaired ability to learn. Thiamine will completely reverse the effects of *WE* but will only partially reverse the symptoms of *KS.*

Nucleic Acid Metabolism

Living cells contain both DNA and RNA. But because the genetic information contained in the DNA of the nucleus is absolutely essential to the long-term survival of a cell, the DNA in the nucleus is never catabolized for energy, even if the cell is dying of starvation. RNA molecules are broken down and replaced regularly, but most nucleotides are recycled rather than broken down further. When the nucleotides *are* broken down, only the sugars, cytosine, and uracil can enter the TCA cycle and be used to generate ATP. Adenine and guanine cannot be catabolized. Instead they are excreted as **uric acid**, a relatively nontoxic waste product that is far less soluble than urea. Urea and uric acid are called *nitrogenous wastes,* because they contain nitrogen atoms.

Nucleic Acid Synthesis

All cells synthesize RNA, but DNA synthesis occurs only in cells that are preparing for mitosis (cell divi-

sion) or meiosis (gamete production). The process of DNA replication was described in Chapter 3. ∞ *p. 73* Messenger RNA (mRNA), transfer RNA (tRNA), and ribosomal RNA (rRNA) are transcribed by different forms of the enzyme RNA polymerase. Messenger RNA is manufactured as needed, when specific genes are activated. Although several ribosomes can read the same message simultaneously, a strand of mRNA has a life span measured in minutes or hours. Molecules of rRNA and tRNA in the cytosol are broken down and replaced regularly. Ribosomes are more durable than mRNA strands—the half-life of a ribosome is just over 5 days. Because each cell contains roughly 100,000 ribosomes, their replacement involves a considerable amount of synthetic activity.

✓ How would a diet deficient in vitamin B₆ affect protein metabolism?

✓ Elevated levels of uric acid in the blood could indicate that the individual has an increased metabolism of which macromolecule?

✓ Why are high-density lipoproteins (HDLs) considered to be beneficial?

A Summary of Cellular Metabolism

Figure 18-7● summarizes the major pathways of cellular metabolism. Although this diagram follows the reactions in a "typical" cell, no one cell can perform all of the anabolic and catabolic operations and interconversions required by the body as a whole. As differentiation proceeds, each cell type develops its own complement of enzymes that determines its metabolic capabilities. In the presence of such cellular diversity, homeostasis can be preserved only when the metabolic activities of tissues, organs, and organ systems are coordinated.

DIET AND NUTRITION

Homeostasis can be maintained indefinitely only if the digestive tract absorbs fluids, organic substrates, minerals, and vitamins at a rate that keeps pace with cellular demands. The absorption of nutrients from food is called **nutrition**.

The individual requirement for each nutrient varies from day to day and from person to person. *Nutritionists* attempt to analyze a diet in terms of its ability to meet the needs of a specific individual. A *balanced diet* contains all of the ingredients necessary to maintain homeostasis, including adequate substrates for energy generation, essential amino acids and fatty acids, minerals, and vitamins. In addition, the diet must include enough water to replace losses in urine, feces, and evaporation. A balanced diet prevents **malnutrition**, an unhealthy state resulting from the inadequate or excessive intake of one or more nutrients.

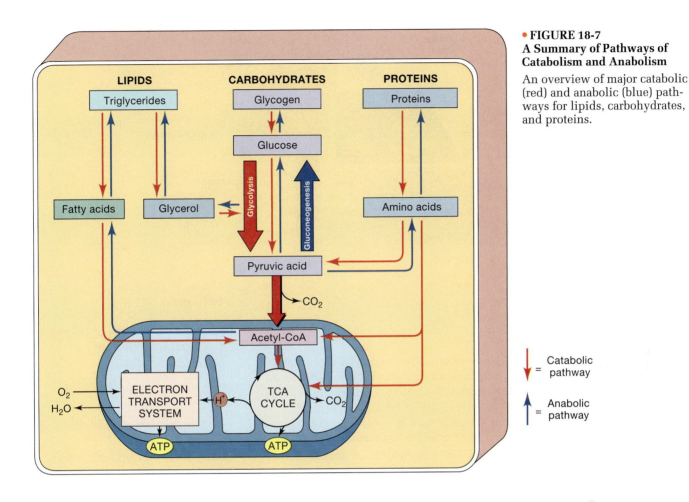

A Summary of Pathways of Catabolism and Anabolism
An overview of major catabolic (red) and anabolic (blue) pathways for lipids, carbohydrates, and proteins.

The Basic Food Groups

For several decades, the traditional American method of avoiding malnutrition was to include in the diet members of each of the four **basic food groups**: the *milk and dairy group*, the *meat group*, the *vegetable and fruit group*, and the *bread and cereal group*. Each group differs from the others in the typical balance of proteins, carbohydrates, and lipids contained, as well as in the amount and identity of vitamins and minerals.

Recently, the four groups have been increased to six by the splitting of the vegetable and fruit group and the establishment of a *fats, oils, and sweets group*. The six groups are now arranged in a *food pyramid*, with the bread and cereal group at the bottom (Figure 18-8●). This arrangement emphasizes the need to restrict dietary fats, oils, and sugar and to increase the consumption of breads, cereals, rice, and pasta, which are rich in complex carbohydrates (polysaccharides such as starch).

Such groupings are artificial at best and misleading at worst. What is important is to obtain nutrients in sufficient *quantity* (adequate to meet energy needs) and

quality (including essential amino acids, fatty acids, vitamins, and minerals). There is nothing magical about the number six—since 1940, the U.S. government has at various times advocated 11, 7, 4, and 6 food groups. The key is to make intelligent choices about what you eat. The wrong selections can lead to malnutrition even if all six groups are represented.

For example, consider the essential amino acids. Some members of the meat and milk groups, such as beef, fish, poultry, eggs, and milk, contain all of the essential amino acids in sufficient quantities. They are said to have *complete proteins*. Many plants contain adequate *amounts* of protein, but they are *incomplete proteins*, deficient in one or more of the essential amino acids. True vegetarians, who restrict themselves to the fruit and vegetable groups (with or without the bread and cereal), must be adept at juggling the constituents of their meals to include a combination of ingredients that will meet all of their amino acid requirements. Even with a proper balance of amino acids, vegetarians face a significant problem, since vitamin B_{12} is obtained only from animal products, fortified cereals, or tofu.

A Guide to Daily Food Choices

Nutrient Group	Provides	Deficiencies
Fats, oils, sweets	Calories	The majority are deficient in most minerals and vitamins
Milk, yogurt, cheese	Complete proteins; fats; carbohydrates; calcium; potassium; magnesium; sodium; phosphorus; vitamins A, B_{12}, pantothenic acid, thiamine, riboflavin	Dietary fiber, vitamin C
Meat, poultry, fish, dry beans, eggs, nuts	Complete proteins; fats; potassium; phosphorus; iron; zinc; vitamins E, thiamine, B_6	Carbohydrates, dietary fiber, several vitamins
Fruits	Carbohydrates; vitamins A, C, E, folacin; dietary fiber; potassium	Many are low in fats, calories, and protein
Vegetables	Carbohydrates; vitamins A, C, E, folacin; dietary fiber; potassium	Many are low in fats, calories, and protein
Bread, cereal, rice, pasta	Carbohydrates; vitamins E, thiamine, niacin, folacin; calcium; phosphorus; iron; sodium; dietary fiber	Fats

Minerals, Vitamins, and Water

Minerals, vitamins, and water are essential components of the diet. The body cannot synthesize minerals, and our cells can generate only a small quantity of water and very few vitamins.

Minerals

Nutritionally, **minerals** are elements other than carbon, hydrogen, oxygen, or nitrogen. Chemically, they are inorganic ions released through the dissociation of electrolytes, such as sodium chloride. Minerals are important for the following reasons:

1. Ions such as sodium and chloride contribute to the osmotic concentration of body fluids. Potassium is important in maintaining the osmotic concentration inside body cells.

2. Ions in various combinations play major roles in important physiological processes, including:

- The maintenance of membrane potentials (Chapters 7 and 8).
- The generation of action potentials (Chapter 8).
- The release of neurotransmitters (Chapters 7 and 8).
- The contraction of muscles (Chapters 7 and 13).
- The construction and maintenance of the skeleton (Chapter 6).
- The transport of respiratory gases (Chapter 16).
- The operation of buffer systems (Chapters 2 and 19).
- The absorption of fluids (Chapter 17).
- The removal of wastes (Chapter 19).

3. Ions are essential to several important enzymatic reactions. For example, the enzyme that breaks down ATP in a contracting skeletal muscle requires the presence of calcium and magnesium ions, and an enzyme required for the conversion of glucose to pyruvic acid needs both potassium and magnesium ions.

The major minerals and a summary of their functions are presented in Table 18-1. Significant reserves of several important minerals in the body help reduce the effects of dietary variations in supply. The reserves are often relatively small, however, and chronic dietary reductions can lead to various clinical problems. Alternatively, because storage capabilities are limited, a dietary excess of mineral ions can prove equally dangerous.

Vitamins

Vitamins (*vita*, life) are essential organic nutrients related to lipids and carbohydrates. They can be assigned to either of two groups, depending on their chemical structure and characteristics: fat-soluble vitamins and water-soluble vitamins.

Fat-Soluble Vitamins. Vitamins A, E, and K are **fat-soluble vitamins**. These vitamins are absorbed primarily from the digestive tract along with the lipid contents of micelles. The term *vitamin D* refers to a group of steroids, including vitamin D_3, or *cholecalciferol*. Unlike the other fat-soluble vitamins, which must be obtained by absorption across the digestive tract, vitamin D_3 can usually be synthesized in adequate amounts by the skin when exposed to sunlight. Current information concerning the fat-soluble vitamins is summarized in Table 18-2.

Because they dissolve in lipids, fat-soluble vitamins normally diffuse into cell membranes and other lipids in the body, including the lipid inclusions in the liver and adipose tissue. The body therefore contains a significant reserve of these vitamins, and normal metabolic operations can continue for several months after dietary sources

---

TABLE 18-1	Minerals and Mineral Reserves				
Mineral	Significance	Total Body Content	Primary Route of Excretion	Recommended Daily Intake
BULK MINERALS				
Sodium	Major cation in body fluids; essential for normal membrane function	110 g, primarily in body fluids	Urine, sweat, feces	0.5–1.0 g
Potassium	Major cation in cytoplasm; essential for normal membrane function	140 g, primarily in cytoplasm	Urine	1.9–5.6 g
Chloride	Major anion in body fluids	89 g, primarily in body fluids	Urine, sweat	0.7–1.4 g
Calcium	Essential for normal muscle and neuron function, bone structure	1.36 kg, primarily in skeleton	Urine, feces	0.8–1.2 g
Phosphorus	As phosphate in high-energy compounds, nucleic acids, and bone matrix	744 g, primarily in skeleton	Urine, feces	0.8–1.2 g
Magnesium	Cofactor of enzymes, required for normal membrane functions	29 g (skeleton, 17 g; cytoplasm and body fluids, 12 g)	Urine	0.3–0.4 g
TRACE MINERALS				
Iron	Component of hemoglobin, myoglobin, cytochromes	3.9 g, 1.6 g stored (ferritin or hemosiderin)	Urine (traces)	10–18 mg
Zinc	Cofactor of enzyme systems, notably carbonic anhydrase	2 g	Urine, hair (traces)	15 mg
Copper	Required as cofactor for hemoglobin synthesis	127 mg	Urine, feces (traces)	2–3 mg
Manganese	Cofactor for some enzymes	11 mg	Feces, urine (traces)	2.5–5 mg

18

TABLE 18-2	The Fat-Soluble Vitamins				
Vitamin	Significance	Sources	Daily Requirement	Effects of Deficiency	Effects of Excess
A	Maintains epithelia; required for synthesis of visual pigments	Leafy green and yellow vegetables	1 mg	Retarded growth, night blindness, deterioration of epithelial membranes	Liver damage, skin peeling, CNS effects (nausea, anorexia)
D (steroids including D₃ or cholecalciferol	Required for normal bone growth, calcium and phosphorus absorption at gut and retention at kidneys	Synthesized in skin exposed to sunlight	None*	Rickets, skeletal deterioration	Calcium deposits in many tissues, disrupting functions
E (tocopherols)	Prevents breakdown of vitamin A and fatty acids	Meat, milk, vegetables	12 mg	Anemia, other problems suspected	None reported
K	Essential for liver synthesis of prothrombin and other clotting factors	Vegetables; production by intestinal bacteria	0.07–0.14 mg	Bleeding disorders	Liver dysfunction, jaundice

*Unless sunlight exposure is inadequate for extended periods and alternative sources (fortified milk products) are unavailable.

have been cut off. As Table 18-2 points out, *too much of a vitamin* can produce effects just as unpleasant as *too little*. **Hypervitaminosis** (hī-per-vī-ta-min-Ō-sis) occurs when the dietary intake exceeds the ability to store, utilize, or excrete a particular vitamin. This condition most often involves one of the fat-soluble vitamins because the excess is retained and stored in body lipids.

Water-Soluble Vitamins. Most of the water-soluble vitamins are components of coenzymes (Table 18-3). Water-soluble vitamins are rapidly exchanged between the fluid compartments and the circulating blood, and excessive amounts are readily excreted in the urine. For this reason, hypervitaminosis involving water-soluble vitamins is relatively uncommon. The intestinal epithelium can easily absorb all of the water-soluble vitamins except B₁₂. The B₁₂ molecule is large, and it must be bound to the *intrinsic factor* secreted by the gastric mucosa before absorption can occur. ∞ *p. 471*

Because these vitamins are not stored in large quantities, insufficient intake can lead to initial symptoms of vitamin deficiency within days to weeks. The condition that results is **avitaminosis** (ā-vī-ta-min-Ō-sis), or a *deficiency disease*. Avitaminosis involving either fat-soluble or water-soluble vitamins can be caused by various factors other than dietary deficiencies. An inability to absorb a vitamin from the digestive tract, inadequate storage, or excessive demand can all produce the same result. The

bacteria that reside in our intestines help prevent deficiency diseases by producing five of the nine water-soluble vitamins, in addition to fat-soluble vitamin K.

Water

Daily water requirements average 2500 ml (10 cups), or roughly 40 ml/kg body weight. The specific requirement varies with environmental and metabolic activities. For example, exercise increases metabolic energy requirements and accelerates water losses due to evaporation and perspiration. The temperature rise accompanying a fever has a similar effect; for each degree the temperature rises above normal, the daily water loss increases by 200 ml. Thus, the advice "drink plenty of fluids" when you are sick has a solid physiological basis.

Most of your daily water ration is obtained by eating or drinking. The food you consume provides roughly 48 percent, and another 40 percent is obtained by drinking fluids. But a small amount of water—called *metabolic water*—is produced in the mitochondria during the operation of the electron transport system. The actual amount produced per day varies with the composition of the diet. A typical mixed diet in the United States contains 46 percent carbohydrates, 40 percent lipids, and 14 percent protein. This diet would produce roughly 300 ml of water per day (slightly more than 1 cup), about 12 percent of the average daily water requirement.

| TABLE 18-3 | The Water-Soluble Vitamins |

Vitamin	Significance	Sources	Daily Requirement	Effects of Deficiency	Effects of Excess
B$_1$ (thiamine)	Coenzyme in decarboxylation reactions	Milk, meat, bread	1.9 mg	Muscle weakness, CNS and cardiovascular problems including heart disease; called *beriberi*	Hypotension
B$_2$ (riboflavin)	Part of FAD	Milk, meat	1.5 mg	Epithelial and mucosal deterioration	Itching, tingling sensations
Niacin (nicotinic acid)	Part of NAD	Meat, bread, potatoes	14.6 mg	CNS, GI, epithelial, and mucosal deterioration; called *pellagra*	Itching, burning sensations, vasodilation, death after large dose
B$_5$ (pantothenic acid)	Part of acetyl-CoA	Milk, meat	4.7 mg	Retarded growth, CNS disturbances	None reported
B$_6$ (pyridoxine)	Coenzyme in amino acid and lipid metabolism	Meat	1.42 mg	Retarded growth, anemia, convulsions, epithelial changes	CNS alterations, perhaps fatal
Folacin (folic acid)	Coenzyme in amino acid and nucleic acid metabolism	Vegetables, cereal, bread	0.1 mg	Retarded growth, anemia, gastrointestinal disorders	Few noted except at massive doses
B$_{12}$ (cobalamin)	Coenzyme in nucleic acid metabolism	Milk, meat	4.5 μg	Impaired RBC production causing *pernicious anemia*	Polycythemia (elevated hematocrit)
Biotin	Coenzyme in decarboxylation reactions	Eggs, meat, vegetables	0.1–0.2 mg	Fatigue, muscular pain, nausea, dermatitis	None reported
C (ascorbic acid)	Coenzyme; delivers hydrogen ions, antioxidant	Citrus fruits	60 mg	Epithelial and mucosal deterioration; called *scurvy*	Kidney stones

Diet and Disease

Diet has a profound influence on general health. We have already considered the effects of too many and too few nutrients—hypervitaminosis and avitaminosis, respectively—and above-normal or below-normal concentrations of minerals. More subtle, long-term problems can occur when the diet includes the wrong proportions or combinations of nutrients. The average American diet contains too many calories, and lipids provide too great a proportion of those calories. This diet increases the in-cidence of obesity, heart disease, atherosclerosis, hypertension, and diabetes in the U.S. population.

✓ In terms of servings per day, which of the six food groups is most important?

✓ What is the difference between foods described as complete proteins and those described as incomplete proteins?

✓ How would a decrease in the amount of bile salts in the bile affect the amount of vitamin A in the body?

18

BIOENERGETICS

When chemical bonds are broken, energy is released. Inside cells, some of that energy may be captured as ATP, but much of it is lost to the environment as heat. The unit of energy measurement is the **calorie (c)** (KAL-o-rē), the amount of energy required to raise the temperature of 1 g of water one degree centigrade. One gram of water is not a very practical measure when you are interested in the metabolic operations that keep a 70-kg human alive, however, so the **kilocalorie (kc)** (KIL-o-kal-o-rē), or simply **Calorie** (with a capital C), is used instead. Each Calorie represents the amount of energy needed to raise the temperature of 1 kilogram of water one degree centigrade. Dieting guides that give the caloric value of various foods list Calories, not calories.

Food and Energy

In living cells, organic molecules are oxidized to carbon dioxide and water. Oxidation also occurs when something burns, and this process can be experimentally observed and measured. A known amount of food is placed in a chamber, called a *calorimeter* (kal-o-RIM-e-ter), that is filled with oxygen and surrounded by a known volume of water. Once the material is completely burned and only ash remains in the chamber, the number of Calories released can be determined by comparing the water temperatures before and after the test. The burning, or catabolism, of lipids releases a considerable amount of energy, roughly 9.46 Calories per gram (C/g). In contrast, the catabolism of carbohydrates releases 4.18 C/g, and the catabolism of protein releases 4.32 C/g. Most foods are mixtures of fats, proteins, and carbohydrates, and as a result, the values in a "Calorie counter" vary.

Metabolic Rate

It is possible to examine the metabolic state of an individual to determine how many Calories are being utilized. The result can be expressed as Calories per hour, Calories per day, or Calories per unit of body weight per day, but what is actually measured is the sum total of all of the varied anabolic and catabolic processes occurring in the body. This value is the **metabolic rate** of the individual at that time. It will change according to the activity under way—sprinting and sleeping measurements are quite different. In an attempt to reduce the variations, the testing conditions are standardized to determine the **basal metabolic rate (BMR)**. Ideally, the BMR would represent the minimum, resting energy expenditures of an awake, alert person. An average individual has a BMR of 70 C per hour, or about 1680 C per day. Although the test conditions are standardized, uncontrollable factors influence the BMR, including age, sex, physical condition, body weight, and genetic differences such as variations among ethnic groups.

The actual daily energy expenditure for each individual varies with the activities undertaken. For example, a person leading a sedentary life may have near-basal energy demands, but one hour of swimming can increase the daily caloric requirements by 500 C or more. If the daily energy intake exceeds the total energy demands, the excess will be stored, primarily as triglycerides in adipose tissue. If the daily caloric expenditures exceed the dietary supply, there will be a net reduction in the body's energy reserves and a corresponding loss in weight. This relationship accounts for the significance of calorie counting and exercise in a weight-control program.

Thermoregulation

The BMR (basal metabolic rate) is an estimate of the rate of energy use. Our cells capture only a part of that energy as ATP, and the rest is "lost" as heat. However, heat loss serves an important homeostatic purpose. Humans are subject to vast changes in environmental temperatures, but our complex biochemical systems have a major limitation: The enzyme systems will operate over only a relatively narrow range of temperatures. Therefore, our bodies have anatomical and physiological mechanisms that keep body temperatures within acceptable limits, regardless of the environmental conditions. This homeostatic process is called **thermoregulation** (*therme*, heat). Failure to control body temperature can result in a series of physiological changes, as indicated in Figure 18-9•.

Mechanisms of Heat Transfer

Heat exchange with the environment involves four basic processes—*radiation, conduction, convection,* and *evaporation* (Figure 18-10•):

1. **Radiation**. Warm objects lose heat as radiation. When we feel the sun's heat, we are experiencing radiation. Our bodies lose heat the same way, but in smaller amounts. Over half of our heat loss occurs by radiation.

2. **Conduction**. Conduction is the direct transfer of energy through physical contact. When you sit on a cold plastic chair in an air-conditioned room, you are immediately aware of this process. Conduction is usually not an effective mechanism of gaining or losing heat.

3. **Convection**. Convection is the result of conductive heat loss to the air that overlies the surface of the body. Warm air is lighter than cool air, so it rises. As the body conducts heat to the air next to the skin, that air warms and rises; cooler air replaces it, and as it in turn becomes warmed, the cycle repeats.

4. **Evaporation**. When water evaporates, it changes from a liquid to a vapor. This process absorbs rough-

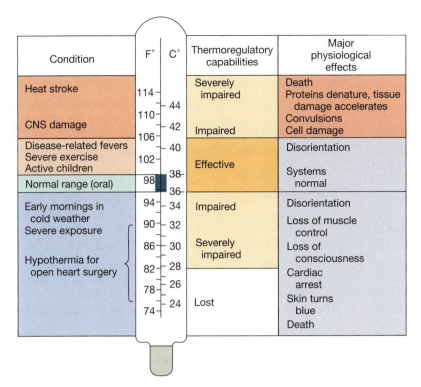

Condition	F°	C°	Thermoregulatory capabilities	Major physiological effects
Heat stroke	114	44	Severely impaired	Death Proteins denature, tissue damage accelerates
CNS damage	110 106	42	Impaired	Convulsions Cell damage
Disease-related fevers Severe exercise Active children	102	40	Effective	Disorientation
Normal range (oral)	98	38 36		Systems normal
Early mornings in cold weather Severe exposure	94 90	34 32	Impaired	Disorientation Loss of muscle control
Hypothermia for open heart surgery	86 82 78 74	30 28 26 24	Severely impaired Lost	Loss of consciousness Cardiac arrest Skin turns blue Death

•**FIGURE 18-9**   **Normal and Abnormal Variations in Body Temperature**

ly 580 calories (0.58 C) per gram of water evaporated. Each hour, 20–25 ml of water crosses epithelia to be evaported from the alveolar surfaces of the lungs and the surface of the skin. This *insensible perspiration* remains relatively constant; at rest it accounts for roughly one-fifth of the average heat loss. The sweat glands responsible for *sensible perspiration* have a tremendous range of activity, from virtual inactivity to secretory rates of 2–4 liters per hour. This is equivalent to an entire day's resting water loss in under an hour. A maximal secretion rate would, if it were completely evaporated, remove 2320 C per hour!

To maintain a constant body temperature, the individual must lose heat as fast as it is generated by metabolic operations. At rest over 50 percent of that loss occurs through radiation, 20 percent through evaporation, 15 percent through convection, and the rest through conduction. Altering these rates requires the coordination of many different systems. These adjustments are made by the **heat-loss center** and **heat-gain center** of the hypothalamus. The heat-loss center adjusts activity in the parasympathetic division of the autonomic nervous system, and the heat-gain center directs its responses through the sympathetic division. The overall effect is to control temperature by influencing two events: the rate of heat production and the rate of heat loss to the environment. These events may be further supported by behavioral changes or modifications, such as the addition or removal of clothing.

Promoting Heat Loss.   When the temperature at the heat-loss center exceeds its thermostat setting, three major results occur:

1. Peripheral blood vessels dilate, and warm blood flows to the surface of the body. The skin takes on a reddish color and rises in temperature; heat loss through radiation and convection increases.
2. Sweat glands are stimulated, and as perspiration flows across the skin, evaporative heat losses accelerate.
3. The respiratory centers are stimulated, and the depth of respiration increases. Often the individual begins respiring through the mouth, increasing evaporative losses through the lungs.

The efficiency of heat loss by evaporation varies with environmental conditions, especially the "relative humidity" of the air. If the air is saturated (100 percent humidity), it holds as much water vapor as it can at that temperature. Under these conditions, evaporation is ineffective as a cooling mechanism. This is why humid, tropical conditions can be so uncomfortable—people perspire continuously but remain warm and wet.

Restricting Heat Loss.   The function of the heat-gain center of the brain is to prevent **hypothermia** (hī-pō-THER-mē-uh), or below-normal body temperature. When body temperature falls below acceptable levels, the heat-loss center is inhibited and the heat-gain center is activated. Blood flow to the skin decreases; with the circulation restricted, it may take on a bluish or pale

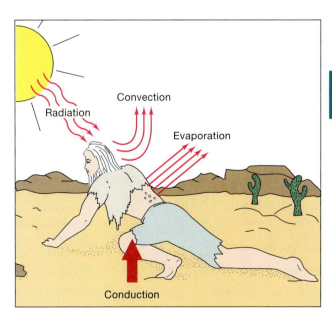

•**FIGURE 18-10**   **Routes of Heat Gain and Loss**

coloration. In addition, the pattern of blood flow changes. In warm weather, blood flows in a superficial venous network. In cold weather, blood is diverted to a network of deep veins that lie beneath an insulating layer of subcutaneous fat.

Promoting Heat Production. In addition to conserving heat, the heat-gain center has two mechanisms for increasing the rate of heat production. In *shivering thermogenesis* (ther-mō-JEN-e-sis), muscle tone is gradually increased until brief, oscillatory skeletal muscle contractions occur. This shivering stimulates energy consumption by skeletal muscles, and it can increase the rate of heat generation by as much as 400 percent.

In *nonshivering thermogenesis*, hormones are released that increase the metabolic activity of all tissues. Epinephrine from the adrenal gland immediately increases the rates of glycolysis in the liver and in skeletal muscles and the rate of aerobic metabolism in most tissues. The heat-gain center also stimulates the release of thyroxine by the thyroid gland, accelerating carbohydrate use and the breakdown of all other substrates. These effects develop gradually over days to weeks.

✓ How would the BMR of a pregnant woman compare with her BMR in the nonpregnant state?

✓ Under what conditions would evaporative cooling of the body be ineffective?

✓ What effect would the vasoconstriction of peripheral blood vessels have on body temperature on a hot day?

AGING AND NUTRITIONAL REQUIREMENTS

Nutritional requirements do not change drastically with age. However, changes in lifestyle, eating habits, and income that often accompany aging can directly affect nutrition and health. For example, current guidelines indicate that dietary calories should come from a mixture of nutrients: Proteins should provide 11–12% of daily calorie intake; carbohydrates, 55–60%; and fats, less than 30%. These percentages do not change with age. Caloric *requirements*, however, do change. For each decade after age 50, caloric requirements decrease by 10 percent. This decrease is associated with changes in metabolic rates, body mass, activity levels, and exercise tolerance.

With age, several factors combine to result in an increased need for calcium. Some degree of osteoporosis is a normal consequence of aging. A sedentary lifestyle contributes to the problem. The rate of bone loss decreases if calcium levels are kept elevated. The elderly are also likely to require supplemental vitamin D_3 if they are to absorb the calcium they need. Many elderly people spend most of their time indoors and avoid the sun when outdoors. This behavior slows sun damage to their skin, which is thinner than that of younger people, but it also eliminates vitamin D_3 production by the skin. ∞ *p. 111* This vitamin is converted to the hormone calcitriol, which stimulates calcium absorption by the small intestine.

Maintaining a healthy diet becomes more difficult with age as a result of changes in the senses of smell and taste and in the structure of the digestive system. With age, the number and sensitivity of olfactory and gustatory receptors decreases. ∞ *p. 298* As a result, food becomes less appetizing, and less food is eaten. Making matters worse, the mucosal lining of the digestive tract becomes thinner as we age, so nutrient absorption becomes less efficient. Thus what food the elderly do eat is not utilized very efficiently. Elderly people on fixed budgets often reduce their consumption of animal protein, which is the primary source of dietary iron. The combination of small quantities plus inefficient absorption makes them prone to iron deficiency, which causes anemia.

1 8

Chapter Review

KEY TERMS

aerobic metabolism, *p. 497*	**glycogen**, *p. 501*	**thermoregulation**, *p. 510*
anaerobic metabolism, *p. 497*	**glycolysis**, *p. 497*	**tricarboxylic (TCA, citric acid, or**
basal metabolic rate (BMR), *p. 510*	**metabolism**, *p. 496*	**Krebs) cycle**, *p. 498*
Calorie, *p. 510*	**metabolic turnover**, *p. 497*	**vitamin**, *p. 507*
electron transport system (ETS),	**nutrient**, *p. 496*	
p. 499	**nutrition**, *p. 504*	

SUMMARY OUTLINE

INTRODUCTION   *p. 496*

1. Cells in the body are chemical factories that break down organic molecules and their building blocks to obtain energy.

CELLULAR METABOLISM   *p. 496*

1. In general, cells will break down excess carbohydrates first, then lipids, while conserving amino acids. Only about 40 percent of the energy released through catabolism is captured in ATP; the rest is released as heat. *(Figure 18-1)*

2. Cells synthesize new compounds (1) to perform structural maintenance and repair, (2) to support growth, and (3) to produce secretions.

Carbohydrate Metabolism   *p. 497*

3. Most cells generate ATP and other high-energy compounds through the breakdown of carbohydrates.

4. **Glycolysis** and **aerobic metabolism** provide most of the ATP used by typical cells. In glycolysis, each molecule of glucose yields two molecules of pyruvic acid and two molecules of ATP. *(Figure 18-2)*

5. In the presence of oxygen, the pyruvic acid molecules enter the mitochondria, where they are broken down completely in the **tricarboxylic acid (TCA) cycle**. The carbon and oxygen atoms are lost as carbon dioxide, and the hydrogen atoms are passed by *coenzymes* to the *electron transport system*. *(Figure 18-3)*

6. *Cytochromes* pass electrons along the electron transport chain of the **electron transport system (ETS)** to generate ATP and water.

7. For each glucose molecule completely broken down by aerobic pathways, a typical cell gains 36 ATP molecules.

Other Catabolic Pathways   *p. 500*

8. Cells can break down other nutrients to provide molecules for the TCA cycle if supplies of glucose are limited. *(Figure 18-4)*

9. **Gluconeogenesis**, the synthesis of glucose, enables a cell to create glucose molecules from other carbohydrates, glycerol, or some amino acids. *Glycogen* is an important energy reserve when the cell cannot obtain enough glucose from the extracellular fluid. *(Figure 18-5)*

Lipid Metabolism   *p. 501*

10. During **lipolysis** (lipid catabolism), lipids are broken down into pieces that can be converted into pyruvic acid or channeled into the TCA cycle.

11. Triglycerides are the most abundant lipids in the body. Triglycerides are split into glycerol and fatty acids. The glycerol enters the glycolytic pathways, and the fatty acids enter the mitochondria for use in the TCA cycle.

12. *Beta-oxidation* is the breakdown of fatty acid molecules into two-carbon fragments. The fragments may be used in the TCA cycle or converted to ketone bodies.

13. Lipids cannot provide large amounts of ATP in a short amount of time. However, cells can shift to lipid-based energy production when glucose reserves are limited.

14. In **lipogenesis**, the synthesis of lipids, almost any organic molecule can be used to form glycerol. **Essential fatty acids** cannot be synthesized and must be included in the diet. *(Figure 18-6)*

15. Lipids circulate as **lipoproteins** (lipid-protein complexes that contain large glycerides, cholesterol, or both) and as **free fatty acids (FFA)** (water-soluble lipids that can diffuse easily across cell membranes).

Protein Metabolism   *p. 502*

16. If other energy sources are inadequate, mitochondria can break down amino acids. In the mitochondria, the amino group may be removed by *transamination* or *deamination*. The resulting carbon skeleton may enter the TCA cycle to generate ATP or be converted to ketone bodies.

17. Protein catabolism is impractical as a quick-energy source.

18. Roughly half of the amino acids needed to build proteins can be synthesized. There are ten essential amino acids that must be acquired through the diet.

Nucleic Acid Metabolism   *p. 504*

19. DNA in the nucleus is never catabolized for energy. RNA molecules are broken down and replaced regularly; usually they are recycled as new nucleic acids.

A Summary of Cellular Metabolism   *p. 504*

20. No one cell can perform all of the anabolic and catabolic operations necessary to support life. Homeostasis can be preserved only when metabolic activities of different tissues are coordinated. *(Figure 18-7)*

DIET AND NUTRITION   *p. 504*

1. **Nutrition** is the absorption of nutrients from food. A *balanced diet* contains all of the ingredients necessary to maintain homeostasis; it prevents **malnutrition**.

The Basic Food Groups   *p. 505*

2. The six **basic food groups** are the milk; meat; vegetable; fruit; fats, oils, and sweets; and bread, cereal, rice, and pasta groups. These are arranged in a *food pyramid* with the bread, cereal, rice, and pasta group forming the base. *(Figure 18-8)*

Minerals, Vitamins, and Water   *p. 506*

3. **Minerals** act as cofactors in various enzymatic reactions. They also contribute to the osmotic concentration of body fluids, and they play a role in membrane potentials, action potentials, neurotransmitter release, muscle contraction, the construction and maintenance of the skeleton, the transport of gases, buffer systems, fluid absorption, and waste removal. *(Table 18-1)*

4. **Vitamins** are needed in very small amounts. Vitamins A, D, E, and K are **fat-soluble vitamins**; taken in excess, they can lead to **hypervitaminosis**. **Water-soluble vitamins** are not stored in the body; a lack of adequate dietary supplies can lead to **avitaminosis** (*deficiency disease*). *(Tables 18-2, 18-3)*

5. Daily water requirements average about 40 ml/kg body weight. Water is obtained from food, drink, and metabolic generation.

Diet and Disease   *p. 509*

6. A balanced diet can improve general health. Most Americans consume too many calories, mostly in the form of lipids.

18

BIOENERGETICS *p. 510*

1. The energy content of food is usually expressed as **Calories** per gram (C/g). Less than half of the energy content of glucose or any other organic nutrient can be captured by our cells.

Food and Energy *p. 510*

2. The catabolism of lipids releases 9.46 C/g, about twice the amount as equivalent weights of carbohydrates and proteins release.

Metabolic Rate *p. 510*

3. The total of all the anabolic and catabolic processes in the body is the **metabolic rate** of an individual. The **basal metabolic rate (BMR)** is the rate of energy utilization at rest.

Thermoregulation *p. 510*

4. The homeostatic regulation of body temperature is **thermoregulation**. Heat exchange with the environment involves four processes: **radiation, conduction, convection,** and **evaporation.** *(Figures 18-9, 18-10)*

5. The hypothalamus acts as the body's thermostat, containing the **heat-loss center** and the **heat-gain center**.

6. Mechanisms for increasing heat loss include physiological mechanisms (superficial blood vessel dilation, increased perspiration and respiration) and behavioral adaptations.

7. Body heat may be conserved by decreased blood flow to the dermis. Heat can be generated by *shivering thermogenesis* and *nonshivering thermogenesis*.

AGING AND NUTRITIONAL REQUIREMENTS *p. 512*

1. Caloric requirements drop by 10 percent per decade after age 50. Changes in the senses of smell and taste and in the digestive system dull appetites and decrease the efficiency of nutrient absorption from the digestive tract.

REVIEW QUESTIONS

LEVEL 1   Reviewing Facts and Terms

Match each item in column A with the most closely related item in column B. Use letters for answers in the spaces provided.

Column A

_____ 1. glucose formation
_____ 2. lipid catabolism
_____ 3. synthesis of lipids
_____ 4. linoleic acid
_____ 5. deamination
_____ 6. phenylalanine
_____ 7. ketoacidosis
_____ 8. A, D, E, K
_____ 9. B complex and vitamin C
_____10. calorie
_____11. uric acid
_____12. hypothermia

Column B

a. gluconeogenesis
b. essential amino acid
c. below-normal body temperature
d. unit of energy
e. fat-soluble vitamins
f. water-soluble vitamins
g. lipolysis
h. nitrogenous waste
i. essential fatty acid
j. removal of an amino group
k. decrease in pH
l. lipogenesis

13. Cells synthesize new organic components to:
    (a) perform structural maintenance and repairs
    (b) support growth
    (c) produce secretions
    (d) a, b, and c are correct

14. During the complete catabolism of one molecule of glucose, a typical cell gains:
    (a) 4 ATP   (b) 18 ATP
    (c) 36 ATP   (d) 144 ATP

15. The breakdown of glucose to pyruvic acid is:
    (a) glycolysis   (b) gluconeogenesis
    (c) cellular respiration (d) beta-oxidation

16. Glycolysis yields an immediate net gain of _____ molecules for the cell.
    (a) 1 ATP   (b) 2 ATP
    (c) 4 ATP   (d) 36 ATP

17. The electron transport chain yields a total of _____ molecules of ATP in the complete catabolism of one glucose molecule.
    (a) 2   (b) 4
    (c) 32   (d) 36

18. The synthesis of glucose from simpler molecules is called:
    (a) glycolysis
    (b) lipolysis
    (c) gluconeogenesis
    (d) beta-oxidation

19. The lipoproteins that transport excess cholesterol from peripheral tissues back to the liver for storage or excretion in the bile are the:
    (a) chylomicrons   (b) FFA
    (c) LDLs   (d) HDLs

20. The removal of an amino group in a reaction that generates an ammonia molecule is called:
    (a) ketoacidosis   (b) transamination
    (c) deamination   (d) denaturation

21. A complete protein contains:
    (a) the proper balance of amino acids
    (b) all the essential amino acids in sufficient quantities
    (c) a combination of nutrients selected from the food pyramid
    (d) N compounds produced by the body

18

22. All minerals and most vitamins:
    (a) are fat-soluble
    (b) cannot be stored by the body
    (c) cannot be synthesized by the body
    (d) must be synthesized by the body because they are not present in adequate amounts in the diet

23. The basal metabolic rate represents the:
    (a) maximum energy expenditure when exercising
    (b) minimum, resting energy expenditure of an awake, alert person
    (c) minimum amount of energy expenditure during light exercise
    (d) muscular energy expenditure added to the resting energy expenditure

24. Over half of the heat loss from our bodies is attributable to:
    (a) radiation   (b) conduction
    (c) convection   (d) evaporation

25. Define the terms *metabolism*, *anabolism*, and *catabolism*.

26. What is a lipoprotein? What are the major groups of lipoproteins, and how do they differ?

27. Why are vitamins and minerals essential components of the diet?

28. What energy yields in Calories per gram are associated with the catabolism of carbohydrates, lipids, and proteins?

29. What is the basal metabolic rate (BMR)?

30. What four mechanisms are involved in thermoregulation?

LEVEL 2   Reviewing Concepts

31. The function of the TCA cycle is to:
    (a) produce energy during periods of active muscle contraction
    (b) break six-carbon chains into three-carbon fragments
    (c) prepare the glucose molecule for further reactions
    (d) remove hydrogen atoms from organic molecules and transfer them to coenzymes

32. During periods of fasting or starvation, the presence of ketone bodies in the circulation causes:
    (a) an increase in blood pH
    (b) a decrease in blood pH
    (c) a neutral blood pH
    (d) diabetes insipidus

33. What happens during the process of glycolysis? What conditions are necessary for this process to take place?

34. Why is the TCA cycle called a cycle? What substance(s) enter(s) the cycle, and what substance(s) leave(s) it?

35. How are lipids catabolized in the body? How is beta-oxidation involved with lipid catabolism?

36. How can the food pyramid be used as a tool to obtain nutrients in sufficient quantity and quality? Why are the dietary fats, oils, and sugars at the top of the pyramid and the breads, cereals, rices, and pastas at the bottom?

37. How is the brain involved in the regulation of body temperature?

38. Articles in popular magazines sometimes refer to "good cholesterol" and "bad cholesterol." To what types and functions of cholesterol might these terms refer? Explain your answer.

LEVEL 3   Critical Thinking and Clinical Applications

39. Why is an individual who is starving more susceptible to infectious disease than an individual who is well nourished?

40. The drug *colestipol* binds bile salts in the intestine, forming complexes that cannot be absorbed. How would this drug affect cholesterol levels in the blood?

ANSWERS TO CONCEPT CHECK QUESTIONS

Page 504

1. Vitamin B_6 (pyridoxine) is an important coenzyme in the processes of deamination and transamination, the first step in processing amino acids in the cell. A deficiency in this vitamin would interfere with the ability to metabolize proteins. 2. Uric acid is the product of the degradation of the nucleotides adenine and guanine in the body. The macromolecules that contain adenine and guanine are the nucleic acids. An increase in uric acid levels could indicate increased breakdown of nucleic acids. 3. HDLs are considered to be beneficial because they reduce the amount of fat (including cholesterol) in the bloodstream by transporting it to the liver for storage or for excretion in the bile.

Page 509

1. In terms of servings per day, the bread, cereal, rice, and pasta group is the most important, with between 6 and 11 per day. 2. Foods that contain all of the essential amino acids in nutritionally required amounts are said to contain complete proteins. Foods that are deficient in one or more of the essential amino acids contain incomplete proteins. 3. Bile salts are necessary for the digestion and absorption of fats and fat-soluble vitamins. Vitamin A is a fat-soluble vitamin. A decrease in the amount of bile salts in the bile would result in a decreased ability to absorb the vitamin A from food and would thus lead to a vitamin A deficiency.

Page 512

1. The BMR of a pregnant woman should be higher than the BMR of the woman in a nonpregnant state because of increased metabolism associated with support of the fetus as well as the added effect of fetal metabolism. 2. Evaporation is ineffective as a cooling mechanism under conditions of high relative humidity, when the air is holding large amounts of water vapor. 3. The vasoconstriction of peripheral vessels would decrease blood flow to the skin and decrease the amount of heat that the body can lose. As a result, the body temperature would increase.

1
8

OVERVIEW

All of the biochemical reactions occurring in the body are referred to as *metabolism.* Living cells use these various chemical reactions to break down organic nutrient molecules in order to obtain energy, usually in the form of *adenosinetriphosphate (ATP).* There are three categories of nutrients: *carbohydrates, proteins,* and *lipids.* Carbohydrates include sugars and starches and are a major source of energy. Complex carbohydrate compounds are usually broken down into simple sugars, most commonly glucose. Glucose is the most frequently used form of carbohydrate. The energy in carbohydrates is obtained through *glycolysis, mitochondrial energy production,* and the *tricarboxylic acid (TCA) cycle,* also called Kreb's Cycle. Lipid molecules can be broken down into pieces that can feed into the TCA cycle thus providing energy. Lipid molecules are important as they provide large amounts of ATP. Proteins are chemical compounds consisting of various amino acids. Like carbohydrates and lipids, proteins can be broken down to yield energy. However, the breakdown of proteins is considerably more complex and is not considered a source of quick energy. This is because proteins are more difficult to break down than are complex lipids and complex carbohydrates. In addition, they produce ammonia, a toxic byproduct that can damage body cells. Finally, proteins are important structural and functional cellular components. Extensive breakdown of proteins can threaten the viability of the cell.

The study of body nutrients and metabolism is referred to as *nutrition.* Persons who study nutrition are *nutritionists.* Nutritionists educate the public on the role that healthy eating habits play in the promotion of wellness and prevention of disease. Nutritionists typically have at least a bachelor's degree in nutrition, although most have a master's degree or Ph.D., especially if they are teaching. Persons who counsel others on nutrition are known as *dietitians.* The American Dietetic Association certifies dietitians who meet their standards. Dietitians may specialize in clinical nutrition, providing nutrition programs for patients. Others may serve in an administrative position planning nutritional programs for institutions or supervising food services. Registered or licensed dietitians must have a bachelor's degree in nutrition or dietetics. Many have graduate degrees.

Some physicians specialize in metabolism, metabolic diseases, and inborn errors of metabolism. Generally, they are pediatricians who take additional training in the diagnosis and treatment of metabolic problems. Most metabolic problems are inherited and are detected early in life. They must be carefully managed in order to prevent growth retardation or developmental defects.

NUTRITION AND EMERGENCY MEDICAL SERVICES

The job demands and scheduling of emergency medical services work make it difficult to eat a balanced diet and obtain adequate exercise. For the most part, EMS work is fairly sedentary. However, at certain times, it can require significant physical exertion and stamina. Because of this, it is essential that emergency personnel eat a balanced diet, obtain moderate aerobic exercise on a regular basis, and maintain normal body weight. Unfortunately, more and more EMS workers can be classified as obese. The definition of obesity varies, but it is generally defined as weighing at least 20 percent or more in excess of your ideal body weight. For example, patients with an ideal body weight of 178 pounds would be considered obese when their weight exceeded 214 pounds. A better measurement of obesity is through determination of the *body mass index (BMI).* The BMI takes the patient's height into consideration and is calculated by dividing the body weight (in kilograms) by the patient's height (in meters). Many of the health problems associated with obesity begin to cause problems when the person's body weight exceeds 120 percent or more of ideal weight. Low back strain, one of the most common on-the-job injuries in EMS, occurs more frequently in personnel who are overweight.

Unfortunately, a few emergency workers can be classified as being morbidly obese. To be labeled as *morbidly obese,* the individuals must weigh more that than two times their ideal body weight. For example, a patients weighing with an ideal body weight of 178 pounds would be considered morbidly obese when their weight exceeds exceeded 356 pounds. People who are morbidly obese have serious risk factors for developing multiple life-threatening problems. Regardless of their overall general health, a morbidly obese person generally cannot perform all of the tasks expected of an EMT or paramedic during the course of routine EMS work.

Many EMS systems have health maintenance programs that identify personnel at risk for illness or injury, including obesity. When an employees is are identified as being obese, they may be asked to participate in developing a plan that will help them to lose weight and restore them to health. Such plans usually include an exercise regimen, dietary counseling, and wellness education. Physical fitness is more ingrained in the fire service, where most fire-based EMS operations have ongoing fitness programs. Although EMS units roll considerably more often than engine and truck companies, the EMS crew can usually get needed exercise over the course of the day. In busy systems, it may be prudent simply to block out time for exercise with the understanding that an MCI or high system usage would require interruption of exercise regimens.

NUTRITION

Many believe that it is impossible to maintain an adequate diet while working in EMS. However, with a little planning and awareness of your options, you can eat sensibly and avoid the fast food habit. Unfortunately, high performance EMS System Status Management systems often requires EMS crews to remain in the ambulance for the entire shift due to "System Status Management." This makes it very difficult to planning meals and eating sensibly very difficult. However, with a little ingenuity and planning, this too can be mastered.

The most difficult part of improving nutrition is altering established bad habits. Changing your behavior requires some commitment and self-discipline, an understanding of the change process, and patience with what will become long-term self-improvement. You must set realistic goals, and understand that backsliding occasionally happens. Whatever your goals may be, such as reducing excess weight, gaining weight, or regularly eating more wholesome foods, it is helpful to be able to analyze your progress by using charts or daily food diaries.

Good nutrition is fundamental to your well-being because your food is your body's fuel. You don't want to be putting diesel fuel into a Ferrari. In addition to eating

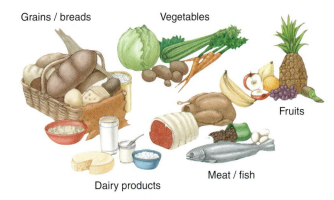

● **FIGURE A18-1   The Major Food Groups**
Preparing and eating a balanced diet is essential. Select from each of the major food groups every day.

balanced meals, you must also eat in moderation, limit fat consumption, and make time for exercise. If you eat and treat yourself poorly, both your short- and long-term well-being will be jeopardized.

The topic of nutrition can seem, at times, overwhelming, but if you rely on sound sources of information and build your knowledge gradually, you will benefit in many ways. One key to eating well is to learn the major food groups and eat a variety of foods from them daily (Figure A18-1●). Those food groups and the recommended number of daily servings are:

- *Grains/breads.* 6–11 servings per day, for complex carbohydrates, B vitamins, and fiber.
- *Vegetables.* 3–5 servings per day, for fiber, iron, vitamins A and C, and folate.
- *Fruits.* 2–4 servings per day, for vitamins A and C, potassium, and fiber.
- *Dairy products.* 2–3 servings per day, for calcium, protein, and vitamins A and D.
- *Meat/fish.* 2–3 servings per day, for protein, zinc, iron, and B vitamins.

Avoid or minimize the intake of fat, salt, sugar, cholesterol, and caffeine. For example, you can avoid a dose of fat by eating lean meat instead of marbled meat. An apple is far more nutritious than a slice of apple pie, which has a filling that is high in sugar and a crust that is saturated with fat. Food labels contain abundant information about nutritional content. Learn to read them. Standardization of food labels has reduced much of the confusion (Figure A18-2●). Be sure to check the serving size to avoid misinterpreting the food's overall nutritional value. In general, aim for a diet that is approximately 40% carbohydrates, 40% protein, and 20% fat.

Food portions also have a significant impact on body weight. Even a well planned, healthy diet can result in weight gain if the portions are too large. Note that snacking is a weight-gain trap. Plan to eat low-calorie snacks, and buy them before you get hungry.

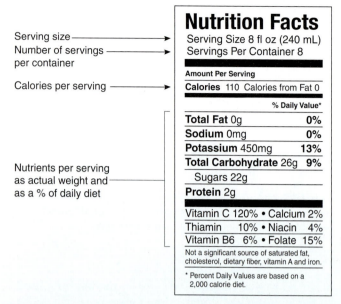

Serving size

Number of servings per container

Calories per serving

Nutrients per serving as actual weight and as a % of daily diet

Nutrition Facts

Serving Size 8 fl oz (240 mL)
Servings Per Container 8

Amount Per Serving

Calories 110 Calories from Fat 0

	% Daily Value*
Total Fat 0g	0%
Sodium 0mg	0%
Potassium 450mg	13%
Total Carbohydrate 26g	9%
Sugars 22g	
Protein 2g	

Vitamin C 120%	•	Calcium	2%
Thiamin 10%	•	Niacin	4%
Vitamin B6 6%	•	Folate	15%

Not a significant source of saturated fat, cholesterol, dietary fiber, vitamin A and iron.

* Percent Daily Values are based on a 2,000 calorie diet.

• **FIGURE A18-2**   **Example of a Standardized Food Label**

TABLE A18-1	Daily Requirements of Essential Vitamins
A	5000 IU
Thiamine	1.5 mg
Riboflavin	1.8 mg
Niacin	20 mg
Ascorbic acid	45 mg
D	400 IU
E	15 IU
K	70 µg
Folic acid	0.4 mg
B_{12}	3 µg
Pyridoxine	2 mg
Pantothenic acid	Unknown

Eating on the run, as EMS providers must often do, can be less detrimental if you plan ahead and carry a small cooler filled with whole-grain sandwiches, cut vegetables, fruit, and other wholesome foods. If you must, stop at a local market instead of the fast-food place next door. Buy fresh fruit, yogurt, and sensible deli selections. They are more nutritious and much cheaper less expensive than "fast foods."

Finally, monitor your fluid intake. Your body needs plenty of fluids to properly maintain the internal environment. Pay attention to what you are drinking. Fill a "go-cup" with fresh ice water when you stop by the emergency department instead of spending your money on soft drinks. Water is more thirst-quenching, cheaper, and much better for you.

VITAMINS

Vitamins are organic compounds needed in small quantities for normal body metabolism. However, they cannot be manufactured by the cells of the body and must be obtained from the diet. Physiological processes that require vitamins include metabolism, growth, development, and tissue repair. The body absorbs most vitamins through the gastrointestinal tract following dietary ingestion. Vitamins are stored in the liver and, to a lesser extent, in the cells. In developed countries, healthy adults usually receive adequate amounts of vitamins and do not need supplements (Table A18-1). Vitamin supplements may, however, be indicated for special populations including pregnant and nursing women, patients with absorption disorders, the chronically ill, surgery patients, alcoholics, and the malnourished. Additionally, people on a strict vegetarian diet may need supplemental vitamins.

Vitamins are classified as either fat-soluble or water-soluble (Table A18-2). The liver stores the fat-soluble vitamins (A, D, E, and K), so the patient will become deficient only after long periods of inadequate vitamin intake. Vitamin D is unique in that the skin produces it with exposure to sunlight. The water-soluble vitamins (C and those in the B complex) must be routinely ingested, as the body does not store them. After short periods of deprivation, patients may begin to experience vitamin deficiency. The B complex vitamins are grouped only because they occur together in foods; otherwise they share no significant characteristics. The individual B vitamins are named for the order in which they were discovered (B_1, B_2, B_6, B_{12}, and so forth). These vitamins also have specific names. For example, B_1 is also known as thiamine, a vitamin that plays a key role in carbohydrate metabolism.

FIRE-GROUND REHABILITATION

Fire fighting is one of the most dangerous and physically demanding occupations today. It is common for EMS personnel to establish and staff rehabilitation units on the fire ground. For years, firefighter rehabilitation at the fire scene consisted of coffee and doughnuts provided by volunteer organizations. However, because it has been recognized that stress- and heat-related emergencies are the primary causes of on-duty firefighter deaths, the concept of *Emergency Incident Rehabilitation (EIR)* was developed. Large fires, such as wildfires, can involve hundreds of firefighters from multiple departments. In these situations, there must be multiple rehab/EIR sectors must be established as a functional part of the Incident Command System (ICS).

TABLE A18-2 Vitamin Sources and Common Vitamin Deficiencies

Vitamin	Problems Resulting from Deficiency	Source
Fat Soluble		
A	Night blindness, skin lesions	Butter, yellow fruit, green leafy vegetables, milk
D	Bone and muscle pain, weakness, softening of bones	Fish, fortified milk, exposure to sunlight
E	Hyporeflexia, ataxia, anemia	Nuts, green leafy vegetables, wheat
K	*Increased bleeding*	*Liver, green leafy vegetables*
Water Soluble		
B₁ (thiamin)	Peripheral neuritis, depression, anorexia, poor memory	Whole grains, beef, pork, peas, beans,
B₂ (riboflavin)	Sore throat, stomatitis, painful or swollen tongue, anemia	Milk, eggs, cheese, green leafy vegetables
B₂ (niacin)	Skin eruptions, diarrhea, enteritis, headache, dizziness, insomnia	Meat, eggs, milk
B₆ (pyridoxine)	Skin lesions, seizures, peripheral neuritis	Liver, meats, eggs, vegetables
B₉ (folic acid)	Megaloblastic anemia	Liver, fresh green vegetables, yeast
B₁₂ (cyanocobalamin)	Irreversible nervous system damage, pernicious anemia	Fish, egg yolk, milk
C	Scurvy	Citrus fruits, tomatoes, strawberries

It is important for all fire-ground personnel to report to the Rehab Sector immediately after any of the following activities:

- Strenuous activity such as forcible entry, advancing hose lines, closed space search and rescue, and/or ventilation
- The use and depletion of two self-contained breathing apparatus (SCBA) bottles
- Thirty (30) minutes of operation within a hazardous/dangerous environment
- Failure of an SCBA unit.

Incoming personnel should be carefully evaluated including vital signs, breath sounds, examination of skin color and condition, and body core temperature. It is important to try and to determine the firefighters' hydration status. Remember, over 60 percent of body weight is water (Table A18-3). Water is the best rehydration agent. Alternatively, water can be mixed with a commercial sport hydration beverage in a 50/50 mixture and administered at about 40 degrees Fahrenheit.

Oral hydration with water is indicated in almost every fire-ground operation, regardless of the season. Large fires, or those occurring during summer months, especially in the South and the Southwest, can cause significant fluid loss. In many cases, firefighting personnel may need several liters of intravenous fluids to restore

TABLE A18-3 Biochemical Content in Grams of a 70-kilogram (154-pound) man

Water	41,400
Fat	12,600
Protein	12,600
Carbohydrate	300
Na	63
K	150
Ca	1,160
Mg	21
Cl	85
P	670
S	112
Fe	3
L	0.014

lost water. There should be established protocols for intravenous hydration in the field. Rehab sector personnel should decide whether a firefighter can return to fire fighting or remain for additional rehabilitation based on protocols (Figure A18-3•). In addition to hydration, personnel should be provided some form of nutrition while in the rehab sector. Cut fresh fruit, such as apples or oranges, are best. Salty products and salt tablets should not be provided.

A18

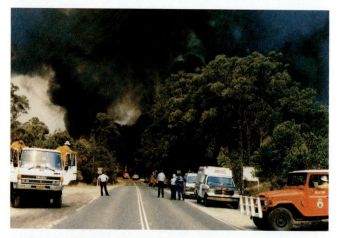

• **FIGURE A18-3   Fire-ground Operations**
Large fires require multiple Rehab Sectors. Firefighting personnel should not be released to return to fire fighting until cleared by Rehab Sector personnel.

Summary

Nutrition is an important component in total patient care. Nutrients are the fuels that drive the various biochemical systems of the body. Because of the nature of the work, EMS personnel often eat at fast food restaurants or eat on the run. Maintaining a balanced diet under such circumstances is difficult. Over time, this can lead to health problems such as obesity, peptic ulcer disease, stress, and many others. EMS personnel should plan ahead and prepare meals that provide a balanced diet, avoiding the high-calorie, high-fat foods found in fast-food restaurants. Although there are short periods of intense physical activity, EMS is a fairly sedentary profession. Because of this, EMS personnel should have an exercise program that promotes flexibility and aerobic conditioning. Long-term survival in EMS is dependent upon long-term care of the body, mind, and spirit.

A1
8

19

The Urinary System

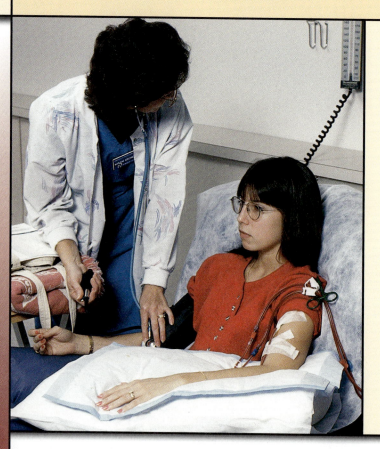

Hemodialysis did not become widely available until the 1960s. Prior to that, persons who developed renal failure simply died. Since then, hemodialysis has been refined so that it provides the most efficient dialysis in the least possible time. Dialysis centers are now located in many neighborhoods, thus preventing the need for patients to drive long distances. Now, many patients can complete hemodialysis at home.

Chapter Outline and Objectives

Vocabulary Development

calyx, a cup of flowers; *minor calyx*
detrudere, to push down; *detrusor muscle*
fenestra, a window; *fenestrated capillaries*
glomus, a ball; *glomerulus*
gonion, angle; *trigone*
juxta, near; *juxtaglomerular apparatus*
micturire, to urinate; *micturition*
nephros, kidney; *nephron*
papillae, small, nipple-shaped projections; *renal papillae*
podon, foot; *podocyte*
ren, kidney; *renal artery*
rectus, straight; *vasa recta*
retro-, behind; *retroperitoneal*
vasa, vessels; *vasa recta*

The human body contains trillions of cells bathed in extracellular fluid. Previous chapters compared these cells to factories that burn nutrients to obtain energy. One can imagine what would happen if real factories were built as close together as cells in the body. Each would generate piles of garbage, and the smoke they produced, together with the depletion of oxygen, would drastically reduce air quality. In short, there would be a serious pollution problem.

Comparable problems do not develop within the body as long as the activities of the digestive, cardiovascular, respiratory, and urinary systems are coordinated. The digestive tract absorbs nutrients from food and excretes solid wastes, and the liver adjusts the nutrient concentration of the circulating blood. The cardiovascular system delivers these nutrients and oxygen from the respiratory system to peripheral tissues. As blood leaves these tissues, it carries the carbon dioxide and cellular waste products to sites of excretion. The carbon dioxide is eliminated at the lungs, as described in Chapter 16. Most of the organic waste products in the blood are removed and excreted in urine produced by the kidneys of the urinary system.

The urinary system performs vital excretory functions and eliminates the dissolved organic waste products generated by cells throughout the body (Figure 19-1●). But it also has other essential functions that are often overlooked. A more complete list includes the following:

- *Regulation of blood volume and blood pressure.* Blood volume and blood pressure are regulated by (a) adjusting the volume of water lost in the urine and (b) releasing the hormones erythropoietin and renin. ∞ *p. 320*
- *Regulation of the concentrations of plasma ions.* The plasma concentrations of sodium, potassium, chloride, and other ions are regulated by controlling the quantities lost in the urine and, for calcium ions, by the synthesis of calcitriol. ∞ *p. 320*

- *Homeostasis of blood pH.* Blood pH is stabilized by controlling the loss of hydrogen ions (H^+) and bicarbonate ions (HCO_3^-) in the urine.
- *Conservation of valuable nutrients.* Valuable nutrients (such as glucose and amino acids) are conserved by preventing their excretion in the urine, while organic waste products, especially the nitrogenous wastes *urea* and *uric acid*, are eliminated.

These activities must be carefully regulated to keep the composition of the blood within acceptable limits. A disruption of any one of these functions will have immediate and potentially fatal consequences. This chapter examines the functional organization of the urinary system and describes the major regulatory mechanisms that control urine production and concentration.

THE ORGANIZATION OF THE URINARY SYSTEM

The components of the urinary system are indicated in Figure 19-1●. The two *kidneys* produce *urine*, a liquid containing water, ions, and small soluble compounds. Urine leaving the kidneys travels along the paired *ureters* to the *urinary bladder* for temporary storage. When *urination* occurs, contraction of the muscular bladder forces the urine through the *urethra* and out of the body.

THE KIDNEYS

The **kidneys** are located on either side of the vertebral column between the last thoracic and third lumbar vertebrae. The right kidney often sits slightly lower than the left (Figure 19-2a●), and both lie between the muscles of the dorsal body wall and the peritoneal lining (Figure 19-2b●). This position is called *retroperitoneal* (re-trō-per-i-tō-NĒ-al; retro-, behind) because the organs are behind the peritoneum.

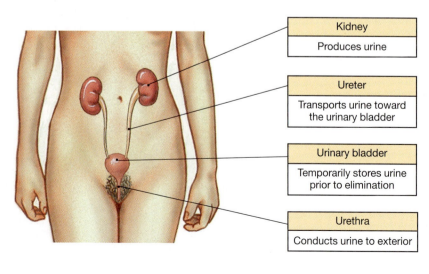

Kidney
Produces urine

Ureter
Transports urine toward the urinary bladder

Urinary bladder
Temporarily stores urine prior to elimination

Urethra
Conducts urine to exterior

●**FIGURE 19-1   The Components of the Urinary System**

The position of the kidneys is maintained by (1) the overlying peritoneum, (2) contact with adjacent organs, and (3) supporting connective tissues. In effect, each kidney is packed in a protective, soft cushion of adipose tissue that prevents the jolts and shocks of day-to-day existence from disturbing normal kidney function. If the kidney is displaced, a condition called a *floating kidney*, the ureters or renal blood vessels may become twisted or kinked, an extremely dangerous condition.

Superficial and Sectional Anatomy

As you might expect, each kidney is shaped like a kidney bean. An indentation called the **hilus** is the point of entry for the renal artery and exit for the *renal vein* and *ureter*. (The adjective "renal" is derived from *ren*, which means kidney in Latin.) The surface of the kidney is covered by a dense, fibrous *renal capsule*. The inner portion of the capsule folds inward at the hilus and lines the *renal sinus*, an internal cavity.

Seen in section (Figure 19-3•), the kidney can be divided into an outer renal **cortex** and an inner renal **medulla**. The medulla contains 6 to 18 conical **renal pyramids**, whose tips, or **papillae**, project into the renal sinus. Renal columns extend from the cortex inward toward the renal sinus between adjacent renal pyramids.

Urine production begins in the renal pyramids and overlying areas of renal cortex. Ducts within each renal papilla discharge urine into a cup-shaped drain, called a **minor calyx** (KĀ-liks; *calyx*, a cup of flowers; plural *calyces*). Four or five minor calyces (KAL-i-sēz) merge to form the **major calyces**, both of which combine to form a large, funnel-shaped chamber, the **renal pelvis**. The renal pelvis is connected to the ureter at the hilus of the kidney.

The Nephron

Urine production begins in the cortex at microscopic structures called **nephrons** (NEF-ronz), the basic functional unit in the kidney. Each nephron consists of a *renal tubule* that is roughly 50 mm long. The tubule has two *convoluted* (coiled or twisted) segments separated

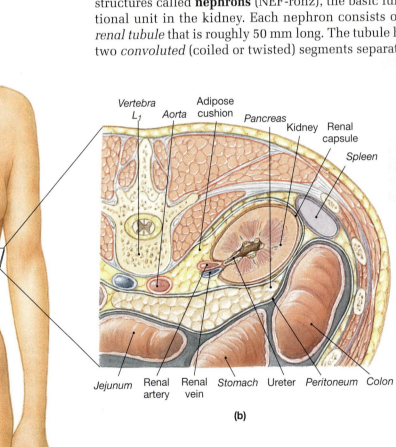

(b)

• **FIGURE 19-2   An Overview of Kidney Anatomy**
(a) An anterior view of the trunk, showing the positions of the kidneys and other components of the urinary system. **(b)** A sectional view at the level indicated in part (a).

(a)

1
9

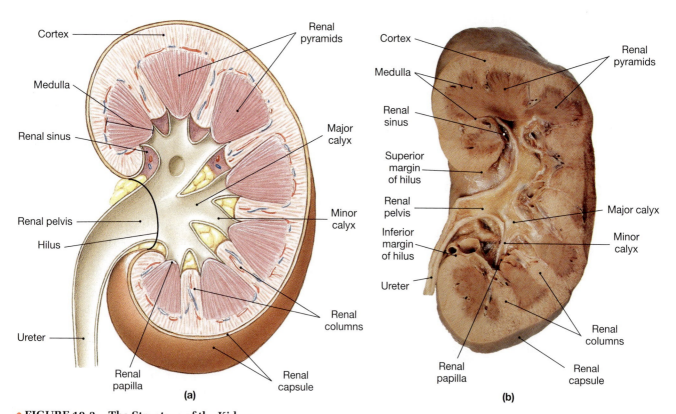

• FIGURE 19-3 The Structure of the Kidney
(a) Diagrammatic and **(b)** sectional views of a frontal section through the left kidney.

by a simple U-shaped tube. The convoluted segments are in the cortex, and the tube extends partially or completely into the medulla. For clarity, the schematic nephron shown in Figure 19-4• has been shortened and straightened out.

An Overview of the Nephron

The nephron begins at a *renal corpuscle* (KOR-pus-l), which contains a capillary knot, or *glomerulus* (glo-MER-ū-lus; *glomus*, a ball) within an expanded chamber. Blood arrives at the glomerulus via the *afferent arteriole* and departs in the *efferent arteriole*. Filtration occurs in the renal corpuscle as blood pressure forces fluid and dissolved solutes out of the capillaries and into the surrounding chamber. This movement produces a protein-free solution known as a **filtrate**.

From the renal corpuscle, the filtrate enters the **renal tubule**, a long passageway that is subdivided into different regions. The major segments are the *proximal convoluted tubule*, the *loop of Henle* (HEN-lē), and the *distal convoluted tubule*. As the filtrate travels along the tubule, its composition gradually changes, and it is then called *tubular fluid*. The changes that occur and the urine that results depend on the specialized activities under way in each segment of the nephron.

Each nephron empties into a *collecting duct*, the start of the **collecting system**. The collecting duct leaves the cortex and descends into the medulla, carrying tubular fluid from many nephrons toward a *papillary duct* that delivers the fluid, now called *urine*, into the renal pelvis.

Functions of the Nephron

Urine is very different from the filtrate produced at the renal corpuscle. The role of each segment of the nephron in the conversion of filtrate to urine is indicated in Figure 19-4•. The renal corpuscle is the site of filtration. During filtration, blood pressure forces water and small solutes across the glomerular walls. The functional advantage of this process is that it is passive and does not require an expenditure of energy. The disadvantage of filtration is that any filter with pores large enough to permit the passage of organic waste products is unable to *prevent* the passage of water, ions, and nutrients such as glucose, fatty acids, and amino acids. These substances, along with most of the water, must be reclaimed, and the waste products must be excreted in a relatively concentrated solution. The segments of the renal tubule are responsible for:

- Reabsorbing all of the useful organic molecules from the filtrate.
- Reabsorbing over 90 percent of the water in the filtrate.
- Secreting into the tubular fluid any waste products that were missed by the filtration process.

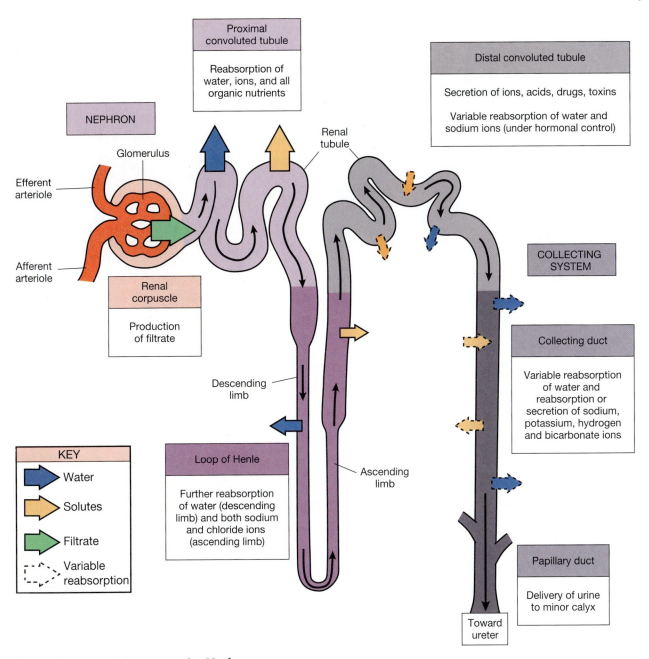

● **FIGURE 19-4   A Representative Nephron**
The major structures and functions of each segment of the nephron and collecting system.

Additional water and salts will be removed in the collecting system before the urine is released into the renal sinus. Table 19-1 summarizes the functions of the different regions of the nephron and collecting system.

The Renal Corpuscle

The **renal corpuscle** consists of (1) the capillary knot of the **glomerulus** and (2) the expanded initial segment of the renal tubule, a region known as **Bowman's capsule** (Figure 19-5●). The glomerulus projects into Bowman's capsule much as the heart projects into the

pericardial cavity (Figure 19-5a●). A *capsular epithelium* lines the wall of the capsule and a *glomerular epithelium* covers the glomerular capillaries. The two are separated by the **capsular space**, which receives the filtrate and empties into the renal tubule. The glomerular epithelium consists of cells called **podocytes** (PŌ-do-sīts, *podon*, foot). Podocytes have long cellular processes that wrap around individual capillaries. A thick basement membrane separates the endothelial cells of the capillaries from the podocytes. The glomerular capillaries are said to be *fenestrated* (FEN-e-strā-ted; *fenestra*, a window) because their endothelial cells contain

**1
9**

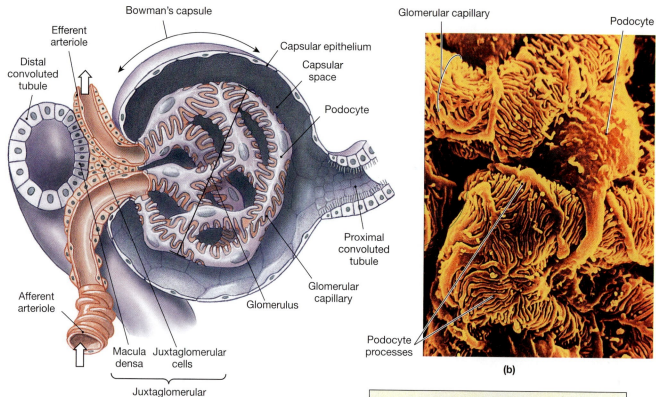

(a)

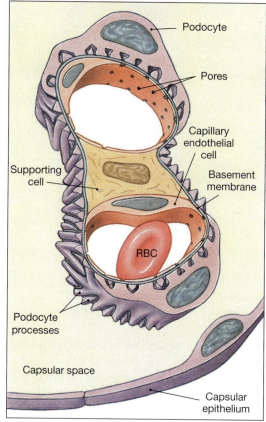

(b)

(c)

TABLE 19-1	The Functions of the Nephron and Collecting System in the Kidney
Region	*Primary Function*
Renal corpuscle	Filtration of plasma to initiate urine formation
Proximal convoluted tubule (PCT)	Reabsorption of ions, organic molecules, vitamins, water
Loop of Henle	Descending limb: reabsorption of water from tubular fluid Ascending limb: reabsorption of ions; helps create the medullary concentration gradient
Distal convoluted tubule (DCT)	Reabsorption of sodium ions; secretion of acids, ammonia, drugs
Collecting duct	Reabsorption of water and of sodium and bicarbonate ions
Papillary duct	Conduction of urine to minor calyx

• **FIGURE 19-5   The Renal Corpuscle**
(a) The renal corpuscle, showing important structural features. **(b)** The glomerular surface, showing individual podocytes and their processes. (SEM × 27,248) **(c)** A section of a glomerulus, showing the composition of the filtration membrane.

pores (Figure 19-5c•). To enter the capsular space, a solute must be small enough to pass through (1) the pores of the endothelial cells, (2) the fibers of the basement membrane, and (3) the slits between the slender processes of the podocytes (Figure 19-5b,c•). The fenestrated capillary, basement membrane, and podocyte processes create a filtration membrane that prevents the passage of blood cells and most plasma proteins but permits the movement of water, metabolic wastes, ions, glucose, fatty acids, amino acids, vitamins, and other solutes into the capsular space. Most of the valuable solutes will be reabsorbed by the proximal convoluted tubule.

The Proximal Convoluted Tubule

The filtrate next moves into the **proximal convoluted tubule (PCT)** (Figures 19-4, 19-5a•). The cells lining the PCT actively absorb organic nutrients, plasma proteins, and ions from the tubular fluid. These materials are then released into the interstitial fluid surrounding the renal tubule. As this transport occurs, the solute concentration of the interstitial fluid increases while that of the tubular fluid decreases. Water then moves out of the tubular fluid by osmosis, reducing the volume of tubular fluid.

The Loop of Henle

The last portion of the proximal convoluted tubule bends sharply and connects to the **loop of Henle** (Figure 19-4•, p. 521). This loop is composed of a *descending limb* that travels toward the renal pelvis and an *ascending limb* that returns to the cortex. The ascending limb, which is impermeable to water and solutes, actively transports sodium and chloride ions out of the tubular fluid. As a result, the interstitial fluid of the medulla contains an unusually high solute concentration. The descending limb is permeable to water, and as it descends into the medulla, water moves out of the tubular fluid by osmosis.

The Distal Convoluted Tubule

The ascending limb of the loop of Henle ends where it bends and comes in close contact with the glomerulus and its vessels. At this point, the **distal convoluted tubule (DCT)** begins, and it passes between the afferent and efferent arterioles (Figure 19-5a•).

The distal convoluted tubule is an important site for (1) the active secretion of ions, acids, and other materials; and (2) the selective reabsorption of sodium ions from the tubular fluid. In the final portions of the DCT, an osmotic flow of water may assist in concentrating the tubular fluid.

The cells of the DCT closest to the glomerulus are unusually tall, and their nuclei are clustered together. This region, diagrammed in Figure 19-5a•, is called the *macula densa* (MAK-ū-la DEN-sa). The cells of the macula densa are closely associated with unusual smooth muscle fibers, the *juxtaglomerular* (*juxta*, near) *cells* in the wall of the afferent arteriole. Together the macula densa and juxtaglomerular cells form the **juxtaglomerular apparatus**, an endocrine structure that secretes two hormones, *renin and erythropoietin*, introduced in Chapter 11. ∞ *p. 320*

The Collecting System

The distal convoluted tubule, the last segment of the nephron, opens into the collecting system. The collecting system consists of collecting ducts and papillary ducts (Figure 19-4•, p. 521). Each **collecting duct** receives tubular fluid from many nephrons, and several collecting ducts merge to form a **papillary duct**, which delivers urine to a minor calyx. In addition to transporting tubular fluid from the nephron to the renal pelvis, the collecting system can make final adjustments to the composition of the urine by reabsorbing water and reabsorbing or secreting sodium, potassium, hydrogen, and bicarbonate ions.

The Blood Supply to the Kidneys

In healthy individuals, about 1200 ml of blood flows through the kidneys each minute, or some 20–25 percent of the cardiac output. This is a phenomenal amount of blood for organs with a combined weight of less than 300 g (10.5 oz)! Figure 19-6a• diagrams the path of blood flow to each kidney. Each kidney receives blood from a *renal artery* that originates from the abdominal aorta. As the renal artery enters the renal sinus, it divides into branches that supply a series of **interlobar arteries** that radiate outward between the lobes. They then turn, arching along the boundary lines between the cortex and medulla as the **arcuate** (AR-kū-āt) **arteries**. Each of the arcuates gives rise to a number of **interlobular arteries** supplying portions of the adjacent lobe.

Blood reaches each glomerulus through an **afferent arteriole** and leaves in an **efferent arteriole** (Figure 19-6c•). It then travels to the **peritubular capillaries** that supply the proximal and distal convoluted tubules. The peritubular capillaries provide a route for the pickup or delivery of substances that are reabsorbed or secreted by these portions of the nephron.

The efferent arterioles and peritubular capillaries are further connected to a series of long, slender capillaries that accompany the loops of Henle into the medulla. These capillaries, known as the **vasa recta** (*rectus*, straight), absorb and transport solutes and water reabsorbed by the loops of Henle or collecting ducts. Under normal conditions, the removal of solutes and water by the vasa recta balances the rates of solute and water reabsorption in the medulla.

Blood from the peritubular capillaries and vasa recta enters a network of venules and small veins that

1 9

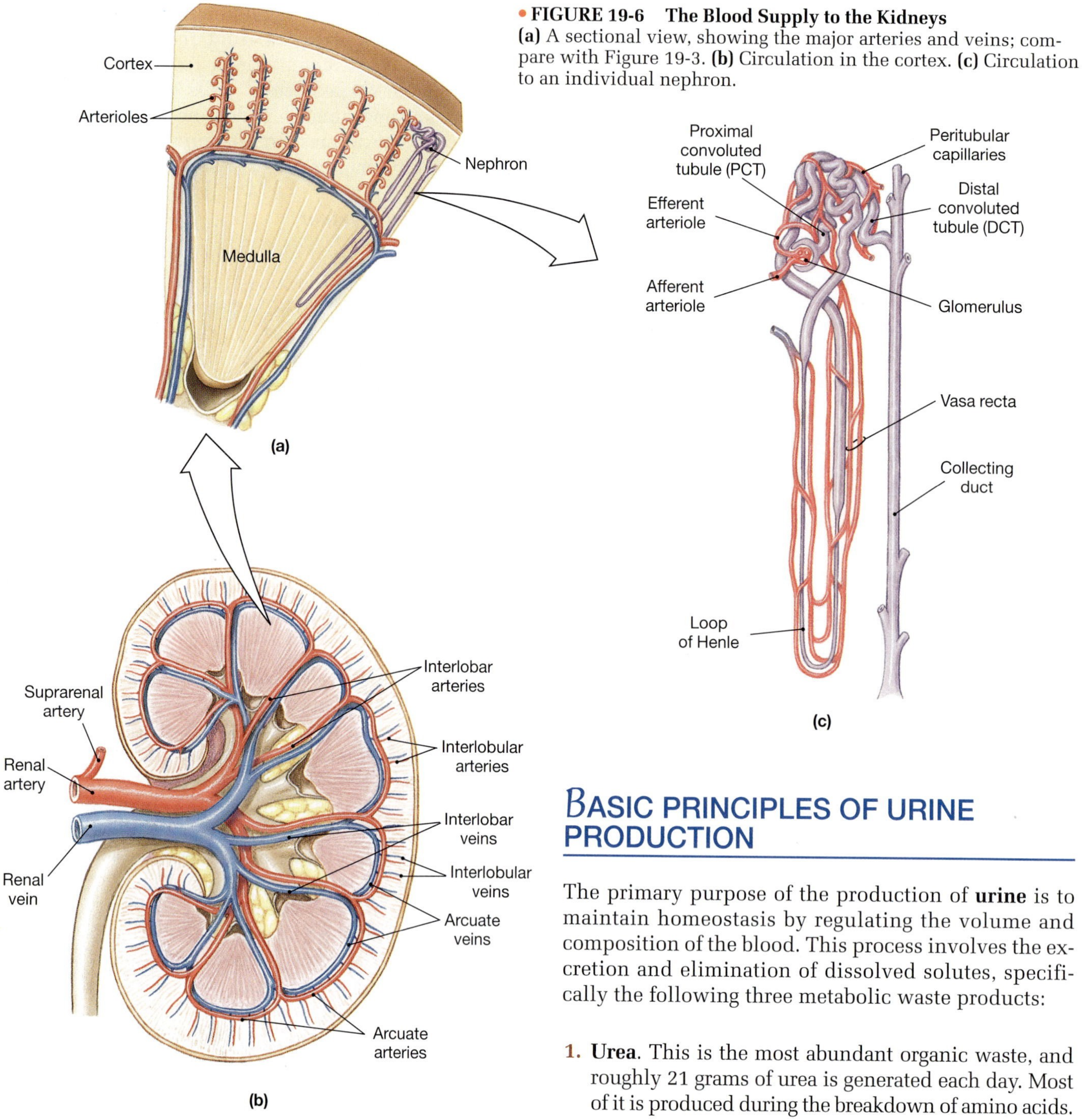

● **FIGURE 19-6   The Blood Supply to the Kidneys**
(a) A sectional view, showing the major arteries and veins; compare with Figure 19-3. **(b)** Circulation in the cortex. **(c)** Circulation to an individual nephron.

BASIC PRINCIPLES OF URINE PRODUCTION

The primary purpose of the production of **urine** is to maintain homeostasis by regulating the volume and composition of the blood. This process involves the excretion and elimination of dissolved solutes, specifically the following three metabolic waste products:

1. **Urea**. This is the most abundant organic waste, and roughly 21 grams of urea is generated each day. Most of it is produced during the breakdown of amino acids.
2. **Creatinine**. Creatinine is generated in skeletal muscle tissue through the breakdown of *creatine phosphate*, a high-energy compound that plays an important role in muscle contraction. The body generates roughly 1.8 g of creatinine each day.
3. **Uric acid**. Approximately 480 mg of uric acid is produced each day during the breakdown and recycling of RNA.

Since these waste products must be excreted in solution, their elimination is accompanied by an unavoidable water loss. The kidneys can minimize this water loss by producing a urine that is four to five times

converge on the **interlobular veins**. In a mirror image of the arterial distribution, blood continues to converge and empty into the **arcuate**, **interlobar**, and **renal veins** (Figure 19-6a●).

✓ How is the position of the kidneys different from other organs in the abdominal region?

✓ Why don't plasma proteins pass into the capsular space under normal circumstances?

✓ Damage to which part of the nephron would interfere with the control of blood pressure?

more concentrated than normal body fluids. If the kidneys could not concentrate the filtrate produced by glomerular filtration, water losses would lead to fatal dehydration in hours. At the same time, the kidneys ensure that the urine excreted does not contain potentially useful organic substrates, such as sugars or amino acids, that are found in blood plasma.

To accomplish these goals, the kidneys rely on three distinct processes:

1. **Filtration**. In filtration, blood pressure forces water across a filtration membrane. Solute molecules small enough to pass through the membrane are carried by the surrounding water molecules.

2. **Reabsorption**. Reabsorption is the removal of water and solute molecules from the filtrate after it enters the renal tubule. This is a selective process, whereas filtration occurs solely on the basis of size. Solute reabsorption may involve simple diffusion or the activity of carrier proteins in the tubular epithelium. Water reabsorption occurs passively, through osmosis. Reabsorbed water and solutes reenter the circulation at the peritubular capillaries and vasa recta.

3. **Secretion**. Secretion is the transport of solutes across the tubular epithelium and into the filtrate. This process is necessary because filtration does not force all of the dissolved materials out of the plasma, and blood entering the peritubular capillaries may still contain undesirable substances.

Together, these processes create a fluid that is very different from other body fluids. Table 19-2 indicates the efficiency of the renal system by comparing the composition of urine and plasma. The kidneys can continue to work efficiently only as long as filtration, reabsorption, and secretion proceed in proper balance. Any disruption in this balance has immediate and potentially disastrous effects on the composition of the circulating blood. If both kidneys fail to perform their assigned roles, death will occur within a few days unless medical assistance is provided.

All segments of the nephron and collecting system participate in the process of urine formation. Most regions perform a combination of reabsorption and secretion, but the balance between the two shifts from one region to another. As indicated in Table 19-1:

- Filtration occurs exclusively in the renal corpuscle, across the capillary walls of the glomerulus.
- Nutrient reabsorption occurs primarily at the proximal convoluted tubule.
- Active secretion occurs primarily at the distal convoluted tubule.
- The loop of Henle and the collecting system interact to regulate the amount of water and the number of sodium and potassium ions lost to the urine.

TABLE 19-2 Significant Differences Between Urinary and Plasma Solute Concentrations

Component	Urine	Plasma
IONS (mEq/l)		
Sodium (Na⁺)	147.5	138.4
Potassium (K⁺)	47.5	4.4
Chloride (Cl⁻)	153.3	106
Bicarbonate (HCO₃⁻)	1.9	27
METABOLITES AND NUTRIENTS (mg/dl)		
Glucose	0.009	90
Lipids	0.002	600
Amino acids	0.188	4.2
Proteins	0.000	7.5 g/dl
NITROGENOUS WASTES (mg/dl)		
Urea	1800	305
Creatinine	150	8.6
Ammonia	60	0.2
Uric acid	40	3

We will now take a closer look at events under way in each of the segments of the nephron and collecting system.

Filtration at the Glomerulus

Filtration Pressure

Chapter 14 introduced the forces acting across capillary walls, and you should consider reviewing that discussion before proceeding. ∞ *p. 381* Blood pressure at the glomerulus tends to force water and solutes out of the bloodstream and into the capsular space. For filtration to occur, this outward force must exceed any opposing pressures, such as the osmotic pressure of the blood. The net force promoting filtration is called the **filtration pressure**. Filtration pressure is higher than capillary blood pressure elsewhere in the body as a result of a difference in the diameters of afferent and efferent arterioles. Because the diameter of the efferent arteriole is slightly smaller, it offers more resistance to blood flow than does the afferent arteriole. As a result, blood "backs up" in the afferent arteriole, increasing the blood pressure in the glomerular capillaries.

The filtration pressure is very low (around 10 mm Hg), and kidney filtration will stop if glomerular blood pressure falls significantly. Reflexive changes in the diameters of the afferent arterioles, the efferent arterioles, and the glomerular capillaries can compensate for minor variations in blood pressure. These changes can occur automatically or in response to sympathetic stimulation. More serious declines in systemic blood pressure can reduce or even stop glomerular filtration. As a result, hemorrhaging, shock, or dehydration can cause a dangerous or even fatal reduction in kidney function. Because the kidneys are more sensitive to blood pressure than are other organs, it is not surprising to find that they control many of the homeostatic mechanisms responsible for regulating blood pressure and blood volume. Examples such as the renin-angiotensin system are considered later in this chapter.

The Glomerular Filtration Rate

Glomerular filtration is the process of filtrate production at the glomerulus; it is driven by the filtration pressure. The **glomerular filtration rate (GFR)** is the amount of filtrate produced in the kidneys each minute. Each kidney contains around 6 square meters of filtration surface, and the GFR averages an astounding *125 ml per minute*. This means that almost 20 percent of the fluid delivered to the kidneys by the renal arteries leaves the bloodstream and enters the capsular spaces. In the course of a single day, the glomeruli generate about 180 liters (50 gal) of filtrate, roughly 70 times the total plasma volume. But as the filtrate passes through the renal tubules, over 99 percent of it is reabsorbed. Tubular reabsorption is obviously an extremely important process. An inability to reclaim the water entering the filtrate, as in *diabetes insipidus*, can quickly cause death by dehydration. (This condition, caused by inadequate ADH secretion, was discussed in Chapter 11.) ∞ *p. 313*

Glomerular filtration is the vital first step essential to all kidney functions. If filtration does not occur, waste products are not excreted, pH control is jeopardized, and an important mechanism for blood volume regulation is eliminated. Filtration depends on adequate circulation to the glomerulus and maintaining normal filtration pressures. If local adjustments fail to maintain acceptable filtration pressures and the GFR declines, hormonal adjustments are initiated by the kidney. The result is a rise in filtration pressures and a restoration of normal glomerular filtration rates.

Hormonal Regulation of the Glomerular Filtration Rate. The *renin-angiotensin system* changes the glomerular filtration rate by its effects on blood pressure and volume. When glomerular blood pressure declines, so does the GFR. Under these conditions, the juxtaglomerular apparatus releases **renin** into the blood. Renin starts a chain reaction that ultimately involves many different systems, bringing about a coordinated

increase in blood volume and blood pressure. ∞ *p. 387* As glomerular blood pressure rises, so do the filtration pressure and the GFR.

Reabsorption and Secretion Along the Renal Tubule

Reabsorption and secretion at the kidney involve a combination of diffusion, osmosis, and carrier-mediated transport. In carrier-mediated transport, a specific substrate binds to a carrier protein that facilitates its movement across the cellular membrane. This movement may or may not require ATP molecules. ∞ *p. 61*

The Proximal Convoluted Tubule

The cells lining the PCT actively absorb organic nutrients, plasma proteins, and ions from the filtrate and transport them into the interstitial fluid. As these materials are absorbed and transported, osmotic forces pull water across the wall of the PCT and into the surrounding interstitial fluid. The PCT usually reclaims 60–70 percent of the volume of filtrate produced at the glomerulus, along with virtually all of the glucose, amino acids, and other organic nutrients. The PCT also actively reabsorbs ions, including sodium, potassium, calcium, magnesium, bicarbonate, phosphate, and sulfate ions. The ion pumps involved are individually regulated and may be influenced by circulating ion or hormone levels. For example, the presence of parathyroid hormone stimulates calcium ion reabsorption. ∞ *p. 318*

Although reabsorption represents the primary function of the PCT, a few substances, such as hydrogen ions, can be actively secreted into the tubular fluid. Active secretion can play an important role in the regulation of blood pH, a topic considered in a later section. A few compounds in the tubular fluid, including urea and uric acid, are ignored by the PCT and by other segments of the renal tubule. As water and other nutrients are removed, the concentration of these waste products gradually rises in the tubular fluid.

The Loop of Henle

Roughly 60–70 percent of the volume of the filtrate produced at the glomerulus has been reabsorbed before the tubular fluid reaches the loop of Henle. In the process, the useful organic molecules, along with many mineral ions, have been reclaimed. The loop of Henle will reabsorb more than half of the remaining water, as well as two-thirds of the sodium and chloride ions remaining in the tubular fluid.

The descending and ascending limbs of the loop of Henle have different permeability characteristics. The descending limb is permeable to water but not to solutes. Thus water can flow in or out by osmosis, but

19

solutes cannot cross the tubular epithelium. The ascending limb is impermeable both to water and to solutes. However, the ascending limb actively pumps sodium and chloride ions out of the tubular fluid and dumps them into the interstitial fluid of the renal medulla. Over time, a *concentration gradient* is created in the medulla, with the highest concentration of solutes (roughly four times that of plasma) near the bend in the loop of Henle. Because the descending limb is freely permeable to water, as tubular fluid flows along that limb, water flows out of the tubular fluid and into the interstitial fluid by osmosis.

Roughly half the volume of filtrate that enters the loop of Henle is reabsorbed in the descending limb, and most of the sodium and chloride ions are removed in the ascending limb. With the loss of the sodium and chloride ions, the solute concentration of the filtrate declines to around one-third that of plasma. However, waste products such as urea now make up a significant percentage of the remaining solutes. In essence, most of the water and solutes have been removed, leaving the waste products behind.

The Distal Convoluted Tubule and the Collecting System

By the time the filtrate reaches the distal convoluted tubule, roughly 80 percent of the water and 85 percent of the solutes have already been reabsorbed. The DCT is connected to a collecting duct that drains into the renal pelvis (Figure 19-7•).

As filtrate passes through the DCT and collecting duct, final adjustments are made in its composition and concentration. Composition depends on the type of solutes present; concentration depends on the volume of water in which they are dissolved. Because the DCT and collecting duct are impermeable to solutes, changes in filtrate composition can occur only through active reabsorption or secretion. The DCT is primarily concerned with active secretion.

Throughout most of the DCT, the tubular cells actively transport sodium ions out of the tubular fluid in exchange for potassium ions or hydrogen ions. The DCT and collecting ducts contain ion pumps that regulate the rates of sodium ion reabsorption and potassium ion secretion in response to the hormone **aldosterone**.

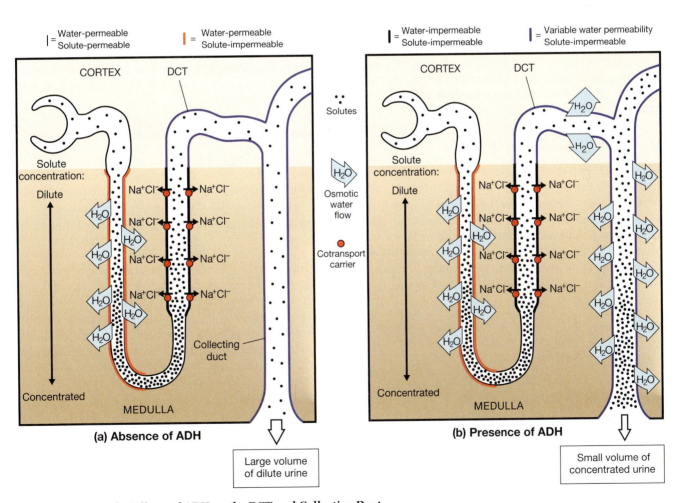

• **FIGURE 19-7   The Effects of ADH on the DCT and Collecting Duct**
(a) Permeabilities and urine production without ADH. **(b)** Permeabilities and urine production with ADH.

Aldosterone secretion occurs (1) in response to circulating ACTH from the anterior pituitary and (2) in response to elevated potassium ion concentrations in the extracellular fluid. The higher the aldosterone levels, the more sodium ions are reclaimed, and the more potassium ions are lost.

The amount of water reabsorbed along the DCT and collecting duct is controlled by circulating levels of *antidiuretic hormone (ADH)*. In the absence of ADH, the distal convoluted tubule and collecting duct are impermeable to water. The higher the level of circulating ADH, the greater the water permeability and the more concentrated the urine. Water moves out of the DCT and collecting duct because in each case the tubular fluid contains fewer solutes than the surrounding interstitial fluid. As noted above, the fluid arriving at the DCT has a solute concentration only around one-third that of the cortex, because the ascending limb of the loop of Henle has removed most of the sodium and chloride ions. The fluid passing along the collecting duct travels into the medulla, where it passes through the concentration gradient established by the loop of Henle.

If circulating ADH levels are low, little water reabsorption will occur, and virtually all of the water reaching the DCT will be lost in the urine (Figure 19-7a●). If circulating ADH levels are high, the DCT and collecting duct will be very permeable to water (Figure 19-7b●). In this case, the individual will produce a small quantity of urine with a solute concentration four to five times that of extracellular fluids.

The Properties of Normal Urine

The general characteristics of normal urine are listed in Table 19-3, but the composition of the 1.2 liters of urine excreted each day depends on the metabolic and hormonal events under way. Because the composition and concentration of the urine vary independently, an individual can produce a small quantity of concentrated urine or a large quantity of dilute urine and still excrete the same amount of dissolved materials. For this rea-

son, physicians often request a 24-hour urine collection rather than a single sample. This enables them to assess both quantity and composition accurately.

The Control of Kidney Function

Renal function is regulated in three ways: (1) by automatic adjustments in glomerular pressures, through changes in the diameters of the afferent and efferent arterioles; (2) through activities of the sympathetic division of the ANS; and (3) through the effects of hormones. The hormonal mechanisms make complex, long-term adjustments in blood pressure and blood volume that stabilize the GFR, in part by regulating transport mechanisms and water permeabilities of the DCT and collecting duct.

The Local Regulation of Kidney Function

Local, automatic changes in the diameters of the afferent arterioles, the efferent arterioles, and the glomerular capillaries can compensate for minor variations in blood pressure. For example, a reduction in blood flow and a decline in glomerular pressure trigger the dilation of the afferent arteriole and glomerular capillaries and the constriction of the efferent arteriole. This combination keeps glomerular blood pressure and blood flow within normal limits. As a result, filtration rates remain relatively constant despite a general decline in arterial blood pressures.

Sympathetic Activation and Kidney Function

Sympathetic activation has three different effects on kidney function. Over the short term, sympathetic activity primarily serves to shift blood away from the kidneys and lower the GFR during a sudden crisis or short-term emergency. Two different mechanisms are involved:

1. *Lowering the glomerular filtration rate by constricting the afferent arterioles and reducing blood flow to the glomerular capillaries.* The sympathetic activation triggered by an acute fall in blood pressure or a heart attack can override the hormonal regulatory mechanisms, and sustained sympathetic stimulation at high levels may cause kidney damage due to reduced blood flow and oxygen starvation.

2. *Changing the regional pattern of blood circulation.* This change can further reduce the GFR. For example, the dilation of superficial vessels in warm weather shunts blood away from the kidneys, and glomerular filtration declines temporarily. The effect becomes especially pronounced during periods of strenuous exercise. As the blood flow increases to the skin and skeletal muscles, it decreases to the kidneys. At maximal levels of exertion, renal blood flow

TABLE 19-3	General Characteristics of Normal Urine
pH	6.0 (range: 4.5–8)
Specific gravity	1.003–1.030
Osmolarity	855–1335 mOsm
Water content	93–97 percent
Volume	1200 ml/day
Color	Clear yellow
Odor	Varies with composition
Bacterial content	Sterile

19

FOCUS   A Summary of Urine Formation

Figure 19-8• summarizes the major steps involved in the reabsorption of water and the production of concentrated urine.

Step 1: Glomerular filtration produces a filtrate resembling blood plasma but containing few plasma proteins. This filtrate has the same solute concentration as plasma or interstitial fluid.

Step 2: In the proximal convoluted tubule, 60–70 percent of the water and almost all of the dissolved nutrients are reabsorbed. The osmolarity of the tubular fluid remains unchanged.

Step 3: In the PCT and descending limb of the loop of Henle, water moves into the surrounding interstitial fluid, leaving a small fluid volume (roughly 20 percent of the original filtrate) of highly concentrated tubular fluid.

Step 4: The ascending limb is impermeable to water and solutes. The tubular cells actively pump sodium and chloride ions out of the tubular fluid. Because only sodium and chloride ions are removed, urea now accounts for a higher proportion of the solutes in the tubular fluid.

Step 5: The final composition and concentration of the tubular fluid will be determined by the events under way in the DCT and the collecting ducts. These segments are impermeable to solutes, but ions may be actively transported into or out of the filtrate under the control of hormones such as aldosterone.

Step 6: The concentration of urine is controlled by variations in the water permeabilities of the DCT and the collecting ducts. These segments are impermeable to water unless exposed to antidiuretic hormone (ADH). In the absence of ADH, no water reabsorption occurs, and the individual produces a large volume of dilute urine. At high concentrations of ADH, the collecting ducts become freely permeable to water, and the individual produces a small volume of highly concentrated urine.

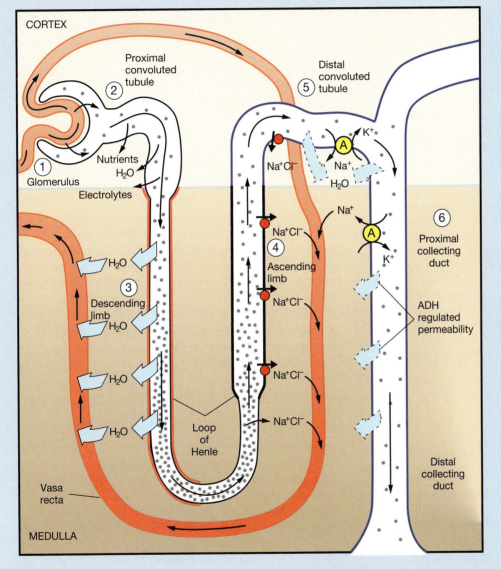

KEY:

•.• = Solutes

H_2O = Osmotic water flow

Membrane permeabilities:

▌ = Water-impermeable and solute-impermeable

▌ = Variable water permeability and solute-impermeable

Transport mechanism:

● = Cotransport carrier

(A) = Aldosterone-regulated exchange pump

▌ = Water-permeable and solute-impermeable

▌ = Water-permeable and solute-permeable

• **FIGURE 19-8   The Major Steps in Urine Production**

19

may be less than one-quarter of normal resting levels. This reduction can create problems for distance swimmers and marathon runners, whose glomerular cells may be damaged by low oxygen levels and the build up of metabolic wastes over the course of a long competition. After such events, protein is commonly lost in the urine, and in some cases, blood appears in the urine. Such problems generally disappear within 48 hours, although a small number of runners experience kidney, or renal, failure and permanent impairment of kidney function.

Over the long term, sympathetic activation stimulates an increase in blood pressure and blood volume by triggering the release of renin by the juxtaglomerular apparatus. After a severe hemorrhage or dehydration, the hormonal response is vital to restoring normal filtration rates and kidney function.

✳ HEMODIALYSIS

Renal failure (RF) can be either *acute (ARF)* or *chronic (CRF)*. ARF is a sudden drop in urine output to less than half a liter per day. It is not uncommon in the very ill, including the victim of multiple trauma. *Emergency hemodialysis* may be initiated. With hemodialysis, the most common type of dialysis, the patient is attached to a machine where their blood comes in contact with a large semipermeable membrane. On the opposite side of the semipermeable membrane is a specialized dialysate solution that is hypo-osmolar for substances that must be removed from the blood. Blood contacts this membrane, and targeted substances diffuse into the dialysate. The net effect of dialysis is the correction of electrolyte abnormalities and blood volume and the removal of toxic substances such as urea or creatinine. For patients requiring chronic hemodialysis, a vascular shunt, capable of handling blood flow of 300–400 mL per minute, is placed between a suitable vein and artery for dialysis access. Typically, the patient will dialyze for 2–3 hours, two or three times per week. Prior to the 1960s, dialysis was unavailable and patients with ARF or CRF died.

The Hormonal Control of Kidney Function

The major hormones involved in regulating kidney function are angiotensin II, ADH, aldosterone, and ANP. These hormones have been discussed in earlier chapters, so only a brief overview will be provided here. ∞ *pp. 313, 318, 320* The secretion of angiotensin II, aldosterone, and ADH is integrated by the *renin-angiotensin system.*

The Renin-Angiotensin System. If the glomerular pressures remain low because of a decrease in blood volume, a fall in systemic pressures, or a blockage in the renal artery or its tributaries, the juxtaglomerular apparatus releases renin into the circulation. Renin converts inactive *angiotensinogen* to *angiotensin I*, which a *converting enzyme* activates to **angiotensin II**. Figure 19-9● diagrams the primary effects of this potent hormone.

Angiotensin II has the following effects:

- *In peripheral capillary beds*, it causes a brief but powerful vasoconstriction, elevating blood pressure in the renal arteries.
- *At the nephron*, it triggers the contraction of the efferent arterioles, elevating glomerular pressures and filtration rates.
- *In the CNS*, it triggers the release of ADH, which in turn stimulates the reabsorption of water and sodium ions and causes the sensation of thirst.
- *At the adrenal gland*, it stimulates the secretion of aldosterone by the cortex and epinephrine and norepinephrine (NE) by the adrenal medullae. The result is a sudden, dramatic increase in systemic blood pressure. At the kidneys, aldosterone stimulates sodium reabsorption along the DCT and collecting system.

ADH. Antidiuretic hormone (1) increases the water permeability of the DCT and collecting duct, stimulating the reabsorption of water from the tubular fluid; and (2) causes the sensation of thirst, leading to the consumption of additional water. ADH release occurs under angiotensin II stimulation; it also occurs independently, when hypothalamic neurons are stimulated by a decrease in blood pressure or an increase in the solute concentration of the circulating blood. The nature of the receptors involved has not been determined, but these specialized hypothalamic neurons are called *osmoreceptors.*

Aldosterone. Aldosterone secretion stimulates the reabsorption of sodium ions and the secretion of potassium ions along the DCT and collecting duct. Aldosterone secretion primarily occurs (1) under angiotensin II stimulation ∞ *p. 387* and (2) in response to a rise in the potassium ion concentration of the blood.

Atrial Natriuretic Peptide. The actions of atrial natriuretic peptide (ANP) oppose those of the renin-angiotensin system (Figure 14-10b●, p. 388). This hormone is released by atrial cardiac muscle cells when blood volume and blood pressure are too high. The actions of ANP that affect the kidneys include (1) a decrease in the rate of sodium ion reabsorption in the DCT, leading to increased sodium ion loss in the urine; (2) the dilation of the glomerular capillaries, which results in increased glomerular filtration and urinary water loss; and (3) the inactivation of the renin-angiotensin system through the inhibition of renin, aldosterone, and ADH secretion. The net result is an accelerated loss of sodium ions and an increase in the volume of urine produced. This combination lowers blood volume and blood pressure.

19

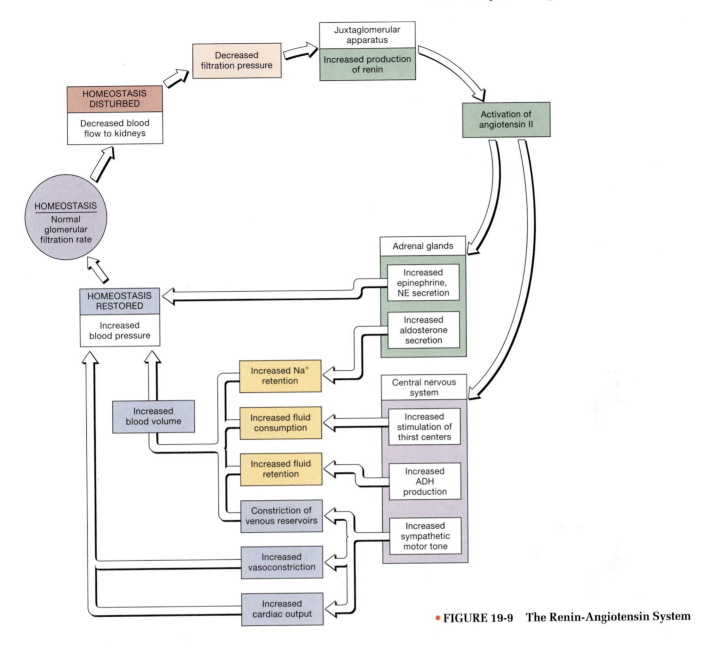

• FIGURE 19-9   The Renin-Angiotensin System

✓ How would a decrease in blood pressure affect the glomerular filtration rate (GFR)?

✓ If the nephrons lacked a loop of Henle, what would be the effect on the volume and solute (osmotic) concentration of the urine they produced?

URINE TRANSPORT, STORAGE, AND ELIMINATION

Filtrate modification and urine production end when the fluid enters the renal pelvis. The rest of the urinary system is responsible for the transport, storage, and elimination of the urine.

The Ureters and Urinary Bladder

The **ureters** (ū-RĒ-terz) are muscular tubes that carry urine from the kidneys to the urinary bladder, a distance of about 30 cm (12 in.) (Figures 19-1, p. 518, and 19-10a•). Like the kidneys, the ureters are retroperitoneal, and they penetrate the posterior wall of the bladder without entering the peritoneal cavity. Under normal conditions, peristaltic contractions begin at the apex of the renal papillae and sweep along the minor and major calyces toward the renal pelvis. Similar contractions move urine out of the renal pelvis and along the ureter to the bladder.

The **urinary bladder** is a muscular, distensible sac that stores urine prior to urination. In males, the base of the urinary bladder lies between the rectum and the

1 9

pubic symphysis (Figure 19-10a•). In females, the urinary bladder sits inferior to the uterus and anterior to the vagina (Figure 19-10b•). Its dimensions vary, depending on the state of distension, but the full urinary bladder can contain up to a liter of urine.

In sectional view, the triangular area bounded by the **ureteral openings** and the entrance to the urethra constitutes the *trigone* (TRĪ-gōn) of the bladder (Figure 19-10c•). The urethral entrance lies at the apex of this triangle, at the lowest point in the bladder. The area surrounding the urethral entrance, called the *neck* of the urinary bladder, contains a muscular sphincter that also extends along the proximal portions of the urethra. This **internal urethral sphincter** provides involuntary control over the discharge of urine from the bladder.

A *transitional epithelium* lines the renal pelvis, the ureters, and the urinary bladder. This stratified epithelium can tolerate a considerable amount of stretching, as indicated in Figure 4-5b•. ∞ *p. 87* The bladder wall contains both longitudinal and circular smooth muscle layers that form the powerful *detrusor* (de-TROO-sor) *muscle* of the bladder. Contraction of this muscle compresses the urinary bladder and expels its contents into the urethra.

The Urethra

In females, the **urethra** is very short, extending 2.5–3.0 cm (about 1 in.) from the bladder to the vestibule. In males, the urethra extends from the neck of the urinary bladder to the tip of the penis, about 18–20 cm (7–8 in.) in length. In both sexes, as the urethra passes through the *urogenital diaphragm*, a circular band of skeletal muscle forms the **external urethral sphincter**. This sphincter consists of skeletal muscle fibers, and its contractions are under voluntary control.

The Micturition Reflex and Urination

Urine reaches the urinary bladder by the peristaltic contractions of the ureters. The process of **urination**, or **micturition** (mik-tu-RI-shun), is coordinated by the **micturition reflex** (Figure 19-11•). Stretch receptors in the wall of the urinary bladder are stimulated as it fills with urine. Afferent sensory fibers in the pelvic nerves carry the resulting impulses to the sacral spinal cord. The increased level of activities by the sensory receptors and the sensory fibers (1) facilitates parasympathetic motor

1
9

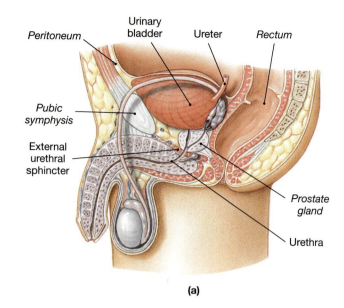

(a)

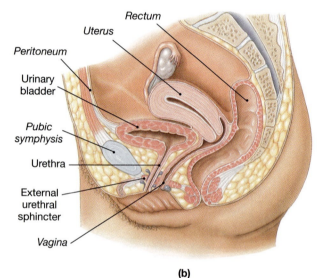

(b)

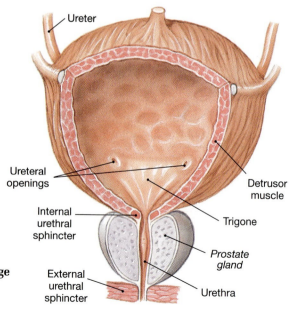

(c)

• **FIGURE 19-10   Organs Responsible for the Conduction and Storage of Urine**
(a) The ureter, urinary bladder, and urethra of a male.
(b) The same organs in a female. **(c)** The urinary bladder of a male.

neurons in the sacral spinal cord and (2) stimulates interneurons that relay sensations to the cerebral cortex. As a result, we become consciously aware of the fluid pressure in the urinary bladder.

The urge to urinate usually occurs when the bladder contains about 200 ml of urine. The micturition reflex begins to function when the stretch receptors have provided adequate stimulation to the parasympathetic motor neurons. At this time, the motor neurons stimulate the smooth muscle in the bladder wall. These commands travel over the pelvic nerves and produce a sustained contraction of the urinary bladder.

This contraction elevates fluid pressures inside the bladder, but urine ejection cannot occur unless both the internal and external sphincters are relaxed. We control the time and place of urination by voluntarily relaxing the external sphincter. When this sphincter relaxes, so does the internal sphincter. If the external sphincter does not relax, the internal sphincter remains closed, and the bladder gradually relaxes. A further increase in bladder volume begins the cycle again, usually within an hour. Each increase in urinary volume leads to an increase in stretch receptor stimulation that makes the sensation more acute. Once the volume of the urinary bladder exceeds 500 ml, the micturition reflex may generate enough pressure to force open the internal sphincter. This opening leads to a reflexive relaxation in the external sphincter, and urination occurs despite voluntary opposition or potential inconvenience. Normally, after micturition, less than 10 ml of urine remain in the bladder.

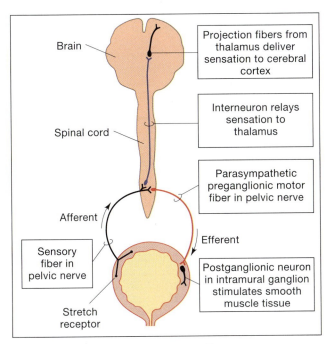

•FIGURE 19-11   The Micturition Reflex
The basic components of the reflex arc involved in the micturition reflex.

Labels in figure:
Brain
Projection fibers from thalamus deliver sensation to cerebral cortex
Spinal cord
Interneuron relays sensation to thalamus
Parasympathetic preganglionic motor fiber in pelvic nerve
Afferent
Efferent
Sensory fiber in pelvic nerve
Postganglionic neuron in intramural ganglion stimulates smooth muscle tissue
Stretch receptor

GENITOURINARY SYSTEM TRAUMA

The *genitourinary (GU)* system is vulnerable to trauma. Isolated trauma to the GU system is uncommon. Most GU injuries occur in conjunction with other injuries.

Renal injury is the most common form of GU trauma. The kidneys are well protected in their retroperitoneal location. Because of this, it takes considerable force to cause significant renal injury. Penetrating injuries are usually secondary to gunshots and stab wounds. Common renal injuries include contusion (bruising), laceration, rupture, renal pedicle injury, and rupture of the renal pelvis.

Bladder injuries are the second most common injury to the GU tract and are usually associated with blunt trauma to the pelvis. The least severe bladder injury is the bladder contusion. In more severe cases, the bladder can rupture, spilling urine. This usually occurs when the bladder is full. Bladder rupture is usually classified as intraperitoneal or extraperitoneal. With intraperitoneal rupture, urine is spilled into the peritoneal cavity. In extraperitoneal rupture, urine spillage occurs into the tissue around the bladder.

Urethral injuries are usually associated with pelvic fractures, but can occur with blunt trauma such as a kick to the groin or a straddle injury. Urethral injury is more common in males due to the increased urethral length.

GU injuries, as a rule, are not life threatening. Treatment of other life-threatening injuries takes precedence over GU injury.

INTEGRATION WITH OTHER SYSTEMS

Along with the urinary system, the integumentary, respiratory, and digestive systems are sometimes considered to form an anatomically diverse *excretory system*:

1. *Integumentary system*. Water and electrolyte losses in perspiration affect plasma volume and composition. The effects are most apparent when losses are extreme, as in maximum sweat production. Small amounts of metabolic wastes are also excreted in perspiration.

2. *Respiratory system*. The lungs excrete the carbon dioxide generated by cells. Small amounts of other compounds, such as acetone and water, evaporate into the alveoli and are eliminated during exhalation.

3. *Digestive system*. Small amounts of metabolic waste products are excreted in liver bile, and a variable amount of water is lost in feces.

These excretory activities affect the composition of body fluids. The respiratory system, for example, is the primary site of carbon dioxide excretion. But the excretory functions of these systems are not regulated as closely as are those of the kidneys, and the effects of integumentary and digestive excretory activities normally are minor compared with those of the urinary system.

Figure 19-12• summarizes the functional relationships between the urinary system and other systems.

1
9

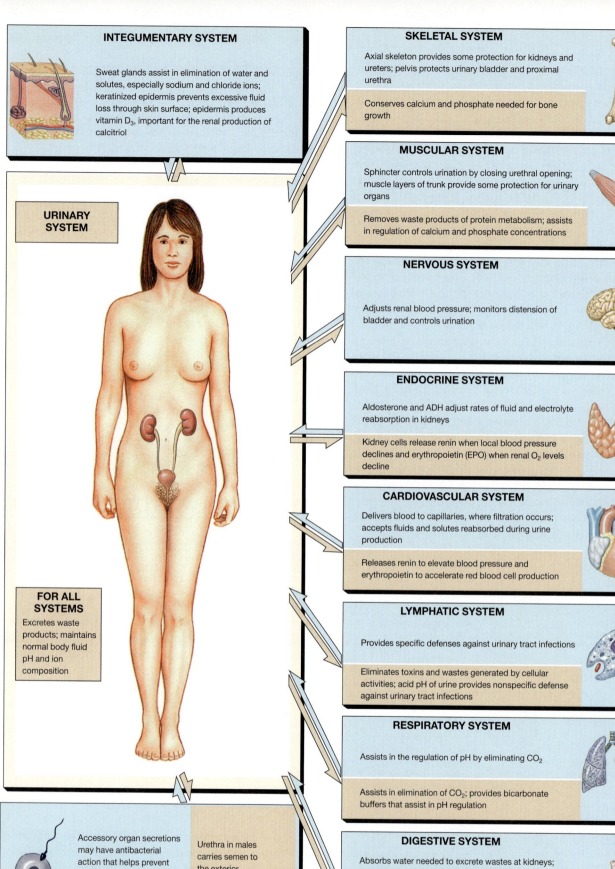

INTEGUMENTARY SYSTEM

Sweat glands assist in elimination of water and solutes, especially sodium and chloride ions; keratinized epidermis prevents excessive fluid loss through skin surface; epidermis produces vitamin D_3, important for the renal production of calcitriol

URINARY SYSTEM

FOR ALL SYSTEMS

Excretes waste products; maintains normal body fluid pH and ion composition

SKELETAL SYSTEM

Axial skeleton provides some protection for kidneys and ureters; pelvis protects urinary bladder and proximal urethra

Conserves calcium and phosphate needed for bone growth

MUSCULAR SYSTEM

Sphincter controls urination by closing urethral opening; muscle layers of trunk provide some protection for urinary organs

Removes waste products of protein metabolism; assists in regulation of calcium and phosphate concentrations

NERVOUS SYSTEM

Adjusts renal blood pressure; monitors distension of bladder and controls urination

ENDOCRINE SYSTEM

Aldosterone and ADH adjust rates of fluid and electrolyte reabsorption in kidneys

Kidney cells release renin when local blood pressure declines and erythropoietin (EPO) when renal O_2 levels decline

CARDIOVASCULAR SYSTEM

Delivers blood to capillaries, where filtration occurs; accepts fluids and solutes reabsorbed during urine production

Releases renin to elevate blood pressure and erythropoietin to accelerate red blood cell production

LYMPHATIC SYSTEM

Provides specific defenses against urinary tract infections

Eliminates toxins and wastes generated by cellular activities; acid pH of urine provides nonspecific defense against urinary tract infections

RESPIRATORY SYSTEM

Assists in the regulation of pH by eliminating CO_2

Assists in elimination of CO_2; provides bicarbonate buffers that assist in pH regulation

DIGESTIVE SYSTEM

Absorbs water needed to excrete wastes at kidneys; absorbs ions needed to maintain normal body fluid concentrations; liver removes bilirubin

Excretes toxins absorbed by the digestive epithelium; excretes bilirubin and nitrogenous wastes produced by the liver

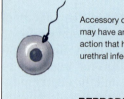

Accessory organ secretions may have antibacterial action that helps prevent urethral infections in males

Urethra in males carries semen to the exterior

REPRODUCTIVE SYSTEM

•FIGURE 19-12   Functional Relationships Between the Urinary System and Other Systems

19

Many of these relationships will be explored further in the next section, which considers fluid, pH, and electrolyte balance.

✓ What process is responsible for the movement of urine from the kidney to the urinary bladder?

✓ An obstruction of a ureter by a kidney stone would interfere with the flow of urine between what two points?

✓ The ability to control the micturition reflex depends on your ability to control which muscle?

FLUID, ELECTROLYTE, AND ACID-BASE BALANCE

The next time you see a small pond, take a moment to think about the fish it contains. They live out their lives totally dependent on the quality of their isolated environment. If evaporation removes too much of the pond water, oxygen and food supplies run out, and the fish suffocate or starve. Most of the fish in a freshwater pond will die if the water becomes too salty; those in a saltwater pond will be killed if their environment becomes too dilute. The pH of the pond water, too, is a vital factor—water that is too acidic or too alkaline will also kill the fish in the pond.

The cells of our bodies live in a pond whose shores are the exposed surfaces of the skin. Most of the weight of the human body is water. Water accounts for up to 99 percent of the volume of extracellular fluid (ECF) and is an essential ingredient of cytoplasm. All of a cell's operations rely on water as a diffusion medium for the distribution of gases, nutrients, and waste products. If the water content of the body changes, cellular activities are jeopardized. For example, when the water content of the body reaches very low levels, proteins denature, enzymes cease functioning, and cells ultimately die.

The ionic concentrations and pH of the body's water are as important as its absolute quantity. If concentrations of calcium or potassium ions in the ECF become too high, cardiac arrhythmias develop, and the individual's life is in jeopardy. A pH outside the normal range can lead to a variety of dangerous problems. Low pH is especially dangerous because hydrogen ions break chemical bonds, change the shapes of complex molecules, disrupt cell membranes, and impair tissue functions.

This section considers the dynamics of exchange between the various body fluids, such as blood plasma and interstitial fluid, and between the body and the external environment. Several different but interrelated types of homeostasis are involved:

- A person is in *fluid balance* when the amount of water gained each day is equal to the amount lost to the environment. Maintaining normal fluid balance involves regulating the content and distribution of water in the body.
- *Electrolyte balance* exists when there is neither a net gain nor a net loss of any ion in body fluids.
- *Acid-base balance* exists when the production of hydrogen ions precisely offsets their loss. While acid-base balance exists, the pH of body fluids remains within normal limits.

This section provides an overview that integrates earlier discussions of fluid, electrolyte, and acid-base balance in the body. Few other chapters have such wide-ranging clinical importance: *Treatment of any serious illness affecting the nervous, cardiovascular, respiratory, urinary, or digestive system must always include steps to restore normal fluid, electrolyte, and acid-base balance.*

Fluid and Electrolyte Balance

Figure 19-13• illustrates the distribution of water in the body. Nearly two-thirds of the total body water content is found inside living cells, as the fluid medium of the intracellular fluid (ICF), introduced in Chapter 3. ∞ *p. 65* The extracellular fluid (ECF) contains the rest of the body water. The largest subdivisions of the ECF are (1) the *tissue fluid*, or *interstitial fluid*, in peripheral tissues and (2) the *plasma* of the circulating blood. Minor components of the ECF include lymph, cerebrospinal fluid (CSF), synovial fluid, serous fluids (pleural, pericardial, and peritoneal fluids), aqueous humor, perilymph, and endolymph.

Exchange between these subdivisions of the ECF occurs primarily across the endothelial lining of capillaries. Fluid may also travel from the interstitial spaces to the plasma by way of the channels of the lymphatic system. Although there are regional variations in the identity and quantity of dissolved electrolytes, proteins, nutrients, and waste products within the ECF, these variations are relatively minor compared with the compositional differences *between* the ECF and the ICF.

In many respects, the ICF and ECF behave as distinct entities, and they are often called **fluid compartments**. As noted in earlier chapters, the principal ions in the ECF are sodium, chloride, and bicarbonate. The ICF contains an abundance of potassium, magnesium, and phosphate ions, plus large numbers of negatively charged proteins.

Despite these differences in the concentration of specific substances, the intracellular and extracellular osmolarities are identical. The cell membranes are freely

1 9

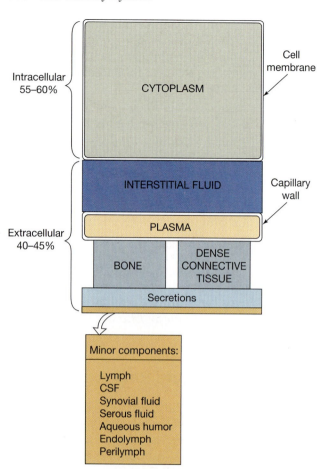

•FIGURE 19-13   Body Fluid Compartments
The major body fluid compartments in a healthy adult. For information concerning the chemical composition of body fluids, see Appendix IV.

permeable to water, and osmosis eliminates any minor concentration differences almost at once.

Fluid Balance

Water circulates freely within the extracellular fluid compartment. At capillary beds throughout the body, capillary blood pressure forces water out of the plasma and into the interstitial spaces. Some of that water is reabsorbed along the distal portion of the capillary bed, and the rest circulates into lymphatic vessels for transport to the venous circulation (see Figure 14-5•, p. 382).

Water moves back and forth across the epithelial surfaces lining the peritoneal, pleural, and pericardial cavities and through the synovial membranes lining joint capsules. The flow rate is significant; for example, roughly 7 liters of peritoneal fluid is produced and reabsorbed each day. Water also moves between the blood and the cerebrospinal fluid, the aqueous and vitreous humors of the eye, and the perilymph and endolymph of the inner ear.

Roughly 2500 ml of water is lost each day through urine, feces, and perspiration. The losses due to per-

spiration vary, depending on the activities undertaken, but the additional deficits can be considerable, reaching well over 4 liters an hour. ∞ *p. 114* Water losses are normally balanced by the gain of fluids through eating (48 percent), drinking (40 percent), and metabolic generation (12 percent).

Fluid Shifts

Water movement between the ECF and ICF is called a *fluid shift*. Fluid shifts occur relatively rapidly, reaching equilibrium within a period of minutes to hours. These shifts occur in response to changes in the osmotic concentration, or *osmolarity*, of the extracellular fluid.

- If the ECF becomes more concentrated (hypertonic) with respect to the ICF, water will move from the cells into the ECF until osmotic equilibrium is restored.
- If the ECF becomes more dilute (hypotonic) with respect to the ICF, water will move from the ECF into the cells, and the volume of the ICF will increase accordingly.

In summary, if the osmolarity of the ECF changes, a fluid shift between the ICF and ECF will tend to oppose the change. Because the volume of the ICF is much greater than that of the ECF, the ICF acts as a "water reserve." In effect, instead of a large change in the composition of the ECF, there are smaller changes in both the ECF and the ICF.

Electrolyte Balance

An individual is in electrolyte balance when the rates of gain and loss are equal for each of the individual electrolytes in the body. Electrolyte balance is important for the following reasons:

- *A gain or loss of electrolytes can cause a gain or loss in water.*
- *The concentrations of individual electrolytes affect a variety of cell functions.* Many examples of ion effects on cell function were described in earlier chapters. For example, the effects of high or low calcium and potassium ion concentrations on cardiac muscle tissue were noted in Chapter 13. ∞ *p. 370*

Two cations, sodium and potassium, merit special attention because (1) they are major contributors to the osmolarities of the ECF and ICF, and (2) they have direct effects on the normal functioning of living cells. Regulatory mechanisms involving a third important ion, calcium, were discussed in Chapters 6 and 11. ∞ *p. 127, 316*

Sodium is the dominant cation within the extracellular fluid. Because more than 90 percent of the osmolarity of the ECF results from the presence of sodium salts, principally sodium chloride ($NaCl$) and sodium bicarbonate ($NaHCO_3$), alterations in the osmolarity of extracellular fluids usually reflect changes in the concentration of sodium ions. Potassium is the dominant cation in the intracellular fluid; extracellular potassium concentrations are normally low. In general:

- *The most common problems with electrolyte balance are caused by an imbalance between sodium gains and losses.*
- *Problems with potassium balance are less common but significantly more dangerous than those related to sodium balance.*

Sodium Balance. The amount of sodium in the ECF represents a balance between sodium ion absorption at the digestive tract and sodium ion excretion at the kidneys and other sites. The rate of uptake varies directly with the amount included in the diet. The kidneys are responsible for regulating sodium ion losses, in response to circulating levels of aldosterone (decreased sodium loss) and ANP (increased sodium loss).

Whenever the rate of sodium intake or output changes, a corresponding gain or loss of water tends to keep the sodium concentration constant. For example, eating a heavily salted meal will not raise the sodium ion concentration of body fluids, because as sodium chloride crosses the digestive epithelium, osmosis brings additional water into the body. (This is why individuals with high blood pressure are told to restrict their salt intake; dietary salt will be absorbed, and because "water follows salt," the blood volume and blood pressure will increase.)

Potassium Balance. Potassium ions are the primary cations of the intracellular fluid. Roughly 98 percent of the potassium content of the body lies within the ICF. The potassium concentration of the ECF, which is relatively low, represents a balance between (1) the rate of potassium ion entry across the digestive epithelium and (2) the rate of loss into the urine. The rate of entry is proportional to the amount of potassium in the diet. Urinary potassium losses are controlled by adjusting the rate of active secretion along the distal convoluted tubules of the kidneys. The secondary rate is primarily determined by aldosterone levels. The ion pumps sensitive to this hormone reabsorb sodium ions from the filtrate in exchange for potassium ions from the interstitial fluid. When potassium levels rise in the ECF, aldosterone levels climb, and additional potassium ions are lost in the urine. When potassium levels fall in the ECF, aldosterone levels fall and potassium ions are conserved.

✓ How would eating a salty meal affect the amount of fluid in the intracellular fluid compartment?

✓ What effect would being lost in the desert for a day without water have on your blood osmolarity?

Acid-Base Balance

The pH of body fluids represents a balance between the acids, bases, and salts in solution. This pH normally remains within relatively narrow limits, usually from 7.35 to 7.45. Any deviation outside the normal range is extremely dangerous because changes in hydrogen ion concentrations disrupt the stability of cell membranes, alter protein structure, and change the activities of important enzymes.

When the pH falls below 7.35, a state of **acidosis** exists. **Alkalosis** exists if the pH exceeds 7.45. These conditions affect virtually all systems, but the nervous system and cardiovascular system are particularly sensitive to pH fluctuations. For example, severe acidosis can be deadly because (1) CNS function deteriorates, and the individual becomes comatose; (2) cardiac contractions grow weak and irregular, and symptoms of heart failure develop; and (3) peripheral vasodilation produces a dramatic drop in blood pressure, possibly causing circulatory collapse.

Although acidosis and alkalosis are both dangerous, in practice, problems with acidosis are much more common than problems with alkalosis because several different types of acids are generated by normal cellular activities.

Acids in the Body

Carbon dioxide concentration is the most important factor affecting the pH in body tissues. In solution, carbon dioxide interacts with water to form molecules of carbonic acid (H_2CO_3). As noted in Chapter 16, the carbonic acid molecules then dissociate to produce hydrogen ions and bicarbonate ions. ∞ *p. 453* The complete reaction sequence is:

$$CO_2 + H_2O \leftrightarrow H_2CO_3 \leftrightarrow H^+ + HCO_3^-$$

This reaction occurs spontaneously in body fluids, but it occurs very rapidly in the presence of *carbonic anhydrase*, an intracellular enzyme found in red blood cells, liver and kidney cells, parietal cells of the stomach, and in many other cell types.

Because most of the carbon dioxide in solution is converted to carbonic acid, and most of the carbonic acid dissociates, there is a direct relationship between the P_{CO_2} and the pH (Figure 19-14•). ∞ *p. 455* When carbon dioxide concentrations rise, additional hydrogen ions and bicarbonate ions are released, and the pH

19

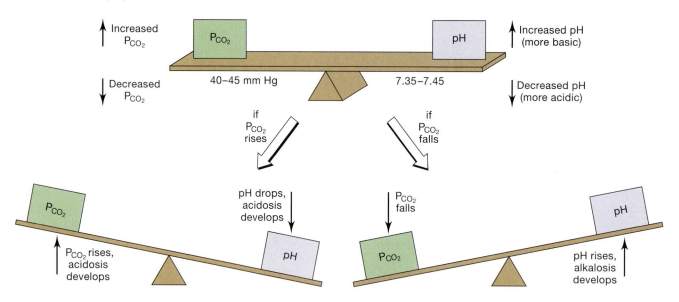

• **FIGURE 19-14** **Basic Relationships Between Carbon Dioxide and Plasma pH**

goes down. (Remember that the smaller the pH value, the greater the acidity.)

At the alveoli, carbon dioxide diffuses into the atmosphere, the number of hydrogen ions and bicarbonate ions declines, and the pH rises. This process, which effectively removes hydrogen ions from solution, will be considered in more detail later in the chapter.

Metabolic acids are generated during normal metabolism. Some are generated during the catabolism of amino acids, carbohydrates, or lipids. Examples are lactic acid produced during anaerobic metabolism and ketone bodies produced when breaking down fatty acids. Under normal conditions, metabolic acids are recycled or excreted rapidly, and significant accumulations do not occur.

Buffers and Buffer Systems

The acids discussed above, produced in the course of normal metabolic operations, must be controlled by the buffers and buffer systems in body fluids. *Buffers*, introduced in Chapter 2, are dissolved compounds that can provide or remove hydrogen ions and thereby stabilize the pH of a solution. ∞ *p. 37* Buffers include *weak acids* that can donate hydrogen ions and *weak bases* that can absorb them. A **buffer system** consists of a combination of a weak acid and its dissociation products: a hydrogen ion (H^+) and an anion. There are three major buffer systems, each with slightly different characteristics and distribution: the *protein buffer system*, the *carbonic acid–bicarbonate buffer system*, and the *phosphate buffer system*.

Protein buffer systems contribute to the regulation of pH in the ECF and ICF. Protein buffer systems depend on the ability of amino acids to respond to alterations in pH by accepting or releasing hydrogen ions. If

the pH climbs, the carboxyl group ($-COOH$) of the amino acid can dissociate, releasing a hydrogen ion. If the pH drops, the amino group ($-NH_2$) can accept an additional hydrogen ion, forming an $-NH_3^+$ group.

The plasma proteins and hemoglobin in red blood cells make substantial contributions to the buffering capabilities of the blood. In the interstitial fluids, extracellular protein fibers and dissolved amino acids also help regulate pH. In the intracellular fluids of active cells, structural and other proteins provide an extensive buffering capability that prevents destructive pH changes when organic acids are produced by cellular metabolism.

The **carbonic acid–bicarbonate buffer system** is an important buffer system in the ECF. Carbon dioxide generation occurs in all living tissues. As detailed earlier, most of it is converted to carbonic acid, which then dissociates into a hydrogen ion and a bicarbonate ion. The net effect is that $CO_2 + H_2O \leftrightarrow H^+ + HCO_3^-$. The carbonic acid and its dissociation products form the carbonic acid–bicarbonate buffer system. If hydrogen ions are removed, they will be replaced through the combination of water and carbon dioxide; if hydrogen ions are added, most will be removed through the formation of carbon dioxide and water.

The primary role of the carbonic acid–bicarbonate buffer system is to prevent pH changes caused by metabolic acids. The hydrogen ions released through the dissociation of these acids combine with bicarbonate ions, producing water and carbon dioxide. The carbon dioxide can then be excreted at the lungs. This buffering system can cope with large amounts of acid because body fluids contain an abundance of bicarbonate ions, primarily in the form of dissolved molecules of *sodium bicarbonate*, $NaHCO_3$. This readily available supply of bicarbonate ions is known as the *bicarbonate reserve*. When hydrogen ions enter the ECF, the bicarbonate ions that combine with them are replaced by the bicarbonate reserve.

The **phosphate buffer system** consists of an anion, $H_2PO_4^-$, that is a weak acid. In solution, it reversibly dissociates into a hydrogen ion and HPO_4^{2-}. In the ECF, the phosphate buffer system plays only a supporting role in the regulation of pH, primarily because the concentration of bicarbonate ions far exceeds that of phosphate ions. However, the phosphate buffer system is quite important in buffering the pH of the intracellular fluids, where the concentration of phosphate ions is relatively high.

Maintaining Acid-Base Balance

The maintenance of acid-base balance involves controlling hydrogen ion losses and gains. In this process, the pulmonary and renal mechanisms support the buffer systems by (1) secreting or absorbing hydrogen ions, (2) controlling the excretion of acids and bases, and, when necessary, (3) generating additional buffers. It is the *combination* of buffer systems and these pulmonary and renal mechanisms that maintains pH within narrow limits. Table 19-4 summarizes the major classes of acid-base disorders by their characteristic pH values, general causes, and treatments.

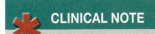

CLINICAL NOTE   DISTURBANCES OF ACID-BASE BALANCE

The maintenance of normal *acid-base balance* is one of the body's most important homeostatic functions. A problem with acid-base balance can constitute a serious medical emergency requiring immediate treatment.

The body's pH is tightly regulated. Changes in pH seldom exceed 0.1 pH units. However, in disease, significant pH shifts can occur. Normal pH is considered 7.35 to 7.45. A pH less than 7.35 is considered *acidosis,* while a pH greater than 7.45 is considered *alkalosis.* The body controls pH principally through three systems: the *buffer systems,* the *respiratory system,* and the *renal system.*

The buffer systems remove hydrogen ions preventing a significant change in pH. The three major buffer systems are the *protein buffer system, the carbonic acid-bicarbonate buffer system,* and the *phosphate buffer system.* The buffer systems react immediately to changes in pH.

The respiratory system compensates for changes in pH by increasing or decreasing respirations. It is primarily controlled by changes in the carbon dioxide (PCO_2) level. An increase in the PCO_2 stimulates respirations causing the removal of CO_2 molecules. Likewise, a decrease in PCO_2 inhibits respirations, causing CO_2 molecules to accumulate.

The renal system reacts to changes in pH by producing more acidic or more alkaline urine. When the body's pH falls, the distal tubule of the kidney begins excreting hydrogen ions into the urine and reabsorbing bicarbonate. Likewise, when the body's pH rises, the distal tubule slows hydrogen ion secretion and reabsorbs less bicarbonate.

Acid-base disorders are classified based upon the source of the problem. Disorders due to an abnormality in the level of CO_2 in the body are termed *respiratory disorders. Metabolic disorders* are caused by the generation of organic or fixed acids. They can also be caused by conditions that affect the concentration of bicarbonate ions in the body.

- *Respiratory acidosis.* Respiratory acidosis is due to a decrease in alveolar ventilation resulting in CO_2 retention (*hypercapnia*). The excess CO_2 is converted to carbonic acid, which decreases the pH. Causes of respiratory acidosis include sedative drugs, brain stem trauma, respiratory

muscle paralysis, and disorders of the chest wall. Disorders of the lung parenchyma, such as pneumonia, asthma, emphysema, pulmonary edema, and bronchitis, can also cause respiratory acidosis. Respiratory acidosis can be either acute or chronic. Chronic respiratory acidosis is seen in chronic obstructive pulmonary disease (COPD) and deformities of the chest wall. In chronic respiratory acidosis, the renal system ultimately compensates by increasing hydrogen ion excretion. Treatment of respiratory acidosis involves increasing ventilation and correcting the underlying cause.

- *Respiratory alkalosis.* Respiratory alkalosis occurs when alveolar ventilation is increased resulting in excess elimination of CO_2 (*hypocapnia*) and an increase in pH. Oftentimes, stimulation of ventilation is due to *hypoxemia* (low oxygen levels) from problems such as pulmonary disease, congestive heart failure, high altitudes, fever, and early salicylate intoxication. A common cause of hyperventilation and subsequent respiratory alkalosis is *hysteria* (hyperventilation). Treatment of respiratory alkalosis involves correcting the underlying cause. In selected cases, hyperventilation from hysteria can be remedied by having a patient rebreathe into a paper bag, thus increasing CO_2 levels.

- *Metabolic acidosis.* In metabolic acidosis, there is an accumulation of noncarbonic acids or a loss of bicarbonate. Causes include lactic acidosis (from poor perfusion), renal failure, or diabetic ketoacidosis. The buffer systems attempt to compensate. Respirations are increased as the pH falls, resulting in elimination of CO_2. The renal system secretes excess hydrogen ions. Treatment is directed at correcting the underlying causes. In severe cases, administration of sodium bicarbonate ($NaHCO_3$) may be required to aid in buffering the excess acids.

- *Metabolic alkalosis.* Metabolic alkalosis is due to an increase in bicarbonate or to excessive loss of metabolic acids. Causes include prolonged vomiting, gastrointestinal suctioning, excessive bicarbonate intake, or diuretic therapy. Vomiting and gastrointestinal suctioning can cause loss of gastric acids ultimately leading to metabolic alkalosis. Treatment is directed at correcting the underlying cause.

19

TABLE 19-4	Acid-Base Disorders		
Disorder	*pH (normal = 7.35–7.45)*	*Remarks*	*Treatment*
Respiratory acidosis	Decreased (below 7.35)	Usually caused by hypoventilation and CO_2 buildup in tissues and blood	Improve ventilation, in some cases, with bronchodilation and mechanical assistance
Metabolic acidosis	Decreased (below 7.35)	Caused by organic or fixed acid buildup, impaired H^+ excretion at kidneys, or bicarbonate loss in urine or feces	Administration of bicarbonate (gradual) with other steps as needed to correct primary cause
Respiratory alkalosis	Increased (above 7.45)	Usually caused by hyperventilation and reduction in plasma CO_2 levels	Reduce respiratory rate, allow rise in P_{CO_2}
Metabolic alkalosis	Increased (above 7.45)	Usually caused by prolonged vomiting and associated gastric acid loss	pH below 7.55, no treatment; pH above 7.55 may require administration of ammonium chloride

Pulmonary Contributions to pH Regulation.   The lungs contribute to pH regulation by their effects on the carbonic acid–bicarbonate buffer system. Increasing or decreasing the rate of respiration can have a profound effect on the buffering capacity of body fluids by lowering or raising the P_{CO_2}. Changes in P_{CO_2} have a direct effect on the concentration of hydrogen ions in the plasma, since the additional carbon dioxide molecules will form carbonic acid, which immediately dissociates.

Mechanisms responsible for controlling the respiratory rate were discussed in Chapter 16 ∞ *p. 454*, and only a brief summary will be presented here. A rise in P_{CO_2} stimulates chemoreceptors in the carotid and aortic bodies, and within the CNS; a fall in the P_{CO_2} inhibits them. Stimulation of the chemoreceptors leads to an increase in the respiratory rate. As the rate of respiration increases, more CO_2 is lost at the lungs, and the P_{CO_2} returns to normal levels. When the P_{CO_2} of the blood or CSF declines, respiratory activity becomes depressed, the breathing rate falls, and the P_{CO_2} in the extracellular fluids rises.

Changes in respiratory rate affect pH because when the P_{CO_2} rises, the pH declines, and when the P_{CO_2} decreases, the pH increases (Figure 19-14●). A change in the respiratory rate that helps stabilize pH is called **respiratory compensation.**

Renal Contributions to pH Regulation.   Glomerular filtration puts hydrogen ions, carbon dioxide, and the other components of the carbonic acid–bicarbonate and phosphate buffer systems into the filtrate. The kidney tubules then modify the pH of the filtrate by secreting hydrogen ions or reabsorbing bicarbonate ions. A change in the rates of hydrogen ion and bicarbonate ion secretion or absorption in response to changes in plasma pH is called **renal compensation**.

✓ What effect would a decrease in the pH of the body fluids have on the respiratory rate?

✓ How would a prolonged fast affect the body's pH?

✓ Why can prolonged vomiting produce alkalosis?

AGING AND THE URINARY SYSTEM

In general, aging is associated with an increased incidence of kidney problems. Age-related changes in the urinary system include:

1. *A decline in the number of functional nephrons.* The total number of kidney nephrons drops by 30–40 percent between ages 25 and 85.

2. *A reduction in the GFR.* This results from decreased numbers of glomeruli, cumulative damage to the filtration apparatus in the remaining glomeruli, and reductions in renal blood flow.

3. *Reduced sensitivity to ADH.* With age, the distal portions of the nephron and collecting system become less responsive to ADH. Less reabsorption of water and sodium ions occurs, and more potassium ions are lost in the urine.

4. *Problems with the micturition reflex.* Several factors are involved in such problems:

1
9

- The sphincter muscles lose muscle tone and become less effective at voluntarily retaining urine. Loss of muscle tone leads to problems with incontinence, often involving a slow leakage of urine.
- The ability to control micturition is often lost after a stroke, Alzheimer's disease, or other CNS problems affecting the cerebral cortex or hypothalamus.
- In males, **urinary retention** may develop secondary to enlargement of the prostate gland. In this condition, swelling and distortion of surrounding prostatic tissues compress the urethra, restricting or preventing the flow of urine.

5. *A gradual decrease of total body water content with age.* Between ages 40 and 60, total body water content averages 55 percent for males and 47 percent for females. After age 60, the values decline to roughly 50 percent for males and 45 percent for females. Among other effects, this decrease results in concentrating waste products, toxins, and administered drugs.

6. *A net loss in body mineral content in many people over age 60 as muscle mass and skeletal mass decrease.* This loss can, at least in part, be prevented by a combination of exercise and increased dietary mineral supply.

Chapter Review

KEY TERMS

SUMMARY OUTLINE

INTRODUCTION *p. 518*

1. The functions of the urinary system include the (1) elimination of organic waste products, (2) regulation of plasma ion concentrations, (3) regulation of blood volume and pressure by adjusting the volume of water lost and releasing hormones, (4) homeostasis of blood pH, and (5) conservation of nutrients.

THE ORGANIZATION OF THE URINARY SYSTEM *p. 518*

1. The urinary system includes the kidneys, the ureters, the urinary bladder, and the urethra. The kidneys produce urine (a fluid containing water, ions, and soluble compounds); during urination urine is forced out of the body. *(Figure 19-1)*

THE KIDNEYS *p. 518*

1. The left **kidney** extends superiorly slightly more than the right kidney. Both lie in a *retroperitoneal* position. *(Figure 19-2)*

Superficial and Sectional Anatomy *p. 519*

2. The **hilus** provides entry for the *renal artery* and exit for the *renal vein* and *ureter*.

3. The ureter communicates with the **renal pelvis**. This chamber branches into two **major calyces**, each connected to four or five **minor calyces**, which enclose the **renal papillae**. *(Figure 19-3)*

The Nephron *p. 519*

4. The **nephron** (the basic functional unit in the kidney) includes the *renal corpuscle* and a **renal tubule**, which empties into the **collecting system** through a *collecting duct*. From the renal corpuscle, the filtrate travels through the *proximal convoluted tubule*, the *loop of Henle*, and the *distal convoluted tubule*. *(Figure 19-4)*

5. Nephrons are responsible for the (1) production of **filtrate**, (2) reabsorption of nutrients, and (3) reabsorption of water and ions.

6. The renal tubule begins at the **renal corpuscle**. It includes a knot of intertwined capillaries called the **glomerulus** surrounded by the **Bowman's capsule**. Blood arrives via the *afferent arteriole* and departs in the *efferent arteriole*. *(Figure 19-5)*

7. At the glomerulus, **podocytes** cover the basement membrane of the capillaries that project into the **capsular space**. The processes of the podocytes are separated by narrow slits. *(Figure 19-5)*

8. The **proximal convoluted tubule (PCT)** actively reabsorbs nutrients, plasma proteins, and electrolytes from the filtrate. They are then released into the surrounding interstitial fluid. *(Figure 19-4)*

9. The **loop of Henle** includes a *descending limb* and an *ascending limb*. The ascending limb is impermeable to water and solutes; the descending limb is permeable to water. *(Figure 19-4)*

19

10. The ascending limb delivers fluid to the **distal convoluted tubule (DCT)**, which actively secretes ions and reabsorbs sodium ions from the urine. The **juxtaglomerular apparatus**, which releases renin and erythropoietin, is located at the start of the DCT. *(Figure 19-5a)*

11. The **collecting ducts** receive urine from nephrons and merge into a **papillary duct** that delivers urine to a minor calyx. The collecting system makes final adjustments to the urine by reabsorbing water or reabsorbing or secreting various ions.

The Blood Supply to the Kidneys *p. 523*

12. The blood vessels of the kidneys include the **interlobar**, **arcuate**, and **interlobular arteries**, and the **interlobar**, **arcuate**, and **interlobular veins**. Blood travels from the **efferent arteriole** to the **peritubular capillaries** and the **vasa recta**. Diffusion occurs between the capillaries of the vasa recta and the tubular cells through the interstitial fluid that surrounds the nephron. *(Figure 19-6)*

BASIC PRINCIPLES OF URINE PRODUCTION *p. 524*

1. The primary purpose in **urine** production is the excretion and elimination of dissolved solutes, principally metabolic waste products, such as **urea**, **creatinine**, and **uric acid**.

2. Urine formation involves **filtration**, **reabsorption**, and **secretion**. *(Tables 19-1, 19-2)*

Filtration at the Glomerulus *p. 525*

3. Glomerular filtration occurs as fluids move across the wall of the glomerulus into the capsular space, in response to blood pressure in the glomerular capillaries. The **glomerular filtration rate (GFR)** is the amount of filtrate produced in the kidneys each minute. Any factor that alters the **filtration (blood) pressure** will change the GFR and affect kidney function.

4. Dropping filtration pressures stimulate the juxtoglomerular apparatus to release *renin*. Renin release increases blood volume and blood pressure.

Reabsorption and Secretion Along the Renal Tubule *p. 526*

5. The cells of the PCT normally reabsorb 60–70 percent of the volume of the filtrate produced in the renal corpuscle. The PCT generally reabsorbs sodium and other ions, water, and almost all of the nutrients in the filtrate. It also secretes various substances.

6. Water and ions are reclaimed from the filtrate by the loop of Henle. The ascending limb reabsorbs sodium and chloride ions, and the descending limb reabsorbs water. A concentration gradient in the medulla encourages the osmotic flow of water out of the filtrate and into the interstitial fluid. As water is lost by osmosis and the filtrate volume decreases, the urea concentration rises.

7. The DCT performs final adjustments by actively secreting or absorbing materials. Sodium ions are actively absorbed in exchange for potassium and hydrogen ions discharged into the filtrate. **Aldosterone** secretion increases the rate of sodium reabsorption and potassium loss.

8. The amount of water in the urine of the collecting ducts is regulated by the secretion of *antidiuretic hormone (ADH)*.

In the absence of ADH, the DCT, collecting tubule, and collecting duct are impermeable to water. The higher the ADH level in circulation, the more water is absorbed and the more concentrated the urine. *(Figure 19-7)*

9. More than 99 percent of the filtrate produced each day is reabsorbed before reaching the renal pelvis. Yet the water content of normal urine is 93–97 percent. *(Table 19-3)*

10. Each segment of the nephron and collecting system contributes to the production of hypertonic urine. *(Figure 19-8)*

The Control of Kidney Function *p. 528*

11. Renal function may be regulated by automatic adjustments in glomerular pressures through changes in the diameters of the afferent and efferent arterioles.

12. Sympathetic activation (1) produces a powerful vasoconstriction of the afferent arterioles, decreasing the GFR and slowing the production of filtrate; (2) alters the GFR by changing the regional pattern of blood circulation; and (3) over the long term, stimulates the release of **renin** by the juxtaglomerular apparatus.

13. Hormones that regulate kidney function include angiotensin II, aldosterone, ADH, and atrial natriuretic peptide (ANP). *(Figure 19-9)*

URINE TRANSPORT, STORAGE, AND ELIMINATION *p. 531*

1. Filtrate modification and urine production end when the fluid enters the renal pelvis. The rest of the urinary system is responsible for transporting, storing, and eliminating the urine.

The Ureters and Urinary Bladder *p. 531*

2. The **ureters** extend from the renal pelvis to the urinary bladder. Peristaltic contractions by smooth muscles move the urine. *(Figures 19-1, 19-10)*

3. Internal features of the **urinary bladder**, a distensible sac for urine storage, include the *trigone*, the neck, and the **internal urethral sphincter**. Contraction of the *detrusor muscle* compresses the bladder and expels the urine into the urethra. *(Figure 19-10)*

The Urethra *p. 532*

4. In both sexes, as the urethra passes through the *urogenital diaphragm*, a circular band of skeletal muscles forms the **external urethral sphincter**, which is under voluntary control. *(Figure 19-10)*

The Micturition Reflex and Urination *p. 532*

5. The process of **urination** is coordinated by the **micturition reflex**, which is initiated by stretch receptors in the bladder wall. Voluntary urination involves coupling this reflex with the voluntary relaxation of the external urethral sphincter, which allows the opening of the internal urethral sphincter. *(Figure 19-11)*

INTEGRATION WITH OTHER SYSTEMS *p. 533*

1. The urinary, integumentary, respiratory, and digestive systems are sometimes considered as an anatomically diverse *excretory system*. The systems' components work together to perform all of the excretory functions that affect the composition of body fluids. *(Figure 19-12)*

FLUID, ELECTROLYTE, AND ACID-BASE BALANCE
p. 535

1. All of our cells' operations depend on water as a diffusion medium for dissolved gases, nutrients, and waste products. Maintenance of normal volume and composition in the extracellular and intracellular fluids is vital to life. Three types of homeostasis are involved: *fluid balance, electrolyte balance*, and *acid-base balance*.

Fluid and Electrolyte Balance *p. 535*

2. The **intracellular fluid (ICF)** contains nearly two-thirds of the total body water; the **extracellular fluid (ECF)** contains the rest. Exchange occurs between the ICF and ECF, but the two **fluid compartments** retain their distinctive characteristics. *(Figure 19-13)*

3. Water circulates freely within the ECF compartment. At capillary beds, hydrostatic pressure forces water from the plasma into the interstitial spaces. Water moves back and forth across the epithelial lining of the peritoneal, pleural, and pericardial cavities; through synovial membranes lining joint capsules; and between the blood and cerebrospinal fluid, the aqueous and vitreous humors of the eye, and the perilymph and endolymph of the inner ear.

4. Water losses are normally balanced by gains through eating, drinking, and metabolic generation.

5. If the ECF becomes hypertonic relative to the ICF, water will move from the ICF into the ECF until osmotic equilibrium has been restored. If the ECF becomes hypotonic relative to the ICF, water will move from the ECF into the cells and the volume of the ICF will increase accordingly. Water movement between the ECF and ICF is called a *fluid shift*.

6. Electrolyte balance is important because total electrolyte concentrations affect water balance and because the levels of individual electrolytes can affect a variety of cell functions. Problems with electrolyte balance generally result from an imbalance between sodium gains and losses. Problems with potassium balance are less common but more dangerous.

7. The rate of sodium uptake across the digestive epithelium is directly proportional to the amount of sodium in the diet. Sodium losses occur mainly in the urine and through perspiration. The rate of sodium reabsorption along the DCT is regulated by aldosterone levels; aldosterone stimulates sodium ion reabsorption.

8. Potassium ion concentrations in the ECF are very low. Potassium excretion increases (1) when sodium ion concentrations decline and (2) as ECF potassium concentrations rise. The rate of potassium excretion is regulated by aldosterone; aldosterone stimulates potassium ion excretion.

Acid-Base Balance *p. 537*

9. The pH of normal body fluids ranges from 7.35 to 7.45; variations outside this relatively narrow range produce **acidosis** or **alkalosis**.

10. Carbonic acid is the most important factor affecting the pH of the ECF. In solution, CO_2 reacts with water to form carbonic acid; the dissociation of carbonic acid releases hydrogen ions. An inverse relationship exists between the concentration of CO_2 and pH. *(Figure 19-14)*

11. Organic acids include metabolic products such as lactic acid and ketone bodies.

12. A buffer system consists of a weak acid and its dissociation products. There are three major buffer systems: (1) *protein buffer systems* in the ECF and ICF; (2) the *carbonic acid–bicarbonate buffer system*, most important in the ECF; and (3) the *phosphate buffer system* in the intracellular fluids and urine.

13. In **protein buffer systems**, the component amino acids respond to changes in H^+ concentrations. Blood plasma proteins and hemoglobin in red blood cells help prevent drastic changes in pH.

14. The **carbonic acid–bicarbonate buffer system** prevents pH changes due to organic acids in the ECF.

15. The **phosphate buffer system** is important in preventing pH changes in the intracellular fluid.

16. In **respiratory compensation**, the lungs help regulate pH by affecting the carbonic acid–bicarbonate buffer system; changing the respiratory rate can raise or lower the P_{CO_2} of body fluids, affecting the buffering capacity.

17. In the process of **renal compensation**, the kidneys vary their rates of hydrogen ion secretion and bicarbonate ion resorption depending on the pH of extracellular fluids.

AGING AND THE URINARY SYSTEM *p. 540*

1. Aging is usually associated with increased kidney problems. Age-related changes in the urinary system include (1) declining number of functional nephrons, (2) reduced GFR, (3) reduced sensitivity to ADH, (4) problems with the micturition reflex (urinary retention may develop in men whose prostate gland is inflamed), (5) declining body water content, and (6) a loss of mineral content.

REVIEW QUESTIONS

LEVEL 1 Reviewing Facts and Terms

Match each item in column A with the most closely related item in column B. Use letters for answers in the spaces provided.

Column A

___ 1. urination

___ 2. renal capsule

___ 3. hilus

___ 4. medulla

___ 5. nephrons

___ 6. renal corpuscle

___ 7. external urethral sphincter

___ 8. internal urethral sphincter

___ 9. aldosterone

___10. podocytes

___11. efferent arteriole

___12. afferent arteriole

___13. vasa recta

___14. ADH

___15. ECF

___16. sodium

___17. potassium

Column B

a. site of urine production

b. capillaries around loop of Henle

c. causes sensation of thirst

d. accelerated sodium reabsorption

e. voluntary control

f. glomerular epithelium

g. fibrous covering

h. blood leaves glomerulus

i. dominant cation in ICF

j. renal pyramids

k. blood to glomerulus

l. interstitial fluid

m. contains glomerulus

n. exit for ureter

o. dominant cation in ECF

p. involuntary control

q. micturition

18. After it leaves the glomerulus, the filtrate empties into the:
    (a) distal convoluted tubule
    (b) loop of Henle
    (c) proximal convoluted tubule
    (d) collecting duct

19. The distal convoluted tubule is an important site for:
    (a) active secretion of ions
    (b) active secretion of acids and other materials
    (c) selective reabsorption of sodium ions from the tubular fluid
    (d) a, b, and c are correct

20. The endocrine structure that secretes renin and erythropoietin is the:
    (a) juxtaglomerular apparatus
    (b) vasa recta
    (c) Bowman's capsule
    (d) adrenal gland

21. The primary purpose of the collecting system is to:
    (a) transport urine from the bladder to the urethra
    (b) selectively reabsorb sodium ions from tubular fluid
    (c) transport urine from the renal pelvis to the ureters
    (d) make final adjustments to the osmotic concentration and volume of urine

22. A person is in fluid balance when:
    (a) the ECF and ICF are isotonic
    (b) there is no fluid movement between compartments
    (c) the amount of water gained each day is equal to the amount lost to the environment
    (d) a, b, and c are correct

23. The primary components of the extracellular fluid are:
    (a) lymph and cerebrospinal fluid
    (b) blood plasma and serous fluids
    (c) interstitial fluid and plasma
    (d) a, b, and c are correct

24. All the homeostatic mechanisms that monitor and adjust the composition of body fluids respond to changes:
    (a) in the ICF
    (b) in the ECF
    (c) inside the cell
    (d) a, b, and c are correct

25. The most common problems with electrolyte balance are caused by an imbalance between gains and losses of:
    (a) calcium ions
    (b) chloride ions
    (c) potassium ions
    (d) sodium ions

26. What is the primary function of the urinary system?

27. What are the structural components of the urinary system?

28. What are fluid shifts? What is their function, and what factors can cause them?

29. What three major hormones mediate major physiological adjustments that affect fluid and electrolyte balance? What are the primary effects of each hormone?

1
9

LEVEL 2   Reviewing Concepts

30. The urinary system regulates blood volume and pressure by:
    (a) adjusting the volume of water lost in the urine
    (b) releasing erythropoietin
    (c) releasing renin
    (d) a, b, and c are correct

31. The balance of solute and water reabsorption in the renal medulla is maintained by the:
    (a) segmental arterioles and veins
    (b) lobar arteries and veins
    (c) vasa recta
    (d) arcuate arteries

32. The higher the plasma concentration of aldosterone, the more efficiently the kidney will:
    (a) conserve sodium ions
    (b) retain potassium ions
    (c) stimulate urinary water loss
    (d) secrete greater amounts of ADH

33. When pure water is consumed:
    (a) the ECF becomes hypertonic with respect to the ICF
    (b) the ECF becomes hypotonic with respect to the ICF
    (c) the ICF becomes hypotonic with respect to the plasma
    (d) water moves from the ICF into the ECF

34. Increasing or decreasing the rate of respiration alters pH by:
    (a) lowering or raising the partial pressure of carbon dioxide
    (b) lowering or raising the partial pressure of oxygen
    (c) lowering or raising the partial pressure of nitrogen
    (d) a, b, and c are correct

35. What interacting controls operate to stabilize the glomerular filtration rate (GFR)?

36. Describe the micturition reflex.

37. Differentiate among fluid balance, electrolyte balance, and acid-base balance, and explain why each is important to homeostasis.

38. Why should a person with a fever drink plenty of fluids?

39. Exercise physiologists recommend that adequate amounts of fluid be ingested before, during, and after exercise. Why is adequate fluid replacement during conditions of extensive sweating important?

LEVEL 3   Critical Thinking and Clinical Applications

40. Why do long-haul trailer truck drivers frequently experience kidney problems?

41. For the past week, Susan has felt a burning sensation in the urethral area when she urinates. She checks her temperature and finds that she has a low-grade fever.

What unusual substances are likely to be present in her urine?

42. Carlos suffers from advanced arteriosclerosis. An analysis of his blood indicates elevated levels of aldosterone and decreased levels of ADH. Explain.

ANSWERS TO CONCEPT CHECK QUESTIONS

Page 524
1. Unlike most other organs, such as those of the digestive system, the kidneys lie beneath the peritoneal lining in a retroperitoneal position. **2.** The slits created by the podocytes are so fine that they will allow only substances smaller than plasma proteins to pass into the capsular space. **3.** Damage to the juxtaglomerular apparatus portion of the nephrons would interfere with the normal control of blood pressure.

Page 531
1. Decreases in blood pressure would reduce the blood hydrostatic pressure within the glomerulus and would decrease the GFR. **2.** If the nephrons lacked a loop of Henle, the kidneys would not be able to form a concentrated urine.

Page 535
1. Under normal conditions, peristaltic contractions move urine along the minor and major calyces toward the renal pelvis, out of the renal pelvis, and along the ureter to the bladder. **2.** An obstruction of the ureters would interfere with the passage of urine from the renal pelvis to the urinary bladder. **3.** To control the micturition reflex, you must be able to control the external urinary sphincter, a ring of skeletal muscle that acts as a valve.

Page 537
1. Consuming a meal high in salt would temporarily increase the osmolarity of the ECF. As a result, some of the water in the ICF would shift to the ECF. **2.** Fluid loss through perspiration, urine formation, and respiration would increase the osmolarity of body fluids.

Page 540
1. A decrease in the pH of body fluids would have a stimulating effect on the respiratory center in the medulla. The resulting increase in the rate of breathing would in turn lead to an elimination of more carbon dioxide, which would tend to cause the pH to increase. **2.** In a prolonged fast, fatty acids are mobilized and large numbers of ketone bodies are formed. These molecules are acids that lower the body's pH. This situation would eventually lead to ketoacidosis. **3.** In vomiting, large amounts of stomach acid are lost from the body. This acid is formed by the parietal cells of the stomach by taking hydrogen ions from the blood. Excessive vomiting would lead to the excessive removal of hydrogen ions from the blood to produce the acid, thus raising the body's pH and causing metabolic alkalosis.

19

OVERVIEW

The urinary system performs a number of vital functions. It maintains blood volume and the proper balance of water, electrolytes, and pH. It also removes a number of toxic waste products. In addition, the urinary system plays a major role in arterial blood pressure regulation and controls the development of red blood cells.

Several urinary system problems that arise may require emergency care. These include kidney infections (pyelonephritis), kidney stones, renal failure, and others. Much of the urinary system is located in the retroperitoneal space and is fairly well protected from trauma. However, penetrating trauma and high-speed motor vehicle collisions can in-

jure the kidneys, ureters, urinary bladder, or urethra. (Figure A19-1●).

The study of urinary system disorders is called *nephrology*. Physicians who specialize in the medical treatment of kidney and related problems are called *nephrologists*. They first train in general internal medicine and then take fellowship training in nephrology. Surgeons who specialize in the surgical treatment of urinary system are referred to as *urologists*. They typically complete a five- to six-year residency program before entering independent practice.

KIDNEY STONES

Kidney stones, or renal calculi (singular, calculus), represent crystal aggregation in the

● **FIGURE A19-1**
Medical Disorders of the Urinary System

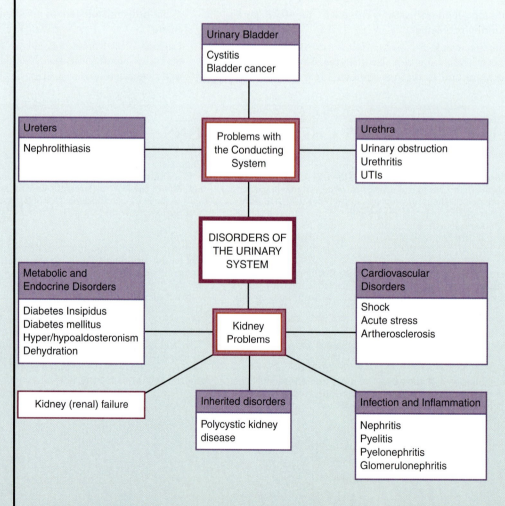

A1
9

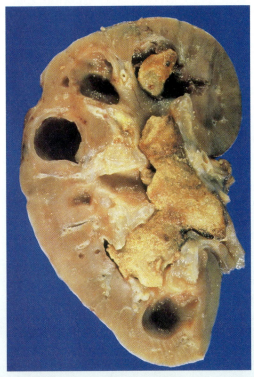

● FIGURE A19-2   Kidney Stones
Cross-section through a kidney showing multiple stones including one "staghorn" stone in the renal pelvis.

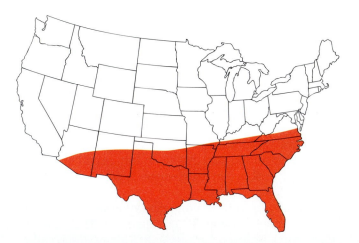

● FIGURE A19-3   The "Kidney Stone Belt"
The incidence of kidney stones is markedly higher in the southern United States.

kidney's collecting system (Figure A19-2●). This condition is also called *nephrolithiasis* (from Greek *lithos,* stone). Kidney stones affect about 500,000 persons each year. Brief hospitalization is common due to the severity of pain as the stone travels from the renal pelvis, through the ureter to the bladder, and is eventually eliminated in urine. If necessary, additional inpatient treatment may include shock-wave lithotripsy, a procedure that uses sound waves to break large stones into smaller ones, and other treatment modalities. Overall morbidity and mortality are low, however, unless a complication such as hemorrhage or urinary tract obstruction results.

Kidney stones occur more frequently in the southern and southeastern United States, a region referred to as the Kidney Stone Belt (Figure A19-3●). North Carolina has more kidney stones per capita than any other state. Several factors appear to be involved in this phenomenon. First, the typical southern diet is high in green vegetables and brewed tea—both of which are high in oxalates, a key ingredient for kidney stones. Another factor is the warm climate, which causes increased sweating and increased loss of body fluids. Finally, modern life styles often reduce the level of physical activity. Together, these risk factors increase the likelihood of kidney stone development.

Stones form more commonly in men than women, although the ratio varies for different types of stones with different compositions. Certain stones also occur in familial patterns, suggesting hereditary factors. Another

risk factor for calculus formation is immobilization due to surgery or injury, with the latter including immobilization secondary to paraplegia or other paralysis syndromes that involve the absence of motor impulses, sensation, or both. Last, the use of certain medications, including anesthetics, opiates, and psychotropic drugs, increases the risk for stones. Historically, about 60 percent of individuals who have experienced one kidney stone will develop another within seven years. Fortunately, with modern therapy, recurrence can be prevented in more than 95 percent of sufferers.

Stones may form in several metabolic disorders including gout or primary hyperparathyroidism, which produce excessive amounts of uric acid and calcium, respectively. More often, they occur when the general balance between water conservation and dissolution of relatively insoluble substances such as mineral ions and uric acid is lost and excessive amounts of the insolubles aggregate into stones. The problem boils down to "too much insoluble stuff" and "too concentrated urine," a situation that may more likely arise with a change in diet, climate, or physical activity.

Stones consisting of calcium salts (namely, calcium oxalate and calcium phosphate) are by far the most common. These compounds are found in 75 to 85 percent of all stones. Calcium stones are from two to three times more common in men than in women, and the average age at onset is between 20 and 30 years. Their formation frequently runs in families, and anyone who has had a calcium stone is at fairly high risk to form another within two to three years.

Struvite stones (chemically denoted $MgNH_4PO_4$) are also common, representing about 10 to 15 percent of all stones. The pathophysiology of struvite stones differs from that of calcium stones. Their formation is associated with chronic urinary tract infection (UTI) or frequent bladder

A19

catheterization. The association with bacterial UTI makes struvite stones much more common in women than in men. These stones can grow to fill the renal pelvis, producing a characteristic "staghorn" appearance on X-rays.

Far less common are stones made of uric acid or cystine. Uric acid stones form more often in men than in women and tend to occur in families; about half of all patients with uric acid stones have gout. Cystine stones are the least common. They are associated with excess levels of the amino acid cystine in filtrate and are probably due at least in part to hereditary factors, as they often run in families.

The largest kidney stone ever reported weighed a fraction under 3 pounds (1.36 kilograms). The smallest stones are the size of grains of sand. Kidney stones come in virtually every color although most are yellow to brown. It is important to try to collect a passed kidney stone for laboratory analysis. Once the chemical composition of the stone has been determined, then prevention strategies can be initiated.

The pain from kidney stones is generally conceded to be among the most painful of human medical conditions. Typically, the patient first notes discomfort as a vague, visceral pain in one flank. Within 30 to 60 minutes it progresses to an extremely sharp pain that may remain in the flank or migrate downward and anteriorly toward the groin. Migrating pain indicates that the stone has passed into the lowest third of the ureter. Kidney stone pain can be colicky in nature. As a rule, kidney-stone patients cannot lie still. They continuously move or pace due to the unrelenting nature of the pain. Stones that lodge in the lowest part of the ureter, within the bladder wall, often cause characteristic bladder symptoms such as frequency during the day or during the night (nocturia), urgency, and painful urination. Because these latter three symptoms far more frequently suggest bladder infection, making the tentative diagnosis may be difficult, particularly in women. Visible blood in the urine (hematuria) is not uncommon in urine specimens taken during passage of a stone. However, hematuria may be microscopic, meaning that it is not visible to the naked eye but can be detected with reagent strips dipped into a urine specimen. Fever, however, is not common unless concomitant infection is present. Whenever kidney stones are suspected, be sure to obtain the patient's personal medical history and family history, because both will often provide useful information.

As mentioned earlier, the patient may be agitated or physically restless; walking sometimes reduces the pain. Vital signs will vary with the level of discomfort experienced by the patient, with highest blood pressure and heart rate associated with the greatest pain. The skin will typically be pale, cool, and clammy. Most patients are nauseated and many vomit because of the severe, unrelenting pain.

Emergency treatment of kidney stones should include hydration and analgesia. Often, the pain is so severe that patients will require large doses of intra-

venous narcotics for pain control (morphine, meperidine, fentanyl). Virtually all patients with a symptomatic kidney stone will be nauseated or vomiting. Administration of medicine to treat nausea and vomiting will also help to increase the effectiveness of the analgesic medications.

In the hospital, kidney stone patients will usually receive intravenous fluids and parenteral analgesics. The kidney stone can be diagnosed with spiral computerized tomography (CT) scanning. Alternatively, physicians can order an intravenous pyelogram (IVP), which involves the intravenous administration of a radiopaque contrast dye. The dye collects in the kidneys allowing the kidneys, ureters, and bladder to be visualized. On occasion, ultrasound can detect a kidney stone.

Many patients will spontaneously pass smaller stones with adequate hydration and analgesia. If the stones do not pass, the urologist can place a stent in the affected ureter and remove the stone with a basket-like device inserted through the cystoscope. Stones that cannot be removed with basket extraction may be treated with other therapies. These include *lithotripsy,* which uses shock waves to break up stones so that they can pass with little problem. Another technology is *lasertripsy,* where a laser is threaded through a cystoscope and, once properly positioned, pulverizes the stone. Another available technology is *electrohydraulic lithotripsy (EHL),* where a special probe breaks up small stones with shock waves generated by electricity. The gravel that remains following lithotripsy or lasertripsy easily passes through the ureters into the bladder.

ACUTE URINARY TRACT INFECTION

Urinary tract infection, or UTI, affects the urethra, bladder, ureter, or kidney, as well as the prostate gland in men. UTIs are extremely common, accounting for over 6 million medical office visits yearly. Almost all UTIs start with pathogenic colonization of the bladder by bacteria that enter through the urethra. Thus, females in general are at higher risk because of their relatively short urethra. Other groups at risk for UTI are paraplegic patients or patients with nerve disruption to the bladder, including some diabetic persons. Any condition that promotes urinary stasis (incomplete urination with urine remaining in the bladder) places a person at increased risk. Pregnant women often have urinary stasis due to pressure from the gravid uterus. People with neurological impairment (some patients with spina bifida or with diabetic neuropathy, for example) also tend to have urinary stasis, which predisposes them to infection. The use of instrumentation in patients who require bladder catheterization places them at even higher risk of developing a UTI.

Associated conditions such as scarring, abscesses, or eventual development of chronic renal failure are most likely in persons with anatomic abnormalities of the urinary system or chronic calculi (the latter acting as a focus for continuing infection and inflammation), those who are immunocompromised, or those who have renal disease due to diabetes mellitus or another condition.

UTIs are generally divided into those of the lower urinary tract, namely, urethritis (urethra), cystitis (bladder), and prostatitis (prostate gland), and those of the upper urinary tract, pyelonephritis (kidney). Lower UTIs are far more common than upper UTIs, for two reasons. First, seeding of infection via the bloodstream is rare. Second, asymptomatic bacterial colonization of the urethra, especially in females, is very common, and can predispose a person to infection by other, pathogenic bacteria. In females, infection may begin when Gram-negative bacteria normally found in the bowel (that is, the enteric floras) colonize the urethra and bladder. Symptomatic urethritis, inflammation secondary to urethral infection, is very uncommon. More often you will see joint symptomatic infection of the urethra and bladder (urethritis and cystitis, respectively). Sexually active females are at higher risk, which may be attributed to use of contraceptive devices or agents, to the introduction of enteric floras (bacteria from the GI tract) during intercourse, or both. Recently, homosexually active men who engage in anal sex have also been found to be at higher risk for bacterial cystitis, possibly due to introduction of enteric bacterial floras during rectal intercourse. In any case, sexually active persons who suffer from urinary stasis are at even higher risk for infection. Persons who urinate after intercourse might lower their risk because voiding eliminates some bacteria. The pathophysiology for persons using bladder catheterization probably differs only in that pathogenic bacteria are introduced directly into the bladder via the catheter. In general, the likelihood that active cystitis will develop, that antibiotic treatment will clear such infections, and that reinfection will occur is determined by the interplay of the pathogen's virulence, the size of its colony, its sensitivity to antibiotic treatment, and the strength of the host's local and systemic immune functions.

Prostatitis, inflammation of the prostate gland, is inflammation of the prostate secondary to bacterial infection, as well as any general inflammatory condition. Men with acute bacterial prostatitis, the closest parallel to acute cystitis in women, also tend to show evidence of associated urethritis, and the same bowel flora tends to be involved. The major difference between acute bacterial prostatitis and acute cystitis is the much lower incidence of prostatitis among men who do not require bladder catheterization.

Upper UTIs usually evolve from infection that spreads upward into the kidney. Pyelonephritis is an infectious inflammation of the renal parenchyma: nephrons, interstitial tissue, or both. Acute pyelonephritis is ten times more common in women than in men. Its incidence is highest in pregnancy and during periods of sexual activity, reflecting the epidemiology of lower UTIs. If the infection of pyelonephritis persists, intrarenal or perinephric abscesses may occur, but these complications are uncommon. Intrarenal abscesses form within the renal parenchyma. If they rupture and spill their contents into the adjacent fatty tissue, perinephric abscesses may result. From 20 to 60 percent of patients who develop perinephric abscesses have a clear predisposing factor such as renal calculi, anatomic abnormalities of the kidney, history of urologic surgery or injury, or diabetic renal disease.

Urinary tract infections may be community-acquired or nosocomial. Among community-acquired infections, Gram-negative enteric bacteria are the most common. In fact, E. coli accounts for roughly 80 percent of infections in persons without the complicating factors of bladder catheterization, renal calculi, or anatomic abnormalities. In nosocomial infections, cases acquired in an inpatient setting or related to catheterization, Proteus, Klebsiella, and Pseudomonas are commonly identified. Less common, but still important, are sexually transmitted pathogens (among women and men) such as Chlamydia and N. gonorrhoeae. Fungi such as Candida are rarely seen except in catheterized or immunocompromised patients or patients with diabetes mellitus.

The symptoms of lower UTI typically include: painful urination, frequent urge to urinate, and difficulty in beginning and continuing to void. Pain often begins as visceral discomfort that progresses to severe, burning pain, particularly during and just after urination. The evolution of pain corresponds roughly to the degree of epithelial damage caused by the pathogen. In both men and women, pain is often localized to the pelvis and perceived as in the bladder (in women) or in the bladder and prostate (in men). The patient may complain of a strong or foul odor in the urine. Many women will give a history of similar episodes, which may or may not have been diagnosed or treated. Patients with pyelonephritis are more likely to feel generally ill or feverish. They typically complain of constant, moderately severe or severe pain in a flank or lower back (just under the rib cage). The pain may be referred to the shoulder or neck. The triad of urgency, pain, and difficulty may or may not be present or included in the past history.

On physical exam, patients with UTI appear restless and uncomfortable. Typically, patients with pyelonephritis appear more ill and are far more likely to have a fever. Skin will often be pale, cool, and moist (in lower UTI) or warm and dry (in febrile upper UTI). Vital signs will vary with the degree of illness and pain, but in an otherwise healthy individual they should not be far from normal. Inspect and auscultate the abdomen to document findings, but neither procedure is likely to be very useful, as visible appearance and bowel sounds are usually within normal limits. Percussion and palpation will probably reveal painful tenderness over the pubis in lower UTI and at the flank in upper UTI. Lloyd's sign, tenderness to percussion of the lower back at the costovertebral angle (CVA), suggests pyelonephritis.

A19

The best prevention technique is hydration to increase blood flow through the kidneys and to produce a more dilute, but voluminous urine. In many cases, this is better accomplished by IV fluid administration, which eliminates the risk of vomiting and satisfies the guidelines for possible surgical cases.

ACUTE RENAL FAILURE

Acute renal failure (ARF) is a deterioration in renal function over hours or days that causes the accumulation of toxic wastes and causes the loss of internal homeostasis. ARF usually results from a decline in renal blood flow. ARF can result from problems in blood flow to the kidney (prerenal failure), a problem within the kidney itself (intrinsic renal failure), or a problem in urine flow (postrenal failure). Depressed renal blood flow and substances that are toxic to the kidney cause renal cell ischemia and death. Damage to the renal tubules can cause a back leak of glomerular filtrate further decreasing perfusion pressure. Finally, the sloughing off of dying cells can obstruct the renal tubules. Recovery depends upon restoration of renal blood flow. In prerenal failure, this involves the replacement of circulating blood volume. Rapid relief of the urinary obstruction in postrenal failure cases will restore glomerular flow as postrenal pressures are reduced. Restoration of renal blood flow and clearance of tubular toxins will aid in correcting intrinsic disease. Once blood supply is restored, the remaining nephrons will increase their filtration rate and eventually hypertrophy. If a critical number of nephrons have been lost, the patient will ultimately deteriorate and develop chronic renal failure requiring hemodialysis.

An all too common complication of multiple trauma is the development of *acute tubular necrosis*. This results from renal ischemia due to prolonged hypotension. If enough nephrons remain functioning, the patient can recover with relatively normal kidney function. If too many nephrons have been lost, then chronic renal failure will eventually develop. Prolonged hypotension due to multiple trauma should be avoided in order to prevent the development of acute tubular necrosis.

RENAL TRAUMA

The renal system is fairly well protected from trauma. Injuries to the genitourinary system occur in only 5 percent or less of all trauma victims. Approximately 10 percent of children with blunt abdominal trauma have renal system injury. Most patients with a kidney injury have other concurrent injuries. The kidneys and ureters are located in the retroperitoneal space and are thus well protected. The bladder is well protected by

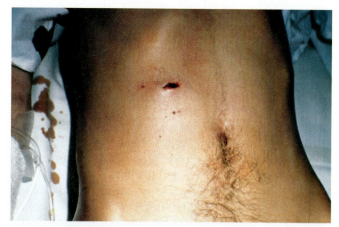

• **FIGURE A19-4   Renal Trauma**
Most cases of renal trauma are due to penetrating injuries. Although this wound is on the anterior abdomen, the right kidney and ureter were lacerated.

the bony structures of the pelvis. In males, the urethra is more vulnerable to trauma due to the anatomy of the penis. Fortunately, renal system injuries are rarely life threatening and usually do not require immediate intervention.

Trauma to the kidneys and ureters usually results from penetrating trauma such as gunshots or stabbings (Figure A19-4•). Rapid deceleration forces may cause injury to the renal pedicle or to the vascular structures. The signs and symptoms of urinary system trauma can be subtle. The most common indicator of renal system trauma is blood in the urine (hematuria). This may be gross (readily visible) or microscopic (seen only with a microscope or detected by urine test strips). Trauma to the prostate and urethra can result in blood at the urethral meatus (or on the underwear). Any of these findings warrant further investigation. In the emergency department, a rectal examination should be carried out. A high-riding or floating prostate indicates the need for further studies. After life-threatening problems have been addressed, the urinary system can be studied with contrast X-rays and CT scanning.

SUMMARY

The urinary system is an important body system. The two most common emergencies related to the urinary system are urinary tract infections and kidney stones. Kidney stones are a frequent reason people seek emergency care. Urinary system trauma usually occurs with other injuries. Fortunately, urinary system injuries are rarely life threatening and can be managed after the patient's other injuries have been stabilized.

20

The Reproductive System

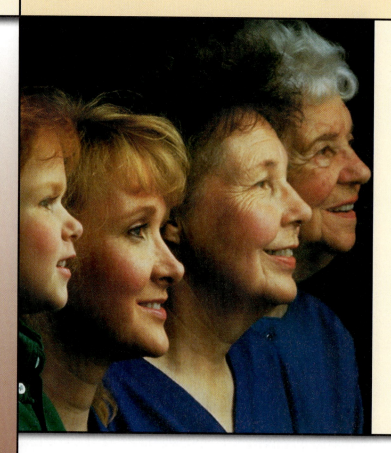

The only organ system not needed for survival is our reproductive system. In a sense, it does not exist for us at all. Instead, it exists for the human species. Modern medicine, along with an absence of major wars and epidemics, has allowed patients to live much longer. Unheard of 100 years ago, it is now possible for four generations to be alive at the same time and enjoy quality life.

Chapter Outline and Objectives

  1 *Describe the components of the male reproductive system.*
  2 *Describe the process of spermatogenesis.*
  3 *Describe the roles the male reproductive tract and accessory glands play in the maturation and transport of spermatozoa.*
  4 *Describe the hormonal mechanisms that regulate male reproductive functions.*

  5 *Describe the components of the female reproductive system.*
  6 *Describe the process of oogenesis in the ovary.*
  7 *Detail the physiological processes involved in the ovarian and menstrual cycles.*

  8 *Discuss the physiology of sexual intercourse as it affects the reproductive system of males and females.*

  9 *Describe the changes in the reproductive system that occur with aging.*

  10 *Explain how the reproductive system interacts with other body systems.*

Vocabulary Development

andro-, male; *androgen*
crypto, hidden; *cryptorchidism*
diplo, double; *diploid*
follis, a leather bag; *follicle*
genesis, generation; *oogenesis*
gyne, woman; *gynecologist*
haplo, single; *haploid*
labium, lip; *labium minus*
lutea, yellow; *corpus luteum*
meioun, to make smaller; *meiosis*
men, month; *menopause*
metra, uterus; *endometrium*
myo-, muscle; *myometrium*
oon, an egg; *oocyte*
orchis, testis; *cryptorchidism*
pausis, cessation; *menopause*
pellucidus, translucent; *zona pellucida*
rete, a net; *rete testis*
tetras, four; *tetrad*

An individual life span can be measured in decades, but the human species has survived for hundreds of thousands of years through the activities of the reproductive system. The entire process of reproduction seems almost magical; many primitive societies even failed to discover the basic link between sexual activity and childbirth and assumed that cosmic forces were responsible for producing new individuals. Although our society has a much clearer view of the reproductive process, a sense of wonder remains. Sexually mature males and females produce individual reproductive cells that are brought together through sexual intercourse. The fusion of these reproductive cells starts a chain of events leading to the appearance of an infant that will mature as part of the next generation.

Chapters 20 and 21 will consider the mechanics of this remarkable process. We will begin by examining the anatomy and physiology of the reproductive system. **Gonads** (GŌ-nadz) are reproductive organs that produce hormones and reproductive cells, or **gametes** (GAM-ēts). Gametes are *sperm* in males and *ova* (Ō-va; singular, *ovum*) in females. The other components of the reproductive system store, nourish, and transport the gametes. The next chapter begins with **fertilization**, the fusion of a sperm from the father and an ovum from the mother. All the cells in the body are the mitotic descendants of a single **zygote** (ZĪ-gōt), the cell created at fertilization. The gradual transformation of that single cell into a functional adult occurs through the process of *development*, the topic of Chapter 21. From fertilization to birth, development occurs within specialized organs of the female reproductive system.

THE REPRODUCTIVE SYSTEM OF THE MALE

The principal structures of the male reproductive system are shown in Figure 20-1•. The male gonads, or *testes* (TES-tēz; singular testis), produce reproductive cells called **sperm**, or *spermatozoa* (sper-ma-tō-ZŌ-a). The spermatozoa leaving each testis travel along the *epididymis* (ep-i-DID-i-mus), the *ductus deferens* (DUK-tus DEF-e-renz), the *ejaculatory* (ē-JAK-ū-la-tō-rē) *duct*, and the urethra before leaving the body. Accessory organs, notably the *seminal* (SEM-i-nal) *vesicles*, the *prostate* (PROS-tāt) *gland*, and the *bulbourethral* (bul-bō-ū-RĒ-thral) *glands*, secrete into the ejaculatory ducts and urethra. The externally visible structures of the reproductive system constitute the *external genitalia* (jen-i-TĀ-lē-a). The external genitalia of the male include the *scrotum* (SKRŌ-tum), which encloses the testes, and the *penis* (PĒ-nis), an erectile organ that surrounds the distal portion of the urethra.

The Testes

The *primary sex organs* of the male system are the **testes**. The testes hang within the **scrotum**, a fleshy pouch suspended below the perineum anterior to the anus. The scrotum is subdivided into two chambers, or scrotal cavities, each containing a testis. Each testis has the shape of a flattened egg roughly 5 cm (2 in.) long, 3 cm (1.2 in.) wide, and 2.5 cm (1 in.) thick. An epithelial lining on the inner surface of the scrotum and

20

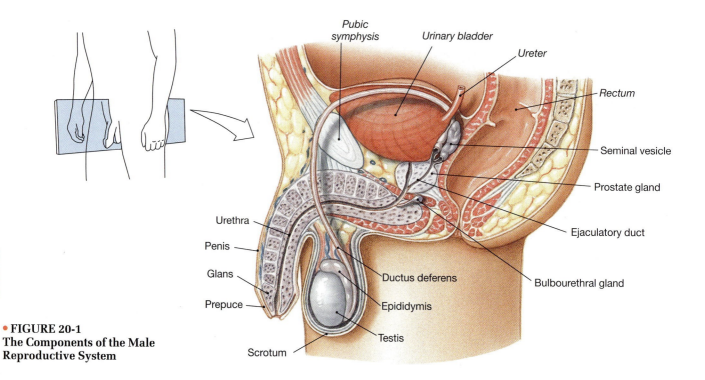

• **FIGURE 20-1**
The Components of the Male Reproductive System

Pubic symphysis · Urinary bladder · Ureter · Rectum · Seminal vesicle · Prostate gland · Ejaculatory duct · Bulbourethral gland · Ductus deferens · Epididymis · Testis · Scrotum · Prepuce · Glans · Penis · Urethra

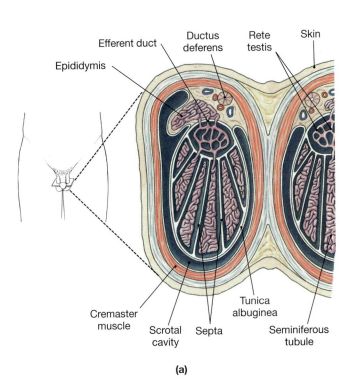

Efferent duct

Epididymis

Ductus deferens

Rete testis

Skin

Cremaster muscle

Scrotal cavity

Septa

Tunica albuginea

Seminiferous tubule

(a)

the outer surface of the testis prevents friction between the opposing surfaces.

The scrotum consists of a thin layer of skin, loose connective tissue, and smooth muscle (Figure 20-2a•). Sustained contractions of the smooth muscle layer, the *dartos* (DAR-tōs), cause the characteristic wrinkling of the scrotal surface. Beneath the dermis is a layer of skeletal muscle, the **cremaster** (kre-MAS-ter) **muscle**, which can contract to pull the testes closer to the body. Normal sperm development requires temperatures around 1.1°C (2°F) below normal body temperature. When environmental temperatures rise, the cremaster relaxes, the testes move away from the body, and excess heat is lost across the surface of the scrotum. When the scrotum is cooled, as in a cold swimming pool, cremasteric contractions pull the testes closer to the body to keep them warm.

Each testis is wrapped in a dense fibrous capsule, the **tunica albuginea** (TŪ-ni-ka al-bū-JIN-ē-a). Collagen fibers from this wrapping extend into the testis, forming partitions, or *septa*, that subdivide the testis into roughly 250 *lobules*. Sperm production occurs in the approximately 800 slender, tightly coiled **seminiferous** (se-mi-NIF-e-rus) **tubules** (Figure 20-2b•) that are distributed among the lobules. Each tubule averages around 80 cm (31 in.) in length, and a typical testis contains nearly half a mile of seminiferous tubules. A maze of passageways known as the **rete** (RĒ-tē; *rete*, a net) **testis** provide passage for sperm cells from the seminiferous tubules to the epididymis.

Seminiferous tubules containing nearly mature spermatozoa about to be released into the lumen

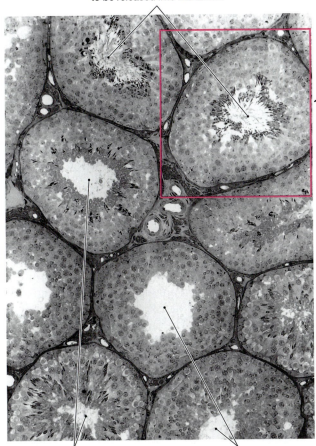

Seminiferous tubules containing late spermatids

Seminiferous tubules containing early spermatids

(b)

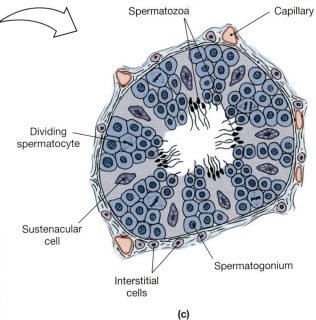

Spermatozoa

Capillary

Dividing spermatocyte

Sustenacular cell

Interstitial cells

Spermatogonium

(c)

•**FIGURE 20-2 The Testes and Seminiferous Tubules**
(a) Anatomical relationships of the testes. **(b)** A section through a coiled seminiferous tubule. **(c)** Cellular organization of a seminiferous tubule.

20

The spaces between the tubules are filled with loose connective tissue, numerous blood vessels, and large **interstitial cells** that produce male sex hormones, or *androgens* (Figure 20-2c•). The steroid **testosterone** is the most important androgen. (Testosterone and other sex hormones were introduced in Chapter 11.) ∞ *p. 322*

Sperm cells, or **spermatozoa**, are produced through **spermatogenesis** (sper-ma-tō-JEN-e-sis). This process begins with stem cells called *spermatogonia* at the outermost layer of cells in the seminiferous tubules (Figure 20-2c•) and proceeds to the central tubular lumen.

Each seminiferous tubule also contains **sustentacular** (sus-ten-TAK-ū-lar) **cells** (*Sertoli cells*). These large cells are attached to the tubular capsule and extend toward the lumen between the spermatocytes and spermatogonia (Figure 20-2c•).

✳ TESTICULAR TORSION

Testicular torsion is a major cause of scrotal pain. It occurs when a testicle twists on the spermatic cord. The testicle almost always torses lateral to medial. This usually compromises blood supply to the testicle resulting in severe scrotal and abdominal pain. If emergency surgery is not performed within six hours, the testicle may be lost. Testicular torsion most often occurs at puberty, but can occur at any age. Often there is a history of an athletic event or strenuous physical exercise prior to the onset. The diagnosis is made by physical exam and by scrotal ultrasound. The scrotal ultrasound will detect any interruptions in blood supply to the testicle. Treatment requires surgical exploration and detorsion of the testicle. The urologist will then secure *(pex)* both testicles so that additional torsions cannot occur.

Spermatogenesis

Spermatogenesis involves three integrated processes:

1. *Mitosis.* Stem cells called **spermatogonia** (sper-ma-to-GŌ-nē-a; singular, *spermatogonium*) undergo mitosis and cell division throughout adult life. (See Chapter 3 for a review of mitosis.) ∞ *p. 73* The cell divisions produce daughter cells that are pushed to the lumen of the tube. These cells differentiate into *spermatocytes* (sper-MA-to-sīts) that prepare to undergo meiosis.

2. *Meiosis.* Meiosis (mī-Ō-sis; *meioun*, to make smaller) is a special form of cell division involved in gamete production. Gametes contain half the number of chromosomes found in other cells. As a result, the fusion of a sperm and an egg yields a single cell with the normal number of chromosomes. In the seminiferous tubules, the meiotic divisions of spermatocytes produce immature gametes called *spermatids*.

3. *Spermiogenesis.* Spermatids are small, relatively unspecialized cells. In *spermiogenesis*, spermatids differentiate into physically mature spermatozoa.

Mitosis and Meiosis. Mitosis and meiosis differ significantly in terms of nuclear events and outcomes. **Mitosis** is part of the process of somatic cell division, which involves one division that produces two daughter cells, each containing the same number and kind of chromosomes as the original cell. In humans, each somatic (nonreproductive) cell contains 23 pairs of chromosomes. Each pair consists of one chromosome provided by the male parent and another by the female parent at the time of fertilization. Because each cell contains both members of each chromosome pair, the daughter cells are described as **diploid** (DIP-loyd; *diplo*, double). **Meiosis** begins with a diploid stem cell. After two divisions, four gametes are produced. Because each of these gametes contains only one member of each chromosome pair, gametes are described as **haploid** (HAP-loyd; *haplo*, single). Meiosis in humans produces haploid gametes that contain 23 individual chromosomes.

Figure 20-3• illllustrates meiosis sperm production. (To make the chromosomal events easier to follow, only 3 of the 23 pairs of chromosomes present in spermatogonia are shown.) The mitotic divisions of spermatogonia produce primary spermatocytes. Like spermatogonia, primary spermatocytes are diploid cells, but they divide by meiosis rather than mitosis. As a primary spermatocyte prepares to begin meiosis, all of the chromosomes in the nucleus replicate themselves as if the cell were to undergo mitosis. As prophase of the first meiotic division, meiosis I, occurs, the chromosomes condense and become visible. As in mitosis, each chromosome consists of two duplicate *chromatids* (KRŌ-ma-tidz).

Each primary spermatocyte contains 46 individual chromosomes, the same as any somatic cell in the body. As prophase ends, the corresponding maternal and paternal chromosomes now come together. This event, known as **synapsis** (sin-AP-sis), produces 23 pairs of chromosomes, each member of the pair consisting of two identical chromatids. A matched set of four chromatids is called a **tetrad** (TET-rad; *tetras*, four). An exchange of genetic material, called *crossing-over*, can occur between the chromatids at this stage of meiosis. This exchange increases genetic variation among offspring.

During metaphase of meiosis I, the nuclear envelope disappears and the tetrads line up along the metaphase plate. As anaphase begins, the tetrads break up, and the maternal and paternal chromosomes separate. This is a major difference between mitosis and meiosis: In mitosis, each daughter cell receives one of the two copies of every chromosome, maternal and paternal, whereas in meiosis, each daughter cell receives both copies of *either* the maternal chromosome or the paternal chromosome from each tetrad.

As anaphase proceeds, the maternal and paternal components are randomly distributed. For example, most of the maternal chromosomes may go to one daughter cell, and most of the paternal chromosomes to the other. As a result, telophase I ends with the for-

chromatids. The duplicates will separate during **meiosis II**. The interphase separating meiosis I and meiosis II is very brief, and the secondary spermatocyte soon enters prophase of meiosis II. The completion of metaphase II, anaphase II, and telophase II produces four **spermatids** (SPER-ma-tidz), each with 23 chromosomes. In summary, for every primary spermatocyte that enters meiosis, four spermatids are produced (Figure 20-3•).

Spermiogenesis. Each spermatid matures into a single **spermatozoon** (sper-ma-tō-ZŌ-on), or sperm cell, through the process of **spermiogenesis**. The entire process, from spermatogonial division to the release of a physically mature spermatozoon, takes approximately 9 weeks.

Sustentacular cells play a key role in spermiogenesis. Because there are no blood vessels inside the seminiferous tubules, all nutrients must enter by diffusion from the surrounding interstitial fluids. The large sustentacular cells control the chemical environment inside the seminiferous tubules and, because they surround the spermatids, provide nutrients and chemical stimuli that promote the production and differentiation of spermatozoa. They also help regulate spermatogenesis by producing *inhibin*, a hormone introduced in Chapter 11. ∞ *p. 322*

Anatomy of a Spermatozoon

A sperm cell has three distinct regions: the head, the middle piece, and the tail (Figure 20-4•). The **head** is a

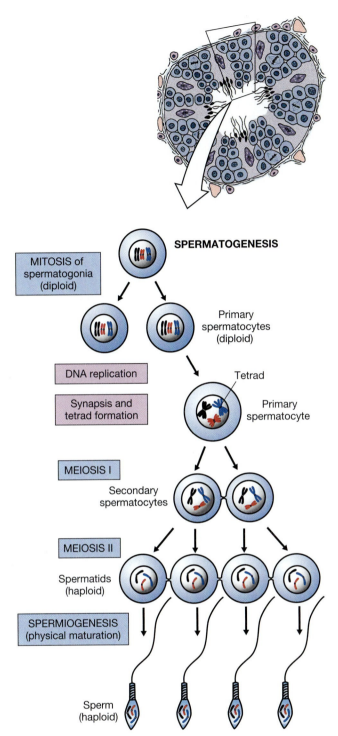

• **FIGURE 20-3** **Meiosis and Spermatozoon Formation**
Each diploid primary spermatocyte that undergoes meiosis produces four haploid spermatids. Each spermatid then differentiates into a spermatozoon.

mation of two daughter cells containing unique combinations of maternal and paternal chromosomes. In the testes, the daughter cells produced by the first meiotic division (meiosis I) are called **secondary spermatocytes**.

Each secondary spermatocyte contains 23 chromosomes. These chromosomes consist of two duplicate

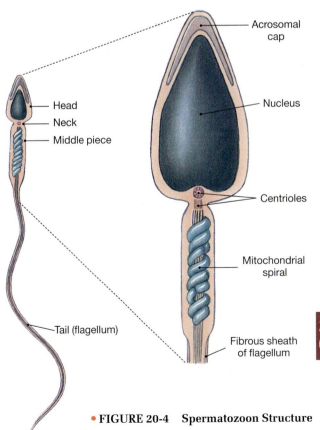

• **FIGURE 20-4** **Spermatozoon Structure**

flattened oval filled with densely packed chromosomes. The tip forms the **acrosomal** (ak-rō-SŌ-mal) **cap**, which contains enzymes essential for fertilization. A very short **neck** attaches the head to the **middle piece**, which is dominated by the mitochondria providing the energy for moving the **tail**. The sperm cell's tail, the only example of a *flagellum* in the human body, moves the cell from one place to another. ∞ *p. 66*

The entire streamlined structure measures only 60 μm in total length. Unlike most other cells, a mature spermatozoon lacks an endoplasmic reticulum, Golgi apparatus, lysosomes, peroxisomes, and inclusions, among other structures. Because the cell does not contain glycogen or other energy reserves, it must absorb nutrients (primarily fructose) from the surrounding fluid.

The Male Reproductive Tract

The testes produce physically mature spermatozoa that are, as yet, incapable of fertilizing an ovum. The other portions of the male reproductive system, sometimes called the *accessory structures*, are concerned with the functional maturation, nourishment, storage, and transport of spermatozoa.

The Epididymis

Late in their development, the spermatozoa become detached from the sustentacular cells and lie within the lumen of the seminiferous tubule. Although they have most of the physical characteristics of mature sperm cells, they are still functionally immature and incapable of coordinated locomotion. At this point, fluid currents transport them into the **epididymis** (see Figure 20-1•, p. 548). This elongate tubule, almost 7 meters (23 ft) long, is so twisted and coiled that it actually takes up very little space. During the 2 weeks that it takes for a spermatozoon to travel through the epididymis, it completes its physical maturation. Damaged or abnormal spermatozoa are recycled, and the epididymis absorbs cellular debris and organic nutrients. Mature spermatozoa then arrive at the ductus deferens.

Although the spermatozoa leaving the epididymus are physically mature, they remain immobile. To become active, motile, and fully functional, they must undergo **capacitation**, and the epididymis secretes a substance that prevents premature capacitation. Capacitation occurs when the spermatozoa (1) mix with secretions of the seminal vesicles and (2) are exposed to conditions inside the female reproductive tract.

The Ductus Deferens

The **ductus deferens**, also known as the *vas deferens*, is 40–45 cm (16–18 in.) long. It extends toward the abdominal cavity within a connective tissue sheath that also encloses the blood vessels, nerves, and lymphat-

ics serving the testis as well as part of the cremaster muscle (Figure 20-5•). The entire complex is called the **spermatic cord**.

After passing through the *inguinal canal*, the components of the spermatic cord go their separate ways. The ductus deferens curves downward alongside the urinary bladder toward the prostate gland (Figures 20-1, p. 548, and 20-5a•). Peristaltic contractions in the muscular walls of the ductus deferens propel spermatozoa and fluid along the length of the duct. The ductus deferens can also store spermatozoa for up to several months. During this period the spermatozoa are in a state of suspended animation, remaining inactive with low metabolic rates.

The junction of the ductus deferens with the duct draining the seminal vesicle creates the **ejaculatory duct**, a relatively short (2 cm, or less than 1 in.) passageway. This duct penetrates the muscular wall of the prostate gland and fuses with the ejaculatory duct from the other side before emptying into the urethra.

The Urethra

The urethra of the male extends from the urinary bladder to the tip of the penis, a distance of 15–20 cm (6–8 in.). The urethra in the male is a passageway used by both the urinary and reproductive systems.

The Accessory Glands

The fluids contributed by the seminiferous tubules and the epididymis account for only about 5 percent of the final volume of *semen*, the fluid that transports and nourishes sperm. The major fraction of seminal fluid is composed of secretions from the *seminal vesicles*, the *prostate gland*, and the *bulbourethral glands*. Primary functions of these glandular organs include: (1) activating the spermatozoa, (2) providing the nutrients spermatozoa need for motility, (3) propelling spermatozoa and fluids along the reproductive tract through peristaltic contractions, and (4) producing buffers that counteract the acidity of the urethral and vaginal contents.

The Seminal Vesicles

Each **seminal vesicle** is a tubular gland with a total length of around 15 cm (6 in.). The body of the gland is coiled and folded into a compact, tapered mass roughly 5 cm by 2.5 cm (2 in. by 1 in.) (Figures 20-1, p. 548, and 20-5a•).

The seminal vesicles contribute about 60 percent of the volume of semen. In particular, their secretions contain relatively high concentrations of fructose, a six-carbon sugar easily metabolized by spermatozoa. The secretions are also slightly alkaline, and alkalinity helps neutralize acids in the prostatic secretions and within the vagina. When mixed with the secretions of the seminal vesicles, previously inactive but mature spermatozoa begin beating their flagella and become highly mobile.

• FIGURE 20-5
The Ductus Deferens

(a) A posterior view of the prostate gland, showing subdivisions of the ductus deferens in relation to surrounding structures. **(b)** Micrographs showing extensive layering with smooth muscle around the lumen of the ductus deferens. (Reproduced from R. G. Kessel and R. H. Kardon, *Tissues and Organs: A Text-Atlas of Scanning Electron Microscopy*, W. H. Freeman & Co., 1979.) (LM × 34; SEM × 42)

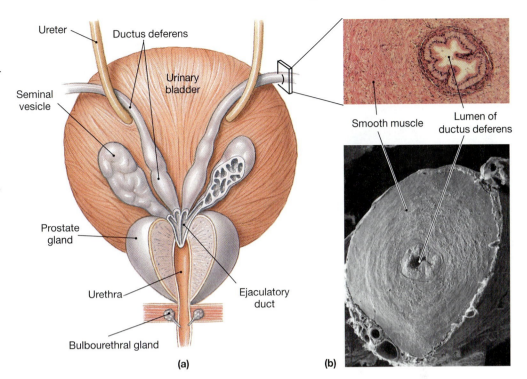

(a) (b)

The Prostate Gland

The **prostate gland** is a small, muscular, rounded organ with a diameter of about 4 cm (1.6 in.). As indicated in Figure 20-5a•, the prostate gland surrounds the urethra as it leaves the urinary bladder. The prostatic wall produces a weakly acidic secretion that contributes about 30 percent of the volume of semen. In addition to several other compounds of uncertain significance, prostatic secretions contain **seminalplasmin** (sem-i-nal-PLAZ-min), an antibiotic that may help prevent urinary tract infections in males. These secretions are ejected into the prostatic urethra by peristaltic contractions of the muscular wall.

✳ PRIAPISM

Priapism is a prolonged, usually painful, penile erection that is not associated with sexual arousal. In many cases, the cause of priapism is unclear *(idiopathic)*. However, it is associated with sickle cell disease, spinal cord injury, spinal anesthesia, leukemia, and drugs. Most cases of priapism result from intracavernous injection of medications to treat impotence. In high spinal cord injury, priapism can occur if there is unopposed parasympathetic stimulation.

The erection seen in priapism is due to engorgement of the *corpora cavernosa*. The *corpora spongiosum* and the *glans* are not engorged as with a normal erection. Priapism is a urological emergency. Treatment within hours is necessary to prevent permanent injury.

The Bulbourethral Glands

The paired **bulbourethral glands**, or *Cowper's glands*, are round, with diameters approaching 10 mm (less than 0.5 in.) (Figure 20-5a•). These glands secrete a thick, sticky, alkaline mucus that has lubricating properties.

Semen

Semen (SĒ-men) is the fluid that contains sperm and the secretions of the accessory glands of the male reproductive tract. In a typical **ejaculation** (ē-jak-ū-LĀ-shun), 2–5 ml of semen is expelled from the body. This volume of fluid, called an **ejaculate**, contains the following:

- *Spermatozoa.* A normal **sperm count** ranges from 20 million to 100 million spermatozoa per milliliter.
- *Seminal fluid.* **Seminal fluid**, the fluid component of semen, is a mixture of glandular secretions with a distinctive ionic and nutrient composition. In terms of total volume, the seminal fluid contains the combined secretions of the seminal vesicles (60 percent), the prostate (30 percent), the sustentacular cells and epididymis (5 percent), and the bulbourethral glands (less than 5 percent).
- *Enzymes.* Several important enzymes are present in the seminal fluid. For example, semen includes a protease that helps dissolve mucous secretions in the vagina, and *seminalplasmin.*

Within a few minutes after ejaculation semen coagulates, liquefying again after a variable period. The function of this clotting is unknown.

The Penis

The **penis** is a tubular organ that surrounds the urethra (see Figure 20-1•). It conducts urine to the exterior and introduces semen into the female vagina during sexual intercourse. As shown in Figure 20-6•, the penis is

20

•FIGURE 20-6   The Penis
(a) The positions of the erectile tissues. **(b)** A frontal section through the penis and associated organs. **(c)** A sectional view through the penis.

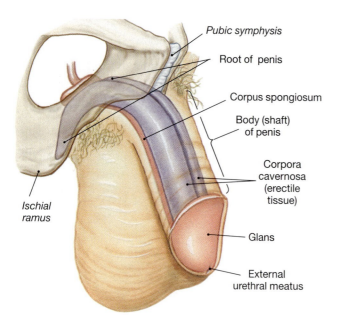

(a) Anterior and lateral view of penis

Labels: Pubic symphysis · Root of penis · Corpus spongiosum · Body (shaft) of penis · Corpora cavernosa (erectile tissue) · Glans · External urethral meatus · Ischial ramus

composed of three regions: (1) the **root**, the fixed portion that attaches the penis to the body wall; (2) the **body (shaft)**, the tubular portion that contains masses of erectile tissue; and (3) the **glans**, the expanded distal end that surrounds the external urethral opening, or *external urethral meatus.*

The skin overlying the penis resembles that of the scrotum. A fold of skin, the **prepuce** (PRĒ-pūs), or *foreskin*, surrounds the tip of the penis. The prepuce attaches to the relatively narrow *neck* of the penis and continues over the glans. *Preputial glands* in the skin of the neck and inner surface of the prepuce secrete a waxy material called *smegma* (SMEG-ma). Unfortunately, smegma can be an excellent nutrient source for bacteria. Mild inflammation and infections in this region are common, especially if the area is not washed frequently. One way of avoiding trouble is *circumcision* (ser-kum-SIZH-un), the surgical removal of the prepuce. In Western societies this procedure is usually performed shortly after birth.

Most of the body, or shaft, of the penis consists of three columns of **erectile tissue** (Figure 20-6b•). Erectile tissue consists of a three-dimensional maze of vascular channels incompletely divided by sheets of elastic connective tissue and smooth muscle. On the anterior surface of the penis, two cylindrical **corpora cavernosa** (KŌR-po-ra ka-ver-NŌ-sa) are bound to the pubis and ischium of the pelvis. The corpora cavernosa extend along as far as the glans of the penis. The relatively slender **corpus spongiosum** (spon-jē-Ō-sum) surrounds the urethra and extends all the way to the tip of the penis, where it forms the glans.

In the resting state, there is little blood flow into the erectile tissue because the arterial branches are constricted. During *arousal*, parasympathetic stimulation

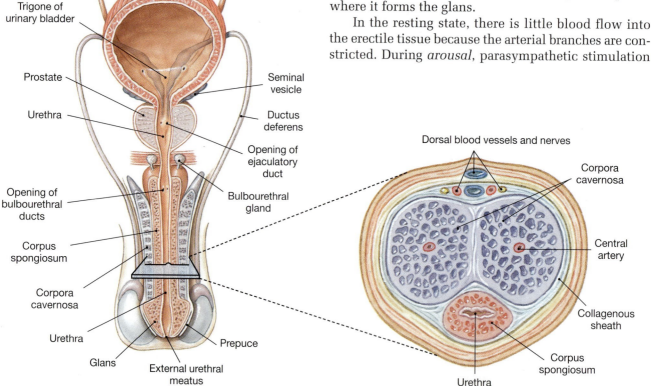

Labels (b): Trigone of urinary bladder · Prostate · Urethra · Opening of bulbourethral ducts · Corpus spongiosum · Corpora cavernosa · Urethra · Glans · External urethral meatus · Prepuce · Ureter · Seminal vesicle · Ductus deferens · Opening of ejaculatory duct · Bulbourethral gland

(b) Frontal section

Labels (c): Dorsal blood vessels and nerves · Corpora cavernosa · Central artery · Collagenous sheath · Corpus spongiosum · Urethra

(c) Section through shaft of penis

dilates the walls of the arterial blood vessels to the erectile tissue, blood flow increases, the penis becomes engorged with blood, and **erection** occurs.

Hormones and Male Reproductive Function

Major reproductive hormones were introduced in Chapter 11, and the hormonal interactions in the male are diagrammed in Figure 20-7●. ∞ *p. 322* The anterior pituitary releases **follicle-stimulating hormone (FSH)** and a second peptide hormone, **luteinizing hormone (LH)**, named after its effects in the female. (This hormone was called *interstitial cell-stimulating hormone, ICSH*, in males before it was known to be identical to the hormone in females.) The pituitary release of these hormones occurs in the presence of **gonadotropin-releasing hormone (GnRH)**, a hormone synthesized in the hypothalamus and carried to the anterior pituitary in the hypophyseal portal system.

FSH and Spermatogenesis

In the male, FSH targets primarily the sustentacular cells of the seminiferous tubules. Under FSH stimulation, and in the presence of testosterone from the interstitial cells, sustentacular cells promote spermatogenesis and spermiogenesis.

The rate of spermatogenesis is regulated by a negative feedback mechanism involving GnRH, FSH, and inhibin. Under GnRH stimulation, FSH promotes spermatogenesis along the seminiferous tubules. As spermatogenesis accelerates, however, so does the rate of inhibin secretion by the sustentacular cells of the testes. Inhibin inhibits FSH production in the anterior pituitary and may also suppress secretion of GnRH at the hypothalamus.

The net effect is that when FSH levels become elevated, inhibin production increases until the FSH levels return to normal. If FSH levels decline, inhibin production falls, and the rate of FSH production then accelerates.

LH and Androgen Production

In the male, LH causes the secretion of testosterone and other androgens by the interstitial cells of the testes. Testosterone, the most important androgen, has numerous functions. It (1) promotes the functional maturation of spermatozoa; (2) maintains the accessory organs of the male reproductive tract; (3) determines the secondary sex characteristics, such as facial hair,

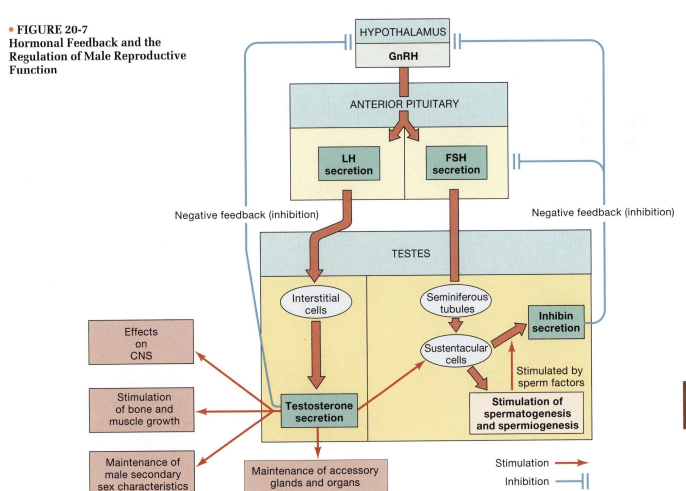

●**FIGURE 20-7**
Hormonal Feedback and the Regulation of Male Reproductive Function

increased muscle mass and body size, and the quantity and location of characteristic adipose tissue deposits; (4) stimulates metabolic operations throughout the body, especially those concerned with protein synthesis and muscle growth; and (5) influences brain development by stimulating sexual behaviors and sexual drive.

Testosterone production begins around the seventh week of embryonic development and reaches a peak after roughly 6 months of development. The early surge in testosterone levels stimulates the differentiation of the male duct system and accessory organs. Testosterone production accelerates markedly at puberty, initiating sexual maturation and the appearance of secondary sex characteristics. In the adult, the level of testosterone is controlled by negative feedback. Above-normal testosterone levels inhibit the release of GnRH by the hypothalamus. This inhibition causes a reduction in LH secretion and lowers testosterone levels.

✓ On a warm day, would the cremaster muscle be contracted or relaxed? Why?

✓ How would the lack of an acrosomal cap affect the ability of a spermatozoon to fertilize an ovum?

✓ What will occur if the arteries serving the penis dilate?

✓ What effect would low levels of FSH have on sperm production?

THE REPRODUCTIVE SYSTEM OF THE FEMALE

A woman's reproductive system must produce sex hormones and gametes, protect and support a developing embryo, and nourish the newborn infant. The primary sex organs of the female reproductive system are the *ovaries*. The internal and external accessory organs include the *uterine tubes*, the *uterus* (womb), the *vagina*, and the components of the external genitalia (Figure 20-8•). As in the male, various accessory glands secrete into the reproductive tract. Physicians specializing in the female reproductive system are called **gynecologists** (gī-ne-KOL-o-jists; *gyne*, woman).

The Ovaries

A typical **ovary** is a flattened oval that measures approximately 5 cm by 2.5 cm by 8 mm (2 in. by 1 in. by 0.33 in.). It has a pale white or yellowish coloration and a nodular consistency that resembles cottage cheese or lumpy oatmeal. The interior of the ovary is composed of a superficial *cortex* and a deep *medulla*. The production of gametes occurs in the cortex, and the arteries, veins, lymphatics, and nerves within the relatively narrow medulla link the ovary with other body systems.

The ovaries are responsible for (1) the production of female gametes, or **ova** (singular *ovum*); (2) the secretion of female sex hormones, including *estrogens*

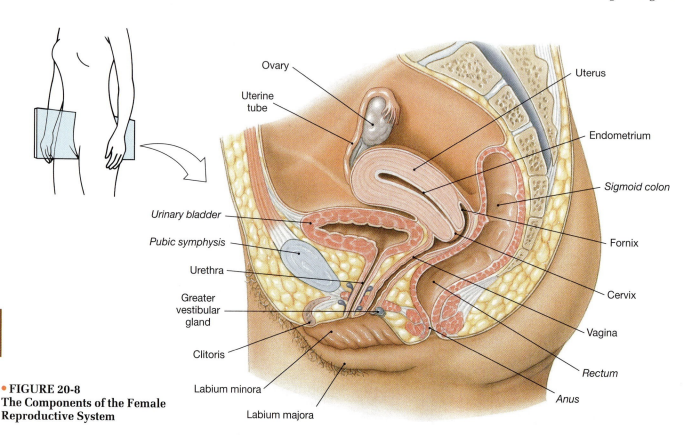

•**FIGURE 20-8**
The Components of the Female Reproductive System

2
0

and *progestins*; and (3) the secretion of inhibin, involved in the feedback control of pituitary FSH production.

Oogenesis

Ovum production, or **oogenesis** (ō-ō-JEN-e-sis; *oon*, egg), begins before birth, accelerates at puberty, and ends at menopause (*men*, month + *pausis*, cessation). Between puberty and menopause, oogenesis occurs monthly, as part of the *ovarian cycle*. Oogenesis is illustrated in Figure 20-9•; as in Figure 20-3• (p. 551) on spermatogenesis, only 3 of the 23 pairs of chromosomes are illustrated.

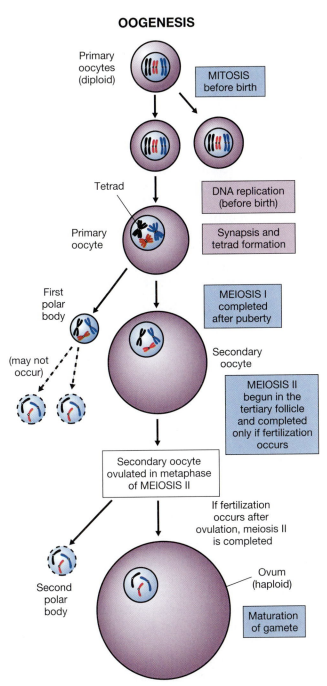

OOGENESIS

Primary oocytes (diploid)

MITOSIS before birth

Tetrad

Primary oocyte

DNA replication (before birth)

Synapsis and tetrad formation

First polar body

MEIOSIS I completed after puberty

(may not occur)

Secondary oocyte

MEIOSIS II begun in the tertiary follicle and completed only if fertilization occurs

Secondary oocyte ovulated in metaphase of MEIOSIS II

If fertilization occurs after ovulation, meiosis II is completed

Second polar body

Ovum (haploid)

Maturation of gamete

•FIGURE 20-9   **Meiosis and Oogenesis**
The production of an ovum.

In the ovaries, stem cells, or **oogonia** (ō-ō-GŌ-nē-a), complete their mitotic divisions before birth. Between the third and seventh months of fetal development, the daughter cells, or **primary oocytes** (Ō-ō-sīts), prepare to undergo meiosis (Figure 20-9•). They proceed as far as prophase of meiosis I, but at that time the process stops. The primary oocytes then remain in a state of suspended development until puberty, awaiting the hormonal signal to complete meiosis. Not all of the primary oocytes in the ovaries at birth survive until puberty. There are roughly 2 million in the ovaries at birth; by the time of puberty, about 400,000 remain. The rest of the primary oocytes degenerate, a process called *atresia* (a-TRĒ-zē-a).

Although the nuclear events under way during meiosis in the ovary are the same as those in the testis, the process differs in two important details.

1. The cytoplasm of the original oocyte is not evenly distributed during the meiotic divisions. Oogenesis produces one functional ovum, containing most of that cytoplasm, and three nonfunctional **polar bodies** that later disintegrate.

2. The ovary releases a *secondary oocyte*, rather than a mature ovum. The second meiotic division does not occur until *after* fertilization.

The Ovarian Cycle

Oogenesis occurs in the cortex within specialized structures called **ovarian follicles** (ō-VAR-ē-an FOL-i-klz). In the outer portions of the cortex, just beneath the capsule, there are clusters of primary oocytes, each surrounded by a layer of follicle cells. The combination is known as a **primordial** (prī-MŌR-dē-al) **follicle**. At puberty, rising levels of FSH begin to activate a different group of primordial follicles each month. This monthly process is known as the **ovarian cycle**. Important steps in the ovarian cycle are shown in Figure 20-10•:

Step 1: *Formation of primary follicles.* The cycle begins as the activated follicles develop into **primary follicles**. The follicle cells divide and form several concentric layers around the oocyte. As the wall of the follicle thickens further, a space opens up between the developing oocyte and the follicular cells. Within this space, called the **zona pellucida** (ZŌ-na pel-LŪ-si-da; *pellucidus*, translucent), microvilli originating at the surface of the oocyte contact those of the follicular cells. These microvilli increase the surface area available for absorption by roughly 35 times, and the follicular cells are continually providing the developing oocyte with nutrients.

Step 2: *Formation of secondary follicles.* Although many primordial follicles develop into primary follicles, usually only a few will take the next step. The transformation begins as the wall of the follicle

2 0

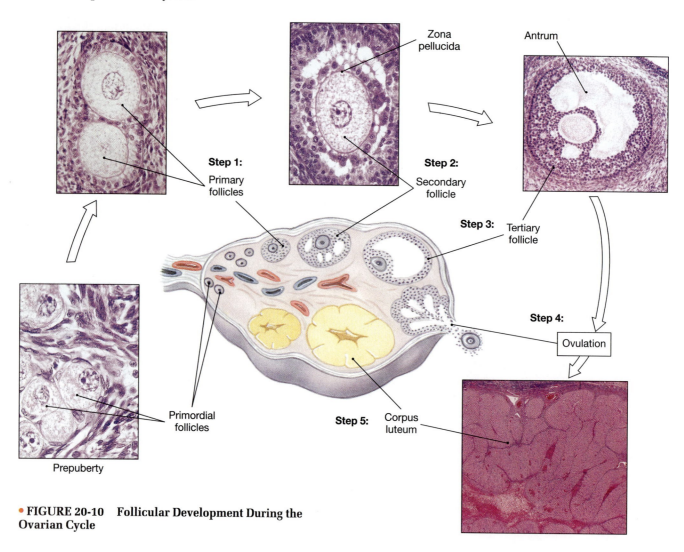

Zona pellucida

Antrum

Step 1: Primary follicles

Step 2: Secondary follicle

Step 3: Tertiary follicle

Step 4: Ovulation

Primordial follicles

Step 5: Corpus luteum

Prepuberty

● **FIGURE 20-10   Follicular Development During the Ovarian Cycle**

thickens and the deeper follicular cells begin secreting small amounts of fluid. This *follicular fluid* accumulates in small pockets that gradually expand and separate the inner and outer layers of the follicle. At this stage, the complex is known as a **secondary follicle**. Although the oocyte continues to grow slowly, the follicle as a whole now enlarges rapidly because of this accumulation of fluid.

Step 3: *Formation of tertiary follicles.* Eight to 10 days after the start of the ovarian cycle, the ovaries usually contain only a single secondary follicle destined for further development. By days 10 to 14 of the cycle, it has formed a mature **tertiary follicle**, or *Graafian* (GRAF-ē-an) *follicle*, roughly 15 mm in diameter. This complex spans the entire width of the ovarian cortex and stretches the ovarian capsule, creating a prominent bulge in the surface of the ovary. The oocyte, surrounded by a mass of follicular cells, projects into the expanded central chamber of the follicle, the **antrum** (AN-trum).

Step 4: *Ovulation.* As the time of egg release, or **ovulation** (ōv-ū-LĀ-shun), approaches, the follicular cells surrounding the oocyte lose contact with the follicular wall, and the oocyte floats within the central chamber. This event usually occurs at day 14 of a 28-day cycle. The follicular cells surrounding the oocyte are now known as the *corona radiata* (ko-RŌ-na rā-dē-A-ta). The distended follicular wall then ruptures, releasing the follicular contents, including the secondary oocyte, into the pelvic cavity. Because the corona radiata has a sticky surface, the oocyte usually attaches to the ovarian surface near the ruptured wall of the follicle. Contact with the entrance to the uterine tube or fluid currents established by its ciliated lining then sweeps the secondary oocyte into the uterine tube.

Step 5: *Formation and degeneration of the corpus luteum.* The empty follicle collapses, and the remaining follicular cells invade the cavity and multiply to create an endocrine structure known as the **corpus luteum** (LOO-tē-um; *lutea*, yellow).

Unless pregnancy occurs, after about 12 days the corpus luteum begins to degenerate. The disintegration marks the end of the ovarian cycle, but almost immediately the activation of another set of primordial follicles begins the next ovarian cycle.

The Uterine Tubes

Each **uterine tube** (*Fallopian tube*, or *oviduct*) measures roughly 13 cm (5 in.) in length. The end closest to the ovary forms an expanded funnel, or **infundibulum** (in-fun-DIB-ū-lum; *infundibulum*, a funnel), with numerous fingerlike projections that extend into the pelvic cavity (Figure 20-11•). The projections, called **fimbriae** (FIM-brē-ē), and the inner surfaces of the infundibulum are carpeted with cilia that beat toward the broad entrance to the uterine tube. Once inside the uterine tube, the ovum is probably transported by ciliary movement and peristaltic contractions. It normally takes 3–4 days for the secondary oocyte to travel from the infundibulum to the uterine chamber. *If fertilization is to occur, the secondary oocyte must encounter spermatozoa during the first 12–24 hours of its passage.* Unfertilized oocytes will degenerate, in the uterine tubes or uterus, without completing meiosis.

✳ PELVIC INFLAMMATORY DISEASE (PID)

Pelvic inflammatory disease (PID) is the most common serious infection among women of reproductive age in the United States. It is caused by organisms ascending the upper female reproductive tract from the vagina and cervix. The most common causative organisms are *Neissera gonorrhoeae* and *Chlamydia trachomatis*. Often, however, multiple organisms are involved.

Risk factors for the development of PID include frequent sexual activity with multiple partners, a history of previous gonococcal infection, adolescence, and use of an intrauterine device. Pregnancy provides protection from PID as the uterus is effectively sealed off from bacterial invasion.

The signs and symptoms of PID are lower abdominal pain, fever, generalized malaise, and a vaginal discharge. With severe infections, even slight movement of the abdomen can cause pain forcing the patient to walk bent over and to take small steps. During the pelvic examination, movement of the cervix causes intense pain. PID can cause the formation of an abscess involving the uterine tubes and ovaries *(tuboovarian abscess).*

The treatment for PID follows guidelines established by the Centers for Disease Control (CDC). Patients with PID that is not complicated by an abscess can be treated with oral antibiotics. More severe cases, and those complicated by an abscess, require hospitalization and intravenous antibiotics.

PID can cause permanent blockage of the uterine tubes, chronic abdominal pain, and infertility. Fifty percent of patients who have more than two episodes of PID are infertile.

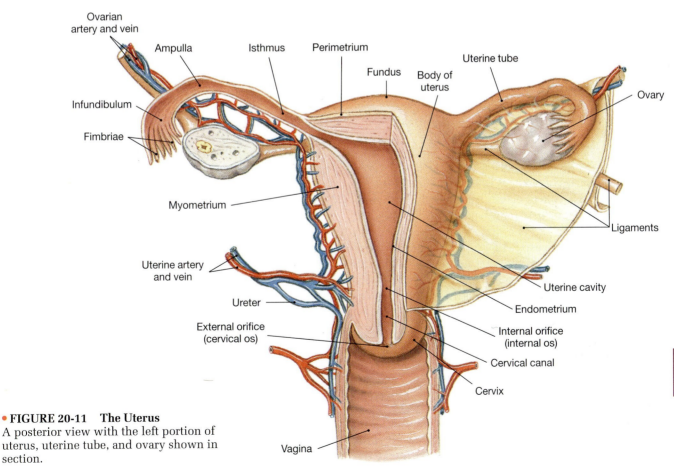

• **FIGURE 20-11   The Uterus**
A posterior view with the left portion of uterus, uterine tube, and ovary shown in section.

2
0

The Uterus

The **uterus** (Ū-ter-us) is a muscular chamber that provides mechanical protection and nutritional support to the developing embryo and fetus (see Figures 20-8, p. 556, and 20-11•). The typical uterus is a small, pear-shaped organ about 7.5 cm (3 in.) in length with a maximum diameter of 5 cm (2 in.). It weighs 30–40 g (1–1.4 oz.) and is stabilized by various ligaments.

The uterus consists of two regions: the body and the cervix. The **body** is the largest division of the uterus. The *fundus* is the rounded portion of the body superior to the attachment of the uterine tubes. The body ends at a constriction known as the **isthmus**. The **cervix** (SER-viks) is the inferior portion of the uterus. The cervix projects a short distance into the vagina, and the **uterine cavity** opens into the vagina at the **external orifice**, or *cervical os.*

The thick uterine wall is made up of an inner **endometrium** (en-dō-MĒ-trē-um) and a muscular **myometrium** (mī-ō-MĒ-trē-um; *myo-*, muscle + *metra*, uterus), covered by the *perimetrium*, a layer of visceral peritoneum (Figure 20-11•). The endometrium of the uterus includes the epithelium lining the uterine chambers and the underlying connective tissues. Uterine glands opening onto the endometrial surface extend deep into the connective tissue layer almost all the way to the myometrium. The myometrium consists of a thick mass of interwoven smooth muscle cells.

The endometrium consists of a superficial *functional zone* and a deeper *basilar zone* that is adjacent to the myometrium. The structure of the basilar layer remains relatively constant over time, but that of the functional zone undergoes cyclical changes in response to sex hormone levels. These alterations produce the characteristic features of the uterine cycle.

The Uterine Cycle

The **uterine cycle**, or *menstrual* (MEN-stroo-al) *cycle,* is a repeating series of changes in the structure of the endometrium. This cycle of events begins with the **menarche** (me-NAR-kē), or first menstrual period at puberty, typically age 11 or 12. The cycles continue until age 45–50, when **menopause** (MEN-ō-paws), the last menstrual cycle, occurs. Over the intervening 3.5–4 decades the regular appearance of menstrual cycles will be interrupted only by unusual circumstances, such as illness, stress, starvation, or pregnancy.

The uterine cycle averages 28 days in length, but it can range from 21 to 35 days in normal individuals. It consists of three stages: *menses*, the *proliferative phase*, and the *secretory phase.*

Menses.   The menstrual cycle begins with the onset of **menses** (MEN-sēz), a period marked by the wholesale destruction of the superficial layer, or *functional zone,* of the endometrium. The process is triggered by the decline in progesterone and estrogen levels as the corpus luteum disintegrates. The endometrial arteries constrict, reducing blood flow to this region, and the secretory glands, epithelial cells, and other tissues of the functional zone die of oxygen and nutrient deprivation. Eventually the weakened arterial walls rupture, and blood pours into the connective tissues of the functional zone. Blood cells and degenerating tissues break away and enter the uterine lumen, to be lost by passage into the vagina. This sloughing of tissue, which continues until the entire functional zone has been lost, is **menstruation** (men-stroo-Ā-shun). Menstruation usually lasts 1 to 7 days, and roughly 35–50 ml of blood is lost. Painful menstruation, or *dysmenorrhea*, may result from uterine inflammation and contraction or from conditions involving adjacent pelvic structures.

The Proliferative Phase.   The **proliferative phase** begins in the days following the completion of menses as the surviving epithelial cells multiply and spread across the surface of the endometrium. This repair process is stimulated by the rising estrogen levels that accompany the growth of another set of ovarian follicles. By the time ovulation occurs, the functional zone is several millimeters thick and its new set of uterine, or endometrial, glands are manufacturing a mucus rich in glycogen. In addition, the entire functional zone is filled with small arteries that branch from larger trunks in the myometrium.

The Secretory Phase.   During the **secretory phase** of the cycle, the endometrial glands enlarge, steadily increasing their rates of secretion as the endometrium prepares for the arrival of a developing embryo. This activity is stimulated by the progestins and estrogens from the corpus luteum. This phase begins at the time of ovulation and persists as long as the corpus luteum remains intact. Secretory activities peak about 12 days after ovulation. Over the next day or two the glandular activity declines, and the uterine cycle comes to a close. A new cycle then begins with the onset of menses and the disintegration of the functional zone.

MENSTRUAL IRREGULARITIES

Menstrual irregularities are common. Normal menstrual flow usually lasts less than a week. On the average, about 35 ml (a little more than an ounce) of blood is lost. A disturbance in the menstruation that results in abnormal uterine bleeding is called *dysfunctional uterine bleeding (DUB).* It is most commonly associated with a cycle where ovulation has not occurred. The absence of a period is termed *amenorrhea.* Pregnancy is the most common cause of amenorrhea, although hormonal factors are also frequently implicated. Pelvic pain associated with the onset of menses is called *dysmenorrhea.* Usually, the discomfort begins shortly before the onset of menstruation and ends by the second day. Dysmenorrhea improves in most women with use of oral contraceptives.

The Vagina

The **vagina** (va-JĪ-na) is a muscular tube extending between the uterus and the external genitalia (Figures 20-8, p. 556, and 20-12•). It has an average length of 7.5–9 cm (3–3.5 in.), but because the vagina is highly distensible, its length and width are quite variable. The cervix of the uterus projects into the vagina. The shallow recess surrounding the cervical protrusion is known as the **fornix** (FŌR-niks). The vagina lies parallel to the rectum, and the two are in close contact. After leaving the urinary bladder, the urethra turns and travels along the superior wall of the vagina.

The vaginal walls contain a network of blood vessels and layers of smooth muscle, and the lining is moistened by the secretions of the cervical glands and by the movement of water across the permeable epithelium. The vagina and vestibule are separated by an elastic epithelial fold, the **hymen** (HĪ-men), which may partially or completely block the entrance to the vagina. The two bulbospongiosus muscles pass on either side of the vaginal orifice, and their contractions constrict the entrance.

The vagina (1) serves as a passageway for the elimination of menstrual fluids; (2) receives the penis during *coitus*, or sexual intercourse, and holds spermatozoa prior to their passage into the uterus; and (3) during childbirth, forms the lower portion of the birth canal through which the fetus passes on its way to an independent existence.

The vagina normally contains resident bacteria supported by the nutrients found in the cervical mucus. As a result of their metabolic activities, the normal pH of the vagina ranges between 3.5 and 4.5, and this acid environment restricts the growth of many pathogenic organisms. An infection of the vaginal canal, known as *vaginitis* (va-jin-Ī-tis), may be caused by fungal, bacterial, or parasitic organisms. In addition to any discomfort that may result, the condition may affect the survival of sperm, thereby reducing fertility.

The External Genitalia

The **perineum**, the muscular floor of the pelvic cavity, includes structures associated with the reproductive system called the **external genitalia**. ∞ p. 192 The perineal region enclosing the female external genitalia is the **vulva** (VUL-va), or *pudendum* (Figure 20-12•). The vagina opens into the **vestibule**, a central space bounded by the **labia minora** (LĀ-bē-a mi-NOR-a; *labia*, lips; singular *labium minus*). The labia minora are covered with a smooth, hairless skin. The urethra opens into the vestibule just anterior to the vaginal entrance. Anterior to the urethral opening, the **clitoris** (KLI-to-ris) projects into the vestibule. The clitoris is the female equivalent of the penis, derived from the same embryonic structures. Internally it contains erectile tissues that become engorged with blood during arousal. A small erectile *glans* sits atop the organ, and extensions of the labia minora encircle the body of the clitoris, forming the *prepuce*.

A variable number of small **lesser vestibular glands** discharge secretions onto the exposed surface of the vestibule, keeping it moist. During **arousal**, a pair of ducts discharges the secretions of the **greater vestibular glands** into the vestibule near the vaginal entrance (Figure 20-8•). These mucous glands resemble the bulbourethral glands of males.

The vulva's outer outer limits are formed by the mons pubis and labia majora. The prominent bulge of the **mons pubis** is created by adipose tissue beneath the skin anterior to the pubic symphysis. Adipose tissue also accumulates in the fleshy **labia majora** (singular *labium majus*), which encircle and partially conceal the labia minora and vestibular structures.

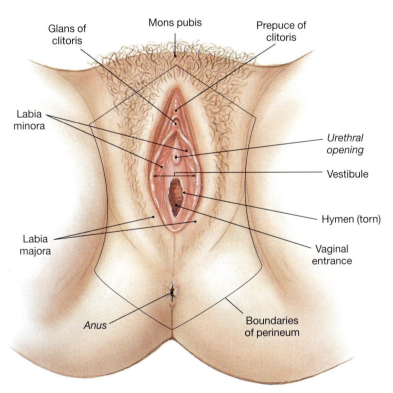

Glans of clitoris
Mons pubis
Prepuce of clitoris
Labia minora
Labia majora
Urethral opening
Vestibule
Hymen (torn)
Vaginal entrance
Anus
Boundaries of perineum

•**FIGURE 20-12   The Female External Genitalia**

The Mammary Glands

A newborn infant cannot fend for itself, and several key systems have yet to complete their development. While adjusting to an independent existence, the infant gains nourishment from the milk secreted by the maternal

2
0

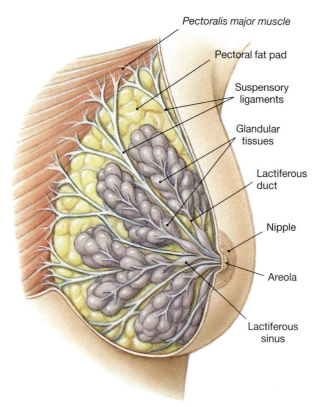

Pectoralis major muscle

Pectoral fat pad

Suspensory ligaments

Glandular tissues

Lactiferous duct

Nipple

Areola

Lactiferous sinus

• **FIGURE 20-13   The Mammary Glands of the Female Breast**

mammary glands. Milk production, or **lactation** (lak-TĀ-shun), occurs in the mammary glands of the **breasts**, specialized accessory organs of the female reproductive system (Figure 20-13•).

The mammary glands lie in the subcutaneous layer beneath the skin of the chest. Each breast bears a small conical projection, the **nipple**, where the ducts of underlying mammary glands open onto the body surface. The skin surrounding each nipple has a reddish brown coloration, and this region is known as the **areola** (a-RĒ-ō-la). Large sebaceous glands beneath the areolar surface give it a granular texture.

The glandular tissue of the breast consists of a number of separate lobes, each containing several secretory lobules. Within each lobe, the ducts leaving the lobules converge, giving rise to a single **lactiferous** (lak-TIF-e-rus) **duct**. Near the nipple, that lactiferous duct expands, forming an expanded chamber called a **lactiferous sinus**. Some 15–20 lactiferous sinuses open onto the surface of each nipple. Dense connective tissue surrounds the duct system and forms partitions that extend between the lobes and lobules. These bands of connective tissue, the *suspensory ligaments of the breast*, originate in the dermis of the overlying skin. A layer of loose connective tissue separates the mammary complex from the underlying muscles, and the two can move relatively independently.

ENDOCRINE'S EFFECTS ON THE BREAST

At puberty, increasing levels of *estrogen* stimulate growth of the breast's *mammary gland.* In pregnancy, the placenta secretes large quantities of estrogens that stimulate growth of the ductal system. Once the ductal system has developed, *progesterone* causes final development of the breasts into milk-secreting glands. While estrogens and progesterone stimulate development of the breasts, they actually inhibit the secretion of milk.

Prolactin causes the production of milk. The prolactin level begins to rise around the fifth week of pregnancy and continues until delivery. When the placenta is delivered, the levels of estrogen and progesterone drop markedly, and the breasts begin to secrete milk. Finally, milk is "let down," or ejected, by the breasts due to stimulation by *oxytocin.* Suckling of the breast by the baby sends sensory impulses to the hypothalamus resulting in oxytocin secretion.

✓ As the result of pelvic inflammatory disease, scar tissue can block the lumen of each uterine tube. How would this blockage affect a woman's ability to conceive?

✓ What is the advantage of the normally acidic pH of the vagina?

✓ Which layer of the uterus is sloughed off during menstruation?

✓ Would blockage of a single lactiferous sinus interfere with delivery of milk to the nipple? Explain.

Hormones and the Female Reproductive Cycle

As in the male reproductive tract, the activity of the female reproductive tract is controlled by both pituitary and gonadal secretions. But the regulatory pattern is much more complicated, for a woman's reproductive system does not just produce functional gametes; it must also coordinate the ovarian and uterine cycles. Circulating hormones control the **female reproductive cycle** to ensure proper reproductive function. For example, it is obvious that a woman who fails to ovulate will be unable to conceive, even if her uterus is perfectly normal. A woman who ovulates normally, but whose uterus isn't ready to support an embryo, will be just as infertile. Because the processes are complex and difficult to study, many of the biochemical details still elude us, but the general patterns are reasonably clear.

Changes in circulating estrogen concentrations are the primary mechanism for coordinating the female reproductive cycle (Figure 20-14•).

Hormones and the Preovulatory Phase

Follicular development begins under FSH stimulation, and each month some of the primordial follicles begin their development into primary follicles. As the follic-

20

• FIGURE 20-14
Hormonal Regulation of Ovarian Activity

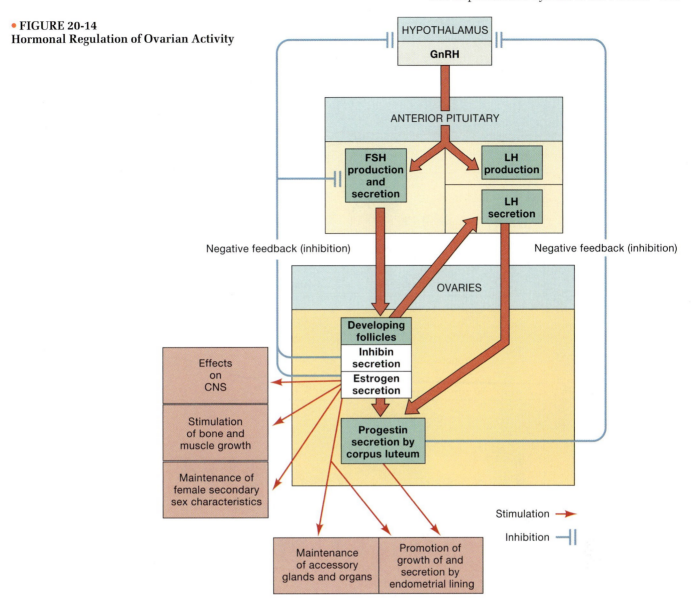

ular cells enlarge and multiply, they release steroid hormones collectively known as **estrogens**. The most important estrogen is **estradiol** (es-tra-DĪ-ol). Estrogens have multiple functions including (1) stimulating bone and muscle growth; (2) maintaining female secondary sex characteristics, such as body hair distribution and the location of adipose tissue deposits; (3) affecting central nervous system activity, including sexual behaviors and drives; (4) maintaining functional accessory reproductive glands and organs; and (5) initiating the repair and growth of the endometrium (Figure 20-14•).

The upper portion of Figure 20-15• summarizes the hormonal events associated with the ovarian cycle. Its cyclic pattern of hormonal regulation differs between the *preovulatory phase* and *postovulatory phase*. As follicular development proceeds, the concentration of circulating estrogens and inhibin rises, for the follicular cells are increasing in number and secretory activity. As estrogen and inhibin concentrations increase, they

inhibit both the hypothalamic secretion of GnRH and the pituitary production and release of FSH. Estrogen also affects the rate of LH secretion. Although the synthesis of LH occurs under GnRH stimulation, the rate of release into the bloodstream depends on the circulating concentration of estrogens. Thus, as the follicles develop and estrogen concentrations rise, the pituitary output of LH gradually increases. Despite a slow decline in FSH concentrations, the combination of estrogens, FSH, and LH continues to support follicular development and maturation.

Estrogen concentrations take a sharp upturn in the second week of the ovarian cycle, as this month's tertiary follicle enlarges in preparation for ovulation. At about day 14, estrogen levels peak, accompanying the maturation of that follicle. The high estrogen concentration then triggers a massive outpouring of LH from the anterior pituitary, which causes the rupture of the follicular wall and ovulation.

20

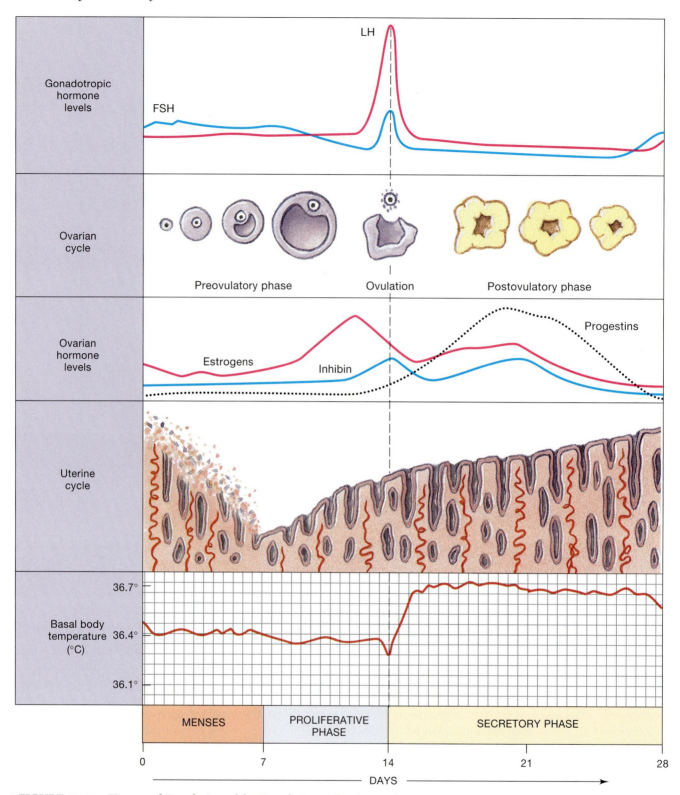

• FIGURE 20-15   Hormonal Regulation of the Female Reproductive Cycle

Hormones and the Postovulatory Phase

After ovulation, LH stimulates the remaining follicular cells to form the corpus luteum, and the yellow color of this mass results from its lipid reserves. These compounds are used to manufacture steroid hormones known as **progestins** (prō-JES-tinz), predominantly the steroid **progesterone** (prō-JES-ter-ōn). Progesterone is the principal hormone of the postovulatory phase. It prepares the uterus for pregnancy by stimulating the growth and development of the blood supply and secretory glands of the endometrium, and it also stimulates metabolic activity and elevates basal body temperature.

Luteinizing hormone levels remain elevated for only 2 days, but that is long enough to stimulate the formation of the functional corpus luteum. Progesterone secretion continues at relatively high levels for the next week. Unless pregnancy occurs, however, the corpus luteum then begins to degenerate. Roughly 12 days after ovulation, the corpus luteum becomes nonfunctional, and progesterone and estrogen levels fall markedly. This decline stimulates the hypothalamic receptors, and GnRH production increases. This increase in turn leads to an increase in the production of both FSH and LH in the anterior pituitary gland, and the entire cycle begins again.

Hormones and the Uterine Cycle

The lower portion of Figure 20-15● follows changes in the endometrium during a single uterine cycle. The sudden declines in progesterone and estrogen levels that accompany the breakdown of the corpus luteum result in menses. The loss of endometrial tissue continues for several days, until rising estrogen levels stimulate the regeneration of the functional zone of the endometrium.

The preovulatory phase continues until rising progesterone levels mark the arrival of the postovulatory phase. The combination of high levels of estrogen and progesterone then causes the enlargement of the endometrial glands as well as an increase in their secretions.

Hormones and Body Temperature

The hormonal fluctuations also cause physiological changes that affect the core body temperature. During the preovulatory phase, when estrogen is the dominant hormone, the resting, or basal, body temperature measured upon awakening in the morning is about 0.3°C (or 0.5°F) lower than it is during the postovulatory phase, when progesterone dominates. At the time of ovulation, basal temperature declines sharply, making the temperature rise over the following day even more noticeable (Figure 20-15●). By keeping records of body temperature over a few menstrual cycles, a woman can often determine the precise day of ovulation. This information can be very important for those wishing to avoid or promote a pregnancy, for pregnancy can occur only if an ovum becomes fertilized within a day of its ovulation.

✓ What changes would you expect to observe in the ovulatory cycle if the LH surge did not occur?

✓ What effect would blockage of progesterone receptors in the uterus have on the endometrium?

✓ What event occurs in the menstrual cycle when the levels of estrogen and progesterone decline?

THE PHYSIOLOGY OF SEXUAL INTERCOURSE

Sexual intercourse, or **coitus** (KŌ-i-tus), introduces semen into the female reproductive tract. The following sections consider the process as it affects the reproductive systems of males and females.

Male Sexual Function

Male sexual function is coordinated by reflex pathways involving both divisions of the ANS. During **arousal**, erotic thoughts or the stimulation of sensory nerves in the genital region increase the parasympathetic outflow over the pelvic nerves and erection occurs. Subsequent stimulation may initiate the secretion of the bulbourethral glands, lubricating the urethra and the surface of the glans.

During intercourse, the sensory receptors in the penis are rhythmically stimulated, eventually resulting in the coordinated processes of emission and ejaculation. **Emission** occurs under sympathetic stimulation. The process begins with peristaltic contractions of the ductus deferens, which push fluid and spermatozoa through the ejaculatory ducts and into the urethra. The seminal vesicles then contract, followed by waves of contraction in the prostate gland. While these contractions are proceeding, sympathetic commands close the sphincter at the entrance to the urinary bladder, preventing the passage of semen into the bladder.

Ejaculation occurs as the *ischiocavernosus* and *bulbospongiosus* muscles, two superficial skeletal muscles of the pelvic floor, contract powerfully and rhythmically. (The positions of these muscles can be seen in Figure 7-15●, p. 194.) Ejaculation is associated with intense pleasurable sensations, an experience known as **orgasm** (ŌR-gazm). Among other changes, heart rate and blood pressure temporarily increase. After ejaculation, blood begins to leave the erectile tissue, and the erection begins to subside. This *detumescence* (de-tū-MES-ens) is mediated by the sympathetic nervous system.

Female Sexual Function

The phases of female sexual function are comparable to those of a male. During sexual arousal, parasympathetic activation leads to an engorgement of the erectile tissues of the clitoris and increased secretion of cervical mucous glands and the greater vestibular glands. Clitoral erection increases its sensitivity to stimulation, and the cervical and vestibular glands provide lubrication for the vaginal walls. A network of blood vessels in the vaginal walls becomes filled with blood at this time, and the vaginal surfaces are also moistened by fluid from underlying connective tissues. Parasympathetic stimulation also causes engorgement of blood vessels at the nipples, making them more sensitive to touch and pressure.

During intercourse, rhythmic contact with the clitoris and vaginal walls, reinforced by touch sensations from the breasts and other stimuli (visual, olfactory, and auditory), provides stimulation that can lead to orgasm. Female orgasm is accompanied by peristaltic contractions of the uterine and vaginal walls and, via impulses over the pudendal nerves, rhythmic contractions of the bulbospongiosus and ischiocavernosus muscles. The latter contractions give rise to the sensations of orgasm.

✳ SEXUALLY TRANSMITTED DISEASES (STDs)

Sexually transmitted diseases (STDs) are infections contracted by intimate, as well as sexual, contact. The causative organism may be bacterial, viral, protozoan, parasitic, or fungal. The incidence of STDs is high. In the United States, the most common STDs are *chlamydia, gonorrhea, syphilis, genital warts,* and *herpes simplex virus, type 2.* These infections primarily affect the genitourinary system. However, STDs such as syphilis and gonorrhea can have systemic effects. Some of the most feared infectious diseases can be sexually transmitted, including *HIV infection (AIDS)* and *hepatitis B (HBV).* The incidence of STDs is highest in adolescents and declines exponentially with age.

AGING AND THE REPRODUCTIVE SYSTEM

The aging process affects the reproductive systems of men and women. The most striking age-related changes in the female reproductive system occur at menopause, whereas changes in the male reproductive system occur more gradually and over a longer period of time.

Menopause

Menopause is usually defined as the time that ovulation and menstruation cease. It typically occurs at age 45–55, but in the preceding years, the ovarian and menstrual cycles become irregular. A shortage of primordial follicles is the underlying cause of these developments; by age 50, often no primordial follicles are left to respond to FSH. In *premature menopause,* this depletion occurs before age 40.

Menopause is accompanied by a sharp and sustained rise in the production of GnRH, FSH, and LH, while circulating concentrations of estrogen and progesterone decline. The decline in estrogen levels leads to reductions in the size of the uterus and breasts, accompanied by a thinning of the urethral and vaginal walls. The reduced estrogen concentrations have also been linked to the development of osteoporosis, presumably because bone deposition proceeds at a slower rate. A variety of neural effects are also reported, including "hot flashes," anxiety, and depression, but the hormonal mechanisms involved are not well understood. In addition, the risk of atherosclerosis and other forms of cardiovascular disease increase after menopause.

The symptoms accompanying and following menopause are sufficiently unpleasant that about 40 percent of menopausal women eventually seek medical assistance. Hormone replacement therapies involving a combination of estrogens and progestins can often prevent osteoporosis and the neural and vascular changes associated with menopause.

The Male Climacteric

Changes in the male reproductive system occur more gradually, over a period known as the **male climacteric**. Circulating testosterone levels begin to decline between ages 50 and 60, coupled with increases in circulating levels of FSH and LH. Although sperm production continues (men well into their eighties can father children), there is a gradual reduction in sexual activity in older men. This reduction may be linked to declining testosterone levels, and some clinicians are now tentatively suggesting the use of testosterone replacement therapy to enhance libido (sexual drive) in elderly men.

✓ The inability to contract the ischiocavernosus and bulbospongiosus muscles would interfere with which part of the male sexual function?

✓ What changes occur in the female during sexual arousal as the result of increased parasympathetic stimulation?

✓ Why does the level of FSH rise and remain high during menopause?

INTEGRATION WITH OTHER SYSTEMS

Figure 20-16• summarizes the relationships between the reproductive system and other physiological systems. Normal human reproduction is a complex process that requires the participation of multiple systems. Hormones play a major role in coordinating these events,

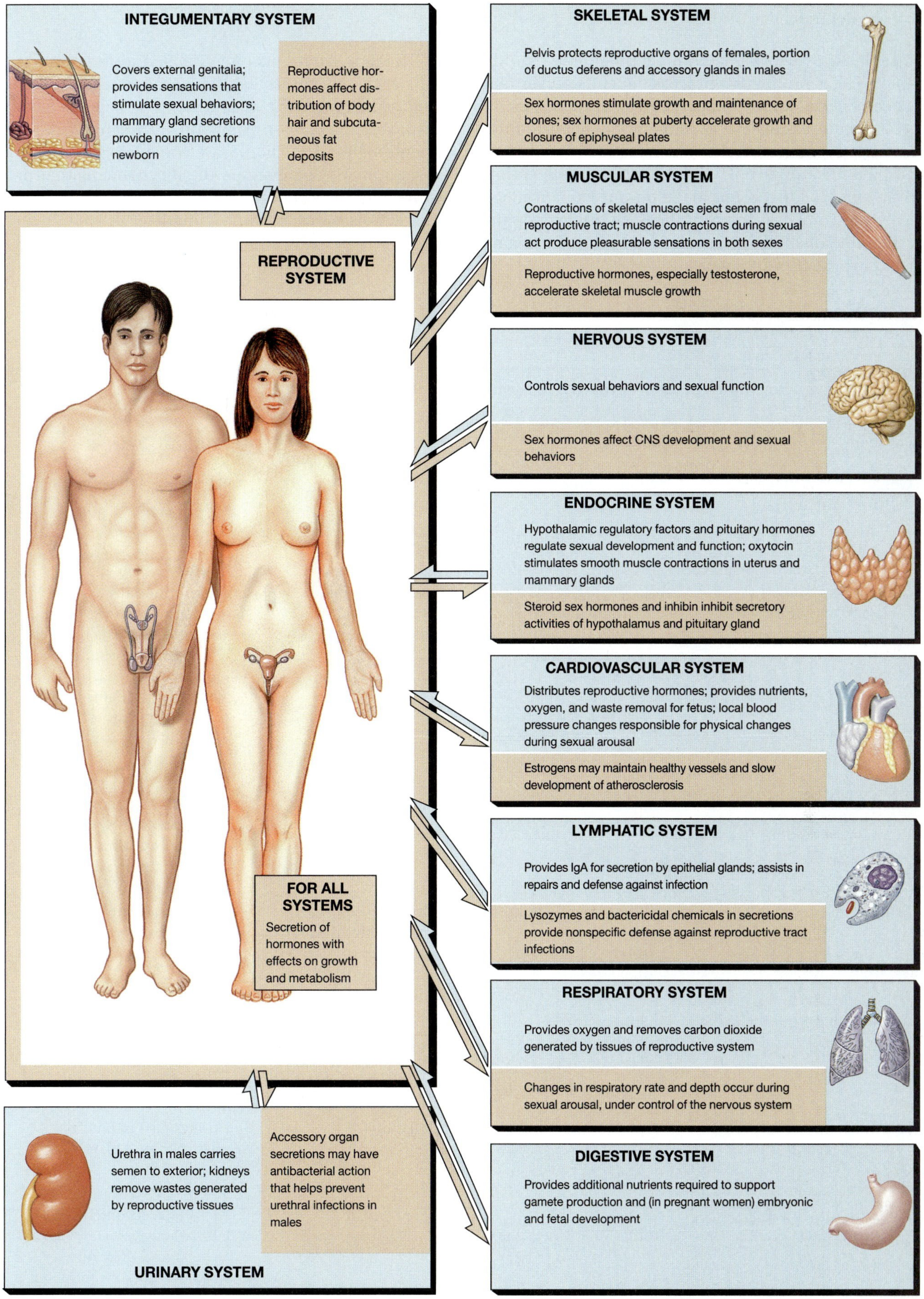

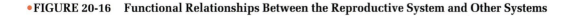

INTEGUMENTARY SYSTEM

Covers external genitalia; provides sensations that stimulate sexual behaviors; mammary gland secretions provide nourishment for newborn

Reproductive hormones affect distribution of body hair and subcutaneous fat deposits

REPRODUCTIVE SYSTEM

FOR ALL SYSTEMS

Secretion of hormones with effects on growth and metabolism

URINARY SYSTEM

Urethra in males carries semen to exterior; kidneys remove wastes generated by reproductive tissues

Accessory organ secretions may have antibacterial action that helps prevent urethral infections in males

SKELETAL SYSTEM

Pelvis protects reproductive organs of females, portion of ductus deferens and accessory glands in males

Sex hormones stimulate growth and maintenance of bones; sex hormones at puberty accelerate growth and closure of epiphyseal plates

MUSCULAR SYSTEM

Contractions of skeletal muscles eject semen from male reproductive tract; muscle contractions during sexual act produce pleasurable sensations in both sexes

Reproductive hormones, especially testosterone, accelerate skeletal muscle growth

NERVOUS SYSTEM

Controls sexual behaviors and sexual function

Sex hormones affect CNS development and sexual behaviors

ENDOCRINE SYSTEM

Hypothalamic regulatory factors and pituitary hormones regulate sexual development and function; oxytocin stimulates smooth muscle contractions in uterus and mammary glands

Steroid sex hormones and inhibin inhibit secretory activities of hypothalamus and pituitary gland

CARDIOVASCULAR SYSTEM

Distributes reproductive hormones; provides nutrients, oxygen, and waste removal for fetus; local blood pressure changes responsible for physical changes during sexual arousal

Estrogens may maintain healthy vessels and slow development of atherosclerosis

LYMPHATIC SYSTEM

Provides IgA for secretion by epithelial glands; assists in repairs and defense against infection

Lysozymes and bactericidal chemicals in secretions provide nonspecific defense against reproductive tract infections

RESPIRATORY SYSTEM

Provides oxygen and removes carbon dioxide generated by tissues of reproductive system

Changes in respiratory rate and depth occur during sexual arousal, under control of the nervous system

DIGESTIVE SYSTEM

Provides additional nutrients required to support gamete production and (in pregnant women) embryonic and fetal development

•FIGURE 20-16   Functional Relationships Between the Reproductive System and Other Systems

2
0

and Table 20-1 reviews the hormones discussed in this chapter. The reproductive process depends on various physical, physiological, and psychological factors, many of which require intersystem cooperation. For example, the male's sperm count must be adequate, the semen must have the correct pH and nutrients, and erection and ejaculation must occur in the proper sequence. For these steps to occur, the reproductive, digestive, endocrine, nervous, cardiovascular, and urinary systems must all be functioning normally.

Even when all else is normal, and fertilization occurs at the proper time and place, a normal infant will not result unless the zygote, a single cell the size of a pinhead, manages to develop into a full-term fetus weighing 3–4 kg. Chapter 21 considers the process of development, focusing on the mechanisms that determine both the structure of the body and the distinctive characteristics of each individual.

TABLE 20-1   Hormones of the Reproductive System

Hormone	Source	Regulation of Secretion	Primary Effects
Gonadotropin-Releasing Hormone (GnRH)	Hypothalamus	*Male:* inhibited by testosterone *Female:* inhibited by estrogens and/or progestins	Stimulates FSH secretion, LH synthesis
Follicle-Stimulating Hormone (FSH)	Anterior pituitary gland	*Male:* stimulated by GnRH, inhibited by inhibin *Female:* stimulated by GnRH, inhibited by estrogens and/or progestins	*Male:* stimulates spermatogenesis and spermiogenesis through effects on sustentacular cells *Female:* stimulates follicle development, estrogen production, and egg maturation
Estrogens (primarily estradiol)	Follicular and interstitial cells of ovaries	Stimulated by FSH	Stimulates LH secretion, maintains secondary sex characteristics and sexual behavior, stimulates repair of endometrium, inhibits secretion of GnRH
Inhibin	Sustentacular cells of testes and follicle cells of ovaries	Stimulated by factors released by developing sperm (male) or developing follicles (female)	Inhibits secretion of FSH and possibly GnRH
Luteinizing Hormone (LH)	Anterior pituitary gland	*Male:* stimulated by GnRH *Female:* production stimulated by GnRH, secretion by estrogens	*Male:* stimulates interstitial cells *Female:* stimulates follicular and interstitial cells
Progestins (primarily progesterone)	Corpus luteum	Stimulated by LH	Stimulates endometrial growth and glandular secretion, inhibits GnRH secretion
Androgens (primarily testosterone)	Interstitial cells of testes	Stimulated by LH	Maintains secondary sex characteristics and sexual behavior, promotes maturation of spermatozoa, inhibits GnRH secretion

20

FOCUS   Birth Control Strategies

For physiological, logistical, financial, or emotional reasons, most adults practice some form of conception control during their reproductive years. When the simplest and most obvious method, sexual abstinence, is unsatisfactory for some reason, another method of contraception must be used to avoid unwanted pregnancies. The selection process can be quite involved, because many methods are available. Each has specific strengths and weaknesses, so the potential risks and benefits must be carefully analyzed.

An estimated 64 percent of U.S. women age 15–44 are practicing some method of contraception; in 1999 an estimated 27 million American women were taking oral birth control pills. There are many different methods of contraception. Only a few will be considered here.

Sterilization makes one unable to provide functional gametes for fertilization. Either sex partner may be sterilized with the same net result. In a **vasectomy** (vaz-EK-to-mē), a segment of the ductus deferens is removed, making it impossible for sperm to pass from the epididymis to the distal portions of the reproductive tract. The surgery can be performed in a physician's office in a matter of minutes. The spermatic cords are located as they ascend from the scrotum on either side, and after each cord is opened, the ductus deferens is severed. After a 1 cm section is removed, the cut ends are usually tied shut (Figure 20-17a●). The cut ends do not reconnect; in time, scar tissue forms a permanent seal. A more recent vasectomy procedure often makes it possible to restore fertility at a later date. In this procedure, the cut ends of the ductus deferens are blocked with silicone plugs that can later be removed. After a vasectomy, the man experiences normal sexual function, for the epididymal and testicular secretions account for only around 5 percent of the volume of the semen. Sperm continue to develop, but they remain within the epididymis until they degenerate. The failure rate for this procedure is 0.08 percent. (A failure is defined as a resulting pregnancy.)

In the female, the uterine tubes can be blocked through a surgical procedure known as a **tubal ligation**

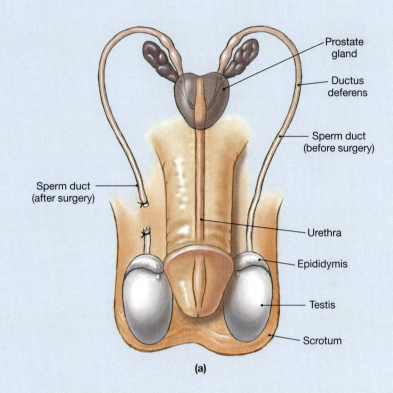

Prostate gland

Ductus deferens

Sperm duct (before surgery)

Sperm duct (after surgery)

Urethra

Epididymis

Testis

Scrotum

(a)

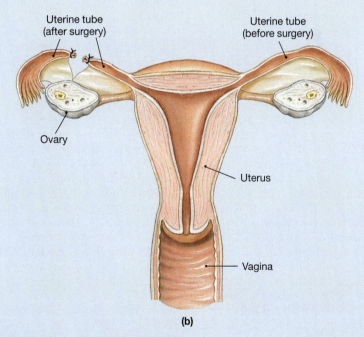

Uterine tube (after surgery)

Uterine tube (before surgery)

Ovary

Uterus

Vagina

(b)

● **FIGURE 20-17   Surgical Sterilization**
(a) In a vasectomy, the removal of a 1 cm section of the male's ductus deferens prevents the passage of sperm cells. **(b)** In a tubal ligation, the removal of a section of the female's uterine tube prevents the passage of sperm and the movement of an ovum or embryo into the uterus.

(Figure 20-17b•). Since the surgery involves entering the adominopelvic cavity, complications are more likely than with vasectomy. As in a vasectomy, attempts may be made to restore fertility after a tubal ligation. The failure rate for this procedure is estimated at 0.45 percent.

Oral contraceptives manipulate the female hormonal cycle so that ovulation does not occur. The contraceptive pills produced in the 1950s contained relatively large amounts of progestins. These concentrations were adequate to suppress pituitary production of GnRH, so FSH was not released and ovulation did not occur. Unpleasant side effects included endometrial bleeding, and most of the oral contraceptive products developed subsequently added small amounts of estrogens. Current combination pills differ significantly from the earlier products because the hormonal doses are much lower, with only one-tenth the progestins and less than half the estrogens. The hormones are administered in a cyclic fashion, beginning 5 days after the start of menses and continuing for the next 3 weeks. Over the fourth week the woman takes placebo pills or no pills at all. Low-dosage combination pills are sometimes prescribed for women experiencing irregular menstrual cycles, for they create a 28-day cycle.

At least 20 brands of combination oral contraceptives are now available, and over 200 million women use them worldwide. In the United States, 25 percent of women under age 45 use the combination pill to prevent conception. The progestin-only "minipill" has proved to be less effective in preventing pregnancy. The failure rate for the combination oral contraceptives, when used as prescribed, is 0.24 percent over a 2-year period.

Birth control pills are not without risks, however. For example, women with severe hypertension, diabetes mellitus, epilepsy, gallbladder disease, heart trouble, or acne may find that their problems worsen when taking the combination pills. Women taking oral contraceptives are also at increased risk for venous thrombosis, strokes, pulmonary embolism, and (for women over 35) heart disease.

Two progesterone-only forms of birth control are now available. *Depoprovera* is injected every 3 months. The Silastic tubes of the *Norplant system* are saturated with progesterone and inserted under the skin. This method provides birth control for a period of approximately 5 years, but to date the relatively high cost has limited the use of this contraceptive method. Both Depoprovera and the Norplant system can cause irregular menstruation and temporary amenorrhea, but they are easy to use and extremely convenient.

The **condom**, also called a *prophylactic*, or "rubber," covers the body of the penis during intercourse and keeps sperm from reaching the female reproductive tract. Synthetic (latex) condoms are also used to prevent the transmission of STDs, such as syphilis, gonorrhea, and AIDS. The condom failure rate has been estimated at over 6 percent.

Vaginal barriers such as the *diaphragm* and *cervical cap* rely on similar principles. A diaphragm, the most popular form of vaginal barrier in use at the moment, consists of a dome of latex rubber with a small metal hoop supporting the rim. Because vaginas vary in size, women choosing this method must be individually fitted. Before intercourse, the diaphragm is inserted so that it covers the external orifice, and it is usually coated with a small amount of spermicidal jelly or cream, adding to the effectiveness of the barrier. The failure rate for a properly fitted diaphragm is estimated at 5–6 percent. The cervical cap is smaller and lacks the metal rim. It, too, must be fitted carefully, but unlike the diaphragm, it may be left in place for several days. The failure rate (8 percent) is higher than that for diaphragm use.

An **intrauterine device (IUD)** consists of a small plastic loop or a T that can be inserted into the uterine chamber. The mechanism of action remains uncertain, but it is known that IUDs stimulate prostaglandin production in the uterus. The net result is an alteration in the chemical composition of uterine secretions, and the changes in the intrauterine environment lower the chances for fertilization and subsequent implantation. IUDs are in limited use today in the United States, but they remain popular in many other countries. The failure rate is estimated at 5–6 percent.

The **rhythm method** involves abstaining from sexual activity on the days ovulation might be occurring. The timing is estimated on the basis of previous patterns of menstruation and sometimes by following changes in basal body temperature. The failure rate for the rhythm method is very high, approaching 25 percent.

Sterilization, oral contraceptives, condoms, and vaginal barriers are the primary contraception methods for all age groups. But the relative proportion of the population using a particular method changes with age. Sterilization is most popular among older women, who may already have had children. Relative availability may also play a role. For example, a sexually active female under age 18 can buy a condom more easily than she can obtain a prescription for an oral contraceptive. But many of the observed changes occur because the relationship between risks and benefits varies for each age group.

When attempting to make a decision about the use and selection of contraceptives, many people simply examine the list of potential complications and make the "safest" choice. For example, media coverage of the potential risks associated with oral contraceptives made many women reconsider their use. But complex decisions should not be made on such a simplistic basis, and the risks associated with contraceptive use must be considered in light of their relative efficiencies.

Pregnancy, although a natural phenomenon, has its risks, and the mortality rate for pregnant women in the United States averages around 8 deaths per 100,000 pregnancies. That average incorporates a broad range; the rate is 5.4 per 100,000 among women under 20, and 27 per 100,000 for women over 40. Although these risks are small, for pregnant women over age 35, the chances of dying from complications related to pregnancy are almost twice as great as the chances of being killed in an automobile accident and many times greater than the risks associated with the use of oral contraceptives. For women in third world countries, the comparison is even more striking. The mortality rate for pregnant women in parts of Africa is approximately 1 per 150 pregnancies. In addition to preventing pregnancy, combination birth control pills have also been shown to reduce the risks of ovarian and endometrial cancers and fibrocystic breast disease.

Before age 35, *any contraceptive method is safer than pregnancy*. In general, over this period the risks are proportional to the failure rates of each method. The notable exception is women taking the pill who also smoke cigarettes. Younger women are more fertile, so despite a lower mortality rate for each pregnancy, they are likely to have more pregnancies. As a result, contraceptive failures imply a higher risk in the younger age groups.

After age 35, the risk of complications associated with oral contraceptive use increases, while the risk from other methods remains relatively stable. Women over age 35 (smokers) or 40 (nonsmokers) are therefore often advised to seek other forms of contraception.

A number of experimental contraceptive methods are being investigated. For example, researchers are attempting to determine whether low doses of inhibin will suppress GnRH release and prevent ovulation. Another approach is to develop a method of blocking human chorionic gonadotropin (hCG) receptors at the cor-

pus luteum. If the corpus luteum was unable to respond to hCG, normal menses would occur despite the implantation of a blastocyst.

Male contraceptives are also under development. *Gossypol*, a yellow pigment extracted from cottonseed oil, produces a dramatic decline in sperm count and sperm motility after 2 months. It can be administered topically, as it is readily absorbed through the skin. Fertility returns within a year after treatment is discontinued. Unfortunately, gossypol has not been approved as yet, because of side effects such as a relatively high risk of permanent sterility (around 10 percent).

Weekly doses of testosterone suppress GnRH secretion over a period of 5 months. The result is a drastic reduction in the sperm count. The combination of a testosterone implant, comparable to that used in the Norplant system, with a GnRH antagonist, *cetrorelix*, effectively suppresses spermatogenesis. A new synthetic form of testosterone, called *alpha-methyl-nortestosterone (MENT)*, appears even more effective than testosterone in suppressing GnRH production.

A drug used to control blood pressure appears to cause a temporary, reversible sterility in males. This drug is now being evaluated to see if low dosages will affect fertility in normal males without affecting blood pressure.

If contraceptive methods fail, options exist to either prevent implantation or terminate the pregnancy.

Morning-after pills contain estrogens or progestins. They may be taken within 72 hours of intercourse, and they appear to act by altering the transport of the zygote or preventing its attachment to the uterine wall. The drug known as *RU-486 (Mifepristone)* blocks the action of progesterone at the endometrial lining. The result is a normal menses, and the degeneration of the endometrium whether or not a pregnancy has occurred.

Abortion refers to the termination of a pregnancy. Most clinicians discriminate between spontaneous, therapeutic, and induced abortions. *Spontaneous abortions*, or *miscarriages*, occur naturally because of some developmental or physiological problem. *Therapeutic abortions* are performed when continuing the pregnancy represents a threat to the life and health of the mother. *Induced abortions* ("elective abortions") are performed at the request of the individual. Each year there are approximately 1.5 million induced abortions in the United States, roughly 1 abortion for every 3 births. Most involve unmarried or adolescent women. The ratio between abortions and deliveries for married women averages 1:10; for unmarried women and adolescents, there are nearly twice as many abortions as deliveries. Induced abortions are currently legal during the first 3 months after conception, and many states permit abortions, sometimes with restrictions, until the fifth or sixth developmental month.

Chapter Review

KEY TERMS

ductus deferens, *p. 552*	**ovarian follicles**, *p. 557*	**spermatogenesis**, *p. 550*
endometrium, *p. 560*	**ovary**, *p. 556*	**spermatozoa**, *p. 550*
estrogens, *p. 563*	**ovulation**, *p. 558*	**testes**, *p. 548*
lactation, *p. 562*	**perineum**, *p. 561*	**testosterone**, *p. 550*
meiosis, *p. 550*	**prepuce**, *p. 554*	**vulva**, *p. 561*
menses, *p. 560*	**progesterone**, *p. 565*	
oogenesis, *p. 557*	**seminiferous tubules**, *p. 549*	

20

SUMMARY OUTLINE

INTRODUCTION *p. 548*

1. The human reproductive system, including the **gonads** (reproductive organs) produces, stores, nourishes, and transports functional **gametes** (reproductive cells). **Fertilization** is the fusion of a *sperm* from the father and an *ovum* from the mother to create a **zygote** (fertilized egg).

THE REPRODUCTIVE SYSTEM OF THE MALE *p. 548*

1. In males, the *testes* produce **sperm** cells. The *spermatozoa* travel along the *epididymis*, the *ductus deferens*, the *ejaculatory duct*, and the *urethra* before leaving the body. Accessory organs (notably, the *seminal vesicles, prostate gland,* and *bulbourethral glands*) secrete into the ejaculatory ducts and urethra. The *scrotum* encloses the testes, and the *penis* is an erectile organ. *(Figure 20-1)*

The Testes *p. 548*

2. The **testes**, the primary sex organ of males, hang within the **scrotum**. The *dartos* muscle layer gives the scrotum a wrinkled appearance. The skeletal **cremaster muscle** pulls the testes closer to the body. The **tunica albuginea** surrounds each testis. Septa extend from the tunica albuginea to subdivide each testis into a series of lobules. **Seminiferous tubules** within each lobule are the sites of sperm production. Between the seminiferous tubules there are **interstitial cells**, which secrete sex hormones. *(Figure 20-2)*

3. Seminiferous tubules contain **spermatogonia**, stem cells involved in **spermatogenesis**, and **sustentacular cells**, which sustain and promote the development of spermatozoa. *(Figure 20-3)*

4. Each spermatozoon has a **head, middle piece,** and **tail.** *(Figure 20-4)*

The Male Reproductive Tract *p. 552*

5. From the testis, the spermatozoa enter the **epididymis**, an elongate tubule that monitors and adjusts the composition of the tubular fluid and serves as a recycling center for damaged spermatozoa. Spermatozoa leaving the epididymis are functionally mature, yet immobile.

6. The **ductus deferens**, or *vas deferens*, begins at the epididymis and passes through the *inguinal canal* as one component of the **spermatic cord**. The junction of the base of the seminal vesicle and the ductus deferens creates the **ejaculatory duct**, which penetrates the prostate gland and empties into the urethra. *(Figure 20-5)*

7. The **urethra** extends from the urinary bladder to the tip of the penis and serves as a passageway used by both the urinary and reproductive systems.

The Accessory Glands *p. 552*

8. Each **seminal vesicle** is an active secretory gland that contributes about 60 percent of the volume of semen; its secretions contain fructose, which is easily metabolized by spermatozoa. The **prostate gland** secretes fluid that makes up about 30 percent of seminal fluid. Alkaline mucus secreted by the **bulbourethral glands** has lubricating properties. *(Figure 20-5)*

Semen *p. 553*

9. A typical **ejaculation** releases 2–5 ml of semen (an **ejaculate**), which contains 20–100 million sperm per milliliter.

The Penis *p. 553*

10. The skin overlying the **penis** resembles that of the scrotum. Most of the body of the penis consists of three masses of **erectile tissue**. Beneath the superficial layers are two **corpora cavernosa** and a single **corpus spongiosum**, which surrounds the urethra. Dilation of the erectile tissue with blood produces an **erection**. *(Figure 20-6)*

Hormones and Male Reproductive Function *p. 555*

11. Important regulatory hormones of males include **follicle-stimulating hormone (FSH)**, **luteinizing hormone (LH)**, and **gonadotropin-releasing hormone (GnRH)**. Testosterone is the most important *androgen*. *(Figure 20-7)*

THE REPRODUCTIVE SYSTEM OF THE FEMALE *p. 556*

1. Principal organs of the female reproductive system include the *ovaries, uterine tubes, uterus, vagina,* and *external genitalia*. *(Figure 20-8)*

The Ovaries *p. 556*

2. The **ovaries** are the primary sex organs of females. Ovaries are the site of **ovum** production, or **oogenesis**, which occurs monthly in **ovarian follicles** as part of the **ovarian cycle**. As development proceeds, **primordial, primary, secondary,** and **tertiary follicles** form. At **ovulation**, an oocyte and the surrounding follicular walls of the **corona radiata** are released through the ruptured ovarian wall. *(Figures 20-9, 20-10)*

The Uterine Tubes *p. 559*

3. Each **uterine tube** has an **infundibulum**, a funnel that opens into the pelvic cavity. For fertilization to occur, the secondary oocyte must encounter spermatozoa during the first 12–24 hours of its passage from the infundibulum to the uterine cavity. *(Figure 20-11)*

The Uterus *p. 560*

4. The **uterus** provides mechanical protection and nutritional support to the developing embryo. It is stabilized by various ligaments. Major anatomical landmarks of the uterus include the **body, cervix, external orifice,** and **uterine cavity**. The uterine wall consists of an inner **endometrium**, a muscular **myometrium**, and a superficial perimetrium. *(Figure 20-11)*

5. A typical 28-day **uterine cycle**, or *menstrual cycle*, begins with the onset of **menses** and the destruction of the *functional zone* of the endometrium. This process of **menstruation** continues from 1 to 7 days.

6. After menses, the **proliferative phase** begins, and the functional zone undergoes repair and thickens. During the **secretory phase**, the endometrial glands are active and the uterus is prepared for the arrival of an embryo. Menstrual activity begins at **menarche** and continues until **menopause**.

The Vagina *p. 561*

7. The **vagina** is a muscular tube extending between the uterus and the external genitalia. A thin epithelial fold, the **hymen**, partially blocks the entrance to the vagina.

20

The External Genitalia p. 561

8. The components of the **vulva**, or female external genitalia, include the **vestibule**, the **labia minora**, the **clitoris**, the **labia majora**, and the **lesser** and **greater vestibular glands**. *(Figure 20-12)*

The Mammary Glands p. 561

9. A newborn infant gains nourishment from milk secreted by maternal **mammary glands**. **Lactation** is the process of milk production. *(Figure 20-13)*

Hormones and the Female Reproductive Cycle p. 562

10. Regulation of the **female reproductive cycle** involves the coordination of the ovarian and uterine cycles by circulating hormones.

11. **Estradiol**, one of the estrogens, is the dominant hormone of the preovulatory phase. Ovulation occurs in response to peak levels of estrogen and LH. *(Figure 20-14)*

12. The hypothalamic secretion of GnRH triggers the pituitary secretion of FSH and the synthesis of LH. FSH initiates follicular development, and activated follicles and ovarian interstitial cells produce estrogens. **Progesterone**, one of the steroid hormones called **progestins**, is the principal hormone of the postovulatory phase. Hormonal changes are responsible for the maintenance of the menstrual cycle. *(Figure 20-15)*

THE PHYSIOLOGY OF SEXUAL INTERCOURSE p. 565

Male Sexual Function p. 565

1. During **arousal** in males, erotic thoughts, sensory stimulation, or both lead to parasympathetic activity that produces erection. Stimuli accompanying **coitus** (sexual intercourse) lead to **emission** and ejaculation. Strong muscle contractions are associated with **orgasm**.

Female Sexual Function p. 565

2. The phases of female sexual function resemble those of the male, with parasympathetic arousal and muscular contractions associated with orgasm.

AGING AND THE REPRODUCTIVE SYSTEM p. 566

Menopause p. 566

1. Menopause (the time that ovulation and menstruation cease in women) typically occurs around age 50. Production of GnRH, FSH, and LH rise, while circulating concentrations of estrogen and progesterone decline.

The Male Climacteric p. 566

2. During the **male climacteric**, between ages 50 and 60, circulating testosterone levels decline, while levels of FSH and LH rise.

INTEGRATION WITH OTHER SYSTEMS p. 566

1. Hormones play a major role in coordinating reproduction. *(Table 20-1)*

2. In addition to the endocrine and reproductive systems, reproduction requires the normal functioning of the digestive, nervous, cardiovascular, and urinary systems. *(Figure 20-16)*

REVIEW QUESTIONS

LEVEL 1   Reviewing Facts and Terms

Match each item in column A with the most closely related item in column B. Use letters for answers in the spaces provided.

Column A

___ 1. gametes
___ 2. gonads
___ 3. interstitial cells
___ 4. seminal vesicles
___ 5. prostate gland
___ 6. bulbourethral glands
___ 7. prepuce
___ 8. corpus luteum
___ 9. endometrium
___10. myometrium
___11. dysmenorrhea
___12. menarche
___13. clitoris
___14. lactation
___15. coitus

Column B

a. production of androgens
b. outer muscular uterine wall
c. high concentration of fructose
d. female erectile tissue
e. secretes thick, sticky, alkaline mucus
f. painful menstruation
g. sexual intercourse
h. uterine lining
i. reproductive cells
j. female puberty
k. milk production
l. secretes antibiotic
m. reproductive organs
n. foreskin of penis
o. endocrine structure

16. Perineal structures associated with the reproductive system are collectively known as:
    (a) gonads
    (b) sex gametes
    (c) external genitalia
    (d) accessory glands

17. Meiosis in males produces four spermatids, each of which contains:
    (a) 23 chromosomes
    (b) 23 pairs of chromosomes
    (c) the diploid number of chromosomes
    (d) 46 pairs of chromosomes

18. Erection of the penis occurs when:
    (a) sympathetic activation of penile arteries occurs
    (b) arterial branches are constricted, and muscular partitions are tense
    (c) the vascular channels become engorged with blood
    (d) a, b, and c are correct

19. In males, the primary target of FSH is the:
    (a) sustentacular cells of the seminiferous tubules
    (b) interstitial cells of the seminiferous tubules
    (c) prostate gland
    (d) epididymis

20. The ovaries in females are responsible for:
    (a) the production of female gametes
    (b) the secretion of female sex hormones
    (c) the secretion of inhibin
    (d) a, b, and c are correct

21. Ovum production, or oogenesis, begins:
    (a) before birth
    (b) after birth
    (c) at puberty
    (d) after puberty

22. In females, meiosis is not completed:
    (a) until birth
    (b) until puberty
    (c) unless and until fertilization occurs
    (d) until uterine implantation occurs

23. If fertilization is to occur, the ovum must encounter spermatozoa during the first _____ of its passage.
    (a) 1 to 5 hours
    (b) 6 to 11 hours
    (c) 12 to 24 hours
    (d) 25 to 36 hours

24. The part of the endometrium that undergoes cyclical changes in response to sexual hormonal levels is the:
    (a) serosa
    (b) basilar zone
    (c) muscular myometrium
    (d) functional zone

25. A sudden surge in LH concentration causes:
    (a) the onset of menses
    (b) the rupture of the follicular wall and ovulation
    (c) the beginning of the proliferative phase
    (d) the end of the uterine cycle

26. At the time of ovulation, the basal body temperature:
    (a) is not affected
    (b) increases noticeably
    (c) declines sharply
    (d) may increase or decrease a few degrees

27. Menopause is accompanied by:
    (a) sustained rises in GnRH, FSH, and LH
    (b) declines in circulating levels of estrogen and progesterone
    (c) thinning of the urethral and vaginal walls
    (d) a, b, and c are correct

28. Which reproductive structures are common to both males and females?

29. Which accessory organs and glands contribute to the composition of semen? What are the functions of each?

30. What are the primary functions of the epididymis in males?

31. What are the primary functions of the ovaries in females?

32. What are the three major functions of the vagina?

LEVEL 2   Reviewing Concepts

33. How does the human reproductive system differ functionally from all other systems in the body?

34. How is meiosis involved in the development of the spermatozoon and the ovum?

35. Using an average uterine cycle of 28 days, describe each of the three phases of the menstrual cycle.

36. Describe the hormonal events associated with the uterine cycle.

37. How does the aging process affect the reproductive systems of men and women?

LEVEL 3   Critical Thinking and Clinical Applications

38. Diane has peritonitis (an inflammation of the peritoneum), which her physician says resulted from a urinary tract infection. Why could this situation occur in females but not in males?

39. Rod injures the sacral region of his spinal cord. Will he still be able to achieve an erection? Explain.

40. Women bodybuilders and women suffering from eating disorders such as anorexia nervosa often cease having menstrual cycles, a condition known as amenorrhea. What does this relationship suggest about the role of body fat and menstruation? What benefit might there be in the discontinuance of menstruation under such circumstances?

20

ANSWERS TO CONCEPT CHECK QUESTIONS

Page 556

1. The cremaster muscle as well as the dartos muscle would be relaxed on a warm day, so the scrotal sac could descend away from the warmth of the body and could cool the testes.   **2.** The acrosomal cap contains the enzymes necessary for fertilizing the ovum. Without an acrosomal cap (and therefore without enzymes), fertilization would not occur.   **3.** The dilation of the arteries serving the penis will result in erection.   **4.** The hormone FSH is required for maintaining a high level of testosterone available to support spermatogenesis. Low levels of FSH would lead to low levels of testosterone in the seminiferous tubules and thus a lower rate of sperm production and a low sperm count.

Page 562

1. A blockage of the uterine tube would cause sterility.   **2.** The acidity of the vagina helps prevent bacterial, fungal, and protozoal infections in this area.   **3.** The functional layer of the endometrium is sloughed off during menstruation.   **4.** The blockage of a single lactiferous sinus would not interfere with the movement of milk to the nipple, because each breast usually has between 15 and 20 lactiferous sinuses.

Page 565

1. If the LH surge did not occur during an ovulatory cycle, ovulation and the subsequent formation of the corpus luteum would not take place.   **2.** Progesterone is responsible for the functional maturation and secretion of the endometrial lining. A blockage of progesterone receptors would inhibit endometrial development and make it unsuitable for implantation.   **3.** A sudden decline in the levels of estrogen and progesterone during the menstrual cycle signals the beginning of menses.

Page 566

1. The inability to contract the ischiocavernosus and bulbospongiosus muscles would interefere with a male's ability to ejaculate and to experience orgasm.   **2.** As the result of parasympathetic stimulation in females during sexual arousal, there is engorgement of the erectile tissues of the clitoris, increased secretion of cervical and vaginal glands, increased blood flow to the walls of the vagina, and engorgement of the blood vessels in the nipples.   **3.** At menopause, circulating estrogen levels begin to drop. Estrogen has an inhibitory effect on GnRH and FSH; as the level of estrogen declines, the levels of these two hormones rise and remain elevated.

20

OVERVIEW

The reproductive system differs significantly between men and women. In the female, all of the reproductive system is located within the pelvic cavity, while in the man, many of the reproductive structures are located outside of the body. The reproductive system, like most body systems, is vulnerable to trauma and infections. Infections, which are often sexually transmitted. Trauma and infections can be more difficult to diagnose in the female because of the internal location of the reproductive organs. Trauma to the reproductive system is most common in the male. Blunt trauma to the penis or scrotum is the most common cause of reproductive system injuries. Reproductive system injuries in the female result from sexual assault or straddle injuries.

Physicians who specialize in the treatment of diseases and injuries of the female reproductive system are called *gynecologists.* Gynecologists complete a four-year program that includes obstetrics. Some gynecologists will take fellowship training in such areas as gynecological oncology. Urologists usually treat reproductive system injuries in the male.

TRAUMA DURING PREGNANCY

Trauma is the number-one killer of pregnant females. Penetrating abdominal trauma alone accounts for as much as 36 percent of overall maternal mortality. Gunshot wounds to the abdomen of the pregnant female also account for fetal mortality rates of between 40 and 70 percent. In blunt trauma, auto collisions are the leading cause of maternal and fetal mortality and morbidity. Proper seat belt placement can significantly reduce injury to the pregnant mother and fetus, while improper placement increases the incidence of both uterine rupture and separation of the placenta from the wall of the uterus. Unrestrained mothers in serious auto collisions are four times more likely to suffer fetal mortality than those who are restrained.

The physiologic changes associated with pregnancy protect both the mother and her abdominal organs. With the increasing size of the uterus, most of the abdominal organs are displaced higher in the abdomen (Figure A20-1●).

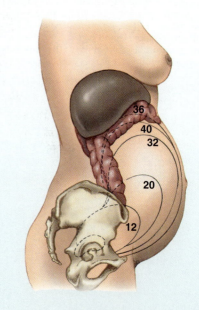

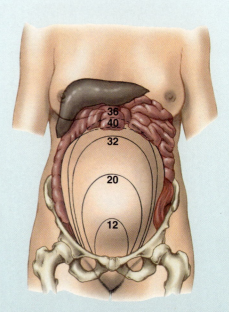

● **FIGURE A20-1** **Expansion of the Gravid Uterus by Weeks**
Note that the other abdominal organs are displaced until the uterus becomes the largest organ in the abdomen.

This generally protects them unless blunt or penetrating trauma impacts the upper abdomen. If that happens, then the injury may involve numerous organs with increased morbidity and mortality. Direct penetrating injury to the central and lower abdomen of the late-pregnancy mother often spares her from serious injury; the resulting injury, however, often damages the uterus and endangers the fetus.

The female in the later part of her pregnancy is at additional risk of vomiting and possible aspiration. Increasing uterine size increases intra-abdominal pressure, while the hormones of pregnancy relax the cardiac sphincter (the valve that prevents reflux of the stomach contents). The bladder is displaced superiorly early in pregnancy and then becomes more prone to injury and, when injured, bleeds more heavily.

The increasing size and weight of the uterus and its contents have several effects on the mother, especially when trauma strikes. The uterus of a supine patient in late pregnancy may compress the inferior vena cava and reduce the venous return to the heart. This may induce hypotension in the uninjured patient and have severe consequences in the hemorrhaging trauma patient (Figure A20-2•). The increased intra-abdominal pressure, along with the compression of the inferior vena cava by the gravid uterus, can raise venous pressure in the pelvic region and the lower extremities. This pressure engorges the vessels and increases the rate of venous hemorrhage from pelvic fractures or lower extremity wounds.

The increased maternal vascular volume (up by 45 percent) helps protect the mother from hypovolemia. However, this protection does not extend to the fetus because fetal blood flow is affected well before there are changes in the maternal blood pressure or pulse rate. In fact, changes in maternal blood pressure or heart rate may not become evident until maternal blood loss reaches between 30 and 35 percent. Therefore, it becomes very important to assure early and aggressive resuscitation of the potentially hypotensive pregnant mother.

In the pregnant female, the thick and muscular uterus contains both the developing fetus and amniotic fluid. This container is strong, distributing the forces of trauma uniformly to the fetus and thereby reducing chances for injury. Significant blunt trauma may cause the uterus to rupture, or penetrating trauma may perforate or tear it. The dangers of severe maternal hemorrhage and disruption of the blood supply to the fetus threaten the lives of the mother and the fetus. The potential release of amniotic fluid into the abdomen is also of great concern. The risk of uterine and fetal injury increases with the length of gestation and is greatest during the third trimester of pregnancy.

If an open wound to the uterus does occur, there may be added risk to the mother, in addition to hemorrhage, if she is Rh negative and the fetus is Rh positive. Penetrating or severe blunt trauma may permit some fetal/maternal blood mixing and lead to compatibility problems. Frank uterine rupture is a rare complication of trauma, but it does occur with severe blunt impact, pelvic fracture, and—very infrequently—with stab or shotgun wounds.

Blunt trauma to the uterus may cause the rather inelastic placenta to detach from the very flexible uterine wall. This condition, called *abruptio placentae,* presents a life-threatening risk to both mother and fetus because the separation causes both maternal and fetal hemorrhage (Figure A20-3•). More frequently than not, this hemorrhage is contained within the uterus and does not extend to the vaginal outlet. Blunt trauma may also cause the premature rupture of the amniotic sac (breaking of the "membranes" or "bag of waters") and may induce an early labor.

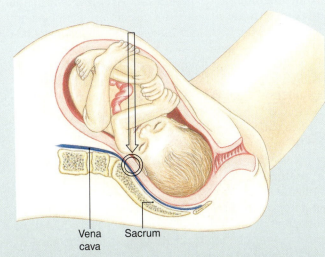

• FIGURE A20-2   Supine Hypotensive Syndrome
When the mother lies flat on her back as the pregnancy nears term, the weight of the gravid uterus compresses the inferior vena cava. This markedly reduces cardiac preload leading to hypotension. The situation can be corrected by having the patient turn on her side or tilt the backboard to the left.

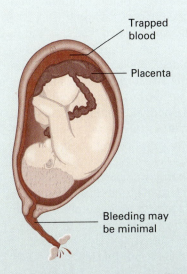

• FIGURE A20-3   Abruptio Placenta
Premature separation of the placenta from the wall of the uterus can result from trauma and threatens the life of both the mother and the fetus.

DATE RAPE

Date rape, also called acquaintance rape, is defined as forced, unwanted intercourse with a person known by the victim. Sometimes, physical force or threats are used to force the victim to cooperate. In many instances, the victim is given a sedative drug that allows the assailant to carry out the assault.

One of the most frequently used drugs in date rape is the benzodiazepine *flunitrazepam.* Also known as *Rohypnol,* or "roofies," flunitrazepam is used in the short-term management of insomnia and as a sedative-hypnotic and preanesthetic medication. It has pharmacological effects similar to those of diazepam (Valium), although Rohypnol is approximately 10 times more potent. The effects begin within 30 minutes and peak within 2 hours. It has significant amnestic properties, similar to those seen with the sedative midazolam (Versed). Rohypnol is neither manufactured nor sold legally in the United States. It is produced and sold by prescription in Europe and Latin America. It is supplied in 1- and 2-milligram tablets. Rohypnol enters the United States through several routes. It is transported across the Mexican border to Texas and then delivered to other parts of the country. It also enters South Florida from Columbia via international mail services or commercial airlines.

The effects of Rohypnol can be reversed with flumazenil (Romazicon) if needed. Because of Rohypnol's amnestic properties, victims may not even remember the assault. They may wake up in a strange place with their clothing in disarray. Many are too embarrassed to seek help after the assault.

PELVIC INFLAMMATORY DISEASE

Probably the most common cause of nontraumatic gynecological pain is pelvic inflammatory disease (PID). PID is an infection of the female reproductive tract that can be caused by bacteria, viruses, or fungi. The organs most commonly involved are the uterus, fallopian tubes, and ovaries. Occasionally the adjoining structures, such as the peritoneum and intestines, also become involved. PID is the most common cause of abdominal pain in women in the childbearing years, occurring in one percent of that population. The highest rate of infection occurs in sexually active women ages 15 to 24. The most common causes of PID are gonorrhea (*Neisseria gonorrhoeae*) or chlamydia (*Chlamydia trachomatis*), although rarely streptococcus or staphylococcus bacteria may cause it. Commonly, gonorrhea or chlamydia progresses undetected in a female until frank PID develops (Figure A20-4●).

Predisposing factors include multiple sexual partners, prior history of PID, recent gynecological procedure, or an IUD. Postinfection damage to the fallopian tubes is a common cause for infertility. PID may be either acute or chronic. If it is allowed to progress untreated, sepsis may

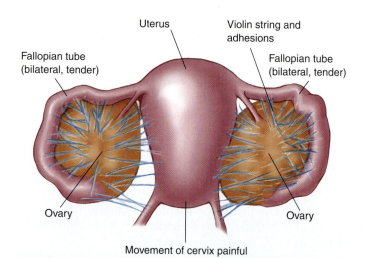

● **FIGURE A20-4   Pelvic Inflammatory Disease**
PID is an infection of the female reproductive organs. It typically causes adhesions on all affected organs.

develop. Additionally, PID may cause adhesions, in which the pelvic organs "stick together." These adhesions are a common cause of chronic pelvic pain and increase the frequency of infertility and ectopic pregnancies.

While it is possible for a patient with pelvic inflammatory disease to be asymptomatic, most patients with PID complain of abdominal pain. It is often diffuse and located in the lower abdomen. It may be moderate to severe, which occasionally makes distinguishing it from appendicitis difficult. Pain may intensify either before or after the menstrual period. It may also worsen during sexual intercourse (dypareunia), as movement of the cervix tends to cause increased discomfort. Patients with PID tend to walk with a shuffling gait, since walking often intensifies their pain. In severe cases, fever, chills, nausea, vomiting, or even sepsis may accompany PID. Occasionally, patients have a foul-smelling, often yellow, vaginal discharge, as well as irregular menses. Midcycle bleeding is common also.

The patient with PID may appear acutely ill or toxic. The blood pressure is normal, although the pulse rate may be slightly increased. Fever may or may not be present. Palpation of the lower abdomen generally elicits moderate to severe pain. In the emergency department, the patient will undergo a pelvic examination. In PID, movement of the cervix causes severe pain, which is referred to as a "chandelier sign" as the patient reaches for the ceiling when the cervix is moved. It is often difficult to distinguish PID from appendicitis in young females.

The primary treatment for PID is antibiotics. Toxic patients may require antibiotics administered intravenously. Once the causative organism is determined, the sexual partner may also require treatment.

RUPTURED OVARIAN CYSTS

Cysts are fluid-filled pockets. When they develop in the ovary, they can rupture and be a source of abdominal pain. When an egg is released from the ovary, a cyst, known as a corpus luteum cyst, is often left in its place. Occasionally, cysts develop independent of ovulation. When the cysts rupture, a small amount of blood spills into the abdomen. Because blood irritates the peritoneum, it can cause abdominal pain and rebound tenderness. Ovarian cysts may be found during a routine pelvic examination. In the field setting, however, your patient is likely to complain of moderate to severe unilateral abdominal pain, which may radiate to her back. She may also report a history of dyspareunia, irregular bleeding, or a delayed menstrual period. It is not uncommon for patients to rupture ovarian cysts during intercourse or physical activity. This often results in immediate, severe abdominal pain causing the patient to immediately stop intercourse or other physical activity. Ruptured ovarian cysts may be associated with vaginal bleeding.

MITTELSCHMERZ

Occasionally, ovulation is accompanied by midcycle abdominal pain known as mittelschmerz. It is thought that this pain is related to peritoneal irritation due to follicle rupture or bleeding at the time of ovulation. The unilateral lower quadrant pain is usually self-limited and may be accompanied by midcycle spotting. While some women may report a low-grade fever, it should be noted that body temperature normally increases at the time of ovulation and remains elevated until the day prior to the onset of the menstrual period. Treatment is symptomatic.

ENDOMETRITIS

An infection of the uterine lining called *endometritis* is an occasional complication of miscarriage, childbirth, or gynecological procedures such as dilatation and curettage (D and C). Commonly reported signs and symptoms include mild to severe lower abdominal pain; a bloody, foul-smelling discharge; and fever (101° to 104° F). The onset of symptoms is usually 48 to 72 hours after the gynecological procedure or miscarriage. These infections often mimic the presentation of PID and can be quite serious if not quickly treated with the appropriate antibiotics. Complications of endometritis may include sterility, sepsis, or even death.

ENDOMETRIOSIS

Endometriosis is a condition in which endometrial tissue is found outside of the uterus. Most commonly it is found in the abdomen and pelvis, although it has been found virtually everywhere in the body, including the central nervous system and lungs. Regardless of its site, the tissue responds to the hormonal changes associated with the menstrual cycle and thus bleeds cyclically. This bleeding causes inflammation, scarring of adjacent tissues, and the subsequent development of adhesions, particularly in the pelvic cavity.

Endometriosis is usually seen in women between the ages of 30 and 40 and is rarely seen in postmenopausal women. The exact cause is unknown. The most common symptom is dull, cramping pelvic pain that is usually related to menstruation. Dyspareunia and abnormal uterine bleeding are also commonly reported. Painful bowel movements have also been reported when the endometrial tissue has invaded the gastrointestinal tract. Endometriosis is commonly diagnosed when the patient is being evaluated for infertility. Definitive treatment may include medical management with hormones, analgesics, and anti-inflammatory drugs, and/or surgery to remove the excessive endometrial tissue or adhesions from other organs.

DERMOID CYSTS

An interesting class of tumors of the female reproductive system is the teratomas. Teratomas are divided into three categories: (1) mature (benign), (2) immature (malignant), and (3) monodermal, or highly specialized. The vast majority of benign teratomas are cystic and are more commonly referred to as *dermoid cysts.* These cysts are lined by skin and are usually filled with a sebaceous cheesy substance. Often, matted hair and teeth can be found within the cyst. The cyst wall arises from stratified squamous epithelium. In more complex cysts, layers of germ cells can give rise to cartilage, bone, thyroid tissue, or organoid formation.

The origination of dermoid tumors has been a matter of fascination for centuries. Some common beliefs blamed witches, nightmares, or adultery with the devil as possible causes. Interestingly, the karyotype of all benign ovarian teratomas is 46,XX (normal human female). Dermoid tumors are usually easily removed sparing the ovary and uterine tube.

MALE GENITAL TRAUMA

The male genitalia are, for the most part, located outside of the body. Despite this, they are rarely injured. The testicles are highly mobile within the scrotum, and the external capsule of the testicle (tunica albuginea) is very tough. These features protect the testes from injury. The most common cause of testicular injury is a direct blow. Most testicular injuries are contusions, although ruptures can occur.

Injuries to the penis can result from several causes. Zippers can trap the penile skin causing pain and bleeding. Mineral oil and ice can aid in removing the entrapped skin. In severe cases, a local anesthetic must be injected so that a wire cutter can be used to open the zipper.

Self-inflicted injuries of the penis can range from the common to the bizarre. Vacuum cleaners can cause extensive injury to the glans penis. Blade injuries can cause lacerations or even amputations. Amputation of the penis is best managed by replantation, if possible.

Traumatic rupture of the corpus cavernosum of the penis, also called a fracture of the penis, occurs when the erect penis impacts forcibly on a hard object, receives a direct blow, or is subjected to abnormal bending. A cracking sound may be heard. This is usually followed by penile pain, loss of the erection, rapid swelling, discoloration, and deformity. Penile ruptures must be carefully managed surgically to avoid permanent loss of function.

TESTICULAR CANCER

Although cancer of the testicle is relatively rare in men overall, it is the most common cancer in men from 15 to 35 years old. Testicular cancer is highly treatable and usually curable. It is generally divided into seminoma and nonseminoma types for treatment planning because seminomas are more sensitive to radiation therapy. The cure rate for patients with seminoma-type cancers exceeds 90 percent. The cure rate for nonseminoma type cancers approaches 100 percent. Men who have an undescended testicle (cryptorchidism) are at a higher risk of developing cancer of the testicle than those where the testicle has descended properly. This is true even if surgery was performed to place the testicle at the appropriate place in the scrotum.

Treatment of testicular cancer includes surgery, chemotherapy, radiation therapy, and/or bone marrow transplantation. Typically, both testicles are surgically re-moved. The lymph nodes in the abdomen are often sampled during surgery. Radiation therapy is used to kill cancer cells and shrink tumors. Chemotherapy kills cancer cells that are located outside of the testicle. Autologous bone marrow transplantation is a newer type of treatment. Bone marrow is taken from the patient and treated with drugs to kill any cancer cells. The marrow is then frozen while the patient is given high-dose chemotherapy, either with or without radiation therapy, to destroy all of the remaining marrow. Following this, the marrow previously removed and treated is thawed and given back to the patient, replacing the marrow that was destroyed. The marrow grows and begins to function producing essential blood cells.

The best treatment for testicular cancer is prevention. The earlier testicular cancer is detected, the better are the chances of obtaining a cure. All men should perform testicular self-examination at least once a month. This is especially important in the 15- to 40-year-old age group. The American Cancer Society and the National Cancer Institute have several tapes and brochures detailing this safe and easy examination.

SUMMARY

Trauma to the reproductive system is fairly uncommon. However, infections and medical conditions are common. In the male, infections and cancers are the most common problems affecting the reproductive structures. In females, problems related to pregnancy, infection, and hormonal problems are most frequently encountered. Reproductive system emergencies can sometimes be embarrassing for patients, and they must sometimes be gently coaxed to provide essential information.

A20

21

Development and Inheritance

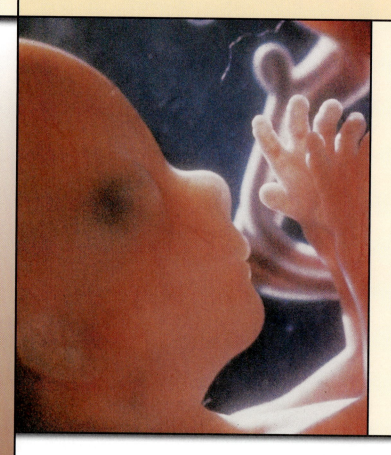

Many physiological processes may last only a fraction of a second. Others may take several hours at most. But some important processes in life are measured in months, years, or decades. A human being develops in the womb for 9 months, grows to maturity in 15 to 20 years, and may live the better part of a century. Birth, growth, maturation, aging, and death are all parts of a single continuous process. In addition, that process may not end with death. Human beings can pass at least some of their characteristics on to a new generation that will repeat the same cycle. Such is the circle of life.

Chapter Outline and Objectives

Vocabulary Development

allanto-, sausage; *allantois*
amphi, two-sided; *amphimixis*
blast, precursor; *trophoblast*
gestare, to bear; *gestation*
heteros, other; *heterozygous*
homos, same; *homozygous*
karyon, nucleus; *karyotyping*
koiloma, hollow; *blastocoele*
meros, part; *blastomere*
meso-, middle; *mesoderm*
mixis, mixing; *amphimixis*
morula, mulberry; *morula*
phainein, to display; *phenotype*
praegnans, with child; *pregnant*
tropho-, food; *trophoblast*
typos, mark; *phenotype*
vitro, glass; *in vitro*

The process of **development** is the gradual modification of physical and physiological characteristics during the period from conception to physical maturity. The changes are truly remarkable—what begins as a single cell slightly larger than the period at the end of this sentence becomes an individual whose body contains trillions of cells organized into tissues, organs, and organ systems. The creation of different cell types in this process is called **differentiation**. Differentiation occurs through selective changes in genetic activity. As development proceeds, some genes are turned off and others turned on. The identities of these genes vary from one cell type to another.

A basic understanding of development provides important insights into anatomical structures. In addition, many of the mechanisms of development and growth (an increase in size) are similar to those responsible for the repair of injuries. This chapter will focus on major aspects of development and consider highlights of the developmental process. We will also consider the regulatory mechanisms and how developmental patterns can be modified—for good or ill.

AN OVERVIEW OF TOPICS IN DEVELOPMENT

Development involves (1) the division and differentiation of cells and (2) the changes that produce and modify anatomical structures. Development begins at fertilization, or **conception**, and can be divided into periods characterized by specific anatomical changes. **Embryology** (em-brē-OL-ō-jē) considers the developmental events that occur in the first 2 months after fertilization. During this period, the developing organism is called an **embryo**. After 2 months, the developing embryo becomes a **fetus**, and **fetal development** begins at the start of the ninth week and continues up to the time of birth. Embryological and fetal development are sometimes referred to collectively as **prenatal development**, the primary focus of this chapter. **Postnatal development** commences at birth and continues to maturity.

Although all human beings go through the same developmental stages, differences in genetic makeup produce distinctive individual characteristics. **Inheritance** refers to the transfer of genetically determined characteristics from generation to generation. **Genetics** is the study of the mechanisms responsible for inheritance. This chapter considers basic genetics as it applies to the appearance of inherited characteristics such as sex, hair color, and various diseases.

FERTILIZATION

Fertilization is the fusion of two haploid gametes, producing a *zygote* containing the normal diploid number of chromosomes (46). ∞ *p. 548* The functional roles of the spermatozoon and the ovum are very different. The spermatozoon simply delivers the paternal chromosomes to the site of fertilization. It is the ovum that must provide all of the nourishment and genetic programming to support embryonic development for nearly a week after conception. The volume of the ovum is therefore much greater than that of the sperm. At the time of fertilization, the diameter of the secondary oocyte is over twice the length of the spermatozoon. The relationship between oocyte and sperm volumes is even more striking, on the order of 2000 to 1 (Figure 21-1a•).

The sperm arriving in the vagina are already motile, but they cannot fertilize an egg until they undergo **capacitation**. ∞ *p. 552* This activation process, necessary for fertilization, is inhibited in the male reproductive tract until emission and ejaculation occur. Capacitation therefore normally takes place in the female reproductive tract.

Fertilization usually occurs in the upper one-third of the uterine tube within a day of ovulation. Contractions of the uterine musculature and ciliary currents in the uterine tubes aid the passage of sperm to the fertilization site. Of the 200 million spermatozoa introduced into the vagina in a typical ejaculate, only around 10,000 make it past the uterus, and fewer than 100 actually reach the secondary oocyte. A male with a sperm count below 20 million per milliliter will usually be sterile, because too few sperm survive to reach the oocyte. One or two spermatozoa cannot accomplish fertilization, because of the layer of cells surrounding the oocyte at ovulation.

The Oocyte at Ovulation

Figure 21-1b• diagrams the steps in the fertilization process:

Step 1: *Oocyte at ovulation.* At ovulation, the secondary oocyte leaving the follicle is in metaphase of the second meiotic division. The cell's metabolic operations have been discontinued, and the oocyte drifts in a sort of suspended animation, awaiting the stimulus for further development. If fertilization does not occur, the secondary oocyte disintegrates without completing meiosis.

Step 2: *Fertilization and oocyte activation.* When it leaves the ovary, the secondary oocyte is surrounded by the *corona radiata*, a layer of follicle cells. The corona radiata protects the oocyte as it passes through the ruptured follicular wall and into the infundibulum of the uterine tube. Although the physical process of fertilization requires only a single sperm in contact with the oocyte membrane, that spermatozoon must first penetrate the corona radiata. The acrosomal cap contains *hyaluronidase* (hī-al-u-RON-a-dās), an enzyme that breaks down the intercellular cement between adjacent cells of

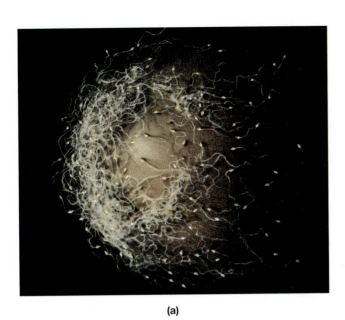

(a)

the corona radiata. Apparently, there must be at least a hundred or more sperm thrashing around, bumping into the corona and releasing hyaluronidase, before the connections between the follicular cells begin to break down. No matter how many sperm slip through the gap, only a single spermatozoon will accomplish fertilization. When that sperm contacts the oocyte, their cell membranes fuse and the sperm's nucleus enters the cytoplasm of the oocyte. This event initiates **oocyte activation**.

Activation of the oocyte involves a series of metabolic changes. For example, the metabolic rate of the oocyte increases rapidly, and meiosis is completed. At the same time, the exocytosis of vesicles releases enzymes that prevent an abnormal process called polyspermy, fertilization by additional sperm cells. Polyspermy produces a zygote incapable of normal development.

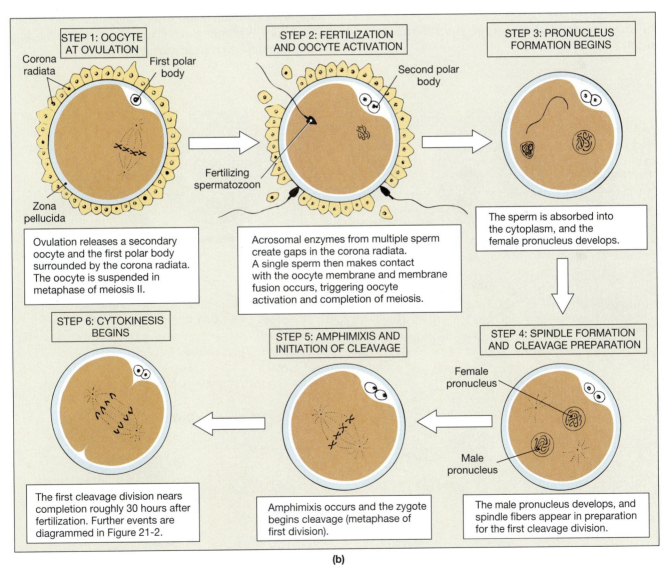

(b)

•**FIGURE 21-1** **Fertilization**
(a) An oocyte at the time of fertilization. Notice the difference in size between the gametes. **(b)** Fertilization and the preparations for cleavage.

Step 3: *Pronucleus formation.* Once meiosis has been completed and the sperm is absorbed, the nuclear material of the ovum reorganizes into a *female pronucleus.*

Step 4: *Spindle formation and cleavage preparation.* The absorbed sperm reorganizes into a *male pronucleus.* Spindle fibers form as the cell prepares for the first of a series of mitotic cell divisions called *cleavage.*

Step 5: *Amphimixis and initiation of cleavage.* The male pronucleus and female pronucleus fuse in a process called **amphimixis** (am-fi-MIK-sis). The zygote now has the normal complement of 46 chromosomes and begins preparing for mitotic cell division. Fertilization is now complete.

Step 6: *Cytokinesis begins.* The first division of cleavage is completed roughly 30 hours after fertilization has occurred.

Further events in fertilization are illustrated in Figure 21-2•.

A Preview of Prenatal Development

The process of prenatal development occurs within the uterus over a period of 9 months. This interval is the duration of **gestation** (jes-TĀ-shun), or *pregnancy.* For convenience, prenatal development is usually considered to consist of three integrated **trimesters**, each 3 months in duration:

1. The **first trimester** is the period of embryonic and early fetal development. During this period, the basic components of each of the major organ systems appear.

2. In the **second trimester**, the organs and organ systems complete most of their development. The body proportions change, and by the end of the second trimester the fetus looks distinctively human.

3. The **third trimester** is characterized by rapid fetal growth. Early in the third trimester most of the major organ systems become fully functional, and an infant born 1 month or even 2 months prematurely has a reasonable chance of survival.

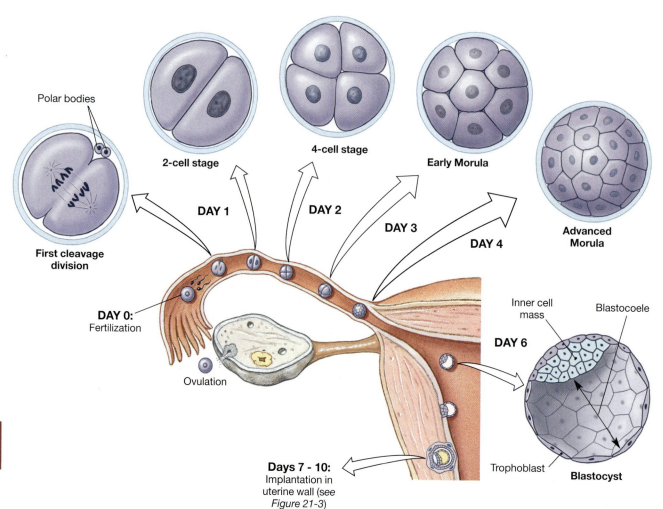

•**FIGURE 21-2   Cleavage and Blastocyst Formation**

THE FIRST TRIMESTER

The events that occur in the first trimester are complex and vital to the survival of the embryo. Because accidents often happen, *the first trimester is the most dangerous period in life.* Only about 40 percent of conceptions produce embryos that survive the first trimester, and some surviving fetuses enter the second trimester already doomed or deformed by some developmental mistake. For this reason, pregnant women are usually warned to take great care to avoid drugs or other disruptive stresses during the first trimester. We will focus on four general processes that occur during this period: *cleavage, implantation, placentation,* and *embryogenesis.*

Cleavage and Blastocyst Formation

Cleavage (KLĒV-ij) is a series of cell divisions that subdivide the cytoplasm of the zygote, producing smaller and smaller cells (Figure 21-2•). The first cleavage division produces two identical cells, called **blastomeres** (BLAS-tō-mērz; *blast,* precursor + *meros,* part). The first division is completed roughly 30 hours after fertilization, and subsequent cleavage divisions occur at intervals of 10–12 hours.

After several cycles of division, the embryo is a solid ball of cells, resembling a mulberry. This stage is called the **morula** (MOR-ū-la; morula, mulberry). After 5 days of cleavage, the blastomeres form a hollow ball, the **blastocyst**, with an inner cavity known as the *blastocoele* (BLAS-tō-sēl; *koiloma,* cavity). At this stage, differences between the cells of the blastocyst become visible. The outer layer of cells, separating the outside world from the blastocoele, is called the **trophoblast** (TRŌ-fō-blast). The function is implied by the name: *tropho,* food + *blast,* precursor. These cells will be responsible for providing food to the developing embryo. A second group of cells, the **inner cell mass,** lies clustered at one end of the blastocyst. In time, the inner cell mass will form the embryo.

Implantation

At fertilization, the zygote is still 4 days away from the uterus. It arrives in the uterine cavity as a morula, and over the next 2–3 days, blastocyst formation occurs. Over this period, the blastomeres are gaining nutrients from the fluid within the uterine cavity. This glycogen-rich fluid is secreted by the endometrial glands. When fully formed, the blastocyst contacts the endometrium, usually in the body or fundus of the uterus, and implantation occurs. Stages in the implantation process are diagrammed in Figure 21-3•; you may find it helpful to review the structure of the uterus at this time (Figure 20-11•, p. 559).

Implantation begins as the surface of the blastocyst closest to the inner cell mass touches and adheres to the uterine lining (Day 7, Figure 21-3•). In this area, the superficial cells undergo rapid divisions, making the trophoblast several layers thick. Near the endometrial wall, the cell membranes separating the trophoblast

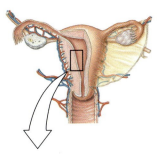

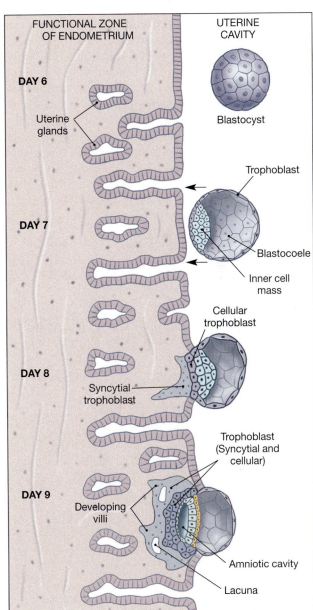

• **FIGURE 21-3   Stages in the Implantation Process**

cells disappear, creating a layer of cytoplasm containing multiple nuclei called the *syncytial trophoblast* (Day 8). The underlying cells remain intact and form a layer called the *cellular trophoblast*. The syncytial trophoblast erodes a path through the uterine epithelium. At first, this erosion creates a gap in the uterine lining, but the division and migration of epithelial cells soon repair the surface. With the conclusion of these repairs, the blastocyst loses contact with the uterine cavity, and further development takes place entirely within the functional zone of the endometrium.

Implantation usually occurs at the endometrial surface lining the uterine cavity. The precise location varies, although most often it is in the body of the uterus. In an *ectopic pregnancy*, implantation occurs somewhere other than within the uterus.

As implantation proceeds, the syncytial trophoblast continues to enlarge into the surrounding endometrium (Day 9). The digestion of uterine gland cells releases quantities of glycogen and other nutrients that are absorbed by the trophoblast and distributed by diffusion to the inner cell mass. These nutrients provide the energy needed to support the early stages of embryo formation. Trophoblastic extensions grow around endometrial capillaries, and as the capillary walls are destroyed, maternal blood begins to percolate through trophoblastic channels known as *lacunae*. Fingerlike villi extend away from the trophoblast into the surrounding endometrium, and these extensions gradually increase in size and complexity as development proceeds.

The Formation of the Blastodisc

By the time of implantation, the inner cell mass is beginning to separate from the trophoblast. The separa- tion gradually increases, creating a fluid-filled chamber called the **amniotic** (am-nē-OT-ik) **cavity**. The amniotic cavity can be seen in Day 9 of Figure 21-3•, and additional details from Days 10–12 are shown in Figure 21-4•. At this stage, the inner cell mass is organized into an oval, two-layered sheet of cells called a **blastodisc** (BLAS-tō-disk).

✳ TERATOGENICITY

The developing fetus is most vulnerable to birth defects during the first 60 days of pregnancy. The first stage of gestation, *embryogenesis,* begins at conception and continues to day 18. Exposure to a *teratogen* during this time can threaten the entire embryo. (A teratogen is a chemical or disease that causes malformation of a fetus.) The second stage of gestation, *organogenesis,* extends from day 18 to day 60. This is the stage when the fetus is most susceptible to teratogens and when most gross anatomical malformations develop. The third stage, the *fetal period,* extends from day 60 to birth. Exposure during this stage can cause abnormal cell growth and differentiation.

Gastrulation and Germ Layer Formation

A few days later, a third layer of cells begins forming through the process of **gastrulation** (gas-troo-LĀ-shun) (Day 12, Figure 21-4•). During gastrulation, cells on the blastodisc surface move toward the center line of the blastodisc, to a region called the *primitive streak*, where they leave the surface to form a third, central layer. This movement creates three distinct embryonic layers with markedly different fates. The superficial layer in contact with the amniotic cavity is called the **ectoderm**, the layer facing the blastocoel is known as the **endoderm**, and the intervening, poorly organized layer is the **mesoderm** (*meso-*, middle).

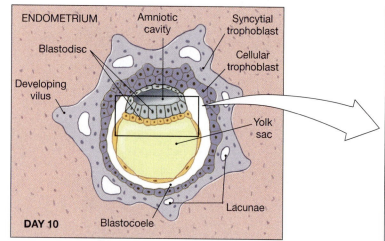

The blastodisc begins as two layers. The migration of cells around the amniotic cavity is the first step in the formation of the amnion. The migration of cells facing the blastocoele creates a sac that hangs below the blastodisc. This is the first step in yolk sac formation.

•FIGURE 21-4 Blastodisc Organization and Gastrulation

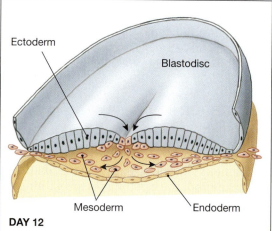

The migration of cells gives the blastodisc a third layer. From the time this process, called gastrulation, begins, the surface facing the amniotic cavity is called the *ectoderm*, the layer facing the yolk sac is called the *endoderm*, and the migrating cells form the *mesoderm*.

2 1

Table 21-1 lists the contributions each of these three **germ layers** makes to the body systems described in earlier chapters.

The Formation of Extraembryonic Membranes

Germ layers also participate in the formation of four extraembryonic membranes: the *yolk sac*, the *amnion*, the *allantois*, and the *chorion*. Although these membranes support embryonic and fetal development, they leave few traces of their existence in adult systems. Figure 21-5• (p. 584) details stages in the development of the extraembryonic membranes.

Yolk Sac. The first extraembryonic membrane to appear is the **yolk sac**, which is already present 10 days after fertilization (Figure 21-4•). As gastrulation proceeds, mesodermal cells migrate around this pouch and complete the formation of the yolk sac (Figure 21-5a•). Blood vessels soon appear within the mesoderm, and the yolk sac becomes an important site of blood cell formation.

Amnion. The **amnion** (AM-nē-on) is completed when ectodermal and mesodermal cells spread over the inner surface of the amniotic cavity. As the embryo and later the fetus enlarges, the amnion continues to expand, increasing the size of the amniotic cavity. The amnion encloses fluid that surrounds and cushions the developing embryo and fetus (Figure 21-5c–e•).

The Allantois. The **allantois** (a-LAN-tō-is) is a sac of endoderm and mesoderm that extends away from the embryo. The base of the allantois later gives rise to the urinary bladder. The allantois accumulates some of the small amount of urine produced by the kidneys during embryonic development.

The Chorion. The **chorion** (KOR-ē-on) is created as migrating mesodermal cells form a layer underneath the trophoblast (Figure 21-5a,b•). Blood vessels then begin to develop within the mesoderm of the chorion, creating a rapid-transit system linking the embryo with the trophoblast. This system provides the nutrients and

TABLE 21-1	The Fates of the Primary Germ Layers
Primary Germ Layer	*Developmental Contributions to the Body*
Ectoderm	*Integumentary system:* epidermis, hair follicles and hairs, nails, and glands communicating with the skin (apocrine and merocrine sweat glands, mammary glands, and sebaceous glands) *Skeletal system:* pharyngeal cartilages of the embryo develop into portions of sphenoid and hyoid bones, auditory ossicles, and styloid processes of temporal bones *Nervous system:* all neural tissue, including brain and spinal cord *Endocrine system:* pituitary gland and the adrenal medullae *Respiratory system:* mucous epithelium of nasal passageways *Digestive system:* mucous epithelium of mouth and anus, salivary glands
Mesoderm	*Skeletal system:* all components except some pharyngeal derivatives *Muscular system:* all components *Endocrine system:* adrenal cortex, endocrine tissues of heart, kidneys, and gonads *Cardiovascular system:* all components, including bone marrow *Lymphatic system:* all components *Urinary system:* the kidneys, including the nephrons and the initial portions of the collecting system *Reproductive system:* the gonads and the adjacent portions of the duct systems *Miscellaneous:* the lining of the body cavities (pleural, pericardial, peritoneal) and the connective tissues supporting all organ systems
Endoderm	*Endocrine system:* thymus, thyroid, and pancreas *Respiratory system:* respiratory epithelium (except nasal passageways) and associated mucous glands *Digestive system:* mucous epithelium (except mouth and anus), exocrine glands (except salivary glands), liver, and pancreas *Urinary system:* urinary bladder and distal portions of the duct system *Reproductive system:* distal portions of the duct system, stem cells that produce gametes

21

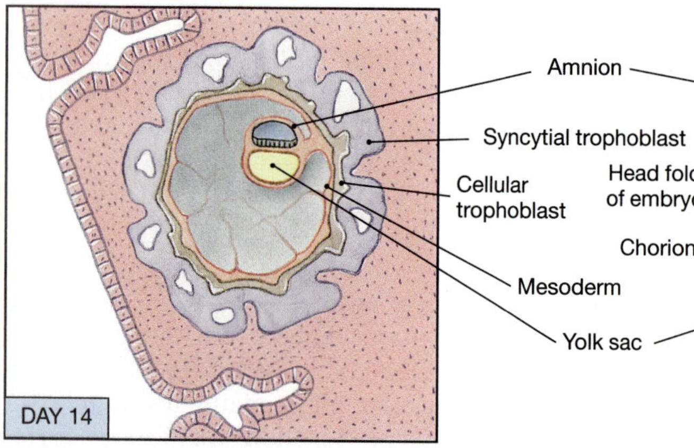

(a) The migration of the mesoderm around the inner surface of the trophoblast creates the chorion. Mesodermal migration around the outside of the amniotic cavity, between the ectodermal cells and the trophoblast, creates the amnion. Mesodermal migration around the endodermal pouch below the blastodisc creates the definitive yolk sac.

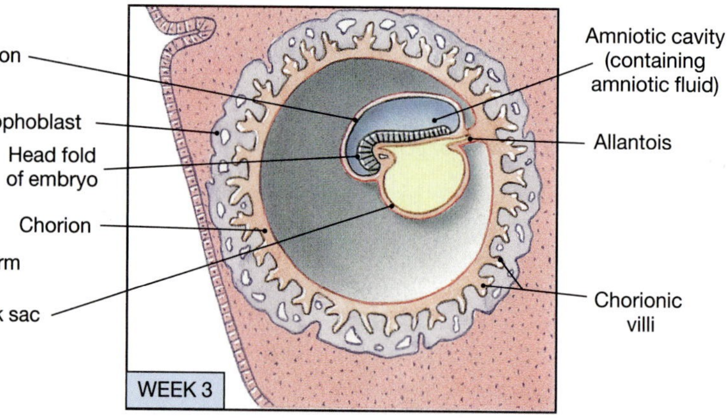

(b) The developing embryo bulges into the amniotic cavity at the head fold. The allantois, an endodermal extension surrounded by mesoderm, extends toward the trophoblast.

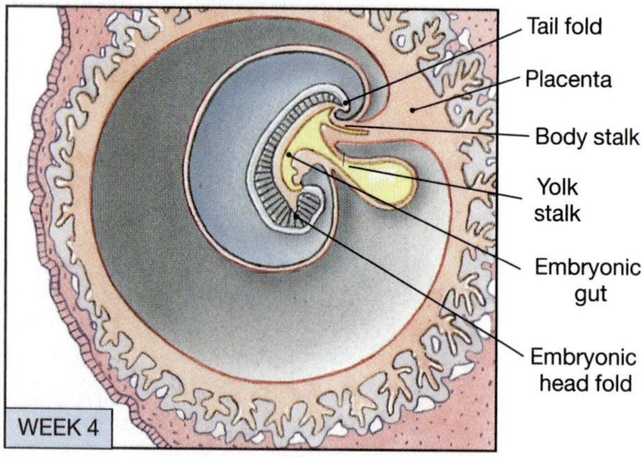

(c) The embryo now has a head fold and a tail fold. Constriction of the connection between the embryo and the surrounding trophoblast constricts the yolk stalk and body stalk.

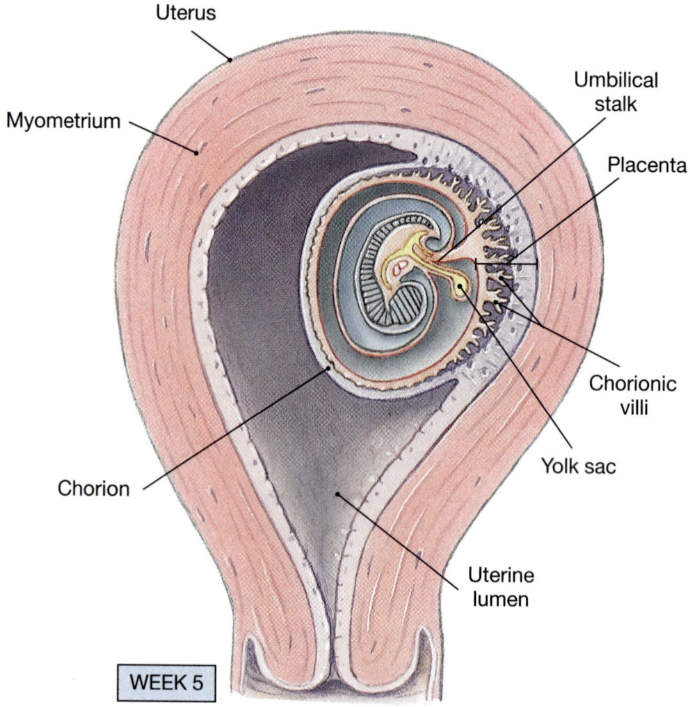

(d) The developing embryo and extraembryonic membranes bulge into the uterine cavity. The trophoblast pushing out into the uterine lumen remains covered by endometrium but no longer participates in nutrient absorption and embryo support. The embryo moves away from the placenta, and the body stalk and yolk stalk fuse to form an umbilical stalk.

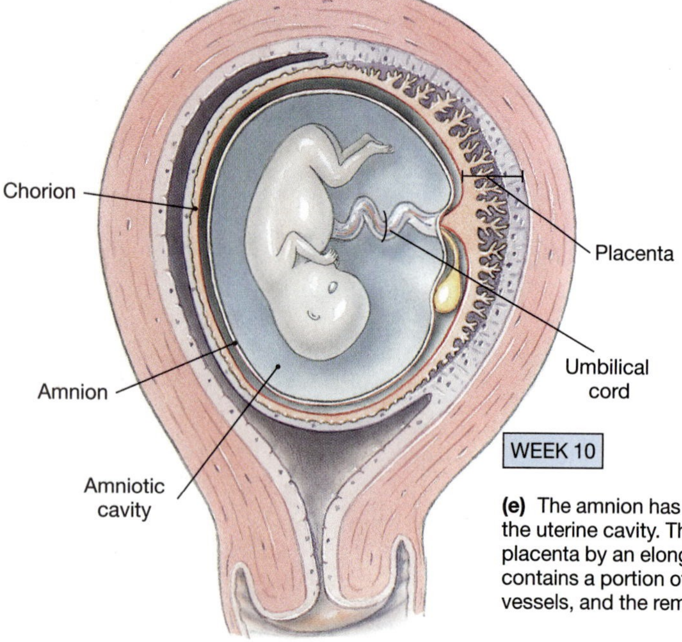

(e) The amnion has expanded greatly, filling the uterine cavity. The fetus is connected to the placenta by an elongate umbilical cord that contains a portion of the allantois, blood vessels, and the remnants of the yolk stalk.

• FIGURE 21-5
Extraembryonic Membranes and Placenta Formation

oxygen needed for continued embryonic growth and development.

Placentation

The **placenta** is a temporary structure in the uterine wall that provides a site for diffusion between the fetal and maternal circulatory systems. **Placentation** (pla-sen-TĀ-shun), or placenta formation, takes place when blood vessels form in the chorion around the periphery of the blastocyst (see Figure 21-5a–e●). By the third week of development, the mesoderm extends along each of the trophoblastic villi, forming *chorionic villi* in contact with maternal tissues (Figure 21-5b●). Embryonic blood vessels develop in each villus, and circulation through these chorionic vessels begins early in the third week, when the heart starts beating. These villi continue to enlarge and branch, forming an intricate network within the endometrium. Blood vessels continue to be eroded, and maternal blood flows slowly through the lacunae. Chorionic blood vessels pass close by, and exchange between the embryonic and maternal circulations occurs by diffusion across the trophoblast layers.

At first, the entire blastocyst is surrounded by chorionic villi. The chorion continues to enlarge, expanding like a balloon within the endometrium, and by the fourth week, the embryo, amnion, and yolk sac are suspended within an expansive, fluid-filled chamber (Figure 21-5c●). At this stage, the yolk sac and its associated blood vessels, which form the *yolk stalk*, are separate from the allantois and blood vessels of the *body stalk*, which develops where mesoderm cells first came into contact with the inner wall of the trophoblast. The body stalk is the only connection between the embryo and the chorion.

As the end of the first trimester approaches, the fetus moves farther away from the placenta. The yolk stalk and body stalk begin to fuse, forming an *umbilical stalk*, which contains placental blood vessels (Figure 21-5d●). By week 10, the fetus floats free within the amniotic cavity (Figure 21-5e●). The fetus remains connected to the placenta by the elongate **umbilical cord**, which contains the allantois, umbilical blood vessels, and the yolk sac.

Placental Circulation

Figures 21-5e and 21-6● indicate the extent of the fetal circulation at the placenta near the end of the first trimester. Blood flows to the placenta through the paired **umbilical arteries** and returns in a single **umbilical vein**. The chorionic villi provide the surface area for active and passive exchange between the fetal and maternal bloodstreams.

Placental Hormones

In addition to its role in providing nutrition to the fetus, the placenta acts as an endocrine organ. Hormones are synthesized by the syncytial trophoblast and are released into the maternal circulation. The placental hormones produced include *human chorionic gonadotropin, human placental lactogen, placental prolactin, relaxin, progestins,* and *estrogens.*

Human chorionic (kō-rē-ON-ik) **gonadotropin (hCG)** appears in the maternal bloodstream soon after implantation has occurred. The presence of hCG in blood or urine samples is a reliable indication of pregnancy, and home pregnancy tests detect this hormone. Because of the hCG, the corpus luteum persists for 3–4 months and maintains its production of progesterone. As a result, the endometrial lining remains perfectly functional, and menses does not occur and terminate the pregnancy.

The decline in the corpus luteum does not trigger the return of menstrual periods, because by the end of the first trimester, the placenta is secreting sufficient amounts of progestins to maintain the endometrial lining and the pregnancy. As the end of the third trimester approaches, estrogen production accelerates. The rising estrogen levels play a role in stimulating labor and delivery.

During the second trimester, the placenta also secretes the hormones **human placental lactogen (hPL)** and **placental prolactin**, which help prepare the mammary glands for milk production. The conversion of the mammary glands to active status requires the presence of placental hormones (hPl, placental prolactin, estrogen, and progestins) as well as several maternal hormones (growth hormone, prolactin, and thyroid hormones).

Relaxin is a hormone secreted by the placenta as well as by the corpus luteum. Relaxin (1) increases the flexibility of the pubic symphysis, permitting the expansion of the pelvis during delivery; (2) causes the dilation of the cervix, making it easier for the fetus to enter the vaginal canal; and (3) suppresses the release of oxytocin by the hypothalamus, delaying the onset of labor contractions.

Embryogenesis

After gastrulation begins, the folding and differential growth of the embryonic disc produce projecting bulges into the amniotic cavity. One of these bulges is called the *head fold* (Figure 21-5b●), and the other is called the *tail fold* (Figure 21-5c●). By this time, the orientation of the embryo can be seen, complete with dorsal and ventral surfaces and left and right sides. The changes in proportions and appearance that occur between the second developmental week

21

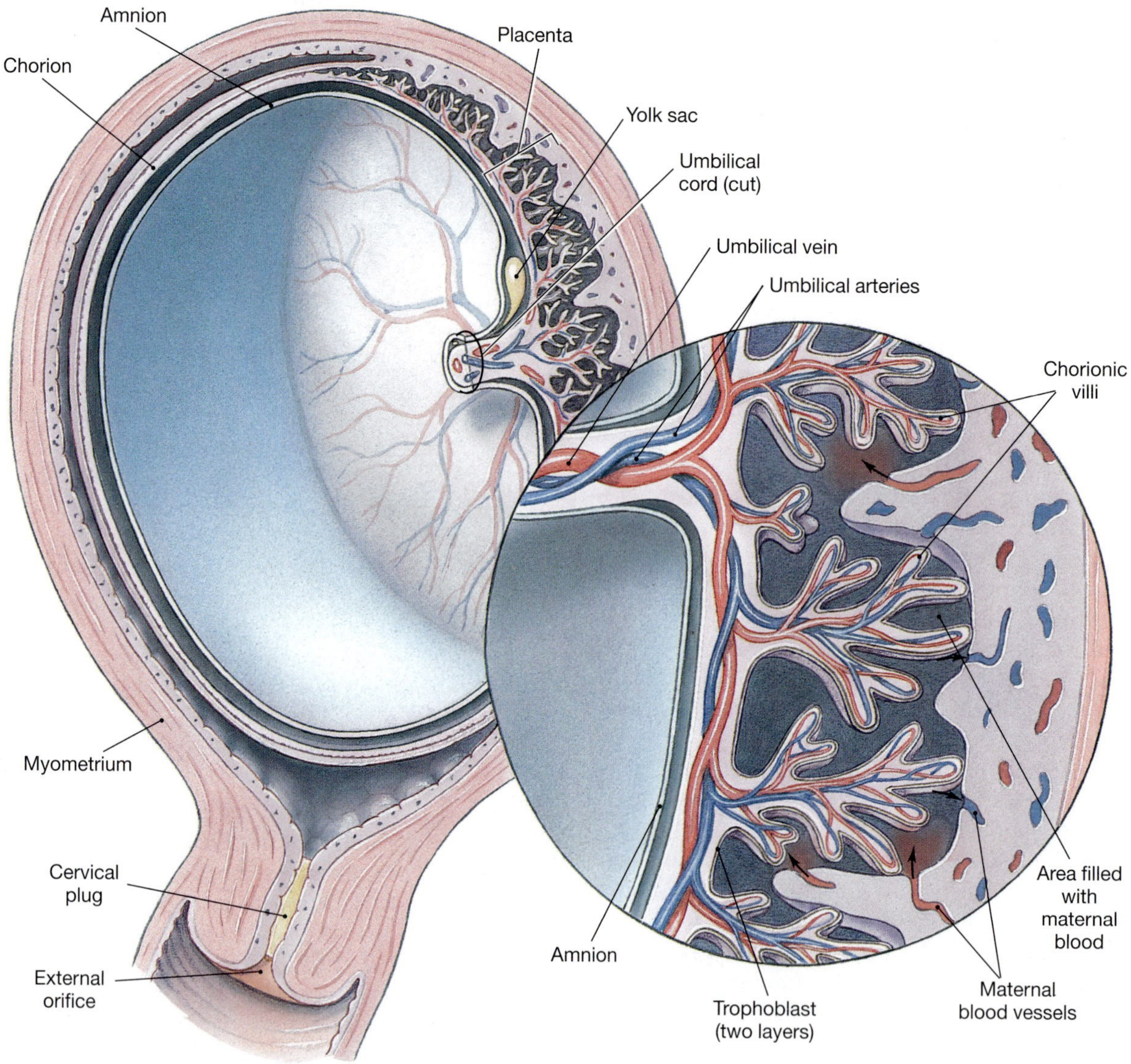

● **FIGURE 21-6   A Three-Dimensional View of Placental Structure**
For clarity, the uterus is shown after the embryo has been removed and the umbilical cord cut. Blood flows into the placenta through ruptured maternal blood arteries. It then flows around chorionic villi that contain fetal blood vessels. Fetal blood arrives over paired umbilical arteries and leaves over a single umbilical vein. Maternal blood reenters the venous system of the mother through the broken walls of small uterine veins. No mixing of maternal and fetal blood occurs.

and the end of the first trimester are summarized in Figure 21-7●.

Embryogenesis (em-brē-ō-JEN-e-sis) is the formation of a viable embryo. The first trimester is a critical period for development, because events during the first 12 weeks establish the basis for **organogenesis**, or organ formation. Table 21-2 (pp. 588–589) includes important developmental milestones during the first trimester.

✓ What would happen if a spermatozoon did not become capacitated in the vagina?

✓ What is the ultimate fate of the inner cell mass of the blastocyst?

✓ Sue's physician tells her that her pregnancy test indicates elevated levels of the hormone hCG (human chorionic gonadotropin). Is Sue pregnant?

✓ What are two important functions of the placenta?

Future head
of embryo

Axis of future
spinal cord

Neural
folds

Cut wall of
amniotic cavity

Future tail
of embryo

Somites (blocks
of tissue that will
form vertebral
column and axial
muscles)

Thickened
neural plate
of ectoderm
(will form brain)

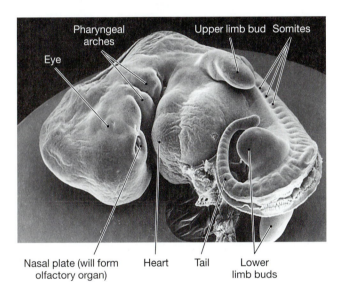

(a) 2 Weeks

● **FIGURE 21-7   The First Trimester**
(a) A superior view of an SEM of an embryo at
2 weeks. **(b)** An SEM and a fiber-optic view of
the lateral surface of embryos at 4–5 weeks.
(c) A fiber-optic view of an embryo at 8 weeks.
(d) A fiber-optic view of an embryo at 12 weeks.

Pharyngeal
arches

Upper limb bud   Somites

Eye

Nasal plate (will form
olfactory organ)

Heart

Tail

Lower
limb buds

Somites

Heart

Medulla

Ear

Upper
limb

Pharyngeal
arches

Forebrain

Eye

Body
stalk

Tail

Lower
limb

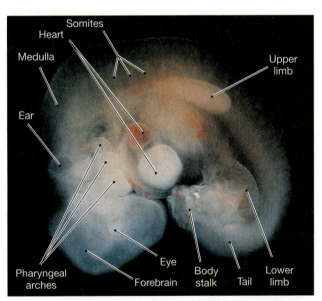

(b) 4 Weeks

Placenta

Umbilical
cord

Amnion

Chorionic
villi

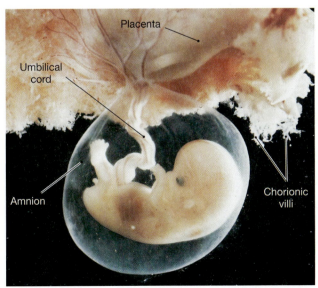

(c) 8 Weeks

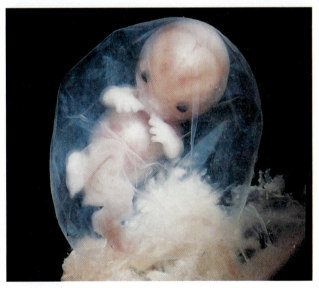

(d) 12 Weeks

21

TABLE 21-2	An Overview of Prenatal and Early Postnatal Development

Gestational Age (Months)	Length and Weight	Integumentary System	Skeletal System	Muscular System	Nervous System	Special Sense Organs
1	5 mm 0.02 g		(b) Somite formation	(b) Somite formation	(b) Neural tube	(b) Eye and ear formation
2	28 mm 2.7 g	(b) Nail beds, hair follicles, sweat glands	(b) Axial and appendicular cartilage formation	(c) Rudiments of axial musculature	(b) CNS, PNS organization, growth of cerebrum	(b) Taste buds, olfactory epithelium
3	78 mm 26 g	(b) Epidermal layers appear	(b) Ossification centers spreading	(c) Rudiments of appendicular musculature	(c) Basic spinal cord and brain structure	
4	133 mm 150 g	(b) Hair, sebaceous glands (c) Sweat glands	(b) Articulations (c) Facial and palatal organization	Fetus starts moving	(b) Rapid expansion of cerebrum	(c) Basic eye and ear structure (b) Peripheral receptor formation
5	185 mm 460 g	(b) Keratin production, nail production			(b) Myelination of spinal cord	
6	230 mm 823 g			(c) Perineal muscles	(b) CNS tract formation (c) Layering of cortex	
7	270 mm 1492 g	(b) Keratinization, nail formation, hair formation				(c) Eyelids open, retina sensitive to light
8	310 mm 2274 g		(b) Epiphyseal plate formation			(c) Taste receptors functional
9	346 mm 2912 g					
Postnatal development		Hair changes in consistency and distribution	Formation and growth of epiphyseal plates continue	Muscle mass and control increase	Myelination, layering, CNS tract formation continue	

Note: (b) = beginning to form; (c) = completed

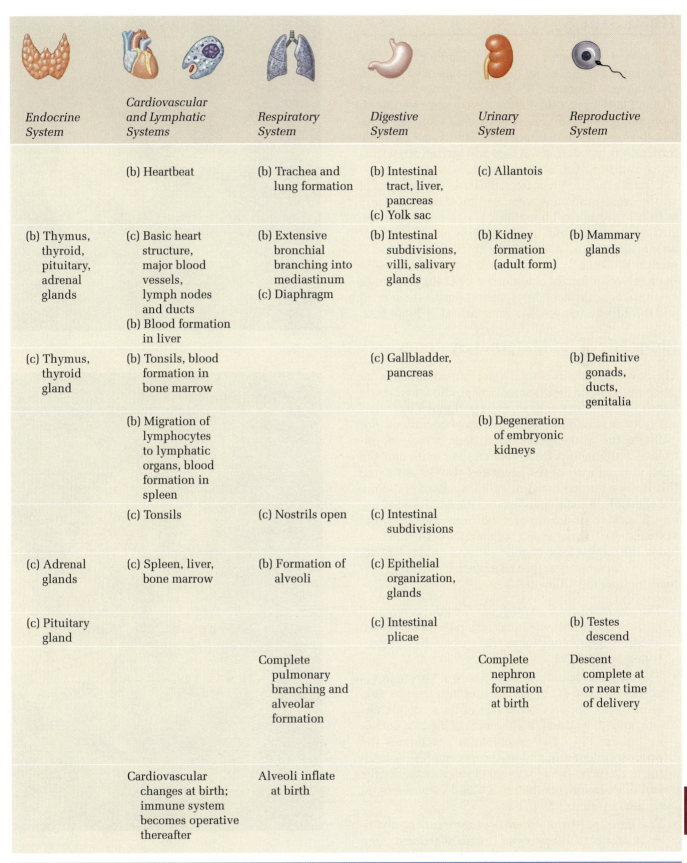

Endocrine System	Cardiovascular and Lymphatic Systems	Respiratory System	Digestive System	Urinary System	Reproductive System
	(b) Heartbeat	(b) Trachea and lung formation	(b) Intestinal tract, liver, pancreas (c) Yolk sac	(c) Allantois	
(b) Thymus, thyroid, pituitary, adrenal glands	(c) Basic heart structure, major blood vessels, lymph nodes and ducts (b) Blood formation in liver	(b) Extensive bronchial branching into mediastinum (c) Diaphragm	(b) Intestinal subdivisions, villi, salivary glands	(b) Kidney formation (adult form)	(b) Mammary glands
(c) Thymus, thyroid gland	(b) Tonsils, blood formation in bone marrow		(c) Gallbladder, pancreas		(b) Definitive gonads, ducts, genitalia
	(b) Migration of lymphocytes to lymphatic organs, blood formation in spleen			(b) Degeneration of embryonic kidneys	
	(c) Tonsils	(c) Nostrils open	(c) Intestinal subdivisions		
(c) Adrenal glands	(c) Spleen, liver, bone marrow	(b) Formation of alveoli	(c) Epithelial organization, glands		
(c) Pituitary gland			(c) Intestinal plicae		(b) Testes descend
		Complete pulmonary branching and alveolar formation		Complete nephron formation at birth	Descent complete at or near time of delivery
	Cardiovascular changes at birth; immune system becomes operative thereafter	Alveoli inflate at birth			

2
1

THE SECOND AND THIRD TRIMESTERS

By the start of the second trimester (Figure 21-7d●), the rudiments of all the major organ systems have formed. Over the next 3 months, the fetus will grow to a weight of about 0.64 kg (1.4 lb). Figure 21-8● shows a 4-month fetus as viewed with a fiber-optic endoscope and a 6-month fetus as seen in ultrasound. The changes in body form that occur during the first and second trimesters are shown in Figure 21-9●.

During the third trimester, the basic components of all the organ systems appear, and most become ready to fulfill their normal functions. The rate of growth begins to decrease, but in absolute terms, the largest weight gain takes place in the third trimester. In 3 months the fetus puts on around 2.6 kg (5.7 lb), reaching a full-term weight of about 3.2 kg (7 lb). Important events in organ system development during the second and third trimesters are also summarized in Table 21-2.

Pregnancy and Maternal Systems

The developing fetus is totally dependent on maternal organ systems for nourishment, respiration, and waste removal. These functions must be performed by maternal systems in addition to their normal operations. For example, the mother must absorb enough oxygen, nutrients, and vitamins for herself and her fetus, and she must eliminate all of the generated wastes. Although this is not a burden over the initial weeks of gestation, the demands become significant as the fetus grows larger. To survive under these conditions, the maternal systems must make major adjustments. In practical terms, the mother must breathe, eat, and excrete for two.

The major changes that take place in maternal systems include the following:

- *The respiratory rate goes up and the tidal volume increases.* As a result, the lungs obtain the extra oxygen required and remove the excess carbon dioxide generated by the fetus.

- *The maternal blood volume increases.* This increase occurs because (1) blood flowing into the placenta reduces the volume in the rest of the systemic circuit, and (2) fetal activity lowers the blood P_{O_2} and elevates the P_{CO_2}. The combination stimulates the production of renin and erythropoietin (EPO), leading to an increase in maternal blood volume. By the end of gestation, the maternal blood volume has increased by almost 50 percent.

- *The maternal requirements for nutrients and vitamins climb 10–30 percent.* Pregnant women, who must "eat for two," are often hungry.

- *The glomerular filtration rate increases by roughly 50 percent.* This increase corresponds to the increase

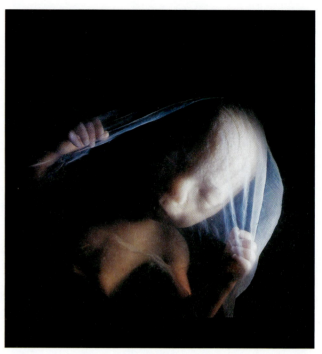

(a)

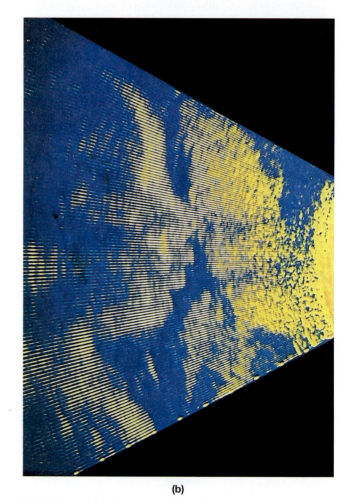

(b)

● FIGURE 21-8 The Second and Third Trimesters
(a) A 4-month fetus seen through a fiber-optic microscope.
(b) A 6-month fetus seen with ultrasound equipment.

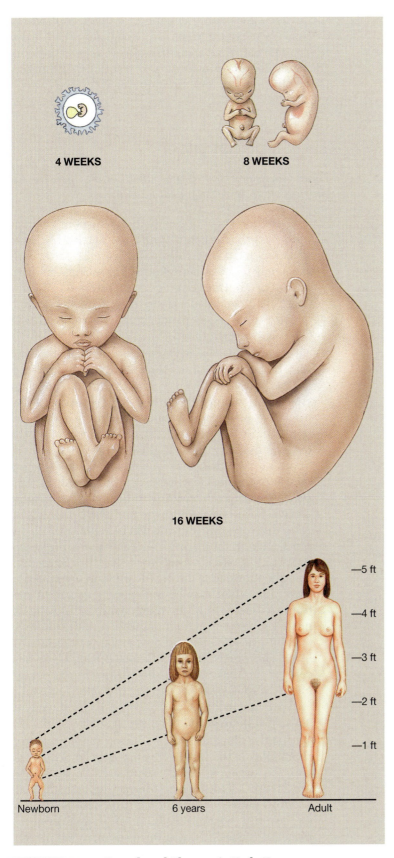

• **FIGURE 21-9   Growth and Changes in Body Form**
The views at fetal ages 4, 8, and 16 weeks are presented at actual size. Notice the changes in body form and proportions as development proceeds. These changes do not stop at birth. For example, the head, which contains the brain and sense organs, is relatively large at birth.

in blood volume, and it accelerates the excretion of metabolic wastes generated by the fetus. Because (1) the volume of urine produced increases and (2) the weight of the uterus presses down on the urinary bladder, pregnant women need to urinate frequently.

- *The uterus undergoes a tremendous increase in size.* Structural and functional changes in the expanding uterus are so important that we will discuss them in a separate section.
- *The mammary glands increase in size and secretory activity begins.* By the end of the sixth month of pregnancy, the mammary glands begin producing secretions that are stored in the duct system.

Structural and Functional Changes in the Uterus

At the end of gestation, a typical uterus will have grown from 7.5 cm (3 in.) in length and 60 g (2 oz.) in weight to 30 cm (12 in.) in length and 1100 g (2.4 lb) in weight. It may then contain almost 5 liters of fluid, giving the organ with contents a total weight of roughly 10 kg (22 lb). This remarkable expansion occurs by the enlargement and elongation of existing cells (especially smooth muscle cells) rather than by an increase in the total number of cells in the uterus.

The tremendous stretching of the myometrium is associated with a gradual increase in the rates of spontaneous smooth muscle contractions. In the early stages of pregnancy, the contractions are weak, painless, and brief in duration. There are indications that the progesterone released by the placenta has an inhibitory effect on the uterine smooth muscle, preventing more extensive and powerful contractions.

Three major factors oppose the calming action of progesterone:

1. *Rising estrogen levels.* Estrogens, also produced by the placenta, increase the sensitivity of the uterine smooth muscles and make contractions more likely. Throughout pregnancy, progesterone exerts the dominant effect, but as the time of delivery approaches, estrogen production accelerates and the myometrium becomes more sensitive to stimulation.

2. *Rising oxytocin levels.* Rising oxytocin levels stimulate an increase in the force and frequency of uterine contractions. Oxytocin release is stimulated by high estrogen levels and by distortion of the cervix.

21

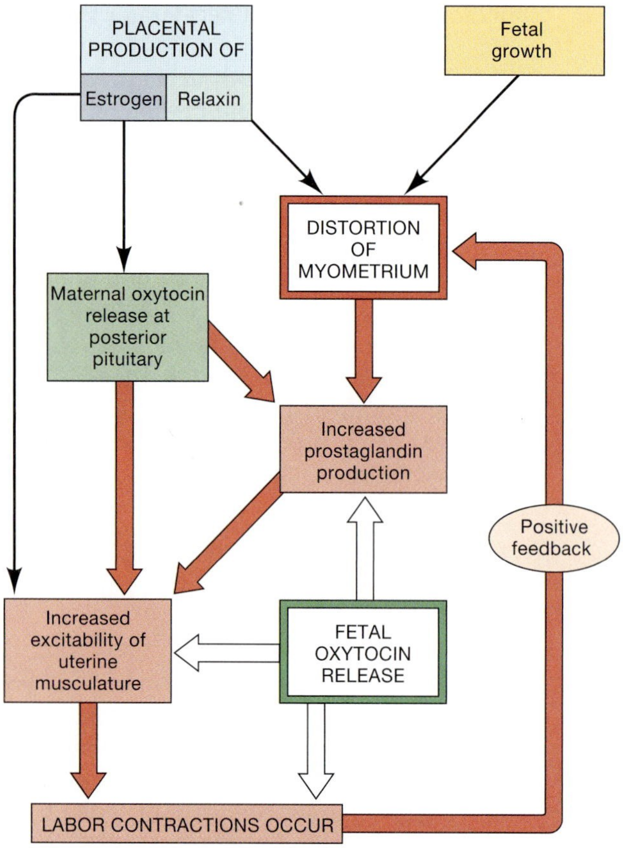

• FIGURE 21-10   Interacting Factors during Labor and Delivery

3. *Prostaglandin production.* In addition to estrogens and oxytocin, uterine tissues late in pregnancy produce prostaglandins that stimulate smooth muscle contractions.

After 9 months of gestation, multiple factors interact to produce **labor contractions** in the myometrium of the uterine wall. Once begun, a positive feedback mechanism operates to ensure that the contractions continue until delivery has been completed.

Figure 21-10• diagrams important factors that stimulate and sustain labor. The actual trigger for the onset of labor may be events in the fetus rather than the mother. At the time labor begins, the fetal pituitary secretes oxytocin, which is released into the maternal bloodstream at the placenta. The resulting increase in myometrial contractions and prostaglandin production, on top of maternal estrogens and oxytocin, finally initiates labor and delivery.

LABOR AND DELIVERY

The goal of labor is the forcible expulsion of the fetus, a process known as **parturition** (par-tū-RISH-un), or birth. During labor, each contraction begins near the top of the uterus and sweeps in a wave toward the cervix. These contractions are strong and occur at regular intervals. As parturition approaches, the contractions increase in force and frequency, changing the position of the fetus and moving it toward the cervical canal.

The Stages of Labor

Labor consists of three stages: the *dilation stage*, the *expulsion stage*, and the *placental stage*.

1. The **dilation stage** begins with the onset of labor, as the cervix dilates completely and the fetus begins to slide down the cervical canal (Figure 21-11a•). This stage may last 8 or more hours, but during this period, labor contractions occur at intervals of once every 10–30 minutes. Late in the process the amnion usually ruptures, an event sometimes referred to as "having the water break."

2. The **expulsion stage** begins as the cervix dilates completely, pushed open by the approaching fetus (Figure 21-11b•). Expulsion continues until the fetus has completely emerged from the vagina, a period that usually lasts less than 2 hours. The arrival of the newborn infant into the outside world represents the birth, or **delivery**. If the vaginal entrance is too small to permit the passage of the fetus and there is acute danger of perineal tearing, the entryway may be temporarily enlarged by making an incision (**episiotomy**; e-pēz-ē-OT-o-mē) through the perineal musculature. After delivery, this incision can be repaired with sutures, a much simpler procedure than dealing with a potentially extensive perineal tear. If unexpected complications arise during the dilation or expulsion stage, the infant may be removed by **cesarean section**, or "C-section." In such cases, an incision is made through the abdominal wall, and the uterus is opened just enough to allow passage of the infant's head. This procedure is performed during 15–25 percent of the deliveries in the United States—more often than necessary according to some studies. Efforts are now being made to reduce the frequency of both episiotomies and cesarean sections.

3. During the **placental stage** of labor, the muscle tension builds in the walls of the partially empty uterus, and the organ gradually decreases in size (Figure 21-11c•). This uterine contraction tears the connections between the endometrium and the placenta. Usually within an hour after delivery, the placental stage ends with the ejection of the placenta, or "afterbirth." The disruption of the placenta is accompanied by a loss of blood, perhaps as much as 500–600 ml, but because the maternal blood volume has increased during pregnancy, the loss can be easily tolerated.

• **FIGURE 21-11** **The Stages of Labor**

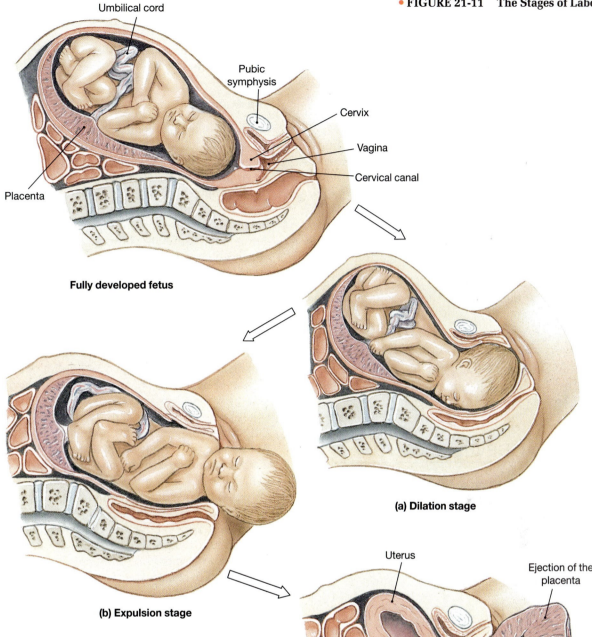

Umbilical cord

Pubic symphysis

Cervix

Vagina

Cervical canal

Placenta

Fully developed fetus

(a) Dilation stage

(b) Expulsion stage

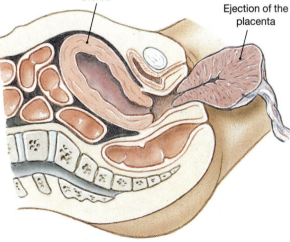

Uterus

Ejection of the placenta

(c) Placental stage

Premature Labor

Premature labor occurs when true labor begins before the fetus has completed normal development. The newborn's chances of survival are directly related to the infant's body weight at delivery. Newborns weighing less than 400 g (14 oz) will not survive, primarily because their respiratory, cardiovascular, and urinary systems are unable to support life. As a result, the dividing line between spontaneous abortion and immature delivery is usually set at 500 g (17.6 oz), the normal weight near the end of the second trimester. A **premature delivery** produces a newborn weighing over 1 kg (35.2 oz). Its chances of survival range from fair to excellent. Infants between 500 g and 1 kg have less than a 50:50 chance of survival, and most survivors have developmental abnormalities.

2
1

Multiple Births

Multiple births (twins, triplets, quadruplets, and so forth) may occur for several reasons. The ratio of twin to single births in the U.S. population is 1:89. About 70 percent of all twins are **fraternal**, or **dizygotic** (dī-zī-GOT-ik). Fraternal twins develop when two eggs are fertilized at the same time, forming two separate zygotes. Fraternal twins can be of the same or different sexes.

Identical, or **monozygotic**, twins result from the separation of blastomeres early in cleavage or from the splitting of the inner cell mass before gastrulation. In either event, the genetic makeup and sex of the pair are identical because both twins formed from the same pair of gametes. Identical twins occur in about 30 percent of all twin births. Triplets and larger multiples can result from the same processes that produce twins.

✓ Why does a mother's total blood volume increase during pregnancy?

✓ What effect would a decrease in progesterone have on the uterus during late pregnancy?

✓ During pregnancy, the uterus increases greatly in size and weight. What process do the uterine cells undergo to produce this change?

POSTNATAL DEVELOPMENT

Developmental processes do not cease at delivery. The newborn infant has few of the anatomical, functional, or physiological characteristics of mature adults. In postnatal development, each individual passes through a number of **life stages**—*neonatal, infancy, childhood, adolescence,* and *maturity*—each with a distinctive combination of characteristics and abilities.

The Neonatal Period, Infancy, and Childhood

The **neonatal period** extends from the moment of birth to 1 month thereafter. **Infancy** then continues to 2 years of age, and **childhood** lasts until puberty commences. Two major events are under way during these developmental stages:

1. The major organ systems, other than those associated with reproduction, become fully operational and gradually acquire the functional characteristics of adult structures.

2. The individual grows rapidly, and significant changes in body proportions take place.

Pediatrics is the medical specialty that focuses on this period of life, from birth through childhood, and also adolescence. Infants and young children often cannot clearly describe the problems they are experiencing, so pediatricians and parents must be skilled observers. Standardized testing procedures assess an individual's developmental progress relative to normal values.

The Neonatal Period

A variety of physiological and anatomical alterations occur as the fetus completes the transition to the status of a newborn infant, or **neonate**. Prior to delivery, the transfer of dissolved gases, nutrients, waste products, hormones, and immunoglobulins occurred across the placenta. At birth, the newborn infant must become relatively self-sufficient, with the processes of respiration, digestion, and excretion performed by its own specialized organs and organ systems. The changes in the cardiovascular and respiratory systems at birth were discussed in Chapter 14. ∞ *p. 402* Typical heart rates of 120–140 beats per minute and respiratory rates of 30 breaths per minute in neonates are considerably higher than those of adults.

Before birth, the digestive system remains relatively inactive, although it does accumulate a mixture of bile secretions, mucus, and epithelial cells. This collection of debris is excreted in the first few days of life. Over that period the newborn infant begins to nurse.

As waste products build up in the arterial blood, they are removed at the glomeruli of the kidneys. Glomerular filtration is normal, but the tubular fluid cannot be concentrated to any significant degree. As a result, urinary water losses are high and neonatal fluid requirements are greater than those of adults.

The neonate has little ability to control body temperature, particularly in the first few days after delivery. For this reason, newborn infants are usually kept bundled up in warm coverings. As the infant grows larger and increases the thickness of its insulating adipose "blanket," its metabolic rate also rises and thermoregulatory abilities improve. Nevertheless, daily and even hourly alterations in body temperature continue throughout childhood.

Lactation and the Mammary Glands. By the end of the sixth month of pregnancy, the mammary glands are fully developed, and the gland cells begin producing a secretion known as **colostrum** (ko-LOS-trum). Provided to the infant during the first 2 or 3 days of life, colostrum contains relatively more proteins and far less fat than milk. Many of the proteins are antibodies that help the infant ward off infections until its own immune system becomes fully functional. As colostrum production declines, milk production increases. Milk consists of a mixture of water, proteins, amino acids, lipids, sugars, and salts. It also contains large quantities of lysozymes, enzymes with antibiotic properties.

The actual secretion of the mammary glands is triggered when the infant begins to suck on the nipple. Stimulation of tactile receptors there leads to the release of

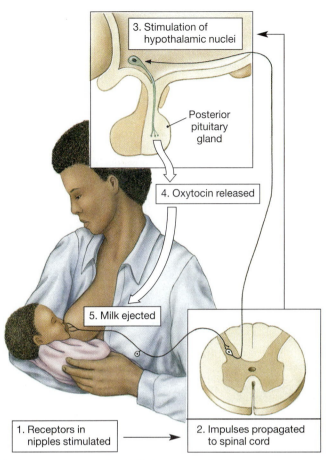

3. Stimulation of hypothalamic nuclei

Posterior pituitary gland

4. Oxytocin released

5. Milk ejected

1. Receptors in nipples stimulated

2. Impulses propagated to spinal cord

•FIGURE 21-12   The Milk Let-Down Reflex

of body growth. **Adolescence** begins at puberty, when three events interact to promote increased hormone production and sexual maturation:

1. The hypothalamus increases its production of gonadotropin-releasing hormone (GnRH).
2. The anterior pituitary becomes more sensitive to the presence of GnRH, and there is a rapid elevation in the circulating levels of FSH and LH.
3. Ovarian or testicular cells become more sensitive to FSH and LH. These changes initiate gametogenesis and the production of male or female sex hormones that stimulate the appearance of secondary sex characteristics and behaviors.

In the years that follow, the continued background secretion of estrogens or androgens maintains these sex characteristics. In addition, the combination of sex hormones and growth hormone, adrenal steroids, and thyroxine leads to a sudden acceleration in the growth rate. The timing of the growth spurt varies between the sexes, corresponding to different ages at the onset of puberty. In girls, the growth rate is maximum between ages 10 and 13; boys grow most rapidly between ages 12 and 15. Growth continues at a slower pace until ages 18 to 21, when most of the epiphyseal plates close. ∞ *p. 125*

The boundary between adolescence and maturity is very hazy, for it has physical, emotional, behavioral, and legal implications. **Maturity** is often associated with the end of growth in the late teens or early twenties. Although development ends at maturity, physiological changes continue. These changes are part of the process of aging, or **senescence**. Aging reduces the efficiency and capabilities of the individual, and even in the absence of other factors will ultimately lead to death.

oxytocin at the posterior pituitary. Oxytocin causes cells within the lactiferous ducts and sinuses to contract. This contraction results in the ejection of milk (Figure 21-12•). This *milk let-down reflex* continues to function until weaning occurs, typically 1–2 years after birth.

Infancy and Childhood

The most rapid growth occurs during prenatal development, and after delivery the relative rate of growth continues to decline. Postnatal growth during infancy and childhood occurs under the direction of circulating hormones, notably growth hormone from the pituitary, adrenal steroids, and thyroid hormones. These hormones affect each tissue and organ in specific ways, depending on the sensitivities of the individual cells. As a result, growth does not occur uniformly, and the body proportions gradually change (see Figure 21-9•, p. 591).

Adolescence and Maturity

Puberty is the period of time between the appearance of secondary sex characteristics and the completion

GENETICS, DEVELOPMENT, AND INHERITANCE

Every somatic cell in the body carries copies of the original 46 chromosomes present in the fertilized egg or zygote. Those chromosomes and their component genes represent the individual's **genotype** (JĒN-ō-tīp). Through development and differentiation, the instructions contained within the genotype are expressed in many different ways. No single living cell or tissue makes use of all the information and instructions contained within the genotype. For example, in muscle fibers the genes important for excitable membrane formation and contractile proteins are active, while a different set of genes is operating in the cells of the pancreatic islets. But the instructions contained within the genotype determine the anatomical and physiological characteristics of each person. Those visible characteristics are known as the individual's **phenotype** (FĒN-ō-tīp; *phainein*, to display + *typos*, mark).

21

Your genotype is derived from those of your parents, but not in a simple way. You are not an exact copy of either parent, nor are you an easily identifiable mixture of their characteristics. Our discussion will begin with the basic patterns and their implications. Then we will examine the mechanisms responsible for regulating the activities of the genotype during subsequent prenatal development.

Genes and Chromosomes

Chromosome structure and the functions of genes were introduced in Chapter 3. ∞ *pp. 69, 70* Chromosomes contain DNA, and genes are segments of DNA. Each gene carries the information needed to direct the synthesis of a specific polypeptide or protein.

Every somatic cell contains 23 pairs of chromosomes. One member of each pair was contributed by the sperm, and the other by the ovum. The members of each pair are known as **homologous** (hō-MOL-o-gus) **chromosomes**. Twenty-two of those pairs are known as **autosomal** (aw-to-SŌ-mal) **chromosomes**. The chromosomes of the twenty-third pair are called the *sex chromosomes* because they differ in the two sexes.

Autosomal Chromosomes

The two chromosomes in an autosomal pair have the same structure and carry genes that affect the same traits. If one member of the pair contains three genes in a row, with number 1 determining hair color, number 2 eye color, and number 3 skin pigmentation, the other chromosome will carry genes affecting the same traits and in the same sequence.

The various forms of any one gene are called **alleles** (a-LĒLS; *allelon*, of one another). If both chromosomes of a homologous pair carry the same allele of a particular gene, the individual is **homozygous** (hō-mō-ZĪ-gus; *homos*, same) for that trait. For example, if a zygote receives a gene for curly hair from the sperm and one for curly hair from the egg, the individual will be homozygous for curly hair. If you are *homozygous for a particular trait, your phenotype will have that characteristic.* Usually about 80 percent of an individual's total set of genes consists of homozygous alleles. Because the chromosomes of a homologous pair have different origins, one paternal and the other maternal, they need not carry the same alleles. An individual who has two different alleles carrying different instructions is **heterozygous** (het-er-ō-ZĪ-gus; *heteros*, other) for that trait. In that case, the phenotype will be determined by the interactions between the corresponding alleles:

- If an allele is **dominant**, it will be expressed in the phenotype *regardless of any conflicting instructions carried by the other allele.*

- If an allele is **recessive**, it will be expressed in the phenotype only if it is present on both chromosomes of a homologous pair. For example, the albino skin condition is characterized by an inability to synthesize the yellow-brown pigment *melanin*. A single dominant allele determines normal skin coloration; two recessive alleles must be present to produce albinism.

Predicting Inheritance. Not every allele can be neatly characterized as dominant or recessive. Some that can are included in Table 21-3. If you restrict attention to these alleles, it is possible to predict the characteristics of individuals on the basis of those of their parents.

Dominant traits are traditionally indicated by capitalized abbreviations, and recessives are abbreviated in lower case. For a given trait, the possibilities are indicated by *AA* (homozygous dominant), *Aa* (heterozygous), or *aa* (homozygous recessive). The gametes involved in fertilization each contribute a single allele for a given trait. That allele must be one of the two contained by all other

TABLE 21-3	The Inheritance of Selected Phenotypic Characteristics

DOMINANT TRAITS

One allele determines phenotype, and the other is suppressed

  Normal skin coloration

  Brachydactyly (short fingers)

  Ability to taste phenylthiocarbamate (PTC)

  Free earlobes

  Curly hair

  Color vision

  Presence of Rh factor on red blood cell membranes

Both dominant alleles may be expressed (codominance)

  Presence of A or B antigens on red blood cell membranes

  Structure of serum proteins (albumins, transferrins)

  Structure of hemoglobin molecule

RECESSIVE TRAITS

  Albinism

  Blond hair

  Red hair (expressed only if individual is also homozygous for blond hair)

  Lack of A, B agglutinogens (Type O blood)

  Inability to roll the tongue into a U-shape

SEX-LINKED TRAITS

  Color blindness

  Hemophilia

POLYGENIC TRAITS

  Eye color

  Hair colors other than pure blond or red

cells in the parental body. Consider, for example, the offspring of an albino mother and a normal father. Because albinism is a recessive trait, the maternal alleles can be abbreviated *aa*. No matter which of her oocytes gets fertilized, it will carry the recessive *a* gene. The father has normal coloration, and this is a dominant trait. He may therefore be homozygous or heterozygous for this trait, since *AA* or *Aa* will give rise to the same phenotype.

A simple box diagram known as a *Punnett square* lets us predict the probabilities that the children will have particular characteristics by giving the possible combinations of parental alleles they can inherit. In the Punnett square in Figure 21-13•, the maternal alleles are listed along the horizontal axis and the paternal ones along the vertical axis. The possible combinations are indicated in the small boxes. Figure 21-13a• shows the possible offspring of an *aa* mother and an *AA* father. All of the children must have the genotype *Aa*, and they will all have normal skin color. Compare these results with those of Figure 21-13b•, for a heterozygous father (*Aa*). The heterozygous individual produces two types of gametes, *A* and *a*, and either one may fertilize the oocyte. As a result, there is a 50 percent probability that a child of such a father will inherit the genotype *Aa* and thus have normal skin color. The probability of inheriting the genotype *aa*, and thus having the albino phenotype, is also 50 percent.

The Punnett square can also be used in reverse, to draw conclusions about the identity and genotype of a parent. For example, a man with the genotype *AA* cannot be the father of an albino child (*aa*).

Simple Inheritance.   In **simple inheritance**, phenotypic characteristics are determined by interactions between a single pair of alleles. The frequency of appearance of an inherited disorder resulting from simple inheritance can be predicted using a Punnett square. Although they are rare disorders in terms of overall numbers, more than 1200 different inherited conditions have been identified that reflect the presence of one or two abnormal alleles for a single gene. A partial listing is included in Table 21-4, along with the location where additional information can be obtained.

Polygenic Inheritance.   **Polygenic inheritance** involves interactions between alleles on several genes. Because multiple alleles are involved, the frequency of occurrence cannot easily be predicted using a simple Punnett square. Several important adult disorders, including hypertension and coronary artery disease, fall within this category. Many of the developmental disorders responsible for fetal mortalities and congenital malformations also result from multiple genetic interactions. In these cases, the particular genetic composition of the individual does

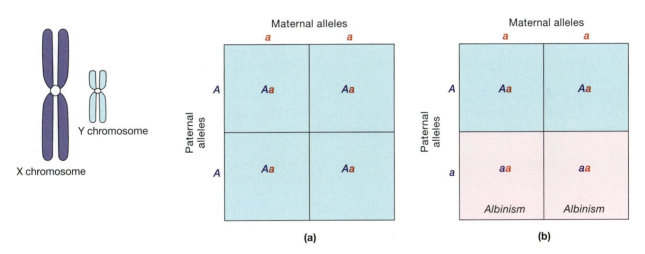

•FIGURE 21-13   **Predicting Phenotypes**
In the X and Y chromosomes above, notice the differences in size and shape. **(a)** The offspring of a homozygous dominant father and a homozygous recessive mother will all be heterozygous for that trait. Their phenotype will be the same as that of the father. **(b)** The offspring of a heterozygous father and a homozygous recessive mother will either be heterozygous or homozygous for the recessive trait. In this example, half of the offspring will have normal skin coloration and the other half will be albinos. **(c)** The inheritance of color blindness, a sex-linked trait. A color-blind father and a heterozygous mother will produce daughters with normal vision, but half of the sons will be color-blind.

2
1

TABLE 21-4	Relatively Common Inherited Disorders
Disorder	*Page in Text*
AUTOSOMAL DOMINANTS	
Marfan's syndrome	p. 92
Huntington's disease	p. 260
AUTOSOMAL RECESSIVES	
Deafness	p. 298
Albinism	p. 111
Sickle-cell anemia	p. 338
Cystic fibrosis	p. 440
Phenylketonuria	p. 502
X-LINKED	
Duchenne's muscular dystrophy	p. 172
Hemophilia (one form)	p. 350
Color blindness	p. 287

not by itself determine the onset of the disease. Instead, the conditions regulated by these genes establish a susceptibility to particular environmental influences. This means that not every individual with the genetic tendency for a particular condition will actually develop it. It is therefore difficult to track polygenic conditions through successive generations. However, because many inherited polygenic conditions are likely but not *guaranteed* to occur, steps can be taken to prevent a crisis. For example, hypertension can be prevented or reduced by controlling diet and fluid volume, and coronary artery disease can be prevented by lowering serum cholesterol concentrations.

Sex Chromosomes

The chromosomes of the twenty-third pair are called the **sex chromosomes** because they determine the biological sex of the individual. Unlike other chromosomal pairs, the sex chromosomes are not necessarily identical in appearance and gene content. There are two different sex chromosomes, an **X chromosome** and a **Y chromosome**. The Y chromosome is considerably smaller than the X chromosome and contains fewer genes, but among those genes are dominant alleles that specify that an individual with that chromosome will be a male. The normal male chromosome pair is *XY*, and the female pair is *XX*. The ova produced by a woman will always carry *X*, and sperm may carry *X* or *Y*.

The X chromosome also carries genes that affect somatic structures. These characteristics are called **X-linked** because in most cases there are no corresponding alleles on the Y chromosome. They are also

known as *sex-linked traits* because the responsible genes are located on the sex chromosomes. The best-known X-linked characteristics are associated with noticeable diseases or defects that are caused by single alleles.

The inheritance of color blindness, a condition discussed in Chapter 10, exemplifies the differences between sex-linked and autosomal inheritance. ∞ *p. 287* A relatively common form of color blindness is associated with the presence of a dominant or recessive gene on the X chromosome. Normal color vision is determined by the presence of a dominant gene, *C*, and color blindness results from the presence of the recessive gene *c*. A woman, with her two X chromosomes, can be either homozygous, *CC*, or heterozygous, *Cc*, and still have normal color vision. She will be color-blind only if she carries two recessive alleles, *cc*. But a male has only one X chromosome, so whatever that chromosome carries will determine whether he has normal color vision or is color-blind. A Punnett square for an X-linked trait, as in Figure 21-13c●, reveals that the sons produced by a normal father and a heterozygous mother will have a 50 percent chance of being color-blind, while the daughters will all have normal color vision.

A number of other clinical disorders are X-linked traits, including certain forms of *hemophilia, diabetes insipidus,* and *muscular dystrophy*. In several instances, molecular genetics techniques have enabled researchers to locate specific genes on the X chromosome. One technique provides a relatively direct method of screening for the presence of a particular condition before the symptoms appear, and even before birth.

The Human Genome Project

Few of the genes responsible for inherited disorders have been identified or even localized to a specific chromosome. However, that situation is changing rapidly, owing to the attention devoted to the **Human Genome Project (HGP)**. This project, funded by the National Institutes of Health and the Department of Energy, is attempting to transcribe the entire human genome, chromosome by chromosome and gene by gene. The project began in October 1990 and was expected to take 10–15 years. Progress has been more rapid than expected, so the project should be completed by 2003.

The first step in understanding the human genome is to prepare a map of the individual chromosomes. **Karyotyping** (KAR-ē-ō-tī-ping; *karyon*, nucleus + *typos*, mark) is the determination of an individual's chromosome complement. Figure 21-14● (p. 600) shows a set of normal human chromosomes. Each chromosome has characteristic banding patterns, and segments can be stained with special dyes. The banding patterns are useful as reference points when more-detailed genetic maps are prepared. The banding patterns themselves can be

CLINICAL NOTE   INHERITED DISORDERS: EMERGENCY IMPLICATIONS

Inherited diseases are those diseases that are passed from parents to child through the genetic material (DNA). Many diseases are thought to have an inheritable component. It is clear that some disease processes, such as heart disease, diabetes, asthma, and Alzheimer's disease, tend to cluster in families. However, some diseases are inherited directly. While they are somewhat uncommon, several of them develop conditions requiring emergency treatment.

- *Marfan syndrome.* Marfan syndrome (MS) is a connective tissue disease that is transmitted through autosomal dominant inheritance. MS is characterized by long, thin extremities that are frequently associated with other skeletal changes; reduced vision due to dislocation of the lenses; and aortic aneurysms. Most persons with MS are tall and thin (some historians have suggested that Abraham Lincoln had MS). Dilation and rupture of an aortic aneurysm is the cause of death in many patients with MS and often occurs in the third or fourth decade of life.

- *Huntington disease.* Huntington disease (HD), also called *Huntington's chorea,* is a debilitating disease that is transmitted by autosomal dominant patterns. HD develops at about 35–40 years of age and is characterized by progressive dementia and involuntary movements. The disease advances slowly, with death occurring, on average, 15–20 years after the onset of symptoms. HD accounts for many of the nursing home admissions of patients in their fourth or fifth decade of life.

- *Sickle cell disease.* Sickle cell disease (SCD) is a group of disorders characterized by the presence of an abnormal form of hemoglobin *(hemoglobin S).* It is inherited in an autosomal recessive pattern. Patients who receive the gene for SCD from only one parent tend to develop *sickle cell trait (SCT).* SCT occurs in 7–13 percent of black Americans. In East Africa, the incidence of SCT may be as high as 45 percent. It appears that SCT may provide protection against lethal forms of malaria. Persons who receive the gene for SCD from both parents develop SCD. SCD causes the red blood cells to *sickle* (assume a crescent shape) due to the abnormal hemoglobin. Sickling causes the clinical signs and symptoms of SCD. Patients with SCD are often frequent visitors to hospital emergency departments as they periodically develop sickle cell crisis, where blood flow to small blood vessels in organs such as the bones and spleen become occluded. Sickle cell crisis can be extremely painful, requiring high doses of narcotics to achieve pain control.

- *Cystic fibrosis.* Cystic fibrosis (CF) is an autosomal recessive disease of the exocrine glands that causes production of excess, thick mucus that obstructs the gastrointestinal system and lungs. One of the classic signs of CF is elevated concentrations of sodium chloride in the sweat and other secretions. The excess mucus coagulates in the ducts of organs or in the airways, causing dilation and obstruction. Bronchial obstruction predisposes the patient to the development of lung infection, primarily with *Staphylococcal aureus* and *Pseudomonas aeruginosa.* Often the CF patient becomes permanently colonized with one of these bacteria. Progressive obstruction of the respiratory system eventually leads to respiratory failure. CF also impacts the pancreas, causing obstruction and destruction of the exocrine glands. The mean life expectancy of the CF patient is about 30 years. The need for medical intervention increases significantly as the patient ages.

- *Muscular dystrophy.* Muscular dystrophy (MD) is a group of disorders that cause degeneration of skeletal muscle fibers. The major type of MD is *pseudohypertrophic MD,* often called *Duchenne's MD,* which causes an abnormality in the intracellular metabolism of the muscle fibers. Duchenne's MD is usually detected in children around 3 years of age. Muscle weakness begins at the pelvic girdle and spreads. Eventually, the pulmonary and cardiovascular systems are affected. Duchenne's MD follows an X-linked recessive pattern and is thought to be caused by a single-gene defect.

- *Hemophilia.* Hemophilia is a disease characterized by abnormal bleeding due to a genetic deficiency in one of the coagulation factors. The most common form of hemophilia is *hemophilia A (classic hemophilia).* It causes a deficiency in factor VIII and is inherited as an X-linked recessive disorder that affects males and is transmitted by females. *Hemophilia B,* also called Christmas disease, is due to a deficiency in factor IX. It too is an X-linked recessive trait and is clinically indistinguishable from hemophilia A. *Hemophilia C* is an autosomal recessive disease that causes a factor XI deficiency. It occurs equally in males and females. *Von Willebrand disease* is an autosomal dominant trait that causes a defect in factor VIII that differs from the defect caused by hemophilia A. The hemophilias cause bleeding. Spontaneous bleeding into a joint (hemarthrosis) is not uncommon and is a frequent reason for hemophiliacs to seek emergency care.

---

useful, as abnormal banding patterns are characteristic of some genetic disorders and several cancers, including a form of leukemia.

As of 1999, HGP progress includes the following:

- Ten chromosomes—chromosomes 3, 7, 11, 12, 16, 17, 19, 21, 22, and the Y chromosome—have been mapped completely, and preliminary maps have been made for all other chromosomes.

- Over 38,000 genes have been identified—nearly one-third to one-half of the estimated 60,000 to 100,000 genes in the human genome. Of that number, approximately 7800 have been assigned to specific locations on individual chromosomes.

- The genes responsible for about 100 inherited disorders have been identified, including many of the disorders listed in Table 21-4. Genetic screening can now be done for many of these conditions.

2 1

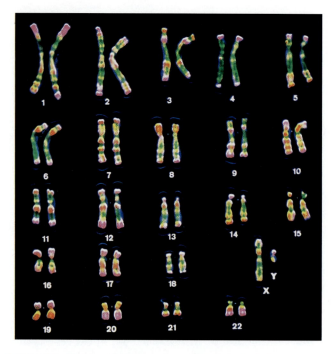

• **FIGURE 21-14** **Chromosomes of a Normal Male**

The Human Genome Project is attempting to determine the normal genetic composition of a "typical" human being. Yet we are all variations on a basic theme. As we improve our ability to manipulate our own genetic foundations, we will face troubling ethical and legal decisions. For example, few people object to the insertion of a "correct" gene into somatic cells to cure a specific disease. But what if we could insert that modified gene into a gamete and change not only that individual but all his or her descendants? And what if the gene did not correct or prevent a disorder, but "improved" the individual by increasing intelligence, height, vision—or altering some other phenotypic characteristic? These and other difficult questions will not go away, and in the years to come, we will have to find answers with which we all can live.

✓ Curly hair is an autosomal dominant trait. What would be the phenotype of a person who is heterozygous for this trait?

✓ Joe has three daughters and complains that it's his wife's "fault" that he has no sons. What would you tell him?

Chapter Review

KEY TERMS

amnion, p. 582	**gestation**, p. 580	**parturition**, p. 592
blastocyst, p. 581	**heterozygous**, p. 596	**phenotype**, p. 595
embryo, p. 578	**homozygous**, p. 596	**placenta**, p. 585
fetus, p. 587	**implantation**, p. 581	**trimester**, p. 580
genotype, p. 595	**neonate**, p. 594	**trophoblast**, p. 581

SUMMARY OUTLINE

INTRODUCTION *p. 578*

1. **Development** is the gradual modification of physical and physiological characteristics from conception to maturity. The creation of different cell types is **differentiation**.

AN OVERVIEW OF TOPICS IN DEVELOPMENT *p. 578*

1. **Prenatal development** occurs before birth; **postnatal development** begins at birth and continues to maturity, when senescence (aging) begins. **Inheritance** refers to the transfer of genetically determined characteristics from generation to generation. **Genetics** is the study of the mechanisms of inheritance.

FERTILIZATION *p. 578*

1. **Fertilization** normally occurs in the uterine tube within a day after ovulation. Sperm cannot fertilize an egg until they have undergone **capacitation**.

The Oocyte at Ovulation *p. 578*

2. The acrosomal caps of the spermatozoa release *hyaluronidase*, an enzyme that separates cells of the *corona radiata* and exposes the oocyte membrane. When a single spermatozoon contacts that membrane, fertilization occurs and **oocyte activation** follows.

3. During activation, the secondary oocyte completes meiosis, and the penetration of additional sperm is prevented.

4. After activation, the *female pronucleus* and *male pronucleus* fuse in a process called **amphimixis**. *(Figure 21-1)*

A Preview of Prenatal Development *p. 580*

5. The 9-month **gestation**, or *pregnancy*, period can be divided into three **trimesters**.

THE FIRST TRIMESTER *p. 581*

1. The **first trimester** is the most dangerous period of prenatal development. The processes of *cleavage, implantation,*

placentation, and *embryogenesis* take place during this critical period.

Cleavage and Blastocyst Formation *p. 581*

2. Cleavage subdivides the cytoplasm of the zygote into cells called **blastomeres** through a series of mitotic divisions. The zygote becomes a hollow ball of blastomeres called a **blastocyst**. The blastocyst consists of an outer **trophoblast** and an **inner cell mass**. *(Figure 21-2)*

Implantation *p. 581*

3. During **implantation**, the blastocyst burrows into the uterine endometrium. Implantation occurs about 7 days after fertilization. *(Figure 21-3)*

4. As the trophoblast enlarges and spreads, maternal blood flows through open *lacunae*. After the resulting **blastodisc** undergoes **gastrulation**, it is composed of **endoderm**, **ectoderm**, and an intervening **mesoderm**. It is from these three **germ layers** that the body systems differentiate. *(Figure 21-4; Table 21-1)*

5. The germ layers help form four **extraembryonic membranes**: the *yolk sac, amnion, allantois,* and *chorion*. *(Figure 21-5)*

6. The **yolk sac** is an important site of blood cell formation. The **amnion** encloses fluid that surrounds and cushions the developing embryo. The base of the **allantois** later gives rise to the urinary bladder. Circulation within the vessels of the **chorion** provides a rapid-transport system linking the embryo with the trophoblast.

Placentation *p. 585*

7. Placentation occurs as blood vessels form around the blastocyst and the **placenta** appears. *Chorionic villi* extend outward into the maternal tissues, forming an intricate, branching network through which maternal blood flows. As development proceeds, the **umbilical cord**, or *umbilical stalk*, connects the fetus to the placenta. *(Figure 21-6)*

8. The placenta synthesizes **human chorionic gonadotropin (hCG)**, estrogens, progestins, **human placental lactogen (hPL)**, **placental prolactin**, and **relaxin**.

Embryogenesis *p. 585*

9. The first trimester is critical because both **embryogenesis** and **organogenesis** (organ formation) occur during this period. *(Figure 21-7; Table 21-2)*

THE SECOND AND THIRD TRIMESTERS *p. 590*

1. In the **second trimester**, vital organ systems are near functional completion. During the **third trimester**, these organ systems become functional. *(Figures 21-8, 21-9; Table 21-2)*

Pregnancy and Maternal Systems *p. 590*

2. The developing fetus is totally dependent on maternal organs for nourishment, respiration, and waste removal. Maternal adaptations include increased blood volume, respiratory rate, tidal volume, nutrient intake, and glomerular filtration.

Structural and Functional Changes in the Uterus *p. 591*

3. Progesterone produced by the placenta has an inhibitory effect on uterine muscles; its calming action is opposed by estrogens, oxytocin, and prostaglandins. At some point, multiple factors interact to produce **labor contractions** in the uterine wall. *(Figure 21-10)*

LABOR AND DELIVERY *p. 592*

1. The goal of labor is **parturition**, the forcible expulsion of the fetus.

Stages of Labor *p. 592*

2. Labor consists of three stages: the **dilation stage**, **expulsion stage**, and **placental stage**. *(Figure 21-11)*

Premature Labor, *p. 593*

3. Premature labor results in the delivery of a newborn that has not completed normal development.

Multiple Births, *p. 594*

4. Fraternal, or **dizygotic**, **twins** develop from two different zygotes. **Identical**, or **monozygotic**, twins result when the blastomeres of an early embryo or portions of the inner cell mass separate during early development.

POSTNATAL DEVELOPMENT *p. 594*

1. Postnatal development involves a series of **life stages**, including the *neonatal period, infancy, childhood, adolescence,* and *maturity*. *Senescence* begins at maturity and ends in the death of the individual.

The Neonatal Period, Infancy, and Childhood *p. 594*

2. The **neonatal period** extends from birth to 1 month of age. **Infancy** then continues to 2 years of age, and **childhood** lasts until puberty commences. During these stages, major organ systems (other than reproductive) become fully operational and gradually acquire adult characteristics, and the individual grows rapidly.

3. In the transition from fetus to **neonate**, the respiratory, circulatory, digestive, and urinary systems begin functioning independently. The newborn must also begin thermoregulating.

4. Mammary glands produce protein-rich **colostrum** during the infant's first few days and then convert to milk production. These secretions are released as a result of the *milk let-down reflex*. *(Figure 21-12)*

Adolescence and Maturity *p. 595*

5. Adolescence begins at **puberty** when (1) the hypothalamus increases its production of GnRH, (2) circulating levels of FSH and LH rise rapidly, and (3) ovarian or testicular cells become more sensitive to FSH and LH. These changes initiate gametogenesis, production of sex hormones, and a sudden acceleration in growth rate.

6. Maturity, the end of growth, occurs by the early twenties. Postmaturity changes in physiological processes are part of aging, or **senescence**.

GENETICS, DEVELOPMENT, AND INHERITANCE *p. 595*

1. Every somatic cell carries copies of the original 46 chromosomes in the zygote; these represent the individual's **genotype**. The physical expression of the genotype is the **phenotype** of the individual.

Genes and Chromosomes *p. 596*

2. Every somatic human cell contains 23 pairs of chromosomes; each pair consists of **homologous chromosomes**; 22 pairs are **autosomal chromosomes**, and the twenty-third pair of chromosomes is called the *sex chromosomes* because the chromosomes differ in the two sexes.

3. Chromosomes contain DNA, and genes are functional segments of DNA. The various forms of a gene are called **alleles**. If both homologous chromosomes carry the same allele of a particular gene, the individual is **homozygous**; if they carry different alleles, the individual is **heterozygous**.

4. Alleles are considered **dominant** or **recessive** depending on how their traits are expressed. *(Table 21-3)*

5. Combining maternal and paternal alleles in a *Punnett square* allows us to predict the probability of a particular phenotype among the offspring. *(Figure 21-13)*

6. In **simple inheritance**, phenotypic characters are determined by interactions between a single pair of alleles. **Poly-**

genic inheritance involves interactions among alleles on several chromosomes. *(Table 21-4)*

7. The two types of **sex chromosomes**: are **X chromosome** and **Y chromosomes**. The normal male sex chromosome complement is *XY*; that of females, *XX*. The X chromosome carries **X-linked** genes, which affect somatic structures but have no corresponding alleles on the Y chromosome.

The Human Genome Project *p. 598*

8. The **Human Genome Project** has identified over 38,000 of our estimated 100,000 genes, including some of those responsible for inherited disorders. *(Figure 21-14; Table 21-4)*

REVIEW QUESTIONS

LEVEL 1   Reviewing Facts and Terms

Match each item in column A with the most closely related item in column B. Use letters for answers in the spaces provided.

Column A

____ 1. gestation
____ 2. cleavage
____ 3. gastrulation
____ 4. chorion
____ 5. human chorionic gonadotropin
____ 6. birth
____ 7. episiotomy
____ 8. afterbirth
____ 9. senescence
____10. neonate
____11. phenotype
____12. homozygous recessive
____13. heterozygous
____14. male genotype
____15. female genotype
____16. trisomy 21

Column B

a. blastocyst formation
b. ejection of placenta
c. germ-layer formation
d. indication of pregnancy
e. embryo-maternal circulatory exchange
f. visible characteristics
g. time of prenatal development
h. *aa*
i. Down syndrome
j. newborn infant
k. *Aa*
l. *XY*
m. *XX*
n. parturition
o. process of aging
p. perineal musculature incision

17. The gradual modification of anatomical structures during the period from conception to maturity is:
  (a) development
  (b) differentiation
  (c) embryogenesis
  (d) capacitation

18. Human fertilization involves the fusion of two haploid gametes, producing a zygote containing:
  (a) 23 chromosomes
  (b) 46 chromosomes
  (c) the normal haploid number of chromosomes
  (d) 46 pairs of chromosomes

19. The secondary oocyte leaving the follicle is in:
  (a) interphase
  (b) metaphase of the first meiotic division
  (c) telophase of the second meiotic division
  (d) metaphase of the second meiotic division

20. The process that establishes the foundation of all major organ systems is:
  (a) cleavage   (b) implantation
  (c) placentation   (d) embryogenesis

21. The zygote arrives in the uterine cavity as a:
  (a) morula   (b) trophoblast
  (c) lacuna   (d) blastomere

22. The surface that provides for active and passive exchange between the fetal and maternal bloodstreams is the:
  (a) yolk stalk   (b) chorionic villi
  (c) umbilical veins   (d) umbilical arteries

23. Milk let-down is associated with:
  (a) events occurring in the uterus
  (b) placental hormonal influences
  (c) circadian rhythms
  (d) reflex action triggered by suckling

24. If an allele must be present on both the maternal and paternal chromosomes to affect the phenotype, the allele is said to be:
    (a) dominant
    (b) recessive
    (c) complementary
    (d) heterozygous

25. Summarize the developmental changes that occur during the first, second, and third trimesters.

26. Identify the three stages of labor, and describe the events that characterize each stage.

27. Identify the three life stages that occur between birth and approximately age 10. Describe the characteristics of each stage and when it occurs.

LEVEL 2   Reviewing Concepts

28. Relaxin is a peptide hormone that:
    (a) increases the flexibility of the symphysis pubis
    (b) causes dilation of the cervix
    (c) suppresses the release of oxytocin by the hypothalamus
    (d) a, b, and c are correct

29. During adolescence, the events that interact to promote increased hormone production and sexual maturation result from activity of the:
    (a) hypothalamus
    (b) anterior pituitary
    (c) ovaries and testicular cells
    (d) a, b, and c are correct

30. In addition to its role in the nutrition of the fetus, what are the primary endocrine functions of the placenta?

31. Discuss the changes that occur in maternal systems during pregnancy. Why are these changes functionally significant?

32. During labor, what physiological mechanisms ensure that uterine contractions continue until delivery has been completed?

33. To what does the phrase "having the water break" refer during the process of labor?

34. What would you conclude about a trait in each of the following situations?
    (a) Children who exhibit this trait have at least one parent who exhibits the same trait.
    (b) Children exhibit this trait even though neither of the parents exhibits it.
    (c) The trait is expressed more frequently in sons than in daughters.
    (d) The trait is expressed equally in both daughters and sons.

35. Explain why more men than women are color-blind. Which type of inheritance is involved?

36. Explain the goals and possible benefits of the Human Genome Project.

LEVEL 3   Critical Thinking and Clinical Applications

37. Hemophilia A, a condition in which the blood does not clot properly, is a recessive trait located on the X chromosome (X^h). A woman heterozygous for the trait marries a normal male. What is the probability that this couple will have hemophiliac daughters? What is the probability that this couple will have hemophiliac sons?

38. Explain why the normal heart and respiratory rates of neonates are so much higher than those of adults, even though adults are so much larger.

39. Sally gives birth to a baby with a congenital deformity of the stomach. She swears that it is the result of a viral infection that she suffered during the third trimester of pregnancy. Do you think this is a possibility? Explain.

ANSWERS TO CONCEPT CHECK QUESTIONS

Page 586
1. A spermatozoon cannot fertilize an ovum unless the sperm has undergone capacitation in the female reproductive tract.   **2.** The inner cell mass of the blastocyst eventually develops into the embryo.   **3.** After fertilization, the developing trophoblasts—and later, the placenta—produce and release the hormone hCG. She is pregnant.   **4.** Placental functions include (1) supplying the developing fetus with a route for gas exchange, nutrient transfer, and waste product elimination, and (2) producing hormones that affect maternal systems.

Page 594
1. During pregnancy, blood flow through the placenta reduces the volume of blood in the systemic circuit, and the fetus adds carbon dioxide to the shared circulatory system. The result is the release of renin and EPO, which stimulate an increase in maternal blood volume.   **2.** Progesterone reduces uterine contractions. A decrease in the progesterone level at any time during the pregnancy can lead to uterine contractions and, in late pregnancy, labor.   **3.** The expansion of the uterus during gestation is a result of the enlargement of the uterine cells, primarily smooth muscle cells.

Page 600
1. A person who is heterozygous for curly hair would have one dominant gene and one recessive gene. The person's phenotype would be "curly hair."   **2.** There are two types of sex chromosomes: an X chromosome and a Y chromosome. The normal male chromosome pair is XY, and the normal female pair is XX. The ova produced during meiosis by Joe's wife will always carry X, and the sperm produced during meiosis by Joe may carry X or Y. As a result, the sex of Joe's children depends on which type of sperm cell fertilizes the ovum.

2
1

OVERVIEW

Problems related to pregnancy are among the more common problems encountered in young women. Pregnancy has significant physical and hormonal effects on the body that must be considered when evaluating a pregnant patient. Several conditions related to pregnancy are potentially life threatening, including spontaneous abortion, ectopic pregnancy, and others. It is essential to have a high index of suspicion for these problems in order to detect them early.

The medical specialty that deals with pregnancy, childbirth, and diseases of women is called obstetrics. Physicians who limit their practice primarily to the care of and delivery of pregnant women are called *obstetricians.* Most obstetricians also practice gynecology and are referred to as *obstetrician/gynecologists* or OB/Gyns for short. Many women use obstetricians as their primary health care provider. Obstetricians usually complete a four-year residency program that teaches the medical and surgical care of pregnancy and problems with the female reproductive tract. Some obstetricians will take fellowship training in special areas of obstetrics or gynecolo-

gy. A common obstetrical subspecialty is *maternal-fetal medicine.* These doctors monitor and manage high-risk pregnancies such as those that occur in diabetics, in mothers with significant prior health problems, or in situations where a fetal abnormality is suspected.

PHYSIOLOGIC CHANGES OF PREGNANCY

The physiologic changes associated with pregnancy are due to an altered hormonal state, the mechanical effects of the enlarging uterus and its significant vascularity, and the increasing metabolic demands on the maternal system. Paramedics must understand the physiologic changes associated with pregnancy in order to better assess pregnant patients.

• *Reproductive System.* Understandably, the most significant pregnancy-related changes occur in the uterus. In its nonpregnant state, the uterus is a small pear-shaped organ weighing about 60 g (2 ounces) with a capacity of approximately 10 cc. By the end of pregnancy, its weight has increased to 1000 g (slightly more than 2 pounds), while its capacity is now approximately

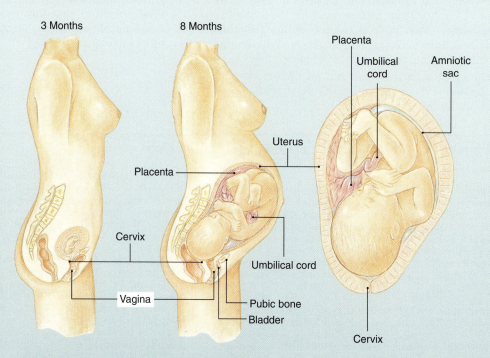

3 Months   8 Months

Placenta
Umbilical cord   Amniotic sac

Uterus

Placenta

Cervix

Umbilical cord

Vagina

Pubic bone

Bladder

Cervix

● **FIGURE A21-1   Uterus During Pregnancy**
Significant uterine changes are associated with pregnancy. By term, the uterus is the largest organ in the abdomen.

A2
1

● **FIGURE A21-2   The Hemodynamic Changes Associated with Pregnancy** Pregnancy causes the heart rate to be faster and the blood pressure to be lower. These findings can easily be interpreted as early signs of shock if unaware of the physiological changes of pregnancy.

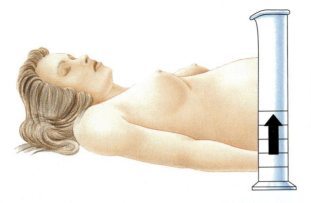

Blood volume usually increases by about 45%. Dilution resulting from the disproportionate increase of plasma volume over the red cell mass is responsible for the so-called "anemia of pregnancy."

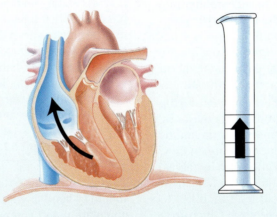

Cardiac output increases by 1.0 to 1.5 L/min during the 1st trimester, reaches 6 to 7 L/min by the late 2nd trimester, and is maintained essentially at this level until delivery.

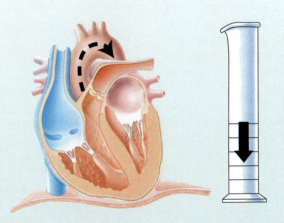

The stroke volume progressively declines to term following a rise early in pregnancy. Heart rate, however, increases by an average of 10 to 15 beats/min.

5,000 mL (Figure A21-1●). Another notable change is that during pregnancy the vascular system of the uterus contains about one-sixth (16 percent) of the mother's total blood volume. Other changes occurring in the re-productive system include the formation of a mucous plug in the cervix that protects the developing fetus and helps to prevent infection. This plug will be ex-pelled when cervical dilation begins prior to delivery. Estrogen causes the vaginal mucosa to thicken, vagi-nal secretions to increase, and the connective tissue to loosen to allow for delivery. The breasts enlarge and become more nodular as the mammary glands increase in number and size in preparation for lactation.

- *Respiratory System.* During pregnancy, maternal oxy-gen demands increase. To meet this need, progesterone causes a decrease in airway resistance. This results in a 20 percent increase in oxygen consumption and a 40 percent increase in tidal volume. There is only a slight increase in respiratory rate. The enlarging uterus pushes up the diaphragm resulting in flaring of the rib margins to maintain intrathoracic volume.
- *Cardiovascular System.* Many changes take place in the cardiovascular system during pregnancy (Figure A21-2●). Cardiac output increases throughout preg-nancy, peaking at 6–7 liters/minute by the time the fetus is fully developed. The maternal blood volume

A21

increases by 45 percent, and although both red blood cells and plasma increase, there is slightly more plasma, resulting in a relative anemia. To combat this anemia, pregnant women receive supplemental iron to increase the oxygen-carrying capacity of their red blood cells. Due to the increase in blood volume, the pregnant female may suffer an acute blood loss of 30–35 percent without a significant change in vital signs. The maternal heart rate increases by 10–15 beats/minute. Blood pressure decreases slightly during the first two trimesters of pregnancy and then rises to near nonpregnant levels during the third trimester.

- *Gastrointestinal System.* Nausea and vomiting are common in the first trimester of pregnancy as a result of varying hormone levels and changed carbohydrate needs. Peristalsis is slowed, so delayed gastric emptying is likely and bloating or constipation is common. As the uterus enlarges, abdominal organs are compressed, and the resulting compartmentalization of abdominal organs makes assessment difficult.

- *Urinary System.* Renal blood flow increases during pregnancy. The glomerular filtration rate increases by nearly 50 percent in the second trimester and remains elevated throughout the remainder of the pregnancy. As a result, the renal tubular absorption also increases. Occasionally glucosuria (large amounts of sugar in the urine) may result from the kidney's inability to reabsorb all of the glucose being filtered. Glucosuria may be normal or may indicate the development of gestational diabetes. The urinary bladder gets displaced anteriorly and superiorly, increasing the potential for rupture. Urinary frequency is common, particularly in the first and third trimesters, due to uterine compression of the bladder.

- *Musculoskeletal System.* Loosened pelvic joints caused by hormonal influences account for the waddling gait that is often associated with pregnancy. As the uterus enlarges and the mother's center of gravity shifts, posture changes to compensate for anterior growth, often causing low back pain.

Fetal Development

Fetal development begins immediately after fertilization and is quite complex. The time at which fertilization occurs is called *conception*. Since conception occurs approximately 14 days after the first day of the last menstrual period (LMP), it is possible to calculate, with fair accuracy, the approximate date the baby should be born. This estimate is usually made during the mother's first prenatal visit. The normal duration of pregnancy is 40 weeks from the first day of the mother's last menstrual period. This is equal to 280 days, which is 10 lunar months or roughly, 9 calendar months. This estimated birth date is commonly called the due date. Medically, it is known as the *estimated date of confinement (EDC)*.

Generally, pregnancy is divided into trimesters. Each trimester is approximately 13 weeks, or 3 calendar months, long.

Several different terms are used to describe the stages of fetal development during the course of pregnancy. The *preembryonic stage* covers the first 14 days following conception; the *embryonic stage* begins at day 15 and ends at approximately 8 weeks; and the *fetal stage* lasts from 8 weeks of age until delivery. Emergency personnel should be familiar with some of the significant developmental milestones that occur during these three periods (Table A21-1). During normal fetal development, the sex of the infant can usually be determined by 16 weeks gestation. By the 20th week, fetal heart tones (FHTs) can be detected by stethoscope. The mother also has generally felt fetal movement. By 24 weeks, the baby may be able to survive if born prematurely. Fetuses born after 28 weeks have an excellent chance of survival. By the 38th week the baby is considered term, or fully developed. Most of the fetus's organ systems develop during the first trimester. Therefore, this is when the fetus is most vulnerable to the development of birth defects.

Obstetrical Terminology

The field of obstetrics has its own unique terminology. You should be familiar with this terminology, since patient documentation and communications with other health care workers and physicians often require it (Figure A21-3●).

antepartum	time interval prior to delivery of the fetus
postpartum	time interval after delivery of the fetus
prenatal	time interval prior to birth, synonymous with antepartum
natal	relating to birth or the date of birth
gravidity*	number of times a woman has been pregnant
parity*	number of pregnancies carried to full term
primigravida	woman who is pregnant for the first time
primipara	woman who has given birth to her first child
multigravida	woman who has been pregnant more than once
nulligravida	woman who has not been pregnant
multipara	woman who has delivered more than one baby
nullipara	woman who has yet to deliver her first child
grand multiparity	woman who has delivered at least seven babies
gestation	period of time for intrauterine fetal development

*Gravidity and parity are expressed in the following shorthand: G_4P_2. G refers to gravidity, and P refers to parity. The woman in this example would have had four pregnancies and two births.

TABLE A21-1	Significant Fetal Development Milestone
Pre-embryonic Stage	
2 weeks	Rapid cellular multiplication and differentiation
Embryonic Stage	
4 weeks	Fetal heart begins to beat
8 weeks	All body systems and external structures are formed
	Size: approximately 3 centimeters (1.2 inches)
Fetal stage	
8–12 weeks	Fetal heart tones audible with Doppler
	Kidneys begin to produce urine
	Size: 8 centimeters (3.2 inches), weight about 1.6 ounces
	Fetus most vulnerable to toxins
16 weeks	Sex can be determined visually
	Swallowing amniotic fluid and producing meconium
	Looks like a baby, although thin
20 weeks	Fetal heart tones audible with stethoscope
	Mother able to feel fetal movement
	Baby develops schedule of sucking, kicking, and sleeping
	Hair, eyebrows, and eyelashes present
	Size: 19 centimeters (8 inches), weight approximately 16 ounces
24 weeks	Increased activity
	Begins respiratory movement
	Size: 28 centimeters (11.2 inches), weight 1 pound 10 ounces
28 weeks	Surfactant necessary for lung function is formed
	Eyes begin to open and close
	Weighs 2 to 3 pounds
32 weeks	Bones are fully developed but soft and flexible
	Subcutaneous fat being deposited
	Fingernails and toenails present
38–40 weeks	Considered to be full-term
	Baby fills uterine cavity
	Baby receives maternal antibodies

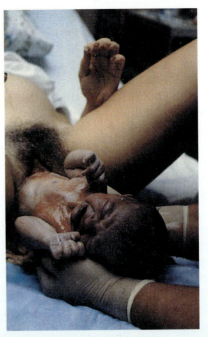

• FIGURE A21-3   Childbirth
The field of obstetrics has its own unique terminology. Emergency personnel should be familiar with this system, as they must interact with other members of the health care team.

ABORTION

Abortion, the expulsion of the fetus prior to 20 weeks gestation, is the most common cause of bleeding in the first and second trimesters of pregnancy. The terms *abortion* and *miscarriage* can be used interchangeably. Generally, the lay public thinks of *abortion* as termination of pregnancy at maternal request and of miscarriage as an accident of nature. Medically, the term abortion applies to both kinds of fetal loss. Spontaneous abortion, the naturally occurring termination of pregnancy that is often called *miscarriage,* is most commonly seen between the 12th and 14th weeks of gestation. It is estimated that 10 to 20 percent of all pregnancies end in spontaneous abortion. If the pregnancy has not yet been confirmed, the mother often assumes she is merely having a period with unusually heavy flow.

About half of all abortions are due to fetal chromosomal anomalies. Other causes include maternal reproductive system abnormalities, maternal use of drugs, placental defects, or maternal infections. Although many people believe that trauma and psychological stress can cause abortion, research does not support that belief.

Since you will be interacting with other health care professionals, you should be familiar with the variety of terms used to describe the classifications of abortion.

- *Complete Abortion.* Abortion in which all of the uterine contents including the fetus and placenta have been expelled.

- *Incomplete Abortion.* Abortion in which some, but not all, fetal tissue has been passed. Incomplete abortions are associated with a high incidence of infection.
- *Threatened Abortion.* Potential abortion characterized by unexplained vaginal bleeding during the first half of pregnancy in which the cervix is slightly open and the fetus remains in the uterus and is still alive. In some cases of threatened abortion, the fetus still can be saved.
- *Inevitable Abortion.* Potential abortion characterized by vaginal bleeding accompanied by severe abdominal cramping and cervical dilatation, in which the fetus has not yet passed from the uterus, but the fetus cannot be saved.
- *Spontaneous Abortion.* Naturally occurring expulsion of the fetus prior to viability, generally as a result of chromosomal abnormalities. Most spontaneous abortions occur before the twelfth week of pregnancy. Many occur within two weeks after conception and are mistaken for menstrual periods. Commonly called a miscarriage.
- *Elective Abortion.* Abortion in which the termination of pregnancy is desired and requested by the mother. Elective abortions during the first and second trimesters of pregnancy have been legal in the United States since 1973. Most elective abortions are performed during the first trimester. Some clinics perform second-trimester abortions. Second-trimester abortions have a higher complication rate than first-trimester abortions. Third-trimester elective abortions are generally illegal in this country.
- *Criminal Abortion.* Intentional termination of a pregnancy under any condition not allowed by law. It is usually the attempt to destroy a fetus by a person who is not licensed or permitted to do so. Criminal abortions are often attempted by amateurs and they are rarely performed in aseptic surroundings.
- *Therapeutic Abortion.* Termination of a pregnancy deemed necessary by a physician, usually to protect maternal health and well being.
- *Missed Abortion.* Abortion in which fetal death occurs but the fetus is not expelled. This poses a potential threat to the life of the mother if the fetus is retained beyond six weeks.
- *Habitual Abortion.* Spontaneous abortions that occur in three or more consecutive pregnancies.

The patient experiencing an abortion is likely to report crampy abdominal pain and a backache. She is also likely to report vaginal bleeding, which is often accompanied by the passage of clots and tissue. If the abortion was not recent, then frank signs and symptoms of infection may be present. Any tissue or large clots should be retained and given to emergency department personnel. If the abortion occurs during or after the late first trimester, a fetus may be passed.

ECTOPIC PREGNANCY

The fertilized egg normally is implanted in the endometrial lining of the uterine wall. The term *ectopic pregnancy* refers to the abnormal implantation of the fertilized egg outside of the uterus. Approximately 95 percent of ectopic pregnancies are implanted in the fallopian tube. Occasionally (less than 1 percent), the egg is implanted in the abdominal cavity. Current research indicates that the incidence of ectopic pregnancy is one for every 44 live births. Improved diagnostic technology is credited with an increased incidence, as most are detected between the 2nd and 12th weeks. Ectopic pregnancy accounts for approximately 10 percent of maternal mortality.

Predisposing factors in the development of ectopic pregnancy include scarring of the fallopian tubes due to pelvic inflammatory disease (PID), a previous ectopic pregnancy, or previous pelvic or tubal surgery, such as a tubal ligation. Other factors include endometriosis or use of an intrauterine device (IUD) for birth control.

Ectopic pregnancy most often presents as abdominal pain, which starts as diffuse tenderness and then localizes as a sharp pain in the lower abdominal quadrant on the affected side. This pain is due to rupture of the fallopian tube when the fetus outgrows the available space. The woman often reports that she missed a period or that her LMP occurred 4 to 6 weeks ago, but with decreased menstrual flow that was brownish in color and of shorter duration than usual. As the intra-abdominal bleeding continues, the abdomen becomes rigid and the pain intensifies and is often referred to the shoulder on the affected side. The pain is often accompanied by syncope, vaginal bleeding, and shock.

Assume that any female of childbearing age with lower abdominal pain is experiencing an ectopic pregnancy. Ectopic pregnancy poses a significant life threat to the mother. Surgery is required to resolve the situation.

POSTNATAL DEVELOPMENT

Developmental processes do not end at delivery. The newborn has few of the anatomical or physiological characteristics of mature adults. In postnatal development, the individual passes through several life stages. These include: *neonatal, infancy, childhood, adolescence,* and *maturity.* The neonatal period extends from birth to 1 month of age. Infancy is the period from 1 month of age to 2 years of age. Childhood lasts from two years of age until the onset of puberty.

Neonates typically lose up to 10 percent of their birth weight as they adjust to extrauterine life. However, this weight is usually recovered within 10 days. Infants should have doubled their birth weight by 5 or 6 months of age. Development occurs in a cephalo-caudal direction with muscle control beginning at the head and later spreading toward the lower extremities. The personality begins to develop in early infancy and definite behaviors and characteristics are present by 5 to 6 months of age (Figure A21-4●).

It is important for emergency personnel to be familiar with many of the anatomical and physiological differences of children as they can affect patient care. Table A21-2 illustrates important anatomical and physiological characteristics of infants and children.

SUMMARY

The development and birth of a child is usually a normal and happy event. However, problems can arise. It is important that emergency personnel be familiar with the normal effects of pregnancy on the mother. Also, several emergency problems related to pregnancy that may arise can be life threatening. Among the most common of these is ectopic pregnancy. It is essential to detect this problem early, as delay can be catastrophic. There are several developmental milestones, especially during infancy and early childhood. Knowledge of these can help determine the age of the child, but can also help identify children who are developmentally delayed.

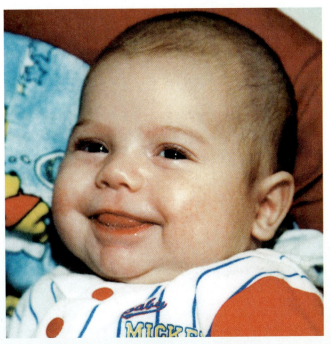

● FIGURE A21-4   Early Infancy
The period from 1 month to 2 years of age is a time of rapid development. The birth weight usually doubles, the infant exhibits improved muscle control, and the personality begins to develop.

TABLE A21-2	Anatomical and Physiological Characteristics of Infants and Children

Differences in Infants and Children as Compared to Adults	Potential Effects That May Impact Assessment and Care
Tongue proportionately larger	More likely to block airway
Smaller airway structures	More easily blocked
Abundant secretions	Can block the airway
Deciduous (baby) teeth	Easily dislodged; can block the airway
Flat nose and face	Difficult to obtain good face mask seal
Head heavier relative to body and less-developed neck structures and muscles	Head may be propelled more forcefully than body producing a higher incidence of head injury in trauma
Fontanelle and open sutures (soft spots) palpable on top of young infant's head	Bulging fontanelle can be a sign of increased intracranial pressure (but may be normal if infant is crying); shrunken fontanelle may indicate dehydration
Thinner, softer brain tissue	Susceptible to serious brain injury
Head larger in proportion to body	Tips forward when supine; possible flexion of neck, which makes neutral alignment of airway difficult
Shorter, narrower, more elastic (flexible) trachea	Can close off trachea with hyperextension of neck
Short neck	Difficult to stabilize or immobilize
Abdominal breathers	Difficult to evaluate breathing
Faster respiratory rate	Muscles easily fatigue, causing respiratory distress
Newborns breathe primarily through the nose (obligate nose breathers)	May not automatically open mouth to breathe if nose is blocked; airway more easily blocked
Larger body surface relative to body mass	Prone to hypothermia
Softer bones	More flexible, less easily fractured; traumatic forces may be transmitted to internal organs, causing injuring without fracturing the ribs; lungs easily damaged with trauma
Spleen and liver more exposed	Organ injury likely with significant force to abdomen

A21

Appendix *I*

Answers to Chapter Review Questions

CHAPTER 1

Level 1: Reviewing Facts and Terms

1. g 2. d 3. a 4. j 5. b 6. l 7. n 8. f 9. h 10. e
11. c 12. o 13. k 14. i 15. m 16. c 17. d 18. b 19. c
20. c 21. b

Level 2: Reviewing Concepts

22. responsiveness, adaptability, growth, reproduction, movement, metabolism, absorption, respiration, excretion
23. molecules–cell–tissues–organs–organ systems—organisms
24. Homeostatic regulation refers to adjustments in physiological systems that are responsible for the preservation of homeostasis.
25. In negative feedback, a variation outside normal ranges triggers an automatic response that corrects the situation. In positive feedback, the initial stimulus produces a response that exaggerates the stimulus.
26. The body is erect and the hands are at the sides with the palms facing forward.
27. Stomach. (You would cut the pericardium to access the heart.)
28. (a) dorsal cavity (b) ventral cavity (c) thoracic cavity (d) abdominopelvic cavity

Level 3: Critical Thinking and Clinical Applications

29. Since calcitonin is controlled by negative feedback, it should bring about a decrease in blood calcium level, thus decreasing the stimulus for its release.
30. To see a complete view of the medial surface of each half of the brain, midsagittal sections are needed.

CHAPTER 2

Level 1: Reviewing Facts and Terms

1. f 2. c 3. i 4. g 5. a 6. l 7. d 8. k 9. b 10. e
11. h 12. j 13. a 14. d 15. a
16. Enzymes are specialized protein catalysts that lower the activation energy of chemical reactions. Enzymes speed up chemical reactions but are not used up or changed in the process.
17. carbon, hydrogen, oxygen, nitrogen, calcium, phosphorus
18. carbohydrates, lipids, proteins, nucleic acids
19. support: structural proteins; movement: contractile proteins; transport: transport proteins; buffering; metabolic regulation; coordination and control; defense

Level 2: Reviewing Concepts

20. b   21. a   22. a
23. (1) covalent bond: equal sharing of electrons (2) polar covalent bond: unequal sharing of electrons (3) ionic bond: loss and/or gain of electrons
24. A solution such as pure water with a pH of 7 is neutral because it contains equal numbers of hydrogen and hydroxyl ions.
25. A nucleic acid. Carbohydrates and lipids do not contain the element nitrogen. Although both proteins and nucleic acids contain nitrogen, only nucleic acids contain phosphorus.

Level 3: Critical Thinking and Clinical Applications

26. The number of neutrons in an atom is equal to the atomic weight minus the atomic number. In the case of sulfur, this would be $32 - 16 = 16$ neutrons. Since the atomic number of sulfur is 16, the neutral sulfur atom contains 16 protons and 16 electrons. The electrons would be distributed as follows: 2 in the first level, 8 in the second level, and 6 in the third level. To achieve a full 8 electrons in the third level, the sulfur atom could accept 2 electrons in an ionic bond or share 2 electrons in a covalent bond. Since hydrogen atoms can share 1 electron in a covalent bond, the sulfur atom would form 2 covalent bonds, 1 with each of 2 hydrogen atoms.
27. If a person exhales large amounts of carbon dioxide, the equilibrium will shift to the left and the level of hydrogen ion in the blood will decrease. A decrease in the amount of hydrogen ion will cause the pH to rise.

CHAPTER 3

Level 1: Reviewing Facts and Terms

1. e 2. d 3. h 4. a 5. f 6. b 7. g 8. c 9. m 10. k
11. q 12. i 13. o 14. j 15. l 16. n 17. p 18. b 19. d
20. c 21. d 22. c 23. a 24. c
25. physical isolation; regulation of exchange with the environment; sensitivity; structural support
26. diffusion; filtration; carrier-mediated transport; vesicular transport
27. synthesis of proteins, carbohydrates, and lipids; storage of absorbed molecules; transport of materials
28. prophase; metaphase; anaphase; telophase

Level 2: Reviewing Concepts

29. b   30. b   31. c   32. c
33. similarities: both processes utilize carrier proteins; differences:

Facilitated diffusion	Active transport
passive	active
no ATP expended	ATP expended
concentration gradient	no concentration gradient

34. Cytosol has a high concentration of K^+; interstitial fluid has a high concentration of Na^+. Cytosol also contains a high concentration of suspended proteins, small quantities of carbohydrates, and large reserves of amino acids and lipids. Cytosol may also contain insoluble materials known as inclusions.
35. In transcription, RNA polymerase uses genetic information to assemble a strand of mRNA. In translation, ribosomes use information carried by the mRNA strand to assemble functional proteins.
36. Prophase: Chromatin condenses and chromosomes become visible; centrioles migrate to opposite poles of the cell and spindle fibers develop; nuclear membrane disintegrates. Metaphase: Chromatids attach to spindle fibers and line up along the metaphase plate. Anaphase: Chromatids separate and migrate toward opposite poles of the cell. Telophase: The nuclear membrane re-forms; chromosomes disappear as chromatin relaxes; nucleoli reappear.
37. Cytokinesis is the cytoplasmic movement that separates two daughter cells, thereby completing mitosis.

Level 3: Critical Thinking and Clinical Applications

38. Facilitated transport, which requires a carrier molecule but not cellular energy. The energy for the process is provided by the diffusion gradient for the substance being transported. When all of the carriers are actively involved in transport, the rate of transport plateaus and cannot be increased further.

39. Solution A must have initially had more solutes than solution B. As a result, water moved by osmosis across the semipermeable membrane from side B to side A, increasing the fluid level on side A.

CHAPTER 4

Level 1: Reviewing Facts and Terms

1. g   2. d   3. j   4. i   5. a   6. f   7. c   8. e   9. b   10. h
11. l   12. k   13. a   14. c   15. c   16. d   17. d   18. c   19. a
20. b   21. b   22. a
23. provide physical protection; control permeability; provide sensations; produce specialized secretions
24. simple, stratified, transitional
25. specialized cells, extracellular protein fibers, fluid ground substance
26. fluid connective tissues: blood and lymph; supporting connective tissues: bone and cartilage
27. mucous, serous, cutaneous, synovial
28. Neurons and neuroglia. The neurons transmit electrical impulses. The neuroglia comprise several kinds of supporting cells and play a role in providing nutrients to neurons.

Level 2: Reviewing Concepts

29. a
30. Holocrine secretion destroys the gland cell. During holocrine secretion, the entire cell becomes packed with secretory products and then bursts, releasing the secretion but killing the cell. The gland cells must be replaced by the division of stem cells.
31. Exocrine secretions are secreted onto a surface or outward through a duct. Endocrine secretions are secreted by ductless glands into surrounding tissues. The secretions are called hormones, which usually diffuse into the blood for distribution to other parts of the body.
32. Tight junctions block the passage of water or solutes between cells. In the digestive tract, these junctions keep enzymes, acids and wastes from damaging delicate underlying tissues.
33. The extensive connections between cells formed by tight junctions, intercellular cement, and physical interlocking hold skin cells together and can deny access to chemicals or pathogens that may cover their free surfaces. If the skin is damaged and the connections are broken, infection can easily occur.
34. Cutaneous membranes are thick, relatively waterproof, and usually dry.

Level 3: Critical Thinking and Clinical Applications

35. Since animal intestines are modified for absorption, you would look for a slide that shows a single layer of epithelium lining the cavity. The cells would be cuboidal or columnar and would probably have microvilli on the surface to increase surface area. With the right type of microscope, you could also see tight junctions between the cells. Since the esophagus receives undigested food, it would have a stratified epithelium consisting of squamous cells to protect it against damage.
36. Step 1: Check for striations. (If striations are present, the choices are skeletal muscle or cardiac muscle. If striations are absent, the tissue is smooth muscle.) Step 2: Check for the presence of intercalated discs. (If the discs are present, the tissue is cardiac muscle. If they are absent, the tissue is skeletal muscle.)

CHAPTER 5

Level 1: Reviewing Facts and Terms

1. f   2. g   3. i   4. j   5. a   6. e   7. b   8. d   9. c   10. h
11. a   12. d   13. b   14. c   15. a   16. a
17. carotene and melanin
18. Papillary layer: consists of loose connective tissue and contains capillaries and sensory neurons; reticular layer: consists of dense irregular connective tissue and bundles of collagen fibers. The reticular and papillary layers of the dermis contain blood vessels, lymphatic vessels, and nerve fibers.
19. apocrine sweat glands and merocrine sweat glands

Level 2: Reviewing Concepts

20. Substances that are lipid soluble pass through the permeability barrier easily, because the barrier is composed primarily of lipids surrounding the epidermal cells. Water-soluble drugs are hydrophobic to the permeability barrier.
21. A tan is a result of the synthesis of melanin in the skin. Melanin helps prevent skin damage by absorbing ultraviolet radiation before it reaches the deep layers of the epidermis and dermis. In the epidermal cells, melanin concentrates around the outer membrane of the nucleus, so it absorbs the UV light before it can damage the nuclear DNA.
22. The subcutaneous layer is not highly vascular and does not contain major organs; thus this method reduces the potential for tissue damage.
23. The dermis becomes thinner and the elastic fiber network decreases in size, weakening the integument and causing loss of resilience.

Level 3: Critical Thinking and Clinical Applications

24. The child probably has a fondness for vegetables high in carotene, such as sweet potatoes, squash, and carrots. It is not uncommon for parents to feed a baby foods that he or she prefers to eat. If the child consumes large amounts of carotene, the yellow-orange pigment will be stored in the skin, producing a yellow-orange skin color.
25. Like most elderly people, Vanessa's grandmother has poor circulation to the skin. As a result, the temperature receptors in the skin do not sense as much warmth as when there is a rich blood supply. The sensory information is relayed to the brain. The brain interprets this as being cool or cold, thus causing Vanessa's grandmother to feel cold.

CHAPTER 6

Level 1: Reviewing Facts and Terms

1. i   2. h   3. m   4. l   5. j   6. k   7. f   8. c   9. o   10. b
11. g   12. n   13. d   14. a   15. e   16. b   17. a   18. c   19. b
20. d   21. a   22. a   23. a   24. a   25. b   26. c   27. d   28. b
29. c
30. support, storage of minerals and lipids, blood cell production, protection, leverage
31. In intramembranous ossification, bone develops from fibrous connective tissue. In endochondral ossification, bone develops from a cartilage model.
32. The hyoid is the only bone in the body that does not articulate with another bone.
33. (1) It protects the heart, lungs, thymus, and other structures in the thoracic cavity. (2) It serves as an attachment point for muscles involved with respiration, the position of the vertebral column, and movements of the pectoral girdle and upper extremities.
34. the acromion and coracoid processes

Level 2: Reviewing Concepts

35. The osteons are parallel to the long axis of the shaft, which does not bend when forces are applied to either end. An impact to the side of the shaft can lead to a fracture.

A I

36. The chondrocytes of the epiphyseal plate enlarge and divide, increasing the thickness of the plate. On the shaft side, the chondrocytes become ossified, "chasing" the expanding epiphyseal plate away from the shaft.

37. The lumbar vertebrae have massive bodies and carry a large amount of weight—both causative factors related to rupturing a disc. The cervical vertebrae are more delicate and have small bodies, increasing the possibility of dislocations and fractures in this region, compared with other regions of the vertebral column.

38. The clavicles are small and fragile, so fractures are quite common. Their position also makes them vulnerable to injury and damage.

39. The pelvic girdle consists of the coxae. The pelvis is a composite structure that includes the coxae of the appendicular skeleton and the sacrum and coccyx of the axial skeleton.

40. Articular cartilages do not have perichondrium, and their matrix contains more water than do other cartilages.

41. The slight movability of the pubic symphysis joint facilitates childbirth, by spreading the pelvis to ease movement of the baby through the birth canal.

Level 3: Critical Thinking and Clinical Applications

42. The fracture might have damaged the epiphyseal plate. Even though the bone healed properly, the damaged plate did not produce as much cartilage as the undamaged plate in the other leg. The result would be a shorter bone on the side of the injury.

43. The virus could have been inhaled through the nose and passed by way of the cribriform plate of the ethmoid bone into the cranium.

44. The large bones of a child's cranium are not yet fused; they are connected by areas of connective tissue called fontanels. By examining the bones, the archaeologist could readily see if sutures had formed yet. By knowing approximately how long it takes for the various fontanels to close and by determining the sizes of the fontanels, she could make a good estimation of the child's age.

45. Frank may have suffered a shoulder dislocation, which is quite a common injury due to the weak nature of the scapulohumeral joint.

46. Ed has a sprained ankle. This condition occurs when ligaments are stretched to the point at which some of the collagen fibers are torn. Stretched ligaments in joints can cause the release of synovial fluid, which results in swelling and pain in the affected area.

CHAPTER 7

Level 1: Reviewing Facts and Terms

1. f 2. i 3. d 4. p 5. l 6. c 7. h 8. n 9. b 10. k
11. o 12. a 13. m 14. j 15. g 16. e 17. d 18. d

19. produce skeletal movement, maintain body posture and body position, support soft tissue, guard entrances and exits, maintain body temperature

20. Step 1: active site exposure. Step 2: cross-bridge attachment. Step 3: pivoting of myosin head (power stroke). Step 4: cross-bridge attachment. Step 5: myosin head activation (cocking)

21. ATP, creatine phosphate, glycogen

22. aerobic metabolism and glycolysis

23. The axial musculature positions the head and spinal column and moves the rib cage, assisting in the movements that make breathing possible. The appendicular musculature stabilizes or moves components of the appendicular skeleton.

Level 2: Reviewing Concepts

24. b

25. Acetylcholine released by the motor neuron at the neuromuscular junction changes the permeability of the cell membrane at the motor end plate. The permeability change allows the influx of positive charges, which in turn triggers an electrical event called an action potential. The action potential spreads across the entire surface of the muscle fiber and into the interior via the T tubules. The cyto-

plasmic concentration of calcium ions (released from sarcoplasmic reticulum) increases, triggering the start of a contraction. The contraction ends when the ACh has been removed from the synaptic cleft and motor end plate by AChE.

26. Metabolic turnover is rapid in skeletal muscle cells. The genes contained in multiple nuclei direct the production of enzymes and structural proteins required for normal contraction, and the presence of multiple gene copies speeds up the process.

27. The spinal column does not need a massive series of flexors because many of the large trunk muscles flex the spine when they contract. In addition, most of the body weight lies anterior to the spinal column and gravity tends to flex the spine.

28. The urethral and anal sphincter muscles are usually in a constricted state, preventing the passage of urine and feces. The muscles are innervated by nerves that are under conscious control, so the sphincters normally relax to allow the passage of wastes only when the individual decides so.

29. flexion of the leg and extension of the hip

Level 3: Critical Thinking and Clinical Applications

30. Since organophosphates block the action of the enzyme acetylcholinesterase, acetylcholine released into the neuromuscular cleft would not be inactivated. This would allow the acetylcholine to continue to stimulate the muscles, causing a state of persistent contraction (spastic paralysis). If this were to affect the muscles of respiration (which is likely), Terry would die of suffocation. Prior to death, the most obvious symptoms would be uncontrolled tetanic contractions of the skeletal muscles.

31. In rigor mortis, the muscles lock in the contracted position, making the body extremely stiff. The membranes of the dead muscle cells are no longer selectively permeable and calcium leaks in, triggering contraction. Contraction persists because the dead cells can no longer make ATP, which is necessary for cross-bridge detachment from the active sites. Rigor mortis begins a few hours after death and lasts until 15 to 25 hours later, when the lysosomal enzymes released by autolysis break down the myofilaments.

32. Jeff should do squatting exercises. If he places a weight on his shoulders as he does these, he will notice better results, since the quadriceps muscles would work against a greater resistance.

CHAPTER 8

Level 1: Reviewing Facts and Terms

1. f 2. g 3. p 4. k 5. m 6. a 7. b 8. j 9. h 10. c
11. d 12. o 13. e 14. q 15. l 16. i 17. n 18. c 19. a
20. a 21. b 22. d 23. b 24. b 25. a 26. b

27. (1) The conduction of one or more action potentials along an axon and (2) the chemical transmission of signals across one or more synapses.

28. The properties of the action potential are independent of the relative strength of the depolarization stimulus.

29. generating conscious thought processes, providing sensations, intellectual functions, memory storage and retrieval, and forming complex motor patterns

Level 2: Reviewing Concepts

30. d   31. c

32. Collaterals enable a single neuron to innervate several other cells—a process called divergence.

33. Since the ventral roots contain axons of motor neurons, those muscles controlled by the neurons of the damaged root would be paralyzed.

34. the feeding and thirst centers of the hypothalamus

35. centers in the medulla oblongata

36. Action potentials travel faster in myelinated fibers. Destruction of the myelin sheath slows the time it takes for motor neurons to communicate with their effector muscles. This delay can result in vary-

ing degrees of uncoordinated muscle activity and paralysis. Cumulative sensory and motor losses may eventually lead to generalized sensory deficiencies and muscular paralysis.

Level 3: Critical Thinking and Clinical Applications

37. Brain tumors result from uncontrolled division of neuroglial cells. Unlike neurons, neuroglial cells are capable of cell division. In addition, cells of the meningeal membranes can give rise to tumors.

38. A major reason that newborn infants cannot roll over, sit, or walk is that a large number of peripheral neurons are not yet myelinated. Without myelination, information concerning limb movement and body position moves slowly to the brain, and motor responses move slowly to the muscles. In other words, by the time the brain is aware of limb movement or position and issues a motor command, the limb has already changed its movement or position. When the motor response reaches the skeletal muscle, the response is no longer appropriate. As the peripheral neurons gradually become myelinated, information flow and processing speed up, and we see improved balance, coordination, and capabilities.

39. The officer is testing the function of Bill's cerebellum. Many drugs, including alcohol, have pronounced effects on the function of the cerebellum. A person who is under the influence of alcohol is not able to anticipate properly the range and speed of limb movement because of slow processing and correction by the cerebellum. As a result, Bill would have a difficult time performing simple tasks such as walking a straight line or touching his finger to his nose.

CHAPTER 9

Level 1: Reviewing Facts and Terms

1. i   2. c   3. g   4. f   5. a   6. j   7. h   8. b   9. d   10. l
11. k   12. e   13. m   14. a   15. d   16. c   17. a   18. c
19. a

20. N I: olfactory; N II: optic; N III: oculomotor; N IV: trochlear; N V: trigeminal; N VI: abducens; N VII: facial; N VIII: vestibulocochlear; N IX: glossopharyngeal; N X: vagus; N XI: accessory; N XII: hypoglossal

21. Pyramidal cells are neurons of the primary motor cortex that direct voluntary movements by controlling somatic motor neurons in the brain stem and the spinal cord.

22. The sympathetic preganglionic fibers emerge from the thoracolumbar area (T_1 through L_2) of the spinal cord. The parasympathetic fibers emerge from the brain stem and the sacral region of the spinal cord (craniosacral).

Level 2: Reviewing Concepts

23. a

24. Transmission across a chemical synapse always involves a synaptic delay, but with only one synapse (monosynaptic), the delay between stimulus and response is minimized. In a polysynaptic reflex, the length of delay is proportional to the number of synapses involved.

25.

	Sympathetic	Parasympathetic
mental alertness	increased	decreased
metabolic rate	increased	decreased
digestive/ urinary function	inhibited	stimulated
use of energy reserves	stimulated	inhibited
respiratory rate	increased	decreased
heart rate/ blood pressure	increased	decreased
sweat glands	stimulated	inhibited

26. Preganglionic fibers entering the adrenal gland proceed to the adrenal medulla, where they synapse on neuroendocrine cells that release the neurotransmitters norepinephrine (NE) and epinephrine (E) into the general circulation.

27. Due to stimulation of sympathetic nervous activity, you would experience an increased respiratory rate, speeding up gas exchange; an increase in the vasoconstriction of peripheral blood vessels, causing an increase in blood pressure; an increase in heart rate and force of contraction, causing an increased rate of blood delivery; and an increase in the release of glucose into the blood, increasing the nutrient supply for energy metabolism.

Level 3: Critical Thinking and Clinical Applications

28. Stress-induced stomach ulcers are due to excessive sympathetic stimulation. The sympathetic division causes the vasoconstriction of vessels supplying the digestive organs, leading to an almost total shutdown of blood supply to the stomach. Lack of blood leads to tissue death and necrosis, which causes the ulcers.

29. the radial nerve

30. A damaged femoral nerve. Since this nerve also supplies the sensory innervation of the skin on the anteromedial surface of the thigh and medial surfaces of the leg and foot, Ramon may also experience numbness in these regions.

CHAPTER 10

Level 1: Reviewing Facts and Terms

1. k   2. c   3. a   4. e   5. f   6. j   7. i   8. b   9. h   10. m
11. g   12. l   13. n   14. d   15. b   16. d   17. b   18. d   19. b
20. b   21. d   22. a   23. c   24. b   25. b   26. a   27. d

28. tactile receptors, baroreceptors, and proprioceptors

29. free nerve endings: sensitive to touch and pressure; root hair plexuses: monitor distortions and movements across the body surface; Merkel's discs: fine touch and pressure receptors; Meissner's corpuscles: fine touch and pressure sensation; Pacinian corpuscles: most sensitive to pulsing or vibrating stimuli (deep pressure); Ruffini corpuscles: -sensitive to pressure and distortion of the skin

30. (a) the sclera and the cornea (b) provides mechanical support and some degree of physical protection; serves as an attachment site for the extrinsic muscles; contains structures that assist in focusing

31. iris, ciliary body, and choroid

32. Step 1: Sound waves arrive at the tympanum. Step 2: Movement of the tympanum causes displacement of the auditory ossicles. Step 3: Movement of the stapes at the oval window establishes pressure waves in the perilymph of the vestibular duct. Step 4: The pressure waves distort the basilar membrane on their way to the round window of the tympanic duct. Step 5: Vibration of the basilar membrane causes hair cells to vibrate against the tectorial membrane. Step 6: Information concerning the region and intensity of stimulation is relayed to the CNS over the cochlear branch of N VIII.

Level 2: Reviewing Concepts

33. c   34. c

35. The general senses include somatic and visceral sensation. The special senses are those whose receptors are confined to the head.

36. Regardless of the type of stimulus, the CNS receives the sensory information in the form of action potentials.

37. The olfactory system has extensive limbic-system connections, accounting for its effect on memories and emotions.

38. A visual acuity of 20/15 means that Jane can discriminate images at a distance of 20 feet, whereas someone with "normal" vision must be 5 feet closer (15 ft.) to see the same details. Jane's visual acuity is better than the acuity of someone with 20/20 vision.

Level 3: Critical Thinking and Clinical Applications

39. As you turn to look at your friend, your medial rectus muscles will contract, directing your gaze more medially. In addition, your pupils will constrict and the lenses will become more spherical.

40. The loud noises from the fireworks have transferred so much energy to the endolymph in the cochlea that the fluid continues to move for a long period of time. As long as the endolymph is moving, it will vibrate the tectorial membrane and stimulate the hair cells. This stimulation produces the "ringing" sensation that Millie perceives. She

A I

finds it difficult to hear normal conversation because the vibrations associated with it are not strong enough to overcome the currents already moving through the endolymph, so the pattern of vibrations is difficult to discern against the background "noise."

41. The rapid descent in the elevator causes the maculae in the saccule of the vestibule to slide upward, producing the sensation of downward vertical motion. When the elevator abruptly stops, the maculae do not. Because of their relatively large inertia, it takes a few seconds for them to come to rest in the normal position. As long as the maculae are displaced, the perception of movement will remain.

CHAPTER 11

Level 1: Reviewing Facts and Terms

1. h 2. e 3. g 4. l 5. b 6. k 7. c 8. a 9. j 10. i 11. f 12. d 13. d 14. a 15. c 16. d 17. b 18. d 19. c 20. b

21. thyroid-stimulating hormone (TSH), adrenocorticotropic hormone (ACTH), follicle-stimulating hormone (FSH), luteinizing hormone (LH), prolactin (PRL), growth hormone (GH), melanocyte-stimulating hormone (MSH)

22. The overall effect of calcitonin is to decrease the concentration of calcium ions in body fluids. The overall effect of parathyroid hormone is to cause an increase in the concentration of calcium ions in body fluids.

23. (a) The GAS includes alarm, resistance, and exhaustion phases. (b) Epinephrine is the dominant hormone of the alarm phase. Glucocorticoids are the dominant hormones of the resistance phase.

Level 2: Reviewing Concepts

24. In communication by the nervous system, the source and destination are quite specific and the effects are short-lived. In endocrine communication, the effects are slow to appear and often persist for days. A single hormone can alter the metabolic activities of multiple tissues and organs simultaneously.

25. Hormones direct the synthesis of an enzyme (or other protein) that is not already present in the cytoplasm. They also turn an existing enzyme "on" or "off" and increase the rate of synthesis of a particular enzyme or other protein.

26. The two hormones may have opposing, or antagonistic, effects; the hormones may have additive or synergistic effects; one hormone may have a permissive effect on another (the first hormone is needed for the second to produce its effect); the hormones may produce different but complementary effects in specific tissues and organs.

27. Phosphodiesterase is the enzyme that converts cAMP to AMP, thus inactivating it. If this enzyme were blocked, the effect of the hormone would be prolonged.

Level 3: Critical Thinking and Clinical Applications

28. Extreme thirst and frequent urination are characteristics of both diabetes insipidus and diabetes mellitus. To distinguish between the two, glucose levels in the blood and urine could be measured. A high glucose concentration would indicate diabetes mellitus.

29. Julie should exhibit elevated levels of parathyroid hormone in her blood. Her poor diet does not supply enough calcium for her developing fetus. The fetus removes large amounts of calcium from the maternal blood, lowering the mother's blood calcium levels. This would lead to an increase in the blood level of parathyroid hormone and increased mobilization of stored calcium from the maternal skeletal reserves.

CHAPTER 12

Level 1: Reviewing Facts and Terms

1. f 2. k 3. a 4. l 5. c 6. j 7. e 8. h 9. g 10. b 11. d 12. i 13. c 14. c 15. a 16. c 17. d 18. a 19. d 20. d 21. b

22. transportation of dissolved gases, nutrients, hormones, and metabolic wastes; regulation of pH and electrolyte composition of interstitial fluids throughout the body; restriction of fluid losses through damaged vessels or at other injury sites; defense against toxins and pathogens; stabilization of body temperature

23. Albumins maintain osmotic pressure of plasma and important in transport of fatty acids. Transport globulins bind small ions, hormones or compounds that might otherwise be filtered out of the blood at the kidneys or have very low solubility in water, and immunoglobulins attack foreign proteins and pathogens. Fibrinogen functions in blood clotting.

24. (a) anti-B agglutinins (b) anti-A agglutinins (c) neither anti-A nor anti-B agglutinins (d) anti-A and anti-B agglutinins

25. amoeboid movement: extension of a cellular process; diapedesis: squeezing between adjacent endothelial cells in the capillary wall; positive chemotaxis: attraction to specific chemical stimuli

26. The common pathway begins when thromboplastin from either the extrinsic or intrinsic pathway appears in the plasma.

27. An embolus is a drifting blood clot. A thrombus is a blood clot that sticks to the wall of an intact blood vessel.

Level 2: Reviewing Concepts

28. a   29. d   30. c   31. d

32. Red blood cells are biconcave discs that lack mitochondria, ribosomes, and nuclei and contain a large amount of the protein hemoglobin.

Level 3: Critical Thinking and Clinical Applications

33. After donating a pint of blood (or after any other loss of blood), you would expect to see a substantial increase in the number of reticulocytes. Since there is not enough time for large numbers of erythrocytes to mature, the bone marrow releases large numbers of reticulocytes (immature cells) in an effort to maintain a constant number of formed elements.

34. In many cases of kidney disease, the cells responsible for producing erythropoietin are either damaged or destroyed. The reduction in erythropoietin levels leads to reduced erythropoiesis and fewer red blood cells, resulting in anemia.

CHAPTER 13

Level 1: Reviewing Facts and Terms

1. i 2. e 3. g 4. h 5. a 6. b 7. k 8. l 9. d 10. f 11. c 12. j 13. c 14. b 15. b 16. a 17. a 18. b 19. a

20. During ventricular contraction, tension in the papillary muscles and chordae tendineae braces the atrioventricular valve cusps and keeps them from swinging into the atrium. This action prevents the backflow, or regurgitation, of blood into the atrium as the ventricle contracts.

21. The atrioventricular (AV) valves prevent backflow of blood from the ventricles into the atria. The right AV valve is the tricuspid valve, and the left AV valve is the bicuspid (mitral) valve. The pulmonary and aortic semilunar valves prevent the backflow of blood from the pulmonary trunk and aorta into the right and left ventricles.

22. SA node → AV node → AV bundle (bundle of His) → R and L bundle branches → Purkinje fibers (into the mass of ventricular muscle tissue)

23. (a) A single cardiac cycle is the period between the beginning of one heartbeat and the beginning of the next heartbeat. (b) [1] the relaxation of ventricles (diastole); the contraction of the atria (systole) draws blood from the atria into the ventricles; and [2] the contraction of the ventricles (systole) forces blood through semilunar valves into major blood vessels; the relaxation of atria (diastole), the collection of incoming blood.

Level 2: Reviewing Concepts

24. c   25. d   26. a

27. The right atrium receives blood from the systemic circuit and passes it to the right ventricle. The right ventricle discharges blood

into the pulmonary circuit. The left atrium collects blood. Contraction of the left ventricle ejects blood into the systemic circuit.

28. Listening to the heart sounds (auscultation) is a simple, effective method of cardiac diagnosis. The first and second heart sounds accompany the action of the heart valves. The first sound ("lubb") marks the start of ventricular contraction and is produced as the AV valves close and the semilunar valves open. The second sound ("dupp") occurs at the beginning of ventricular filling when the semilunar valves close.

29. (a) Sympathetic activation causes the release of norepinephrine by postganglionic fibers and the secretion of norepinephrine and epinephrine by the adrenal medullae. These compounds stimulate cardiac muscle fiber metabolism and increase the force and degree of contraction. (b) Parasympathetic stimulation causes the release of ACh at membrane surfaces, where it produces hyperpolarization and inhibition. The result is a decrease in the heart rate and in the force of cardiac contractions.

Level 3: Critical Thinking and Clinical Applications

30. This patient has second-degree heart block, a condition in which not every signal from the SA node reaches the ventricular muscle. In this case, for every two action potentials generated by the SA node, only one is reaching the ventricles. This accounts for the two P waves but only one QRS complex. This condition frequently results from damage to the internodal pathways of the atria or problems with AV node.

31. Blocking the calcium channels in myocardial cells would lead to a decrease in the force of cardiac contraction. Since the force of cardiac contraction is directly proportional to the stroke volume, you would expect a reduced stroke volume.

CHAPTER 14

Level 1: Reviewing Facts and Terms

1. d   2. l   3. a   4. j   5. i   6. h   7. k   8. f   9. e   10. c
11. g   12. b   13. d   14. b   15. b   16. a   17. d   18. b   19. c
20. b   21. c   22. b   23. d   24. c   25. b   26. c   27. c

28. (a) Fluid leaves the capillary at the arterial end primarily in response to hydrostatic pressure. (b) Fluid returns to the capillary at the venous end primarily in response to osmotic pressure.

29. The cardiac output decreases due to parasympathetic stimulation and inhibition of sympathetic activity, and peripheral vasodilation is widespread due to the inhibition of excitatory neurons in the vasomotor center.

30. changes in the carbon dioxide, oxygen, or pH levels in the blood and cerebrospinal fluid

31. When an infant takes its first breath, the lungs expand, and so do the pulmonary vessels. The smooth muscles in the ductus arteriosus contract, isolating the pulmonary and aortic trunks, and blood begins flowing through the pulmonary circuit. As pressure rises in the left atrium, the valvular flap closes the foramen ovale, completing the circulatory remodeling.

32. blood: decreased hematocrit, formation of thrombin, and valvular malfunction; heart: reduction in maximum cardiac output and changes in the activities of the nodal and conducting fibers, reduction in the elasticity of the fibrous skeleton, progressive atherosclerosis, and replacement of damaged cardiac muscle fibers by scar tissue; blood vessels: progressive inelasticity in arterial walls, deposition of calcium salts on weakened vascular walls, and formation of thrombi at atherosclerotic plaques

Level 2: Reviewing Concepts

33. d   34. c   35. b

36. Artery walls are generally thicker. They contain more smooth muscle and elastic fibers, enabling them to resist and adjust to the pressure generated by the heart. Venous walls are thinner and the pressure in the veins is less than that in the arteries. Arteries constrict more than veins do when not expanded by blood pressure, due to a greater degree of elastic tissue. In addition, the endothelial lining of an artery has a pleated appearance because it forms folds, being unable to contract. The lining of a vein looks like a typical endothelial layer.

37. Capillaries are only one cell thick. Small gaps between adjacent endothelial cells permit the diffusion of water and small solutes into the surrounding interstitial fluid but prevent the loss of blood cells and plasma proteins. Some capillaries also contain pores that permit very rapid exchange of fluids and solutes between the interstitial fluid and the plasma. Conversely, the walls of arteries and veins are several cell layers thick and are not specialized for diffusion.

38. The brain receives arterial blood via four arteries. Because these arteries form anastomoses inside the cranium, interruption of any one vessel will not compromise the circulatory supply to the brain.

39. The accident victim is suffering from shock and acute circulatory crisis characterized by hypotension and inadequate peripheral blood flow. The hypotension results from the loss of blood volume and decreased cardiac output. Her skin is pale and cool due to peripheral vasoconstriction; the moisture results from the sympathetic activation of sweat glands. Falling blood pressure to the brain causes confusion and disorientation. If you took her pulse, you would find it to be rapid and weak, reflecting the heart's response to reduced blood flow and volume.

Level 3: Critical Thinking and Clinical Applications

40. Three factors contribute to Bob's elevated blood pressure. (1) The loss of water through sweating increases blood viscosity. The number of red blood cells remains about the same, but because there is less plasma volume, the concentration of red cells is increased, thus increasing the blood viscosity. Increased viscosity increases peripheral resistance and contributes to increased blood pressure. (2) To cool Bob's body, blood flow to the skin is increased. This in turn increases venous return which increases stroke volume and cardiac output (Frank-Starling's law of the heart). The increased cardiac output can also contribute to increased blood pressure. (3) The heat stress that Bob is experiencing leads to increased sympathetic stimulation (the reason for the sweating). Increased sympathetic stimulation of the heart will increased heart rate and stroke volume, thus increasing his cardiac output and blood pressure.

41. Antihistamines and decongestants are drugs that have the same effects on the body as stimulating the sympathetic nervous system. In addition to the desired effects of counteracting the symptoms of the allergy, these medications can produce an increased heart rate, stroke volume, and peripheral resistance, all of which will contribute to elevating blood pressure. If a person has hypertension (high blood pressure), these drugs will aggravate this condition, with potentially hazardous consequences.

42. When Gina rapidly moved from a lying position to a standing position, gravity caused her blood volume to move to the lower parts of her body away from the heart, decreasing venous return. The decreased venous return resulted in a decreased volume of blood at the end of diastole, which lead to a decreased stroke volume and cardiac output. These resulted in decreased blood flow to the brain, where the diminished oxygen supply caused her to be light-headed and feel faint. This usually does not occur, because as soon as the pressure drops due to blood moving inferiorly, the baroreceptor reflex should be triggered. Normally, a rapid change in blood pressure is sensed by baroreceptors in the aortic arch and carotid sinus. Action potentials from these areas are carried to the medulla oblongata, where appropriate responses are integrated. In this case, we would expect an increase in peripheral resistance to compensate for the decreased blood pressure. If this doesn't compensate enough for the drop, then an increase in heart rate and force of contraction would occur. In healthy individuals, these responses occur so quickly that no changes in pressure are noticed after body position is changed.

A I

CHAPTER 15

Level 1: Reviewing Facts and Terms

1. h 2. k 3. b 4. g 5. d 6. c 7. j 8. a 9. i 10. l
11. f 12. e 13. c 14. d 15. c 16. c 17. b 18. a 19. c
20. a 21. a 22. d 23. d 24. c

25. Left thoracic duct: collects lymph from the body below the diaphragm and from the left side of the body above the diaphragm; right thoracic duct: collects lymph from the right side of the body above the diaphragm.

26. (a) responsible for cell-mediated immunity, which defends against abnormal cells and pathogens inside living cells (b) stimulate the activation and function of T cells and B cells (c) inhibit the activation and function of both T cells and B cells (d) produce and secrete antibodies (e) recognize and destroy abnormal cells (f) interfere with viral replication inside the cell and stimulate the activities of macrophages and NK cells (g) provide cell-mediated immunity (h) provide antibody-mediated immunity, which defends against antigens and pathogenic organisms in the body (i) enhance nonspecific defenses and increase T cell sensitivity and stimulate B cell activity

27. physical barriers, phagocytic cells, immunological surveillance, interferon, complement, inflammation, and fever

Level 2: Reviewing Concepts

28. c   29. d

30. Specificity: The immune response is triggered by a specific antigen, and defends against only that antigen. Versatility: The immune system can differentiate from among tens of thousands of antigens it may encounter during a normal lifetime. Memory: The immune response following second exposure to a particular antigen is stronger and lasts longer. Tolerance: Some antigens, such as those on an individual's own cells, do not elicit an immune response.

31. The antigen may be destroyed by neutralization, agglutination and precipitation, activation of complement, attraction of phagocytes, stimulation of inflammation, or prevention of bacterial and viral adhesion.

32. destruction of target cell membranes, stimulation of inflammation, attraction of phagocytes, and enhancement of phagocytosis

Level 3: Critical Thinking and Clinical Applications

33. IgA immunoglobulins are found in body secretions such as tears, saliva, semen, and vaginal secretions but not in blood plasma. Blood plasma contains IgM, IgG, IgD, and IgE of immunoglobulins. By testing for the presence or absence of IgA and IgG antibodies, the lab could determine whether the sample was blood plasma or semen.

34. It appears that Ted has contracted the disease. On initial contact with a virus, the first type of antibody to be produced is IgM. The response is fairly rapid but short-lived. About the time IgM peaks, IgG levels are beginning to rise. IgG plays the more important role in eventually controlling the disease. The fact that Ted's blood sample has an elevated level of IgM antibodies would indicate that he is in the early stages of a primary response to the measles virus.

CHAPTER 16

Level 1: Reviewing Facts and Terms

1. h 2. f 3. i 4. c 5. b 6. d 7. j 8. e 9. a 10. l
11. g 12. k 13. c 14. b

Level 2: Reviewing Concepts

15. a   16. d

17. With less cartilaginous support in the lower respiratory passageways, the amount of tension in the smooth muscles has a greater effect on bronchial diameter and on the resistance to air flow.

18. The nasal cavity is designed to cleanse, moisten, and warm inspired air, whereas the mouth is not. Air entering through the mouth is drier and as a result can irritate the trachea, causing soreness of the throat.

19. The walls of bronchioles, like the walls of arterioles, are dominated by smooth muscle tissue. Varying the diameter (bronchodilation or bronchoconstriction) of the bronchioles provides control over the amount of resistance to air flow and over the distribution of air in the lungs, just as vasodilation and vasoconstriction of the arterioles regulate blood flow/distribution.

20. The surfactant cells produce surfactant, which reduces surface tension in the fluid coating the alveolar surface. The alveolar walls are very delicate; without surfactant, the surface tension would be so high that the alveoli would collapse.

Level 3: Critical Thinking and Clinical Applications

21. An increase in ventilation will increase the movement of venous blood back to the heart. (Recall the respiratory pump.) Increasing venous return would in turn help increase the blood pressure (according to the Frank-Starling law of the heart).

22. While you were sleeping, the air that you were breathing was so dry it absorbed more than the normal amount of moisture as it passed through the nasal cavity. The loss of moisture made the mucous secretions quite viscous and harder for the cilia to move. Your nasal epithelia continued to secrete mucus, but very little of it moved. This ultimately produced the nasal congestion. After the shower and juice, more moisture was transferred to the mucus, loosening it and making it easier to move, thus clearing up the problem.

CHAPTER 17

Level 1: Reviewing Facts and Terms

1. c 2. k 3. g 4. a 5. i 6. h 7. j 8. d 9. f 10. b
11. l 12. e 13. d 14. d 15. b 16. c 17. b 18. d 19. d
20. a 21. d 22. d

23. ingestion, mechanical processing, secretion, digestion, absorption, and excretion

24. The folds increase the surface area available for absorption and may permit expansion of the lumen after a large meal.

25. muscosa: This innermost layer is a mucous membrane consisting of epithelia and loose connective tissue (the lamina propria); submucosa: This layer, which surrounds the mucosa, contains blood vessels, lymphatics, and neural tissue (which helps control and regulate smooth muscle tissue in the lamina propria and glandular secretions into the mucosa); muscularis externa: This layer is made up of two layers of smooth muscle tissue—longitudinal and circular—whose contractions agitate and propel materials along the digestive tract; serosa: This outermost layer is a serous membrane that protects and supports the digestive tract inside the peritoneal cavity.

26. analysis of material before swallowing; mechanical processing through the actions of the teeth, tongue, and palatal surfaces; lubrication by mixing with mucus and salivary secretions; limited digestion of carbohydrates and lipids

27. incisors: clipping or cutting; cuspids: tearing or slashing; bicuspids: crushing, mashing and grinding; molars: crushing and grinding

28. duodenum, jejunum, and ileum

29. The pancreas provides digestive enzymes as well as buffers that assist in the neutralization of acid chyme. The liver and gallbladder provide bile, a solution that contains additional buffers and bile salts that facilitate the digestion and absorption of lipids. The liver is responsible for metabolic regulation, hematological regulation, and bile production. It is the primary organ involved in regulating the composition of the circulating blood.

30. resorption of water and compaction of chyme into feces; absorption of important vitamins liberated by bacterial action; storage of fecal material prior to defecation

31. The rate of epithelial stem cell division declines; smooth muscle tone decreases; the effects of cumulative damage become apparent; cancer rates increase; and changes in other systems have direct or indirect effects on the digestive system.

Level 2: Reviewing Concepts

32. d   33. d   34. a

35. Peristalsis consists of waves of muscular contractions that move along the length of the digestive tract. During a peristaltic movement, the circular muscles contract behind the digestive contents. Longitudinal muscles contract next, shortening adjacent segments. A wave of contraction in the circular muscles then forces the materials in the desired direction. Segmentation movements churn and fragment the digestive materials, mixing the contents with intestinal secretions. Because they do not follow a set pattern, segmentation movements do not produce directional movement of materials along the tract.

36. The stomach performs four major functions: the bulk storage of ingested food, the mechanical breakdown of ingested food, the disruption of chemical bonds through the actions of acids and enzymes, and the production of intrinsic factor.

37. The cephalic phase begins with the sight or thought of food. Directed by the CNS, this phase prepares the stomach to receive food. The gastric phase begins with the arrival of food in the stomach. The gastric phase is initiated by distension of the stomach, an increase in the pH of the gastric contents, and the presence of undigested materials in the stomach. The intestinal phase begins when chyme starts to enter the small intestine. This phase controls the rate of gastric emptying and ensures that the secretory, digestive, and absorptive functions of the small intestine can proceed at reasonable efficiency.

Level 3: Critical Thinking and Clinical Applications

38. If the gallstone is small enough, it can pass through the common bile duct and block the pancreatic duct. Enzymes from the pancreas will not be able to reach the small intestine; as they accumulate, they will irritate the duct and ultimately the exocrine pancreas, producing pancreatitis.

39. The small intestine, especially the jejunum and ileum, are probably involved. Regional inflammation is the cause of Barb's pain. The inflamed tissue will not absorb nutrients; this accounts for her weight loss. Among the nutrients that are not absorbed are iron and vitamin B_{12}, which are necessary for formation of hemoglobin and red blood cells; this accounts for her anemia.

CHAPTER 18

Level 1: Reviewing Facts and Terms

1. a   2. g   3. l   4. i   5. j   6. b   7. k   8. e   9. f   10. d
11. h   12. c   13. d   14. c   15. a   16. b   17. c   18. c   19. d
20. c   21. b   22. c   23. b   24. a

25. Metabolism is all of the chemical reactions occurring in the cells of the body. Anabolism is those chemical reactions resulting in the synthesis of complex molecules from simpler reactants. Anabolic products are used for maintenance/repair, growth, and secretion. Catabolism is the breakdown of complex molecules into their building block molecules, resulting in the release of energy for the synthesis of ATP and related molecules.

26. Lipoproteins are lipid-protein complexes that contain large insoluble glycerides and cholesterol, with a superficial coating of phospholipids and proteins. The major groups are chylomicrons (the largest lipoproteins, which are 95% triglyceride and carry absorbed lipids from the intestinal tract to the circulation), very low-density lipoproteins (VLDLs, which consist of triglyceride, phospholipid, and cholesterol and function in transporting triglycerides to peripheral tissues), intermediate-density lipoproteins (IDLs, which are intermediate in size and composition between VLDLs and LDLs), low-density lipoproteins (LDLs, which are mostly cholesterol and function in delivering cholesterol to peripheral tissues; sometimes this cholesterol gets deposited in arteries, hence the designation of LDLs as "bad cholesterol"), and high-density lipoproteins (HDLs, which are known as "good cholesterol," contain equal parts protein and lipid—cholesterol and phospholipids—and function in transporting excess cholesterol back to the liver for storage or excretion in the bile).

27. Most vitamins and all minerals must be provided in the diet because the body can not synthesize these nutrients.

28. carbohydrates: 4.18 C/g; lipids: 9.46 C/g; proteins: 4.32 C/g

29. The BMR is the minimum, resting energy expenditures of an awake, alert person.

30. radiation (heat loss as infrared waves), conduction (heat loss to surfaces in physical contact), convection (heat loss to the air), and evaporation (heat loss with water becoming gas)

Level 2: Reviewing Concepts

31. d   32. b

33. Glycolysis results in the breakdown of glucose to pyruvic acid through a series of enzymatic steps. 4 ATP and 2 NADH are also produced. Glycolysis requires glucose, specific cytoplasmic enzymes, ATP and ADP, inorganic phosphates, and NAD (nicotinamide adenine dinucleotide), a coenzyme.

34. The TCA reaction sequence is a cycle because the 4-carbon starting compound (oxaloacetic acid) is regenerated at the end. Acetyl-CoA and oxaloacetic acid enter the cycle and CO_2, NADH, ATP, $FADH_2$, and oxaloacetic acid leave the cycle.

35. A triglyceride is hydrolyzed, yielding glycerol and fatty acids. Glycerol is converted to pyruvic acid and enters the TCA cycle. Fatty acids are broken into 2-carbon fragments by beta-oxidation, a process that occurs inside mitochondria. The 2-carbon compounds then enter the TCA cycle.

36. The food pyramid indicates the relative amounts of each food group an individual should consume per day to ensure adequate intake of nutrients and calories. The placement of fats, oils, and sugars at the top of the food pyramid indicates that such foods are to be consumed very sparingly, whereas carbohydrates, represented at the bottom of the pyramid as the bread, cereal, rice, and pasta group, is to be consumed in largest relative quantities.

37. The brain contains the "thermostat" of the body, a region known as the hypothalamus. The hypothalamus regulates the ANS control of such mechanisms as sweating and shivering thermogenesis, via negative feedback homeostatic mechanisms.

38. These terms refer to the HDL and LDL, lipoproteins in the blood that transport cholesterol. HDL ("good cholesterol") transports excess cholesterol to the liver for storage or breakdown, whereas LDL ("bad cholesterol") transports cholesterol to peripheral tissues, which unfortunately may include the arteries. The buildup of cholesterol in the arteries is linked to cardiovascular disease.

Level 3: Critical Thinking and Clinical Applications

39. During starvation, the body must use fat and protein reserves to supply the energy necessary to sustain life. Some of the protein that is metabolized for energy is the gamma globulin fraction of the blood, which is mostly composed of antibodies. This loss of antibodies coupled with a lack of amino acids to synthesize new ones, as well as protective molecules such as interferon and complement proteins, renders an individual more susceptible to contracting a disease and less likely to recover from it.

40. The drug colestipol would lead to a decrease in the plasma levels of cholesterol. Bile salts are necessary for the absorption of fats. If the bile salts cannot be absorbed, the amount of fat absorption, namely cholesterol and triglycerides, will decrease. This would in turn lead to a decrease in cholesterol from a dietary source as well as a decrease in fatty acids that could be used to synthesize new cholesterol. In addition, the body will have to replace the bile salts that are being lost with the feces. Since bile salts are formed from cholesterol, this will also contribute to a decline in cholesterol levels.

CHAPTER 19

Level 1: Reviewing Facts and Terms

1. q   2. g   3. n   4. j   5. a   6. m   7. e   8. p   9. d   10. f
11. h   12. k   13. b   14. c   15. l   16. o   17. i   18. c   19. d

A
I

20. a 21. d 22. c 23. c 24. b 25. d
26. The urinary system performs vital excretory functions and eliminates the organic waste products generated by cells throughout the body.
27. The urinary system includes the kidneys, ureters, urinary bladder, and urethra.
28. A fluid shift is a water movement between the ECF and ICF; this movement helps prevent drastic variations in the volume of the ECF. Changes in the osmolarity of the ECF can cause fluid shifts. If the ECF becomes more concentrated (hypertonic) with respect to the ICF, water will move from the cells into the ECF until equilibrium is restored. If the ECF becomes more dilute (hypotonic), water will move from the ECF into the cells. Changes in osmolarity can result from water loss (such as excessive perspiration, dehydration, vomiting, or diarrhea), from water gain (drinking pure water, administering hypotonic solutions through an IV), or from changes in electrolyte concentrations (such as sodium).
29. antidiuretic hormone: stimulates the thirst center and water conservation at the kidneys; aldosterone: determines the rate of sodium absorption along the DCT and collecting system of the kidneys; atrial natriuretic peptide: reduces thirst and blocks the release of ADH and aldosterone

Level 2: Reviewing Concepts

30. d   31. c   32. a   33. b
34. a
35. autoregulation at the local level; hormonal regulation initiated by the kidneys; autonomic regulation, (sympathetic division of the ANS)
36. The urge to urinate usually appears when the bladder contains about 200 ml of urine. The micturition reflex begins to function when the stretch receptors have provided adequate stimulation to the parasympathetic motor neurons. The activity in the motor neurons generates action potentials that reach the smooth muscle in the bladder wall. These efferent impulses travel over the pelvic nerves, producing a sustained contraction of the urinary bladder.
37. Fluid balance is a state in which the amount of water gained each day is equal to the amount lost to the environment. The water content of the body must remain stable, because water is an essential ingredient of cytoplasm and accounts for about 99% of the volume of extracellular fluid. Electrolyte balance exists when there is neither a net gain nor a net loss of any ion in body fluids. The ionic concentrations in body water must remain within normal limits; if levels of calcium or potassium become too high, for instance, cardiac arrhythmias can develop. Acid-base balance exists when the production of hydrogen ions precisely offsets their loss. The pH of body fluids must remain within a relatively narrow range; variations outside this range can be life threatening.
38. "Drink plenty of fluids" is physiologically sound advice because the temperature rise accompanying a fever can also increase water losses. For each degree the temperature rises above normal, the daily water loss increases by 200 ml.
39. Since sweat is usually hypotonic, the loss of a large volume of sweat causes hypertonicity in body fluids. The loss of fluid volume is primarily from the interstitial space, which leads to a reduction in plasma volume and an increase in the hematocrit. Severe dehydration can cause the blood viscosity to increase substantially, resulting in an increased workload on the heart, ultimately increasing the probability of heart failure.

Level 3: Critical Thinking and Clinical Applications

40. Truck drivers may not urinate as frequently as they should. Resisting the urge to urinate can result in urine backing up into the kidneys. This puts pressure on the kidney tissues, which can lead to tissue death and ultimately to kidney failure.
41. Susan may have a urinary tract infection; her urine may contain blood cells and bacteria. She is more likely to have this problem than her husband, because the urethral orifice in females is closer to the anus, and the urethral canal is short and opens near the vagina. Both regions normally harbor bacteria, which can easily reach the urethral entrance (often during sexual intercourse).
42. Arteriosclerosis contributes to hypertension (high blood pressure). The hypertension would trigger a baroreceptor reflex that would lead to a decrease in the level of ADH in the blood. Assuming that the arteriosclerosis is affecting all of Carlos' large arteries, including the renal arteries, the stiffening of the vessels would decrease the blood flow to the kidneys, thus triggering the release of renin from the juxtaglomerular apparatus. The renin would catalyze the conversion of angiotensinogen into angiotensin I, which would be converted into angiotensin II. The angiotensin II would stimulate the secretion of aldosterone which would increase sodium and water reabsorption thus increasing blood volume. The increase in blood volume would add to the hypertension, further decreasing the levels of ADH.

CHAPTER 20

Level 1: Reviewing Facts and Terms

1. i 2. m 3. a 4. c 5. l 6. e 7. n 8. o 9. h 10. b
11. f 12. j 13. d 14. k 15. g 16. c 17. a 18. c 19. a
20. d 21. a 22. c 23. c 24. d 25. b 26. c 27. d
28. The reproductive system of both males and females includes reproductive organs (gonads) that produce gametes and hormones, ducts that receive and transport gametes, accessory glands and organs that secrete fluids into these or other excretory ducts, and perineal structures collectively known as external genitalia.
29. The accessory organs and glands include the seminal vesicles, prostate gland, and the bulbourethral glands. The major functions of these glands are activating the spermatozoa, providing the nutrients sperm need for motility, propelling sperm and fluids along the reproductive tract, and producing buffers that counteract the acidity of the urethral and vaginal contents.
30. monitors and adjusts the composition of the tubular fluid, acts as a recycling center for damaged spermatozoa, and stores spermatozoa and facilitates their functional maturation
31. produces female gametes (ova); secretes female sex hormones, including estrogens and progestins; and secretes inhibin, involved in the feedback control of pituitary FSH production
32. serves as passageway for the elimination of menstrual fluids; receives the penis during sexual intercourse and holds spermatozoa prior to their passage into the uterus; and, in childbirth, forms the lower portion of the birth canal through which the fetus passes during delivery

Level 2: Reviewing Concepts

33. The reproductive system is the only physiological system that is not required for the survival of the individual.
34. Meiosis is the two-step nuclear division resulting in the formation of 4 haploid cells from 1 diploid cell. In males, 4 sperm are produced from each diploid cell, whereas in females only 1 ovum (plus 3 polar bodies) is produced from each diploid cell.
35. Menses: This phase is marked by the degeneration and loss of the functional zone of the endometrium; usually lasts 1 to 7 days, when approximately 35–50 ml of blood is lost. Proliferative phase: Growth and vascularization result in the complete restoration of the functional zone; lasts from the end of the menses until the beginning of ovulation around day 14; also called the preovulatory, or follicular, phase. Secretory phase: The endometrial glands enlarge, accelerating their rates of secretion; the arteries elongate and spiral through the tissues of the functional zone, under the combined stimulatory effects of progestins and estrogens from the corpus luteum; begins at the time of ovulation and persists as long as the corpus luteum remains intact; sometimes called the postovulatory, or luteal, phase.
36. In the degeneration of the corpus luteum a decline in progesterone and estrogen levels results in endometrial breakdown of menses. After menses, rising levels of FSH, LH, and estrogen stimu-

late the repair and regeneration of the functional zone of the endometrium. During the postovulatory phase, the combination of estrogen and progesterone cause the enlargement of the endometrial glands and an increase in their secretory activity.

37. In women, menopause is defined as the time that ovulation and menstruation cease. Menopause is accompanied by a sharp and sustained rise in the production of GnRH, FSH, and LH, while concentrations of circulating estrogen and progesterone decline. The decline in estrogen levels leads to reductions in the size of the uterus and breasts, accompanied by a thinning of the urethral and vaginal walls. In addition to a variety of neural and cardiovascular effects, reduced estrogen concentrations have been linked to the development of osteoporosis, presumably because bone deposition proceeds at a slower rate. During the male climacteric, circulating testosterone levels begin to decline between ages 50 and 60, coupled with increases in circulating levels of FSH and LH. Although sperm production continues in older men, there is a gradual reduction of sexual activity as age increases.

Level 3: Critical Thinking and Clinical Applications

38. There is no direct entry into the abdominopelvic cavity in males as there is in females. In females, the urethral opening is in close proximity to the vaginal orifice; therefore, infectious organisms can exit from the urethral meatus and enter the vagina. They can then proceed through the vagina to the uterus, then into the uterine tubes and finally into the peritoneal cavity.

39. The sacral region of the spinal cord contains the parasympathetic centers that control the genitals. Damage to this area of the spinal cord would interfere with the ability to achieve an erection by way of parasympathetic stimuli. However, erection can also occur by way of sympathetic centers in the lower thoracic region of the spinal cord. Visual, auditory, or cerebral stimuli can result in decreased tone in the arteries serving the penis. This results in increased blood flow and erection. Tactile stimulation of the penis, however, would not generate an erection.

40. It appears that a certain amount of body fat is necessary for uterine cycles to occur. The ratio of body fat to muscle tissue is somehow monitored by the nervous system; when the ratio falls below a certain set point, menstruation ceases. The actual mechanism appears to be a change in the levels of hypothalamic releasing hormone and pituitary gonadotrophins. Possibly without proper fat reserves, a woman could not have a successful pregnancy. To avoid damage to the female body and death of a fetus, the body prevents pregnancy from occurring by shutting down the ovarian cycle and thus the uterine cycle. When appropriate energy reserves are available, the cycles begin again.

CHAPTER 21

Level 1: Reviewing Facts and Terms

1. g   2. a   3. c   4. e   5. d   6. n   7. p   8. b   9. o   10. j
11. f   12. h   13. k   14. l   15. m   16. i   17. a   18. b   19. d
20. d   21. a   22. b   23. d   24. b

25. First trimester: The rudiments of all major organ systems appear. Second trimester The organs and organ systems complete most of their development, and the body proportions change to become more human. Third trimester: The fetus grows rapidly, and most of the major organ systems become fully functional.

26. Dilation stage: This begins with the onset of true labor, as the cervix dilates and the fetus begins to slide down the cervical canal. Late in this stage, the amnion usually ruptures. Expulsion stage: This stage begins as the cervix dilates completely and continues until the fetus has completely emerged from the vagina (delivery). Placental stage: The uterus gradually contracts, tearing the connections between the endometrium and the placenta and ejecting the placenta.

27. Neonatal period (birth to 1 month): The newborn becomes relatively self-sufficient and begins performing respiration, digestion,

and excretion for itself. Heart rates and fluid requirements are higher than those of adults. Neonates have little ability to thermoregulate. Infancy (1 month to 2 years): Major organ systems (other than those related to reproduction) become fully operational and start to take on the functional characteristics of adult structures. Daily, even hourly, variations in body temperature continue throughout childhood. Childhood (2 years to puberty): The child continues to grow, and significant changes in body proportions occur.

Level 2: Reviewing Concepts

28. d   29. d

30. The placental hormone human chorionic gonadotropin (HCG) resembles LH, in function, because it maintains the integrity of the corpus luteum and promotes the continued secretion of progesterone, which keeps the endometrial lining perfectly functional. The placental hormone human placental lactogen (HPL) helps prepare the mammary glands for milk production. The conversion from the resting state of the mammary glands to active status requires the presence of HPL and another placental hormone, placental prolactin, as well as several maternal hormones. The placental hormone relaxin is a peptide hormone that increases the flexibility of the symphysis pubis, causes the dilation of the cervix, and suppresses the release of oxytocin by the hypothalamus, delaying the onset of labor contractions.

31. The respiratory rate and tidal volume increase, allowing the lungs to obtain the extra oxygen and to remove the excess carbon dioxide generated by the fetus. Maternal blood volume increases, compensating for blood that will be lost during delivery. Requirements for nutrients and vitamins climb 10–30 percent, reflecting the fact that part of the mother's nutrients must nourish the fetus. The glomerular filtration rate increases by about 50 percent, corresponding to the increased blood volume and accelerates the excretion of metabolic wastes generated by the fetus.

32. Positive feedback mechanisms ensure that labor contractions continue until delivery is complete.

33. The amnion generally ruptures late in the dilation stage of labor.

34. (a) dominant (b) recessive (c) X-linked (d) autosomal

35. The trait of color blindness is carried on the X chromosome. Men are thus more likely to inherit it, because they have only one X chromosome. So whatever that chromosome carries will determine whether he is color blind or has normal vision. Since women have two X chromosomes, they will be color blind only if they are homozygous-recessive. This is an X-linked inheritance.

36. The Human Genome Project is attempting to determine the normal genetic composition of a "typical" human being. The project will help identify the genes responsible for inherited disorders and will localize the specific chromosomes involved.

Level 3: Critical Thinking and Clinical Applications

37. None of the couple's daughters will be hemophiliacs, since each will receive a normal allele from her father. There is a 50 percent chance that a son will be hemophiliac since there is a 50 percent chance of receiving either the mother's normal allele or her recessive allele.

38. The fact that the adults are larger is precisely why their rates are lower. Heat is lost across the skin. In infants, the surface-area-to-volume ratio is high, so they lose heat very quickly. To maintain a constant body temperature in the face of the heat loss, cellular metabolism must be high. Cellular metabolism requires oxygen, thus increased metabolism demands an increased respiratory rate. There must also be an increase in cardiac output to move the blood from the lungs to the tissues. Since the range of contraction in the neonate heart is limited, the greatest increase in cardiac output is achieved by increased heart rate.

39. The baby's condition is almost certainly not the result of a virus contracted during the third trimester. The development of organ systems occurs during the first trimester. By the end of the second trimester, almost all of the organ systems are fully formed. During the third trimester, the fetus undergoes tremendous growth but very little new organ formation.

A Periodic Chart of the Elements

The **periodic table** presents the known elements in order of their atomic weights. Each horizontal row represents a single electron shell. The number of elements in that row is determined by the maximum number of electrons that can be stored at that energy level. The element at the left end of each row contains a single electron in its outermost electron shell; the element at the right end of the row has a filled outer electron shell. Organizing the elements in this fashion highlights similarities that reflect the composition of the outer electron shell. These similarities are evident when you examine the vertical columns. All the gases of the right-most column—helium, neon, argon, krypton, xenon, and radon—have full electron shells; each is a gas at normal atmospheric temperature and pressure, and none reacts readily with other elements. These elements, highlighted in blue, are known as the *noble*, or *inert*, *gases*. In contrast, the elements of the left-most column—lithium, sodium, potassium, and so forth—are silvery, soft metals that are so highly reactive that pure forms cannot be found in nature. The fourth and fifth electron levels can hold 18 electrons. Table inserts are used for the *lanthanide* and *actinide series* to save space, as higher levels can store up to 32 electrons. Elements of particular importance to our discussion of human anatomy and physiology are highlighted in pink.

Atomic number — 1 — Chemical symbol
H — Hydrogen — Element name
Atomic weight — 1.01

1 H																		2 He
Hydrogen 1.01																		Helium 4.00
3 Li Lithium 6.94	4 Be Beryllium 9.01											5 B Boron 10.81	6 C Carbon 12.01	7 N Nitrogen 14.01	8 O Oxygen 16.00	9 F Fluorine 19.00	10 Ne Neon 20.18	
11 Na Sodium 22.99	12 Mg Magnesium 24.31											13 Al Aluminum 26.98	14 Si Silicon 28.09	15 P Phosphorus 30.97	16 S Sulfur 32.07	17 Cl Chlorine 35.45	18 Ar Argon 39.95	
19 K Potassium 39.10	20 Ca Calcium 40.08	21 Sc Scandium 44.96	22 Ti Titanium 47.88	23 V Vanadium 50.94	24 Cr Chromium 52.00	25 Mn Manganese 54.94	26 Fe Iron 55.85	27 Co Cobalt 58.93	28 Ni Nickel 58.69	29 Cu Copper 63.55	30 Zn Zinc 65.39	31 Ga Gallium 69.72	32 Ge Germanium 72.61	33 As Arsenic 74.92	34 Se Selenium 78.96	35 Br Bromine 79.90	36 Kr Krypton 83.80	
37 Rb Rubidium 85.47	38 Sr Strontium 87.62	39 Y Yttrium 88.91	40 Zr Zirconium 91.22	41 Nb Niobium 92.91	42 Mo Molybdenum 95.94	43 Tc Technetium (98)	44 Ru Ruthenium 101.07	45 Rh Rhodium 102.91	46 Pd Palladium 106.42	47 Ag Silver 107.87	48 Cd Cadmium 112.41	49 In Indium 114.82	50 Sn Tin 118.71	51 Sb Antimony 121.76	52 Te Tellurium 127.60	53 I Iodine 126.90	54 Xe Xenon 131.29	
55 Cs Cesium 132.91	56 Ba Barium 137.33	57 La* Lanthanum 138.91	72 Hf Hafnium 178.49	73 Ta Tantalum 180.95	74 W Tungsten 183.85	75 Re Rhenium 186.21	76 Os Osmium 190.2	77 Ir Iridium 192.22	78 Pt Platinum 195.08	79 Au Gold 196.97	80 Hg Mercury 200.59	81 Tl Thallium 204.38	82 Pb Lead 207.2	83 Bi Bismuth 208.98	84 Po Polonium (209)	85 At Astatine (210)	86 Rn Radon (222)	
87 Fr Francium (223)	88 Ra Radium 226.03	89 Ac† Actinium 227.03	104 Db Dubnium (261)	105 Jl Joliotium (262)	106 Rf Rutherfordium (263)	107 Bh Bohrium (262)	108 Hn Hahnium (265)	109 Mt Meitnerium (266)	110 Unnamed (269)	111 Unnamed (272)	112 Unnamed (272)							

*Lanthanide series

58 Ce Cerium 140.12	59 Pr Praseodymium 140.91	60 Nd Neodymium 144.24	61 Pm Promethium (145)	62 Sm Samarium 150.36	63 Eu Europium 151.96	64 Gd Gadolinium 157.25	65 Tb Terbium 158.93	66 Dy Dysprosium 162.50	67 Ho Holmium 164.93	68 Er Erbium 167.26	69 Tm Thulium 168.93	70 Yb Ytterbium 173.04	71 Lu Lutetium 174.97

†Actinide series

90 Th Thorium 232.04	91 Pa Protactinium 231.04	92 U Uranium 238.03	93 Np Neptunium 237.05	94 Pu Plutonium (244)	95 Am Americium (243)	96 Cm Curium (247)	97 Bk Berkelium (247)	98 Cf Californium (251)	99 Es Einsteinium (252)	100 Fm Fermium (257)	101 Md Mendelevium (258)	102 No Nobelium (259)	103 Lr Lawrencium (260)

Appendix III

Weights and Measures

Accurate descriptions of physical objects would be impossible without a precise method of reporting the pertinent data. Dimensions such as length and width are reported in standardized units of measurement, such as inches or centimeters. These values can be used to calculate the **volume** of an object, a measurement of the amount of space it fills. **Mass** is another important physical property. The mass of an object is determined by the amount of matter it contains. On earth the mass of an object determines its weight.

Most U.S. readers describe length and width in inches, feet, or yards; volumes in pints, quarts, or gallons; and weights in ounces, pounds, or tons. These are units of the **U.S. system** of measurement. Table 1 summarizes terms used in the U.S. system. For reference, this table also includes a definition of the "household units," popular in recipes. The U.S. system can be very difficult to work with, because there is no logical relationship between the various units. For example, there are 12 inches in a foot, 3 feet in a yard, and 1760 yards in a mile. Without a clear pattern of organization, converting feet to inches or miles to feet can be confusing and time-consuming. The relationships between ounces, pints, quarts, and gallons or ounces, pounds, and tons are no more logical.

In contrast, the **metric system** has a logical organization based on powers of 10, as indicated in Table 2. For example, a **meter (m)** is the basic unit for the measurement of size. For measuring larger objects, data can be reported in **dekameters** (*deka,* ten), **hectometers** (*hekaton,* hundred), or **kilometers (km;** *chilioi,* thousand); for smaller objects, data can be reported in **decimeters** (0.1 m; *decem,* ten), **centimeters (cm =** 0.01 m; *centum,* hundred), **millimeters** (**mm** = 0.001 m; *mille,* thousand), and so forth. Notice that the same prefixes are used to report weights, based on the **gram (g)**, and volumes, based on the **liter (l)**.

This text reports data in metric units, usually with U.S. equivalents. Use this opportunity to become familiar with the metric system, because most technical sources report data only in metric units, and most of the rest of the world uses the metric system exclusively. Conversion factors are included in Table 2.

The U.S. system and metric system also differ in their methods of reporting temperature: In the United States, temperature is usually reported in degrees Fahrenheit (°F), whereas scientific literature and individuals in most other countries report temperature in degrees centigrade (or degrees Celsius, °C). The relationship between temperature in degrees Fahrenheit and temperature in degrees centigrade is given in Table 2.

TABLE 1	The U.S. System of Measurement		
Physical Property	Unit	Relationship to Other U.S. Units	Relationship to Household Units
Length	inch (in.)	1 in. = 0.083 ft	
	foot (ft)	1 ft = 12 in. = 0.33 yd	
	yard (yd)	1 yd = 36 in. = 3 ft	
	mile (mi)	1 mi = 5280 ft = 1760 yd	
Volume	fluidram (fl dr)	1 fl dr = 0.125 fl oz	
	fluid ounce (fl oz)	1 fl oz = 8 fl dr	= 6 teaspoons (tsp)
		= 0.0625 pt	= 2 tablespoons (tbsp)
	pint (pt)	1 pt = 128 fl dr = 16 fl oz = 0.5 qt	= 32 tbsp = 2 cups (c)
	quart (qt)	1 qt = 256 fl dr = 32 fl oz = 2 pt = 0.25 gal	= 4 c
	gallon (gal)	1 gal = 128 fl oz = 8 pt = 4 qt	
Mass	grain (gr)	1 gr = 0.002 oz	
	dram (dr)	1 dr = 27.3 gr = 0.063 oz	
	ounce (oz)	1 oz = 437.5 gr = 16 dr	
	pound (lb)	1 lb = 7000 gr = 256 dr = 16 oz	
	ton (t)	1 t = 2000 lb	

A III

TABLE 2   The Metric System of Measurement

Physical Property	Unit	Relationship to Standard Metric Units	Conversion to U.S. Units	
Length	nanometer (nm)	1 nm = 0.000000001 m (10^{-9})	= 4×10^{-8} in.	25,000,000 nm = 1 in.
	micrometer (µm)	1 µm = 0.000001 m (10^{-6})	= 4×10^{-5} in.	25,000 mm = 1 in.
	millimeter (mm)	1 mm = 0.001 m (10^{-3})	= 0.0394 in.	25.4 mm = 1 in.
	centimeter (cm)	1 cm = 0.01 m (10^{-2})	= 0.394 in.	2.54 cm = 1 in.
	decimeter (dm)	1 dm = 0.1 m (10^{-1})	= 3.94 in.	0.25 dm = 1 in.
	meter (m)	standard unit of length	= 39.4 in.	0.0254 m = 1 in.
			= 3.28 ft	0.3048 m = 1 ft
			= 1.09 yd	0.914 m = 1 yd
	dekameter (dam)	1 dam = 10 m		
	hectometer (hm)	1 hm = 100 m		
	kilometer (km)	1 km = 1000 m	= 3280 ft	
			= 1093 yd	
			= 0.62 mi	1.609 km = 1 mi
Volume	microliter (µl)	1 µl = 0.000001 l (10^{-6}) = 1 cubic millimeter (mm^3)		
	milliliter (ml)	1 ml = 0.001 l (10^{-3}) = 1 cubic centimeter (cm^3 or cc)	= 0.03 fl oz	5 ml = 1 tsp
				15 ml = 1 tbsp
				30 ml = 1 fl oz
	centiliter (cl)	1 cl = 0.01 l (10^{-2})	= 0.34 fl oz	3 cl = 1 fl oz
	deciliter (dl)	1 dl = 0.1 l (10^{-1})	= 3.38 fl oz	0.29 dl = 1 fl oz
	liter (l)	standard unit of volume	= 33.8 fl oz	0.0295 l = 1 fl oz
			= 2.11 pt	0.473 l = 1 pt
			= 1.06 qt	0.946 l = 1 qt
Mass	picogram (pg)	1 pg = 0.000000000001 g (10^{-12})		
	nanogram (ng)	1 ng = 0.000000001 g (10^{-9})		
	microgram (µg)	1 µg = 0.000001 g (10^{-6})	= 0.000015 gr	66,666 mg = 1 gr
	milligram (mg)	1 mg = 0.001 g (10^{-3})	= 0.015 gr	66.7 mg = 1 gr
	centigram (cg)	1 cg = 0.01 g (10^{-2})	= 0.15 gr	6.7 cg = 1 gr
	decigram (dg)	1 dg = 0.1 g (10^{-1})	= 1.5 gr	0.67 dg = 1 gr
	gram (g)	standard unit of mass	= 0.035 oz	28.35 g = 1 oz
			= 0.0022 lb	453.6 g = 1 lb
	dekagram (dag)	1 dag = 10 g		
	hectogram (hg)	1 hg = 100 g		
	kilogram (kg)	1 kg = 1000 g	= 2.2 lb	0.453 kg = 1 lb
	metric ton (mt)	1 mt = 1000 kg	= 1.1 t	
			= 2205 lb	0.907 mt = 1 t

Temperature	Centigrade	Fahrenheit
Freezing point of pure water	0°	32°
Normal body temperature	36.8°	98.6°
Boiling point of pure water	100°	212°
Conversion	°C → °F: °F = (1.8 × °C) + 32	°F → °C: °C = (°F − 32) × 0.56

The figure below spans the entire range of measurements that we will consider in this book. Gross anatomy traditionally deals with structural organization as seen with the naked eye or with a simple hand lens. A microscope can provide higher levels of magnification and reveal finer details. Before the 1950s, most information was provided by *light microscopy*. A photograph taken through a light microscope is called a **light micrograph (LM)**. Light microscopy can magnify cellular structures about 1000 times and show details as fine as 0.25 μm. The symbol μm stands for *micrometer*; 1 μm = 0.001 mm, or 0.00004 inch. With a light microscope, we can identify cell types, such as muscle cells or neurons, and see large structures within the cell. Because individual cells are relatively transparent, thin sections taken through a cell are treated with dyes that stain specific structures, making them easier to see.

Although special staining techniques can show the general distribution of proteins, lipids, carbohydrates, and nucleic acids in the cell, many fine details of intracellular structure remained a mystery until investigators began using *electron microscopy*. This technique uses a focused beam of electrons, rather than a beam of light, to examine cell structure. In *transmission electron microscopy*, electrons pass through an ultrathin section to strike a photographic plate. The result is a **transmission electron micrograph (TEM)**. Transmission electron microscopy shows the fine structure of cell membranes and intracellular structures. In *scanning electron microscopy*, electrons bouncing off exposed surfaces create a **scanning electron micrograph (SEM)**. Scanning microscopy cannot achieve as much magnification as transmission microscopy, but it provides a three-dimensional perspective of cell structure, whereas transmission microscopy gives a two-dimensional view.

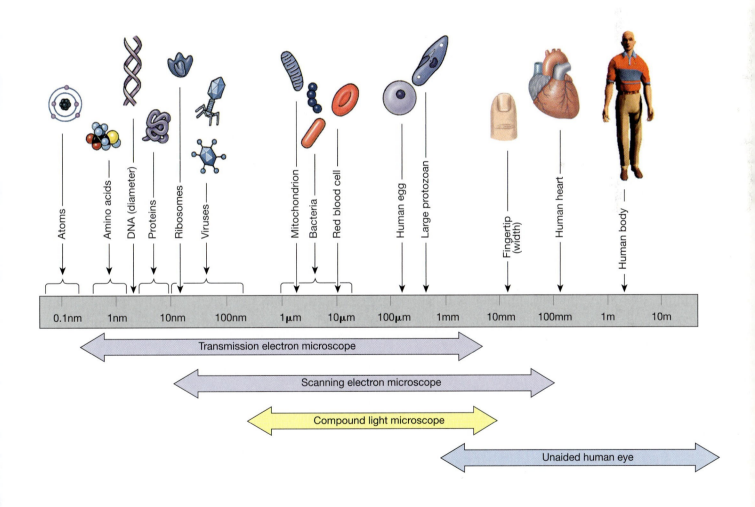

Appendix IV

A
IV

Normal Physiological Values

Tables 3 and 4 present normal averages or ranges for the chemical composition of body fluids. These values should be considered approximations rather than absolute values, as test results vary from laboratory to laboratory owing to differences in procedures, equipment, normal solutions, and so forth. Sources used in the preparation of these tables are indicated on p. A-15. Blanks indicate tests for which data were not available.

TABLE 3	The Chemistry of Blood, Cerebrospinal Fluid, and Urine		
	Normal Ranges		
Test	*Blood*[a]	*CSF*	*Urine*
pH	S: 7.38–7.44	7.31–7.34	4.6–8.0
OSMOLARITY (mOsm/l)	S: 280–295	292–297	500–800
ELECTROLYTES	(mEq/l unless noted)		(urinary loss per 24-hour period[b])
Bicarbonate	P: 21–28	20–24	
Calcium	S: 4.5–5.3	2.1–3.0	6.5–16.5 mEq
Chloride	S: 100–108	116–122	120–240 mEq
Iron	S: 50–150 µg/l	23–52 µg/l	40–150 µg
Magnesium	S: 1.5–2.5	2–2.5	4.9–16.5 mEq
Phosphorus	S: 1.8–2.6	1.2–2.0	0.8–2 g
Potassium	P: 3.8–5.0	2.7–3.9	35–80 mEq
Sodium	P: 136–142	137–145	120–220 mEq
Sulfate	S: 0.2–1.3		1.07–1.3 g
METABOLITES	(mg/dl unless noted)		(urinary loss per 24-hour period[c])
Amino acids	P/S: 2.3–5.0	10.0–14.7	41–133 mg
Ammonia	P: 20–150 µg/dl	25–80 µg/dl	340–1200 mg
Bilirubin	S: 0.5–1.2	<0.2	0.02–1.9 mg
Creatinine	P/S: 0.6–1.2	0.5–1.9	1.01–2.5
Glucose	P/S: 70–110	40–70	16–132 mg
Ketone bodies	S: 0.3–2.0	1.3–1.6	10–100 mg
Lactic acid	WB: 5–20[d]	10–20	100–600 mg
Lipids (total)	S: 400–1000	0.8–1.7	0–31.8 mg
Cholesterol (total)	S: 150–300	0.2–0.8	1.2–3.8 mg
Triglycerides	S: 40–150	0–0.9	
Urea	P/S: 23–43	13.8–36.4	12.6–28.6
Uric acid	S: 2.0–7.0	0.2–0.3	80–976 mg
PROTEINS	(g/dl)	(mg/dl)	(urinary loss per 24-hour period[c])
Total	S: 6.0–7.8	20–4.5	47–76.2 mg
Albumin	S: 3.2–4.5	10.6–32.4	10–100 mg
Globulins (total)	S: 2.3–3.5	2.8–15.5	7.3 mg (average)
Immunoglobulins	S: 1.0–2.2	1.1–1.7	3.1 mg (average)
Fibrinogen	P: 0.2–0.4	0.65 (average)	

[a] *S = serum, P = plasma, WB = whole blood*

[b] *Because urinary output averages just over 1 liter per day, these electrolyte values are comparable to mEq/l.*

[c] *Because urinary metabolite and protein data approximate mg/l or g/l, they must be divided by 10 for comparison with CSF or blood concentrations.*

[d] *Venous blood sample*

| TABLE 4 | The Composition of Minor Body Fluids |

Test	Perilymph	Endolymph	Synovial Fluid	Sweat	Saliva	Semen
pH			7.4	4–6.8	6.4[a]	7.19
SPECIFIC GRAVITY			1.008–1.015	1.001–1.008	1.007	1.028
ELECTROLYTES (mEq/l)						
Potassium	5.5–6.3	140–160	4.0	4.3–14.2	21	31.3
Sodium	143–150	12–16	136.1	0–104	14[a]	117
Calcium	1.3–1.6	0.05	2.3–4.7	0.2–6	3	12.4
Magnesium	1.7	0.02		0.03–4	0.6	11.5
Bicarbonate	17.8–18.6	20.4–21.4	19.3–30.6		6[a]	24
Chloride	121.5	107.1	107.1	34.3	17	42.8
PROTEINS (mg/dl)						
Total	200	150	1.72 g/dl	7.7	386[b]	4.5 g/dl
METABOLITES (mg/dl)						
Amino acids				47.6	40	1.26 g/dl
Glucose	104		70–110	3.0	11	224 (fructose)
Urea				26–122	20	72
Lipids, total	12		20.9	[d]	25–500[c]	188

Normal Averages or Ranges (spanning Perilymph through Semen)

[a] *Increases under salivary stimulation*
[b] *Primarily alpha-anylase, with some lysozomes*
[c] *Cholesterol*
[d] *Not present in eccrine secretions*

Sources

Ballenger, John Jacob. 1977. *Diseases of the Nose, Throat, and Ear.* Philadelphia: Lea and Febiger.

Davidsohn, Israel, and John Bernard Henry, eds. 1969. *Todd-Sanford Clinical Diagnosis by Laboratory Methods,* 14th ed. Philadelphia: W. B. Saunders.

Diem, K., and C. Lenter, eds. 1970. *Scientific Tables,* 7th ed. Basel, Switzerland: Ciba-Geigy.

Halsted, James A. 1976. *The Laboratory in Clinical Medicine: Interpretation and Application.* Philadelphia: W. B. Saunders.

Harper, Harold A. 1987. *Review of Physiological Chemistry.* Los Altos, Calif.: Lange Medical Publications.

Isselbacher, Kurt J., Eugene Braunwauld, Robert G. Petersdorf, Jean D. Wilson, Joseph B. Martin, Anthony S. Fauci, and Dennis L. Kaspar, eds. 1994. *Harrison's Principles of Internal Medicine,* 13th ed. New York: McGraw-Hill.

Lentner, Cornelius, ed. 1981. *Geigy Scientific Tables,* 8th ed. Basel, Switzerland: Ciba-Geigy.

Glossary/Index

A

A band, 171
Abdomen, A1-7–A1-8
Abdominal aortic aneurysm, A14-2
Abdominal cavity, 21, 466, A1-8
Abdominal pain, 474
Abdominopelvic cavity, A1-8
Abdominopelvic cavity: Portion of the ventral body cavity that contains abdominal and pelvic subdivision, 21
Abdominopelvic quadrants, 18
Abdominopelvic regions, 18
Abducens nerves (N VI), 253–254
Abduction: Movement away from the midline, 151, 152
Abortion, 571, A21-4–A21-5
Abrasion, 115, A5-8
Abruptio placentae, A20-2
Absence seizures, A8-3
Absorption: The active or passive uptake of gases, fluids, or solutes, 464, 475–476, 477–478, 485–488
of electrolytes, 487
in the large intestine, 484
of lipids, 486
malabsorption syndromes, 488
of nutrients, 485–487
of proteins, 486
of vitamins, 487
of water, 487
Accessory nerve (N XI), 255
Accessory sex organs, 13
Accommodation: Alteration in the curvature of the lens to focus an image on the retina; decrease in receptor sensitivity or perception following chronic stimulation, 285–286
Acetabulum (a-se-TAB-ū-lum): Fossa on lateral aspect of pelvis that accommodates the head of the femur, 146
Acetic acid, A9-1
Acetone, 502
Acetylcholine, A9-1
Acetylcholine (ACh) (as-ē-til-KŌ-lēn): Chemical neurotransmitter in the brain and PNS; dominant neurotransmitter in the PNS, released at neuromuscular junctions and synapses of the parasympathetic division, 172, 173, 225–226, 262, 369–370
Acetylcholinesterase, A9-1
Acetylcholinesterase (AChE): Enzyme found in the synaptic cleft, bound to the postsynaptic membrane, and in tissue fluids; breaks down and inactivates ACh molecules, 172, 225–226
Acetyl-CoA: An acetyl group bound to coenzyme A, a participant in the anabolic and catabolic pathways for carbohydrates, lipids, and many amino acids, 498, 500–501
Acetyl group: $CH_3C=O$
Achilles tendon, 148, 204
Aching and burning pain (slow pain), 272
Acid: A compound whose dissociation in solution releases a hydrogen ion and an anion; an acid solution has a pH below 7.0 and contains an excess of hydrogen ions, 36
amino, 42–43, 71–73, 306–307, 316, 502–504
arachidonic, 307, 502
ascorbic (vitamin C), 509

carbonic, 453, 537
fatty, 39–41, 57, 307, 476, 501–503
folic (folacin), 509
gamma aminobutyric, 225
hydrochloric, 471
inorganic, 38
lactic, 38, 180–181
linoleic, 501–502
linolenic, 502
metabolic, 538
nicotinic (niacin), 509
nucleic, 45–46
organic, 38
pantothenic (vitamin B_5), 509
pyruvic, 180, 181, 497–498
structure and function, 48
uric, 504, 524
weak, 538
Acid-base balance, 537–540
Acidic, A2-2
Acidic solution, 36
Acidosis (a-sid-Ō-sis): An abnormal physiological state characterized by a plasma pH below 7.35, 537, 539, 540
Acinus/acini (AS-i-nī): Histological term referring to a blind pocket, pouch, or sac.
Acini, pancreatic, 448
Acne, 113
Acquired immune deficiency syndrome (AIDS), 426, 445
Acquired immunity, 421, A15-2
Acquired immunodeficiency syndrome (AIDS), 566
Acromion, 143–144
Acrosomal cap, 552, 578
ACTH (adrenocorticotropic hormone), 312, 315
Actin: Protein component of microfilaments; form thin filaments in skeletal muscles and produce contractions of all muscles through interaction with thick (myosin) filaments, 65, 97, 99, 171. *See also* **Sliding filament theory**
Action, muscle, 184
Action potential: A conducted change in the membrane potential of excitable cells, initiated by a change in the membrane permeability to sodium ions. *See also* **Nerve impulse**
cardiac muscle, 361, 363–364
muscle fiber, 172
nervous system, 222–224, 225–226
sensory information and, 272
Activase, A12-3
Activation energy, 43–44
Active immunity, 421, 430, A15-2
Active site
actin, 171, 172
enzyme, 44
Active transport: The ATP-dependent absorption or excretion of solutes across a cell membrane, 62, 64
Acuity, visual, 286
Acute: Sudden in onset, severe in intensity, and brief in duration.
Acute angle-closure glaucoma, A10-4
Acute arterial occlusion, A14-3
Acute coronary syndrome, A12-3, A13-2–A13-3
Acute fulminate cardiovascular beriberi, 504
Acute glaucoma, A10-4
Acute ischemic stroke, A12-3
Acute myocardial infarction, 174

Acute pancreatitis, 478
Acute pulmonary embolism, A14-2–A14-3
Acute renal failure (ARF), A19-5, 530
Acute tubular necrosis, A19-5
Acute urinary tract infection, A19-3–A19-5
Adaptability, 4
Adaptation, 272
Addison's disease, A11-8–A11-9
Adduction: Movement toward the axis or midline of the body as viewed in the anatomical position, 148, 151, 152, A1-3
Adductor brevis muscle, 201–203
Adductor longus muscle, 201–203
Adductor magnus muscle, 201–203
Adenine: One of the nitrogenous bases in the nucleic acids RNA and DNA, 45–46, 70, 71–72
Adenocarcinoma, A16-5
Adenoids: The pharyngeal tonsil, 415
Adenosine: A nucleoside consisting of adenine and a five-carbon sugar, 46
Adenosine diphosphate (ADP): Adenosine with two phosphate groups attached, 46
Adenosine phosphate (AMP): A nucleotide consisting of adenosine plus a phosphate group (PO_4^{3-}); also known as *adenosine monophosphate,* 46
Adenosine triphosphate (ATP): A high-energy compound consisting of adenosine with three phosphate groups attached; the third is attached by a high-energy bond. *See* **ATP (adenosine triphosphate)**
Adenosinetriphosphate (ATP), A18-1
Adenylate cyclase: An enzyme bound to the inner surfaces of cell membranes that can convert ATP to cyclic–AMP; also called *adenyl cyclase* or *adenylyl cyclase,* 308
ADH. *See* **Antidiuretic hormone (ADH)**
Adipocyte (AD-i-pō-sīt): A fat cell, 90
Adipose tissue: Loose connective tissue dominated by adipocytes, 91, 92, 561
Adolescence, 595, A21-5
ADP (adenosine diphosphate), 46
Adrenal cortex: Superficial portion of adrenal gland that produces steroid hormones, 318
Adrenal gland: Small endocrine gland secreting hormones, located superior to each kidney, 10, 307
cortex, 318
innervation, ANS, 265
medulla, 262, 319–320
Adrenal glands, disorders of, A11-8–A11-9
Adrenal insufficiency, A11-8–A11-9
Adrenal medulla: Core of the adrenal gland; a modified sympathetic ganglion that secretes hormones into the blood following sympathetic activation, 262, 319–320
Adrenergic (ad-ren-ER-jik): A synaptic terminal that releases norepinephrine when stimulated, 225
Adrenergic synapses, A9-1
Adrenocorticotropic hormone (ACTH): Hormone that stimulates the production and secretion of glucocorticoids by the adrenal cortex; released by the anterior pituitary, 312, 315
Adventitia (ad-ven-TISH-a): Superficial layer of connective tissue surrounding an internal organ; fibers are continuous with those of surrounding tissues, providing support and stabilization, 466

GI

Antibody-mediated immunity. *See* **Humoral immunity**

Anticoagulant: Compound that slows or prevents clot formation by interfering with the clotting system, 350

Anticodon: Triplet of nitrogenous bases on a tRNA molecule that interacts with an appropriate codon on a strand of mRNA, 72

Antidiuretic hormone (ADH) (an-tī-dī-ū-RET-ik): Hormone synthesized in the hypothalamus and secreted at the posterior pituitary; causes water retention at the kidneys and an elevation of blood pressure, 307, 309, 313, 315, 387, 528, 529, 530, 540

Antigen: A substance capable of inducing the production of antibodies, 414, 422

Antigen-antibody complex: The combination of an antigen and a specific antibody, 425

Antigen exposure, 427

Antigen recognition, 422

Antigenic determinant site: A portion of an antigen that can interact with an antibody molecule.

Anti-inflammatory compounds, 318

Antioxidants, 323

Antiplatelets, 350

Antrum (AN-trum): A chamber or pocket, 558

Anus: External opening of the anorectal canal, 484

Aorta: Large, elastic artery that carries blood away from the left ventricle and into the systemic circuit, 392, 394, 396–397

Aorta, rupture of, A14-5

Aortic bodies, 275, 276, 386, 456

Aortic reflex: Baroreceptor reflex triggered by increased aortic pressures; leads to a reduction in cardiac output and a fall in systemic pressure.

Aortic sinuses, 274, 275, 385

Aortic valve, 359, 360, 361

Apex
of heart, 357
of sacrum, 140

Aphasia: Inability to speak, 238, A8-2

Apheresis, A12-2

Apocrine secretion: Mode of secretion in which the glandular cell sheds portions of its cytoplasm, 88, 89

Apocrine sweat glands, 113–114

Apoidea, A15-5

Aponeurosis/aponeuroses (ap-ō-nū-RŌ-sēz): A broad tendinous sheet that may serve as the origin or insertion of a skeletal muscle.

Apoptosis, 423

Appendicitis, 482, A17-1–A17-2

Appendicular muscles. *See* **Muscular system**

Appendicular skeleton, 8, 130, 142–149
lower limb, 147–149
pectoral girdle, 142–144
pelvic girdle, 145–147
upper limb, 144–145

Appendix: A blind tube connected to the cecum of the large intestine, 415, 416, 482

Appositional growth: Enlargement by the addition of cartilage or bony matrix to the outer surface, 125

Aqueous humor: Fluid similar to perilymph or CSF that fills the anterior chamber of the eye, 280, 284

Arachidonic acid, 307, 502

Arachnoid (a-RAK-noyd): The middle meninges that encloses CSF and protects the central nervous system, 229

Arachnoid granulations, 235

Arcuate (AR-kū-āt): Curving.

Arcuate arteries, 523, 524

Arcuate veins, 524

Areola (a-RĒ-ō-la): Pigmented area that surrounds the nipple of a breast, 562

Areolar: Containing minute spaces, as in areolar connective tissue, 92

Arm, A1-2

Arm. *See* **Upper limb**

Arousal, sexual, 554, 561, 565

Arrector pili (a-REK-tōr PĪ-lī): Smooth muscles whose contractions cause erection of hairs, 112

Arrhythmias (a-RITH-mē-az): Abnormal patterns of cardiac contractions, 367

Art therapist, A4-7

Arterial anastomosis, 379

Arterial blood gas (ABG), 451

Arterial puncture, 335

Arteries: Blood vessels that carries blood away from the heart and toward a peripheral capillary, 10, 93, 356, 376. *See also* **Circulation;** *specific vessels*
arcuate, 523, 524
coronary, 363, 378, 503
elastic, 377
interlobar, 523, 524
interlobular, 523, 524
systemic, 392–397

Arteriole (ar-TĒ-rē-ōl): A small arterial branch that delivers blood to a capillary network, 376

Arteriosclerosis, 378, A13-1

Arteriovenous anastomosis, 379

Arthritis (ar-THRĪ-tis): Inflammation of a joint, 150–151

Articular: Pertaining to a joint.

Articular capsule: *See* **Joint capsule**

Articular cartilage: Cartilage pad that covers the surface of a bone inside a joint cavity.

Articular facet, 138

Articulations, 96. *See also* **Joints**

Artificially acquired immunity, 422, A15-2

Artificial sweeteners, 39

Arytenoid cartilage, 441–442

Ascites, A17-6

Ascending tract: A tract carrying information from the spinal cord to the brain.

Aseptic meningitis, A8-4

Assist control mode ventilation (ACMV), A16-6

Association areas: Cortical areas of the cerebrum responsible for integration of sensory inputs and/or motor commands, 237
visual, 237

Association neuron: *See* **Interneuron**

Asthma (AZ-ma): Reversible constriction of smooth muscles around respiratory passageways, frequently caused by an allergic response, 443, 456, A16-3–A16-4

Astigmatism: Visual disturbance due to an irregularity in the shape of the cornea, 286

Astrocyte (AS-trō-sīt): One of the glial cells in the CNS; responsible for the blood-brain barrier, 218, 219, 230

Ataxia, 243

Atelectasis, 449

Athero-elam, 378

Atherogenesis, A13-1, 378

Atheromatous plaques, 378

Atherosclerosis (ath-er-ō-skle-RŌ-sis): Formation of fatty plaques in the walls of arteries, leading to circulatory impairment, 378, 566, A13-1

Athletic trainer, A4-8

Atlas, 140

Atom: The smallest stable unit of matter, 30–34

Atomic number: The number of protons in the nucleus of an atom, 30

Atomic weight: Roughly, the average total number of protons and neutrons in the atoms of a particular element, 31

ATP (adenosine triphosphate), 46, 66
muscle activity and, 174–176, 179–181
production, 68–69, 179–180, 496–499

Atreptokinase, A12-4

Atresia, 557

Atria: Thin-walled chambers of the heart that receive venous blood from the pulmonary or systemic circuit, 356, 357–358, 359, 364–365, 366, 367

Atrial natriuretic peptide (nā-trē-ū-RET-ik): Hormone released by specialized atrial cardiocytes when they are stretched by an abnormally large venous return; promotes fluid loss and reductions in blood pressure and venous return, 320, 389, 530

Atrial reflex: Reflexive increase in heart rate following an increase in venous return; due to mechanical and neural factors; also called *Bainbridge reflex,* 369

Atrioventricular (AV) node (ā-trē-ō-ven-TRIK-ū-lar): Specialized cardiocytes that relay the contractile stimulus to the AV bundle, the bundle branches, the Purkinje fibers, and the ventricular myocardium; located at the boundary between the atria and ventricles, 364–365

Atrioventricular (AV) valve: One of the valves that prevent backflow into the atria during ventricular systole, 358–361, 368

Atrophy (AT-rō-fē): Wasting away of tissues from lack of use, ischemia, or nutritional abnormalities, 88, 178, A5-3

Attending physicians, A4-2

Attenuated vaccines, A15-2

Audiologist, A4-8

Auditory: Pertaining to the sense of hearing, 440

Auditory ossicles: The middle ear bones: malleus, incus, and stapes, 131, 133, 290

Auditory tubes, 290, 440

Auricle, 357

Autoantibodies, 429

Autodigestion, 478

Autoimmunity: Immune system sensitivity to normal cells and tissues, resulting in the production of autoantibodies, 428–429

Autolysis: Destruction of a cell due to the rupture of lysosomal membranes in its cytoplasm, 68

Automatic transport, A16-6

Automaticity: Spontaneous depolarization to threshold, a characteristic of cardiac pacemaker cells.

Autonomic ganglion: A collection of visceral motor neurons outside the CNS.

Autonomic nerve: A peripheral nerve consisting of preganglionic or postganglionic autonomic fibers.

Autonomic nervous system (ANS): Centers, nuclei, tracts, ganglia, and nerves involved in the unconscious regulation of visceral functions; includes components of the CNS and PNS, 216, 259, 261–265
cardiac effects, 369–370
heart rate, 369
stroke volume, 370
cardiovascular effects of, 386–387
digestive tract and, 464
effects on organs, 265
parasympathetic division, 262–265
sexual function and, 565–566
sympathetic division, 262, 264–265

Autoregulation: Alterations in activity that maintain homeostasis in direct response to changes in the local environment; does not require neural or endocrine control, 377, 384–385

Autosomal (aw-to-SŌ-mal): Chromosomes other than the X or Y chromosomes, 596–598

**G
I**

urinary system, 534
nails, 114–115
sebaceous glands, 113, 114
structure and function, 108–109
subcutaneous layer (hypodermis), 108, 112
sweat glands, 113–114
Intercalated discs (in-TER-ka-lā-ted): Regions where adjacent cardiocytes interlock and where gap junctions permit the movement of ions and action potentials between the cells, 98, 99, 183, 361
Intercellular cement: A combination of protein and carbohydrate molecules, especially hyaluronic acid, between adjacent epithelial cells, 83
Intercellular connections, 83–84
Intercostal muscles, 192, 193, 447–448
Intercourse, physiology of, 565–566
Interferons (in-ter-FĒR-onz): Peptides released by virus-infected cells, especially lymphocytes, that make other cells more resistant to viral infection and slow viral replication, 420, 428
Interleukins (in-ter-LOO-kinz): Peptides released by activated monocytes and lymphocytes that assist in the coordination of the cellular and humoral immune responses, 427, 428
Interlobar arteries, 523, 524
Interlobar veins, 524
Interlobular arteries, 523, 524
Interlobular veins, 524
Intermittent mandatory ventilation (IMV), A16-6
Intestinal wall, 475–476
Intestine
large, 12, 482–485
small, 12, 474–478. See also **Small intestine**
Internal, A1-3
Internal ear: The membranous labyrinth that contains the organs of hearing and equilibrium, 291, 292
Internal hemorrhoids, A17-9
Internal medicine, A4-3
Internal nares: The entrance to the nasopharynx from the nasal cavity, 539
Internal orifice, 560
Interneuron: An association neuron; neurons inside the CNS that are interposed between sensory and motor neurons, 217, 226
Interns, A4-2
Internship, A4-2
Interoceptors: Sensory receptors monitoring the functions and status of internal organs and systems, 217
Interphase: Stage in the life of a cell during which the chromosomes are uncoiled and all normal cellular functions except mitosis are underway, 73, 75, 551
Interstitial cells, 322, 550
Interstitial cell-stimulating hormone (ICSH), 312, 555
Interstitial fluid (in-ter-STISH-al): Fluid in the tissues that fills the spaces between cells, 93, 334, 336, 381, 413
Interstitial fluid colloid osmotic pressure, 381
Interstitial growth: Form of cartilage growth through the growth, mitosis, and secretion of chondrocytes inside the matrix.
Interventional cardiology, A4-3
Interventricular sulcus, 357
Intervertebral articulations, 155
Intervertebral disc: Fibrocartilage pad between the bodies of successive vertebrae that acts as a shock absorber, 139, 140, 155
Intervertebral foramina, 139

Intestinal juice, 476
Intestinal phase of gastric secretion, 474
Intracellular fluid: The cytosol, 535–537
Intracerebral hemorrhage (ICH), A8-7
Intramembranous ossification (in-tra-MEM-bra-nus): The formation of bone within a connective tissue without the prior development of a cartilaginous model, 125
Intramuscular administration, 204
Intraosseous needle placement, A6-6–A6-7
Intrauterine device (IUD), 559, 570
Intrinsic factor: A compound secreted by the parietal cells of the stomach that facilitates the intestinal absorption of vitamin B₁₂, 471, 487, 508
Intrinsic pathway: A pathway of the clotting system that begins with the activation of platelets and ends with the formation of platelet thromboplastin, 349, 350
Invasive cardiologists, A13-1
Inversion: A turning inward, 153
Inversion of the foot, A1-5
Involuntary muscle, 99
Iodine, 30, 316
Ion: An atom or molecule bearing a positive or negative charge due to the acceptance or donation of an electron, 32. See also **Electrolytes**
Ionic bond (ī-ON-ik): Molecular bond created by the attraction between ions with opposite charges, 32, 33
Ionization (ī-on-i-ZĀ-shun): Dissociation; the breakdown of a molecule in solution to form ions, 38
Ion pump, 62, 221, 527
Iris: A contractile structure made up of smooth muscle that forms the colored portion of the eye, 281–282
Iron, 30, 339, 507
Irregular bone, 122–123
Irritability, 4
Ischemia (is-KĒ-mē-a): Inadequate blood supply to a region of the body.
Ischemic stroke, 238, A8-1
Ischiocavernosus muscle, 193–194, 565, 566
Ischium (IS-kē-um): One of the three bones whose fusion creates the coxa, 146–147
Islets of Langerhans, 321
Isoenzymes, 174
Isometric contraction: A muscular contraction characterized by rising tension production but no change in length, 178
Isotonic: A solution having an osmotic concentration that does not result in water movement across cell membranes; of the same contractive strength, 61
Isotonic contraction: A muscular contraction during which tension climbs and then remains stable as the muscle shortens, 178
Isotonic solutions, A3-2
Isotope: Form of an element whose atoms contain the same number of protons but different numbers of neutrons (and thus differ in atomic weight), 31
Isthmus, 560
IUD (intrauterine device), 559, 570
IV fluid therapy, A3-2–A3-5

J

Jaundice, 339, A5-2
Jejunum (je-JOO-num): The middle portion of the small intestine, 474–475
Joint: An area where adjacent bones interact; an articulation, 149–158
cartilage and, 95, 96
classification of, 149–150, 153–155
elbow, 144–145, 156
form and function, 151–155
hip, 146, 157
intervertebral, 155

knee, 150, 151, 157–158
rheumatism and arthritis, 150–151
shoulder, 156
synovial membranes, 96–97
Joint capsule: Dense collagen fiber sleeve that surrounds a joint and provides protection and stabilization; also called articular capsule, 150
Jugular veins, 399
Jugular venous pulse (JVP), 399
Junctions, in epithelia, 83–84
Juxtaglomerular apparatus: The macula densa and the juxtaglomerular cells; a complex responsible for the release of renin and erythropoietin, 522, 523

K

Kaposi's sarcoma, 426
Karyotyping (KAR-ē-ō-tī-ping): The determination of the chromosomal characteristics of an individual or cell, 598
Keloid, A5-2
Keratin (KER-a-tin): Tough, fibrous protein component of nails, hair, calluses, and the general integumentary surface, 110, 112
Keratinization (KER-a-tin-i-zā-shun): The production of keratin by epithelial cells; also called cornification, 110
Kernig's sign, A8-3
Ketone bodies: Organic acids produced during the catabolism of lipids and certain amino acids; acetone is one example, 501, 502–503
Ketosis, 502
Kidney: A component of the urinary system; an organ functioning in the regulation of plasma composition, including the excretion of wastes and the maintenance of normal fluid and electrolyte balance, 10, 12, 518–524
ADH effect on, 313
anatomy, superficial and sectional, 519, 520
blood supply, 523–524
control of function, 528, 530–531
endocrine system and, 307, 320
erythropoietin (EPO), 340, 387
nephron, 519–523
position of, 518–519
Kidney stones, A19-1–A19-3
Killer T cells: See T cells
Kilocalorie (KIL-o-kal-o-rē): The amount of heat required to raise the temperature of a kilogram of water 1°C.
Kinesiotherapist, A4-8
Kinetic energy, 34
Klebsiella, A19-4
Knee jerk, 256–257
Knee joint, 95, 150, 151, 157–158
Korotkoff sounds, 383
Korsakoff's psychosis (KP), 504
Korsakoff's syndrome (KS), 504
Kreb's cycle, 498, 499, A18-1
Kupffer cells (KOOP-fer): Stellate reticular cells of the liver; phagocytic cells of the liver sinusoids, 480
Kuru, A8-5
Kwashiorkor, 504
Kyphosis, 138

L

Labia (LĀ-bē-a): Lips; labia majora and minora are components of the female external genitalia, 13, 467
Labia majora, 561
Labia minora, 561
Labor, 313, 592–593
Laboratory testing, in heart attack, 174
Labrum: A lip or rim.

Illustration Credits